Sandra Smith's Review for
NCLEX-RN® TWELFTH EDITION

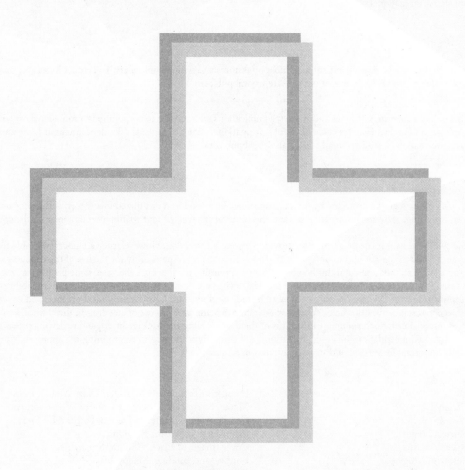

Sandra F. Smith, RN, MS

JONES AND BARTLETT PUBLISHERS

Sudbury, Massachusetts

BOSTON   TORONTO   LONDON   SINGAPORE

World Headquarters
Jones and Bartlett Publishers
40 Tall Pine Drive
Sudbury, MA 01776
978-443-5000
info@jbpub.com
www.jbpub.com

Jones and Bartlett Publishers Canada
6339 Ormindale Way
Mississauga, Ontario L5V 1J2
Canada

Jones and Bartlett Publishers International
Barb House, Barb Mews
London W6 7PA
United Kingdom

Jones and Bartlett's books and products are available through most bookstores and online booksellers. To contact Jones and Bartlett Publishers directly, call 800-832-0034, fax 978-443-8000, or visit our website www.jbpub.com.

Substantial discounts on bulk quantities of Jones and Bartlett's publications are available to corporations, professional associations, and other qualified organizations. For details and specific discount information, contact the special sales department at Jones and Bartlett via the above contact information or send an email to specialsales@jbpub.com.

The authors, editor, and publisher have made every effort to provide accurate information. However, they are not responsible for errors, omissions, or for any outcomes related to the use of the contents of this book and take no responsibility for the use of the products and procedures described. Treatments and side effects described in this book may not be applicable to all people; likewise, some people may require a dose or experience a side effect that is not described herein. Drugs and medical devices are discussed that may have limited availability controlled by the Food and Drug Administration (FDA) for use only in a research study or clinical trial. Research, clinical practice, and government regulations often change the accepted standard in this field. When consideration is being given to use of any drug in the clinical setting, the health care provider or reader is responsible for determining FDA status of the drug, reading the package insert, and reviewing prescribing information for the most up-to-date recommendations on dose, precautions, and contraindications, and determining the appropriate usage for the product. This is especially important in the case of drugs that are new or seldom used.

Production Credits

Publisher: Kevin Sullivan
Acquisitions Editor: Emily Ekle
Acquisitions Editor: Amy Sibley
Editorial Assistant: Patricia Donnelly
Editorial Assistant: Rachel Shuster
Production Editor: Carolyn F. Rogers
Associate Marketing Manager: Ilana Goddess

Interactive Technology Manager: Dawn Mahon Priest
Manufacturing and Inventory Control Supervisor: Amy Bacus
Composition and Interior Design: Forbes Mill Press
Cover Design: Kristin E. Ohlin
Cover Image: © ErickN/ShutterStock, Inc.
Printing and Binding: Malloy, Inc.
Cover Printing: Malloy, Inc.

Library of Congress Cataloging-in-Publication Data
Smith, Sandra Fucci.
  Sandra Smith's review for NCLEX-RN / Sandra F. Smith. — 12th ed.
    p. ; cm.
  Includes bibliographical references and index.
  ISBN 978-0-7637-5601-7 (pbk. : alk. paper)
  1. National Council Licensure Examination for Registered Nurses—Study guides. 2. Nursing—Outlines, syllabi, etc. 3. Nursing—Examinations, questions, etc. I. Title. II. Title: Review for NCLEX-RN.
  [DNLM: 1. Nursing Care—Examination Questions. 2. Nursing Care—Outlines. WY 18.2 S6592s 2009]
  RT52.S34 2009
  610.73076—dc22
                              2008010109

6048

Printed in the United States of America
12 11 10 09 08   10 9 8 7 6 5 4 3 2 1

BRIEF CONTENTS

CONTENTS IN DETAIL

CONTRIBUTORS AND REVIEWERS

CONTRIBUTING AUTHORS

Marianne Barba, RN, MS
Community College of Rhode Island
Bristol Community College
Providence, RI

Shirley Chang, RN, MS, PhD
Evergreen College
San Jose, CA

Debra Denham, RN, MS, PhD
Salinas Valley Medical Center
Salinas, CA

Joseann DeWitt, RN, MSN, BC, CLNC
Legal Nurse Consultant
Vidalia, LA

Donna Duell, RN, MS, ABD
Consultant-ADN Programs
California

Marianne Hultgren, RN, MS
Hawaii Pacific University
Honolulu, HI

Jeanine Tweedie, RN, MSN, CNE
Hawaii Pacific University
Honolulu, HI

Susan Yadro, RN, MS
University of Wisconsin
Madison, WI

REVIEWERS

Lynn Clark Callister, RN, PhD
Brigham Young University

Pattie Garrett Clark
Abraham Baldwin College

Maureen Cluskey, RN, DNSc
Bradley University

Normajean Colby, RN, MSN
Widener University

Amy Hudson, RN, MSN
Phillips Community College
  of the University of Arkansas

Viginia Lester, RN, MSN
Angelo State University

Mercy M. Popoola, RN, CNS, PhD
Georgia Southern University

Rosalie Tierney-Gumaer, RN, MSN, MPH
University of Texas Health Science Center San Antonio

Daryle Wane, APRN, BC
Pasco–Hernando Community College

Susan Yadro, RN, MS, MA
University of Wisconsin—Madison

CONTRIBUTORS TO THE CD-ROM

Donald Anderson, RN, EdD
Regis College
Weston, MA

Audrey Bopp
St. John Fisher College
Rochester, NY

Vera Dauffenbach
University of Wisconsin
Green Bay, WI

Linda Dunaway
Maysville Community College
Maysville, KY

Angie Grabau
University of Nebraska Medical Center
Lincoln, NE

Sammie Justesen
Internet Communications Corporation of America
Logan, UT

Susan Kangas-Packett
Creighton University
Omaha, NE

Kim Kendall
Maysville Community College
Maysville, KY

Sandra Liming
North Seattle Community College
Seattle, WA

Patricia O'Connor
Mariam College
Fond Du Lac, WI

Teresa Shellenbarger
Indiana University of Pennsylvania
Indiana, PA

Jacqueline Thayer
North Seattle Community College
Seattle, WA

PREFACE

Passing the National Council Licensure Examination (NCLEX®) is a crucial step in your nursing career. ***Sandra Smith's Review for NCLEX-RN,*** ® written to assist you to prepare for and pass this examination, summarizes in concise outline format the essential nursing content that you must know to pass the NCLEX. The content is supplemented by practice questions, providing you the opportunity to test your mastery over nursing theory, principles, and interventions.

The twelfth edition of this popular book includes all the material that has been incorporated into prior editions with revisions, updates, deletions, and new, expanded material including a new chapter on Emergency Nursing. It also reflects the author's university teaching experience and feedback from many candidates who used earlier editions for NCLEX success.

Chapter 1 presents useful material on NCLEX background, study and review guidelines, and test-taking strategies.

- The NCLEX description summarizes the current test plan's overall purpose and basic framework. We assist you to understand the test plan, client needs, critical thinking, and the nursing process. Cognitive levels are also included, with examples to assist you in identifying the various levels at which questions are written on NCLEX.

- The study and review guidelines suggest how you can design your personal plan for NCLEX preparation, how to use this book effectively, and why testing yourself repeatedly is an important complement to, but not a replacement for, concentrated study of the outline content.

- The test-taking strategies are common-sense, but often overlooked, methods of responding to multiple-choice questions. In this edition, new priority decision-making strategies, with examples, are included.

- While the majority of questions are straightforward multiple choice, as of 2005 several variations of questions called "Alternate Item Format Questions" have been included in the examination. Examples of the different question formats are in Chapter 1 and in various sections of this edition.

Chapter 2 covers essential management issues, an increasingly important subject on NCLEX, and legal/ethical concerns. This will enable you to understand NCLEX questions that deal with these issues.

The major portion of the book consists of a comprehensive nursing content review organized by clinical area: general nursing concepts, medical–surgical, maternal–newborn, pediatric, psychiatric, and gerontological nursing. Additional chapters focus on other important subjects, such as pharmacology, laboratory tests, oncology, infection control, nutrition, management principles, and legal issues. A unique chapter, Disaster Nursing: Bioterrorism, is included with a new section on natural disasters. This edition also presents a new chapter, Emergency Nursing, with additional content that brings into focus current trends in health care.

To assist your review process to be efficient and effective, the nursing content is presented in an outline format. This enables the author to identify and prioritize essential clinical information clearly and concisely. As you progress from subject to subject, you will note that the consistent page design allows you to easily recognize the main topics and their subtopics. Many boxes of information, tables and charts include supplemental data to enhance learning.

Nursing content in each chapter is organized using the nursing process as the basic framework. The author emphasizes the assessment and implementation steps. The NCLEX will require you to demonstrate your ability to effectively assess a situation and then implement appropriate nursing interventions by including many questions that require you to choose the first or priority action. Making clinical judgments is what the NCLEX asks you to do.

Throughout the text, a special icon (✦) directs your attention to important content for NCLEX preparation. If the icon appears near a major section of content, it means that the entire section is important. Another icon may appear under the same heading indicating especially important material. The NCLEX draws upon a test pool containing thousands of questions when selecting the items for your test. Any material in this book could be phrased as a question, so focusing your review exclusively on the icon topics would not be a wise preparation strategy.

Finally, this text is now in its successful twelfth edition. Each edition has been revised with the assistance of feedback from candidates who have taken the NCLEX; thus, there is little extraneous or useless information included.

Practice questions follow each chapter throughout the book to enable you to check your level of understanding of each chapter's contents or, in the medical–surgical chapter, each section's contents. The answers with rationales are included, along with coding for nursing process, client need, clinical area, and cognitive level.

Review the material, spending a little extra time on the icon areas; answer the practice questions that follow each section or chapter, and then review content again if you identify areas of weakness. Then, take the comprehensive tests at the end of the book. Use the questions on the CD-ROM as a final step in your preparation for NCLEX. All of the questions in the book also appear on the CD-ROM. There are also an additional 1700 questions on the CD that do not exist in the book. The goal of the CD is to give you experience with answering questions in an electronic format—just like the NCLEX. This is one of the most comprehensive NCLEX CDs on the market, so please use it!

The three simulated NCLEX examinations at the back of this book and the additional practice questions on the CD-ROM provide you with substantial opportunities to measure your mastery of the subject matter. The answer rationales throughout the book and on the CD-ROM will reinforce your understanding of the principles that underlie each question. Studying rationales for questions that you answered correctly as well as incorrectly will reinforce your knowledge and understanding. As your understanding increases, so will your confidence.

ACKNOWLEDGMENTS

I wish to thank all of the contributing authors and reviewers who assisted with the development of this and the earlier editions. Because of their contributions, this review package will continue to be a valuable resource for RN licensure candidates.

PHOTO CREDITS

Figures 8-3, 8-4, and 8-5 are from *Arrhythmia Recognition: The Art of Interpretation,* courtesy of Tomas B. Garcia, MD.

The NCLEX-RN® and Test-Taking Strategies

1

® NCLEX and NCLEX-RN are registered trademarks of the
National Council of State Boards of Nursing, Inc.

INTRODUCTION TO THE NCLEX®

The National Council Licensure Examination for Registered Nurses, commonly abbreviated to NCLEX®, measures the licensure candidate's competence to perform safe and effective entry-level nursing practice. This important screening test is designed and administered by the National Council of State Boards of Nursing, Inc., known as the National Council. All 50 states, the District of Columbia, and all U.S. territories are members of the Council and utilize the NCLEX as an integral part of their licensure process. The NCLEX licensure procedures define common entry-level nursing standards throughout the United States while providing healthcare protection to consumers. Licensed nurses have reciprocity from state to state, an additional benefit provided by a national licensure system.

Developing the NCLEX-RN®

The National Council contracts with clinical nurses and nurse educators to write questions (referred to as test items) that test your ability to apply your knowledge of nursing. The test questions focus on job tasks normally performed by entry-level RNs during their first 6 to 12 months on the job. The National Council identifies these tasks by conducting extensive surveys, called RN practice analyses, about every three years. It is possible that your RN program may have included instruction on certain tasks that are not considered to be entry level by the National Council's job surveys. It is also possible that your program may not have provided you with instruction on some of the tasks about which questions have been included in the current test pool.

The practice analysis activities are analyzed by frequency of their performance, priority and their impact on maintaining client safety. The results guide the development of the NCLEX-RN Test Plan framework based upon specific client needs. On a continuing basis, the practice analysis studies are also used to help validate the current Test Plan and to provide the basis for selecting subjects to be covered by NCLEX.

The Test Plan serves as a guide for examination development and candidate preparation. Each test reflects the knowledge, skills, and abilities necessary for each nurse to safely meet client needs for the promotion, maintenance, and restoration of health.

CLIENT NEEDS

The basic framework for the NCLEX is Client Needs. The health needs of clients are organized into four major categories and six subcategories. This section reviews Client Needs so that you can understand how NCLEX is structured and what material you need to master to pass this examination. The NCLEX questions are proportional according to a survey conducted every three years by the National Council. Table 1-1 lists the categories and subcategories and provides the percentage of questions for each. You should concentrate your study and review on the categories that are emphasized most by the NCLEX.

Safe Effective Care Environment (21–33%)

To meet the client's needs for safe, effective care, the nurse must be able to provide nursing care in the following areas:

- *Management of Care*—providing and directing nursing care to protect clients, family, significant others, and healthcare personnel. The related content encompasses advance directives, management and delegating, and legal responsibilities. There are a total of 19 subcategories of Management of Care.
- *Safety and Infection Control*—protecting clients, family, significant others and healthcare personnel from environmental hazards. Related content includes topics such as accidents and disasters, asepsis, safety, and Standard Precautions.

Health Promotion and Maintenance (6–12%)

The nurse provides and directs nursing care for the client and family/significant others that incorporates the knowledge of expected growth and development principles, prevention and/or early detection of health problems, and strategies to achieve optimal health. Related content includes such topics as aging and newborn care, family disease prevention and health promotion activities.

Psychosocial Integrity (6–12%)

The nurse provides and directs nursing care that promotes and supports the emotional, mental and social well-being of the client and family/significant others experiencing stressful events as well as clients with acute or chronic mental illness. Related content includes but **is not limited** to such topics as chemical dependency, crisis, family dynamics, psychopathology, and therapeutic communication.

Physiological Integrity (43–67%)

The final category is the largest and applies to an average of 50% of the questions. This category relates to meeting the client's needs for physiological integrity—including acute and/or chronically recurring physiological conditions, as well as potential complications.

- *Basic Care and Comfort*—providing comfort and assistance in the performance of activities of daily living.
- *Pharmacological and Parenteral Therapies*—providing care related to the administration of medication and parenteral therapies.
- *Reduction of Risk Potential*—reducing the likelihood that clients will develop complications or health problems related to existing conditions, treatments, or procedures.
- *Physiological Adaptation*—providing care to clients with acute, chronic, or life-threatening physical health conditions.

Adapted from *Test Plan for the National Council Licensure Examination for Registered Nurses*, National Council of State Boards of Nursing, Chicago, 2006.

Integrated Processes

The following processes, fundamental to the practice of nursing, are integrated throughout the four major Client Needs categories. NCLEX questions will reflect these processes. They include:
- *Nursing Process*—a scientific problem-solving approach to client care.
- *Caring*—interaction of the nurse and client in an atmosphere of mutual respect and trust.
- *Communication and Documentation*—verbal and nonverbal interactions between the nurse and the client, the client's significant others and other members of the healthcare team.
- *Teaching/Learning*—knowledge, skills and attitudes promoting a change in behavior.

Because the NCLEX-RN Test Plan centers on the categories of Client Needs, you may wish to visit the National Council's Web site at *www.ncsbn.org.* Detailed information will help guide your review process, as it lists specific nursing actions in relation to Client Needs in each of the Nursing Process categories.

NURSING PROCESS

The National Council no longer provides a percentage breakdown of questions according to the individual phases of the Nursing Process. However, the Nursing Process continues to be an integral foundation for nursing education, clinical training, and textbooks. Therefore, it is appropriate for you to understand the concepts and to be able to relate NCLEX questions to the Nursing Process as you apply your knowledge of nursing to select the correct answers.

The five phases of the Nursing Process are Assessment, Analysis, Planning, Implementation, and Evalu-

Table 1-1. CATEGORIES OF CLIENT NEEDS	
Categories	**Percentage of Test Questions**
A. Safe Effective Care Environment	
• Management of Care	13–19%
• Safety and Infection Control	8–14%
B. Health Promotion and Maintenance	6–12%
C. Psychosocial Integrity	6–12%
D. Physiological Integrity	
• Basic Care and Comfort	6–12%
• Pharmacological and Parenteral Therapies	13–19%
• Reduction of Risk Potential	13–19%
• Physiological Adaptation	11–17%

ation. The Nursing Process is a frequently used, but often misunderstood, term. By definition, a *process* is a series of actions that lead toward a particular result. When attached to *nursing*, the term *Nursing Process* becomes a general description of a nurse's job: assessing, analyzing, planning, implementing, and evaluating. Ideally, this process of decision making results in optimal health care for the clients. While the five steps can be described separately and in logical order, in practice the steps will overlap and events may not always occur in the order listed above, especially when the unexpected happens.

Assessment

The assessment phase refers to the establishment of a database for a specific client. Assessment requires skilled observation, reasoning and a theoretical knowledge base to gather and differentiate data, verify data and document findings. The nurse gathers information relevant to the client and then assigns meaning to these data. Assessment is a very critical phase because all other steps in the Nursing Process depend on the accuracy and reliability of the assessment process.

Analysis/Nursing Diagnosis

The analysis phase focuses on the comprehension and the interpretation of data collected during assessment for the purpose of goal formulation. This phase includes identifying client needs, choosing the appropriate nursing diagnosis and setting goals. Developing a plan of action for goal achievement follows this.

Planning

Based on data collected, the planning phase refers to setting goals for meeting client needs and identifying nursing actions (strategies) to achieve the goals of care. This phase of the Nursing Process also includes nursing measures for the delivery of care. Clients may be involved in the planning phase.

Implementation

The fourth phase of the Nursing Process is implementation, or intervention. It explicitly describes the action component of the Nursing Process. This phase involves initiating and completing those nursing actions necessary to accomplish the identified client goals. Implementation includes performing basic therapeutic and preventive nursing measures, providing a safe and effective environment, recording and reporting specific information, and assisting the client to understand the care plan. Implementation of the plan involves giving direct care to accomplish the specified goal.

Evaluation

The final phase of the Nursing Process is evaluation, or determining the extent to which identified goals were achieved. Evaluation is the examination of the outcome of the nursing interventions. This process is extremely important, because without this step, the nursing plan cannot be evaluated and adapted to the client's ongoing needs.

CRITICAL THINKING

All nurses are required to use critical thinking skills. Critical thinking competencies are the cognitive processes that a nurse employs to make clinical judgments, including diagnostic reasoning and decision making. The Nursing Process is the framework for critical thinking competency in nursing.

- **Assessment:** Obtaining, classifying and organizing data is a principle component of critical thinking.
- **Analysis/Nursing Diagnosis:** The nurse critically analyzes, synthesizes, clusters and interprets all the collected data before formulating a Nursing Diagnosis.
- **Planning:** Defining realistic goals (both short and long term) and prioritizing these goals also requires critical thinking. The nurse must sort through the available information, evaluate the goals, determine the probable outcomes (which must be time specific), and prioritize them. This is a key step in the critical thinking process.
- **Implementation:** The fourth component of critical thinking is based on strategies designed to achieve

positive outcomes. Deciding on the appropriate actions (after considering all those possible), while examining the risks and consequences of each action, completes this step in the process.
- **Evaluation:** Critical analysis of each of the client outcomes is the final step. Was the goal achieved? If not, the plan is revised.

THE NCLEX-RN TEST PLAN

To plan an efficient and effective study and review program, it is important that you understand both the purpose and framework of the NCLEX. This examination is designed to measure your ability to practice entry-level nursing in a safe, competent manner. NCLEX questions are designed to require you to apply your knowledge of nursing care and procedures to specific clinical situations. When you take the NCLEX, you will complete a brief computer tutorial, which includes examples of the various types of questions that you may encounter. The tutorial is accessible at *www.vue.com/nclex.*

NCLEX Question Types and Examples

Simple Multiple Choice

The vast majority of test items are presented as straightforward multiple-choice questions containing four answer options with only one correct answer.

> The nurse is assigned a client undergoing chronic peritoneal dialysis. The priority assessment is
>
> 1. Pulmonary embolism.
> 2. Hypotension.
> 3. Dyspnea.
> 4. Peritonitis.
>
> Peritonitis (4) is a potentially life-threatening complication with peritoneal dialysis.

Alternate Item Formats

✦ Multiple-response questions may offer as many as six possible answers, and you must choose all that apply. Your answer must include all that apply to be scored "correct."

> A client has been placed on a low-potassium diet. List the following high-potassium foods that he should avoid.
>
> 1. Butter.
> 2. Shellfish.
> 3. Milk.
> 4. Frozen vegetables.
> 5. Orange juice.
> 6. Dried dates.
>
> The correct answer is 3, 5, 6. Milk (3), orange juice (5) and dried dates (6) are high in potassium. The other foods are high in sodium.

✦ Fill-in-the-blank questions require the candidate to complete a calculation and type in the correct answer.

> The orders are to give warfarin (Coumadin) 12.5 mg. On hand are 5 mg tablets. The nurse should give the client _____ tablets.

> The answer is 2.5 tablets. This computation uses the formula D (dose desired) ÷ H (dose on hand) x Q (quantity of dose on hand): 12.5 ÷ 5 x 1 = 2.5 tablets.

✦ Drag and drop questions involve putting a list into proper sequence. You will use the computer mouse to move items from the left box to the right as shown below.

> When removing an isolation gown, place in order the steps the nurse will complete to follow infection control protocol.

Unordered Options	Blank Option Box	Options in Correct Order
Remove gloves. Untie neck ties. Untie front waist strings. Wash hands Remove gown.		Untie front waist strings. Remove gloves. Untie neck ties. Remove gown. Wash hands.

> Place cursor on each option. Drag to right box and place in correct sequence.

✦ Hotspot questions also require using the mouse. You will be asked to identify an area on a drawing or other graphic by placing the cursor on the spot and clicking the mouse.

> The nurse is completing a cardiac assessment by listening to S2 heart sounds. Locate the pulmonic area where S2 sounds can be detected.

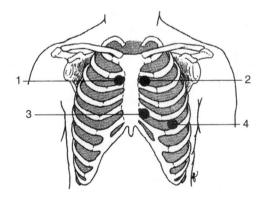

The pulmonic area (2) is one the two best positions to hear S2 heart sounds. The other position is the aortic (1).

LEVELS OF COGNITIVE ABILITY

Cognitive levels are defined in taxonomy as "the orderly classification of data into appropriate categories on the basis of relationships between them." The practice of nursing requires application of knowledge at various lev-

els of cognitive domain underlying theory, skills and ability. The majority of the NCLEX-RN questions are written at the more advanced levels of application and analysis rather than at the lower levels of knowledge or comprehension. The taxonomy of cognitive levels is as follows.

- **Knowledge:** Recall or recognize theoretical principles or facts of nursing content. Questions ask the nurse to define, identify, recognize, or select the appropriate data.
- **Comprehension:** Understand the information presented. Questions ask the nurse to explain, interpret, predict, or distinguish data.
- **Application:** Apply or use information in a new or different manner. Questions ask the nurse to problem solve, change or manipulate data, or use the information appropriately.
- **Analysis:** Separate parts of the whole or determine relationships between parts for a new understanding. Questions ask the nurse to analyze, differentiate, evaluate, or interpret data from a variety of sources.
- **Synthesis:** The highest level of cognitive functioning, which puts information together in a totally new and meaningful way.

The questions in this book have been coded according to cognitive levels. While all levels are represented, most questions are written at the application and analysis levels. Understanding this component of the test is important because as a licensure candidate, you cannot expect to simply memorize data and recall it for the examination (knowledge level) or interpret data (comprehension level). Rather, most questions will require that you apply your knowledge to clinical problems. This requires application of the data.

Examples of Cognitive Level Questions

Knowledge Level

> One of the primary developmental tasks of adolescence is
>
> 1. Feeling independent.
> 2. Finding one's identity.
> 3. Experiencing intimacy.
> 4. Achieving generativity.
>
> Correct answer is (2). Early adolescence has the primary task of finding one's identity and moving out of role diffusion. The task from later adolescence to young adulthood is to experience intimacy (3), not independence and isolation (1). Adults should achieve generativity (4) versus stagnation.

This is a knowledge base question that requires the nurse to recognize or recall knowledge or information learned (i.e., the developmental tasks of adolescents).

Comprehension Level

A mother brings her six-week-old infant to the clinic for a well-baby exam. The nurse, when teaching about infant nutrition, would inform the mother that

1. Whole eggs are a good source of iron and can be introduced at six months.
2. Solid foods can be introduced in the sixth week of life.
3. Rice cereal is the least allergenic of the cereals for infants.
4. Only one new food should be introduced per day.

Correct answer is (3.) Rice cereal is the least allergenic food. The latest research indicates that solid food (2) should not be given until the child is six months old. This may prevent allergies later in life, and the infant's digestive system has had time to mature. Egg yolks, not whole eggs (1), can be introduced because the whites of the egg may cause an allergy. Only one new food should be added each week, not each day (4).

Comprehension involves understanding information (infant nutrition) and being able to explain it effectively in the right context.

Application Level

A nurse is assigned to take two clients' vital signs, complete a focus assessment, provide hygienic care, and administer medications, as well as complete a dressing change for a third client with an abdominal wound. Which task will have priority with this assignment?

1. Take vital signs and provide hygienic care on the first client.
2. Administer medications to both clients.
3. Complete the dressing change on the third client.
4. Take vital signs on the two clients.

Correct answer is (4). Taking vital signs on the two clients would be the priority nursing action to determine if there are any emergent problems. Even if one of the clients had TB, the nurse could don gloves and a HEPA filter mask to complete the assignment. Next, the nurse would give the meds (2) that need to be given within a certain time frame. Because changing the dressing (3) might also involve a pain assessment, this would take more time and should probably be done last.

Application is the ability to apply knowledge. In this example, understanding that taking vital signs would reveal any problems is correct application of knowledge.

Analysis Level

A nurse is assessing a client with a radiation implant and observes that the implant has been dislodged. The nurse cannot immediately locate the implant. The first nursing action is to

1. Search for the implant in the bed covers and place it in a lead container.
2. Call the physician and bar all visitors from the room.
3. Pick up the source with a foot-long applicator.
4. Notify the radiation safety team.

Table 1-2. CODING FOR QUESTIONS AND ANSWERS IN THIS BOOK*	
Nursing Process	**NP**
Assessment	A
Analysis	AN
Planning	P
Implementation	I
Evaluation	E
Client Needs	**CN**
Safe, Effective Care Environment	S
Health Promotion and Maintenance	H
Psychosocial Integrity	PS
Physiological Integrity	PH
Content Area	**CA**
(will be included only for those questions included in the comprehensive tests).	
Medical Nursing	M
Surgical Nursing	S
Maternity Nursing	MA
Pediatric Nursing	P
Psychiatric Nursing	PS
Cognitive Level	**CL**
Knowledge	K
Comprehension	C
Application	A
Analysis	AN

*Each answer will be coded and the reference code will appear at the beginning of each answer section.

The correct answer is (2). The first nursing action is to bar all visitors from the room and notify the physician. It is important not to contaminate yourself by searching for the implant (1). The physician will notify the radiation team and make decisions about reimplanting the radiation source in the client.

Analysis requires the nurse to analyze or evaluate data, and then make a determination for nursing action. This example requires the nurse to analyze the situation and then problem solve to a conclusion, or nursing intervention.

NCLEX APPLICATION PROCEDURES

As a candidate for RN licensure, you will deal with several organizations as you complete your application procedures to take the NCLEX. The key organization is the board of nursing in the state or jurisdiction where you plan to practice. Each state board of nursing sets education and other eligibility requirements for RN licensure. Fortunately, all states and territories accept the NCLEX as the standard licensure examination. Assuming you qualify, the state board will send you an Authorization to Test (ATT). Now you are authorized to contact a Pearson Professional Center of your choice to schedule your test session. The center does not have to be located in the state where you plan to practice. As a first-time test taker, you should be able to schedule your test within 30 days of receiving your ATT.

When you receive your ATT from the board of nursing, note its expiration date. You must take the NCLEX before the ATT expires, or you will have to reapply and pay the filing fees again. You should also be aware that the Pearson Professional Centers are highly booked at certain times of the year, especially May through July, so plan your testing date accordingly.

The NCLEX Candidate Bulletin contains a description of computerized adaptive testing and important information regarding NCLEX registration, scheduling, and other important procedures. Published by the National Council of State Boards of Nursing, this useful resource is available via the Internet at *www.ncsbn.org.*

Candidates whose applications for licensure have been approved are eligible for an interim permit to practice under the direct supervision of a registered nurse. However, this permit is not renewable and is in effect until its expiration date or until the results of NCLEX are mailed to you. These procedures give you strong incentive to pass the NCLEX on your first attempt.

TAKING THE NCLEX

Upon arriving at the Pearson Professional Center, you will present your Authorization to Test and two forms of identification, both signed and one with a photo. A driver's license, school or employee ID, and passport are the most accepted forms. At check-in, you will be photographed and thumb printed. Before commencing the test questions, you will complete a brief computer tutorial to make certain that you are comfortable with the testing procedures. The National Council advises that no prior computer experience is necessary for Computer Adaptive Testing (CAT). The CD-ROM accompanying this book allows you to practice and become comfortable with CAT procedures.

TESTING PROCEDURES

Two categories of questions appear on NCLEX. The *real* questions test your competency and safety and provide the basis for your pass or fail score. The *tryout* questions are unscored items being field-tested for future NCLEX exams. You have no way of knowing the difference between *real* and *tryout* questions.

The minimum number of questions for each candidate is 75. The maximum number of questions that a candidate may answer during the exam period is 265.

Computer Adaptive Testing does not allow you to skip questions or go back to look at or change questions already answered. Each question has an assigned degree of difficulty. Based on your prior answers—correct or incorrect—the computer selects the next question. Therefore, you must answer each question as it is presented. Because the computer draws from a large pool of questions, each candidate's test is unique. There is no absolute passing score in terms of the number or percentage of questions that you must answer correctly to pass.

Although there is no minimum amount of time for your test, the maximum allowable time is six hours. This includes your computer tutorial, sample questions and rest breaks.

Because the number of questions is flexible, from a minimum of 75 to a maximum of 265, there is no optimal amount of time you should spend per question. However, because you won't know how long it will take you to reach the point where the computer stops presenting questions, it is not wise to spend too much time on any one question. If you don't know the answer, guess and move on, rather than risk becoming immobilized. When you answer questions correctly, the CAT software presents you with more difficult items. As you answer questions incorrectly, you will receive easier items.

Your test continues until the computer software calculates with a 95% degree of confidence that you fall into the safe/competent group or that you do not. The total number of questions answered does not indicate whether you have passed or failed.

Getting Your Test Results

NCLEX test results are available only from the state board of nursing to which you applied for approval to take the NCLEX. Do not request feedback from the Pearson Professional Center or the National Council. You can expect to receive your results within one month after taking the exam, but often in less time. A failure notice is accompanied by a performance report to help the candidate identify areas of weakness. Most state boards of nursing require that candidates who fail must wait a minimum of 45 to 91 days, depending on the state, before retaking the exam.

GUIDELINES FOR NCLEX REVIEW

How to Use This Book

Sandra Smith's Review for NCLEX-RN® summarizes extensive nursing content to which you have been introduced during your RN education. The material is organized into 15 chapters and presented in outline format for your review.

Nursing theory and practical applications of this theory are included for each major subject area. Nursing theory includes pathophysiology, signs and symptoms of diseases, diagnosis and treatment of medical conditions, and appropriate nursing care. Tables and appendices are distributed throughout the book to assist you to efficiently review factual material. Familiarize yourself with how the contents are organized in each chapter and how the Nursing Process is integrated throughout the book.

Other features to note for further reference include three simulated NCLEX exams at the back of the book, a detailed index, and a CD-ROM attached to the inside of the back cover with additional NCLEX-type questions.

The multiple-choice questions that follow various content review sections are similar in format, subject matter, length, and degree of difficulty to those contained in the NCLEX-RN. The answer and rationale sections provide you with additional learning. If you understand the basic principles of nursing content, you can transfer that knowledge to the clinical situations and questions on the NCLEX.

The CD-ROM contains the questions printed in the book. They can be accessed for each chapter by clicking on the chapter title. This provides you with the opportunity to gain computer experience while you assess and review. Also, the CD contains more than 1700 additional questions not printed in the book, for a total of more than 2500 questions.

How to Design Your Personal Review Program

Ideally, you will begin your review process several months prior to NCLEX. If you choose to allocate only a few weeks to prepare for this exam, however, it is important that you conduct the review process in an efficient manner. The following recommendations are offered to help you achieve maximum results for the amount of time invested.

A. Schedule regular periods for study and review.
   1. Arrange to study when mentally alert. Studying during periods of mental and physical fatigue reduces your efficiency.
   2. Allow short breaks at relatively frequent intervals. Breaks used as rewards for hard study serve as incentives for continued concentrated effort. A 10- to 15-minute break is recommended after each hour of concentrated study.
B. Familiarize yourself with the examination format.
   1. Review the NCLEX Test Plan description so that you understand the Client Needs categories. Notice which areas have the greater

---

NCLEX-RN CAT Quick Reference
Test Location: Pearson Professional Centers
Minimum Number of Questions: 75
Maximum Number of Questions: 265
Minimum Testing Time: None
Maximum Testing Time: 6 hours

---

number of questions and allocate more review time to these topics. Refer to Table 1-1 for the allocation of questions among the subcategories of Client Needs.
   2. Study the format used for NCLEX questions. You must know how to read, evaluate, and respond to multiple-choice questions similar to those in this book and on the CD-ROM.
C. Identify your strengths and weaknesses.
   1. Assess your past performance on classroom tests and written material (clinical pathways or nursing care plans).
   2. Learn from your past errors and weaknesses by looking up and studying the appropriate material in this book.
D. Systematically study the material contained in each chapter of this book.
   1. First, gain a general impression of the content unit to be reviewed. Skim over the entire section and identify the main ideas.
   2. Note the tables, glossaries, and appendices.
   3. The special icon (✦) that appears throughout the book's review sections identifies nursing content that is particularly important or involves critical decision making. If an entire section is marked by an icon, then assume that all of this material is important. Do not, however, limit your study to only the icon-marked content; use the icon to help you focus and prioritize. Mark key material that you do not thoroughly understand.
E. Follow up on your priority areas.
   1. Set priorities for specific material to be learned or reviewed. Identify the most crucial sections and underline the essential thoughts.
   2. Review what you have read. Think of examples that illustrate the main points you have studied.
   3. To be sure that you have learned the material, write down the main ideas or explain the major points to another person.
F. Test and retest.
   1. Complete the clinical practice questions presented at the conclusion of each chapter as well as on the CD-ROM. Study the rationale for missed questions so that you understand why

you missed them. Refer back to the content outline preceding the questions to study content relating to the topics contained in the questions. Study the rationale for the questions that you answered correctly because this will reinforce your understanding of those topics and increase your confidence about material you firmly understand.

2. After you have worked your way through the clinical questions, take the first simulated NCLEX test at the back of the book. Analyze your results by noting the category of each question missed in terms of Nursing Process, Client Needs, and clinical area (*see* Table 1-2). This will help you identify your weaker areas. Refer to the appropriate content for further study and review.

3. Take the second and third simulated NCLEX tests. Repeat the same process of analysis and review. If you studied the content relating to questions you missed, you should see improvement. In addition to the questions printed in the book (and also contained on the CD-ROM), you can utilize the CD-ROM to answer more than 1700 additional practice questions (drawn at random or by clinical area). Upon answering these questions, you will receive immediate feedback—correct or incorrect—as well as the rationale. This is an excellent assessment and learning experience.

4. After you have completed the practice questions and simulated tests in the book, utilize the CD-ROM for additional practice and review. The key to this process is to use the content outline in the various chapters as a learning vehicle to strengthen your grasp of the material. This, in turn, will increase your ability to apply what you know to specific clinical situations tested in the NCLEX.

TEST-TAKING STRATEGIES

The following test-taking strategies will provide you with useful guidelines when answering NCLEX questions. These strategies are neither absolute nor foolproof; they are intended to guide you in choosing the best response for each question.

A. Carefully read each question. Determine what the question is really asking. Some details may not be important. Mentally note important factors; pay attention to key terms and phrases. Read the question as it is presented, not as you would like it to be stated.

B. When answering multiple-choice questions, an effective strategy is to first eliminate the answers that you know are wrong, and then focus on deciding among the remaining answers. If you are not sure about any of the four possible answers, you will have to make an educated guess. Remember, you are not allowed to skip a question, nor will you be able to change any answers that you have selected on previous questions.

C. Your first "hunch" is usually correct. Many candidates have a first impression, choose an answer, and, upon reflection, change their mind. Sensing that a particular alternative is correct has some basis. Your brain has made rapid connections. You came to an immediate conclusion based on your knowledge and experience. The fact that you did not go through the logical steps of arriving at the correct solution does not indicate that your choice is incorrect.

D. Be alert for a question that requires you to identify which answer is **not** correct, or a question that asks for a negative response; for example, "Which of the following interventions is inappropriate?"

E. Evaluate the answers in relation to the stem (the question), not to other answers. Choose the answer that best fits the question, rather than an answer that appears to be a correct statement but may not fit the question.

F. The most comprehensive answer is often the best choice. For example, if two alternatives seem reasonable but one answer includes the other (i.e., it is more detailed, extends the first answer, or is more comprehensive), then this answer may be the best choice.

G. Eliminate answers that are obviously different from what is logically right, such as an answer given in grams when other choices are given in milligrams.

H. Do not look for a pattern to the answers. The questions are chosen at random, and the same number may be the correct answer to several consecutive questions.

I. The test administrator will provide you with erasable note boards and a writing implement for your use during the test session. You are not allowed to bring your own notes, scratch paper, or writing implements into the test center.

Guidelines for Making Priority Decisions

Priority decision making is an important test-taking skill. NCLEX places increasingly greater emphasis on requiring candidates to analyze and evaluate information and then to make decisions. The following examples are presented as guidelines to help you recognize and answer priority-based NCLEX questions.

Most Life-Threatening

If you are asked which sign or symptom would you respond to first, or which nursing diagnosis would you identify as the priority intervention, you should determine which is the most life-threatening. Always choose the critical intervention—airway, breathing, circulation (ABC)—if one is listed as an option.

A client diagnosed with rheumatic heart disease has been admitted to the hospital due to cardiac arrhythmias. The registered nurse develops the nursing care plan. The nursing diagnosis to be given the highest priority is

1. Excess fluid volume.
2. Deficient fluid volume.
3. Ineffective tissue perfusion.
4. Ineffective breathing pattern.

Correct answer is (4). Because the atria do not empty fully in atrial fibrillation, the ventricles are not able to pump normal cardiac output. The client, therefore, may exhibit shortness of breath. Ineffective breathing pattern is the most life-threatening condition of the four answer selections. The client may also show signs of heart failure and decreased cerebral flow, but these symptoms would not be the *most* life-threatening.

First-Priority Nursing Intervention

When a question focuses on which intervention you would perform *first*, consider which is the most immediate for the well-being of the client. For example, you would suction the client before administering a routine medication (providing it was not nitroglycerin), because medications can be given up to 30 minutes before or after the ordered time.

A client in the labor room is lying comfortably on her back after receiving an epidural injection 30 minutes earlier. The nurse checks the fetal heart rate and finds the fetal rate is 100 per minute. The first nursing action is to

1. Administer oxygen by mask.
2. Turn the client onto her left side.
3. Notify the physician immediately.
4. Take the client's blood pressure.

Correct answer is (2). All of the interventions will be carried out; however, the first action is to turn the client onto her side to reduce the pressure of the uterus on the vena cava. Oxygen administration should be initiated after turning the client onto her side. Fetal heart rate should then be checked and rechecked frequently.

Safety Issue

The answer choices that involve a safety issue for the client will always take priority over other concerns. For example, monitoring the oxygen level in an incubator of a premature infant is a safety issue. If the oxygen level goes above 40% for the premature fetus, it could damage the retinas and lead to blindness. The oxygen level for an adult would not be a serious safety issue unless the client has COPD.

After assessing that a blood transfusion allergic reaction has occurred, the first nursing intervention is to

1. Place the client in high-Fowler's position.
2. Call the physician.
3. Slow the rate of infusion to "keep open" rate.
4. Turn off the transfusion.

Correct answer is (4). If the nurse suspects an allergic reaction, the blood transfusion IV should be turned off immediately. Then, the physician should be notified and the client placed in a position to facilitate breathing. While in actual practice some nurses advocate slowing the IV rate to "keep open," NCLEX would view this as a safety issue. To be safe, the transfusion should be turned off to prevent a more serious reaction.

Computer Testing Tips

A. When taking the NCLEX, you must answer each question that appears on the computer screen. If you do not recognize a correct answer among the four choices, use your test-taking skills or, if necessary, make your best guess.
B. Be certain of your answer selection before confirming your choice.
C. Take your time and carefully read each question and answer choices.
D. Do not become immobilized by any one question. Spending five minutes or more on a question will probably make you more nervous and less attentive as you proceed.
E. Maintain a steady pace of allocating about one minute per question. This strategy will allow you to complete the examination within the required time of six hours should you need to answer 265 questions.

Final Preparation

A. The night before the test.
   1. Assemble materials that you will take with you to the test center, such as your ATT, identifications and other items as specified in the *NCLEX Candidate Bulletin.* Do not bring textbooks, notes or any NCLEX study aids to the test center.
   2. Get a good night's sleep. Do not stay up all night trying to learn new material.
   3. Avoid the use of stimulants or depressants, either of which may affect your ability to think clearly during the test.
   4. Approach the test with confidence and the determination to do your best. Think positively and concentrate on all that you do know rather than on what you think you do not know.

B. The day of the test.
   1. Eat a high-protein, no-sugar breakfast. Do not rush.
   2. Allow ample time to travel to your testing site, including time to park, and to present your Authorization to Test at least 30 minutes before your scheduled testing time.
   3. You may wish to take a light, energizing snack and bottled water to have available for your breaks. Secure storage will be provided for your personal items.

The Importance of a Confident Attitude

Anxiety, a forceful deterrent to test-taking success, interferes with your ability to think clearly. Anxiety blocks the search and retrieval process so that you cannot access the knowledge held in your "memory bank." Fear of the unknown is a major source of anxiety. This fear can be overcome by diligent review. As you gain mastery over the nursing content, your self-confidence increases. It is also important to understand test construction and test-taking strategies. This introduction is designed to reduce many of the unknowns associated with the NCLEX-RN and to provide you with helpful review guidelines and effective test-taking techniques.

These strategies are guidelines, not absolutes. Always use your own judgment, knowledge, and nursing experience. These assets will serve you well.

WEB SITES

For additional information on NCLEX testing procedures and current policies, contact the National Council of State Boards of Nursing at *www.ncsbn.org*.

To register online to take the NCLEX or to obtain information on Pearson Professional Center locations, contact Pearson at *www.vue.com/nclex*.

For information on NCLEX review aids by Sandra F. Smith, RN, MS, contact Jones and Bartlett Publishers at *www.jbpub.com*.

To download the *NCLEX Candidate Bulletin*, or to complete the Online Tutorial for NCLEX, visit *www.vue.com/nclex*.

Management Principles and Legal Issues

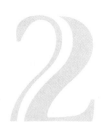

✦ The icon denotes content of special importance for NCLEX.

LEGAL ASPECTS OF NURSING

Board of Registered Nursing (BRN)

A. Each state has a Board of Registered Nursing (or its equivalent) organized within the executive branch of the state government. Primary responsibilities of the BRN include administration of the state Nurse Practice Act as applied to registered nurses.

✦ B. Functions of each state's Board of Registered Nursing.
  1. Establishes and oversees educational standards.
  2. Establishes professional standards.
  3. Monitors examinations for licensure (NCLEX).
  4. Registers and renews nurses' licenses.
  5. Conducts investigations of violations of the statutes and regulations.
  6. Issues citations.
  7. Holds disciplinary hearings for possible suspension or revocation of the license.
  8. Imposes penalties following disciplinary hearings.
  9. Establishes and oversees diversion programs in some states.

Authorization to Practice Nursing

✦ A. To legally engage in the practice of nursing, an individual must hold an active license issued by the state in which he or she intends to work.

B. The licensing process.
  ✦ 1. The applicant must pass a licensing examination administered by the state Board of Registered Nursing, or the BRN may grant reciprocity to an applicant who holds a current license in another state.
  ✦ 2. The applicant for RN licensure examination must have attended a state accredited school of nursing, must be a qualified related nursing

Table 2-1. STANDARDS OF CLINICAL NURSING PRACTICE	
Standards of Care	**Standards of Professional Performance**
Assessment	Quality of Care
Diagnosis	Performance Appraisal
Outcome Identification	Education
Planning	Collegiality
Implementation	Ethics
Evaluation	Collaboration
	Research
	Resource Utilization

professional or para-professional, or must meet specified prerequisites if licensed in a foreign country.
  3. Boards of Registered Nursing contract with the National Council of State Boards of Nursing, Inc., for use of the National Council Licensure Examination (abbreviated as NCLEX).

LEGAL ASPECTS OF MANAGEMENT

Nurse Practice Act

✦ A. A series of statutes enacted by each state legislature to regulate the practice of nursing in that state.

✦ B. Subjects covered by the Nurse Practice Act in each state include definition of scope of practice, education, licensure, grounds for disciplinary actions, and related topics.
  1. Provides legal authority for nursing practice, including delegation of nursing tasks.
  2. Many boards of nursing also provide decision trees or delegation checklists.

C. The Nurse Practice Acts are quite similar throughout the United States, but the professional nurse is held legally responsible for the specific requirements for licensure and regulations of practice as defined by the state in which he or she is working.

D. Responsibilities of the professional nurse involve a level of performance for a defined range of healthcare services.
  1. Provide direct and indirect client care services.
  2. Perform and deliver basic healthcare services.
  3. Implement testing and prevention procedures.
  4. Observe signs and symptoms of illness.
  5. Administer treatments per physician's order.
  6. Observe treatment reactions and responses.
  7. Administer medications per physician's order.
  8. Observe medication responses and any side effects.
  9. Observe general physical and mental conditions of individual clients.
  10. Provide client and family teaching.
  11. Act as a client advocate when needed.
  12. Document nursing care.
  13. Supervise allied nursing personnel.
  14. Coordinate members of the healthcare team.

Legal Issues

A. Legal issues and regulations play a dominant role in nursing practice today.

1. The law provides a framework for establishing nursing actions in the care of clients.
2. Laws determine and set boundaries and maintain a standard of nursing practice.

◆ B. The Nurse Practice Act defines professional nursing.
  ◆ 1. Recommends those actions that the nurse can take independently.
  ◆ 2. Recommends those actions that require a physician's order before completion.

C. Each state has the authority to regulate as well as *administrate* healthcare professionals.
  1. Provisions of Nurse Practice Acts are quite similar from state to state.
  2. The nurse must know the licensing requirements and the grounds for license revocation defined by the state in which he or she works.

◆ D. Legal and ethical standards for nurses are complicated by a myriad of federal and state statutes and the continually changing interpretation of them by the courts of law. Nurses today are faced with the threat of legal action based on negligence, malpractice, invasion of privacy, and other grounds.

MANAGEMENT PRINCIPLES

RN Management Duties

A. Responsibilities.
  ◆ 1. Performance, for compensation, of a defined range of healthcare services, including assessment, planning, implementation, and evaluation of nursing actions as well as teaching and counseling.
  ◆ 2. Administration of medications and treatments as prescribed by a licensed physician or other designated licensed professional.
  ◆ 3. Supervision of other nursing personnel; RN assigns, directs, monitors, and evaluates care performed by other personnel.
    ◆ a. The RN delegates or assigns duties and tasks to LVN/LPNs, licensed caregivers.
    ◆ b. The RN delegates or assigns tasks to unlicensed assistive personnel (UAPs) or certified nurse assistants (CNAs).
    c. UAPs are individuals employed in healthcare settings to augment client care—persons without licensure under state Nurse Practice Acts.
    d. CNAs have received minimal training (a few weeks) and have earned a certificate.

B. Requirements: specialized skills taught by and acquired at an accredited nursing school.

UNUSUAL OCCURRENCE—INCIDENT REPORT

There are three purposes
- Help document quality of care.
- Identify where in-service education is needed.
- Record details of an incident for legal reference.

Report must include specific details
- Details of the incident.
- Client's response.
- Nursing action or reaction.
- List of personnel who were aware of the incident.
- Report forwarded to unit manager, nursing administration, hospital legal department.

Useful tool for documenting quality of care
- Identify areas of practice that need improvement (i.e., increase in number of client falls).
- Plan classes or educational seminars to improve deficient areas.

◆ C. Standards of competent performance.
  1. A registered nurse shall be considered competent when he/she consistently demonstrates the ability to transfer scientific knowledge from social, biological, and physical sciences in applying the nursing process.
  2. *Incompetence* means lacking possession of or failure to exercise that degree of learning, skill, care, and experience ordinarily possessed and exercised by a competent registered nurse.

D. Professional functions of the RN (denoted by state).
  1. Formulates a nursing diagnosis through observation of the client's physical condition and behavior, and through interpretation of information obtained from the client and others, including the health team.
  2. Formulates a care plan, in collaboration with the client, which ensures that nursing care services provide for the client's safety, comfort, hygiene, and protection, and for disease prevention and restorative measures.
  3. Performs skills essential to the kind of nursing action to be taken, explains the health treatment to the client and family, and teaches the client and family how to care for the client's health needs.
  4. Delegates tasks to subordinates based on the legal scope of practice of the subordinate and on the preparation and capability needed in the tasks to be delegated, and effectively supervises nursing care being given by subordinates.
  5. Evaluates the effectiveness of the care plan through observation of the client's physical condition and behavior, signs and symptoms of illness, reactions to treatment, and through

communication with the client and health team members, modifies the plan as needed.

6. Acts as the client's advocate, as circumstances require, by initiating action to improve health care or change decisions or activities that are against the interests or wishes of the client, and by giving the client the opportunity to make informed decisions about health care before it is provided.

Management Decisions

A. Understaffed units force RNs to prioritize and even ration their caregiving.
   1. Should the nurse give care to those who need it most?
   2. Should the nurse care for those for whom she/he can do the most good?
B. Any one of these options lessens the quality of care for the other clients.
C. Value of care extenders (UAPs, PCTs, CNAs).
   1. Alleviate or lessen nursing workload and stress.
   2. Perform tasks that enable the professional staff to do more complex tasks.
   3. Provide cost-effective quality client care.
   4. Provide extra hands to get the work completed in a timely manner.

Risk Management

✦ A. Nurses are responsible to advise hospital authorities of unsafe nursing situations.
✦ B. Document unsafe staffing practices in an unusual occurrence and internal memo.
   1. Provides legal protection.
   2. These actions may be viewed as mitigating factor if you are sued.
✦ C. The ANA's Code for Nurses states that the nurse is the client's advocate and must take action if the rights or best interests of the client are in jeopardy.
D. ANA takes the position that nurses have a professional obligation to refuse assignments that put licenses or clients "in serious jeopardy."

DELEGATION PRINCIPLES

RN Delegation

A. Delegation is defined as "transferring to a competent individual the authority to perform a selected nursing task in a selected situation" (*Source:* National Council of State Boards of Nursing).
B. State licensing laws designate that nurses are legally accountable for quality of care.
✦ C. RNs are responsible for direct client care.

1. RNs decide which tasks to delegate and under what circumstances.
2. RNs must know what is safe delegation of nursing care tasks.
✦ 3. RNs must supervise (monitor and evaluate) outcomes for all delegated tasks.
✦ D. RNs must know legal scope of practice of other licensed providers.
✦ E. RNs must know competency of licensed and unlicensed personnel, as well as the tasks that may be delegated.
   1. Some states identify tasks that may *not ever* be delegated (such as applying a sterile dressing by unlicensed personnel).
   2. Review individual state rulings regarding tasks that may be legally delegated.
   ✦ 3. RNs may *not* delegate assessment, evaluation, or nursing judgment functions.
F. Tasks may be assigned to UAPs if the client is *not* medically fragile and/or performance of the task will not cause potential harm.
G. RNs and LVNs must check with their own states' laws and regulations to determine which activities may *not* be performed by UAPs or CNAs. Examples of these tasks follow:
   1. Administration of medications.
   2. Venipuncture or intravenous therapy.
   3. Parenteral or tube feedings.
   4. Invasive procedures including inserting NG tubes, inserting catheters, or tracheal suctioning.
   5. Assessment of the client's condition.
   6. Educating clients and their families concerning healthcare problems, including postdischarge care.
   7. Moderate-complexity laboratory tests.

✦ RN Responsibilities That Cannot Be Delegated

A. Data entry into clients' charts for all unlicensed personnel to whom tasks are delegated.
B. Initial health assessments (only by RN).
C. Care plan objectives—checked by RN if completed by LVN.
D. Review data obtained by other healthcare workers.
E. Complete referral form for additional client services.
F. Receive reports of client conditions and any unexpected findings from delegated activities.
G. Identify parameters for which worker is to notify nurse.
H. Carry out pain management activities (epidural narcotic analgesia done only by RN).
I. Check advance directives in client's chart.
J. Organ donation—RN or LVN responsible for carrying out hospital policies.
K. Complete discharge teaching plan.

Activity Delegation to the LVN/LPN

+ A. Determine which tasks may be delegated.
    1. Client diagnosis.
    2. Legal limits of delegation to the LVN. (Does this state allow an LVN to administer IV drugs?)
    3. Amount of judgment and experience needed to perform task or skill.
    4. Predictability of outcome of task.
    5. Whether assistant is capable of performing task.
  B. Delegation and responsibility.
    1. The RN is legally responsible for client care.
        + a. The LVN works with the RN, who initiates the nursing care plan; LVN may update care plan.
        + b. RN completes initial assessment; RN validates assessment changes noted by LVN.
    + 2. RN initiates client teaching and evaluates the results.
        a. LVNs may not initiate client teaching with exception of using standard care plan.
        b. LVNs may reinforce client teaching.
    3. Intravenous administration parameters vary by state.
        a. RN may initiate IVs and add medications.
        b. LVNs, depending on each state's standards, may or may not add medications to an IV, do IV push, or administer piggy-back solutions.
        c. LVNs may add vitamins and minerals in most states.
        d. LVNs may initiate IVs after completing IV course.

Delegation Policies and Regulations for Unlicensed Assistive Personnel and Certified Nurse Assistants

  A. The term *UAP* refers to healthcare workers who are not licensed to perform nursing tasks; this group also refers to those workers who are trained and certified, but not licensed.
  B. Many boards of nursing have enacted laws to protect clients in acute care settings.
+ C. Basic principles of staffing should be based on several criteria:
    1. Client care needs.
    2. Severity of the client's condition.
    3. Services needed.
    4. Complexity surrounding these conditions.
  D. These policies further state that unlicensed personnel cannot be assigned in lieu of a registered nurse.
    1. The nurse must determine which tasks may be performed by the UAP or CNA.

    2. The nurse must assess real or potential harm to the client by assigning certain tasks to the UAP or CNA.
    3. The nurse must "effectively supervise" other healthcare workers, taking into account:
        a. Client safety.
        b. Competency to perform task.
        c. Number and acuity of clients.
        d. Number and complexity of tasks.
        e. Staffing patterns.
+ E. Unlicensed personnel may not perform functions (even under the direct clinical supervision of an RN) that require a specific amount of scientific knowledge and technical skills.

+ ## Potential Problems in Delegation

  A. Delegating too much responsibility.
  B. Client welfare in jeopardy as a result of UAP and CNA activity.
    1. Poorly supervised and monitored.
    2. Unequipped to perform tasks.
  C. CNAs and UAPs given responsibility beyond the legal limit specified.
  D. Professional staff use UAPs in ways for which they are not prepared—also underutilizing these staff.
  E. Inappropriate delegation leads to unsafe client situations.
  F. Inability to recognize inappropriate delegation and unsafe client situations.
  G. Signs are overlooked that indicate the client's condition is deteriorating and the UAPs do not report it.

Appropriate Delegation to UAPs and CNAs

+ A. Use of assistive personnel.
    1. Evaluate specific client needs.
    2. Judge assistant's competence to perform assigned tasks.
    3. Communicate expectations.
    4. Provide instructions and active monitoring.
    5. Monitor progress in client care through feedback, evaluate outcomes, and follow-up on identified problems.
+ B. Determining appropriate delegation to an unlicensed healthcare worker—ask these questions:
    1. Can the UAP legally do this procedure according to the Nurse Practice Act in that state?
    2. Has the UAP been trained to perform this procedure?
    3. Can the UAP demonstrate this procedure safely and consistently?
    4. Is the client status stable, and does this client require frequent assessment during the procedure?
    5. Is the client response predictable?

6. When performing this task or activity, can the UAP or CNA obtain the same or similar results as the RN?
7. Can the UAP or CNA understand the rationale behind each task?

◆ C. Parameters of delegation: many state boards of nursing have identified the parameters of delegation. Examples of these **"rights of delegation"**:

1. **Right task**—a task that can be legally delegated to an LVN/LPN, CNA, PCT, or UAP. Check the state Nurse Practice Act to determine if the caregiver is trained to perform the task. Judge if the UAP or LVN is competent to perform the task.

2. **Right circumstance**—the LVN, CNA, PCT, or UAP understands the elements of the procedure and the RN is assured that the UAP can perform the procedure safely in an appropriate setting. Caregiver is able to collect the right supplies to perform the procedure.

3. **Right person**—the right person (RN or LVN) delegates the right task (legally can be delegated to a CNA or UAP) to the right person (legally can perform the task) on the right client (stable with predictable outcomes).

4. **Right communication**—person delegating the task (RN or LVN) has described the task clearly including directions, special steps of the task, and the expected outcomes.

5. **Right supervisor**—the RN or LVN delegating the activity answers the CNA's or UAP's questions and is available to problem solve if necessary (the task cannot be completed or the client's condition changes). The CNA, PCT, or UAP performing the task reports its completion and the client response to the nurse who delegated the activity.

Modified from the National Council of State Boards of Nursing.

D. Duties commonly delegated to unlicensed assistive personnel.
1. Take vital signs.
2. Obtain height and weight.
3. Assist a client to bed.
4. Escort a client out of the hospital.
5. Bathe and make beds.
6. Daily care activities.
7. Personal hygiene activities.
8. Move and turn clients and reposition.
9. Transfer clients.
10. Assigned to clients requiring infection control precautions.
11. Record drainage from an NG tube.
12. Serve a food tray and feed a client.
13. Provide oral hygiene.

14. Obtain specimens that are nonsterile and non-invasive.
15. Monitor specific gravity.
16. Check urine glucose.
17. Administer disposable enema or tap water enema.
18. Apply elastic hosiery.
19. Perform range-of-motion exercises.
20. Initiate CPR or perform Heimlich maneuver (with CPR certification).
21. Work with a dying client.
22. Give postmortem care.

LEGAL ISSUES: NATURE OF THE LAW

Definition: A system of principles and processes by which people who live in a society deal with their disputes and problems. Laws are rules of human conduct. Our legal system is continually changing as it responds to and is shaped by our society and its expectations and demands. The types of law that most directly affect nurses and their practice are civil and criminal.

Types of Law

A. Civil. (*See* Table 2-2.)
1. The harm is against an individual, and guilt requires proof by a preponderance of the evidence.
2. Civil law covers contracts, labor issues, and, among other areas, tort law (normally involved in malpractice claims). (*See* Table 2-3.)

Table 2-2. NURSING LIABILITY	
Civil Law	**Criminal Law**
Contract	Assault
Unintentional Tort	Battery
Intentional Tort	Murder
Negligence	Manslaughter

Table 2-3. CLASSIFICATIONS OF LAW RELATED TO NURSING	
Classification	**Example**
Constitutional	Clients' rights to equal treatment
Administrative	Licensure and the state BRN
Labor Relations	Union negotiations
Contract	Relationship with employer
Criminal	Handling of narcotics
Tort	
Medical Malpractice	Reasonable and prudent client care
Product Liability	Warranty on medical equipment

3. Punishment is generally the payment of monetary compensation.

B. Criminal.
   1. The harm is against society, and guilt requires proof beyond a reasonable doubt.
   2. Crimes are classified as misdemeanors (lesser) or felonies (serious).
   3. Examples are falsification of narcotics records, withholding life support from terminally ill clients, and administration of drugs that hasten a client's death.
   4. Punishment may be a payment of compensation and/or imprisonment.

KEY LEGAL TERMS

Liability

✦ A. A nurse has a personal, legal obligation to provide a standard of client care expected of a reasonably competent professional nurse.
✦ B. Professional nurses are held responsible (liable) for harm resulting from their negligent acts or omission to act.

Respondeat Superior

A. Legal doctrine that holds an employer liable for negligent acts of employees in the course and scope of employment.
B. Physicians, hospitals, clinics, and other employers may be held liable for negligent acts of their employees.
C. This doctrine does not support acts of gross negligence or acts that are outside the scope of employment.

Negligence

✦ A. The doctrine of negligence rests on the duty of every person to exercise due care in his or her conduct toward others from which injury may result.
✦ B. Liability results from
   1. A duty to provide care on the part of the nurse and a causal relationship between damage or harm to the client.
   2. An act or an omission to act by the nurse.
C. **Gross negligence** is the intentional failure to perform a duty in reckless disregard of the consequences affecting the client—a gross lack of care to such a level as to be considered willful and wanton.
✦ D. **Criminal negligence** consists of a duty on the part of the nurse and an act that is the proximate cause of the injury or death of a client.

PROVING NEGLIGENCE

- To prove negligence against a nurse, these four elements must be present:
  a. Failed a duty to provide a standard of care to the client.
  b. Failed to adhere to the standard of care.
  c. Failure to adhere to the standard of care caused injury to the client.
  d. Client suffered damages as a result of the nurse's negligent action.
- Documentation in the client's chart must show that the nurse met the standard of care.

---

   1. Usually defined by statute and punishable as a crime.
   2. The act being punished would be a flagrant and reckless disregard for the safety of others and/or a willful disregard for the injury liable to follow.
   3. The act is converted to a crime when it results in personal injury or death.
E. A nurse is considered "negligent" if he or she fails to provide a client with the standard of care that a reasonably prudent nurse would exercise under similar circumstances.

Malpractice

✦ A. Any professional misconduct that is an unreasonable lack of skill or fidelity in professional duties.
✦ B. Bad, wrong, or injurious treatment of a client.
✦ C. Results of treatment may include injury, unnecessary suffering, or death to a client proceeding from ignorance; carelessness; lack of professional skill; disregard of established rules, protocols, principles, or procedures; neglect; or a malicious or criminal intent.
D. It is the nurse's legal duty to provide competent, reasonable care to clients.
   ✦ 1. To ensure that these standards occur, the nurse must know the standards of care, develop patterns of practice that meet these standards, and document these actions.
   ✦ 2. Nursing actions that constitute a breach of standards of care and lead to client injury can be termed malpractice.
E. Avoiding malpractice litigation:
   1. Do not accept an assignment for which you have not been trained or which you do not feel competent to complete.
   2. Be very careful and vigilant when administering medications.
   3. Document all nursing aspects of interventions, because poor, missing, or incorrect charting could result in legal complications.

4. Do not change charting without following the rules of change. You may never cover up a mistake by changing a chart.

F. Legal doctrine holds that an employer may also be liable for negligent acts of employees in the course and scope of employment.

1. Physicians, hospitals, clinics, and other employers may be held liable for negligent acts of their employees.

2. This doctrine does not support acts of gross negligence or acts that are outside the scope of employment.

Professional Misconduct

A. Nurses must meet certain standards.

B. Any one of the following actions would be considered misconduct.

1. Obtaining an RN license through misrepresentation or fraudulent methods.

2. Giving false information on an application for license.

3. Practicing in an incompetent or grossly negligent manner.

4. Practicing when ability to practice is severely impaired.

5. Being habitually drunk or dependent on drugs.

6. Furnishing controlled substances to himself or herself or to another person.

7. Impersonating another certified or licensed practitioner or allowing another person to use his or her license for the purpose of nursing.

8. Being convicted of or committing an act constituting a crime under federal or state law.

9. Refusing to provide healthcare services on the grounds of race, color, creed, or national origin.

10. Permitting or aiding an unlicensed person to perform activities requiring a license.

11. Practicing nursing while one's license is suspended.

12. Practicing medicine without a license.

13. Procuring, aiding, or offering to assist at a criminal abortion.

14. Holding oneself out to the public as a "nurse practitioner" without being certified by the BRN as a nurse practitioner (in some states).

Risk Areas

A. Certain areas of practice increase the risk of potential liability for the nurse.

B. These areas are increased nursing involvement, potential hazards involved in the nurse's functions, and/or an increased social awareness on the part of clients and their families and associates.

RIGHTS AND CONSENT

A. A right or claim may be moral and/or legal.

1. A legal right can be enforced in a court of law.

2. Within the healthcare system, all clients retain their basic constitutional rights such as freedom of expression, due process of law, freedom from cruel and inhumane punishment, equal protection, and so forth.

B. Client rights may conflict with nursing functions.

1. Key elements of a client's rights with which nurses should be thoroughly familiar include consent, confidentiality, and involuntary commitment.

2. The client's rights may be modified by his or her mental or physical condition as well as by his or her social status.

Client's Right to Privacy (Confidentiality)

✦ A. Confidential information.

1. Clients are protected by law (invasion of privacy) against unauthorized release of personal clinical data such as symptoms, diagnoses, and treatments.

2. Nurses, as well as other healthcare professionals and their employers, may be held personally liable for invasion of privacy, as well as other torts, should litigation arise from unauthorized release of client data.

3. Nurses have a legal and ethical responsibility to become familiar with their employers' policies and procedures regarding protection of clients' information.

4. Confidential information may be released with consent of the client.

5. Information release is mandatory when ordered by a court or when state statutes require reporting child abuse, communicable diseases, or other incidents.

B. Client care: Nurses have an ethical responsibility to protect the client's personal privacy during treatment or hospitalization by means of gowns, screens, closed doors, etc.

C. Medical records.

1. As the key written account of client information such as signs and symptoms, diagnosis, treatment, etc., the medical record fulfills many functions both within the hospital or clinic and with outside parties.

    a. Documents the care given to the client.

    b. Provides an effective means of communication among healthcare personnel.

    c. Contains important data for insurance and other expense claims.

    d.   May be utilized in court in the event of litigation.

2. Nurses have an ethical and legal obligation to maintain complete and timely records, and to sign or countersign only those documents that are accurate and complete.

The Client's Bill of Rights

A. Inform client of his/her specific rights.
1. The client has the right to considerate and respectful care.
2. The client has the right to and is encouraged to obtain from physicians and other direct caregivers relevant, current, and understandable information concerning diagnosis, treatment, and prognosis. In emergencies, the client is entitled to the opportunity to discuss and request information related to specific procedures and/or treatments, the risk involved, and the financial implications of the treatment choices. Clients also have the right to know the identity of healthcare professionals caring for them.
3. The client has the right to make decisions about the plan of care prior to and during the course of treatment, to refuse a recommended treatment or plan of care to the extent permitted by law and hospital policy, and to be informed of the medical consequences of this action.
4. The client has the right to have an advance directive and have the hospital honor the intent of the directive to the extent permitted by law and hospital policy. The institution must advise clients of their rights under state law and hospital policy to make informed medical choices. Hospitals must identify if a client has an advance directive and place it in the client records.
5. The client has the right to every consideration of privacy including examination, treatment, consultation, and case discussion.
6. The client has the right to expect all communications and records pertaining to his/her care be treated as confidential by the hospital, except in cases of suspected abuse and public health hazards.
7. The client has the right to review the records pertaining to his/her medical care and have the information explained or interpreted as necessary, except when restricted by law.
8. The client has the right to expect that, within its capacity and policies, a hospital will make a reasonable response to the request of a client for appropriate and medically indicated care and services.
9. The client has the right to ask and be informed of the existence of business relationships among the hospital, educational institutions, other healthcare providers, or payers that may influence the client's treatment and care.
10. The client has the right to consent to or decline to participate in proposed research studies or human experimentation affecting care and treatment or requiring direct client involvement, and to have those studies fully explained prior to consent.
11. The client has the right to expect reasonable continuity of care when appropriate and to be informed by physicians and other caregivers of available and realistic client care options when hospital care is no longer appropriate.
12. The client has the right to be informed of hospital policies and practices that relate to client care, treatment, and responsibilities, including grievances and conflicts.

B. Originally devised in 1992 and revised in 2003 (American Hospital Association).

Informed Consent [to Receive Health Services]

✦ A. Consent is the client's approval to have his or her body touched by a specific individual (such as doctor, nurse, laboratory technician).
1. Types of consent: expressed or implied—verbal or written.
✦ 2. Informed consent: prior to granting a consent, the client must be fully informed regarding

treatment, tests, surgery, etc., and must understand both the intended outcome and the potentially harmful results.

   3. The client may rescind a prior consent verbally or in writing.

 ✦ B. Authority to consent.

   1. A mentally competent adult client must give his or her own consent.

   2. In emergency situations, if the client is in immediate danger of serious harm or death, action may be taken to preserve life without the client's consent.

   3. Parents or legal guardians may give consent for minors.

   4. Court-authorized persons may give consent for mentally incompetent clients.

  C. Two major forms of consent are signed by clients in a healthcare facility.

   1. The first consent is signed at the time of admission.

     a. The client signs the form in the admissions office or in the emergency department.

     b. This agreement indicates the client will agree to such procedures as medical treatment, x-rays, blood transfusions, and injections.

   2. The second type of consent is for invasive testing procedures, such as biopsies, surgery, or special studies involving dye injection or other procedures where risk is involved.

  D. Nurse's liability.

 ✦ 1. The nurse who asks a client to sign a consent form may be held personally liable if the nurse knows or should know that the client has not been fully informed by the physicians, hospital staff, or others regarding potentially harmful effects of treatments, tests, surgery, and other acts.

   2. Nurses must respect the right of a mentally competent adult client to refuse health care; however, a life-threatening situation may alter the client's right to refuse treatment.

  E. Hospital admissions.

   1. Voluntary admission.

     a. A person freely consents to enter an institution for purposes of receiving medical, surgical, or psychiatric care and treatment.

     b. Clients who enter on a voluntary basis may leave at will.

 ✦ 2. Involuntary admission.

     a. An individual may legally be admitted to an institution without his or her own consent when that individual does not have the mental capacity or competency to under-

---

ADVANCE DIRECTIVES

The Patient Self-Determination Act of 1990 (PSDA) is a federal law that imposes on states and providers of health care certain requirements concerning advance directives as well as an individual's right under state law to make decisions concerning medical care.

 ✦ The Omnibus Budget Reconciliation Act (OBRA) of 1990 requires states to provide advance directives as options for clients. This document should be completed and signed before treatment becomes necessary. The nurse should check with the client's physician to determine that advance directives are on file. Documents include

- Client's choice in continuing medical care when the client is unable to speak or make decisions.
- Living will, power of attorney for health care, or a notarized handwritten document.
- Documents available in client's medical record.
- Documents witnessed by persons other than medical personnel or relatives of the client or heirs to the client's estate.

---

stand his or her own acts and is a danger to self or others.

 ✦ b. Occurs when the client is judged by a court of law to be mentally ill or dangerous to self and others, and to require admission to a psychiatric ward or center.

Advance Directives

 ✦ A. An advance directive is a document that allows clients to make legal decisions about how they wish to receive future medical treatment. It is written and signed before any such care becomes necessary.

   1. It allows clients to participate in choosing healthcare providers (physicians and nurses).

   2. It allows clients to choose the type of medical treatments they desire.

   3. It allows clients to consent to or refuse certain types of medical treatments.

 ✦ B. Within this document, the client may indicate the person or persons he or she wishes to make medical decisions in situations in which the client is unable to do so.

  C. The document needs to be signed and witnessed, and copies should be kept on file in the physician's office and the hospital.

  D. The witness to this document should not be a hospital employee, relative, or heir to the client's estate.

  E. Advance directives vary among states and, therefore, the nurse must be knowledgeable about the use and type of directives in the state in which he or she practices.

LEGAL ISSUES FOR MEDICARE

Medicare recently issued a new ruling to take effect in 2008. Medicare will cease paying for eight preventable hospital-acquired conditions. The new policy will save lives and millions of dollars. Medicare will not reimburse hospitals for specific conditions that could reasonably have been prevented.

The specific hospital-acquired conditions for which Medicare will not reimburse hospitals are

- Blood incompatibility
- Air embolisms
- Objects left in body during surgical procedures
- Pressure ulcers
- Vascular catheter-associated infections
- UTIs related to improper catheter use
- Mediastinitis: post-surgical coronary artery bypass graft
- Injuries, including fractures, dislocations, burns

Medicare is considering adding ventilator-associated pneumonia, *Staphylococcus aureus* septicemia, and even deep-vein thrombosis/pulmonary embolism to the list. This measure will promote quality of care and give hospitals a financial incentive (they cannot bill clients for these conditions) to take steps to prevent hospital-acquired conditions.

✦ LEGAL ASPECTS OF DRUG ADMINISTRATION

A. Nurses must not administer a specific drug unless allowed to do so by the particular state's Nurse Practice Act.
  1. Nurses must not administer any drug without a specific physician's order.
  2. Nurses must not administer a controlled substance if the physician's order is outdated.
B. Nurses are to take every safety precaution in whatever action they perform.
C. Nurses are to be certain that the employer's policy allows them to administer a specific drug.
D. A drug may not lawfully be administered unless all the above items are in effect.
E. General rules for drug dispensing:
  1. Never leave medicines unattended.
  2. Always report errors immediately.
  3. Send labeled bottles that are unintelligible back to the pharmacist for relabeling.
  4. Store internal and external medicines separately if possible.

Living Will

✦ A. A living will is a type of advance directive.
✦ B. The document indicates the client's wishes regarding
  1. Prolonging life using life support measures.
  2. Refusing or stopping medical interventions.
  3. Making decisions about his or her medical care.
✦ C. Living wills are executed while the client is competent and able to make sound decisions.

D. As conditions change, a living will needs to be evaluated for relevance. (States differ in their acceptance of living wills as legal documents.)

Durable Power [of Attorney] for Health Care

A. This is a legal document concerning health care for the client.
  ✦ 1. This document gives power to make healthcare decisions to a designated individual in the event that the client is unable to make competent decisions for himself or herself.
  ✦ 2. It must be prepared and signed while the client is competent.
  ✦ 3. The designated person is obligated to follow the directives outlined in the document.
✦ B. Decisions regarding withdrawing or using life support, organ donation, or consent to treatment or procedures are included in the directives.
  1. As long as the client is competent, the agent does not have the right to make legal decisions.
  2. The major difference between the living will and power of attorney is that the latter is more flexible.

Do Not Resuscitate (DNR)

A. A "Do Not Resuscitate" or DNR order is another type of advance directive.
  1. DNR is a request to not have cardiopulmonary resuscitation (CPR) if the client ceases to breathe or is unable to sustain a heartbeat.
  2. This form can be signed at any time before or during hospitalization.
B. When a DNR order is signed, the physician places a DNR notation in the client's medical chart.

LEGAL ISSUES IN DRUG ADMINISTRATION

Definition: In their daily work, most nurses handle a wide variety of drugs. Failure to give the correct medication or improper handling of drugs may result in serious problems for the nurse due to strict federal and state statutes relating to drugs. (*See* Chapter 5 on pharmacology.)

Regulation

✦ A. The Comprehensive Drug Abuse Prevention Act of 1970 provides the fundamental regulations (federal) for the compounding, selling, and dispensing of narcotics, stimulants, depressants, and other controlled items.
B. Each state has a similar set of regulations for the same purpose.

Violation

A. Each state's pharmacy act provides standards for dispensing drugs.

B. Noncompliance with federal or state drug regulations can result in liability.

✦ C. Violation of the state drug regulations or licensing laws is grounds for BRN administrative disciplinary action.

LEGAL ISSUES IN PSYCHIATRIC NURSING

Statutes of Protection

A. Laws of certain states protect individuals from themselves.
   1. These laws require that such persons be evaluated by competent psychiatric personnel.
   2. The laws protect clients' rights and civil liberties by not allowing psychiatric clients to be hospitalized inappropriately.

B. Laws also protect family members and the general community from persons who are dangerous or severely disturbed.

Admission Procedures

A. There are voluntary and involuntary admissions for psychiatric clients.

✦ B. Voluntary admission occurs when an individual recognizes that he or she needs treatment and signs in to a hospital.
   1. After admission, the client is *not* free to leave before a specified period of time.
   2. Such a client may leave the hospital against the physician's advice if the client gives notice of such intent at least one or two days prior to leaving.
   3. If the physician feels the client is too ill, he can legally assign the client to involuntary status.
   4. A voluntary client loses none of his or her civil rights.

✦ C. Involuntary status occurs when the client is psychiatrically evaluated to be too ill to function outside the hospital.
   1. Admission is not initiated by the client.
   2. When a client is committed, he or she cannot leave the hospital against medical advice.
   3. Family members, a physician, a law officer, or a community member can institute commitment proceedings.
   4. Clients are permitted to leave only when psychiatric evaluation indicates they are able to care for themselves or are not dangerous to themselves or others.

5. A client may retain some, all, or none of his or her civil rights. This depends on the individual state laws.

6. The different classifications include emergency admission (time limited), observational (diagnostic evaluation or short term), and indefinite (formal commitment).

Psychiatric Advance Directives (PAD)

A. PAD is similar to advance directives prepared for end-of-life care.

B. Specific components that may be included in the PAD:
   1. Refusal of specific drugs, surgery, or treatments [e.g., electroconvulsive therapy (ECT)].
   2. Consent for specific psychiatric interventions and conditions under which they may be implemented.
   3. Appointment of a trusted individual who may give consent for the client.
   4. Willingness to participate in research studies.

C. PADs are not accepted in every state. They are popular with mental health providers for providing guidance to family, staff, and the courts.

RESTRAINTS

✦ A. Used as a last resort—legal only to protect the client or others from forseeable harm.
   1. Hospital policy and procedures must be followed when applying restraints.
   ✦ 2. Most states and facilities require a physician's order for restraints.
      a. Orders must specify justification for restraint, type of restraint, length of time, and criteria for removal.
      b. Restraints may *not* be ordered PRN; a nurse may legally restrain a client without an order if essential.
   ✦ 3. Legal implications for the nurse applying restraints.
      a. A nurse may be charged with assault if restraints are used when not needed.
      b. A nurse may be charged with negligence when client injury occurs.

B. Types of restraints.
   ✦ 1. Physical restraints—application of a device to restrict movement.
      a. Prevent client falls.
      b. Discourage client from disconnecting vital equipment.
      c. Prevent client from harming self or others.
   ✦ 2. Chemical restraints—medications given to prevent certain behaviors.

a. Prevent clients from disconnecting vital equipment.

b. Assist in preventing client from harming self or others.

c. Allow staff to care for all clients on a unit.

✦ C. Alternatives to restraints.

1. Encourage family and friends to monitor client; use sitters to monitor client.

2. Use a bed occupancy monitor or similar device to immediately notify nurses when a client is out of bed.

3. Provide appropriate and continuing stimulation and monitoring.

✦ D. Restraint guidelines.

1. Review hospital policy for the use of restraints.

2. Use restraints for the client's protection and to prevent injury, not for the nurse's convenience.

3. Use the least amount of restraint possible. A torso belt is least restrictive, limb restraint is more restrictive, and chemical (medication) is *most* restrictive.

4. Allow clients as much freedom of movement as possible. Use slipknots for quick release. Do not use square knots or bows.

5. Always explain the purpose of the restraint to the client and family. Afford as much dignity to the client as possible.

6. Remember that restraints can cause emotional, mental, and physical deterioration and increase the risk of injury if falls occur.

7. Remember that circulation and skin integrity can be affected by restraints.

8. Special precautions should be taken for adult females in restraints to protect breast tissue.

9. Clients must be observed every 15 minutes and restraints released every 2 hours for at least 5 minutes to inspect tissues and provide joint range of motion and position change to prevent circulatory impairment. When a client is combative, release only one restraint at a time.

10. Assess and provide for client's fluid and elimination needs, pain management, and position change every 2 hours.

11. Pad bony prominences, such as wrists and ankles, beneath a restraint.

12. Attempt to make restraints as inconspicuous as possible for the sake of the client's relatives and friends, who may be upset by seeing restraints.

13. Notify families, significant others, or guardians if restraints are necessary.

14. Clearly document rationale and precautions taken for client safety.

Adapted from Smith, S., Duell, D., & Martin, B. (2008). *Clinical nursing skills* (7th ed.). Upper Saddle River, NJ: Prentice Hall Health.

ORGAN DONATION

✦ A. Legal aspects of donation.

1. The federal Omnibus Budget Reconciliation Act of 1986 states that all facilities receiving Medicare or Medicaid funding must have policies in place to identify potential organ donors and to inform families about the option to donate.

✦ a. Laws do not require the consent of a family member to retrieve organs if the donor has already declared his wish to donate (must be 18 years of age or older).

✦ b. The choice to donate an organ must be a written document—a donor card, a will, or an advance directive signed by the client.

✦ c. Providers are reluctant to act without a family member's permission because of fear of being sued.

✦ d. Some states have limited the family's involvement in the donation process.

2. Legal definition of death.

a. Death is defined legally as cardiac death—total failure of cardiopulmonary system.

b. The second definition is neurologic or brain death—unresponsive to all stimuli, fixed pupils and no brain stem reflexes.

✦ 3. Hospitals are required by law to contact donor team so they may give families the information they need to make an informed decision about organ donation.

4. The Uniform Anatomical Gift Act protects those who are involved in organ procurement from liability, but provider must "act in good faith" and must provide next of kin with complete and accurate information.

✦ B. Allocating organs.

1. United Network for Organ Sharing: Clients awaiting transplant (heart or kidney) are assigned priority according to medical need. (Currently there is a waiting list of more than 80,000 for organs.)

2. Ethical question: Should more desperately ill receive preference or should priority be given to healthier clients? The answer varies according to facility.

C. Organ donor potential.

1. Review specific facility's death criteria.

2. Generally accepted criteria—brain death.

a. Cause of client's injury known.

b. Exhibits no brain stem reflexes.

c. No CNS depressants present.

d. Temperature greater than 90°F.

e. Exhibits no spontaneous responses.

f. Unresponsive to noxious stimuli.

MANAGEMENT PRINCIPLES AND LEGAL ISSUES REVIEW QUESTIONS

MANAGEMENT PRINCIPLES

1. An RN team leader observed an LVN beginning an IV without putting on gloves. When confronted, the LVN replied, "Oh, I was careful and didn't get any blood on me." How should the RN initially respond?

   1. "The regulations state that all of us must wear gloves. If I see you without them, I will place you on report."
   2. "Tell me your understanding of what Standard Precautions for all clients means."
   3. "Well, if you are absolutely sure that you can be careful—but I don't think it is safe nursing practice."
   4. "I think we should clarify this with the charge nurse to see who is right."

2. The RN is very short-staffed because two people did not show up for work. Of the following four clients, which one would the RN care for first?

   1. A client just admitted with acute abdominal pain and possible cholecystitis.
   2. A client with nephrotic syndrome with increasing edema; hourly urine checks and vital signs.
   3. A confused client yelling because he is in soft restraints and cannot get out of bed.
   4. A head-injury client (with an IV) who was just admitted to the unit.

3. The RN has a full workload and must reassign some of her clients to the UAP. The most appropriate client to reassign to the UAP would be a(n)

   1. Client just returning from the recovery room following colostomy surgery.
   2. Cerebrovascular accident (CVA) client who has been hospitalized for 2 days.
   3. Oncology client who is in severe pain controlled by epidural anesthesia.
   4. Newly admitted client with suspected pancreatitis.

4. The RN observes two nurses talking and laughing when in the room of a client in a coma. The appropriate response for the RN is to

   1. Ignore the behavior because the client cannot hear them.

   2. Call the nurses outside the room and ask them to be more professional.
   3. Notify the charge nurse of this unprofessional behavior.
   4. Point out to the nurses, outside the room, that the client might hear them.

5. The RN asked the nursing assistant (NA) to wash the client's hair as part of her assignment. The RN will help the NA to understand that washing the client's hair will

   1. Raise her self-esteem.
   2. Make her feel better.
   3. Improve her physical condition.
   4. Make her more presentable.

6. The nurse suspects a peer is abusing drugs. This suspicion would be based on the behavior of

   1. Always arriving late for work and often taking a sick day.
   2. Socializing with others and bargaining with coworkers to change hours.
   3. Requesting to have clients who are located close to the bathroom.
   4. Offering to dispense meds or to care for clients on pain meds.

7. The RN tells the LPN she is very busy and needs assistance. Which one of the following tasks *cannot* be delegated to an LPN?

   1. Checking the blood glucose level of a client and giving the appropriate insulin dose.
   2. Completing a peripheral vascular assessment that a nursing assistant identified as being different from the earlier assessment.
   3. Completing an initial health assessment on a newly admitted client.
   4. Completing client teaching for a client scheduled for discharge.

The nursing unit is very busy. The nurse has five critically ill clients (none are terminal; all are full codes and have required IV push medications). Seven clients are being discharged and two new clients are being admitted with chest pain who are on lidocaine drips. One of the clients with chest pain had two runs of ventricular tachycardia in the ER. The nurse also has a comatose terminal client with a life expectancy of less than 72 hours. This client has a sump tube, a Foley catheter, and TPN running through a central line. His orders are comfort measures only. Questions 8–10 relate to this scenario.

8. Considering the above, who is the most appropriate person to take care of the critically ill clients?

   1. RN.
   2. LPN.
   3. CNA.
   4. UAP.

9. The most appropriate person to take care of the terminally ill client is the

   1. RN.
   2. LPN/LVN.
   3. CNA.
   4. UAP.

10. The most appropriate person to take care of the clients being discharged who need teaching reinforced would be the

   1. RN.
   2. LPN.
   3. CNA.
   4. UAP.

11. Which client is most critical and should be assessed by the RN?

   1. Diabetic client being discharged and requiring discharge teaching.
   2. Cardiac client with a history of ventricular tachycardia.
   3. Client requiring IV push medication.
   4. Comatose, terminally ill client.

12. The RN in charge of assignments, with limited available staff, must assign the following four clients. Which client would be most appropriate for the UAP?

   1. A recent postsurgical TURP.
   2. A head-injury client with stable intracranial pressure.
   3. A client with heart failure.
   4. A client with acute pancreatitis.

13. A new graduate RN has been assigned to work in a subacute nursing unit. The nurse has the help of two UAPs to care for 15 clients. When delegating client care, what is the most important concept for the nurse to keep in mind?

   1. The length of time it takes to care for each client.
   2. The skill level of the two UAPs.
   3. The length of time each UAP has been on the job.
   4. Which clients the RN has taken care of before.

14. In the presence of the RN, a physician asks the LVN to remove the sutures from the incision before the client is discharged. The initial response to the physician should be

   1. LVNs cannot remove the sutures; the RN will do it.
   2. Please write the order and the sutures will be removed.
   3. We will remove them right away.
   4. The LVN will get the suture removal set for you because he or she is not allowed to remove sutures.

15. A nurse in charge of a unit observes a certified nursing assistant (CNA) listening to breath sounds. Which of these actions by the CNA would require immediate attention by the charge nurse?

   1. Encouraging the client to cough and deep breathe.
   2. Giving the client the incentive spirometer to use.
   3. Administrating Combivent and Serevent to enhance breathing.
   4. Completing pulse oxygenation on the client.

LEGAL ISSUES

1. The civil rights of a client would not be jeopardized in which of the following situations?

   1. Trying to forcibly detain a client who may suffer great harm by leaving the hospital.
   2. Giving emergency medical care to a client without his or her consent or the consent of the family.
   3. Giving a psychiatric client's letters addressed to the President of the United States to his physician.
   4. Giving the client's insurance broker access to his chart.

2. The primary purpose and criteria of licensure is to

   1. Limit practice.
   2. Define the scope of practice.
   3. Protect the public.
   4. Outline legislative action.

3. One of the elements of negligence is breach of the standard of care. *Standard of care* may be defined as

   1. Nursing competence as defined by the state Nurse Practice Act.
   2. The degree of judgment and skill in nursing care given by a reasonable and prudent professional nurse under similar circumstances.
   3. Health services as prescribed by community ordinances.
   4. Giving care to clients in good faith to the best of one's ability.

4. The decision as to whether a nurse can lawfully restrain a client is made by the

   1. Nurse.
   2. Family.
   3. Hospital administrator.
   4. Physician.

5. The physician wrote a medication order for a client. The nurse thought the dosage was incorrect. She questioned the physician, who said it was all right. Still questioning, she asked another nurse, who said it was all right. The nurse gave the medicine, and the client died from an overdose. Who is liable?

   1. The physician and the two nurses.
   2. The physician.
   3. The nurse who gave the medication.
   4. Both the physician and the nurse who gave the medication.

6. Which of the following best describes the function and purpose of the unusual occurrence (incident) report?

   1. A legal part of the chart used to furnish data about the incident.
   2. A hospital record used to record the details of the incident for possible legal reference.
   3. A legal hospital business record that is subject to subpoena and can be used against the hospital personnel.
   4. A hospital record that is entered into the client's chart if he or she dies.

7. If the nurse is involved in a situation in which he or she must countersign the charting of a paraprofessional, which of the following will most aid in decreasing legal liability?

   1. Read the document before signing it.

2. Have personal knowledge of the information contained in the document.
3. Make sure the information is accurate.
4. Check with a second nurse to see if the information is accurate.

8. The nurse transcribing the physician's order finds it difficult to read. Which of the following people should the nurse consult for clarification of the order?

   1. The head nurse who is familar with the physician's writing.
   2. Another nurse working with the nurse.
   3. The physician who wrote the order.
   4. The nursing supervisor.

9. Which of the following would not constitute negligent conduct?

   1. A medication error.
   2. Failure to follow a physician's order.
   3. Failure to challenge a physician's order.
   4. Disagreeing with a physician.

10. The nurse is asked to do a TV commercial for hand lotion. In this commercial she will wear her nurse's uniform and advocate the use of this lotion by nurses in their work setting. In doing this, the nurse is violating

    1. Consumer fraud laws.
    2. The Nurse Practice Act.
    3. The code of ethics for nurses.
    4. None of the above.

11. Nurse Practice Acts include

    1. A definition of nursing practice.
    2. Qualifications for licensure.
    3. Grounds for revocation of a license.
    4. All of the above.

12. Clients' rights are

    1. Specifically written into many laws.
    2. A position paper that was developed by the American Hospital Association.
    3. A declaration of the World Health Organization.
    4. Not supported by statutory law.

13. Which of the following statements concerning nursing liability is true?

    1. A physician may assume personal liability for the negligent acts of the nurse.

2. The nurse is responsible for his or her own negligent acts.
3. The doctrine of respondeat superior always protects the nurse.
4. Malpractice insurance will always cover the damages assessed against the nurse.

14. Which of the following might negate liability on the part of the nurse in a negligent action?

1. The client consented to the act.
2. The harm was not reasonably foreseeable.
3. The nurse had not been taught to do the procedure in nursing school.
4. Other foreseeable acts occurred that added to the client's injury.

15. The nurse's liability in terms of the client's consent to receive health services is to

1. Be certain that the physician has prepared the client.
2. Ensure that the client is fully informed before being asked to sign a consent form.
3. Check that the client understands the details of the surgery.
4. The nurse would not be liable—the physician would be.

MANAGEMENT PRINCIPLES AND LEGAL ISSUES

Answers with Rationale

MANAGEMENT PRINCIPLES

1. (2) The best way to determine what the LVN knows and/or understands or believes is to ask this basic question. Once the RN has baseline data, then teaching about the importance of always using Standard Precautions can be done. When a nurse becomes inconsistent in the use of these Standard Precautions, clients as well as the other healthcare team members are in jeopardy. Standard Precautions are to be used for **all** clients when there is a danger of coming into contact with body fluids.

   NP:I; CN:S; CA:M; CL:AN

2. (4) Head injury would take the first priority because the danger of increasing intracranial pressure must be assessed and, if it is increasing or the level of consciousness is changing, these results must be reported immediately. This client has the most serious and potentially unstable condition; thus the nursing judgment would be to care for him first. The nephrotic client (2) is not in critical condition and the confused client (3) can also wait; the second priority would be the client with possible cholecystitis (1) because of the unstable condition.

   NP:AN; CN:S; CA:M; CL:AN

3. (2) The most appropriate client would be the CVA diagnosis. This client would have been in the hospital for 2 days, so the initial assessment would have been completed. Also, this client does not require immediate intervention, as does the colostomy client (1) (assessing for hemorrhage, vital signs, etc.). The oncology client (3) must be assessed for effectiveness of pain control, and the RN or LVN is the only staff member who can do this. The newly admitted client with suspected pancreatitis (4) also requires a complete health assessment, and the RN is the only person who can complete this task.

   NP:AN; CN:S; CA:M; CL:AN

4. (4) It is the RN's responsibility to teach those on her or his team. The RN should deal with the situation directly and teach the nurses so they understand that the last sense to disappear in a coma client is hearing. The nurses' behavior is not only nontherapeutic, but also unprofessional.

   NP:I; CN:S; CA:M; CL:A

5. (1) Improving a person's physical appearance as well as helping the client to be clean and attractive will raise her self-esteem, which in turn may have a positive effect on her physical condition. It is important to give the NA a rationale for the task assigned so that she will understand the value—it will also raise her self-esteem.

   NP:I; CN:S; CA:M; CL:C

6. (4) If the nurse were abusing drugs, he or she would try to dispense drugs or care for clients on pain medications. The nurse would not want to take days off, because he or she would not be near the drug source.

   NP:AN; CN:S; CA:M; CL:A

7. (3) Completing the initial health assessment on the client is the RN's responsibility according to the legal guidelines. The LPN may update and perform a focus assessment on the client. All of the other interventions may be performed by the LPN.

   NP:P; CN:S; CA:M; CL:C

8. (1) An RN is responsible for the continuous assessment of clients. If they are critically ill, clients will need continuous assessment. These clients are not terminal; if they were, they could be cared for by the LPN.

   NP:P; CN:S; CA:M; CL:A

9. (4) UAP. This client is terminal and requires comfort measures only. The RN can assess and maintain the

---

Coding for Questions/Answers Abbreviations: **Nursing Process: NP,** Assessment: A, Analysis: AN, Planning: P, Implementation: I, Evaluation: E; **Client Needs: CN,** Safe, Effective Care Environment: S, Health Promotion and Maintenance: H, Psychosocial Integrity: PS, Physiological Integrity: PH; **Clinical Area: CA,** Medical Nursing: M, Surgical Nursing: S, Maternal/Newborn Nursing: MA, Pediatric Nursing: P, Psychiatric Nursing: PS; **Cognitive Level: CL,** Knowledge: K, Comprehension: C, Application: A, Analysis: AN.

TPN rate via pump, and irrigate the Foley catheter and sump as needed. The UAP can safely provide the care to keep the client comfortable. Any IV pain medications would be given by the RN.

NP:P; CN:S; CA:M; CL:AN

10. (2)   LPN. The RNs are needed for the other clients on the unit. Reinforcement of the teaching can be safely and effectively done by an LPN or an LVN.

NP:P; CN:S; CA:M; CL:AN

11. (2)   The cardiac client requires constant assessment with the possibility of immediate life support intervention should he have another run of ventricular tachycardia. Given the instability of the client's situation, the cardiac client is the most critical.

NP:P; CN:S; CA:M; CL:AN

12. (3)   The most appropriate choice, although not an ideal one, would be the heart failure client. The TURP client (1) must be assessed for hemorrhage; the head-injury client (2) must be monitored for a change in ICP; and the client with acute pancreatitis (4) requires vital signs, monitoring every 15 minutes, and frequent assessment for complications.

NP:AN; CN:S; CA:M; CL:AN

13. (2)   There are two UAPs who probably have different skill levels. It is important to consider their abilities and skill level (as well as the legal parameters for which tasks they can perform) when assigning clients and tasks. The other variables are important, but should be taken into account after the skill level has been evaluated.

NP:P; CN:S; CA:M; CL:A

14. (2)   LVN/LPNs may remove sutures; however, both nurses must make sure that the physician has written the order to do so. A verbal order would not be sufficient in this situation.

NP:I; CN:S; CA:S; CL:A

15. (3)   The CNA does not have the knowledge, skills, or ability to assess lung sounds and make judgments based on this high level of assessment. In addition, CNAs do not administer medications.

NP:P; CN:S; CA:M; CL:AN

LEGAL ISSUES

1. (2)   Key elements of a client's rights are consent, confidentiality, and involuntary commitment.

NP:AN; CN:S; CL:A

2. (3)   The primary purpose of licensing nurses, both RN and LVN, is to safeguard the public by determining that the nurse is a safe and competent practitioner.

NP:AN; CN:S; CL:K

3. (2)   Nursing actions are evaluated against a set of standards referred to as standards of performance.

NP:AN; CN:S; CL:K

4. (4)   To administer any form of restraint, there must be a physician's order.

NP:P; CN:S; CL:A

5. (4)   The professional nurse and the physician who wrote the order are held responsible (liable) for harm resulting from their negligent acts.

NP:AN; CN:S; CL:AN

6. (2)   The most accurate answer is (2). The other purposes are to help document the quality of care and to identify areas where more in-service education is needed.

NP:AN; CN:S; CL:K

7. (2)   To sign a document without having personal knowledge of what occurred would open the possibility of liability.

NP:P; CN:S; CL:C

8. (3)   Because the nurse will be responsible (and liable) if she transcribes the order incorrectly, the physician who wrote the order should be consulted.

NP:P; CN:S; CL:A

9. (4)   Because the nurse is a licensed professional with an education based on a defined body of knowledge, he or she had the right—indeed, the responsibility—to disagree with the physician. This is especially so when the health and welfare of the client is involved.

NP:AN; CN:S; CL:K

10. (3)   The code of ethics is a set of formal guidelines for governing professional action. This situation is not illegal—it is unethical.

NP:AN; CN:S; CL:C

11. (4)   The Nurse Practice Act is a series of statutes enacted by a state to regulate the practice of nursing in that state. It includes all of these plus education.

NP:AN; CN:S; CL:K

12. (1)   All but 10 states have some provision for the rights of clients written into a law, and these rights can be enforced by the law.

    NP:AN; CN:S; CL:K

13. (2)   The nurse is responsible for her or his own negligent acts; however, legal doctrine holds that an employer is also liable for negligent acts of employees.

    NP:AN; CN:S; CL:C

14. (2)   If basic rules of human conduct are not violated, the elements of liability may not exist. There must be certain elements of liability present; for example, there must exist a causal relationship between harm to the client and the act by the nurse. There must be some damage or harm sustained by the client and there must be a legal basis—such as statutory law—for finding liability.

    NP:AN; CN:S; CL:A

15. (2)   The client must be fully informed of potentially harmful effects of the treatment. If this is not done, it could result in the nurse's being personally liable.

    NP:P; CN:S; CL:C

Nursing Concepts

✦ The icon denotes content of special importance for NCLEX.

STRESS AND ADAPTATION

Homeostasis

✦ *Definition:* The maintenance of a constant state in the internal environment through self-regulatory techniques that preserve the organism's ability to adapt to stresses.
  A. Dynamics of homeostasis.
    1. Danger or its symbols, whether internal or external, result in the activation of the sympathetic nervous system and the adrenal medulla.
    ✦ 2. The organism prepares for *fight or flight* (attack–withdrawal; one's immediate response to stress—an archaic and often inappropriate response, but part of our biological heritage).
  B. Adaptation factors.
    1. Age—adaptation is greatest in youth and young middle life, and least at the extremes of life.
    2. Environment—adequate supply of required materials is necessary.
    3. Adaptation involves the entire organism.
    4. The organism can more easily adapt to stress over a period of time than suddenly.
    5. Organism flexibility influences survival.
    6. The organism usually uses the adaptation mechanism that is most economical in terms of energy.
    7. Illness decreases the organism's capacity to adapt to stress.
    8. Adaptation responses may be adequate or deficient.
    9. Adaptation may cause stress and illness (i.e., ulcers, arthritis, allergy, asthma, and overwhelming infections).

Stress

  A. Definitions of stress.
    ✦ 1. A physical, chemical, or emotional factor that causes bodily or mental tension and that may be a factor in disease causation; a state resulting from factors that tend to alter an existing equilibrium.
    2. Selye's definition of stress.
      a. The state manifested by a specific syndrome that consists of all the nonspecifically induced changes within the biologic system.
      b. The body is the common denominator of all adaptive responses.
      c. Stress is manifested by the measurable changes in the body.
      d. Stress causes a multiplicity of changes in the body.

    3. Wolff's theory of stress.
      a. Poor adaptation to a life situation may lead to a breakdown in homeostasis with subsequent development of disease.
      b. Wolff believed that a person's total life situation (with its positive as well as negative aspects) affects a person's susceptibility to disease.
      c. Disease may result from attempts to restore homeostasis.
  ✦ B. General aspects of stress.
    1. Body responses to stress are a self-preserving mechanism that automatically and immediately becomes activated in times of danger.
      a. Caused by physical or psychological stress: disease, injury, anger, or frustration.
      b. Caused by changes in internal and/or external environment.
    2. There are a limited number of ways an organism can respond to stress (for example, a cornered amoeba cannot fly).

Stress and Disease

  A. Stress and individual methods of coping are associated with heart disease, cancer and other diseases.
  B. Actual physical changes occur with high stress levels.
    1. Increased release of adrenalin, cortisol and other hormones lead to increased heart rate, blood pressure and platelet stickiness which may accelerate atherosclerosis and other causes of heart disease.
    2. Changes in immune system may interfere with individual ability to recognize and destroy cancer cells.
  C. Stress can be both positive and negative. Individual must have adaptive mechanism to cope with stress to increase health and avoid risk for disease.

Selye's Theory of Stress

  A. General adaptive syndrome (GAS).
    1. Alarm stage (call to arms).
      a. Shock: the body translates it as sudden injury, and the GAS becomes activated.
      b. Countershock: the organism is restored to its preinjury condition.
    2. Stage of resistance: the organism is adapted to the injuring agent.
    3. Stage of exhaustion: if stress continues, the organism loses its adaptive capability and goes into exhaustion, which is comparable to shock.

DANGER SIGNALS OF STRESS

- Depression, lack of interest in life
- Uncontrolled hyperactive behavior
- Lack of concentration, inability to focus
- Feelings of unreality, feelings of dread
- Loss of control, emotional instability
- Pervasive high anxiety level
- Physical manifestations
  - Irregular heartbeats
  - Tremors, tics
  - Gastrointestinal disturbance
  - Skin disturbance
  - Changes in respiratory patterns
- Insomnia
- Disease
- Increased dependence on alcohol, drugs

Adapted from Smith, S. F., Duell, D. J., & Martin, B. C. (2008). *Clinical nursing skills* (7th ed.). Upper Saddle River, NJ: Prentice Hall Health.

B. Local adaptive syndrome (LAS).
   1. Selective changes within the organism.
   2. Local response elicits general response.
   3. Example of LAS: a cut, followed by bleeding, followed by coagulation of blood.
   4. The ability of parts of the body to respond to a specific injury is impaired if the whole body is under stress.
C. Whether the organism goes through all the phases of adaptation depends on both its capacity to adapt and the intensity and continuance of the injuring agent.
   1. Organism may return to normal.
   2. Organism may overreact; stress decreases.
   3. Organism may be unable to adapt or maintain adaptation, a condition that may lead to death.
✦ D. Objective of stress response.
   1. To maintain stability of the organism during stress.
   2. To repair damage.
   3. To restore body to normal composition and activity. (*See* Table 3-1.)

Psychological Stress

Definition: All processes that impose a demand or requirement upon the organism, the resolution or accommodation of which necessitates work or activity of the mental apparatus.

Characteristics

A. May involve other structures or systems, but primarily affects mental apparatus.
   1. Anxiety is a primary result of psychological stress.

2. Causes mental mechanisms to attempt to reduce or relieve psychological discomfort.
   a. Attack/fight.
   b. Withdrawal/flight.
   c. Play dead/immobility.
B. Causes of psychological stress.
   1. Loss of something of value.
   2. Injury/pain.
   3. Frustrations of needs and drives.
   4. Threats to self-concept.
   5. Many illnesses cause stress.
      a. Disfigurement.
      b. Sexually transmitted diseases (STDs).
      c. Long-term or chronic diseases.
      d. Cancer.
      e. Heart disease.
   6. Conflicting cultural values (i.e., the American values of competition and assertiveness vs. the need to be dependent).
   7. Future shock: physiological and psychological stress resulting from an overload of the organism's adaptive systems and decision-making processes brought about by too rapidly changing values and technology.
   8. Cultural shock: stress developing in response to transition of the individual from a familiar environment to unfamiliar one.
      a. Involves unfamiliarity with communication, technology, customs, attitudes, and beliefs.
      b. Examples: individual moving to new area from foreign country or individual placed in hospital environment.
   9. Social stress: stress that develops as a result of social rather than psychological problems.
      a. Personal relationships may be a source of stress.
      b. A sense of not belonging or lack of identification with a social group or friends.
      c. Feelings of isolation or separation from others.
      d. Social pressure of being pushed to join group activities or engage in social behaviors that make one uncomfortable.

Assessment

A. Assess increased anxiety, anger, helplessness, hopelessness, guilt, shame, disgust, fear, frustration, or depression.
B. Evaluate behaviors resulting from stress.
   1. Apathy, regression, withdrawal.
   2. Crying, demanding.
   3. Physical illness.
   4. Hostility, manipulation.
   5. Senseless violence, acting out.

Table 3-1. SELYE'S STRESS ADAPTATION SYNDROME

Stage	Function	Interpersonal	Behavioral	Affective	Cognitive	Physiological
1. Alarm reaction	Mobilization of body defenses	Interpersonal communication effectiveness decreases	Task-oriented Increased restlessness Apathy, regression Crying	Feelings of anger, suspiciousness, helplessness Anxiety level increases	Alert Thinking becomes narrow and concrete Symptoms of thought blocking, forgetfulness, and decreased productivity	Muscle tension Increase in epinephrine and cortisone Stimulation of adrenal cortex and lymph glands Increase in blood pressure, heart rate, and blood glucose
2. Stage of resistance	Adaptation to stresses Resistance increases	Interpersonal communication is self-oriented Uses interpersonal relationships to meet own needs	Automatic behaviors Self-oriented behaviors Fight or flight behavior apparent	Increased use of defense mechanisms Emotional responses may be automatic or exaggerated	Thought processes more habitual than problem-solving oriented	Hormonal levels return to prealarm stage if adaptation occurs All physiological responses return to normal or are channeled into psycho-somatic symptoms
3. Stage of exhaustion	Depletion or exhaustion of organs and resources Loss of ability to resist stress	Disintegration of personal interactions Communication skills are ineffective and disorganized Self-oriented	Restless, withdrawn, agitated; may become violent or self-destructive Diminished productivity	Depressed, flat, or inappropriate affect Exaggerated or inappropriate use of defense mechanisms Decreased ability to cope	Thought disorganization, hallucinations, preoccupation Reduced intellectual processes	Exhaustion, with increased demands on organism Adrenal cortex hormone depletion Death, if stress is continuous and excessive

Implementation

A. Gather information about client's internal and external environment.
B. Modify external environment so that adaptation responses are within the capacity of client.
C. Support the efforts of client to adapt or to respond.
D. Provide client with the materials required to maintain constancy of internal environment.
E. Understand body's mechanisms for accommodating stress.
F. Prevent additional stress.
G. Reduce external stimuli.
H. Reduce or increase physical activity depending on the cause of and response to stress.

DEVELOPMENT THROUGH THE LIFE CYCLE*

Early Adolescence

A. Physical development.
   1. Exhibits further development of secondary sex characteristics.
   2. Shows poor posture.

*For infancy to adolescence, *see* Pediatric Nursing, Chapter 13.

3. Exhibits rapid growth and becomes awkward and uncoordinated.
4. Shows changes in body size and development.
B. Social development.
 1. Needs social approval of peer group.
 2. Strives for independence from family.
 3. Has one or two very close friends in peer group.
 4. Becomes more interested in opposite sex.
 5. Period of upheaval: displays confusion about body image.
 6. Must again learn to control strong feelings (love, aggression).
C. Counseling guidelines.
 1. Provide adult understanding when adolescent deals with social, intellectual, and moral issues.
 2. Allow some financial independence.
 3. Provide limits to ensure security.
 4. Provide necessary assurance to help adolescent accept changing body image.
 5. Show flexibility in adjusting to emotional and erratic mood swings.
 6. Be calm and consistent when dealing with an adolescent.
D. Developmental tasks.
 1. Finds identity; moves out of role diffusion.
  a. Integrates childhood identifications with basic drives.
  b. Expands concept of social roles.
 2. Moves toward heterosexuality.
 3. Begins separation from family.
 4. Integrates personality.

Adolescence to Young Adulthood

A. Physical development.
 1. Completes sexual development.
 2. Exhibits signs of slowing down of body growth.
 3. Is capable of reproduction.
 4. Shows more energy after growth spurt tapers off.
 5. Exhibits increased muscular ability and coordination.
B. Menstruation.
 1. Menstruation is the sloughing off of the endometrium that occurs at regular monthly intervals if conception fails to take place. The discharge consists of blood, mucus, and cells, and it usually lasts for four to five days.
 2. Menarche—onset of menstruation—usually occurs between the ages of 11 and 14.
 3. Discomforts associated with menstruation.
  a. Breast tenderness and feeling of fullness.
  b. Tendency toward fatigue.
  c. Temperament and mood changes—because of hormonal influence and

Table 3-2. PIAGET'S COGNITIVE DEVELOPMENT	
Age	**Developmental Level**

Infancy–2 years	Sensorimotor
	   Development of intellect through
	     sensory–motor apparatus
	   Simple problem solving

2–7 years
  2–4 years
	Preoperational Thought
	   Preconceptual Phase
	     Use of symbols—language
	     Imitative play to understand the
	       world

4–7 years	Intuitive Phase
	     Egocentric and stage of "moral
	       realism"
	     Beginning use of symbols for cognition
	     Asks questions

7–12 years	Concrete Operational Thought
	   Wide use of symbols
	   Observes relationships between
	     objects
	   Understands cause and effect
	   Visualizes conclusions

12+ years	Formal Operational Thought
	   Abstract thinking processes
	   Conceptualization
	   Ability to test hypotheses

decreased levels of estrogen and progesterone.
  d. Discomfort in pelvic area, lower back, and legs.
  e. Retained fluids and weight gain.
 4. Abnormalities of menstruation.
  a. Dysmenorrhea (painful menstruation).
   (1) May be caused by psychological factors: tension, anxiety, preconditioning (menstruation is a "curse" or should be painful).
   (2) Physical examination is usually done to rule out organic causes.
  b. Treatment.
   (1) Oral contraceptives—produce anovulatory cycle.
   (2) Mild analgesics such as aspirin.
   (3) Urge client to carry on normal activities to occupy her mind.
   (4) Dysmenorrhea may subside after childbearing.
  c. Amenorrhea (absence of menstrual flow).
   (1) Primary—over the age of 17 and menstruation has not begun.
    (a) Complete physical necessary to rule out abnormalities.
    (b) Treatment aimed at correction of underlying condition.

Table 3-3. ERIKSON'S EIGHT STAGES OF PERSONALITY DEVELOPMENT—INFANT TO ADULT

Stage	Approx. Age	Psychological Crises	Significant Persons	Accomplishments
Infant	0–1 yrs.	Basic trust vs. mistrust	Mother or maternal figure	Tolerates frustration in small doses Recognizes mother as separate from others and self
Toddler	1–3 yrs.	Autonomy vs. shame and doubt	Parents	Begins verbal skills Begins acceptance of reality vs. pleasure principle
Preschool	3–6 yrs.	Initiative vs. guilt	Basic family	Asks many questions Explores own body and environment Differentiates between sexes
School	6–12 yrs.	Industry vs. inferiority	Neighborhood school	Gains attention by accomplishments Explores things Learns to relate to own sex
Puberty and adolescence	12–20 yrs.	Identity vs. role diffusion	Peer groups External groups	Moves toward heterosexuality Begins separation from family Integrates personality (e.g., altruism)
Young adult	18–25 yrs.	Intimacy and solidarity vs. isolation	Partners in friendship; sexual partners	Is ablue to form lasting relationships with others, committed to work
Adulthood	25–65 yrs.	Generativity vs. stagnation		Creative, productive life, caring for others
Late adulthood, elderly	65–death	Ego integrity vs. despair		Acceptance of worth and value of one's life

Based on Erikson, E. H. (1963). *Childhood and society* (2nd ed.). New York: Norton.

(2) Secondary—occurs after menarche; does not include pregnancy and lactation.
   (a) Causes include psychological upsets or endocrine conditions.
   (b) Evaluation and treatment by physician is necessary.
  d. Menorrhagia (excessive menstrual bleeding)—may be due to endocrine disturbance, tumors, or inflammatory conditions of the uterus.
  e. Metrorrhagia (bleeding between periods)—symptom of disease process, benign tumors, or cancer.

✦ 5. Counseling guidelines.
  a. Provide education about the physiology of normal menstruation and correct misinformation.
  b. Provide education about abnormal conditions associated with menstruation—absence of menstruation, bleeding between menstrual periods, etc.
  c. Provide education related to normal hygiene during menstruation.
   (1) Importance of cleanliness.
   (2) Use of perineal pads and tampons.
   (3) Continuance of normal activities.

C. Social development.
  1. Is less attached to peers.
  2. Shows increased maturity.
  3. Exhibits more interdependence with family.
  4. Begins romantic love affairs.
  5. Increases mastery over biologic drives.
  6. Develops more mature relationship with parents.
  7. Values fidelity, friendship, and cooperation.
  8. Begins vocational development.

D. Counseling guidelines.
  1. Assist adolescent in making a vocational choice.
  2. Provide safety education, especially regarding driving and drugs.
  3. Encourage positive attitudes toward health in issues of nutrition, drugs, smoking, and drinking.
  4. Attempt to understand own (parental) difficulties in accepting transition of the adolescent to independence and adulthood.

E. Developmental tasks.
  1. Intimacy and solidarity versus isolation.

a.   Moves from security of self-involvement to insecurity of building intimate relationships with others.

b.   Becomes less dependent and more self-sufficient.

2.   Able to form lasting relationships with others.

3.   Learns to be productive and creative.

4.   Handles hormonal changes of developmental period.

ADULTHOOD

Developmental Tasks

✦ A.   Achieves goal of generativity versus stagnation or self-absorption.

1.   Shows concern for establishing and guiding next generation.

2.   Exhibits productiveness, creativity, and an attitude of looking forward to the future.

3.   Stagnation results from the refusal to assume power and responsibility of the goals of middle age.

a.   Suffers pervading sense of boredom and impoverishment.

b.   Undergoes but does not resolve midlife crisis.

B.   Has relaxed sense of competitiveness.

C.   Opens up new interests.

D.   Shifts values from physical attractiveness and strength to intellectual abilities.

E.   Shows productivity (may be most productive years of one's life).

F.   Has more varied and satisfying relationships.

G.   Exhibits no significant decline in learning abilities or sexual interests.

H.   Shifts sexual interests from physical performance to the individual's total sexuality and need to be loved and touched.

I.   Assists next generation to become happy, responsible adults.

J.   Achieves mature social and civic responsibility.

K.   Accepts and adjusts to physiological changes of middle life.

L.   Uses leisure time satisfactorily.

M.   Failure to complete developmental tasks may cause the individual to approach old age with resentment and fear.

1.   Neurotic symptoms may appear.

2.   Increased psychosomatic disorders develop.

Values of Adulthood

A.   Becomes more introspective.

B.   Shows less concern as to what others think.

C.   Identifies self as successful even though all life goals may not be achieved.

D.   Shows less concern for outward manifestations of success.

E.   Lives more day to day and values life more deeply.

F.   Has faced one's finiteness and eventual death.

Parenting in Adulthood

A.   Characteristics.

1.   Tendency toward smaller families.

2.   Career-oriented women who limit family size or who do not want children.

3.   Early sexual experimentation, necessitating sexual education, and contraceptive information.

4.   Tendency toward postponement of children.

a.   To complete education.

b.   Economic factors.

5.   High divorce rates.

6.   Alternative family designs.

a.   Single parenthood.

b.   Communal family.

✦ B.   Family planning.

1.   General concepts.

a.   Dealing with individuals with particular ideas regarding contraception.

b.   No perfect method of birth control.

c.   Method must be suited to individual.

d.   Individuals involved must be thoroughly counseled on all available methods and how they work—including advantages and disadvantages. This includes not only female but also sexual partner (if available).

e.   Once a method is chosen, both parties should be thoroughly instructed in its use.

f.   Individuals involved must be motivated to succeed.

2.   Effectiveness depends on several factors:

a.   Method chosen.

b.   Degree to which couple follows prescribed regimen.

c.   Thorough understanding of the chosen method.

d.   Motivation on part of individuals concerned.

See Contraceptive Methods in Chapter 12.

Physiological Changes

Menopause

A.   Characteristics.

1.   The cessation of menstruation caused by physiologic factors; ovulation no longer occurs.

2.   Menopause usually occurs between the ages of 45 and 55.

B. Mechanisms in menopause.
  1. Ovaries lose the ability to respond to pituitary stimulation and normal ovarian function ceases.
  2. Gradual change due to alteration in hormone production.
     a. Failure to ovulate.
     b. Monthly flow becomes smaller, irregular, and gradually ceases.
  3. Menopause is accompanied by changes in reproductive organs. The vagina gradually becomes smaller; the uterus, bladder, rectum, and supporting structures lose tone, leading to uterine prolapse, rectocele, and cystocele.
  4. Atherosclerosis and osteoporosis are more likely to develop at this time.

See Menopause, p. 347.

Assessment

A. Assess presence of symptoms—varies with individuals and may be mild to severe.
B. Assess feelings of loss as children grow and leave home and aging process continues.
✦ C. Assess presence of physiological symptoms: hot flashes, night sweats, vaginal atrophy, mood swings, and fatigue.

Implementation

A. Refer client to physician who can discuss hormone replacement therapy (HRT), now controversial, versus natural methods of controlling symptoms.
  1. Diet: more vegetarian with essential fatty acids; limiting caffeine, sugar, meat and dairy, and saturated oils.
  2. Herbs: black cohosh, dong quai, fennel, red clover, and other phytoestrogen plants.
  3. Progesterone substitute—skin cream made from the Mexican yam, natural progesterone and natural estrogen (estriol) via a skin patch.
B. Monitor estrogen therapy—usually given on cyclic basis: one pill daily except for five days during the month; progesterone 10–12 days per month.
C. Evaluate need for treatment of psychological problems.

Major Health Problems

A. Heart disease occurs in both male and female clients (more than 250,000 die each year).
B. Diabetes.
C. Hypertension.
D. Accidents.
E. Confrontation with the most acute psychological problems of any age group.
  1. Depression.
  2. Involutional psychosis.
F. Cancer.

Psychosocial Changes

Midlife Crisis

A. A normal stage in the ongoing life cycle in which the middle-aged person reevaluates his or her total life situation in relation to youthful achievements and actual accomplishments.
  1. Struggles to maintain physical attractiveness in relation to younger people.
  2. Feels partner or lover is essential.
  3. Feels he or she has peaked in ability.
  4. Blames environment or others for failure to succeed.
  5. Displays increased interest in sexuality.
  6. Exhibits competitiveness in career plans.
B. Unresolved crisis.
  1. May result in stagnation, boredom, and decreased self-esteem and depression.
  2. Age for crisis varies.
     a. Women usually pass through it at age 35 to 40.
     b. Men usually experience the crisis at age 40 to 45.

Causes of Psychological Problems

A. Fear of losing job.
B. Competition with younger generation.
C. Loss of job.
D. Loss of nurturing functions.
E. Loss of spouse, particularly females.
F. Realization that person is not going to accomplish some of the things that he or she wanted to do.
G. Changes in body image.
H. Illness.
I. Role change within and outside of family.
J. Fear of approaching old age.
K. Physiological changes.

MASLOW'S HIERARCHY OF NEEDS THEORY

- Abraham Maslow identified a hierarchy of human needs. The most basic must be met before the next levels can be fulfilled.
- The most basic needs are bodily drives—hunger, thirst, and physical needs for shelter, sleep, exercise.
- More general needs follow (also necessary for life) and become the focus after essential physical needs.
  1. Feeling safe in the world.
  2. Sense of belonging and love.
  3. Failure to meet these needs negates fulfillment of even higher needs (respect, self-esteem, and self-actualization).
- Nursing implications: use Maslow's hierarchy of needs when you are answering a priority question that involves issues of physiological needs versus needs such as recognition, belonging, and loving. Basic physical needs (such as hunger, and pain) must be met first.

THE AGED*

Developmental Tasks

A. Maintains ego integrity versus despair.
   1. Integrity results when an individual is satisfied with his or her own actions and lifestyle, feels life is meaningful, remains optimistic, and continues to grow.
   2. Despair results from the feeling that he or she has failed and that it is too late to change.
B. Continues a meaningful life after retirement.
C. Adjusts to income level.
D. Makes satisfactory living arrangements with spouse.
E. Adjusts to loss of spouse. (Forty-five percent of women older than age 65 are widowed.)
F. Maintains social contact and responsibilities.
G. Faces death realistically.
H. Provides knowledge and wisdom to assist those at other developmental levels to grow and learn.
I. In the year 2000, there were approximately 40 million people older than age 65 in the United States.

Physiological Changes

A. Decrease in ability to maintain homeostasis.
   1. Decrease in physical strength and endurance.
   2. Decrease in muscular coordination and strength.
B. Changes in bone composition.
   1. Loss of density and increased brittleness.
   2. Increased spine curvatures.
C. Tendency to gain weight.
D. Loss of pigment in hair and elasticity of skin.
E. Diminution of sensory faculties.
   1. Vision decreases.
   2. Loss of hearing occurs.
   3. Smell and taste become dull.
   4. Greater sensitivity to temperature changes occurs with low tolerance to cold.
F. Lowered immune system—decreased resistance to infection and disease.
G. Degenerative changes in the cardiovascular system.
   1. Heart pump action diminishes.
   2. Blood flow decreases—may be due to fat deposits in arteries.
   3. Vascular changes result in less effective oxygenation.
H. Changes in respiratory system.
   1. Blood flow decreases to lungs: contributes to decrease in function.
   2. Less oxygen diffusion so tolerance is less.
I. Changes in gastrointestinal system.

*For more in-depth coverage *see* Chapter 15.

   1. Absorption function impaired.
      a. Body absorbs less nutrients.
      b. Decrease in gastric enzymes affects absorption.
   2. Peristalsis weakens and constipation is common.
J. Changes in urinary system.
   1. Structural and functional changes occur in kidney through degeneration.
   2. Decreased musculature ability leads to atonic bladder.

Major Health Problems

A. All systems are more vulnerable because of the aging process; degeneration can be affected.
   1. Chronic disease and disability.
   2. Nutritional deprivation; dehydration.
   3. Sensory impairment—blindness and deafness.
   4. Organic brain changes.
      a. Not all persons become senile.
      b. Most people have memory impairment.
      c. The change is gradual.
B. Impact of disease on aged.
   1. Diseases may be multiple and chronic (more than 40% have more than one illness concurrently).
   2. Disability results more readily when an aging person becomes ill.
   3. Response to treatment is diminished.
   4. Resistance is lower due to the aging process so person is more susceptible to disease.
   5. The aged have less resistance to stressors—mental, environmental, and physical.
   6. Changes in the neurological system make aged persons more prone to organic brain changes.
   7. Many elderly take numerous medications and are susceptible to drug reactions and side effects.

Psychosocial Changes

A. Developmental process retrogresses.
   1. Exhibits increasing dependency.
   2. Concerns focus increasingly on self.
   3. Displays narrower interests.
   4. Needs tangible evidence of affection.
B. Major fears of the aged.
   1. Physical and economic dependency.
   2. Chronic illness.
   3. Loneliness.
   4. Boredom resulting from not being needed.
C. Major problems of the aged.
   1. Alteration in living style (i.e., nursing home, moving in with children).
   2. Economic deprivation.
      a. Increased cost of living on a fixed income.

Table 3-4. CULTURAL BELIEFS

Ethnic Group	Cultural Beliefs
Asian/Pacific Islander	→ Extended family has strong influence on client.
	Older family members are honored and respected, and their authority is unquestioned.
	Oldest male is decision maker and spokesman.
	Strong emphasis on avoiding conflict and direct confrontation.
	Respect authority and do not disagree with healthcare recommendations; however, they may not follow recommendations.
Chinese	→ Chinese clients will not discuss symptoms of mental illness or depression because they believe this behavior reflects on family; therefore it may produce shame and guilt.
	Use herbalists, spiritual healers, and physicians for care.
Japanese	→ Believe physical contact with blood, skin diseases, and corpses will cause illness.
	Believe improper care of the body, including poor diet and lack of sleep, causes illness.
	Believe in healers, herbalists, and physicians for healing, and energy can be restored with acupuncture and acupressure.
	They use group decision making for health concerns.
Hindu and Muslim	→ Indians and Pakistanis do not acknowledge a diagnosis of severe emotional illness or mental retardation because it reduces the chance of other family members getting married.
Vietnamese	→ Vietnamese accept mental health counseling and interventions, particularly when they have established trust with the healthcare worker.
Hispanic	→ Older family members are consulted on issues involving health and illness.
	Patriarchal family—men make decisions for family.
	Illness is viewed as God's will or divine punishment resulting from sinful behavior.
	Prefer to use home remedies and consult folk healers known as curanderos rather than traditional Western healthcare providers.
African American	→ Family and church oriented.
	Extensive extended family bonds.
	Key family member is consulted for important health-related decisions.
	Illness is a punishment from God for wrongdoing, or is due to voodoo, spirits, or demons.
	Health prevention is through good diet, herbs, rest, cleanliness, and laxatives to clean the system.
	Wear copper and silver bracelets to prevent illness.
Native American	→ Oriented to the present.
	Value cooperation.
	Value family and spiritual beliefs.
	Strong ties to family and tribe.
	Believe a state of health exists when the client lives in total harmony with nature.
	Illness is viewed as an imbalance between the ill person and natural or supernatural forces.
	Use a medicine man or woman known as a shaman.
	Illness is prevented through elaborate religious rituals.

    b.   Increased need for costly medical care.
3. Chronic disease and disability.
4. Social isolation/loneliness.
5. Sensory deprivation (blindness and deafness).
6. Senility, confusion, and lack of awareness.
7. Nutritional deprivation.
8. Series of losses (i.e., relationships, friends, family).
9. Loss of physical strength and agility.

D. Sexuality and aging.
   1. Older people are sexual beings.
   2. There is no particular age at which a person's sexual functioning ceases.

3. Frequency of genital sexual behavior (intercourse) may tend to decline gradually in later years, but capacity for expression and enjoyment continue far into old age.
4. Touching and companionship are of importance for older people and should be encouraged.

CULTURAL SENSITIVITY

A. Demographic shifts influence the direction of health care.

Table 3-5. RELIGIOUS DIVERSITY CONSIDERATIONS

Religious Orientation	Baptism	Death Rituals	Health Crisis	Diet
Adventist	Opposed to infant baptism	No last rites	Communion or baptism may be desirable	No alcohol, coffee, tea, or any narcotic
Baptist	Opposed to infant baptism	Clergy supports and counsels	Some believe in healing and laying on of hands Some sects resist medical help	Condemn alcohol Some do not allow coffee and tea
Islam	No baptism	Prescribed procedures by family for washing body and shrouding after death	No faith healing Ritual washing after prayers every day	Prohibit alcohol and pork
Buddhist	Rites are given after child is mature	Send for Buddhist priest Last rite chanting	Family should request priest to be notified	Alcohol and drugs discouraged; some are vegetarian
Christian Scientist	No baptism	No last rites No autopsy	Deny the existence of health crises Many refuse all medical help, blood transfusions, or drugs	Alcohol, coffee, and tobacco viewed as drugs and not allowed
Episcopalian	Infant baptism mandatory	Last rites not essential for all members	Medical treatment acceptable	Some do not eat meat on Fridays
Jehovah's Witness	No infant baptism	No last rites	Opposed to blood transfusions	Do not eat anything to which blood has been added
Judaism	No baptism but ritual circumcision on eighth day after birth	Ritual washing of body after death	All ill people seek medical care Treatment supersedes dietary restrictions	Orthodox observe kosher dietary laws, which prohibit pork, shellfish, and the eating of meat and milk products at the same time
Methodist	Baptism encouraged	No last rites	Medical treatment acceptable	No restrictions
Mormon	Baptism at eight years or older	Baptism for the dead can be done by proxy	Do not prohibit medical treatment, although they believe in divine healing	Do not allow alcohol, caffeine, tobacco, tea, and coffee
Roman Catholic	Infant baptism mandatory	Last rites required	Sacrament of the sick	Most ill people are exempt from fasting

Note: There may exist circumstances that require a court order to supervene religious practices (e.g., a blood transfusion to save the life of a child).

1. In the United States, 29 percent of the population are people of color and more than 12 percent are of Hispanic origin.
2. In 2000, there were more than 20 million foreign-born Americans and 14 million did not speak English.
3. These statistics create barriers to health care.
   a. The major barrier is language.
   b. The other barriers are poverty, poor nutrition, and poor prevention practices.
4. Reduced access to health care is a major problem for non-English-speaking peoples.

B. It is important for nurses to understand the impact of various cultures on healthcare practices.
C. Cultural diversity implications.
   1. Differences in values, beliefs, customs, folklore, traditions, language and patterns of behavior.
   2. Other aspects of differences are personal space related to culture, gender and group behavior.
D. Cultural assessment—important to include in a complete client assessment.
   1. Cultural background and orientation.
   2. Communication patterns.

3. Nutritional practices.
   a. Cultural/religious beliefs that do not eliminate whole food groups.
   b. Beliefs that interfere with receiving a healthy, balanced diet (such as a macrobiotic diet).
   c. Food practices that do not allow foods to lose all nutrient value during preparation (over-cooking vegetables).
4. Family relationships.
5. Beliefs and perceptions related to health, illness, and treatment.
6. Values related to health.
7. Education.
8. Issues affecting healthcare delivery.

THE GRIEVING PROCESS

✦ Stages of Grief

Definition: A process that an individual goes through in response to the loss of a significant or loved person. The grieving process follows certain predictable phases—classic description originally defined by Dr. Eric Lindeman. The normal grieving process is described by George Engle, M.D., in "Grief and Grieving," *American Journal of Nursing*, September 1964.

A. *Shock and disbelief:* first response is shock and refusal to believe that the loved one is dead.
B. *Developing awareness:* as awareness increases, the bereaved experiences severe anguish.
   1. Crying is common in this stage.
   2. Anger directed toward those people or circumstances thought to be responsible.
C. *Restitution:* mourning is the next stage where the work of restitution takes place.
   1. Rituals of the funeral help the bereaved accept reality.
   2. Support from friends and spiritual guidance comfort the bereaved.
D. *Resolution of the loss:* occurs as the mourner begins to deal with the void.
E. *Idealization:* negative feelings are repressed and only the pleasant memories are remembered.
   1. Characterized by the mourner's taking on certain qualities of the deceased.
   2. This process takes many months as preoccupation with the deceased diminishes.
✦ F. Outcome of the grief process takes a year or more.
   1. Indications of successful outcome are when the mourner remembers both the pleasant and unpleasant memories.
   2. Eventual outcome influenced by:

   a. Importance of the deceased in the life of mourner.
   b. The degree of dependence in the relationship. The amount of ambivalence toward the deceased.
   ✦ c. The more hostile the feelings that exist, the more guilt that interferes with the grieving process.
   d. Age of both mourner and deceased.
   e. Death of a child is more difficult to resolve than that of an aged loved one.
   ✦ f. Number and nature of previous grief experiences. Loss is cumulative.
   g. Degree of preparation for the loss.

Counseling Guidelines

✦ A. Recognize that grief is a syndrome with somatic and psychological symptomatology.
   1. Weeping, complaints of fatigue, digestive disturbance, and insomnia.
   2. Guilt, anger, and irritability.
   3. Restless, but unable to initiate meaningful activity.
   4. Depression and agitation.
B. Be prepared to support the family as they learn of the death.
   1. Know the general response to death by recognizing the stages of the grief process.
   2. Understand that the behavior of the mourner may be unstable and disturbed.
C. Use therapeutic communication techniques.
   1. Encourage the mourner to express feelings, especially through crying.
   2. Attempt to meet the needs of the mourner for privacy, information, and support.
   3. Show respect for the religious and social customs of the family.
D. Recognize the difference between grief and loss.
   1. Grief is the emotion experienced in response to loss.
   2. When one is grieving, he or she is feeling all of the emotions that accompany loss.
      a. Grief is not one emotion, but a combination of feelings.
      b. Grief encompasses all of the initial feelings of loss and moves through the stages to resolution.

DEATH AND DYING

A. The dying process is described in *On Death and Dying*, by Elisabeth Kübler-Ross, New York, Macmillan Publishing Company, Inc., 1969.

B. Stages of dying.
1. *Denial:* individual is stunned at the knowledge he or she is dying and denies it.
2. *Anger:* anger and resentment usually follow as the individual questions, "Why me?"
3. *Bargaining:* with the beginning of acceptance of impending death comes the bargaining stage—that is, bargaining for time to complete some situation in his or her life.
4. *Depression:* full acknowledgment usually brings depression; individual begins to work through feelings and to withdraw from life and relationships.
5. *Acceptance:* final stage is full acceptance and preparation for death.
C. Throughout the dying process, hope is an important element that should be supported but not reinforced unrealistically.
D. Psychosocial clinical manifestations—behaviors and reactions the nurse will expect to observe in clients who are going through the dying process.
1. Depression and withdrawal.
2. Fear and anxiety.
3. Focus is internal.
4. Agitation and restlessness.

The Concept of Death in the Aging Population

A. In American culture, death is very distasteful.
B. Older adults may see death as an end to suffering and loneliness.
C. Death is not feared if the person has lived a long and fulfilled life, having completed all developmental tasks.
D. Religious beliefs and/or philosophy of life is important.

Death and Children

A. Understanding of death for the young child.
1. Death is viewed as a temporary separation from parents, sometimes viewed synonymously with sleep.
2. Child may express fear of pain and wish to avoid it.
3. Child's awareness is lessened by physical symptoms if death comes suddenly.
4. Gradual terminal illness may simulate the adult process: depression, withdrawal, fearfulness, and anxiety.
B. Older children's concerns.
1. Death is identified as a "person" to be avoided.
2. Child may ask directly if he or she is going to die.

3. Concerns center on fear of pain, fear of being left alone, and fear of leaving parents and friends.
C. Adolescent concerns.
1. Death is recognized as irreversible and inevitable.
2. Adolescent often avoids talking about impending death, and staff may enter into this "conspiracy of silence."
3. Adolescents have more understanding of death than adults tend to realize.

Stages of Grief	Stages of Dying
• Shock and disbelief	• Denial
• Developing awareness	• Anger
• Restitution/mourning	• Bargaining
• Resolution	• Depression
• Idealization	• Acceptance
According to George Engle	According to Elisabeth Kübler-Ross

Adapted from Smith, S. F., Duell, D. J., & Martin, B. C. (2008). *Clinical nursing skills* (7th ed.). Upper Saddle River, NJ: Prentice Hall Health.

Nursing Management

Nursing Management of the Dying Adult

A. Minimize physical discomfort.
1. Evaluate pain as the fifth vital sign.
a. Alleviate client's pain according to orders—be the client's advocate for pain relief.
b. Explore all options (drugs and alternative therapy) for achieving pain relief.
See Pain Management on following pages.
2. Attend to all physical needs.
3. Make client as comfortable as possible.
B. Recognize crisis situation.
1. Observe for changes in client's condition.
2. Support client.
C. Be prepared to give the dying client the emotional support needed.
D. Encourage communication.
1. Allow client to express feelings, to talk, or to cry.
2. Pick up cues that client wants to talk, especially about fears.
3. Be available to form a relationship with client.
4. Communicate honestly.
E. Prepare and support the family for their impending loss.
F. Understand the grieving process of client and family.

✦ **Nursing Management of the Dying Child**

A. Always elicit the child's understanding of death before discussing it.

B. Before discussing death with child, discuss it with parents.

C. Parental reactions include the continuum of grief process and stages of dying.

   1. Reactions depend on previous experience with loss.

   2. Reactions also depend on relationship with the child and circumstances of illness or injury.

   3. Reactions depend on degree of guilt felt by parents.

D. Assist parents in expressing their fears, concerns and grief so that they may be more supportive to the child.

E. Assist parents in understanding siblings' possible reactions to a terminally ill child.

   1. *Guilt:* belief that they caused the problem or illness.

   2. *Jealousy:* demand for equal attention from the parents.

   3. *Anger:* feelings of being left behind.

PAIN MANAGEMENT

✦ **Characteristics**

A. Pain now considered the fifth vital sign—must be assessed regularly (Joint Commission) to maintain client's quality of life.

B. The experience of pain.

   1. Pain source—direct causative factor.

   2. Stimulation of pain receptor—mechanical, chemical, thermal, electrical, or ischemic.

   3. Pain pathway.

      a. Sensory pathways through dorsal root, ending on second-order neuron in posterior horn.

      b. Afferent fibers cross over to anterolateral pathway, ascend in lateral spinothalamic tract to thalamus.

      c. Fibers then travel to postcentral gyrus in parietal lobe.

Theories of Pain

A. Specificity theory—certain pain receptors are stimulated by a type of sensory stimulus that sends impulses to the brain.

B. Pattern theory—pain originates in spinal cord and results in receptor stimulation coded in CNS and signifies pain.

C. Gate control theory.

   1. Pain impulses can be modulated by a transmission blocking action within CNS.

   2. Large-diameter cutaneous pain fibers can be stimulated (rubbing, scratching) and may inhibit smaller-diameter excitatory fibers and prevent transmission of that impulse.

   3. Cerebral cortical mechanisms that influence perception and interpretation may also inhibit transmission.

D. Endorphins—the brain produces natural brain opioids that fit (lock) into special receptors. Antilocks, called antagonists, keep endorphins from working.

Assessment

✦ A. Assess for type of pain.

   1. Acute—localized, shorter duration, sharp sensation. Occurs over defined period—6 months or less.

   2. Chronic pain—long duration, diffuse, dull aching quality; associated autonomic responses, musculoskeletal tension, nausea. Occurs over 6-month period or longer.

   3. Malignant—recurrent, acute episodes; also includes chronic varying in intensity—lasts longer than 6 months.

   4. Psychogenic—due to emotional factors without anatomic or physiological explanation.

B. Assess onset of pain.

C. Assess location, where it originates and travels.

D. Evaluate intensity and character of pain.

   1. Select a tool based on client's preferences and cognitive abilities.

   2. Examples of pain scales—verbal descriptor, numeric rating, FACES, and pain thermometer.

E. Quality—searing, dull, sharp, throbbing.

F. Pattern—timing.

G. Check precipitating factors.

H. Assess associated factors.

   1. Nausea and/or vomiting.

   2. Bradycardia/tachycardia.

   3. Hypotension/hypertension.

   4. Profuse perspiration.

   5. Apprehension or anxiety.

I. Assess duration of pain.

J. Evaluate previous experience of pain.

Implementation

A. Assess pain before treating.

B. Give reassurance, reduce anxiety and fears.

C. Offer distraction.

D. Give comfort measures: positioning, rest, elevation, heat/cold applications; protect from painful stimuli.

E. Massage non-surgical area of pain—but never massage calf due to danger of emboli.

IDENTIFYING PAIN IN YOUNG CHILDREN

Unidimensional indicators:
- Increase in heart rate
- Elevations in blood pressure
- Sweating
- Changes in skin color

Multidimensional indicators:
- High-pitched cry
- Baby or child is inconsolable
- Awake continuously—not able to sleep
- Fussy
- Grunting sounds

Behavioral responses:
- Facial movement
- Bulging of area between eyebrows
- Tightly closed eyes
- Rigid mouth and tongue

F. Administer pain medication as needed: monitor therapeutic, toxic dose, and side effects.
G. Monitor alternative methods to control pain.
1. Dorsal column stimulator: stimulation of electrodes at dorsal column of spinal cord by client-controlled device to inhibit pain.
2. Analgesics: alter perception, threshold, and reaction to pain.
3. Anesthesia: block pain pathway.
4. Local nerve block.
5. Neurosurgical procedures: interrupt sensory pathways; usually also affect pressure and temperature pathways.
   a. Neurectomy: interrupt cranial or peripheral nerves.
   b. Sympathectomy: interrupt afferent pathways (ganglia).

JOINT COMMISSION PAIN STANDARDS (2000–2001)

- Healthcare providers must be knowledgeable about pain assessment and management.
- Facilities must have policies in place for analgesics and other pain control therapies.
- Joint Commission standards:
  1. Clients have the right to pain assessment.
     a. Facility must provide pain assessment tools.
     b. If facility (i.e., long-term care) cannot treat client for pain (PCA), client must be referred to a facility that can.
  2. Clients will be treated for pain and involved in their own pain management.
  3. Discharge planning and teaching will include pain management.

HUMAN SEXUALITY

Overview of Human Sexuality

A. Biological sexuality is determined at conception.
1. Male sperm contributes an X or a Y chromosome.
2. Female ovum has an X chromosome.
3. Fertilization results in either an XX (female) or an XY (male).
B. Preparation for adult sexuality originates in the sexual role development of the child.
1. Significant differences between male and female infants are observable even at birth.
2. Biological changes are minimal during childhood, but parenting strongly influences a child's behavior and sexual role development.
3. Anatomical and physiological changes occur during adolescence that establish biological sexual maturation.
4. Learning about sexuality has several stages.
   a. The first stage: person becomes aware that they are sexual beings and accept the fact.
   b. Second stage: person seeks to learn about the sexual self—experiments with bodies and emotions.
   c. Third stage: involves sharing self with a partner.
C. Human sexuality pervades the whole of an individual's life.
1. More than a sum of isolated physical acts.
2. Functions as a purposeful influence in human nature and behavior.
3. Observable in everyday life in endless variations.
D. Each society develops a set of normative behaviors, attitudes, and values in respect to sexuality, which are considered "right" and "wrong" by individuals.
E. Freud described the bisexual (androgynous) nature of the person.
1. Each person has components of maleness–femaleness, masculinity–femininity, and heterosexuality–homosexuality.
2. These components are physiological and psychological in nature.
3. All components influence an individual's sexuality and sexual behavior.
F. Gender identity (identified at birth) refers to whether a person is male or female.
1. Cases of "ambiguous genitalia" are rare (1/3000 births) and require special care for the infant and parents.
2. *Ambiguous genitalia* is a clinical label similar to slang term *morphodite*, or biological term *hermaphrodite*.

G. Sexual object choice is the selection of a mode of outlet for sexual desire, usually with another person.
   1. Generally occurs during adolescence and beyond.
   2. Includes heterosexuality, homosexuality, bisexuality, celibacy, and narcissism/onanism.
H. Sexual object choice has strong influence on a person's lifestyle.
   1. Individual must establish patterns of intimacy and sexual behavior that are acceptable to self, to significant others, and to society to a certain extent.
   2. Psychological demands and expectations throughout life influence an individual's sexual interest, activity, and functional capacity.
   3. Sexual object choice can affect a person's choices in life such as whether to be a parent, where to live, and which career to pursue.

Sexual Behavior

A. Sexual behavior is a composite of developed patterns of intimacy, psychological demands and expectations, and sexual object choice.
   1. Can be genital (sexual intercourse), intimate (holding, hugging), or social (dating, choice of clothing).
   2. Beyond the obvious examples, one never stops "behaving sexually."
   3. Dress, communication, and activity are all expressions of sexuality.
   4. Every person exhibits sexual behavior continually; no one is sexless.
B. *Transvestite* and *transsexual* are two terms that often cause confusion and need definition and differentiation.
   1. Transvestite refers to one who enjoys wearing clothing of the opposite sex; may or may not be homosexual.
   2. Transsexual is a person who chooses sexual reassignment: a complex physical (surgical), psychological, and social process of taking on the gender identity, sex role, sexual object choice, and sexual behavior of the opposite sex.
C. Sexuality, although difficult to define, is pervasive from birth to death, and nurses need to look beyond the framework of reproduction and procreation to understand the influence of sexuality on clients' health and illness.

Characteristics

A. Difficult to define precisely, human sexuality is considered to be a pervasive life force and includes a person's total feelings, attitudes, and behavior.
B. It is related to gender identity, sex-role identity, and sexual motivation.

C. Touching, intimacy, and companionship are factors that have unique meaning for each person's sexuality.
D. Sex role describes whether a person assumes masculine or feminine behaviors, usually a combination of both.
   1. This role is generally considered to be fairly established by age 5.
   2. Usually referred to by the concepts boy/girl and man/woman.

Assessment

A. If necessary, obtain a full sexual history.
B. Include consideration of each client's sexuality in assessing health and illness status.
C. Assess primary sexual concerns.
D. Listen for nonverbal cues of sexual problems.
E. Elicit verbalization of underlying concerns.
F. Identify major problem area.
   1. Be aware that the most common problem is the need for sexual recognition of each client.
   2. Allow sexual expression within appropriate limits.
   3. Assess whether client has correct information or misconceptions about sexuality.
   4. Assess the relationship between each client's health problems and his or her sexuality needs.

Implementation

A. Provide sex education and counseling.
   1. Clients consider nurses to be experts in sexuality.
   2. Intervention requires knowledge and skill.
   3. Nurses need to know referral sources for interventions beyond their ability.
B. Give clients "permission" or acceptance to maintain sexuality and sexual behavior.
C. Be aware of the effect of medications on clients' sexuality and sexual functioning.
   1. Oral contraceptives are considered by some to have played a major role in creating a sense of sexual freedom in contemporary society.
   2. Drugs that decrease sexual drive or potency may act directly on the physiological mechanisms or may decrease interest through a depressant effect on the central nervous system.
   3. Drugs with an adverse effect on sexual activity include antihypertensive drugs, antidepressants, antihistamines, antispasmodics, diuretics, sedatives and tranquilizers, ethyl alcohol, and some hormone preparations and steroids.
D. Medications for sexual dysfunction.
   1. Example—sildenafil (Viagra): oral therapy (25–100 mg) for erectile dysfunction.
      a. Rapidly absorbed, 30–120 minutes, with resulting ability to achieve an erection sufficient for sexual intercourse.

      b.   Appropriate for healthy young and elderly males.

  2. Precautions: any male who is at cardiac risk, has peptic ulcer disease.

✦ E. Be aware of the problems to which nursing personnel should direct themselves in relation to the area of human sexuality.

  ✦ 1. Attitudes.

    a. Nurses should increase their self-awareness of their own attitudes and the effect of these attitudes on the sexual health care of their clients.

    b. Nurses should suppress negative biases and prejudices and/or make appropriate referrals when they cannot give effective or therapeutic sexual health care.

  2. Knowledge.

    a. May have to be actively sought, although nursing programs are increasing the sexuality content in their curricula.

    b. Also available through books, journal articles, classes and workshops, and preparation for sexuality therapy on the graduate level.

  3. Skills.

    a. Primary skills needed are interpersonal techniques such as therapeutic communication, interviewing, and teaching.

    b. As with any skill, practice is needed for proficiency in sexual-history taking, education, and counseling.

Sexual Behaviors Related to Health

A. Masturbation.

  1. A common sexual outlet for many people.

  2. For clients requiring long-term care, masturbation may be the only means for gratifying their sexual needs.

  3. Nurses frequently react negatively to any type of masturbatory activity, especially by male clients.

  ✦ 4. Clients should be allowed privacy; if a nurse walks in on a client masturbating, he or she should leave with an apology for having intruded on the client's privacy.

  5. Frequent or inappropriate masturbation may be harmful to the client's health.

    a. Nurse should use team planning to identify what need the client is attempting to meet.

    b. Limits need to be set to protect client and other clients if behavior is inappropriate.

B. Gender identity issues—homosexuality.

  1. Homosexuality is accepted as a viable lifestyle.

  2. Nurses may have negative attitudes based on incorrect knowledge about homosexuality.

  ✦ 3. A client's homosexual (gay) or lesbian lifestyle should be accepted and respected. These clients should be treated without judgments.

  4. As with any client, visitors should be encouraged as appropriate for the health/illness status, and these people should not be embarrassed or ridiculed.

  5. For chronically ill clients, such as in a nursing home, it is essential that sexuality needs be considered in the total care plan and special efforts be made to have these needs met.

C. Inappropriate sexual behavior.

  1. Difficult to precisely define "inappropriate" sexual behavior.

  2. Sometimes sexual behavior is in reaction to unintentional "seductive" behavior of nurses.

  ✦ 3. Specific nursing interventions.

    a. Set limits to unacceptable behavior immediately.

    b. Interact without rejecting client.

    c. Help client express feelings in an appropriate manner.

    d. Teach alternative behaviors that are acceptable.

    e. Provide acceptable outlets to sexual feelings.

D. Venereal disease.

  1. Based on reported cases, the incidence of gonorrhea and syphilis is increasing slowly.

  ✦ 2. Both syphilis and gonorrhea can be cured with appropriate antibiotic therapy. (Recently there has occurred a strain of syphilis resistant to antibiotic therapy, so prevention is an important teaching concept.)

  ✦ 3. Treatment and care should be given without judgment.

  4. Case finding and treatment are still very difficult, especially for adolescents who may need parental consent to obtain health services.

✦ E. Contraception.*

  1. Nurses are considered experts on forms of birth control.

  2. Nurses should be familiar with different methods and relative effectiveness of each one.

  3. Clients should be assisted to make their own choices as to whether to use contraception and which method is best for them.

*For a more detailed outline of contraception, *see* Chapter 12.

F. Therapeutic abortion.*

  1. Clients need information about resources for and procedures of therapeutic abortions.

  ✦ 2. Clients should be given nonjudgmental assistance and support in decision-making process.

*For a more detailed outline of abortion, *see* Chapter 12.

✦ 3. If nurse cannot in good conscience assist the
    client because of conflicting religious or spiri-
    tual beliefs, referral should be made to someone
    who can.

Sexuality and Disability

A. Physically and developmentally disabled persons are
   sexual beings also.
✦ B. Developmentally disabled persons should be given
   sexuality education and counseling in preparation
   for sexual expression and behavior.
C. After spinal cord injury, the level of the lesion and
   degree of interruption of nerve impulses influence
   sexual functioning; adaptation of previous sexual
   practices may be needed after the injury.
D. Fertility and the ability to bear children are usually
   not compromised in women with spinal cord injury.
✦ E. Nurses working with disabled clients must make
   special effort to include sexuality in total health care
   and services.
   1. Discuss sexual needs openly with client so he or
      she will not feel embarrassed to ask questions.
   2. Discuss previous sexual activity and how current
      needs can be met.
   3. Nurse must maintain a nonjudgmental attitude
      or relationship will be jeopardized.
   4. Support client and partner during sexual adjust-
      ment period.
   5. Refer to therapy support groups for ongoing
      support.

Child Sexual Abuse*

A. There is only a beginning awareness of this problem
   area.
B. Most child sexual abuse involves a male adult and
   female child, but male children can also be victims of
   female or male sexual abusers.
C. The child may need special protection or temporary
   placement outside the home, but often the family
   unit can be maintained.
✦ D. Child sexual abuse or molestation is a form of child
   abuse, and nurses should know local regulations and
   procedures for case finding and reporting.
✦ E. Nursing interventions.
   1. Establish a safe environment for the child.
   2. Allow and encourage child to verbalize or com-
      municate in his or her own way (through
      drawings or play acting).
   3. Observe for appearance of symptoms over time
      (withdrawal, depression, phobias).

* For more detailed information on child abuse, *see* Psychiatric Nursing,
Chapter 14.

4. Encourage ongoing therapy to work through
   trauma.

JOINT COMMISSION CLIENT SAFETY GOALS, 2008

A. JCAHO defines safety goals for client care.
   1. Improve accuracy of client identification.
   2. Improve effectiveness of communication among
      caregivers.
   3. Improve safety of using medications.
   4. Reduce risk of healthcare-associated infections.
   5. Accurately and completely reconcile medica-
      tions across the continuum of care.
   6. Reduce risk of client harm resulting from falls.
   7. Encourage clients' active involvement in their
      own care as a client safety strategy.
   8. Identify safety risks inherent in an
      organization's client population.
B. Goal 3—preventing medication errors—has specific
   guidelines.
   1. Hospitals must limit the number of drug con-
      centrations.
   2. Hospitals must compile a list of at least ten
      look-alike, sound-alike (LASA) drug pairs.
      Examples:
      a. Concentrated liquid morphine (Roxanol)
         and conventional liquid morphine.
      b. Ephedrine and epinephrine.
      c. Hydromorphone (Dilaudid) and morphine
         injection.
      d. Hydroxyzine (Vistaril, Atarax) and
         hydrazine (Apo-hydral, Apresoline).
      e. Vinblastine and vincristine.
   3. Clinicians must label all medications, medica-
      tion containers such as syringes, medicine cups,
      basins, and other solutions on and off the sterile
      field.
C. JCAHO suggests hospitals develop a list of abbreviations, acronyms, and symbols that should not be
   used because of potential misinterpretation. Items
   on this list must be written out. Examples:
   1. U mistaken for O or cc.
   2. IU mistaken for IV or #10.
   3. QD, q.d., or daily for QOD or qod every other
      day.
   4. MS can mean morphine sulfate or magnesium
      sulfate.
   5. MSO$_4$ for MgSo$_4$.
D. The Institute of Medicine's strategies for reducing
   medication errors.
   1. Complete steps to improve communication
      between clients and providers.

2. Improve drug naming, labeling, and packaging.
3. Assign appropriate groups (FDA) to create easy-to-understand drug information for consumers.
4. Write all prescriptions electronically by 2010.
5. Inform clients of clinically significant medication errors made in their care, even if the mistake did not lead to harm.

ALTERNATIVE AND COMPLEMENTARY THERAPIES

A. Alternative or complementary medicine became popular in the early 1990s.
   1. More than 600 million Americans use alternative therapy.
   2. Bills in Congress have authorized healthcare providers to give alternative treatments.
B. There are more than 200 alternative methods available. A short sampling of these treatment modes follows:
   1. *Acupuncture:* Use of sharp needles inserted along energy lines called meridians. Used for pain and to treat diseases caused by blocked or a lack of energy in the body.
   2. *Chiropractic:* Manipulation of bones and muscles to realign the spinal column as well as other areas in the body, thus enabling the body to heal itself.
   3. *Energy Medicine:* Use of varying frequencies of light and sound to heal the body. This mode is based on the premise that the body is made of electronic and magnetic vibrations.
   4. *Herbal Medicine:* Plant-based remedies with a long history of safety and efficacy used as an adjunct or in place of drugs to treat diseases and conditions.
   5. *Homeopathy:* A system of treatment that uses a minute dose of a substance (may be herbal or chemical) that mimics a disease resulting in a positive effect on the body. The principle with this therapy is that "like cures like."
   6. *Massage:* The oldest form of alternative medicine, massage is the application of touch to the skin to relieve stress and tension. This is a non-pharmacological approach to relieve pain.
   7. *Naturopathy:* A more global alternative therapy that includes natural therapies such as nutrition, herbs, homeopathy, massage, body work (Rolfing) and other treatments, all designed to help the body heal itself.
   8. *Relaxation and Visualization:* A form of therapy that uses exercise, visualization and mental imagery to control the autonomic nervous system. These techniques have proven to be beneficial in controlling stress, oxygen consumption, respiratory and heart rate and blood pressure.
C. Other therapies of note in the alternative medicine arena include ayurveda, biofeedback, aromatherapy, kinesiology, reflexology, Tai Chi and yoga.

NURSING CONCEPTS REVIEW QUESTIONS

1. According to Selye's stress theory, when the individual is in the alarm phase of the general adaptive syndrome, the body first responds by

    1. Going into shock and countershock.
    2. Resisting the stressor.
    3. Adapting to the stressor.
    4. Moving to a state of exhaustion.

2. Which of the following danger signals of stress would it be important to identify so that an appropriate intervention can be made?

    1. Lack of concentration.
    2. Depression.
    3. Anxiety.
    4. Skin rash.

3. When the nurse is counseling a couple on family planning, the effectiveness most strongly depends on the

    1. Method and understanding of the contraceptive choice.
    2. Belief in the method of contraception chosen.
    3. Degree to which the couple wishes not to have children.
    4. Degree to which the method suits the individual using it.

4. A 12-year-old can accomplish formal operational thought, according to Piaget. The nurse understands that this statement means that a young person is able to

    1. Ask direct questions.
    2. Use symbols.
    3. Conceptualize.
    4. Understand cause and effect.

5. Erik Erikson's theory of personality explains that a child who was never allowed to function autonomously may, in later life, experience the psychological crisis of

    1. Mistrust.
    2. Inferiority.
    3. Guilt.
    4. Shame and doubt.

6. One of the primary developmental tasks of adolescence is

    1. Feeling independent.
    2. Finding one's identity.
    3. Experiencing intimacy.
    4. Achieving generativity.

7. A client has just received a diagnosis of breast cancer from her physician. When the nurse asks if she would like to talk about the diagnosis, the client replies, "Oh, no, I'm sure they are wrong—I've always had cysts in my breasts." The nurse recognizes that this may be a grief response, which probably means that the client is

    1. Not ready to accept the diagnosis.
    2. In the disbelief stage of the grief process.
    3. Not comfortable in discussing the diagnosis with the nurse.
    4. Mourning the loss she will have to experience.

8. The ultimate outcome, when the grieving process is successfully completed, will be when the bereaved

    1. Is able to think of the deceased without emotion.
    2. Remembers only the pleasures of the relationship.
    3. Is no longer emotionally dependent on the deceased.
    4. No longer feels the need to talk about the deceased.

9. A nurse who is sensitive to his or her client's need to talk about dying would recognize which of the following cues as the "need to talk"?

    1. The client's refusal to talk to anyone.
    2. Constant crying and looking depressed.
    3. The client's asking the nurse to stay a while.
    4. Constantly asking to be released to go home.

10. The registered nurse (RN) observes the nursing assistant (NA) regulating the IV of an oncology client receiving morphine sulfate for pain. A licensed vocational nurse (LVN) on the RN's team is responsible for the client and has assigned the client to the NA. The RN's intervention is to

    1. Inform the LVN so that he or she intervenes to instruct the NA that this action is not within the realm of responsibility of an NA.

2. Immediately inform the charge nurse and fill out an incident report.
3. Call a staff meeting and confront the LVN and the NA.
4. Ask the LVN and the NA to meet with the RN to discuss the responsibility parameters each of them has.

11. A nurse enters the private room of a male client and realizes he is masturbating. The appropriate response is to

1. Set limits on his behavior in the hospital.
2. Apologize for intruding on the client's privacy.
3. Tell the client his behavior is inappropriate.
4. Ignore the behavior and continue with the intervention planned when entering the room.

12. In the area of human sexuality, nurses may encounter problems in relating to their clients. A major barrier or problem the nurse should be aware of is

1. Lack of knowledge about human sexuality.
2. The nurse's personal attitudes toward human sexuality.
3. Lack of appropriate referrals in this area.
4. Lack of proficiency in sexual-history taking.

13. Pain is now considered the fifth vital sign according to the Joint Commission. For a client who is in pain, this change would be important because

1. The nurse is now responsible for monitoring a client's pain level.
2. It helps to maintain the client's quality of life.
3. As a vital sign it will now be monitored every 15 minutes.
4. The client's pain level was often ignored in the past by the nursing staff.

14. The most effective method of evaluating a client's pain level is to

1. Ask the client where he or she feels the pain.
2. Select a tool to measure pain based on the client's preferences and cognitive level.
3. Observe the nonverbal cues to pain level.
4. Determine if the pain medication ordered is actually relieving the client's pain.

NURSING CONCEPTS

Answers with Rationale

1. (1) The first stage is alarm—shock and counter-shock. The body translates the shock as sudden injury and then is restored to preinjury state (countershock). Resistance (2) is the second stage, and exhaustion (4) is the third stage, according to stress theory.

   NP:AN; CN:H; CL:K

2. (2) All of the conditions may be considered danger signals of stress, but depression is the most dangerous owing to the possibility of suicide (which may occur with any degree of depression).

   NP:A; CN:PS; CL:AN

3. (1) The effectiveness of family planning depends most on the method chosen and the degree of understanding of the method. Motivation and the degree to which the couple follow the prescribed regimen also affect the outcome. Belief in the method (2) and the wish to have or not have children (3) do not affect the success of family planning. The degree to which the method suits the person (4) may have some influence, but is not definitive enough as an answer.

   NP:AN; CN:H; CL:C

4. (3) At age 12 years and older, a young person is able to conceptualize and do abstract thinking. Before this age, the young person is only able to think concretely. Using symbols (2) and understanding cause/effect (4) occurs at 7 to 12 years. Answer (1) occurs from 4 to 7 years. This is important theoretical information for the nurse to have when the child is in the hospital, because it will give cues as to how much the child or young adult will understand the diagnosis or instructions.

   NP:AN; CN:H; CL:C

5. (4) Erikson's theory explains that at every age the individual has to go through a psychological crisis period of development. In this case, if the toddler is allowed to gain autonomy, he or she will not experience shame and doubt in later life. If the infant develops trust in the maternal figure, he will not mistrust; if the school-age child is industrious, he will not feel inferior later; and, if the preschooler is allowed to show initiative, in later life he or she will not experience guilt.

   NP:AN; CN:PS; CL:C

6. (2) Early adolescence has the primary task of finding one's identity and moving out of role diffusion. Later adolescence to young adulthood's task is to experience intimacy (3), not isolation. Adults should achieve generativity (4) versus stagnation.

   NP:AN; CN:H; CL:K

7. (2) The first stage of grief is often disbelief, along with shock. The client may also not be ready to accept the diagnosis or wish to discuss it with the nurse. Mourning is a later stage of the grief process.

   NP:AN; CN:H; CL:A

8. (3) When the grieving process is completed, the bereaved will no longer feel emotionally dependent on the person who died. The individual will always feel emotion (1) when thinking of the loved one, but he or she will be able to realistically recall both the good and the bad times. There will always be the need to talk about the loved one (4), even when the grief has been resolved.

   NP:E; CN:PS; CL:C

9. (3) Asking the nurse to stay a while may be a cue that the client is ready to talk about the difficult subject. The other behaviors do not indicate a willingness to talk.

   NP:A; CN:H; CL:AN

Coding for Questions/Answers Abbreviations: **Nursing Process: NP,** Assessment: A, Analysis: AN, Planning: P, Implementation: I, Evaluation: E; **Client Needs: CN,** Safe, Effective Care Environment: S, Health Promotion and Maintenance: H, Psychosocial Integrity: PS, Physiological Integrity: PH; **Clinical Area: CA,** Medical Nursing: M, Surgical Nursing: S, Maternal/Newborn Nursing: MA, Pediatric Nursing: P, Psychiatric Nursing: PS; **Cognitive Level: CL,** Knowledge: K, Comprehension: C, Application: A, Analysis: AN.

10. (4) While regulating or even touching an IV is definitely not within the scope of behaviors that an NA can legally perform, both teaching and clarification of duties are needed in this situation. Before accusing the NA, a nonpunitive environment should be created so that teaching of both the LVN and the NA can occur, and so that this action will not happen again. Unless too much medication was given, an incident report does not need to be filled out (2). Confronting the team member in a staff meeting (3) would not be following good management principles.

    NP:I; CN:S; CL:AN

11. (2) The appropriate response is to apologize, leave the room, and return later. Clients should be allowed privacy, and this is a common sexual outlet for many people. When the behavior is inappropriate, limits should be set (1). The client's behavior is not necessarily inappropriate for him (3). Continuing with the nurse's intended intervention (4) is also inappropriate because it intrudes on the client's privacy.

    NP:I; CN:H; CL:A

12. (2) Negative attitudes, biases, prejudices, or judgments on the part of the nurse can present a major problem for nurses working in the area of sexual health. If these attitudes are negative, the relationship will be compromised. Lack of knowledge (1), referrals (3), or proficiency (4) may all present problems, but do not affect relating to the client.

    NP:P; CN:H; CL:A

13. (2) As a fifth vital sign, pain will be monitored as often as the other vital signs, which will help to maintain the client's quality of life. (1) The nurse has always been responsible for monitoring the pain level. Pain does not have to be monitored every 15 minutes (3). A client's pain level has not been ignored, but this additional reminder will assist the nurse to monitor pain more frequently.

    NP:P; CN:H; CL:C

14. (2) The most effective way to measure pain is with a scale (either zero to five or zero to ten) that the client can understand. This allows the evaluation to be consistent over time. Just asking the client will not yield enough data (1), nor will observing nonverbal cues. This measure will be helpful with a young child or a cognitively impaired adult. Just evaluating the pain medication is not an accurate measure for pain control.

    NP:E; CN:PH; CL:A

Nutritional Management

4

✦ The icon denotes content of special importance for NCLEX.

MACRONUTRIENTS

Carbohydrates

A. Carbohydrates are the chief source of energy and contain carbon, hydrogen, and oxygen.
    1. Carbohydrates include sugars, starches, and cellulose.
    2. Simple sugars, such as fruit sugar, are easily digested.
    3. Starches, which are more complex, require more sophisticated enzyme processes to be reduced to glucose.
    4. One gram of carbohydrate provides 4 kilocalories.
    5. Glucose, which is converted sugar or starch, appears in the body as blood sugar.
        a. It is "burned" as fuel by the tissues.
        b. Some glucose is processed by the liver, converted to glycogen, and stored by the liver for later use.
B. Ingesting too many carbohydrates crowds out other important foods; it prevents the body from receiving the necessary nutrients for healthy maintenance.
C. Ingesting too few carbohydrates leads to loss of energy, depression, ketosis; it also leads to a breakdown of body protein.
D. The amount and kind of carbohydrates that should be consumed for optimal health are determined by several factors.
    1. Differences in body structure; energy expenditure; basal metabolism rate; and general health status.
    2. The average American diet provides 45% of calories from carbohydrates; it is recommended that this proportion be increased to 50–65%.
    3. Simple (refined) sugars should be limited to 10% total calories.

Fats or Lipids

A. Fats or lipids are the second important group of nutrients.
    1. They provide energy.
    2. When oxidized, they are the most concentrated sources of energy.
    3. They furnish the calories necessary for survival; each fat gram provides 9 kilocalories.
B. Fats also act as carriers for the fat-soluble vitamins A, D, E, and K.
C. Consuming too much fat is unhealthy.
    1. The average American diet provides 35–40% of calories from fat.
    2. Fats should account for no more than 20–35% of daily calorie intake.
D. Fatty acids are the basic components of fat, and comprise two main groups.

1. Saturated fatty acids usually come from animal sources. It is recommended to substitute saturated fats with polyunsaturated and monounsaturated fats.
    a. Saturated fats should be less than 10% of calories.
    b. Cholesterol should be limited to 300 mg daily.
2. Unsaturated fatty acids primarily come from vegetables, nuts, or seed sources and are liquid at room temperature.
    a. This group contains three essential fatty acids.
    b. These acids are called *essential* because they are necessary to prevent a specific deficiency disease.
    c. The body cannot manufacture these acids. They are obtained only from the diet.
    d. These acids are called linoleic acid, arachidonic acid, and linolenic acid.
    e. A deficiency in this group would lead to skin problems, illness, and unhealthy blood and arteries.

Proteins

A. Proteins are complex organic compounds that contain amino acids.
B. Protein is critical to all aspects of growth and development of body tissues. It is necessary for the building of muscles, blood, skin, internal organs, hormones, and enzymes.
C. Each gram of protein provides 4 kilocalories.
    1. The RDA for protein is 56 g/day for men and 45 g/day for women.
    2. The optimal diet should be 10–12% protein rather than the 17% most Americans consume.
D. Protein is also a source of energy.
    1. When there is insufficient carbohydrate or fat in the diet, protein is burned.
    2. When protein is spared, it is either used for tissue repair and maintenance or converted by the liver and stored as fat.
E. When proteins are digested and broken down, they form 20 amino acids.
    1. Amino acids are absorbed from the intestine into the bloodstream.
    2. They are carried to the liver for synthesis into the tissues and organs of the body.
F. Amino acids are the chemical basis for life. If just one is missing, protein synthesis will decrease or even stop.
G. All but nine amino acids can be synthesized by the body. Eight are required by all humans; infants require one more—histidine.
    1. These nine must be obtained from the diet.

2. If all nine are present in a particular food, the food is a *complete protein.*
3. Foods that lack one or more essential amino acids are called *incomplete proteins.*
✦ 4. Most meat and dairy products are complete proteins.
5. Most vegetables and fruits are incomplete proteins.
✦ 6. When several incomplete proteins are ingested, they should be combined carefully so that the result will be a balance yielding complete protein. For example, the combination of beans and rice is a complete protein food.

H. Protein deficiency can affect the entire body—organs, tissues, skin, and muscles, as well as certain body processes.

Water

A. While not specifically a nutrient, water is essential for survival.
   1. Water is involved in every body process, from digestion and absorption to excretion.
   2. It is a major portion of circulation and is the transporter of nutrients throughout the body.
B. Body water performs three major functions.
   1. Water gives form to the body, accounting for 50–75% (average 60%) of the body mass.
   2. It provides the necessary environment for cell metabolism.
   3. It maintains a stable body temperature.
C. Almost all foods contain water that is absorbed by the body.
D. The average adult body (male weighing 70 kg) contains approximately 40 L of water and loses about 3 L per day.
   1. If a person suffers severe water depletion, dehydration and salt depletion can result and can eventually lead to death.
   2. A person can survive longer without food than without water.

MICRONUTRIENTS

Vitamins

A. Vitamins are organic food substances and are essential in small amounts for growth, maintenance, and the functioning of body processes.
B. Vitamins are found only in living things—plants and animals—and usually cannot be synthesized by the human body.
C. Vitamins can be grouped according to the substance in which they are soluble.

✦ **Table 4-1. FOODS RICH IN FAT- AND WATER-SOLUBLE VITAMINS**

Foods rich in fat-soluble vitamins

Vitamin A—liver, egg yolk, whole milk, butter, fortified margarine, green and yellow vegetables, fruits
Vitamin D— fortified milk and margarine, fish oils
Vitamin E—vegetable oils and green vegetables
Vitamin K—egg yolk, leafy green vegetables, liver, cheese

Foods rich in water-soluble vitamins

Vitamin C—citrus fruits, tomatoes, broccoli, cabbage
Thiamine (B_1)—lean meat such as beef, pork, liver; whole-grain cereals and legumes
Riboflavin (B_2)—milk, organ meats, enriched grains
Niacin—meat, beans, peas, peanuts, enriched grains
Pyridoxine (B_6)—yeast, wheat, corn, meats, liver, kidney
Cobalamin (B_{12})—lean meat, liver, kidney
Folic acid—leafy green vegetables, eggs, liver

✦ D. The fat-soluble group includes vitamins A, D, E, and K.
E. The water-soluble vitamins include the B-complex vitamins, vitamin C, and the bioflavonoids.
F. Vitamins have no caloric value, but they are as necessary to the body as any other basic nutrient.
   1. Currently, there are about 20 substances identified as vitamins.
   2. Recent research is concerned with identifying even more of these substances because they are so essential to survival.
G. The most commonly used guidelines are the listings of the Recommended Dietary Allowances (RDA), based on standards established by the National Academy of Sciences. (*See* Table 4-1.)

Minerals

A. Minerals are inorganic substances, widely prevalent in nature, and essential for metabolic processes.
B. Minerals are grouped according to the amount found in the body. These are both major minerals and trace minerals.
✦ C. Major minerals include calcium, magnesium, sodium, potassium, phosphorus, sulfur, and chlorine, all of which have a known function in the body.
D. Trace minerals include iron, copper, iodine, manganese, cobalt, zinc, florine, selenium, and molybdenum. Their function in the body remains unclear.
E. There remains another group of trace minerals found in scanty amounts in the body and whose function is also unclear.
✦ F. Minerals form 60–90% of all inorganic material in the body, and are found in bones, teeth, soft tissue, muscle, blood, and nerve cells.

G. Minerals act on organs and in metabolic processes.
  1. They serve as catalysts for many reactions, such as controlling muscle responses, maintaining the nervous system, and regulating acid–base balance.
  2. They assist in transmitting messages, maintaining cardiac stability, and regulating the metabolism and absorption of other nutrients.
H. Even though they are considered separately, all minerals work synergistically with other minerals, and their actions are interrelated.
  1. A deficiency in one mineral will affect the action of others in the body.
  2. Adequate minerals must be ingested because a mineral deficiency can result in severe illness.
  3. Excessive amounts of minerals can throw the body out of balance and may be toxic to the body.
I. Adequate diet can supply sufficient minerals. (*See* Table 4-2.)

ASSIMILATION OF NUTRIENTS

Gastrointestinal Tract

A. The main functions of the gastrointestinal system.
  1. Secretion of enzymes and electrolytes to break down raw materials that are ingested.
  2. Movement of ingested products through the system.
  3. Complete digestion of nutrients.
  4. Absorption of nutrients into the blood.
  5. Storage of nutrients.
  6. Excretion of the end products of digestion.
B. When nutrients reach the stomach, both mechanical and chemical digestive processes occur.
  1. Nutrients are churned, and peristaltic waves move the material through the stomach.
  2. At intervals, with relaxation of the pyloric sphincter, they move into the duodenum.
  3. This chemical action creates hydrochloric acid, which provides a medium for pepsin to split protein into proteoses and peptones.
  4. The digestive process produces other chemical actions.
    a. Lipase, a fat-splitting enzyme.
    b. Rennin, an enzyme that coagulates the protein of milk.
    c. The intrinsic factor, which acts on certain food components to form the antianemic factor.
C. Nutrients then move into the duodenum and the jejunum.
  1. Intestinal juices provide a large number of enzymes.

Table 4-2. ESSENTIAL BODY NUTRIENTS	
Carbohydrates	Monosaccharides
	Glucose, fructose, galactose
	Disaccharides
	Sucrose, lactose, maltose
	Polysaccharides
	Starch, dextrin, glycogen, cellulose, hemicellulose
Fats	Linoleic acid, linolenic acid, arachidonic acid
Proteins	Amino acids
	Phenylalanine, lysine, isoleucine, leucine, methionine, valine, tryptophan, threonine, histidine
Vitamins	Fat-soluble
	Vitamins A, D, E, and K
	Water-soluble
	Vitamins B_1, B_2, B_6, B_{12}, niacin, pantothenic acid, folacin, biotin, choline, mesoinositol, para-aminobenzoic acid, and vitamin C
Minerals	Major elements
	Calcium, chlorine, iron, magnesium, phosphorus, potassium, sodium, sulfur
	Trace elements
Water	

    a. These break down protein into amino acids.
    b. They form and convert maltase to glucose.
    c. They split nucleic acids into nucleotides.
  2. The large intestine provides for the absorption of nutrients and the elimination of waste products.
    a. Vitamins K and B_{12}, riboflavin, and thiamine are formed.
    b. Water is absorbed from the fecal mass.

The Accessory Organs

A. The accessory organs of the gastrointestinal tract play an important role in the utilization of nutrients.
B. The liver plays a major role in the metabolism of carbohydrates, fats, and proteins.
  1. Liver converts glucose to glycogen and stores it.
  2. It reconverts glycogen to glucose when the body requires higher blood sugar.
  3. The process of releasing carbohydrates (end products) into the bloodstream is called glycogenolysis.
  4. Fats are metabolized through the process of oxidation of fatty acids and the formation of acetoacetic acid.

Table 4-3. MAJOR ENZYMES OF DIGESTION

Enzyme	Source/Secretion	Substance Acted on
Ptyalin	Oral/Saliva	Starch
Maltose	Oral/Saliva	Maltose
Pepsin	Gastric	Protein
Lipase	Gastric	Fat
Rennin	Gastric	Casein (protein in milk)
Trypsin	Pancreatic	Protein
Steapsin	Pancreatic	Fat
Amylopsin	Pancreatic	Starch
Amylase	Intestinal	Starch
Maltase	Intestinal	Maltose
Lactase	Intestinal	Lactose
Sucrase	Intestinal	Sucrose
Erepsin	Intestinal	Protein
Enterokinase	Intestinal	Protein

5. Lipoproteins, cholesterol, and phospholipids are formed, and carbohydrates and protein are converted to fats.
6. Proteins are metabolized in the liver, and deamination of amino acids takes place.
7. The formation of urea and plasma proteins is completed.
8. The interconversions of amino acids and other compounds occur in the liver.

C. The gallbladder's primary function is to act as a reservoir for bile.
   1. Bile emulsifies fats through constant secretion.
   2. Secretion rate is 500–1000 mL every 24 hours.
D. The pancreas secretes pancreatic juices that contain enzymes for the digestion of carbohydrates, fats, and proteins.
   1. Enzymes are secreted as inactive precursors that do not become active until secreted into the intestine.
   2. In the intestine, the enzyme trypsin acts on proteins to produce peptones, peptides, and amino acids.
   3. Pancreatic amylase acts on carbohydrates to produce disaccharides.
   4. Pancreatic lipase acts on fats to produce glycerol and fatty acids.

Gastrointestinal Dysfunctions

A. Dysphagia (difficulty swallowing) occurs in 60% of stroke clients and 50% of clients with Parkinson's disease.
   1. Dysphagia may also occur in cerebral palsy, multiple sclerosis, polio, and myasthenia gravis.

2. Most serious complication is aspiration of liquid or food into lungs.
B. Gastrointestinal hemorrhage may cause a rise in serum ammonia, which may lead to altered neurologic function.
C. Intestinal obstruction—cessation of peristalsis (ileus) results in altered GI movement and absorption.

NUTRITIONAL CONCEPTS

Normal and Therapeutic Nutrition

A. Normal nutrition.
   1. A guide for determining adequate nutrition is the U.S. Department of Agriculture recommended daily dietary allowances.
      a. The guide is scientifically designed for the maintenance of healthy people in the United States.
      b. The values of the caloric and nutrient requirements given in the guide are used in assessing nutritional states.
      c. Stress periods in the life cycle, which require alterations in the allowances, should be considered during the planning of menus.
   2. The basic food groups are described in the food pyramid. (*See* Appendix 4-2, Revised Food Pyramid, 2005)
      a. Choices in these food groups are offered to meet the nutrient recommendations during the life cycle. (Caloric requirements are not included.)
      b. The basic nutrients in each food group should be related to dietary needs during the life cycle when menus are planned for each age group.
B. Therapeutic nutrition.
   1. The therapeutic or prescription diet is a modification of the nutritional needs based on the disease condition and/or the excess or deficit nutrition state.
   2. Combination diets, which include alterations in minerals, vitamins, proteins, carbohydrates, and fats, as well as fluid and texture, are prescribed in therapeutic nutrition.
   3. Although not all such diets will be included in this review, study of the selected diet concepts will enable you to combine two or more diets when necessary.
✦ C. Normal and therapeutic nutrition considerations.
   1. Cultural, socioeconomic, and psychological influences, as well as physiological requirements, must be considered for effective nutrition.

2. In any given situation, the nutrition requirements must be considered within the context of the biopsychosocial needs of an individual.

Diet Related to Heart Disease Risk

A. The lipid hypothesis, introduced in the 1950s, suggested diet and cholesterol (especially saturated fat) presented risk for heart disease.
    1. Total cholesterol over 200 and ratio of high-density lipoproteins (HDL), the "good" cholesterol, to low-density lipoproteins (LDL) or "bad" cholesterol, predict risk.
    2. Goal is to reduce saturated fat in diet.
B. High concentration of homocysteine in blood is also associated with risk for heart disease.
    1. An amino acid forms when diet has a high concentration of meat and dairy products.
    2. Excess levels damage artery walls, causing the blood vessel to trap circulating cholesterol.
    3. Increasing daily intake of B vitamins (folic acid, pyridoxine and B_{12}) will reduce homocysteine levels.

Nutritional Problems in the Hospital

A. Nutrition is frequently neglected as a viable component of client management.
B. For clients who seem to be stable on admission and give no history of nutritionally related food problems, the usual hospital diet is adequate.
    ✦ 1. These clients must be reassessed periodically to prevent nutritional problems from developing.
    2. A periodic assessment is especially important for clients hospitalized for a long period of time. (*See* Appendix 4-1, Nutritional Assessment Parameters.)
    3. Studies conducted at various medical centers support the claim that as many as 50% of hospitalized clients suffer from malnutrition and become more malnourished the longer they remain in a hospital.
C. For clients identified as having a nutritional problem, a client care plan must be developed.
    1. The cause of depletion must be determined.
    2. Research indicates that poor food intake is the leading cause of malnutrition.
    ✦ 3. Reasons for poor food intake.
        a. The client may feel fear, anxiety, or depression prior to or during hospitalization.
        b. Some clients may not be capable of feeding themselves or may have poor-fitting dentures.
        c. Treatment and therapy may limit the capability of a client to eat or interfere with a client's appetite.
        d. Although the desire for food is present, shortly after eating a certain food a client may have cramps, pain, gas, or diarrhea or feel nauseous and/or vomit.
D. As clients become more and more malnourished, they lose the ability to handle foodstuffs metabolically.
    1. As intake decreases below nutritional requirements, the body cannot generate the epithelium of the gastrointestinal tract from the crypt cells.
    2. The villi and microvilli needed to metabolize and absorb food flatten and become ineffective.
    3. This condition leads to malabsorption, resulting in malnutrition.
E. Malabsorption—the osmotic gap.
    1. To check client for malabsorption, assess the stool's osmotic gap.
    2. Send a stool specimen to lab and check sodium, potassium levels, and osmolarity.
    3. Calculate gap by combining Na and K values, doubling them, and subtracting osmolarity.
    4. Normal value is 40–100 Osm/kg H_2O. A value above 100 Osm/kg H_2O indicates malabsorption.

Instituting Therapeutic Regimens

A. Check that a complete nutritional assessment has been completed on the client. (*See* Appendix 4-1, Nutritional Assessment Parameters.)
B. Evaluate the status of the client's gastrointestinal tract to determine if modifications in nutrients are necessary.
    1. Can the client split intact protein into the peptides and amino acids needed for absorption?
    2. Can the client tolerate the osmotic load of monosaccharides or disaccharides?
    3. Is the client fat intolerant, or does the client need special fat? Is the client lactose intolerant?
C. Check that therapeutic diet is ordered.
D. Be aware of compliance by the client.
    1. The nurse can best determine the client's actual intake.
    2. The nurse should ensure that the client is not receiving inappropriate foods from other sources.
    3. The nurse should check that the client is actually eating the foods prescribed.
E. If the prescribed diet is not meeting the client's needs, consider an alternative method of feeding.
    1. If oral feedings prove inadequate, then alternative methods such as nasogastric, nasoduodenal, or nasojejunal tube feeding should be considered.

✦ Table 4-4. RECOMMENDED NUTRIENT REQUIREMENTS FOR HEALING*

Total calories

2800 for tissue repair; 6000 for extensive repair

Protein

50–75 g/day early in postoperative period
100–200 g/day if needed for new-tissue synthesis

Carbohydrate

50–65% of calories or sufficient in quantity to meet calorie needs and allow protein to be used for tissue repair

Fat

20–35% or not excessive; it leads to poor tissue healing and susceptibility to infection

Vitamins

Vitamin C—up to 1 g/day
Vitamin B—increased above normal
Vitamin K—normal amounts
Vitamin A—stimulates immune response
Vitamin E—400 U, increases O_2 to tissues

Minerals

Normal amount for tissue repair and healing
   Zinc—tissue repair
   Selenium—cell repair
   Calcium/magnesium—maintains electrical stimulation and relaxes nerves

*Diet will be individualized—depends on assessment of client's needs.

INTAKE MEASUREMENTS

Ice cream cup (3 oz)	90 mL
Jello cup (3 oz)	90 mL
Ice chips (8 oz) melt to 50%	120 mL
Coffee cup (5 oz)	150 mL
Soup bowl (5 oz)	150 mL
Drinking glass (8 oz)	240 mL

2. A variety of delivery systems and methods of enteral feeding are now available for adequate care of the client.
3. When other methods have failed, parenteral nutrition may be the management of choice.
   a. This can be administered peripherally, using isotonic concentrations of glucose, crystalline amino acids, and fats.
   b. It can be administered through a central, high-flow vein in which hypertonic glucose is given, supplemented with crystalline amino acids, fats, electrolytes, vitamins, and trace elements.

F. Be alert to clients' nutritional needs so that no client becomes or remains malnourished or develops any kind of nutritional problem. (*See* Table 4-4.)
1. Elicit food preferences from the client.
2. Send request to the diet kitchen for the specific diet and keep diet sheets or diet rands up to date.
✦ 3. Check all diet trays before serving to ensure the diet provided is the one ordered.
4. Ensure that hot food is hot and cold food is cold.
5. Keep food trays attractive. Avoid spilling liquids on tray.
✦ 6. Position the client in a chair or up in bed (unless otherwise ordered) to assist in feeding.
7. Assist the client with cutting meat and opening milk cartons as needed.
8. Feed the client if necessary.

G. Administer ordered fluids and tabulate fluid intake.

Nutritional Guidelines for Managing Clients

A. An adequate diet must include carbohydrates, fats, proteins, vitamins, and minerals.
1. Carbohydrates are the chief source of energy, and diets not sufficient in carbohydrates lead to a low energy level, use of protein for energy, and ketosis.
2. Fats provide the most concentrated source of energy and are carriers for fat-soluble vitamins.
3. Proteins are essential for building body tissue and are necessary for tissue repair.
4. Vitamins are essential for growth, maintenance, and functioning of body processes.
5. Minerals are essential for metabolic processes.

B. Digestion takes place throughout the gastrointestinal tract.
1. The gastrointestinal system breaks down raw materials through the secretion of enzymes and electrolytes.
2. Mechanical and chemical digestive processes are necessary for nutritional synthesis.
3. Nutrients are absorbed through the large intestine.
4. The liver plays a major role in nutritional metabolism.

C. Nutritional needs are based on a client's disease condition and excess or deficit of a nutritional state.
1. Therapeutic diets are used to alter health status.
2. Combination diets, which include alteration of all the major nutrients, are prescribed for certain disease conditions.

D. Alternative methods of providing nutrients must be instituted when clients are unable to ingest or assimilate foods orally.

1. Enteral feedings provide life-sustaining nutrients when other oral methods cannot be utilized.
2. Parenteral nutrition may be administered peripherally, using isotonic concentrations, or centrally with intravenous catheter placement.

Administering Therapeutic Diets

Restricting Dietary Carbohydrates

✦ A. Hypoglycemia occurs when most of the glucose moves from the blood into the cells and results in abnormally low blood glucose levels (< 70 mg/dL).
   1. Foods prescribed are high protein, moderate-complex carbohydrates in 5 or 6 meals/day.
   2. Foods limited are simple carbohydrates—for example, sugar, syrup, candy. Complex carbohydrates or starches have higher nutritional values and more fiber.

✦ B. Diabetic guidelines.
   1. Nutrition is the cornerstone of disease management.
      a. Normal weight must be maintained and may dramatically reduce symptoms.
      b. Diet together with insulin supplement or oral medication and exercise complete the regimen.
   2. Goal of dietary therapy is to have a well-balanced diet and to count carbohydrates (CHO) because CHO raises blood sugar.
      a. Diabetics do not have to give up their favorite foods; they must learn the amounts that are allowed and substitutions permitted.
   ✦ b. General guidelines for nutrient balance are:

Carbohydrate	50–60 percent (40% from complex CHOs)
Fat	20–30 percent
Saturated fat	10 percent
Cholesterol	Limit to 300 mg or less
Protein	10–20 percent

Consume 20–35 grams of fiber daily (including soluble and insoluble)
      c. Dietary ratio: 5:2:1 carbohydrate to fat to protein (according to the American Dietetic Association).

✦ C. Carbohydrate counting is a nutritional tool used to maintain blood glucose levels.
   1. Count grams of carbohydrates (Type 1 diabetics require more accurate monitoring).
   2. Measure servings or choices (more often used with Type 2 diabetics). 1 carbohydrate serving = 15 g carbohydrate with vegetables is counted as one-third serving of carbohydrate.

Table 4-5. THE GLYCEMIC INDEX OF COMMON FOODS

Low	**Moderate**
(Recommended in abundance)	*(Recommended in moderation)*
Green vegetables	Whole-grain breads
Tomatoes	Whole-grain pasta
Beans and peas	Oatmeal
Dried apricots	Sweet potatoes
Berries	Grapes
Grapefruit	Apples
Nuts	Oranges
Rye and barley	Carrots

High	
(Not recommended at all or very sparingly)	
Most sugars	White potatoes
White breads	Corn
Crackers, rice cakes, and chips	Pineapple
Most cold cereals	Raisins
White rice	Ripe bananas

3. Use the glycemic index, which describes how much the blood glucose level rises with a specific food when compared with an equivalent amount of glucose. Foods with a higher glycemic index enter bloodstream rapidly, causing glucose to spike. (*See* Table 4-5.)
   a. Particular foods (most sugars and items made with white flour) have a higher glycemic index than others.
   b. By combining certain foods, the client may lower the glycemic index and do better at stabilizing blood glucose levels.
   c. Combining a starch with protein or fat will lower the glycemic index.
   d. Eating raw and whole foods and fruit rather than juices will lower glycemic index.
   e. Keeping a chart and building individual glycemic indices by monitoring blood glucose levels after food consumption will improve stabilizing blood glucose levels.
4. The client may choose any method to monitor carbohydrate consumption, but monitoring is essential if blood sugar levels are to remain within normal limits.

D. Level of activity must be assessed to determine energy requirements.
   1. Increased activity uses more carbohydrates.
   2. Most adults require 30 cal/kg of ideal body weight.

✦ Table 4-6. FOODS HIGH IN PROTEIN	
Food	**Protein (Grams)**
Dairy and eggs	
Cottage cheese, ½ cup	14.0
Milk, 1 cup	8.5
Cheddar cheese, 1 oz	7.1
Egg, 1 medium	6.1
Ice cream, ½ cup	2.4
Meat and fish	
Tuna, canned, drained, 4 oz	32.0
Chicken, 4 oz cooked	31.2
Hamburger, 4 oz cooked	30.7
Sirloin steak, 4 oz cooked	26.7
Grains	
Whole-wheat flour, ½ cup	8.0
Spaghetti, 1 cup cooked	6.0
Cornmeal, ½ cup	5.5
Rice, brown, 1 cup cooked	5.0
Rice, white, 1 cup cooked	4.0
Legumes	
Soybeans, ½ cup cooked	12.0
Peanut butter, 1 oz	7.1
Lima beans, ½ cup cooked	6.1
Cashews, 1 oz	4.8

Table 4-7. FOODS HIGH IN PURINE

Meat extracts
Shellfish
Liver and other organ meats
Sardines, mussels, anchovies
Chicken, turkey
Beans, lentils
Peas
Spinach
Cauliflower
Asparagus

✦ Table 4-8. FOODS HIGH IN CHOLESTEROL

Beef liver	Bacon
Organ meats	Chicken
Eggs	Lobster
Sardines	Turkey
Veal	Ice cream
Lamb	Hot dogs
Beef	White fish
Pork	

Restricting Dietary Protein

A. A restricted-protein diet is utilized for renal impairment because protein is processed through the kidneys. (*See* Table 4-6.)
   1. End products (nitrogenous waste) of protein metabolism are controlled by limiting protein intake.
   2. Protein processing uses up calcium reserves.
   3. Conditions utilizing restricted protein diets.
      a. Pyelonephritis.
      b. Glomerulonephritis, if oliguria is present.
      c. Kidney insufficiency.
      d. Dialysis management.
      e. Encepholopathy due to liver failure.
B. A PKU diet is an amino acid metabolism abnormality diet utilized for phenylketonuria (PKU), galactosemia, and lactose intolerance.
   1. Reduce and/or eliminate the offending enzyme in the food intake of protein and utilize substitute nutrient foods.
   2. Avoid milk and milk products as they constitute the main source of enzymes for the three diseases.
   3. Employ substitutes to meet daily allowances.

Low-Purine Diet

A. Prevents uric acid stones; also utilized for gout clients. (*See* Table 4-7.)
B. *Restrict purine*, which is the precursor of uric acid.
C. *Allow foods* such as milk, tea, fruit juices, carbonated beverages, breads, cereals, cheese, eggs, fat, and most vegetables.
D. *Restrict foods* such as glandular meats, gravies, fowl, fish, and high meat quantities.

Restricted Dietary Fat

A. A restricted-cholesterol diet decreases cardiovascular disease risk and diabetes mellitus. (*See* Table 4-8.)
   1. Blood cholesterol level is reduced and/or maintained at a normal level by restricting foods high in cholesterol.
   2. Lipid level goals—cholesterol: 160–200 mg/dL; LDL < 100 mg/dL; HDL > 45 for males and > 55 for females; triglycerides < 150.
      a. Total cholesterol.
         < 200 desirable
         > 240 high
      b. LDL (bad cholesterol).
         < 100 optimal
         160–189 } high
         > 190
      c. HDL (good cholesterol).
         < 40 low
         > 60 high

Table 4-9. MAJOR FOOD SOURCES OF VITAMINS					
Vitamin A	**Vitamin B Group**	**Vitamin C**	**Vitamin D**	**Vitamin E**	**Vitamin K**
Dairy products (milk) Liver Egg yolk Dark green and dark yellow vegetables and fruits: carrots, sweet potato, spinach, cantaloupe, broccoli, watermelon, leaf lettuce	Pork, beef, fish, liver, organ meats Eggs Peanuts, nuts Enriched whole grains Legumes, beans, spinach Green, leafy vegetables Yeast Oatmeal	Fruits and vegetables: citrus (oranges, grapefruit, lemons), strawberries, tomatoes, bell peppers, cantaloupe, broccoli, greens	Foods fortified with vitamin D—milk Egg yolk Fish	Vegetable oils Nuts, seeds Green vegetables, especially leafy vegetables Wheat germ; whole-grain products	Meats Egg yolk Liver Vegetable oils Tomatoes Cauliflower Peas Potatoes Cheese

d.   Triglycerides.
  < 150   normal
  200–499 } high
  > 500 }

3.   Restrict total fat to 30% of calories; restrict saturated fat to 10% (or less) of calories.

✦ 4.   The average person should consume 250–300 mg of cholesterol per day. (One egg has 275 mg of cholesterol; one 3-ounce serving of hamburger has 50 mg of cholesterol.)

5.   Substitute trans fats and saturated fat with monounsaturated fats (found in plant products); increase essential fatty acids.

6.   Decrease high-cholesterol foods found in animal products—for example, egg yolks, shellfish, organs and red meat, and pork.

7.   Encourage low-cholesterol foods, such as vegetable oils, raw or cooked vegetables, fruits, lean meats, and fowl.

B.   A modified-fat diet is utilized according to individual tolerance in specific diseases and conditions and for those wishing to lose weight.
1.   Attempt to lower fat content in diet to reduce irritation of diseased organs and to reduce fat content where there is inadequate absorption.
2.   Modified-fat diets are appropriate for the following conditions:
  a.   Malabsorption syndromes.
  b.   Cystic fibrosis.
  c.   Obstructive jaundice.
  d.   Liver disease.

✦ C.   A polyunsaturated-fat diet is utilized primarily for cardiovascular diseases.
1.   Reduce intake of saturated fats and increase intake of foods rich in polyunsaturated fats. (Physician usually prescribes caloric level as well as restrictions.)
2.   Limit foods originating from animal sources and selected plants, such as peanuts, olives, avocado, coconuts, chocolate, and cashew nuts.
3.   Allow foods originating from vegetable sources (except for those named above), butter substitute, corn/soybean/safflower oil, fresh ground peanut butter, and nuts (except cashews).

Vitamins

A.   An increased-vitamin diet is necessary for treatment of specific vitamin deficiencies.
1.   Provide a high-vitamin diet for clients with burns, healing wounds, raised temperatures, and infections. Also used for pregnant clients. (*See* Table 4-9.)
2.   Evaluate diseases, such as cystic fibrosis and liver disease, that require water-soluble vitamins. (*See* Table 4-1 for water-soluble vitamins.)

B.   Total low-vitamin diets are not generally prescribed, although specific vitamins might be decreased for periods of illness.

Minerals

A.   Sodium restriction.
1.   Correct and/or control the retention of sodium and water in the body by limiting sodium

intake. May be done by restriction of salt in the diet or in combination with medications.

2. Restrict salt in cooking or at the table. In clients requiring dietary modification in salt intake, any product containing sodium, such as soda bicarbonate, may be prohibited.
3. The typical diet provides 4–6 g of sodium per day.
✦ 4. Sodium dietary restrictions. (*See* Table 4-10.)
   a. *Mild:* 2–3 g sodium (no added salt provides 3 g sodium per day).
   b. *Moderate:* 1500 mg sodium.
5. Conditions utilizing low sodium in their management.
   a. Ménière's disease.
   b. Edema in congestive heart failure.
   c. Right ventricular failure.
   d. Hypertension.
   e. Cirrhosis with edema.
   f. Portal hypertension.
   g. Uremia.
   h. Dialysis management.
   i. Pregnancy-induced hypertension.
B. Potassium management.
   1. Replace potassium loss from the body with specific foods high in potassium or a potassium supplement. Severe loss is managed with intravenous therapy. (*See* Table 4-11.)
   2. Avoid no specific foods unless there is a sodium restriction because some foods high in potassium are also high in sodium.
   3. Conditions requiring low potassium.
      a. Glomerulonephritis.
      b. Dialysis management.
   4. Conditions requiring increased potassium.
      a. Diabetic acidosis.
      b. Burns, after the first 48 hours.
      c. Vomiting.
      d. Extended high temperature.
      e. Use of diuretic drugs.
C. Enhanced-calcium diet. (*See* Table 4-12.)
   1. Used to prevent or correct postmenopausal osteoporosis and prevent and treat hypertension.
   2. Increase normal adult intake of 1 g/day to 1.5 g/day.
   3. Recommend use of fortified low-fat and non-fat dairy products.
   4. Lactose-intolerant clients should use green, leafy vegetables and nonliquid dairy products (cheese, yogurt).
D. Iron supplements. (*See* Table 4-13.)
   1. Replace a deficit of iron caused by inadequate intake or chronic blood loss. Women especially tend to be low in iron.

✦ Table 4-10. FOODS HIGH IN SODIUM

Table salt and all prepared salts, such as celery salt
Smoked meats and salted meats
Most frozen or canned vegetables with added salt
Butter, margarines, and cheese
Quick-cooking cereals
Shellfish and frozen or salted fish
Seasonings and sauces
Canned soups
Chocolates and cocoa
Beets, celery, and selected greens (spinach)
Foods with salt added, such as potato chips and popcorn

✦ Table 4-11. FOODS HIGH IN POTASSIUM

Fruit juices such as orange, grapefruit, banana, and apple
Instant, dry coffee powder
Egg, legumes, whole grains
Fish, especially fresh halibut and codfish
Pork, beef, lamb, veal, chicken
Milk, skim and whole
Dried dates, prunes
Bouillon and meat broths
Salt substitute

Table 4-12. FOODS HIGH IN CALCIUM

Milk, cream
Cottage cheese
Mustard greens, turnip greens
Kale
Shrimp, clams, oysters
Salmon
Cheese
Ice cream

Table 4-13. FOODS HIGH IN IRON

Organ meats, especially beef liver
Red meat, turkey, chicken
Fish, shellfish
Blackstrap molasses
Egg yolk
Lima beans, legumes
Sunflower seeds
Almonds, pecans, cashews
Dried fruits, apricots, prunes, raisins
Leafy vegetables, broccoli, Brussels sprouts
Peas
Kidney beans
Brewer's yeast
Cheese—Swiss, ricotta, roquefort
Wild rice
Yogurt
Wheat germ
Bananas

◆ 2. Suggested iron intake is 18 mg/day.
3. Conditions utilizing high iron in their management.
 a. Peptic ulcer disease.
 b. Diverticulosis.
 c. Ulcerative colitis.
 d. Anemias: nutritional, pernicious.
 e. Hemorrhage.
 f. Postgastrectomy syndrome.
 g. Malabsorption syndrome.
 h. Crohn's disease.
 i. Increased for pregnancy and lactation.

Fiber Control

◆ A. A high-fiber (roughage) diet is an important constituent of our diet. The average person eats 20 g of fiber per day; 30–40 g is recommended.
1. High-fiber foods help a person lose weight, keep the heart healthy, and lower the risk of developing cancer of the colon (examples are bran, cereals, beans, fruits, and vegetables).
2. Foods low in carbohydrates are usually high in residue, and vice versa.
B. There are two types of fiber.
1. Insoluble fibers are found in the cell walls of plants; they do not dissolve in water. They speed up elimination of waste products.
2. Soluble fibers (oat bran) dissolve in water. They decrease cholesterol levels and slow absorption of glucose so blood sugar levels are reduced in diabetes.
◆ C. A low-residue diet (foods high in fiber) is utilized for certain diseases and conditions.
1. Low-residue foods include ground meat, fish, broiled chicken without skin, creamed cheeses, limited fat, warm drinks, refined strained cereals, and white bread.
2. Conditions that require a low-residue diet.
 a. Crohn's disease.
 b. Postoperative colon and rectal surgery.
 c. Diverticulitis—while inflammatory period lasts.
 d. Diarrhea and enteritis.

Bland Food Diets

◆ A. A bland diet promotes healing of the gastric mucosa. It eliminates food sources that are chemically and mechanically irritating. (*See* Table 4-14.)
1. Bland diets are presented in stages with the gradual addition of certain foods.
2. Frequent, small feedings during active stress periods are important.
B. Move from bland to regular diet and establish regular meals and food patterns when condition permits.

Table 4-14. BLAND DIET ALLOWANCES

Foods allowed
Milk, butter, eggs (not fried), custard, vanilla ice cream, cottage cheese
Cooked refined or strained cereal, enriched white bread
Jello; homemade creamed, pureed soups
Baked or broiled potatoes

Examples of foods that are eliminated
Spicy and highly seasoned foods
Raw foods
Very hot and very cold foods
Gas-forming foods (varies with individuals)
Coffee, alcoholic beverages, carbonated drinks
High-fat foods (some butter and margarine allowed)

C. Bland diets may be appropriate for the following conditions:
1. Duodenal and gastric ulcers.
2. Chronic pancreatitis.
3. Prostate surgery, postoperative.
4. Stomach surgery, postoperative.

Preoperative and Postoperative Diets

◆ A. A high-protein preoperative diet is essential for the maintenance of normal serum protein levels during and following surgery.
B. This diet also restores nitrogen balance if protein-depleted for burn victims, the elderly, and severely debilitated clients.
1. Provide adequate carbohydrates to maintain liver glycogen and adequate amino acids to promote wound healing.
2. Provide a 2500-calorie diet that is high in carbohydrates, moderate in protein with high-protein supplements.
3. Instruct client that an elemental diet is low in residue and contains a synthetic mixture of CHO, amino acids, and essential fatty acids with added minerals and vitamins. It is bulk free and easily assimilated and absorbed.

Postoperative Surgical Diet

◆ A. Provide 2800 total calories for tissue repair and even more calories for extensive repair.
B. Fluid intake: 2000–3000 mL/day for uncomplicated surgery and 3000–4000 mL/day for sepsis or renal damage. Seriously ill clients with drainage can require more fluid.

Postoperative Diet Progression

◆ A. Nothing by mouth the day of surgery.

♦ Table 4-15. SUMMARY OF DIETARY CONTROL FOR DISORDERS

Malabsorption syndromes

Cystic fibrosis: high calorie, high protein, with vitamin and mineral supplements; if diet has increased fats (not recommended), add extra enzymes

Ulcerative colitis: high protein, high calorie, low lactase, low residue

Crohn's disease: low residue, high protein, and vitamin–mineral supplements

Diverticulosis: high fiber

Constipation: high fiber with liquids

Diarrhea: low residue

Liver, biliary, and pancreatic problems

Liver involvement: high calories, high protein, high carbohydrates, low to moderate fat intake

Gallbladder: low fat and exclude any foods that cause problems (fatty foods, gas-forming vegetables)

Pancreatitis: high protein, high carbohydrate, low fat, and decreased alcohol intake

Genitourinary problems

Urinary tract infection: increase acid ash, reduce alkali ash (citrus, milk, vegetables)

Renal failure: high carbohydrates, limited protein, low potassium

Chronic renal failure: low protein, low salt, restricted fluids

Renal calculi: acid ash diet for stones formed of exalate or phosphate; alkali ash when stones formed of uric acid or cystine; force fluids

Specific disorders

Gout: restrict foods high in purine, increase fluid intake, high carbohydrate, control of calories

Hyperthyroidism: high carbohydrate, high protein, restrict caffeine

Phenylketonuria (PKU): restrict phenylalanine (Phenylalanine is found in all natural protein foods; meat, milk, etc. are eliminated.)

Obesity: restrict calories but nutritionally sound with adequate protein, complex carbohydrates, and limited fat (Fat and carbohydrates are retained to ensure protein utilization.)

B. A clear-liquid diet is 1000–1500 mL/day and composed of water, tea, broth, Jello, and juices (apple, cranberry) or 7-Up. Avoid juices with pulp.

C. A full-liquid diet lacks many nutrients, so it is used temporarily. It includes clear liquids, milk and milk products, custard, puddings, creamed soups, sherbet, ice cream, and any fruit juice.

D. A surgical soft diet is full liquid and, in addition, pureed vegetables, eggs (not fried), milk, cheese, fish, fowl, tender beef, veal, potatoes, and cooked fruit. Do not include gas-formers.

E. General diet: Take into consideration specific alterations necessary for client's health status.

Mechanical Soft Diet

A. A mechanical soft diet is used when clients are edentulous, have poorly fitted dentures, have difficulty chewing, or do not chew food thoroughly.

B. Any food that can be easily broken down can be included in this diet. It allows clients variations in taste that are not allowed on a soft diet (chili beans).

Puree Diet

A. A puree diet provides food that has been mashed or blended to a smooth consistency.
1. Mainly used for clients with dysphagia or who are unable to chew.

2. Often used with small babies.
3. Some hospitals provide this type of diet for gastrostomy feedings.

B. When assisting clients with this type of diet, talk with them about the meal, describing the different foods; when the texture is all the same, distinguishing between foods is difficult.

C. Do not mix all pureed foods together or feed the client out of one bowl or dish. Try to keep foods separate and feed alternately, with dessert being last.

Providing Nutrients through Enteral Feeding

Assessment

A. Assess overall status.
1. Weight change/loss; temperature.
2. Presence of sepsis; trauma.
3. Mental state.
4. Other medically related nutritional problems (e.g., diabetes, hyperlipidemia, alcoholism).
5. For all of the following procedures, identify client using *three* methods.

B. Evaluate oral intake.

C. Assess nutritional requirements.

D. Assess status of GI tract.

E. Assess capacity to chew and swallow; assess risk for aspiration.

A.

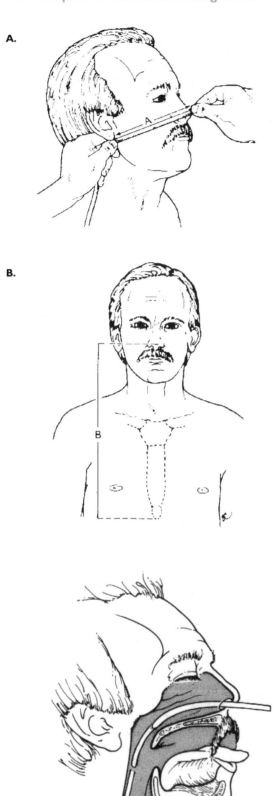

B.

FIGURE 4-1. Nasogastric tube measurement and placement.
A: Tip of nose to ear lobe. **B:** Tip of ear lobe to xiphoid.

F. Assess for presence of gag reflex.
G. Evaluate respiratory or thoracic conditions.
H. Check for renal complications.
I. Check for vomiting and/or diarrhea.
J. With high-protein diets, assess for fluid and electrolyte imbalance.

Implementation

A. Inserting a large bore nasogastric (NG) tube.
    ❖ PROCEDURE ❖
    1. Check order for tube feeding.
    2. Warm feeding to room temperature.
    3. Discuss procedure with the client.
    4. Demonstrate and display items to be used in order to allay the client's fear and to gain cooperation.
    5. Perform hand hygiene and don gloves.
    6. Position the client at 45-degree angle or more.
    7. Examine nostrils and select the more patent.
    8. Measure from tip of nose to earlobe to xiphoid process of sternum (NEX). (*See* Figure 4-1.) If tube is to go below stomach, small flex-tube is used. Mark point on tube with tape.
    9. Lubricate first 10 cm of tube with water-soluble lubricant and stylet if used.
    10. Insert tube through nostril to back of throat and ask client to swallow. Sips of water may aid in pushing tubing past oropharynx.
    11. Instruct client to flex head forward to help prevent tube entering client's airway.
    12. Continue advancing tube until taped mark is reached.
    13. Tape securely to nose and cheek.
    14. Check position of tube.
        a. Inject 10 mL of air through NG tube and listen with the stethoscope over stomach for a rush of air (whoosh sound). This method is not safe to be used alone to check tube placement because it does not tell you where the tube is—lung, esophagus, stomach, or other location.
        b. The most accurate method is to aspirate gastric contents, sometimes difficult with small-bore tubes, and check the pH. If pH is acidic (gastric contents are usually pH 5 or less, greenish to tan or off-white), tube is in the stomach. If NG tube is in respiratory tree, the gastric contents will be pH 6 or more, clear to light yellow.
        c. It is no longer considered safe practice to place proximal end of NG tube in a glass of water and observe for bubbling.
        d. Obtain x-ray to confirm correct placement.
    15. Remain with and talk with client until anxiety is decreased and client is comfortable.

B. Irrigating a nasogastric (NG) tube.
   ❖ PROCEDURE ❖
   1. Obtain a disposable irrigation set or emesis basin for irrigation solution, a 50-mL syringe, and a normal saline irrigation solution.
   2. Perform hand hygiene and don gloves.
   3. Place client in semi-Fowler's position.
   4. Disconnect NG tube from suction, if necessary, and check for tube placement.
   5. Draw up 20–30 mL normal saline into the irrigating syringe.
   6. Gently instill the normal saline into the NG tube. Do not force the solution.
   7. Withdraw the irrigation solution and empty into basin.
   8. Repeat the procedure twice.
   9. Record on I&O sheet the irrigation solution that has not been returned.

✦ C. Administering an enteral feeding (TPN).
   ❖ PROCEDURE ❖
   1. Check order from the physician for appropriate formula (calories and/or amount).
   2. Check early in shift to ensure adequate formula is available.
   3. Warm formula to room temperature—DO NOT use microwave oven.
   4. Assemble feeding equipment. If using bag, fill with ordered amount of formula.
   5. Explain procedure to the client and assure privacy.
   6. Check for presence of bowel sounds.
      a. Now considered to be questionable; instead, assess that client does not have abdominal distention, nausea, or pain.
      b. If client does have flatus or bowel elimination.
   7. Place the client on right side in high-Fowler's position.
   ✦ 8. Aspirate stomach contents to determine amount of residual. If residual volume is greater than 200 mL, further assessment is indicated.
   ✦ 9. Return aspirated contents to stomach to prevent electrolyte imbalance.
   10. Pinch the tubing to prevent air from entering stomach.
   11. Attach syringe to NG tube.
   12. Fill syringe with formula. (If using feeding bag, adjust drip rate to infuse over 30 minutes.)
   13. Hold tubing no more that 39 cm above client.
   ✦ 14. Allow formula to infuse slowly (between 20 to 35 minutes) through the tubing.
   15. Follow tube feeding with water in amount ordered.
   16. Clamp end of the tube.

17. Wash tray and return it to client's bedside—change syringe daily.
18. Give water between feedings if tube feeding is the sole source of nutrition.

D. Administering continuous tube feedings (Dubbhoff, Keofeed tubes). ❖ PROCEDURE ❖
   1. Complete steps 1 through 5 of previous skill.
   2. Elevate head of bed 30 degrees.
   ✦ 3. Check length of exposed tubing—an increase may indicate tube has dislocated upward.
   4. Check patency of existing tube.
   ✦ 5. Irrigate feeding tube with sterile water or saline at least every eight hours.
   6. Administer formula at prescribed infusion rate (usually 60–80 mL/hr). Infusion pumps are used to maintain continuous flow.

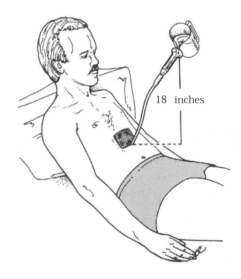

FIGURE 4-2. Gastrostomy feeding—tubing is held straight up from insertion point.

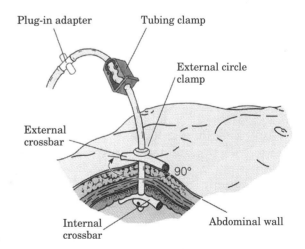

FIGURE 4-3. PEG for gastrostomy feedings. *Source:* Smith, S., Duell, D., & Martin, B. (2008). *Clinical nursing skills* (7th ed.), Upper Saddle River, NJ: Prentice Hall.

7. Avoid keeping formula at room temperature for longer than four hours to prevent spoilage and bacterial contamination.
8. Turn off flow when placing client supine.

E. Administering gastrostomy feeding. (*See* Figures 4-2 and 4-3.) ❖ Procedure ❖

✦ 1. Assess gastric contents to determine amount per intermittent feeding. Further assessment is needed if residual is greater than 200 mL.
2. Return aspirated contents to stomach.
3. Feed slowly (flow by gravity) for intermittent feeding (usually 20–35 minutes). Keep at prescribed rate for continuous feeding.
4. Observe gastrostomy tube insertion site for signs of dislodging or infection.
5. Provide site care; wash area with warm water and soap.
6. Apply skin protective barrier. Cover area with sterile dressing.

Total Nutritional Alimentation (TNA) via Central Venous Catheter ❖ Procedure ❖

✦ **Assessment**

A. Assess nutritional needs of clients unable to ingest calories normally.
B. Identify the caloric intake necessary to promote positive nitrogen balance, tissue repair, and growth; lipids included in formula.

C. Observe for correct additives in each hyperalimentation bottle.
D. Check label of solution against physician's orders.
E. Check rate of infusion on physician's orders.
F. Assess ability of client to understand instructions during procedure.
G. Ensure patency of central venous line following insertion.
H. Observe catheter insertion site for signs of infection, thrombophlebitis, or possible infiltration.
I. Inspect dressing over central line to ensure a dry, noncontaminated dressing.

Implementation

✦ A. Teach Valsalva's maneuver if client does not have a cardiac disorder. This maneuver prevents air from entering the catheter during catheter insertion or tubing changes.
1. Ask client to take a deep breath and bear down.
2. Apply gentle pressure to the abdomen.
B. Review physician's order for correct hyperalimentation solution additives. (*See* Table 4-16.)
1. TNA bottles come directly from the pharmacy and are numbered sequentially.
2. Each TNA bottle label will include client's name, room number, additives, IV number, start time, date, and stop time.
3. Inspect TNA bottle for cracks, turbidity, or precipitates.

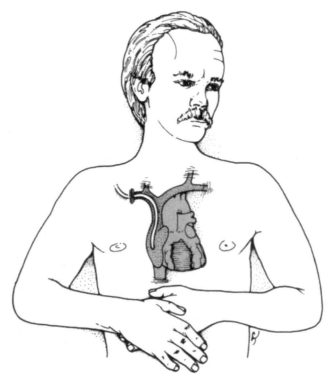

FIGURE 4-4. Central venous catheter insertion for TNA—right subclavian vein is preferred access to right atrium.

Table 4-16. COMPOSITION OF HYPERALIMENTATION SOLUTIONS

Amino acid—Freamine or Aminosol
Carbohydrates—10–35% glucose
Vitamins (become inactive when exposed to light)
Minerals and trace elements
Electrolytes (individualized)
Water
Hyperalimentation solution is prepared in the pharmacy under a laminar flow hood
Lipids

C. Assemble IV system with in-line filter and prime IV tubing and filter with solution.

◆ D. Position client in head-down position with head turned to opposite direction of catheter insertion site. Place a small roll between client's shoulders to expose insertion site.

E. Cleanse insertion area with antimicrobial swabs.

F. Perform hand hygiene, don a mask and sterile gloves, and assist physician as needed during catheter insertion.

G. Instruct client in Valsalva's maneuver when stylet is removed from catheter and when IV tubing is connected to catheter.
   1. After tubing is connected, instruct client to breathe normally.
   2. Tape area between tubing and catheter hub.

◆ H. Turn on IV infusion pump, using normal saline solution at a slow rate of 10 drops/min until x-ray ensures accurate catheter placement. (Flush catheter with saline and heparinize with dilute heparin according to agency policy.)

◆ I. Confirm catheter placement via x-ray and change IV solution to hyperalimentation solution.
   1. Store hyperalimentation solution in refrigerator until 30 minutes before use. This prevents growth of organisms, but should be warmed to room temperature prior to use.
   2. Change solution every 12 to 24 hours to prevent growth of bacterial organisms.

J. Time tape the bottle after adjusting flow rate. Be prepared to document on IV hourly infusion record.

K. Observe for complications with TNA.
   1. Allergic responses to protein (chills, increased temperature, nausea, headache, urticaria, dyspnea).
   2. Air embolism—potentially fatal (respiratory distress, chest pain, dyspnea, hypotension).
   3. Catheter-related infection (sepsis). Symptoms of fever, chills, erythema at insertion site.
   4. Hyperglycemia—elevated glucose levels.
   5. Hypoglycemia—decreased blood glucose levels.

L. Take vital signs every 4 hours.

◆ M. Maintain central vein infusion.
   1. Apply 4 × 4 sterile gauze pad over IV site and occlude dressing with micropore or plastic tape.
   2. Change IV tubing, filter, and infusion pump cassette (if used) every 24 hours.
   3. Change extension tubing every 48 hours. Change solution every 12–24 hours (prevents growth of bacteria when using sugar in solution).
   4. Maintain IV flow rate at prescribed rate.
      a. If rate is too rapid, hyperosmolar diuresis occurs (excess sugar will be excreted); if severe enough, intractable seizures, coma, and death can occur.
      b. If rate is too slow, little benefit will be derived from the calories and nitrogen.
      c. Do not correct an overload or deficit in flow, as doing so could result in complications for the client. Notify physician if this occurs.

◆ N. Check client's finger-stick blood sugar every 6 hours. If necessary, administer Regular insulin according to prescribed "sliding scale."

O. Maintain accurate I&O. Record on special TNA sheet at least every 4 hours.

P. Weigh daily and record on graphic sheet and TNA sheet.

Dressing and Tubing Change ❖ PROCEDURE ❖

◆ A. Maintain sterile technique for both procedures.
   1. Use sterile gloves, mask, drape, and equipment.
   2. Goal is to prevent contamination of site and prevent infection.

B. Observe insertion site for erythema, drainage, etc., then cleanse with povidone–iodine.

C. Change gauze dressings every 48 to 72 hrs. Transparent dressing can be changed every 72 to 96 hrs.

D. Change tubing every 24 hours.
   1. Loosen tubing at catheter hub.
   2. Tell client to hold breath and bear down while new tubing is inserted to prevent air from entering catheter causing air embolism.
   3. Observe for signs of respiratory distress: air embolism, pneumothorax.
      a. Cyanosis.
      b. Hypotension.
      c. Rapid, weak pulse.
      d. Alterations in heart sounds.
      e. Elevated central venous pressure (CVP).
   4. Check vital signs frequently, including temperature.
   5. If respiratory distress occurs—suspect air embolism.
      a. Place client in Trendelenburg's position with right chest uppermost and left chest down.

b.   Inform physician.

c.   Administer oxygen at 6 L/min via nasal prongs.

Hyperalimentation for Children

A.   Examine solution.

✦ 1.   Generally, there is a higher concentration of calcium, phosphorus, magnesium, and vitamins.

2.   Usually, a 10% solution of dextrose with 2% amino acids is started—it can be increased to 25% if tolerated.

B.   Monitor patency of catheter (usually placed through internal or external jugular or scalp veins). Stopcocks are never used. Monitor constant infusion pump and filter.

✦ C.   Obtain finger-stick blood samples. Sugar level will rise, but usually exogenous insulin is not required as the pancreas adapts to high glucose loads.

D.   Change the dressing every 96 hours and the tubing every 24 hours using aseptic technique.

1.   Stockinette can be used to keep scalp dressing secure.

2.   Tight-fitting T-shirt can keep chest site secure.

E.   Monitor for accurate rate of infusion.

1.   Do not "catch up" if infusion is behind.

2.   Positive pressure pumps can be used to maintain infusion rates, particularly when small amounts of solution are being infused.

F.   Observe the child when ambulating for accidents such as twisting or kinking the tubing, getting the tubing caught in the crib, or stepping on it.

Appendix 4-1. NUTRITIONAL ASSESSMENT PARAMETERS

Clinical Assessment	Normal	Abnormal
Dietary Data		
Appetite	Remains unchanged	Increased or decreased recently Particular cravings
Nutritional intake	Adequate foods and fluids to supply body nutrients Nonallergic response to major food groups	Elimination of certain food categories that results in limited nutrients Emphasis on some food groups (sugar) to the exclusion of others (vegetables) Allergic response to certain foods
Caloric intake	Average 28 kcal/kg/day	Constant use of fad diets to lose weight Use of drugs or chemicals that interfere with appetite or nutrient assimilation
Meal patterns	3–6 home-prepared meals/day Adequate time and calm atmosphere for meals	Fast-food or packaged foods Missed meals, constant snacking, or overeating Eating "on the run" or hurried
General Appearance		
	Alert, responsive, healthy-appearing eyes and skin	Listless, dull, nonresponsive Skin and eyes appear unhealthy
Physical factors	Adequate chewing and swallowing capability Mouth and gums healthy so food can be ingested Physical exercise adequate for calorie intake	Teeth or gums in poor condition or ill-fitting dentures Swallowing impairs ingestion Inadequate physical exercise to burn calories
Presence of disease	No disease process that interferes with nutrient assimilation No congenital condition or postsurgery condition that interferes with nutrient assimilation	Disease present that interferes with ingestion, digestion, assimilation, or excretion Congenital condition, rehabilitation phase, or postsurgery condition that interferes with food assimilation
Elimination schedule	Regular, adequate elimination of foods Absence of constant flatus, discharge or mucus	Irregular or painful elimination Presence of constant flatus Presence of discharge, blood, or mucus

Appendix 4-1. NUTRITIONAL ASSESSMENT PARAMETERS *(Continued)*

Clinical Assessment	Normal	Abnormal
Anthropometric Measurements		
Height	For bedridden patients, measure arm span —fully extend arms at a 90° angle to body and measure from tip of one middle finger to the tip of other middle finger for estimated height	Loss of 2–3 inches in height may indicate osteoporosis
Weight—compared to ideal and usual body weight	Ideal body weight 100 lb (female); 106 lb (male) for 5 feet height + 5 lb for each 1 inch over 5 feet (female) and 6 lb for each 1 inch over 5 feet (male) Small frame minus 10% Large frame plus 10%	Changed—markedly increased or decreased recently: important indicator of changed nutritional status Loss of more than 10% weight for prior 6 months should be clinically evaluated
Body mass index (ratio of weight in kilograms and height in meters)	19–24.9	Less than 19—underweight 25 to 29—overweight 30 to 39—obese
Triceps skinfold measurement (mm)	Standard values—male to female 12.5–16.5	If values change over months, may indicate a chronic condition
Circumference of upper arm (cm)	29.3–28.5	
Midarm muscle circumference (cm)	25.3–23.2	Hydration status may influence results
Biochemical Assessments*		Examples of possible disease conditions:
Serum albumin	3.5–5.0 g/dL	Decrease signifies lowered nutritional status—protein deficient
Serum transferrin binds iron to plasma and transports to bone marrow	200–430 mg/dL	Reduced levels may indicate chronic diseases and protein deficiency Elevated levels—anemias, liver damage, lead toxicity
Hemoglobin	Male—13.5–17 g/dL Female—12–15 g/dL	Decrease related to iron deficiency (anemias and leukemia)
Prealbumin (PA) serum	20–50 mg/dL	Decreased—protein wasting diseases, malnutrition (< 10.7 indicates severe nutritional deficiency) Elevated—Hodgkin's disease
Blood urea nitrogen/creatinine	10:1–20:1	Nitrogen imbalance, inadequate renal functioning
24-hour urinary nitrogen	Positive balance	Inadequate protein intake

*Laboratory test parameters differ among laboratories. Check the reference range for the specific lab where the patient's blood or urine was tested.

Appendix 4-2.   REVISED FOOD PYRAMID, 2005

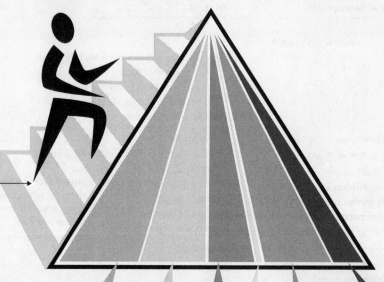

New food pyramid
Pyramid now symbolizes a personalized approach to eating healthy and exercise.

Physical activity
Figure is a reminder on the importance of physical activity. Amount needed:

Minimum: At least 30 minutes most days of the week

To prevent weight gain: 60 minutes

To sustain weight loss: 60 to 90 minutes

Estimating daily calorie needs		
Females	**Sedentary**	**Active**
9–13 years	1600	2200
14–18	1800	2400
19–30	2000	2400
31–50	1800	2200
51+	1600	2200
Males		
9–13 years	1800	2600
14–18	2200	3200
19–30	2400	3000
31–50	2200	3000
51+	2000	2800

Food groups	Grains	Vegetables	Fruits	Oils	Milk	Meat and beans
The five food groups and oils are color-coded for easy identification	At least half should be whole grains	Fresh, frozen, canned, dried, juices	Fresh, frozen, canned, dried, juices	Liquid, not solid	Low- or no-fat, calcium-rich types	Lean meat, poultry, fish; eggs; beans, nuts, seeds; tofu; peanut butter
Daily amount of food from each group by calorie level:						
2000 calories Moderately active women 26–50	6 oz* (170 g)	2.5 cups	2 cups	6 tsp	3 cups	5.5 oz** (720 g)
2600 calories Moderately active men 26–45	9 oz* (280 g)	3.5 cups	2 cups	8 tsp	3 cups	6.5 oz** (200 g)

Milk

Foods Included: milk: low- or no-fat, calcium-rich types

Contribution to Diet: Milk is a leading source of calcium, which is needed for bones and teeth. It also provides a high-quality protein, riboflavin, vitamin A (if milk is whole or fortified), and other nutrients.

Amounts Recommended: Three cups.

Cheese may replace part of the milk. To substitute, figure the amount on the basis of calcium content. Common portions of various kinds of cheese and ice cream and their milk equivalents in calcium are

2.5-cm cube cheddar-type cheese	= ½ cup milk
½ cup cottage cheese	= ⅓ cup milk
2 tablespoons cream cheese	= 1 tablespoon milk
½ cup ice cream or ice milk	= ⅓ cup milk

Meat and Beans

Foods Included:
- Lean meats
- Poultry and eggs
- Fish and shellfish
- Beans, dry peas, lentils, nuts, seeds, tofu, peanut butter

Contribution to Diet: Foods in this group are valued for their protein, which is needed for growth and repair of body tissues, muscle, organs, blood, skin, and hair. These foods also provide iron, thiamine, riboflavin, and niacin.

Amounts Recommended: Choose 5.5 to 6.5 oz every day. *Count as a serving:* 62–93 g (not including bone weight) cooked lean meat, poultry, or fish. Count as alternates for ½ serving meat or fish: 1 egg, ½ cup cooked dry beans, dry peas, or lentils, or 2 tablespoons peanut butter.

Vegetables and Fruits

Foods Included: all vegetables and fruit: fresh, frozen, canned, dried, juices. This guide emphasizes those that are valuable as sources of vitamin C and vitamin A.

Sources of Vitamin C

Foods Included:

Good sources: grapefruit or grapefruit juice, orange or orange juice, cantaloupe, guava, mango, papaya, raw strawberries, broccoli, Brussels sprouts, green pepper, sweet red pepper.

Fair sources: honeydew melon, lemon, tangerine or tangerine juice, watermelon, asparagus tips, raw cabbage, cauliflower, collards, garden cress, kale, kohlrabi, mustard greens, potatoes and sweet potatoes cooked in the jacket, rutabagas, spinach, tomatoes or tomato juice, turnip greens.

Sources of Vitamin A

Foods Included: dark-green and deep-yellow vegetables and a few fruits—namely, apricots, broccoli, cantaloupe, carrots, chard, collards, cress, kale, mango, persimmon, pumpkin, spinach, sweet potatoes, turnip greens and other dark-green leaves, winter squash.

Contribution to Diet: Fruits and vegetables are valuable chiefly because of the vitamins and minerals they contain. In this plan, this group is counted on to supply nearly all of the vitamin C needed and more than half of the vitamin A. Vitamin C is needed for healthy gums and body tissues. Vitamin A is needed for growth, normal vision, and healthy condition of skin and other body surfaces.

Amounts Recommended: Choose 2.5 cups vegetables and 2 cups fruit.

Count as one serving: $\frac{1}{2}$ cup of vegetable or fruit; or one medium apple, banana, orange, or potato, $\frac{1}{2}$ medium grapefruit, a slice of cantaloupe, or the juice of one lemon.

Grains (At least half should be whole grains.)

Foods Included: All breads and cereals that are whole grain, enriched, or restored; check labels to be sure. Specifically, this group includes whole wheat and rye breads, cooked cereal, ready-to-eat whole-grain cereal, cornmeal, crackers, rolled oats, grains (wheat, corn, millet, oats, brown rice), whole-grain or enriched flour.

Contribution to Diet: Foods in this group furnish worthwhile amounts of protein, iron, several of the B vitamins, and energy.

Amounts Recommended: Choose 6 oz or more every day. If no cereals are chosen, include an extra serving of whole-grain bread or baked goods, which will make at least 6 oz from this group daily.

Count as a serving: one slice of bread; 31 g ready-to-eat cereal; $\frac{1}{2}$ to $\frac{3}{4}$ cup cooked cereal, cornmeal, grits, macaroni, noodles, rice, or spaghetti.

Oils (Liquid, not solid.)

Foods Included: vegetable oils that have no trans fats (e.g., olive oil, flax seed oil, cod liver oil)

Contribution to Diet: Major source of vitamin E and polyunsaturated fatty acids, including essential fatty acids omega-3 and -6).

Amounts Recommended: 6–8 tsp/day.

Source: MyPyramid.gov; USDA, 2005.

NUTRITIONAL MANAGEMENT REVIEW QUESTIONS

1. Evaluating the teaching plan for a client recently placed on a low-sodium diet by her physician, the nurse will know the client understands the plan when she states that she will

   1. Call the dietitian if she cannot remember it.
   2. Look at the list of foods she can have.
   3. Read the label on the food product.
   4. Cook without adding salt to the food.

2. The nurse asks a client to list the snacks he likes that are allowed on his low-fat, low-sodium, low-cholesterol diet. The nurse realizes that further dietary teaching is necessary when one of his choices is

   1. Buttermilk.
   2. A jam sandwich.
   3. An apple.
   4. Applesauce.

3. A client's physician has placed him on a low-potassium diet. Of the following foods, which ones should he avoid because they are high in potassium? List all that apply.

   1. Butter.
   2. Shellfish.
   3. Milk.
   4. Frozen vegetables.
   5. Orange juice.
   6. Dried dates.

4. The nurse will know that her teaching has been effective when the client responds that a low-fiber diet allows the inclusion of

   1. Whole-grain breads, seeds, and legumes.
   2. Fresh fruits and vegetables.
   3. Bran and whole-grain cereals.
   4. Cooked vegetables, fruits, and refined breads.

5. The nurse questions the dietary department about the lunch delivered for a client with the diagnosis of cirrhosis when she finds on his tray

   1. A tuna sandwich.
   2. French fries.
   3. A ham sandwich.
   4. A milkshake.

6. Clients with a history of pancreatitis have dietary restrictions. While evaluating diet history with these clients, the nurse will determine that they understand food restrictions when they avoid

   1. Noodles.
   2. Vegetable soup.
   3. Baked fish fillet.
   4. Cheddar cheese sandwiches.

7. A 28-year-old client has just learned that her pregnancy test is positive. The nurse will reinforce nutritional counseling by telling the client that her diet should

   1. Maintain iron intake and increase calorie intake by 500 calories.
   2. Increase iron and folic acid as well as calorie intake by 300 calories.
   3. Increase iron and multivitamins but maintain calorie intake.
   4. Decrease iron but increase calorie intake by 200 to 300 calories.

8. A client with cirrhosis and ascites is placed on a sodium-restricted diet to help control the ascites. For this plan to be effective, it is important that the client also

   1. Restrict his fluid intake.
   2. Increase his potassium intake.
   3. Increase his fluid intake.
   4. Decrease his potassium intake.

9. A client with acute pancreatitis required NG intubation due to persistent vomiting and paralytic ileus. Following NG tube removal, the feeding schedule would start with a diet that is

   1. NPO for 12 hours.
   2. High in protein.
   3. High in carbohydrates.
   4. Clear liquid.

10. The most appropriate sweetener for the insulin-dependent diabetes mellitus, Type 1 (IDDM) client is

    1. Corn sugar.
    2. Honey.
    3. Sugar substitute.
    4. Fructose.

11. The diabetic client understands her diet when she says that she should obtain the greatest percentage of calories from

1. Fats.
2. Complex carbohydrates.
3. Simple carbohydrates.
4. Protein.

12. When a client is in early prehepatic coma, the dietary regimen will be changed to include how much protein per day?

1. 20 to 40 g.
2. 50 to 70 g.
3. 75 to 95 g.
4. 100 to 120 g.

13. The nurse will know the client understands his low-purine diet when he states

1. "I will need to limit the number of fruit servings each day."
2. "Organ meats must be eliminated from my diet."
3. "I can drink only white wine because red wine is high in purine."
4. "Beef, chicken, and pork are high in purine; therefore, I can have them only once in a while."

14. Which of the following statements would be correct when counseling a client about the postoperative diet he would receive following a simple surgical procedure?

1. A client undergoing major surgery may have a soft diet the day of surgery.
2. Approximately 2800 calories is required daily for general tissue repair, so this will be his caloric intake.
3. Daily fluid intake should be 1500 mL for an uncomplicated surgical procedure.
4. A mechanical, soft diet should be given the first postoperative day.

15. The nurse's diet instructions for a client with a colostomy will be

1. According to his own individual needs and similar to his preoperative diet.
2. Low in fiber with a large amount of fluids.
3. High in fiber with large amounts of fluids and supplemental vitamin K.
4. Elimination of milk products.

16. Discharge planning for a client with a partial colectomy will include which one of the following dietary principles?

1. High residue, force fluids.
2. Low residue, no dairy products.
3. High fiber, no spices.
4. Regular, no dairy products.

17. The nurse will know that the client understands presurgical instructions for hemorrhoid surgery if her diet is

1. Low roughage.
2. High fiber.
3. High carbohydrate.
4. Low fiber.

18. A client with chronic lymphocytic leukemia is started on chemotherapy. Many clients suffer nausea and vomiting with these drugs. The nurse should counsel the client to try a diet of

1. No liquid just before the treatments.
2. Low-calorie foods that are high in bulk and fiber.
3. High protein and fat.
4. Fruits and vegetables.

19. The nurse's discharge teaching for a client with acute pancreatitis will include advising him to take

1. Vitamin K.
2. Fat-soluble vitamins.
3. Vitamin C.
4. Vitamin B_{12}.

20. A 54-year-old client has been diagnosed as having lung cancer. The tumor is inoperable, and she will undergo radiation therapy. Because of the gastrointestinal (GI) complications associated with radiation, the client will be placed on a diet of

1. High protein, high carbohydrate, low residue.
2. High protein, high residue.
3. High protein, high residue, low sodium.
4. Low protein, low residue, high calcium.

21. A 53-year-old client with Crohn's disease is placed on total nutritional alimentation (TNA). The fluid in the present TNA bottle should be infused by 8 AM. At 7 AM the nurse observes that it is empty and another TNA bottle has not yet arrived on the unit. The nursing action is to attach a bag of

1. D_{25} and water.
2. D_5 and water.
3. D_{10} and water.
4. D_{45} and water.

22. A client has injured both eyes with a chemical and must have eye patches in place for several weeks. When her food tray arrives, the most helpful nursing intervention would be to

    1. Feed the client or assign a nursing assistant to feed her.
    2. Explain that her tray is here and put her hands on it.
    3. Tell her to think of a clock and describe which food is where and put the fork in her hand.
    4. Ask her if she would prefer a liquid diet.

23. A client will have a central vein infusion to maintain nutritional status while his GI tract is being bypassed. The nurse would expect that the site of catheter insertion for a protein and glucose concentration of 15% would be in the

    1. Jugular vein.
    2. Right subclavian vein.
    3. Right subclavian artery.
    4. Left arm artery access.

24. A client's physician has ordered intralipid therapy for his client. In carrying out this order, the nurse understands that monitoring for side effects is important. Which of the following side effects would necessitate that the nurse immediately notify the physician?

    1. Dyspnea and chills.
    2. Hyperlipemia.
    3. Eczema-like rash and dry, scaly skin.
    4. Erythema and edema at the insertion site.

25. A client has had abdominal surgery and the physician has ordered a bland diet 3 days postsurgery. Which of the following diet trays would have portions removed because it does not adhere to the dietary regimen?

    1. Scrambled eggs, cereal, and white toast.
    2. Baked potato, cottage cheese, and coffee.
    3. Cream soup, Jello, and white toast.
    4. Cooked cereal, boiled egg, and milk.

NUTRITIONAL MANAGEMENT

Answers with Rationale

1. (3) Clients should be instructed to read labels before purchasing canned, frozen, or processed foods because they are usually very high in sodium. A list of foods (2) will provide guidance, but she should know the sodium content of food. Not adding salt to foods (4) when cooking is also important, but not as critical as (3).

   NP:E; CN:PH; CA:M; CL:C

2. (1) Buttermilk contains large amounts of fat and must be avoided. Fruits and whole grains are encouraged.

   NP:E; CN:PS; CA:M; CL:A

3. The answer is *3 5 6—milk (3), orange juice (5), and dried dates (6).* All are high in potassium, while the other three foods are high in sodium.

   NP:P; CN:H; CA:M; CL:A

4. (4) Cooked vegetables and fruits as well as refined breads are included in a low-fiber diet. Bran, fresh fruits, and whole grains and seeds are included in a high-fiber diet.

   NP:E; CN:PH; CA:M; CL:C

5. (3) Ham is high in sodium and can increase fluid retention, leading to edema. Cirrhosis clients are prone to edema as the osmotic pressures change due to a decrease in plasma albumin.

   NP:I; CN:PH; CA:M; CL:AN

6. (4) Clients with this condition must not consume foods high in fat content because there are inadequate pancreatic enzymes to digest the fat. High fat content also causes pain two to four hours after ingestion. Suggested diet is high in calories and protein.

   NP:E; CN:PH; CA:M; CL:A

7. (2) During pregnancy, iron supplements and folic acid must be added to the diet. Studies have found that pregnant women cannot assimilate enough iron from their regular diet and they need folic acid to prevent neural tube defect. Calories are increased by 300 to be certain that the mother-to-be and fetus have enough nutritional intake.

   NP:I; CN:PH; CA:MA; CL:K

8. (1) It is important that fluids be restricted as well, because unrestricted fluid intake leads to a progressive decrease in serum sodium from dilution. Electrolyte imbalance with potential neurologic complications could result.

   NP:P; CN:PH; CA:M; CL:AN

9. (3) Foods that are high in carbohydrate are given, because those with high protein or fat content stimulate the pancreas. Alcohol is forbidden. There is no need for the client to be NPO.

   NP:P; CN:PH; CA:M; CL:A

10. (3) Sugar substitute is the only calorie-free sweetener listed; the others are nutritive, with their average caloric value being 20 kcal per teaspoon. When an equal volume of honey and sugar are compared, honey provides about $1\frac{1}{3}$ times as many kcal as does table sugar.

    NP:P; CN:PH; CA:M; CL:K

11. (2) The diabetic's diet should be between 50 and 65 percent carbohydrate calories with only 5 percent of these being sucrose. Fat recommendation is less than 30 percent of calories and protein should be 0.8 mg/kg per day.

    NP:E; CN:PH; CA:M; CL:C

Coding for Questions/Answers Abbreviations: **Nursing Process: NP,** Assessment: A, Analysis: AN, Planning: P, Implementation: I, Evaluation: E; **Client Needs: CN,** Safe, Effective Care Environment: S, Health Promotion and Maintenance: H, Psychosocial Integrity: PS, Physiological Integrity: PH; **Clinical Area: CA,** Medical Nursing: M, Surgical Nursing: S, Maternal/Newborn Nursing: MA, Pediatric Nursing: P, Psychiatric Nursing: PS; **Cognitive Level: CL,** Knowledge: K, Comprehension: C, Application: A, Analysis: AN.

12. (1) In the early stages, protein intake will be reduced to 20 to 40 g because high protein intake elevates blood ammonia. Protein will need to be reduced further if the coma state progresses.

    NP:P; CN:PH; CA:M; CL:A

13. (2) Organ meats, wine, yeast, scallops, and mussels are all high in purine and must be eliminated from the diet of the client who has gout.

    NP:E; CN:PH; CA:M; CL:A

14. (2) A daily intake of 2800 calories is required for usual/general tissue repair, whereas 6000 calories may be required for extensive tissue repair. Fluid intake is 2000 to 3000 mL/day for uncomplicated surgery. The diet progresses from nothing by mouth on the day of surgery to a general diet within a few days.

    NP:I; CN:PH; CA:S; CL:C

15. (1) Diets are individualized and clients are generally able to eat the same foods they enjoyed preoperatively. Fresh fruits may cause diarrhea in some, but not all, individuals.

    NP:I; CN:PH; CA:S; CL:A

16. (2) The low-residue diet will put less strain on the colon, and eliminating dairy products initially is important because these products cause mucus.

    NP:P; CN:PH; CA:S; CL:C

17. (2) A high-fiber diet produces a soft stool without mechanically irritating the hemorrhoidal area. Foods include bran and complex carbohydrates.

    NP:E; CN:PH; CA:S; CL:A

18. (1) Fluids given just before treatments may cause nausea and vomiting. Because of possible problems with constipation, the foods need to be high in bulk and fiber and high in protein and calories because of the weight loss (a side effect of chemotherapy). Fat in the diet may not be appealing with anorexia.

    NP:I; CN:PH; CA:M; CL:A

19. (2) Because the client will be on a low-fat diet to decrease pancreatic activity, he will need supplements of the fat-soluble vitamins. A well-balanced diet should meet the other nutritional needs.

    NP:P; CN:PH; CA:M; CL:A

20. (1) Clients undergoing external radiation therapy may develop GI irritation and can bleed. They need calories and protein but not rough, high-residue foods, as they can further irritate the GI tract.

    NP:P; CN:PH; CA:S; CL:AN

21. (3) So that the client will not experience a sudden drop in blood sugar, the solution nearest most TNA solution concentrations is $D_{10}W$. $D_{25}W$ and $D_{45}W$ could cause osmotic diuresis or fluid overload.

    NP:I; CN:PH; CA:M; CL:AN

22. (3) The most helpful intervention is to assist the client to help herself, allowing her to be as independent as possible. Feeding her or changing the diet to liquid would not be as therapeutic.

    NP:I; CN:H; CA:M; CL:A

23. (2) The most common placement site is the right subclavian vein. The jugular vein might be used as an alternative for high-concentration IV infusions, but it is more difficult to access. The arm is used for insertion of an arterial line for arterial blood gas samples and monitoring.

    NP:P; CN:PH; CA:M; CL:K

24. (1) Dyspnea, chills, fever, and cyanosis are all side effects that necessitate stopping the infusion and notifying the physician. It may be an allergic reaction or the client's inability to tolerate the lipid infusion. Answer (2) is a liver function test and the physician should be notified if results are abnormal, but this would occur after the infusion. Eczema and dry skin are signs of fatty acid deficit. Erythema and edema need to be monitored and perhaps the IV insertion site changed.

    NP:E; CN:PH; CA:M; CL:AN

25. (2) Coffee is one food eliminated from a bland diet because it is chemically irritating to the stomach. All of the other foods are allowed on a bland diet. Other foods eliminated are raw, spicy, gas-forming, very hot or very cold foods; alcohol; and carbonated drinks.

    NP:AN; CN:PH; CA:M; CL:N

*Pharmacology** 5

*Please note: All drugs/medications with actions, expected outcomes
and side effects are included at the end of each section in the Medical–
Surgical section and at the end of each chapter.

✦ The icon denotes content of special importance for NCLEX.

DRUG METABOLISM

Stages of Metabolism

Definition: Drug metabolism in the human body is accomplished in four basic stages—absorption, transportation, biotransformation, and excretion. For a drug to be completely metabolized, it must first be given in sufficient concentration to produce the described effect on body tissues. When this critical drug concentration level is achieved, body tissues change.

A. Absorption.
   1. The first stage of metabolism refers to the route a drug takes from the time it enters the body until it is absorbed in the circulating fluids.
   ✦ 2. Drugs are absorbed by the mucous membranes, the gastrointestinal tract, the respiratory tract, and the skin.
      a. The mucous membranes are one of the most rapid and effective routes of absorption because they are highly vascular.
      b. Drugs are absorbed through these membranes by diffusion, infiltration, and osmosis.
   3. Drugs given by mouth are absorbed in the gastrointestinal (GI) tract.
      a. Portions of these drugs dissolve and absorb in the stomach.
      b. The rate of absorption depends on the pH of the stomach's contents, the food contained in the stomach at the time of ingestion, and the presence of disease conditions.
      c. Most of the drug concentrate dissolves in the small intestine, where the large vascular surface and moderate pH level enhance the process of dissolution.
   4. Methods of administration include intradermal, subcutaneous, intravenous, and intra-arterial injections.
      a. Parenteral methods are the most direct, reliable, and rapid route of absorption.
      b. The actual administration site will depend on type of drug, its action, and the client.
   5. Another route of administration is inhalation or nebulization through the respiratory system.
      a. This method is not as rapid as parenteral injections but faster than the GI tract.
      b. Drugs administered through the respiratory tract must be made up of small particles that can pass through to the alveoli in the lungs.
   6. The final mode of absorption is the skin.
      a. Most drugs, when applied to the skin, produce a local rather than a systemic effect.
      b. The degree of absorption will depend on the strength of the drug as well as location where it is applied on the body surface.
B. Distribution.
   ✦ 1. The second stage of metabolism refers to the way in which a drug is transported from the site of introduction to the site of action.
   2. First a drug enters or is absorbed by the body.
      a. The drug binds to plasma protein in the blood.
      b. Then the drug is transported through circulation to all parts of the body.
   3. As a drug moves from the circulatory system, it crosses cell membranes and enters the body tissues.
      a. Some of the drug is distributed to and stored in fat and muscle.
      b. Greater masses of tissue (such as fat and muscle) attract the drug.
   ✦ 4. The amount of drug that is distributed to body tissues depends on the permeability of the membranes and the blood supply to the absorption area.
   5. A drug that first accumulates in the brain may move into fat and muscle tissue and then back to the brain because the drug is still chemically active.
      a. The drug is released in small quantities from the tissues and travels back to the brain.
      b. Equal drug and blood concentration levels in the body are maintained.
C. Metabolism or biotransformation.
   1. The third stage of metabolism takes place as the drug—a foreign substance in the body—is converted by enzymes into a less active and harmless agent that can be easily excreted.
   ✦ 2. Most of this conversion occurs in the liver.
      a. Both synthetic and biochemical reactions take place.
      b. Some conversion does take place in the kidney, plasma, and intestinal mucosa.
   3. Synthetic reactions: liver enzymes conjugate the drug with other substances to make it less harmful for the body.
   4. Biochemical reactions: drugs are oxidized, reduced, hydrolyzed, and synthesized so they become less active and more easily eliminated from the body.
D. Excretion.
   1. The final stage in metabolism takes place when the drug is changed into an inactive form or excreted from the body.

2. The kidneys are the most important route of excretion.

✦ 3. The kidneys eliminate both the pure drug and the metabolites of the parent drug.
   a. During excretion these two substances are filtered through the glomeruli.
   b. They are then secreted by the tubules.
   c. Finally, they are reabsorbed through the tubules or directly excreted.

4. Other routes of excretion include the lungs (which exhale gaseous drugs), feces, saliva, tears, and mother's milk.

Factors That Affect Drug Metabolism

A. Personal attributes.
   1. Body weight.
   2. Age.
   3. Sex.
B. Physiological factors.
   1. State of health.
   2. Disease processes.
C. Acid–base and fluid and electrolyte balance.
D. Permeability.
E. Diurnal rhythm.
F. Circulatory capability.
G. Genetic and immunologic factors.
H. Drug tolerance.
I. Cumulative effect of drugs.
J. Other factors.
   1. Psychological.
   2. Emotional.
   3. Environmental.
K. Responses to drugs vary.
   1. Responses depend on the speed with which the drug is absorbed into the blood or tissues.
   2. Responses depend on the effectiveness of the body's circulatory system.

✦ Factors That Affect Drug Absorption

A. Absorption factors.
   1. Solubility of the drug.
   2. Route of administration: oral, subcutaneous, topical, sublingual, or intramuscular.
   3. Client's sex, age, and health status.
      a. Females absorb IM injections slower than males because they have increased adipose tissue and a smaller blood supply.
      b. Older clients respond slower—often related to lower gastric acid in the stomach.
      c. Certain diseases decrease tissue perfusion.
B. Distribution factors.
   1. Cardiac output and circulation influence how the drug reaches the target tissues.

✦ 2. If drug is attached to serum proteins and the protein level is low, there would be more free drug in the bloodstream; this condition indicates that dosage should be decreased with certain drugs (warfarin, Dilantin, and barbiturates).

✦ 3. Drug half-life is the time it takes for a half-dose of the drug to be eliminated from the body.
   a. Four to five half-lives are required to reach a steady state of equilibrium in the bloodstream.
   b. For a blood sample to reflect therapeutic action of a drug, there must be a half-life times four or five.

✦ C. Clients with impaired liver function or liver disease may lose much of the therapeutic value of a drug.
   1. Drugs that pass through the liver (called first-pass effect) before being absorbed into the bloodstream may be affected by the liver status.
   2. Certain drugs that go from the GI tract to the portal vein to the liver may need to have their oral dosages adjusted upward to compensate for partial deactivation (lidocaine, morphine, propranolol, verapamil).

D. Kidneys also play a role in drug absorption— depends on tissue perfusion, disease and urinary pH.
   1. Renal disease interferes with renal clearance, and drugs (potassium chloride or digoxin) can reach toxic levels in the bloodstream.
   2. The more alkaline the urine, the faster certain drugs are excreted (salicylates, barbiturates, and sulfonamides). Sodium bicarbonate will make urine more alkaline.
   3. Some drugs are excreted faster when urine is acidic (amphetamines and ephedrine). Vitamin C will make urine more acidic.

ORIGIN AND NOMENCLATURE OF DRUGS

Common Sources

A. Plant sources.
   1. Roots, bark, sap, leaves, flowers, and seeds from medicinal plants can be used as drug components.
   2. Component substances.
      a. Alkaloid.
         (1) Alkaline (base) in reaction.
         (2) Bitter in taste.
         (3) Physiologically powerful in activity.

b.   Glycoside: a compound containing a carbo-hydrate molecule.

c.   Resin: soluble in alcohol; insoluble in water.

d.   Gum.

(1)   Mucilaginous (gelatinlike) excretion.

(2)   Used in bulk laxatives; may absorb water.

(3)   Used in skin preparations as a soothing effect (e.g., Karaya gum).

e.   Oil.

(1)   Fixed oil: does not evaporate on warming; occurs as a solid, semisolid, or liquid (e.g., castor oil).

(2)   Volatile oil: evaporates readily; occurs in aromatic plants (e.g., peppermint).

B.   Animal sources.

1.   Processed from an organ, from organ secretion, or from organ cells.

2.   Insulin, as an example, is a derivative from the pancreas of sheep, cattle, or hogs.

C.   Mineral sources.

1.   Inorganic elements occurring in nature, but not of plant or animal origin; may be metallic or nonmetallic.

2.   Usually form a base or acid salt in food.

3.   Dilute hydrochloric acid (HCl), as an example, is diluted in water and then taken through a straw to prevent damage to teeth by acid.

D.   Synthetic sources.

1.   A pure drug made in a laboratory from chemical, not natural, substances.

2.   Many drugs—sulfonamides, for example—are synthetics.

Methods of Naming Drugs

A.   Chemical name.

1.   Precise description of chemical constituents with the exact placement of atom groupings.

2.   "N-methyl-4-carbethoxypiperidine hydrochloride" is an example of a chemical name.

B.   Generic name.

1.   Reflects chemical name of the drug, but is simpler.

2.   It is never changed and used commonly in medical terminology.

3.   The synthetic narcotic "meperidine" is an example of a generic name.

C.   Trademark name (brand name, proprietary name).

1.   Appears in literature with the sign ® (e.g., Demerol®).

2.   The sign indicates the name is registered; use of the name is restricted to the manufacturer that is its legal owner.

3.   Trademark name is capitalized or shown in parentheses if generic name stated.

DRUG CLASSIFICATION

Classification by Action

✦ A.   Anti-infectives.

1.   Antiseptics.

a.   *Action*—inhibit growth of microorganisms (bacteriostatic).

b.   *Purpose*—application to wounds and skin infections, sterilization of equipment, and hygienic purposes.

2.   Disinfectants.

a.   *Action*—destroy microorganisms (bactericidal).

b.   *Purpose*—destroy bacteria on inanimate objects (not appropriate for living tissue).

✦ B.   Antimicrobials.

1.   Sulfonamides.

a.   *Action*—inhibit the growth of microorganisms.

b.   *Usage*—reduce or prevent infectious process, especially for urinary tract infections.

2.   Antibiotics (e.g., penicillin).

a.   *Action*—interfere with microorganism metabolism.

b.   *Usage*—reduce or prevent infectious process.

c.   Specific drug and dosage based on culture and sensitivity of organism.

✦ C.   Metabolic drugs.

1.   Hormones obtained from animal sources, found naturally in foods and plants.

2.   Synthetic hormones.

D.   Diagnostic materials.

1.   *Action*—dyes and opaque materials ingested or injected to allow visualization of internal organs.

2.   *Purpose*—to analyze organ status and function.

E.   Vitamins and minerals.

1.   *Action*—necessary to obtain healthy body function.

2.   Found naturally in food or through synthetic food supplements.

✦ F.   Vaccines and serums.

1.   *Action*—prevent disease or detect presence of disease.

2.   Types.

a.   Antigenics produce active immunity.

(1)   Vaccines—attenuated suspensions of microorganisms.

(2)   Toxoids—products of microorganisms.

b. Antibodies—stimulated by microorganisms or their products.
(1) Antitoxins.
(2) Immune serum globulin.
c. Allergens—agents for skin immunity tests.
(1) Extracts of materials known to be allergenic.
(2) Can be used to relieve allergies.
d. Antivenins—substances that neutralize venom of certain snakes and spiders.
✦ G. Antifungals—check growth of fungi.
✦ H. Antihistaminics.
1. *Action*—prevent histamine action.
2. *Purpose*—relieve symptoms of allergic reaction.
✦ I. Antineoplastics—prevent growth and spread of malignant cells.

Classification by Body System

Central Nervous System

A. Drugs affect CNS by either inhibiting or promoting the actions of neural pathways and centers.
1. Action-promoting drug groups (stimulants).
a. Antidepressants—psychic energizers used to treat depression.
b. Caffeine—increases mental activity and lessens drowsiness.
c. Ammonia—used for revival for fainting spell (client smells cap, not contents of bottle).
2. Action-inhibiting drug groups (depressants).
✦ a. Analgesics—reduce pain by interfering with conduction of nerve impulses.
(1) Narcotic analgesics—opium derivatives may depress respiratory centers; must be used with caution and respiratory rate above 12.
(a) A narcotic antagonist drug counteracts depressant drugs.
(b) Such antagonist drugs include Lorfan, Narcan, and Nalline.
(2) Nonnarcotic antipyretics—reduce fever and relieve pain.
(3) Antirheumatics—analgesics given to relieve arthritis pain; may reduce joint inflammation.
✦ b. Alcohol—stimulates appetite when given in small doses but is classified as a depressant.
✦ c. Hypnotics—sedatives that induce sleep; common form is the barbiturates.
✦ d. Antispasmodics—relieve skeletal muscle spasms; anticonvulsants prevent muscle spasms or convulsions.

✦ e. Tranquilizers.
(1) Relieve tension and anxiety, preoperative and postoperative apprehension, headaches, menstrual tension, chronic alcoholism, skeletal muscle spasticity, and other neuromuscular disorders.
(2) Tranquilizers and analgesics frequently given together (in reduced dosage); the one drug enhances the action of the other (synergy).
f. Anesthetics—produce the state of unconsciousness or conscious sedation painlessly.
✦ B. Precautions to be taken with CNS drugs.
1. Drugs that act on CNS may potentiate other CNS drugs.
2. Client may be receiving other medications; find out drug name and dosage.
3. Dependence on CNS drugs may occur.

Autonomic Nervous System

A. This system governs several body functions so that drugs that affect the ANS will at the same time affect other system functions.
B. The ANS is made up of two nerve systems—the sympathetic and parasympathetic.
1. Sympathetic—the protective emergency system.
2. Parasympathetic—the stabilizing system.
C. Each system has a separate basic drug group acting on it.
✦ 1. Adrenergics—mimic the actions of sympathetic system.
a. Vasoconstrictors—stimulants such as Adrenalin.
(1) Action is to constrict peripheral blood vessels, thereby increasing blood pressure.
(2) Dilate bronchial passages.
(3) Relax gastrointestinal tract.
b. Vasodilators—depressants such as nicotinic acid.
(1) Antagonists of epinephrine and similar drugs.
(2) Vasodilate blood vessels.
(3) Increase tone of GI tract.
(4) Reduce blood pressure.
(5) Relax smooth muscles.
(6) *Caution:* If drug is to be stopped, reduce dosage gradually over a period of a week; do not stop it suddenly.
✦ 2. Cholinergics—mimic actions of parasympathetic system.
a. Cholinergic stimulants (e.g., Prostigmin or neostigmine).

(1) Decrease heart rate.

(2) Contract smooth muscles.

(3) Contract pupil in eye.

(4) Increase peristalsis.

(5) Increase gland secretions.

b. Cholinergic inhibitors (anticholinergics).

(1) Decrease gland secretion.

(2) Relax smooth muscle.

(3) Dilate pupil in eye.

(4) Increase heart action.

Gastrointestinal System

A. Drugs affecting GI system act on muscular and glandular tissues.

✦ B. Antacids—counteract excess acidity.

1. Have alkaline base.

2. Used in the treatment of ulcers.

3. Neutralize hydrochloric acid in the stomach.

4. Given frequently (2-hour intervals or more often).

5. May be given with water.

6. May cause constipation, depending on type of medication.

7. Baking soda is a systemic antacid which disturbs the pH balance in the body. Most other antacids coat the mucous membrane and neutralize hydrochloric acid.

C. Emetics—produce vomiting (emesis).

✦ D. H_2-receptor antagonists—block gastric acid secretion (e.g., cimetidine, ranitidine).

✦ E. Antiulcer drugs—sucralfate; give 1 hour AC and at HS; nonsystemic.

F. Digestants—relieve enzyme deficiency by replacing secretions in digestive tract.

G. Antidiarrheics—prevent diarrhea.

H. Cathartics—affect intestine and produce defecation.

1. Provide temporary relief for constipation.

2. Rid bowel of contents before surgery, and prepare viscera for diagnostic studies.

3. Counteract edema.

4. Treat diseases of GI tract.

5. Are contraindicated when abdominal pain is present.

6. Classifications.

a. By degree of action.

(1) Laxative—mild action.

(2) Cathartic—moderate action.

(3) Purgative—severe action.

b. By method of action.

Respiratory System

A. Drugs that act on respiratory tract, tissues, and cough center.

B. Action is to suppress, relax, liquefy, and stimulate depth and rate of respiration.

✦ C. Bronchodilators—relax smooth muscle of trachea and bronchi.

1. Sympathomimetics.

a. Taken PO or inhaled (fewer side effects).

b. Beta$_2$ agonists preferred (e.g., albuterol, metaproterenol).

2. Anticholinergics (e.g., atropine sulfate by nebulizer or metered dose inhaler).

3. Theophyllines.

a. Monitor serum levels.

b. Examples: theophylline PO, aminophylline IV.

4. Anti-inflammatory agents—reduce bronchospasm.

a. Mast cell inhibitor (e.g., cromolyn sodium).

b. Corticosteroids (PO, IV, or inhaled).

Urinary System

A. Drugs that act on kidneys and urinary tract.

B. Action is to increase urine flow, destroy bacteria, perform other important body functions.

✦ 1. Diuretics.

a. Rid body of excess fluid and relieve edema.

b. Some drugs that act on the GI tract and circulatory system also are diuretic in action.

2. Urinary antiseptics.

3. Acidifiers and alkalinizers—certain foods will also increase body acidity and alkalinity.

Circulatory System

A. Drugs that act on heart, blood, and blood vessels.

B. Action is to change heart rhythm, rate, and force and to dilate or constrict vessels.

✦ 1. Cardiotonics—used for heart-strengthening.

a. Direct heart stimulants that speed heart rate (e.g., caffeine, Adrenalin).

b. Indirect heart stimulants (e.g., digitalis).

(1) Stimulate vagus nerve.

(2) Slow heart rate and strengthen it.

(3) Improve heart action, thereby improving circulation.

(4) Do not administer if apical pulse below 60.

✦ 2. Cardioprotective drugs.

a. Beta-adrenergic blockers.

b. Calcium-entry blockers.

✦ 3. Antiarrhythmic drugs—used clinically to convert irregularities to a normal sinus rhythm.

✦ 4. Drugs that alter blood flow.

a. Anticoagulants—inhibit blood clotting action (e.g., heparin, Coumadin).

b. Thrombolytic agents (streptokinase, urokinase).

c. Platelet-inhibiting agents (aspirin, dipyridamole).

    d.   Vasodilators.
    e.   Hemorrheologic agents [e.g., pentoxifylline (Trental)].
  5.   Blood replacement.

DOSAGE AND PREPARATION FORMS

Solids

A. Extract—obtained by dissolving drug in water or alcohol and allowing solution to evaporate; residue is the extract.
B. Powder—finely ground drugs.
C. Pill—common term for tablet; made by rolling drug and binder into a sphere.
D. Suppository.
  1.   Contains drugs mixed with a firm base.
  2.   Liquefies at body temperature when inserted into orifice.
  3.   Releases drug to produce a local or systemic effect.
E. Ointment—semisolid mixture of drugs with a fatty base.
F. Lozenge—flavored flat tablet that releases drug slowly when held in mouth.
G. Medication patch.
  1.   Premeasured medication paper (also called transdermal medication).
  2.   Check manufacturer's directions for application.
H. Capsule.
  1.   Drugs in small, cylindrical gelatin containers that disguise the taste of the drug.
  2.   Capsule can be opened and drug mixed with food or jam to mask taste.
I. Tablets.
  1.   Dried, powdered drugs that are compressed into a small disk, which easily disintegrates in water.
  2.   Enteric coated—tablet does not dissolve until reaching intestines, where release of drug occurs.

Liquids

A. Fluid extract.
  1.   Concentrated fluid preparation of drugs produced by dissolving crude plant drug in a solvent.
  2.   Strength of extract is such that 1 mL (about ¼ teaspoon or 15 to 16 gtt) represents 1 g of the drug at 100 percent strength.
B. Tincture.
  1.   Diluted alcoholic extract of a drug.
  2.   Varies in strength from 10 to 20 percent.
C. Spirit—preparation of volatile (easily vaporized) substances dissolved in alcohol.

D. Syrup—drug contained in a concentrated sugar solution.
E. Elixir—solution of drug made with alcohol, sugar, and some aromatic or pleasant-smelling substance.
F. Suspension.
  1.   Undissolved, finely divided particles of drug dispersed in a liquid.
  2.   Gels and magma are other forms of suspensions.
  3.   Shake all bottles of suspension well before giving.
G. Emulsion—suspension of unmixed oils, fats, or petrolatum in water.
H. Liniment and lotion—liquid suspension of medication applied to the skin.

Packaging Methods and Dispensing

A. Unit dosage package method.
  1.   Package contains premeasured amount of drug in proper form for administering.
  2.   Pharmacy may deliver the daily needs for each client to the floor.
  3.   Procedures for delivery and storage vary from hospital to hospital.
  4.   Nurse administers the medication to the client.
B. Traditional method.
  1.   Nurse prepares medication on the unit.
  2.   Supplies come from stock or bulk on the ward or from client's multiple-dose bottle.
C. The nurse is responsible for accuracy of the medication given, regardless of the packaging or dispensing method used.

ROUTES OF ADMINISTRATION

Oral Route

A. Ingested (swallowed).
B. Sublingual (under tongue).
C. Buccal (on mucous membrane of cheek or tongue).

Rectal Route

A. Suppository.
B. Liquid (retention enema).

✦ Parenteral Route

A. Intravenous.
  1.   The response is fast and immediate.
  2.   More than 5 mL medication can be given.
  ✦ 3.   Drug *must be* given slowly and usually in diluted form.
  4.   Check medication leaflets to determine if medication route is IM or IV.

B. Intradermal.
   1. Injected into skin; usual site is inner aspect of forearm or scapular area of back.
   2. A short bevel 26-gauge, 1-cm needle is used.
   ✦ 3. Needle should be inserted with bevel up.
   4. This route is usually used to inject antigens for skin or tuberculin tests.
   5. Amount injected ranges from 0.01 to 0.1 mL.
C. Subcutaneous.
   1. A 25-gauge, 1.3- to 1.6-cm needle is used.
   2. Injection site is the fatty layer under skin.
      a. Abdomen at navel.
      b. Lateral upper arm or thigh.
   ✦ 3. This route usually used for injecting medication that is to be absorbed slowly with a sustained effect.
   4. Amount injected ranges from 0.5 to 1.5 mL.
   5. If repeated doses are necessary, as with insulin for a diabetic person, rotate the injection sites.
D. Intramuscular.
   1. Needle gauge and length will vary with site.
      a. Deltoid—located by having client raise arm.
         (1) A 23- to 25-gauge, 1.6- to 2.5-cm needle is used.
         (2) Administer no more than 2 mL.
      ✦ b. Thigh and buttock.
         (1) Needle must be long enough to reach muscle; may vary from 2 to 8 cm.
         (2) Needle gauge depends upon substance of medication.
         (3) Oil bases require 20 gauge; water bases require 22 gauge.
   2. Absorption rate of IM medication dependent on circulation of person injected.
   3. This route usually used for systemic effect of an irritating drug.
   ✦ 4. Amount of medication must not be over 5 mL, as absorption would be difficult and painful.
   5. Techniques for lessening pain for the client using an IM medication.
      a. Encourage relaxation of area to be injected; request client to lie on side with flexed knee or flat on abdomen, if giving injection in buttock.
      b. Reduce puncture pain by "darting" needle.
      c. Prevent antiseptic from clinging to needle during insertion by waiting until skin antiseptic is dry.
      d. If medication must be drawn through a rubber stopper, use a new needle for injection.
      e. Avoid sensitive or hardened body areas.
      f. After needle is under skin, aspirate to be certain that needle is not in a blood vessel.

NURSE PRACTICE ACT GUIDELINES FOR DRUG ADMINISTRATION

✦ **Nurses must not administer a specific drug unless allowed to do so by the particular state's Nurse Practice Act.**
- Nurses must not administer any drug without a specific physician order.
- Nurses are to take every safety precaution in whatever they are doing.
- Nurses are to be certain that employer's policy allows them to administer a specific drug.
- Nurses must not administer a controlled substance if the physician's order is outdated.
- A drug may not lawfully be administered unless all the above items are in effect.
- Nurses are not permitted to fill prescriptions and in most states cannot write prescriptions.

✦ **General rules for drug dispensing**
- Never leave prepared medicines unattended.
- Always report errors immediately.
- Send labeled bottles or packages that are unintelligible back to pharmacist for relabeling.
- Store internal and external medicines separately if possible.

---

      g. Inject slowly.
      h. Maintain grasp of syringe.
      i. Withdraw needle quickly after injection.
      j. Massage relaxed muscle gently to increase circulation and to distribute medication.
   6. Observe for side effects of medication following action.

Other Routes

A. Inhalation route.
B. Topical route.

MEDICATION ADMINISTRATION

Basic Guidelines for Medication Administration

✦ A. Determine the correct dosage, actions, side effects, and contraindications of any medication before administration.
B. Determine if medications ordered by the physician are appropriate for client's condition. This is part of the nurse's professional responsibility.
C. Question the physician about any medication orders that are incomplete, illegible, or inappropriate for the client's condition.
   ✦ 1. Remember, the nurse may be liable if a medication error is made.

2. Report every medication error to the physician and nursing administrator.

3. Complete a medication incident report.

D. Check to determine if the medication ordered is compatible with the client's condition and with other medications prescribed.

E. Ascertain what the client has been eating or drinking before administering a medication.

1. Determine what effect the client's diet has on the medication.

2. Do not administer medication if contraindicated by diet. For example, do not give a monoamine oxidase (MAO) inhibitor to a client who has just ingested cheddar cheese or wine.

F. Check that calculated drug dosage is accurate for young children, elderly people, or for very thin or obese clients. These age and weight groups require smaller or larger dosages.

DOCUMENTATION OF MEDICATIONS

Medication Orders

✦ A. Medication administered to client must have a physician's order or prescription before it can be legally administered.

B. Physician's order is a verbal or written order, recorded in a book or file or in client's chart.

C. If order is given verbally over the telephone, nurse must write a verbal order in client's chart for the physician to sign at a later date.

D. Written orders are safer—they leave less room for potential misunderstanding or error.

✦ E. Drug order should consist of seven parts.
1. Name of the client.
2. Date the drug was ordered.
3. Name of the drug.
4. Dosage.
5. Route of administration and any special rules of administration.
6. Time and frequency the drug should be given.
7. Signature of the individual who ordered the drug.

Types of Medication Schedules

A. Routine orders.
1. Administered according to instructions until it is canceled by another order.
2. Can also be used for PRN drugs.
   a. Administered when client needs the medication.
   b. Not given on a routine time schedule.

> ### THE SIX RIGHTS OF MEDICATION ADMINISTRATION
>
> 1. **Right medication.**
>   a. Compare drug card with drug label three times.
>   b. Know general purpose or action, dosage, method of administration.
>   c. Know side effects of drug.
> 2. **Right client.** Check ID band and have client state name. Use two client identifiers other than room number.
> 3. **Right time.** Give medication 30 minutes before or after ordered time.
> 4. **Right method or route of administration.**
> 5. **Right dose.**
>   a. Check all calculations of divided dosages with another nurse.
>   b. Check heparin, insulin, and IV digitalis doses with another nurse.
> 6. **Documentation** is now considered the sixth right. Document the drug name, dose, route and time of administration. Client's reaction to the medication may also be included.

3. Continued validity of any routine order should be assessed—physicians occasionally forget to cancel an order when it is no longer appropriate for client's condition.

B. One-time orders.
1. Administered as stated, only one time.
2. Given at a specified time or "STAT," which means immediately.

Legal Implications of Medication Errors

✦ A. Nurse who prepares a medication must also give it to client and chart it.
1. If client refuses drug, chart that medication was refused—report this information to the physician.
2. When charting medications, use the correct abbreviations and symbols.

✦ B. If error in a drug order is found, it is the nurse's responsibility to question the order.
1. If order cannot be understood or read, verify with the physician.
2. Do not guess at the order as this constitutes gross negligence.
3. In many hospitals it is the pharmacist's responsibility to contact physicians when medication orders are unclear.
4. Even when drug dose is prepared by pharmacy, it is the nurse's responsibility to know correct drug and dose.

C. Always report medication errors to the physician immediately.
1. This action minimizes potential danger to the client.

2. Measures can be taken immediately to assess and evaluate the client's status.
3. A plan of action can be implemented to reverse the effects of the medication.

D. Errors in medication are documented in an unusual occurrence or incident report and on the client's record.
   1. This action is necessary for both legal reasons and nursing audits.
   2. Nursing audits are conducted to determine problems in medication administration.
      a. A particular source of problems.
      b. A range of problems that seem to have no connection.

ADMINISTERING MEDICATIONS

Oral Medication

Assessment

A. Assess that oral route is the most efficient means of medication administration.
B. Check medication orders for their completeness and accuracy.
C. Research unfamiliar drugs.
D. Review client's record for allergies, lab data, etc.
◆ E. Assess client's physical ability to take medication as ordered.
   1. Swallow reflex present.
   2. State of consciousness.
   3. Signs of nausea and vomiting.
   4. Uncooperative behavior.
F. Check client's MAR with previous day's MAR to make sure you have the correct medication for the client.
G. Assess correct dosage when calculation is needed.

Implementation

A. Preparing oral medications.
   1. Obtain client's medication record (MAR). Medication record may be a drug card, medication sheet, or drug Kardex, depending on the method of dispensing medications in the hospital.
   2. Compare the MAR with the most *recent* physician's order.
   3. Perform hand hygiene.
   4. Gather necessary equipment.
   5. Retrieve the medication.
   6. Compare the label on the bottle or drug package to the MAR.
   7. Correctly calculate dosage if necessary and check the dosage to be administered.
   8. Pour the medication from the bottle into the lid of the container and then into the medicine cup. With unit dosage, take drug package from medication cart and place in medication cup. Do not remove drug from drug package.
   9. Check medication label again to ensure correct drug and dosages if drug is not prepackaged.
  10. Place medication cup on a tray, if not using medication cart.
  11. Return the multidose vial bottle to the storage area. If medication to be given is a narcotic, sign out the narcotic record sheet with your name.

B. Administering oral medications to adults.
   1. Take medication tray or cart to client's room; check room number against medication card or sheet.
   2. Place client in sitting position, if not contraindicated by his or her condition.
   3. Tell the client what type of medication you are going to give and explain the actions this medication will produce.
◆ 4. Check the client's Identaband and ask client to state name so that you are sure you have correctly identified him or her.
   5. If prepackaged medication is used, read label, take medication out of package, and put into medication cup.
   6. Give the medication cup to the client.
   7. Offer a fresh glass of water or other liquid to aid swallowing, and give assistance with taking medications.
   8. Make sure the client swallows the medication.
   9. Discard used medicine cup.
  10. Position client for comfort.
  11. Record the medication on the appropriate forms.

C. Administering oral medications to children.
◆ 1. Follow the procedures for the previous intervention, keeping the following guidelines in mind.
      a. Play techniques may help to elicit a young child's cooperation.
      b. Remember, the smaller the quantity of diluent (food or liquid), the greater the ease in eliciting the child's cooperation.
      c. Never use a child's favorite food or drink as an enticement when administering medication because the result may be the child's refusal to eat or drink anything.
      d. Be honest and tell the child that you have medicine, not candy.
   2. Assess child for drug action and possible side effects.
   3. Explain medication action and side effects to parents.

Narcotic Medication

A. Check medication sheet for narcotic orders.

B. Check dose and time last narcotic administered.

C. Unlock and open narcotic drawer and find appropriate narcotic container.

D. Count number of pills, ampules, or injectable cartridges in container.

✦ E. Check narcotic sign-out sheet and check that number of narcotics matches number of sign-out sheets.

F. Rectify situation before proceeding with narcotic administration if narcotics and sign-out sheets do not coincide.

G. Sign out for narcotic on narcotic sheets, after taking narcotic out of drawer or cupboard.

H. Lock drawer or cupboard after taking out medication.

I. Sign out narcotics on MAR according to usual procedure.

J. For unit narcotic stock, check narcotics every 8 hours.
   1. One off-going and one on-going nurse check the narcotics.
   2. Number of sign-out sheets must match remaining number of narcotics.
   3. Each narcotic sheet is checked for accuracy.

K. Return empty counter (if used) to pharmacy with completed narcotic sign-out sheet when sheet is filled.
   1. A new narcotic supply and narcotic check sheet are signed out in pharmacy.
   2. The nurse receiving narcotics signs drug record receipt.

L. For automated dispensing system, enter ID code number and user password and continue with dispensing process.

✦ Patient-Controlled Analgesia (PCA)

A. Advantages of PCA.
   1. Method provides consistent level of pain control.
   2. Allows client to self-administer pain medication.
   3. Allows client to feel in control of pain management.

B. Procedure.
   1. PCA infuser pump is prepared and attached to IV.
   2. Morphine sulfate or hydromorphone (Dilaudid) is delivered in loading dose as ordered and initiates pain management.
   3. Client is instructed in PCA use and continues to self-administer narcotic.
   4. Dose calculation.
      a. PCA infuser delivers in milliliters.
      b. Maximum rate of administration 20 mL/hour.
      c. Four-hour limit is set for infuser—5- to 30-mL increments.

Parenteral Medications

Assessment

A. Determine appropriate method for administration of drug.
   1. Intradermal (intracutaneous): injection is made below surface of the skin; 25–27-gauge, $\frac{3}{8}$–$\frac{1}{2}$-inch needle; 0.01 to 0.1 mL.
   2. Subcutaneous: small amount of fluid is injected beneath the skin in the loose connective tissues; 25–29-gauge, $\frac{3}{8}$–$\frac{5}{8}$-inch needle; to 2 mL.
   3. Intramuscular: larger amount of fluid is injected into large muscle masses in the body; 23–25-gauge, $\frac{5}{8}$–1-inch needle; up to 5 mL; 21–22 gauge ($1\frac{1}{2}$) needles may be used for deep IM.
   4. Intravenous: medication is injected or infused directly into a vein—route used when immediate drug effect is desired.

B. Evaluate condition of administration site for presence of lesions, rash, inflammation, lipodystrophy, ecchymosis, and other problems.
   1. Ventrogluteal site (client side-lying).
   2. Dorsogluteal site (client in prone position).
   3. Vastus lateralis site (supine with thigh available).
   4. Deltoid site (exposed upper arm).

C. Assess for tissue damage from previous injections.

✦ D. Assess client's level of consciousness.
   1. *For client in shock:* certain methods (subcutaneous) will not be used.
   2. *For presence of anxiety:* make sure client is allowed to express his or her fear of injections and offer explanations of ways in which injections will be less frightening.

✦ E. Check client's written and verbal history for past allergic reactions. Do *not* rely solely on client's chart.

F. Review client's chart noting previous injection sites, especially insulin and heparin administration sites.

G. Check label on medication bottle to determine if medication can be administered via route ordered.

Implementation

A. Preparing medications.
   1. Perform hand hygiene.
   2. Obtain equipment for injection: safety needle and syringe, antimicrobial wipes, medication cart or dispenser.

3. Select the appropriate size needle, considering the size of the client's muscle mass and the viscosity of the medication.

4. Open the wipe and cleanse top of vial or break top of ampule.

5. Remove the needle guard.

6. Pull back on barrel of syringe to markings where medication will be inserted.

7. Pick up vial, insert needle into vial, and inject air in an amount equal to the solution to be withdrawn by pushing barrel of syringe down. If using an ampule, break off top at colored line, insert syringe, but do not inject air into ampule as it causes a break in the vacuum and possible loss of medication through leakage.

8. Extract the desired amount of fluid. Remove needle from container and cover needle with guard. Needle should be changed to prevent tracking medication on skin and subcutaneous tissue if drug is caustic.

9. Double-check drug and dosage against drug card or medication sheet and vial or ampule.

10. Place syringe on tray.

11. Check label and drug card or medication sheet for accuracy before returning multidose vial to correct storage area.

12. Return multidose vial to correct storage area or discard used vial or ampule.

B. Administering intradermal injections.

1. Take medication to client's room. Check room number against medication card or sheet.

2. Explain the medication's action and the procedure for administration to client.

✦ 3. Check client's Identaband and ask client to state name.

4. Perform hand hygiene and don gloves.

5. Select the site of injection.

6. Cleanse the area with an antimicrobial wipe, wiping in circular area from inside to outside.

7. Take off needle guard.

8. Grasp client's forearm from underneath and gently pull the skin taut.

9. Insert the needle at 10- to 15-degree angle with the bevel of needle facing up. (*See* Figure 5-2.)

10. Inject medication slowly. Observe for wheals and blanching at the site.

11. Withdraw the needle, wiping the area gently with a dry 2 × 2 bandage to prevent dispersing medication into the subcutaneous tissue.

12. Return the client to a comfortable position.

13. Activate safety needle and discard supplies in appropriate area.

14. Chart the medication and site used.

C. Administering subcutaneous (sub q) injections.

1. Take medication to client's room.

2. Set tray on a clean surface, not the bed.

3. Check client's Identaband and ask client to state name.

4. Explain action of medication and procedure of administration.

5. Provide privacy when injection site is other than on the arm.

6. Perform hand hygiene and don gloves.

7. Select site for injection by identifying anatomical landmarks. Remember to alternate sites each time injections are given.

8. Cleanse area with antimicrobial wipe. Using a circular motion, cleanse from inside outward.

9. Take off needle guard.

10. Express any air bubbles from syringe.

11. Insert the needle at a 45- or 90-degree angle. (*See* Figure 5-1.)

12. Aspirate by pulling back on the plunger.

13. Inject the medication slowly.

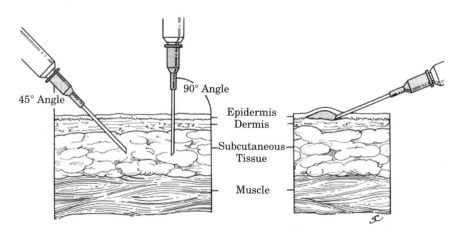

FIGURE 5-1. Insert needle at 45- or 90-degree angle for subcutaneous injection.

FIGURE 5-2. Insert needle at 15-degree angle under the epidermis for intradermal injection.

14. Withdraw needle quickly and massage area with wipe to aid absorption and lessen bleeding. Do not massage after administering certain drugs, i.e., heparin, insulin. Put on Band-Aid if needed.
15. Activate needle safety feature and discard in puncture-proof container.
16. Return client to a position of comfort.
17. Chart the medication and site used.
✦ D. Administering insulin injections.
   1. Gather equipment and check medication orders and injection site. Opened insulin does not need to be refrigerated.
   2. Perform hand hygiene and don gloves.
   3. Obtain specific insulin syringe for strength of insulin being administered (U100).
   4. Rotate insulin bottle between hands to bring solution into suspension.
   5. Wipe top of insulin bottle with antimicrobial swab.
   6. Take off needle guard.
   7. Pull plunger of syringe down to desired amount of medication and inject that amount of air into the insulin bottle.
   8. Draw up ordered amount of insulin into syringe.
   9. Expel air from syringe.
  10. Replace needle guard.
  11. Check medication card, bottle, and syringe with another RN for accuracy.
  12. Take medication to client's room.
  13. Double-check site of last injection with client.
✦ 14. Rotating injection site from one body area to another is no longer recommended due to variation in insulin absorption and action.
     a. Move injection site one inch from previous site.
     b. Absorption is most predictable in abdomen.
     c. Avoid injecting into extremity.
  15. Provide privacy.
  16. Perform hand hygiene.
  17. Follow protocol for administration of medications by subcutaneous injections.
✦ E. Administering intramuscular (IM) injections.
   1. Take medication to client's room. Check room number against medication card or sheet.
   2. Set tray on a clean surface, not the bed.
   3. Explain the procedure to client.
   4. Check client's Identaband and have client state name.
   5. Provide privacy for client.
   6. Perform hand hygiene and don gloves.
   7. Select the site of injection by identifying anatomical landmarks. (*See* Figures 5-3 and 5-4.) Remember to alternate sites each time injections are given.

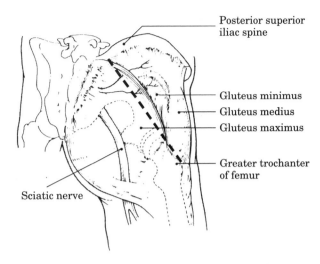

FIGURE 5-3. Place injection in ventrogluteal site (preferred over dorsogluteal) above and outside the diagonal line for intramuscular injections.

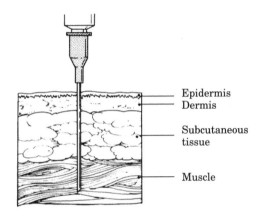

FIGURE 5-4. Insert needle at 90-degree angle and deep into muscle tissue for intramuscular injections.

   8. Cleanse the area with antimicrobial wipe. Using a circular motion, cleanse from inside outward.
   9. Hold the syringe; take off needle cover.
  10. Express air bubbles from syringe. Some clinicians suggest leaving a small air bubble at the tip so that all medicine will be expelled.
  11. Insert the needle at 90-degree angle. (*See* Figure 5-4.)
  12. Pull back on plunger. If blood returns, you know you have entered a blood vessel; textbooks advocate discarding all equipment and medication.
  13. Inject the medication slowly.
  14. Withdraw the needle, activate safety feature, and apply pressure to area while massaging with alcohol wipe. Put on a Band-Aid, if needed.
  15. Return client to a comfortable position.
  16. Discard supplies in appropriate area.
  17. Chart the medication and site used.

HERB–DRUG INTERACTIONS

A. Mixing herbs with traditional medicines may increase or decrease the effects—in some cases this can be dangerous.
   1. Unlike prescription medicines, herbal products are not regulated by the FDA.
   2. More than 60 million Americans spend $4 billion annually on herbs; more than 15 million adults are at risk for potential drug–herb interactions.
   3. Table 5-1 lists some of the most popular herbs and their interactions with specific drugs.

B. On the whole, herbal medicine is safe and a gentle form of therapy. However, if the health problem is serious or the person is taking strong orthodox medications, teaching is indicated.
C. Client teaching with herbs.
   1. When completing a nursing history, ask about taking herbs.
   2. Educate yourself about herbs—check for known side effects, drug interactions, and potential risk with certain drugs.
   3. Remind the client to tell his or her physician about any herbs being taken.

Table 5-1. ALTERNATIVE NURSING: HERB–DRUG INTERACTIONS

Herb	Action	Side Effects	Drug Interaction	Drugs Affected
Black cohosh	An herb for females, especially during menopause for hot flashes —maintains healthy levels of luteinizing hormone Decreases menstrual discomfort Sedative, diuretic Lowers blood pressure	Overdose may cause nausea, vomiting, headache, dizziness, tremors and depressed heart rate	Increases effects of drugs— especially synthetic hormones **Congestive heart failure clients and pregnant women should not use this herb**	Hormone replacement therapy (HRT) Contraceptives Heart/cardiac medications
Echinacea	Immunostimulant Treatment for colds (URIs) and influenza Bladder infections Blood purifier Helps preserve white cells during radiation treatment	Possible, but not common: diarrhea, heartburn, intestinal upset, skin rash	Stimulates immune system may alter effect of certain drugs **Do not use if clients are taking immunosuppressants or have AIDS, or if they are pregnant**	Anabolic steroids Amiodarone Methotrexate Ketocomazole
Ephedra (ma huang)	Promotes weight loss and acts as a stimulant (asthma) Considered toxic by FDA	Stimulant, insomnia, headaches, nervousness, seizures, death	Heart attack, seizure or death Additive effect; increased thermogenesis (related to stimulants/coffee) Elevation of BP (related to MAO inhibitors) Reduces drug action—may cause arrhythmias Increased steroid drug clearance/may reduce effectiveness	Decongestants (Actifed, Dristan, Sinutab, Sudafed) Stimulants—caffeine MAO inhibitors Beta blockers Cardiac glycosides Steroids (anti-inflammatories)
Feverfew	Eases pain and nausea of migraine headaches Prevents blood vessel spasms Interferes with action of platelets (which clump together to form clots) Lowers blood pressure	Nervousness, insomnia, and tiredness Gastrointestinal symptoms	Severe bleeding **Pregnant women, children under age two, and people taking drugs as listed should not take this herb**	Warfarin Aspirin NSAIDs (ibuprophen)
Garlic	Contains allicin, a natural antibiotic—effective against bacteria and viruses	Intestinal problems— upset stomach, heartburn, strong garlic odor	Excessive thinning of blood (bleeding) when used with blood thinners	Warfarin Coumadin Aspirin Antihypertensives NSAIDS

Table 5-1. ALTERNATIVE NURSING: HERB–DRUG INTERACTIONS (Continued)

Herb	Action	Side Effects	Drug Interaction	Drugs Affected
Garlic (continued)	Lowers total cholesterol and increases HDL Reduces blood pressure Reduces blood clot formation (when arteries are narrowed)			**Clients who have blood disorders should use this herb with caution**
Ginger	Relieves nausea associated with seasickness, motion sickness, or anesthesia Digestive aid; increased secretion of bile Reduces side effects of chemotherapy Reduces congestion and fevers Supports cardiovascular system	Heartburn	Excessive thinning of blood (bleeding) when used with blood thinners Interferes with platelet action Increases gut absorption (may increase drug bioavailability)	Warfarin Take cautiously with all cardiac or diabetic medications; blood pressure therapy
Ginkgo biloba	Improves circulation by thinning blood Enhances flow of oxygen and blood to brain Improves memory and mental function May delay progression of Alzheimer's disease (jury still out) Asthma, peripheral vascular disease	Headache Indigestion, nausea Nervousness Allergic skin reactions	Anticoagulant effect and may cause spontaneous or excessive bleeding **Those with blood clotting disorders should not take this drug**	Aspirin NSAIDs Cox-2 inhibitors Coumadin Warfarin Vitamin K antagonists Diuretics
Siberian ginseng	Tonic, boosts energy and stamina Reduces stress Improves sexual performance, regulates hormones Strengthens immune system Raises "good" cholesterol, HDL Protects against heart attacks Preventive for aging	Insomnia, hypertension Low blood glucose Affects insulin level Allergy symptoms Increased alcohol clearance Diarrhea	Increases anticoagulant effect and bleeding Headache, manic behavior Monitoring effect of drug may be difficult—may increase digoxin levels Stimulates alcohol metabolism **Those who have blood-clotting problems, high blood pressure, asthma or emphysema, and children and pregnant women should not take this herb** Improves blood sugar and diabetic symptoms (could reduce amount of insulin needed)	Warfarin Coumadin Aspirin NSAIDs Nardil (MAO inhibitor) Digoxin (Lanoxin) Alcohol Insulin Antidepressants (phenelzine sulfate)
Kava kava	Sedative effect to treat anxiety	GI problems, liver problems (even failure has been reported) Allergic skin reaction	Sedation, and even coma when taken with certain drugs	Alprazolam Sleeping meds Antipsychotics Alcohol Xanax (antidepressant) Drugs treating Parkinson's disease

Continues

Table 5-1. ALTERNATIVE NURSING: HERB–DRUG INTERACTIONS *(Continued)*				
Herb	**Action**	**Side Effects**	**Drug Interaction**	**Drugs Affected**
Licorice root	Helps steroid drug withdrawal Helps to heal gastric ulcers Diuretic effect	Raises blood pressure Headache Lethargy Cardiac dysfunction	Potentiates drug levels and offsets effects of NSAIDs Antibiotics reduce herb activity Diuretic effect could result in decreased potassium leading to toxicity, electrolyte imbalance Increased sensitivity to digoxin or other cardiac glycosides **Pregnant and nursing women, and those with glaucoma, hypertension, stroke, and heart disease should not take this herb**	Corticosteroids Thiazides Oral contraceptives Antibiotics
Saw palmetto	Supports health of prostate gland—benign prostatic hypertrophy Improves urine flow Maintains healthy testosterone metabolism Anti-inflammatory	Relatively few: mild nausea, gastrointestinal disturbance, hypertension, headache	The safety profile of this herb is very good—no known drug interactions	
Silymarin (milk thistle)	Increases liver detoxification capacity Supports liver function Protects liver from drug damage	Nausea, GI disturbance	Reduces drug toxicity to liver and protects liver from drug damage Reduces toxic side effects of chemotherapy Potentially dangerous for transplant clients—reduces levels of immunosuppressives	Aspirin Alcohol Chemotherapy
St. John's wort	Relieves mild to moderate depression by countering monamine oxidase (avoid same foods—tyramine—as if taking an MAO inhibitor) Immune stimulating properties—useful with AIDS because it is antiviral Helps bruises and hemorrhoids	Dry mouth, dizziness, fatigue, digestive problems (fewer side effects than prescription antidepressants) Sensitivity to light	Decreases immunosuppressant therapy Additive serotonin-like effects—serotonin syndrome (serious condition: fever, dizziness, sweating) Could affect action of epilepsy drugs **Clients with hypertension and those on immunosuppressive therapy should not use this herb**	Tetracyclines Cyclosporin Digoxin Oral contraceptives Zoloft and antidepressants Other SSRIs Anticonvulsants Warfarin
Valerian	Quiets and calms neurological system Promotes sleep Used for headache, anxiety and nervousness	Restlessness, headache, giddiness, nausea, and blurred vision	Use may be affected by alcohol or barbiturates—use cautiously Not for children younger than 2 years Effect may be enhanced with sleeping tablets Additive effect—may be used to wean off drugs (diazepam)	Alcohol Barbiturates Sleeping tablets Benzodiazepines

D. The top five herbs clients take but do not tell their physicians about.
   1. Black cohosh.
   2. Echinacea.
   3. Ginkgo biloba.
   4. Saw palmetto.
   5. St. John's wort.

Source: Crock, R. (September 2003). Herbal medicine consultant.

GOVERNING LAWS

Federal Food, Drug, and Cosmetic Act of 1938

A. The act is an update of the Food and Drug Act first passed in 1906.
B. It designates *United States Pharmacopeia* and *National Formulary* as official standards.
C. The government has the power to enforce standards.
D. Provisions of the act.
   1. Drug manufacturer must provide adequate evidence of drug's safety.
   2. Correct labeling and packaging of drugs.
E. Amended in 1952 to include control of barbiturates by restricting prescription refills.
F. Amended in 1962 to require substantial investigation of drug and evidence that drug is effective in terms of labeling claims.

Harrison Narcotic Act of 1914

A. Provisions of the act.
   1. Regulates manufacture, importation, and sale of opium, cocaine, and their derivatives.
   2. Amendments have added addictive synthetic drugs to the regulated drug listing.
B. Applications of the act.
   1. Individuals who produce, sell, dispense (pharmacists), and prescribe (dentists, physicians) these drugs must be licensed and registered; prescriptions must be in triplicate.
   2. Hospitals order drugs on special blanks that bear hospital registry number. The following information is recorded for each dose.
      a. Name of drug.
      b. Amount of drug.
      c. Date and time drug obtained.
      d. Name of physician prescribing drug.
      e. Name of client receiving drug.
      f. Nurse's signature and type of license (RN, LVN, or LPN).

Controlled Substance Act of 1970

A. Provisions of the act.
   1. Regulates potentially addictive drugs as to prescription, use, and possession.
      a. Regulations refer to use in hospital, office, research, and emergency situations.
      b. Regulations cover narcotics, cocaine, amphetamines, hallucinogens, barbiturates, and other sedatives.
   2. Controlled drugs are placed in five different schedules or categorical listings, each governed by different regulations.
      a. The regulations govern manufacture, transport, and storage of the controlled drugs.
      b. The use of the drugs is controlled as to prescription, authorization, the mode of dispensation, and administration.
B. Application of the act for use of controlled drugs in hospitals.
   1. The nurse is to keep the stock supply of controlled drugs under lock and key.
      a. Nurse must sign for each dose (tablet, mL) of drug.
      b. Key is held by the nurse responsible for administration of medication.
      c. At the end of each shift, nurse must account for all controlled drugs in the stock supply.
   2. Violations of the Controlled Substance Act.
      a. Violations are punishable by fine, imprisonment, or both.
      b. Nurses, upon conviction of violation, are subject to losing their licenses to practice nursing.

Prescription and Medication Orders

A. A prescription is a written order for dispensation of drugs that can be used only under a physician's supervision.
B. Prescriptions outside the hospital.
   1. Formula to pharmacist for dispensing drugs to client.
   2. Consists of four parts.
      a. Superscription (symbolized by Rx, meaning "take").
         (1) Client's name.
         (2) Client's address (required only for controlled drugs).
         (3) Age (required only if age is a factor in the dose preparation).
         (4) Date (must *always* be included).
      b. Inscription.
         (1) Specifies ingredients and their quantities.
         (2) May specify other ingredients necessary to a specific drug form.

    c.   Subscription—directions to the pharmacist as to method of preparation.

    d.   Signature—consists of two parts.

        (1) Accurate instructions to client as to when, how, and in what quantities to take medication; typed on label.

        (2) Physician's signature and refill instructions.

C. Orders inside the hospital.

    1. Physician writes medication order in book, file, or client's chart; if given over phone, nurse writes verbal order which physician later signs.

    2. An order consists of six parts.

      a.   Name of drug.

      b.   Dosage.

      c.   Route of administration with time drug was or is to be given.

      d.   Reason drug is required (not always included).

      e.   Length of time client is to receive drug (not always included).

      f.   Signature of individual who ordered drug.

Example: Aspirin gr × PO q3h for pain for 3 days.

                                     D. Smith, M.D.

Informational Resources

Official Publications

A. A drug listed in the following publications is designated as official by the Federal Food, Drug, and Cosmetic Act (FDC).

    1. *United States Pharmacopeia* (USP).

    2. *National Formulary* (NF).

    3. *Homeopathic Pharmacopeia of the United States.*

B. These publications establish standards of purity and other criteria for product acceptability; these standards are binding according to law.

C. Publications contain information on each drug entry.

    1. Source.

    2. Chemical and physical composition.

    3. Method of storage.

    4. General type or category.

    5. Range of dosage and usual therapeutic dosage.

Other Publications

A. *American Hospital Formulary* is a publication indexed by generic and proprietary names.

B. *Physicians' Desk Reference* (PDR).

    1. Annual publication with quarterly supplements.

    2. Handy source of information about dosage and drug precautions.

Miscellaneous Resources

A. Package inserts from manufacturers that accompany the product.

B. Pharmacist.

C. Physician.

D. Nursing journals.

E. Pharmaceutical and medical treatment texts.

Appendix 5-1. SYSTEMS OF MEASUREMENT

Apothecary System

A. Older system based on unrelated, arbitrary units of measure; gradually being replaced by metric system.
   1. Portions of a unit of measurement designated by common fractions (e.g., one-fourth grain, written as gr $\frac{1}{4}$).
   2. Symbols for ounces and drams are similar in form and must be written clearly (e.g., ℨ is dram, ℥ is ounce).
   3. Symbols and abbreviations are placed before Roman numerals (5 grains written as gr v).
B. Common apothecary measures and symbols.

drop	gtt
minim	m
dram	ℨ
ounce	℥
pint	pt
grain	gr

C. Equivalents.

1 drop	= 1 minim
15 drops	= 1 grain
60 minims	= 1 fluid dram
8 fluid drams	= 1 fluid ounce
16 fluid ounces	= 1 pint

Metric System

A. French-invented system based on rationally and related derived units.
   1. Developed in the eighteenth century.
   2. Basic units of measure used in drug administration are the gram and liter.
   3. Other units are decimal, fractions, and Arabic numerals.
   4. Number and fraction placed before symbol.
B. Common metric measures and symbols.

gram	g, gm, *or* G
kilogram	kg
milligram	mg
milliliter	mL
liter	L *or* l

C. Weight and volume equivalents with corresponding symbols.

1 gram = 1000 milligrams	1 g = 1000 mg
1 liter = 1000 milliliters	1 L = 1000 mL

Household System

A. System based on familiar measures used in the home.
   1. Most measures not sufficiently accurate for measure of medicines.
   2. Pints and quarts also used in apothecary system.
B. Common household measures and their abbreviations.

pint	pt	tablespoon	T
teaspoon	t	quart	qt

Appendix 5-2. MATHEMATIC CONVERSIONS

Approximate Equivalents

A. The metric system is the universal system of weights and measures.
B. Apothecary and metric do not use same size units; denominations of one system not compatible with the other.
C. Conversion (Equivalency) Tables established to list measurement denominations of one system in terms of another. (*See* Appendix 5-4.)
   1. Conversion from one system to another can be computed, but is not equivalent in absolute terms.
   2. If there is occasion to compute, have computations checked by another licensed nurse.
      a. Do not compute unless allowed to do so by your state's Nurse Practice Act.
      b. Check hospital policy for further guidelines.

Computation

A. Drugs are not always labeled clearly as to number of tablets to administer, so computation may be necessary. Always have your computation checked by another licensed nurse.

B. Method.
   1. Both desired (ordered) dose and dose on hand must be in same unit of measurement (e.g., grains, grams, milligrams).
   2. If not the same, convert so that unit of measure is the same.
      a. Refer to Conversion Table (Appendix 5-4).
      b. To convert one measure unit to another, basic equivalencies must be memorized.
   3. After converting, divide desired dose by dose on hand to find amount to administer.

✦ Calculation of Dosages

A. Using equivalent tables to calculate drug dosages.
   1. To make conversions from the metric system to the apothecary or household system, it is necessary to memorize or refer to equivalency tables.
   2. To convert milligrams to grains, use the following formula:
   Example: Convert 180 milligrams to grains.

   $$\frac{1 \text{ gr}}{\text{mg in gr}} = \frac{\text{dose desired}}{\text{dose on hand}}$$

Continues

Appendix 5-2. MATHEMATIC CONVERSIONS *(Continued)*

$$\frac{1}{60} = \frac{x}{180}$$

$$60x = 180$$
$$x = 3 \text{ grains}$$

3. You may also make this conversion as a ratio:

1 gr:60 mg: :x gr:180 mg $60x = 180$
$$x = 3 \text{ grains}$$

4. Check equivalency tables in the drug supplement.

B. Calculating oral dosages of drugs.

1. To calculate oral dosages, use the following formula:

$$\frac{D}{H} = x$$

where D = dose desired
H = dose on hand
x = dose to be administered

Example: Give 500 mg of ampicillin when the dose on hand is in capsules containing 250 mg.

$$\frac{500 \text{ mg}}{250 \text{ mg}} = 2 \text{ capsules}$$

2. To calculate oral dosages of liquids, use the following formula:

$$\frac{D}{H} \times Q = x$$

where D = dose desired
H = dose on hand
Q = quantity
x = dose to be administered

Example: Give 375 mg of ampicillin when it is supplied as 250 mg/5 mL.

$$\frac{375 \text{ mg}}{250 \text{ mg}} \times 5$$

$$1.5 \times 5 = 7.5 \text{ mL}$$

You can also set up a direct proportion and, following the algebraic principle, cross multiply:

$$\frac{375 \text{ mg}}{x} = \frac{250 \text{ mg}}{5 \text{ mL}}$$

$$250x = 1875$$
$$x = 7.5 \text{ mL (of strength 250 mg/5 mL)}$$

C. Calculating parenteral dosages of drugs.

1. To calculate parenteral dosages, use the following formula:

$$\frac{D}{H} \times Q = x$$

Example: Give the client 40 mg gentamicin. On hand is a multidose vial with a strength of 80 mg/2 mL.

$$\frac{40}{80} \times 2 = 1 \text{ mL}$$

2. Check your calculations before drawing up the medication.

♦ **Calculation of Solutions**

A. Types of solutions.

1. Volume to volume (v/v): a given volume of solute is added to a given volume solvent.

2. Weight to weight (w/w): a stated weight of solute is dissolved in a stated weight of solvent.

3. Weight to volume (w/v): a given weight of solute is dissolved in a given volume of solvent, which results in the proper amount of solution.

B. Preparing solutions.

1. Solutions of varying strengths.

a. Determine the strength of the solution, the strength of the drug on hand, and the quantity of solution required.

b. Use this formula for preparing solutions:

$$\frac{D}{H} \times Q = x$$

where D = desired strength
H = strength on hand
Q = quantity of solution desired
x = amount of solute

2. *Example:* You have a 100% solution of hydrogen peroxide on hand. You need a liter of 50% solution.

$$\frac{(D)\ 50\%}{(H)\ 100\%} \times (Q)\ 1000 \text{ mL} = (x)\ 500 \text{ mL (solute)}$$

Add 500 mL of the solute to an additional 500 mL of desired solvent to make 1 liter of 50% solution.

C. If the strength desired and strength on hand are not in like terms, you need to change one of the terms.

1. *Example:* You have 1 liter of 50% solution on hand. You need a liter of 1:10 solution. 1:10 solution is the same as 10%.

$$\frac{10\%}{50\%} \times 1000 \text{ mL} = 200 \text{ mL}$$

Add 200 mL of the drug to 800 mL of the solvent to make 1 liter of 10% solution.

2. Volume to volume solutions. Use the formula:

$$\frac{D}{H} \times Q = x$$

where x = amount of stock solution used

Appendix 5-2. MATHEMATIC CONVERSIONS *(Continued)*

Example: Prepare 1 liter of 5% solution from a stock solution of 50%.

$$\frac{5\%}{50\%} \times 1000 \text{ mL} = 100 \text{ mL}$$

Add 100 mL to 900 mL of diluent to make 1 liter of 5% solution.

3. Solutions from tablets.
   a. Use the formula:

   $$\frac{D}{H} \times Q = x$$

   where x = amount/number of tablets used

   Example: Prepare 1 liter of a 1:1000 solution, using 10-grain tablets.

   $$\frac{1/1000}{10 \text{ gr}} \times 1000 \text{ mL} = x$$

   b. First convert 10 grains to grams so the numerator and the denominator are in the same unit of measure. 1 g = 15 gr; therefore, 10 g = 2/3 g. Now substitute the new numbers in the formula and solve for x.

   $$\frac{1/1000}{2/3} \times \frac{1000}{1} \text{ mL} = x$$

   $$\frac{3}{2000} \times \frac{1000}{1} \text{ mL} = x$$

   $x = {}^{3}\!/_{2}$ or $1{}^{1}\!/_{2}$ tablets

   Place $1{}^{1}\!/_{2}$ tablets into the 1 liter of solution and dissolve.

Appendix 5-3. ABBREVIATIONS AND SYMBOLS FOR ORDERS, PRESCRIPTIONS, AND LABELS

aa	of each	oz or ℥	ounce
AC	before meals	PC	after meals
ad lib	freely, as desired	per	by, through
Ba	barium	PO	by mouth
BID	twice each day	PRN	whenever necessary
c̄	with	QH	every hour
C	carbon	QID	four times each day
Ca	calcium	qs	as much as required
Cl	chlorine	q2h	every two hours
d or ʒ	dram	q3h	every three hours
et	and	q4h	every four hours
GI	gastrointestinal	Rx	treatment, "take thou"
gt or gtt	drop(s)	s̄	without
H_2O	water	s̄s̄	one-half ($^{1}\!/_{2}$)
H_2O_2	hydrogen peroxide	STAT	immediately
IM	intramuscular	TID	three times a day
in	inch	tsp	teaspoon
K	potassium	WBC	white blood cell
lb or #	pound	°	degree
m	minimum (a minim)	−	minus, negative, alkaline reaction
Mg	magnesium	+	plus, positive, acid reaction
N	nitrogen, normal	%	percent
Na	sodium	v	Roman numeral five
NPO	nothing by mouth	vii	Roman numeral seven
OD	every day	ix	Roman numeral nine
oob	out of bed	xiii	Roman numeral thirteen
os	mouth		

Appendix 5-4. CONVERSION TABLES

Table A. HOUSEHOLD EQUIVALENTS (Volume)

Metric	Apothecary	Household
0.06 mL	1 minim	1 drop
5(4) mL	1 fluid dram	1 teaspoonful
15 mL	4 fluid drams	1 tablespoonful
30 mL	1 fluid ounce	2 tablespoonfuls
180 mL	6 fluid ounces	1 teacupful
240 mL	8 fluid ounces	1 glassful

Table B. APOTHECARY EQUIVALENTS (Volume)

Metric		Apothecary
1.0	mL	= 15 minims
0.06	mL	= 1 minim
4.0	mL	= 1 fluid dram
30.0	mL	= 1 fluid ounce
500.0	mL	= 1 pint
1000.0	mL (1 L)	= 1 quart

Table C. APOTHECARY EQUIVALENTS (Weight)

Metric		Apothecary
4 g		1 dr
30 g		1 oz
1 kg		2.2 lb
1.0	g or 1000 mg	gr xv
0.65	g or 600 mg	gr x
0.5	g or 500 mg	gr viiss
0.33	g or 330 mg	gr v
0.2	g or 200 mg	gr iii
0.1	g or 100 mg	gr 1½
0.06	g or 60 mg	gr 1
0.05	g or 50 mg	gr ¾
0.03	g or 30 mg	gr ½
0.015	g or 15 mg	gr ¼
0.010	g or 10 mg	gr ⅛
0.008	g or 8 mg	gr ⅛

Appendix 5-5. MOST COMMONLY USED DRUGS*

Medical–Surgical Nursing

- Acetaminophen
- Amiodarone hydrochloride
- Diltiazem hydrochloride
- Dopamine hydrochloride
- Enalapril maleate
- Epinephrine hydrochloride
- Furosemide
- Heparin sodium
- Insulin
- Levofloxacin
- Lorazepam
- Metoprolol tartrate
- Morphine sulfate
- Nitroglycerin
- Potassium chloride

Maternity Nursing

- Acetaminophen/codeine
- Acetaminophen/oxycodone
- Dinoprostone
- Ibuprofen
- Magnesium sulfate
- Nalbuphine hydrochloride
- Oxytocin
- Penicillin
- Promethazine hydrochloride
- Terbutaline sulfate

Pediatric Nursing

- Albuterol
- Amoxicillin/clavulanate potassium
- Amoxicillin trihydrate
- Cetirizine hydrochloride
- Co-trimoxazole
- Fluticasone propionate
- Gentamicin sulfate
- Hydrocortisone (topical)
- Methylphenidate hydrochloride
- Montelukast sodium

Psychiatric Nursing

- Carbamazepine
- Clonazepam
- Divalproex sodium
- Escitalopram oxalate
- Lithium carbonate
- Olanzapine
- Paroxetine hydrochloride
- Risperidone
- Sertraline hydrochloride
- Venlafaxine hydrochloride

* Because these are the most commonly used drugs in each speciality area, be sure you are familiar with their action, side effects, and the average dosage. NCLEX focuses 13–19% of the test questions on this particular client need.

Adapted from: *2005 Nursing Spectrum drug handbook.* Available at *www.nursesdrughandbook.com.* Accessed October 12, 2004.

PHARMACOLOGY REVIEW QUESTIONS

1. Following surgery, a client has an order for nalbuphine HCl (Nubain) for moderate to severe pain. The assessment for possible adverse reactions should include observing for

   1. Blurred vision, palpitations, and urinary retention.
   2. Increased pulse rate, drowsiness, and nausea.
   3. Increased confusion, tachycardia, and anorexia.
   4. Irregular pulse, hypotension, and oliguria.

2. The nurse is assigned to a client who is receiving mydriatic eye drops. Which of the following symptoms indicates a systemic anticholinergic effect?

   1. Complaints of lightheadedness and headache.
   2. Respirations becoming more shallow.
   3. Sweating and blurred vision.
   4. Decreased pulse and blood pressure.

3. A female client with a history of multiple sclerosis has orders for dantrolene sodium (Dantrium). The nurse will know the client understands the action of the drug when she says

   1. "I need to use a sunscreen when I go outside."
   2. "I can't take any other medications when I'm on this drug."
   3. "I take this drug only when my spasms are bad."
   4. "I should see a marked change in my muscle strength within two to three days."

4. Bethanechol chloride (Urecholine) is ordered PRN for a client following a transurethral resection (TUR). Which of the following conditions would need to be present for the nurse to administer this drug?

   1. Complaints of bladder spasms.
   2. Complaints of severe pain.
   3. Inability to void.
   4. Frequent episodes of painful urination.

5. Which one of the statements is most accurate about the drug cimetidine (Tagamet) and should be discussed with clients who take the medication?

   1. Tagamet should be taken with an antacid to decrease GI distress, a common occurrence with the drug.
   2. Tagamet should be used cautiously with clients on Coumadin because it could inhibit the absorption of the drug.

   3. Tagamet should be taken on an empty stomach for better absorption.
   4. Tagamet is usually prescribed for long-term prevention of gastric ulcers.

6. You are caring for a client who is to receive 2000 units of heparin by IV push. The vial contains heparin 5000 U/mL. The client will receive _____ mL.

7. A client is receiving lithium carbonate for manic behavior. Administration of this medication should be guided by

   1. Maintaining a therapeutic dose of 900 mg TID.
   2. Encouraging regular blood studies (serum lithium levels) until the maintenance dose is stabilized.
   3. Telling the client that a lag of 7 to 10 days can be expected between the initiation of lithium therapy and the control of manic symptoms.
   4. Telling the client that muscle weakness indicates severe toxicity and the physician should be notified.

8. Some clients with severely active lupus erythematosus are managed with steroids. A positive response to steroid therapy would be evidenced by

   1. An increase in platelet count.
   2. A normal gamma globulin count.
   3. A decrease in anti-DNA titer.
   4. Negative syphilis serology.

9. A client in liver failure from cirrhosis with ascites is receiving spironolactone. The expected outcome when this drug is given is

   1. Increased urine sodium.
   2. Increased urinary output.
   3. Decreased potassium excretion.
   4. Prevention of metabolic alkalosis.

10. A client with a fractured right hip has Buck's traction applied and orders for prophylactic anticoagulant therapy. The nurse anticipates that the physician will order

    1. Aspirin.
    2. Dextran.
    3. Heparin.
    4. Coumadin.

11. A client with a urinary tract infection is given an aminoglycoside (gentamicin) antimicrobial therapy. The nurse understands that this drug is more active when the urine is

    1. Concentrated.
    2. Dilute.
    3. Alkaline.
    4. Acid.

12. A client with the diagnosis of systemic lupus erythematosus is placed on Plaquenil, an antimalarial drug, to reduce skin inflammation. A toxic reaction to this drug that the nurse will teach the client to report is

    1. Muscle cramps.
    2. Decreased visual acuity.
    3. Cardiac arrhythmias.
    4. Joint pain.

13. A client with thrombophlebitis has orders for continuous heparin infusion. What is the antidote that must be available?

    1. Vitamin K.
    2. Protamine sulfate.
    3. Mephyton.
    4. Calcium gluconate.

14. The physician orders dexamethasone (Decadron) to be administered to a client with a head injury. Based on nursing knowledge of this medication, the nurse would question the physician if he did not order which of the following additional medications?

    1. Morphine sulfate.
    2. Sodium bicarbonate.
    3. Cimetidine.
    4. Levophed.

15. A male client is currently taking Digitalis 0.25 mg daily, Lasix 100 mg daily, Acyclovir 10 mg QID, and Tagamet 300 mg QID. Which one of the following drugs has potential side effects that are the most life-threatening?

    1. Digitalis.
    2. Lasix.
    3. Acyclovir.
    4. Tagamet.

16. A client with the diagnosis of multiple sclerosis has the drug Baclofen ordered. The most accurate information the nurse should tell him about the drug is that he should

    1. Not drive a car until he knows if any CNS effects occur with the use of the drug.

    2. Take the medication on an empty stomach for better absorption.
    3. Notify the physician if diarrhea occurs.
    4. Notify the physician if any side effects occur.

17. Which of the following actions is *not* accurate or safe when administering a medication using the Z-track method?

    1. Placing 0.3 to 0.5 mL of air into the syringe.
    2. Using a 2- to 3-inch needle.
    3. Inserting the needle and injecting medication without aspirating.
    4. Pulling skin laterally away from the injection site before inserting the needle.

18. A 68-year-old client has an IV infusing at 50 mL per hour. The IV administration set delivers 15 gtt/mL. When adjusting the flow rate, the nurse would regulate the rate at _____ drops per minute.

19. After a client begins taking a prescribed antianxiety agent, the nurse would observe her for side effects of

    1. Sedation and slurred speech.
    2. Photosensitivity and muscular rigidity.
    3. Tremors and hypertension.
    4. A paradoxical reaction and hypoactivity.

20. When administering a one-time dose of Valium (a benzodiazepine drug) to a client, the nurse needs to inform the client that

    1. Valium has sedative properties.
    2. There are no important side effects to consider because it is a one-time dose.
    3. Valium should never be mixed with foods containing tyramine.
    4. Valium directly affects the blood pressure as a vasoconstrictor.

21. The drug that will most likely be used in the treatment of malignancy of the prostate is

    1. Human chorionic gonadotropin (HCG).
    2. Cytoxan.
    3. Diethylstilbestrol (DES).
    4. Nitrogen mustard.

22. A 65-year-old with the diagnosis of organic brain syndrome has orders for Seconal at bedtime. The nurse's understanding of this drug is that it has the effect on the body of

    1. Tranquilization.
    2. Sedation.

3. Mood elevation.
4. Stimulation.

23. A client has developed agranulocytosis as a result of medications he is taking. In counseling the client, the nurse knows that one of the most serious consequences of this condition is

1. The potential danger of excessive bleeding, even with minor trauma.
2. Generalized ecchymosis on exposed areas of the body.
3. High susceptibility to infection.
4. Extreme prostration.

24. The instructions to a client whose physician recently ordered nitroglycerin are that this medication should be taken

1. Every two to three hours during the day.
2. Before every meal and at bedtime.
3. At the first indication of chest pain.
4. Only when chest pain is not relieved by rest.

25. The nurse is counseling a client taking corticosteroids who has developed an infectious process. How would the infection affect the medication dosage?

1. Corticosteroid dose would be increased.
2. Corticosteroid dose would be discontinued.
3. Corticosteroid dose would be decreased.
4. There would be no change in dosage.

26. You have just admitted a client and you observe that he brought a bottle of ginkgo biloba with him to the hospital. When you ask, he says that he takes it every day to help his brain. The next question you should ask is

1. What does this do for your brain?
2. Did your physician prescribe this?
3. Which medications are you taking?
4. What are the side effects of ginkgo biloba?

27. You are admitting a pregnant woman with a diagnosis of pneumonia. She is six weeks pregnant. When taking her history, she tells you she is taking the herb feverfew for migraine headaches. You counsel her to

1. Continue with the herb.
2. Discontinue the herb while pregnant.
3. Ask her physician about taking the herb.
4. Go to her herbalist and ask about taking the herb while pregnant.

Please note that many questions on specific drugs, side effects, and other issues, are integrated throughout the text and relate to specific conditions or diseases.

PHARMACOLOGY

Answers with Rationale

1. (1)   These are symptoms associated with adverse reactions to Nubain. Drowsiness, nausea, confusion, bradycardia, and anorexia are also adverse reactions. Tachycardia (3), irregular pulse, and hypotension (4) are not symptoms associated with adverse effects of Nubain.

    NP:E; CN:PH; CA:S; CL:C

2. (3)   Sweating and blurred vision are signs of a systemic anticholinergic effect. In addition to these symptoms, the client may experience loss of sight, difficulty breathing, flushing, or eye pain. If these symptoms occur, the medication must be discontinued and the physician notified.

    NP:E; CN:PH; CA:M; CL:A

3. (1)   This drug has the potential for photosensitivity; therefore, the client should protect her skin by wearing a hat and using sunscreen.

    NP:E; CN:PH; CA:M; CL:A

4. (3)   Urecholine stimulates the parasympathetic nervous system. It increases the tone and motility of the smooth muscles of the urinary tract. It is used frequently following a TUR when the client has a lack of muscle tone and is unable to void. Bladder spasms can be relieved with belladonna or opium suppositories.

    NP:A; CN:PH; CA:S; CL:AN

5. (2)   Tagamet can interfere with the absorption of Coumadin and several other drugs such as Dilantin, Lidocaine, or Inderal; therefore, the serum levels of the drugs should be monitored closely. Tagamet should not be taken within one hour of an antacid, because this will interfere with the absorption (1). It is best to take the drug with food (3). Tagamet is usually ordered for short-term treatment of duodenal and active gastric ulcers (4).

    NP:AN; CN:PH; CA:M; CL:A

6. The answer is *0.4 mL.* Divide 5000 units into 2000 units and the answer is 0.4 mL.

    NP:P; CN:PH; CA:M; CL:A

7. (3)   There will be 7 to 10 days before the client will experience a decrease in the manic symptoms. A therapeutic dose is 300 mg TID (1); regular blood studies must be continued throughout drug therapy (2); muscle weakness is an expected side effect and does not indicate toxicity (4).

    NP:P; CN:PH; CA:PS; CL:A

8. (3)   Anti-DNA antibody levels correlate most specifically with lupus disease activity. A positive response to steroids would show a decrease in these levels. Twenty percent of clients with lupus develop a positive syphilis serology (4), and many have hypergamma-globulinemia (2) and a decreased platelet count (1).

    NP:E; CN:PH; CA:M; CL:A

9. (1)   The primary action of spironolactone is to increase urine sodium and thereby cause diuresis. It is also potassium sparing (3) and helps counteract metabolic alkalosis (4) by this mechanism.

    NP:E; CN:PS; CA:M; CL:AN

10. (3)   Anticoagulant prophylaxis would be initiated with intermittent heparin therapy, which is effective immediately. Dextran (2) is frequently given postoperatively, and aspirin (1) is used in the recovery period during hospitalization to prevent venous thrombosis.

    NP:P; CN:PH; CA:S; CL:C

11. (3)   Aminoglycoside antibiotics are more active when the urine is alkaline, and the client may receive soda bicarbonate to accomplish creating this environment.

    NP:AN; CN:PH; CA:M; CL:A

Coding for Questions/Answers Abbreviations: **Nursing Process: NP,** Assessment: A, Analysis: AN, Planning: P, Implementation: I, Evaluation: E; **Client Needs: CN,** Safe, Effective Care Environment: S, Health Promotion and Maintenance: H, Psychosocial Integrity: PS, Physiological Integrity: PH; **Clinical Area: CA,** Medical Nursing: M, Surgical Nursing: S, Maternal/Newborn Nursing: MA, Pediatric Nursing: P, Psychiatric Nursing: PS; **Cognitive Level: CL,** Knowledge: K, Comprehension: C, Application: A, Analysis: AN.

12. (2) Retinal damage can occur with the use of Plaquenil; the client should be assessed regularly for visual acuity.

NP:E; CN:PH; CA:M; CL:C

13. (2) The heparin antidote is protamine sulfate. Answers (1) and (3) are antidotes to coumarin derivatives. Calcium gluconate is given for hypocalcemia (4).

NP:I; CN:PH; CA:M; CL:A

14. (3) Dexamethasone (Decadron) is an anti-inflammatory corticosteroid used in the treatment and prevention of cerebral edema. It is a very potent drug, often prescribed preoperatively and continued postoperatively for the neurosurgery client. Because the drug is irritating to the GI tract, it should be administered with antacids such as Maalox or Mylanta, or with drugs used to reduce gastric secretions such as cimetidine (Tagamet) (3) or rantidine (Zantac). The nurse must be alert for signs of toxic side effects associated with steroid administration. In particular, the nurse must know that the drug must never be abruptly withdrawn and a gradual tapering of the dose is necessary.

NP:E; CN:PH; CA:M; CL:AN

15. (2) Although each of these drugs has significant side effects, Lasix has the potential for life-threatening cardiac arrhythmias. Potassium is lost as a result of the drug use. Because 100 mg is a large dose, a low serum potassium level could easily occur, leading to ventricular arrhythmias.

NP:E; CN:PH; CA:M; CL:AN

16. (1) Several CNS-related side effects are common, including drowsiness, dizziness, headache, and confusion. Therefore, until the client knows if he will experience these side effects, he should not drive a car. The drug causes nausea and GI distress, so it should be taken with milk or meals (2). Constipation is a common side effect (3) and, therefore, a mild laxative should also be ordered.

NP:I; CN:PH; CA:M; CL:A

17. (3) This is not accurate or safe because the nurse should pull back on the plunger, or aspirate. This would ensure that the needle had not entered a blood vessel. This action would be included in the Z-track method.

NP:I; CN:PH; CA:M; CL:C

18. The answer is *12 drops per minute*. To calculate the drip factor, multiply the hourly rate times the drop factor (50 mL × 15). Divide the answer by 60 minutes (750/60 = 12.5 gtt/min). Round off the answer to 12.

NP:I; CN:PH; CA:M; CL:A

19. (1) Sedation and slurred speech are the primary side effects. Photosensitivity, an increased susceptibility to sunlight and sunburn, is a common side effect of antipsychotic medications. Muscular rigidity (2) is not a side effect of these medications; in fact, the antianxiety agents often act as muscle relaxants.

NP:A; CN:PH; CA:PS; CL:A

20. (1) Valium has sedative properties, and the client needs to be warned about possible side effects. For example, driving while taking Valium is dangerous. Also important is to inform the client about the life-threatening danger of mixing this drug with alcohol.

NP:AN; CN:PH; CA:PS; CL:A

21. (3) DES is used to treat cancer of the prostate. It antagonizes the androgens required by the androgen-dependent neoplasm. HCG (1) is used for treatment of undescended testicles in young boys. Cytoxan (2) and nitrogen mustard (4) are used in Hodgkin's disease.

NP:P; CN:PH; CA:M; CL:K

22. (2) Seconal is a common barbiturate used for sleeplessness. It has a sedative effect on the CNS. Its use should be monitored because of potential addiction or overdose, especially with the elderly.

NP:E; CN:PH; CA:PS; CL:C

23. (3) Agranulocytosis is characterized by neutropenia (decreased number of lymphocytes), which lowers the body defenses against infection. Granulocytes are the first barrier to infection in the body.

NP:AN; CN:PH; CA:M; CL:A

24. (3) Nitroglycerin should be taken whenever the client feels a full, pressure feeling or tightness in his chest, not waiting until chest pain is severe. It can also be taken prophylactically before engaging in an activity known to cause angina in order to prevent an anginal attack.

NP:I; CN:PH; CA:M; CL:A

25. (1) Infectious processes increase the body's need for steroids. During times of stress (infection), the dose needs to be increased to prevent adrenal insufficiency in previously steroid-dependent clients.

NP:AN; CN:PH; CA:M; CL:AN

26. (3) You would immediately want to know what medications he is taking because ginkgo biloba interferes with the action of Coumadin, aspirin, NSAIDs, digoxin, and insulin. The herb is also dangerous for anyone with blood clotting problems, high blood pressure, asthma or emphysema. Answers (1) and (4) are not as important, and answer (2) would be asked after option (1).

NP:AN; CN:PH; CA:M; CL:AN

27. (2) She should immediately discontinue taking feverfew because it interferes with platelet action. Her physician may not be aware that she is taking herbs, so it is important when taking any client's history to ask about medicinal herbs the client is taking, and check them against the prescribed medications.

NP:I; CN:PH; CA:MA; CL:A

Infection Control

✦ The icon denotes content of special importance for NCLEX.

INFECTION

The Infectious Process

A. For an infection to occur, a process involving six links or steps must be present.
1. If any links are missing, the infection will not occur.
2. Infection control measures can interrupt the process by eliminating one or more of the steps.
✦ B. Six links form the chain of infection.
1. Infectious agent (microorganism): bacteria, virus, fungi, etc.
    a. Capability of producing an infection depends on
        (1) Virulence and number of organisms present.
        (2) Susceptibility of host.
        (3) Existence of portal of entry.
        (4) Affinity of host to harbor micro-organism.
    b. The circumstances above must be present to produce an infection.
2. Reservoir: people, equipment, water, etc., provides survival for organism.
    a. Appropriate environment for growth and multiplication of microorganism must be present.
    b. Reservoirs include respiratory, gastro-intestinal, reproductive and urinary tracts, and the blood.
3. Portal of exit: allows the microorganism to move from reservoir to host (includes excretions, secretions, skin, droplets).
✦ 4. Route of transmission of microorganisms: five routes. Three primary (contact, droplet and airborne); two lesser routes [vehicle (contaminated items such as food, water, and devices) and vector (e.g., mosquitoes, fleas, rats)].
    a. *Contact*—most frequent source of nosoco-mial infection.
        (1) Direct contact—transmission body to body and physical transmission (sexual intercourse, kissing or touch).
        (2) Indirect contact—contact with con-taminated intermediate object (needle, dressing, dirty hands).
    b. *Droplet*—transmission of large particle droplets (larger than 5 microns); diphthe-ria, pertussis, pneumonia, etc.
    c. *Airborne*—transmission of small particle droplets or residue of 5 microns (measles, varicella, TB).
    d. Two lesser routes.
        (1) *Common vehicle:* transmission by con-taminated items such as food, water, devices.
        (2) *Vector borne:* mosquitoes, fleas, rats, etc.
5. Portal of entry: mucous membrane, gastroin-testinal (GI) tract, genitourinary (GU) tract, respiratory tract, and nonintact skin.
6. Susceptible host: a host who is immunosup-pressed, fatigued, malnourished, weakened by other diseases, elderly, stressed, or hospitalized with wounds, IVs, and catheters is at high risk.

Barriers to Infection

✦ A. The primary barrier to infection is the individual's general health and immunologic system (defense mechanisms).
B. Factors that contribute to infection susceptibility.
1. Disease states.
2. Altered nutritional status.
3. Stress and fatigue.
4. Metabolic function.
5. Age.
6. Medications.
✦ C. The body's protection against infection.
1. The immune process.
    a. Natural immunity is inherited.
    b. Acquired immunity comes from disease exposure or vaccinations.
2. Anatomic barriers (skin and mucous membranes).
    a. Integrity of the skin and mucous membrane—when integrity is broken, bac-teria can enter the body.
    b. How quickly a wound heals depends on the degree of vascularization in the injured area.
3. The inflammatory process.
    a. When an area is inflamed, cells activate the plasmin, clotting, and kinin systems to release histamine.
    b. Histamine creates increased vascular per-meability at the injured site.
    c. Phagocytes are summoned to the site to combat the infection.
D. Assessing the probability of infection.
1. Considering the numbers of organisms, viru-lence and resistance of the host, the client's risk factors can be evaluated.
2. Combining these variables with the client's general health and immune status, the probabil-ity of nosocomial infection can be assessed.
✦ E. Conditions predisposing client to infection.
1. Surgical wounds.
2. Alterations in the respiratory or genitourinary tracts (most common sites for nosocomial infections).

3. Invasive devices such as central lines or venipuncture sites.
4. Implanted prosthetic devices—cardiac valves, grafts, shunts, or orthopedic joints or pins.

CDC GUIDELINES

Principles of Precautions

✦ A. Risk reduction.
   1. Standard Precautions—hand hygiene is primary method.
   2. Follow procedures to recognize and reduce risks.
   3. Assign infection control practitioner for every 250 beds.
   4. Have hospital epidemiologist on site.
   5. Program of surveillance for nosocomial infections with appropriate interventions.
B. The CDC guidelines, revised in 1994, contain two tiers of precautions.
✦ C. First-tier *Standard Precautions* blend the major features of universal precautions (blood and body fluids precautions) and body substance isolation into a single set of precautions.
   1. Used for the care of all clients in hospitals regardless of diagnosis or infection status.
   2. Applies to blood, all body fluids, secretions, and excretions, whether or not they contain visible blood; nonintact skin; and mucous membranes.
   3. Standard Precautions are designed to reduce the risk of transmission of both recognized and unrecognized sources of infection in hospitals.
   4. As a result of the new category of Standard Precautions, clients with diseases or conditions that previously required category-specific or disease-specific precautions are now covered under this category and do not require additional precautions.
✦ D. Second tier *Transmission-Based Precautions* are designed only for the care of specified clients. They reduce the disease-specific precautions into three sets of precautions based on routes of transmission.
   1. Categories designed for clients documented or suspected to be infected or colonized with highly transmissible or epidemiologically important pathogens for which additional precautions must be used to interrupt transmission to others in the hospital.
   ✦ 2. Three types of transmission-based precautions include airborne precautions, droplet precautions, and contact precautions.
      a. *Airborne precautions* reduce the risk of airborne transmission of infectious agents, such as measles, varicella, and tuberculosis.
      b. *Droplet precautions* are used to prevent the transmission of diseases such as meningitis, pneumonia, scarlet fever, diphtheria, rubella, and pertusis.
      c. *Contact precautions* are used for clients known or suspected to have serious illnesses easily transmitted by direct contact, such as herpes simplex, staphylococcal infections, hepatitis A, respiratory syncytial virus, and wound or skin infections.
   3. All three types of precautions may be used at one time when multiple routes of transmission are suspected in a client. These precautions are always used in conjunction with Standard Precautions. Table 6-1 outlines recommendations for transmission-based precautions.
E. Transmission-based precautions are used (in addition to Standard Precautions) when a client is infected with microorganisms or communicable disease.
   ✦ 1. Airborne precautions.
      a. Implemented when infections can spread through the air (TB, chickenpox, rubeola).
      b. Pathogens can be suspended in air for long periods and are transmitted when a person inhales particles that contain the pathogen.
      c. Healthcare workers should wear HEPA (high-efficiency particulate air) filter respirators when working with clients who have TB.
   ✦ 2. Droplet precautions.
      a. This system used when caring for clients who have infections that spread by large-particle droplets containing microorganisms (includes rubella, diphtheria, mumps, pertussis, influenza).
      b. Clients with this type of infection should be in a private room or with another client with same disease.
      c. Healthcare workers should wear a surgical mask for protection when coming within 3 feet of client.
   ✦ 3. Contact precautions.
      a. These precautions are used when caring for clients infected or colonized by microorganisms that spread by direct contact (skin to skin) or indirect contact (touch) with a contaminated object.
      b. Client requires private room or room with another client with same illness.
      c. Wear gloves when entering room and change gloves as needed during care. Remove gloves and wash hands when leaving client's room.

Table 6-1. HICPAC* RECOMMENDATIONS FOR TRANSMISSION-BASED PRECAUTIONS

	Contact	Droplet	Airborne
Purpose	Prevent transmission of known or suspected infected or colonized microorganisms by direct hand or skin-to-skin contact that occurs when providing direct client care. Conditions in which contact precautions are required: diphtheria, herpes simplex, scabies, *Staphylococcus* infection, hepatitis A, and respiratory syncytial virus wound or skin infection	Prevent transmission of large-particle droplets, larger than 5 microns (μm) (i.e., diphtheria, pertussis, streptococcal pharyngitis, pneumonia, scarlet fever, meningitis, rubella)	Prevent transmission of small-particle residue of 5 microns (μm) or smaller droplets (i.e., measles, varicella, tuberculosis)
Client placement	• Private room • Can be placed in room of client with same microorganism	• Private room • Can be placed in room of client with same diagnosis	• Private room • Can be placed in room of client with same diagnosis • Monitor negative air pressure • Keep door closed • Keep client in room
Respiratory protection	• Mask not necessary	• Use mask when working within 3 feet of client	• Respiratory protective equipment • Do not enter room of clients with rubeola or varicella if susceptible to these infections
Gloves and gown	• Wear gloves when entering room • Change gloves after contact with infective material, such as wound drainage or fecal material • Wash hands immediately after removing gloves • Wear gown when working with clients with diarrhea, ostomies, or wound drainage not contained in dressing • Wear gown if contact with client or environment will occur	• Follow Standard Precautions	• Follow Standard Precautions
Client transport	• Transport only if essential • Ensure precautions are maintained to minimize risk of transmission	• Transport only if essential • Place mask on client when outside room	• Transport only if essential • Place mask on client when outside room
Client care items	• Client care items and environmental surfaces are cleaned daily • Dedicate equipment to single client use (i.e., stethoscope, thermometer)		

*Hospital Infection Control Practices Advisory Committee.

Source: Adapted from Department of Health and Human Services: CDC, *Federal Register*, "Guidelines for Isolation Precautions in Hospitals."

d. Wear gown if clothing may come into contact with clients, environmental surfaces, or items in client's room, if client has diarrhea, wound drainage, or GI surgery.

e. Use dedicated equipment when a client has multiple-resistant microorganisms.

✦ F. Transmission guidelines.

1. Infections and conditions fall into two categories because microorganisms are transmitted in more than one way.

a. Chickenpox and zoster can spread through both airborne and contact routes.

b. Adenovirus infection can spread through droplet and contact.

2. If client's infection spreads through two transmission routes, institute both precautions and hang both signs on client's door.

✦ G. Transmission-based precautions and client transfer.

1. When client is transferred to another unit or area for testing, client must wear a mask and impervious dressing.

2. Transporter takes necessary precautions and wears appropriate barriers.

3. Staff in receiving area have been notified and understand precautions.

✦ H. Methods of infection prevention.

1. Vaccinations.

a. Currently more than 25 vaccines licensed in United States.

b. Preventive vaccines: smallpox, measles, mumps, rubella, polio, diphtheria, pertussis, and tetanus.

c. Goal of vaccines—prevent specific infectious diseases in a specific population.

2. Education.

Standard Precautions

✦ A. The term *Standard Precautions* incorporates universal blood and body fluid precautions.

✦ B. Apply Standard Precautions to all clients regardless of diagnosis or infection status.

✦ C. The following guidelines are recommended by the Centers for Disease Control and Prevention (CDC) for use with all clients (whether identified as infectious or not) to prevent transmission of infections. Please follow these guidelines when caring for clients.

1. Hand hygiene—wash hands thoroughly with soap and water or alcohol-based handrub or gel before and after all client contact. Wash hands and change gloves between contact with clients.

2. Wear gloves if there is a possibility of direct contact with blood or bodily secretions (e.g., pus, sputum, urine, feces, blood, saliva).

a. This includes a neonate before first bath.

b. Wash as soon as possible if unanticipated contact with these body substances occurs.

3. Gloves should be worn when in contact with items or surfaces soiled with blood or body fluids.

4. In 2003, the CDC stated that healthcare workers in contact with clients must remove all false fingernails.

5. Protect clothing with gowns or plastic aprons if there is a possibility of being splashed or direct contact with contaminated material.

6. Wear masks and/or goggles or face shields to avoid being splashed, especially during suctioning, irrigations, and deliveries.

7. Do not break needles into receptacles; rather, discard them intact and uncapped into containers.

HEALTHCARE-ASSOCIATED INFECTIONS (HAIs)

Risks of Hospitalization

A. In 2007, the CDC replaced the term "nosocomial infections" with HAI. The term was revised to reflect changes in healthcare development.

✦ B. Major risk—nosocomial infections; leading cause of death in United States.

1. More than 90,000 deaths/year as direct or indirect result of infections (CDC).

2. These infections begin in hospital or healthcare facility—each year 2 million clients in the United States acquire infections in these settings (CDC).

3. Major source of nosocomials: healthcare workers and clients are reservoirs.

4. One-third of all nosocomials could be prevented with effective infection control programs in healthcare facilities.

5. CDC states these figures can be reduced with client education and strict adherence to infection control practices.

6. A CDC study in 2000 showed that infections contracted in hospitals by clients hospitalized for other health reasons cost $5 billion/year.

✦ C. Most common sites for infection.

1. Urinary tract infections most common (80% related to catheterization).

2. Pneumonia second most common nosocomial.

a. Affects 40 percent of all critically ill or immunocompromised clients.

b. Causes 15 percent of all in-hospital deaths.

3. Surgical wound infections—account for 60 percent of additional hospital days.

D. Intravascular devices present increased risk.
  1. Risk of infection related to device itself, site of insertion, and technique of insertion.
  2. *Staphylococcus* is usual cause of infection and bacteremia.

E. Drug-resistant strains of pathogens are increasing nosocomials.
  1. Major organisms: *Clostridium difficile*, *Staphylococcus aureus* (MRSA), and vancomycin-resistant enterococcus (VRE).
  2. Vancomycin-resistant enterococcus (VRE) was a serious development in the 1990s.
    a. *Enterococcus faecium* (called a supergerm) frequently invades surgical wounds, heart valve replacements, and abdominal and urinary tracts.
    b. Enterococcal infections are often impervious to antibiotics—25 percent of these infections in intensive care clients were untreatable.
  3. The most common is *C. difficile*, an anaerobic, gram-positive, spore-forming bacillus associated with infectious diarrhea.
  4. Methicillin-resistant *Staphylococcus aureus* (MRSA).
  5. Resistant strain of *Mycobacterium tuberculosis*.

F. In April 2000, the FDA approved a new super antibiotic called Zyvox, which is a new weapon against drug-resistant infections.
  1. The first entirely new type of antibiotic in 35 years.
  2. Drug should be reserved to fight life-threatening infections that are resistant to other antibiotics.

Basic Infection Control Measures

A. Hand hygiene.
  1. Many nurses believe wearing gloves eliminates the need to wash hands—not so!
    a. Donning gloves with unclean hands can transfer microorganisms to outside of glove. (People carry between 10,000 and 10 million bacteria on each hand.)
    b. It is important to wash hands between client contacts *and* before and after using gloves.
  2. Proper method of washing hands.
    a. Wet hands with warm running water.
    b. Apply soap or antimicrobial agent.
    c. Rub hands together vigorously for at least 10 to 15 seconds—include all surfaces of fingers and hands.
    d. Rinse hands thoroughly under running water to remove all soap.
    e. Dry hands with paper towels removed one at a time from dispenser.
    f. Use paper towel to turn off faucet if there is no foot pedal.
  3. Washing with waterless agents.
    a. Use only if hands are free of obvious dirt.
    b. Apply small amount on palm of hand.
    c. Rub hands together vigorously, covering all surfaces of hands and fingers.
    d. Rub until dry.

B. Gloving: basic infection control measure.
  1. The Occupational Safety and Health Administration (OSHA) stipulates that gloves in all sizes are to be available for healthcare workers.
  2. Gloves necessary for any task or procedure that may result in blood or body fluid exposure to hands.
  3. Important to change gloves *and* wash hands between clients.

C. Latex allergy to gloves.
  1. Affects 8 to 12 percent of healthcare workers.
  2. Assess allergy to avocados, bananas, kiwi fruit or chestnuts. Client may have cross-sensitivity to latex.
  3. Classified as immediate immunological reaction caused by latex proteins.
  4. Reaction may progress to anaphylaxis.
  5. Know symptoms of latex allergy: contact dermatitis, local swelling, itching, hives, redness.
  6. If healthcare worker thinks he or she has latex allergy, they should switch to latex-free gloves *immediately*.

D. Items needed as protective barriers.
  1. Gloves most common barrier protection: protects health workers from mucous membranes, wounds, or infectious body substances.
  2. Face mask: prevents airborne infection. Change mask every 30 minutes or sooner if it becomes damp.
  3. Face shield or goggles: reduces risk of contamination of mucous membranes of eyes. Wear when there is risk of being sprayed or splashed with contaminated body fluids.
  4. Gown: protects clothing from splashed blood or body fluids.

E. Removing protective garb.
  1. Untie ties of gown if tied in front (ties are contaminated).
  2. Remove gloves.
    a. Do not touch outer surface to skin.
    b. Pull first glove down, turning inside out as you pull it off.
    c. Insert two fingers of ungloved hand inside glove edge and pull downward.

d. Discard gloves in paper receptacle.

3. Remove gown: unfasten waist ties (if tied in back), then neck ties. Pull gown off shoulders and over arms, turning gown inside out as it is removed, and discard.

4. Remove face shield or goggles (do not touch face) and discard.

5. Remove mask: untie lower string first, then upper strings, and discard.

6. Complete procedure by washing hands.

✦ F. Isolation protocol.
   1. Prepare for isolation.
      a. Check physician's orders.
      b. Obtain isolation cart.
      c. Place isolation cart at client's door.
      d. Place a linen hamper and trash cans conveniently.
   2. Follow dressing procedure when entering or leaving room.
      a. Gown or wear plastic apron.
      b. Use a mask (HEPA filter recommended).
      c. Use an eyeshield or goggles if appropriate.
   3. Remove items from isolation room by double-bagging (using red biohazard bags).

G. Governmental regulatory agencies.
   ✦ 1. CDC goal is disease reduction.
   ✦ 2. OSHA goal is to reduce risk exposure.
   3. OSHA requires that healthcare facilities have educational protocols in place for prevention of blood-borne pathogens and hepatitis B control.

Healthcare–Associated Infections (Nosocomial Infections)

Definition: Infections acquired while the client is in the hospital—infections that were not present or were incubating at the time of admission.

A. Affects more than 2 million and estimated to cause or contribute to more than 90,000 deaths annually in the United States.

B. Many of these infections are caused by pathogens transmitted from one client to another by healthcare workers.

C. Usually caused by poor or no hand hygiene technique between clients.

Nosocomial Infectious Diarrhea

✦ A. Most common cause is *Clostridium difficile*–associated diarrhea (CDAD) infectious diarrhea.
   1. Anaerobic, gram-positive bacillus—20 to 40 percent of hospitalized clients become colonized within a few days of entering hospital.
   2. Spores and microbes found on hospital toilets, bedpans, floors, and healthcare workers' hands.

HANDLING BIOHAZARD WASTE

Biohazard waste is any solid or liquid waste that presents a threat of infection

- Separate at point of origin or before it leaves client's room—reduces risk of exposure.
- Use impermeable red plastic bag labeled "biohazard." Close securely and double bag.
- Red bags cannot be placed with other they could contaminate all waste.

Storage of biohazard material

- Appropriately sealed. May be stored for 30 days.
- Waste must be restricted, locked up or stored separately.
- Waste must be labeled correctly so tracking may be done.

✦ B. Recognizing signs and symptoms of CDAD.
   1. Diarrhea occurring after antibiotics.
   2. Abdominal pain—crampy pain and abdominal tenderness.
   3. Fever—above 102.2°F (39°C).
   4. Leukocytosis—WBCs can go as high as 50,000/mm^3 (average is 4500 to 11,000).
   5. Lab tests will confirm CDAD with a positive stool assay for toxin A or B and autotoxin neutralization test.

✦ C. Preventive methods.
   ✦ 1. Wash hands before and after client contact *and* after removing gloves with antiseptic soap. *Alert:* The alcohol-based gels do *not* kill *C. difficile*, so soap and water must be used.
   2. In addition to Standard Precautions, institute contact isolation precautions—includes placing client in a private room and always wearing gloves and gown when in direct contact with client.
   3. After removing gloves and gown, do not touch any potentially contaminated surface.
   4. Use dedicated equipment such as stethoscope and BP cuff—*never* use electronic thermometer because of the potential for spreading bacteria.
   5. Dispose of all contaminated items (bed linens, towel) in proper receptacles.
   6. Instruct family and friends to use infection precautions.

D. Treatment.
   1. Antibiotics for a mild case.
   2. For more severe cases, the physician may discontinue the antibiotic and start antimicrobial therapy (metronidazole drug of choice).
   3. CDC has recently advised against using vancomycin to treat CDAD because of vancomycin-resistant enterococcus (VRE).

Nosocomial Pneumonia

✦ A. Second most common infection—affects 40 percent of all critically ill or immunosuppressed clients.
  1. Aspiration of gram-negative bacteria are typically acquired in the hospital.
  2. Gram-positive strain *(Staphylococcus aureus)* is leading cause of condition; develops into methicillin-resistant condition (MRSA).
     a. Vancomycin, drug of choice to treat MRSA, is rapidly losing its effectiveness.
     b. MRSA may occur when food, fluid, or gastric contents enter lung via aspiration.
     c. MRSA may also occur when airborne particles are inhaled through respirations or anesthesia equipment.
  3. Viral pneumonia (causes 20 percent of all nosocomials). Most common are adenoviruses, influenza, and respiratory syncytial viruses (RSV).
  4. Fungal pneumonia *Aspergillus* through contact with unfiltered air system, food, or plants.
✦ B. Preventive measures.
  1. Change ventilator tubing no more frequently than every 48 hours.
  2. Use closed suction system.
  3. Remove pooled secretions above cuff when endotracheal (ET) tube is repositioned.
  4. Provide frequent mouth care.
  5. Provide 100 percent relative humidity at body temperature with all ventilation systems (will help client fight off pneumonia infection).
  6. Recognizing signs and symptoms.
     a. Onset 72 hours after hospital admission.
     b. Crackles in lung and dullness on percussion.
     c. Purulent sputum.
     d. Positive bacterial or fungal culture.
     e. In elderly client, may be confusion and fatigue with no fever.
  C. Treatment.
  1. Administer antibiotics as prescribed.
  2. Observe for dyspnea, respiratory rate, and administer O_2 (as prescribed) to maintain paO_2 at 80 mm Hg plus.
  3. Position client at 45-degree angle.
  4. Encourage fluid intake—good nutrition.
  5. Encourage incentive spirometry.

✦ Nosocomial Bloodstream Infections

  A. Types of infection.
  1. Presence of bacteria in bloodstream.
  2. Fungemia—infection in bloodstream caused by a fungal organism.
✦ B. Two categories of infection.

  1. Primary infection means host has no preexisting infection but there is direct introduction of microorganisms into bloodstream and host becomes infected via external (catheter) or internal means (internal tubing during manipulation).
  2. Secondary infection occurs when host has another site of infection (urinary tract) that enters bloodstream.
✦ C. Preventive measures.
  1. IV therapy increases risk of invasion by harmful microorganisms (invasive devices and venipuncture sites provide route for infection to occur).
  2. Use of impeccable Standard Precaution methods will reduce risk.

Nosocomial Tuberculosis

✦ A. Tuberculosis is an infectious disease caused by the tubercle bacillus *Mycobacterium tuberculosis.*
  1. Currently 100 million afflicted—30 to 40 million will die and 1/3 may be resistant.
  2. Main reservoir for the organism is respiratory tract.
  3. Transmission occurs between individuals through respiratory contact via droplets transmitted through productive coughing.
✦ B. Symptoms.
  1. Occur 4–12 weeks after exposure.
  2. Active disease and symptoms of cough, weight loss, and fever usually occur within first 2 years after infection.
  3. Latent infections (asymptomatic) are not infectious and may last a lifetime.
  4. Without treatment, tuberculosis progresses.
✦ C. Multidrug-resistant tuberculosis (MDR-TB).
  1. Disease can progress from diagnosis to death in 4–15 weeks.
  2. Clients develop resistance to standard drug regimen as a result of noncompliance and/or inappropriate drug therapy.
  3. MDR-TB also caused by person-to-person contact through sneezing or coughing, or from a person with primary drug resistance.
  4. According to the CDC, MDR-TB accounts for 1.2 percent of TB cases.
✦ D. Effective tuberculosis control requirements: early identification, isolation, and treatment of persons with active tuberculosis.
  1. Purified protein derivative (PPD) skin test used to quickly identify infection in the absence of clinical symptoms.
  2. Sputum specimens for acid-fast bacilli (AFB), culture, sensitivity, and chest x-rays.
     a. PPD skin test is read 48–72 hours after the injection.

b. Positive skin test is indicated by an induration of 10 mm or more at site of injection.

c. HIV or immunosuppressed—5 mm or more is considered positive. If positive, chest x-ray will rule out active TB.

✦ 3. CDC recommendation for tuberculosis isolation—directional air-flow, negative-pressure ventilation system in room.

a. Anyone entering the client's room should wear a mask that forms a tight-fitting seal against particulates 1–5 μ.

b. Disposable particulate respirators are suggested by the CDC when adequate ventilation is not available in the room.

Nosocomial Infected Wounds

✦ A. The longer a person is hospitalized prior to the surgical procedure, the greater risk of postsurgical infection.

B. Factors that influence infection rates.
1. Duration of time in the operating room.
2. Time surgery is done (between midnight and 8 AM is period of greatest risk).
3. Whether client has postsurgical drains in place.
4. If the surgery enters a colonized or infected part of the body.

EMERGING VIRUSES

Biology of Infectious Disease

A. Various forms of flora help protect the human from invasion of pathogens, usually microorganisms that can cause disease.

B. Host defenses determine whether infection will occur.
1. Natural barriers: skin and mucous membranes.
2. Nonspecific immune responses: white cells.
3. Specific immune responses: antibodies.

C. Pathogenesis of infection.
1. Toxins: protein molecules that cause development of disease (diphtheria, cholera, tetanus, etc.).
2. Virulence factors: assist pathogens in invasion and resistance of host defense mechanisms (different forms of *H. influenzae*).
3. Microbial adherence: ability to adhere to surfaces to invade tissue (*Escherichia coli* attaching to human cells in GI tract).
4. Antimicrobial resistance: agents that can exert selective pressures on microbial populations allowing bacteria to develop resistance to an antimicrobial agent (MRSA).

Marburg and Ebola Viruses

Definition: Acute infection (perhaps related to exposure to monkeys in Africa or the Philippines) that produces severe illness.

Characteristics

A. Vector is unknown, human to human.
B. Transmission occurs via skin and mucous membrane contact with an infected person.
C. Incubation period is 5–10 days.
D. Mortality rate is 25–90%.

Assessment

A. Fever with myalgia and headache with upper respiratory symptoms.
B. Hemorrhagic symptoms begin within a few days.

Implementation

A. Mask-gown-glove precautions.
B. There is no vaccine or effective antiviral therapy.

Hanta Virus

Definition: Acute infection caused by the hanta virus transmitted to humans from rodents.

Characteristics

A. Transmission is through inhalation of infectious aerosols from rodent excreta.
B. Characterized by acute renal failure or acute pulmonary edema.
C. Incubation period 7–36 days.

Assessment

A. Sudden onset with high fever, headache, backache and abdominal pain.
B. Hemorrhages appear; severe neurological symptoms occur in 1%; severe cases are 10–15%.

Implementation

A. Treatment is ribavirin IV and supportive care.
B. Overall mortality rate is 6–15%.

Lassa Fever

Definition: Systemic arena virus infection that involves visceral organs; spares the CNS.

Characteristics

A. Most human cases result from contamination of food with rodent urine; human to human transmission can occur.
B. Mortality rate between 16–45%.
C. Incubation period 1–24 days.

Assessment

A. Initial symptoms are sore throat, fever, headache, myalgia and malaise.

B. Onset of severe symptoms take several days; severity correlates with amount of virus absorbed and degree of fever.

Implementation

A. Standard Precautions, airborne isolation including high-efficiency mask and negative-pressure room.

B. Ribavirin used to reduce mortality rate, given within 6 days of onset.

C. Supportive care including fluid and electrolyte balance critical.

Dengue Fever

Definition: Acute febrile disease caused by flavivirus transmitted by bite of Aedes mosquito.

Characteristics

A. Occurs mostly in children living where Dengue is endemic (Southeast Asia, China and Cuba).

B. Incubation period is 3–15 days.

Assessment

A. Abrupt onset with chills, headache, aching joints with rapid rise in temperature (104°F) followed by afebrile period for 24 hours.

B. Second rise in temperature follows with rash covering entire body.

Implementation

A. Dengue prophylaxis requires eradication of mosquito vector.

B. Treatment is symptomatic—complete bedrest and acetaminophen (avoid aspirin).

Severe Acute Respiratory Syndrome (SARS)

✦ *Definition:* A respiratory illness of unknown etiology; the first severe and readily transmittable viral disease of the 21st century.

Characteristics

A. First detected in November 2002 in China; in March 2003, the World Health Organization (WHO) announced a global alert. SARS proceeded to be reported in 30 countries.

B. SARS is believed to be caused by a new variety of the coronavirus (the common cold).

✦ C. Transmission of SARS.
   1. Spread by person-to-person contact.
   2. Possibly spread by contact with objects that have been contaminated with infectious droplets.
   3. Disease may have airborne transmission, but this is still undetermined.

D. Incubation period is 2–7 days (or possibly as long as 10 days).

Assessment

✦ A. SARS begins with elevated temperature (> 100.4°F or > 38°C).
   1. Fever may be associated with chills, headache or malaise.
   2. During this prodromal period, client may develop mild respiratory symptoms.

✦ B. After 3 to 7 days, lower respiratory symptoms develop.
   1. Dry, nonproductive cough and dyspnea.
   2. Hypoxemia may develop, as well as respiratory distress syndrome.

C. The last stage of SARS is classified as atypical pneumonia.

D. No definitive diagnostic test for SARS; CDC has serum tests to detect antibodies to the virus but specificity is still being evaluated.

E. Epidemiological criteria: travel (through an airport) within 10 days of onset of symptoms; close contact with a person known or suspected to have SARS.

Implementation

✦ A. Implement immediate infection control measures with a suspected case of SARS.
   1. Use standard hand hygiene (soap and water or alcohol-based gel).
   2. Use contact protection (gloves, gown, and eye shield).
   3. Use airborne protection: N95 disposable respirators; place client in a negative-pressure isolation room.

B. No accepted medical treatment.
   1. A viral drug, Ribavirin (a drug used to treat AIDS clients), may be useful for those younger than age 40.
   2. Elderly clients do not react well to this drug.

C. Give supportive care; in some cases mechanical ventilation is started when normal functioning of the lungs is compromised.

D. Complementary physicians are recommending the herb echinacea because it boosts immune responses and aids clients in fighting the virus.

E. As of 2006, the SARS virus had mutated to a weaker virus that is no longer a threat. It could, however, reverse course in the future.

West Nile Virus

✦ *Definition:* A mosquito-borne viral disease that has been detected in 43 states. It is a single-stranded RNA virus of the family of encephalitis-causing viruses.

Characteristics

A. First cases were identified in New York City in 1999; introduced by an infected host (bird or human) or vector (mosquito).

B. Transmission occurs in summer and early fall when mosquitoes are active.

Assessment

A. Infection occurs 3 to 14 days after infected mosquito bites.
   1. 80% of infections are mild, without symptoms.
   2. 20% develop flu symptoms, lasting less than 1 week.
   3. Less than 1% develop a severe illness—encephalitis or meningitis.

B. Assess for symptoms of severe neurologic disease.
   1. Fever, headache, stiff neck, and mental confusion.
   2. Tremors, muscle weakness and convulsions in about 15% (of the 1%).

C. Symptoms may be confused with (or misdiagnosed) Guillain-Barré.

D. The FDA has approved a rapid West Nile Virus test, called West Nile IgM STATus test.
   1. This test can confirm the diagnosis in 15 minutes.
   2. Early diagnosis and treatment may prevent serious complications.

E. MAC-ELISA is another diagnostic test to detect antibody in serum or cerebrospinal fluid (collected within 8 days of illness onset).

Implementation

A. No treatment is needed for asymptomatic West Nile virus.

B. Clients with symptoms of encephalitis or meningitis require hospitalization.
   1. No specific therapy is available; give supportive therapy.
   2. Airway management, respiratory support (mechanical ventilation) may be ordered to control cerebral edema.
   3. Fluid management.

C. Use Standard Precautions to protect healthcare workers.

D. Teach clients preventive methods.
   1. Avoid mosquito bites.
   2. Use the chemical insect repellent, DEET, which will offer protection. (Studies show DEET lasts 5 hours after application.)

Avian (Bird) Influenza (H5N1)

Characteristics

A. Viral infection caused by the avian influenza virus found in wild birds.
   1. Infected birds carry the virus in their intestines (which does not cause illness). Virus that causes illness is transferred to domesticated birds.
   2. Virus is then transmitted to people who work closely with these birds or eat meat that has been undercooked.

B. Outbreaks of H5N1 occurred in poultry in eight countries during 2003–2004.

C. This virus can result in a pandemic threat—there is a 50-50 chance it could mutate and easily spread from one person to another.

Assessment

A. Symptoms range from fever, cough, and sore throat to eye infections, pneumonia and severe respiratory distress.

B. Humans have little or no immune protection because these viruses do not commonly infect humans.

Implementation

A. The CDC recommends total infection control precautions with airborne precautions to prevent transmission.

B. Isolation precautions for clients who have traveled within 10 days to a country where avian flu has been detected and who are hospitalized with a severe respiratory illness.
   1. Use of a HEPA-filtered negative-pressure isolation room.
   2. Healthcare workers should wear a respirator mask (N95 face piece).

C. The FDA has recently approved a vaccination against H5N1 avian flu.
   1. Vaccine will be stockpiled and sold publicly if the virus acquires the ability to pass from person to person.
   2. Vaccine would be used in the early phase for protection until a specific vaccine that is tailored to the actual strain is developed.

IMMUNOSUPPRESSION

The Immunosuppressed Client

✦ *Definition:* An acquired immune deficiency characterized by a defect in natural immunity against disease. With loss of the immune system, the individual is susceptible to a variety of "opportunistic infections."

Characteristics

A. The immune system—how it functions.
   1. A complex system of organs and cells that work to distinguish foreign invaders from natural components in the body.

a. The body's skin and mucous membranes provide the *first line of defense* against invading organisms.

b. When a foreign organism enters the body, it may be destroyed by circulating white blood cells, macrophages and neutrophils—the *second line of defense.*

✦ 2. The immune system is triggered when an antigen has not been stopped or destroyed by the body's first and second defense system.

a. Lymphocytes then mobilize to defend the body against invaders or antigens.

b. Lymphocytes fall into two classes.
   (1) B cells (30 percent of blood lymphocytes) develop in the bone marrow.
   (2) T cells (70 percent of blood lymphocytes) originate in the bone marrow but complete development in the thymus gland.

✦ B. Etiology of immunosuppression.
   1. Drug treatment protocols.
      a. Cancer chemotherapeutic agents.
      b. Antibiotics such as tetracycline, chloramphenicol, streptomycin, gentamicin inhibit cellular immunity.
      c. Mafenide and silver sulfadiazine inhibit neutrophil movement to the area of inflammation.
      d. Steroids cause temporary lymphocytopenia, increase in neutrophils, decrease in monocytes and eosinophils.
         (1) Chronic use leads to nonresponsive immune system.
         (2) Anergy may lead to susceptibility to opportunistic infections.
   2. Age—the older a client's chronologic age, the more susceptible to infections.
   3. Acute and chronic diseases.
      a. Acquired immune deficiency syndrome (AIDS).
      b. Cancer.
      c. Inflammatory bowel disease.
      d. Diabetes.
      e. Chemical sensitivity.
      f. Chronic fatigue syndrome.
   4. Poor nutritional status.
      a. Protein and calorie depletion lead to lymphocyte suppression.
      b. Iron deficiency causes atrophy of the liver, spleen and bone marrow, and lymphoid tissue.
      c. Zinc deficiency affects thymus gland.
   5. Surgery and anesthesia.
   6. Stress, both specific and generalized.

a. Environmental stress such as pollution, high-intensity sound or noise may create stress that results in immunosuppression.

b. Stressful life events, such as loss of job, marriage, or death, decrease immune function.

7. Psychiatric illness, especially major illness such as schizophrenia, depression or manic episode.

8. Lesions of the central nervous system, especially the hypothalamus, produce changes in the immune response.

Assessment

✦ A. Observe for possible sites of infection.
   1. IV sites and invasive devices (prosthetic devices).
   2. Catheter sites.
   3. Surgical wounds.
   4. All body crevices.
   5. Respiratory tract (lungs) and genitourinary tract.

✦ B. Observe for signs of inflammation or systemic infection.
   1. Changes in temperature—fever may be only sign since signs of inflammation may not appear due to diminished neutrophils.
   2. Changes in white blood cell count and differential count.
   3. Signs of inflammation: pain, redness, swelling, and heat.

C. Assess the lungs for adventitious sounds.

D. Assess nutritional status.
   1. Calorie and protein intake to build immune system.
   2. Adequate vitamins (including vitamins A and C) and minerals (iron and zinc).

Implementation

✦ A. Prevention and early detection of infection.
   ✦ 1. Hand hygiene and gloving are essential for prevention.
      a. Wash hands frequently during the care, and wash thoroughly before and after any contact with an immunosuppressed client. Use antiseptic, not bar soap, or waterless antiseptic.
      b. Wear gloves for any client contact where there is possibility of contact with blood, body secretions, or contaminated surface.
   ✦ 2. Use of aseptic technique when caring for all possible entrance sites for infection: catheters, central lines, endotracheal tubes, pressure-monitoring lines and peripheral IV lines.
   ✦ 3. Be aware of possibility of cross contamination—deliver care first to the immunosuppressed client.

◆ 4. Assign client to private room, if possible.
   a. Keep door closed to prevent transmission of airborne organisms.
   b. Keep room well ventilated.
5. Use masks for all persons with the slightest evidence of upper respiratory or other type of infection.
6. Damp dust with a disinfectant solution when cleaning client's room or objects used in care.
7. Use a humidifier to reduce microorganisms that may thrive in an arid environment.
8. Do not allow water to collect and stagnate; change every 24 hours to prevent breeding of organisms.
◆ 9. Prevent contamination of suctioning equipment.
   a. Use two-glove technique to prevent spread of organisms.
   b. Complete thorough hand hygiene before and after suctioning.
   c. Clean connecting tubes with germicide solution.
   d. Change tubes every 8 hours.
◆ 10. Use strict aseptic technique for every dressing change.
◆ B. Complete impeccable skin care for the immunosuppressed client.
1. Observe all pressure areas for signs of breakdown.
2. Turn frequently, every hour if client is immobile.
3. Complete passive or active range-of-motion exercises when indicated.
4. Change any wet clothing or dressing immediately; wetness will break down skin.
5. Lubricate and massage skin to prevent cracks and stimulate blood circulation to potential areas of breakdown.
◆ C. Perform pulmonary toilet.
1. Assess pulmonary function frequently for lung sounds, coughing, drainage, and ability to breathe.
2. Perform toilet every 2–4 hours.
D. Monitor nutritional status.
1. Provide high-calorie, high-protein diet; without adequate nutrients, client cannot produce enough lymphocytes to fight infection.
2. Malnutrition impairs the humoral system of the immune response.
3. Administer enteral feedings for clients with normal GI functions.
4. Administer total parenteral nutrition (TPN/TNA) if GI tract is not functioning. This achieves high-density caloric support.

E. Assist client to handle stressful conditions.
1. Support accommodation to hospital regimen. Normalize hospital environment as much as possible.
2. Allow client to be as independent as possible.
   a. Support concerns about forced dependency.
   b. Support client taking an active role in care activities.
3. Provide method of dealing with psychological impact of illness—special consultation, extra time to communicate, etc.
4. Provide care that will enhance body image.
   a. Frequent assistance for bathing, hair washing, etc.
   b. Use touch to communicate; do not act as if client is "untouchable."
5. Allow client to make choices and discuss options for care.
6. Allow private time for client and make allowances for family and friends to spend time with client.
F. Present realistic optimism when caring for client—a no-hope attitude on the part of the nurse will be conveyed.

Acquired Immunodeficiency Syndrome (AIDS)

Definition: The most severe form of a continuum of illnesses associated with human immunodeficiency virus (HIV) infection.

Characteristics

◆ A. Normal versus AIDS immune response.
1. In the normal immune system, killer/suppressor and helper/inducer T cells are evenly distributed.
◆ 2. AIDS clients show an acquired defect of immunity.
   a. Helper T cells are depleted which causes a reversal of normal ratio of helper to killer/suppressor T cells.
   b. Client cannot activate effective immune response either to foreign invaders or to cancer cells.
   c. This deficiency leads to the majority of signs and symptoms observed in AIDS clients.
B. HIV is a blood-borne retrovirus and has a different life cycle from a normal virus.
1. Genetic information is usually sequenced by DNA being transcribed into RNA, which is then translated into proteins necessary for life.
2. Retroviruses reverse the sequence: RNA code is transcribed backward into DNA and may be integrated into host cell chromosomes.

TESTING FOR HIV

- The ELISA (enzyme-linked immunosorbent assay) test was developed to screen national donor blood.
  a. This test does not test for AIDS, but rather for antibodies to the HIV virus.
  b. Once exposed to a virus, it takes the body time to produce antibodies. A person may already be infected and if the body has not yet produced antibodies, the ELISA test will be negative.
  c. Test is also imperfect in that it may produce a false positive or false negative.
- All positive results must be retested via ELISA.
- If second test is positive, the Western blot test is given for final confirmation.

3. This retrovirus invades CD4+ T-lymphocyte (immunity) cells, renders them useless, and then duplicates itself (which affects client's immune function so that the disease becomes clinically manifested).
✦ 4. HIV attaches and changes the protein on the surface of the helper T cells.
   a. When helper T cells are affected, they are unable to activate B cells and killer T cells.
   b. The immune system collapses when many helper T cells have been destroyed.
   c. When immune system ceases to function, diseases that may be mild become life-threatening.
   d. Most common illnesses are *Pneumocystis carinii* pneumonia, a parasitic lung infection, and Kaposi's sarcoma, a type of skin cancer.
   e. These illnesses, not AIDS, result in death.
✦ C. Transmission of the HIV virus.
   1. HIV does not appear to be highly contagious.
✦ 2. Transfer of the virus occurs through a transfer of body fluids, either from mother to child during perinatal period or through intimate sexual contact or parenteral exposure. Fluids with HIV transmission potential of the disease are: semen, blood, breast milk, vaginal/cervical secretions.
   3. Body fluids containing infected lymphocytes must enter the bloodstream or body cavity to spread the virus.
   4. The virus exists in tears, saliva, urine, feces, spinal fluid, sputum, pus, and bone marrow; epidemiological evidence has not confirmed transmission through these body fluids.
   ✦ a. High concentrations of HIV found in blood, semen, and cerebrospinal fluid.
      b. Lower concentrations of HIV found in urine, vaginal secretions, saliva, feces, breast milk.
D. HIV statistics.

1. 800,000 to 900,000 Americans are living with HIV—40,000 new infections occur each year. Internationally, an estimated 5 million people were infected with HIV in 2005.
2. The World Health Organization (WHO) estimates that as of 2010, 75 million people in 5 industrial nations will be infected with HIV. 19 million have been killed by AIDS worldwide.
3. AIDS is the second leading killer of young men 24–44 years old and fifth leading killer of young women.
4. Two major risk groups continue to be homosexual (accounting for 47.9 percent of AIDS cases) or bisexual men and IV drug abusers (which make up 85 percent of all AIDS cases).
E. AIDS-related complex (ARC) and AIDS.
   1. The CDC uses a strict surveillance definition to establish an AIDS diagnosis because AIDS symptoms can occur in non-AIDS clients.
   ✦ 2. AIDS is defined by the CDC as an HIV infection in a person with a CD4+ T-lymphocyte count of less than 200 cells/µL of blood or a CD4+ percentage of less than 14.
F. Opportunistic conditions: disease processes that occur as a result of suppressed immune system.
   ✦ 1. *Pneumocystis carinii:* a parasitic infection of the lungs. One of the two rare diseases that affect 85 percent of AIDS clients; similar to other types of pneumonia.
   ✦ 2. Kaposi's sarcoma: a type of cancer usually occurring on the surface of the skin or in the mouth. This disease may also spread to internal organs.
   3. Dementia with AIDS virus: a clinical syndrome in which there is acquired persistent intellectual impairment, in this case caused by the HIV virus.

Assessment

A. Assess for chronic fatigue.
   1. Activity level and need for support.
   2. Alterations in sleep patterns.
   3. Pulmonary insufficiency.
   4. Degree of anxiety associated with pulmonary problems.
B. Assess for presence of diarrhea.
   1. Intractable or intermittent.
   2. Degree of dehydration.
   3. Electrolyte imbalance; observe blood chemistries.
   4. Malnutrition due to GI malabsorption and intractable diarrhea.
C. Assess for skin breakdown and mucous membrane involvement.
   1. Lesions and Kaposi's sarcoma.
   2. Degree of excoriation or pressure sores.

3. Presence of *Candida* or genital/anal herpes.
4. Mouth for bleeding or lesions.

D. Assess for persistent elevated temperature.
1. Check temperature every 4 hours or more as needed.
2. Assess need for cooling measures such as ice packs, alcohol rubs, cooling blankets.

E. Assess for degree of pain.
1. Character, intensity, or dramatic changes in pain.
2. Need for medication and effects of drug regimen.

F. Assess nutritional status.
1. Malnutrition.
   a. Severe weight loss.
   b. Weakness and fatigue.
   c. Decreased serum proteins.
   d. Decreased intake of foods and fluids.
2. Intake and output.
3. Dehydration.
   a. Decreased skin turgor.
   b. Dry mucous membranes.
   c. Weight loss.
4. Need for antiemetics.

G. Assess presence of neurologic symptoms.
1. Memory lapses and confusion.
2. Seizure activity.
3. Confusion and disorientation.
4. Infection of the optic nerve.
   a. Visual changes.
   b. Blindness.
5. Symptoms of dementia.

H. Assess degree of pulmonary involvement.

I. Assess client for potential injury.
1. Identify risk factors.
   a. Weakness.
   b. Sedation.
   c. Mental confusion, dementia.
   d. Orthostatic hypotension.
2. Assess physical status for degree of independence.
   a. Ability to be mobile without assistance.
   b. Amount of medication that interferes with alertness.

Implementation

A. New therapies have extended the life span of AIDS clients.
1. Trends of both AIDS cases and deaths are declining.
2. Decrease is thought to be related to prevention efforts targeted at high-risk populations and new medications.

B. Twenty antiretroviral drugs have been approved by the FDA. There are 4 classes:

1. Nucleoside reverse transcriptase inhibitors (NRTIs).
2. Non-nucleoside reverse transcriptase inhibitors.
3. Protease inhibitors (PIs).
4. Fusion inhibitors.

✦ C. CDC recommends aggressive antiviral therapy—viral suppression is the goal.
1. HAART (highly active antiretroviral therapy)—one protease inhibitor and two non-nucleoside reverse transcriptase inhibitors is recommended.
2. Compliance is a problem due to number of meds and dose schedule.
3. Combination therapy (HIV cocktail) is now the standard of care for these clients.

✦ D. Maintain nutritional status of client.
1. Administer fluids PO to maintain hydration status, minimum 1500 to 2000 mL/day.
2. Provide dietary planning for client.
   a. Allow client to participate in menu planning.
   b. Suggest family members bring in food from home.
3. Provide dietary supplements—high-protein, high-calorie nutritional supplements, vitamin supplements.
4. Administer antiemetics to minimize anorexia and nausea.
5. Administer IV fluids if necessary.
   a. Examine IV site every shift for infection, inflammation.
   b. Change dressings as needed; do not allow dressing to remain wet.
6. Provide good oral hygiene.
   a. Use soft toothbrush, lemon glycerine swabs.
   b. Use dilute H_2O_2 several times a day as a mouthwash.
7. Suggest anesthetic solution (viscous lidocaine) before meals to assist in swallowing.
8. Administer nasogastric tube feedings as ordered.
9. Evaluate status for Total Nutritional Alimentation (TNA); institute before nutritional status has severely deteriorated.

E. Provide oxygen and maintain pulmonary function.
1. Monitor pulmonary status from baseline data to determine changes that require medical management.
2. Maintain bedrest if condition indicates (dyspnea upon any exertion).
3. Provide oxygen if indicated.
4. Monitor vital signs; pulse, BP, respirations, skin color.

F. Provide comfort measures for fatigue.
1. Periods of rest during the day, especially before meals.
2. Provide oxygen on exertion or continuously, if indicated.
3. Administer medications to assist in adequate sleep.
4. Teach relaxation methods to assist in coping with anxiety (which can be debilitating).
5. Assist with activities of daily living (ADLs) as necessary.
6. Increase activity levels as tolerated. Suggest PT, OT, etc.

G. Provide excellent skin care.
1. Keep skin clean and free of moisture.
2. Change soiled or wet linen immediately.
3. Provide bath if condition indicates.
4. Massage with lotion to increase tissue perfusion.
5. Wash and air perineum and anal area regularly.
6. Administer pressure ulcer treatment as indicated.
   a. Prescribed ointments.
   b. Op-Site treatment.
7. Assist with position changes as necessary; for client on bedrest, turn every 2 hours.
   a. Maintain functional body alignment.
   b. Provide appropriate beds: Clinitron, air mattress, etc.

H. Provide supportive care for elevated temperature.
1. Administer antipyretics (acetaminophen and/or nonsteroidal anti-inflammatory) as ordered.
2. Monitor temperature every 4 hours; note pattern of temperature spikes.
3. Change linen for night sweats.
4. Provide cooling measures as necessary (alcohol rubs, cooling blankets).
5. Encourage fluid intake; consider need for IV fluids.

I. Administer appropriate care for diarrhea.
1. Administer prescribed antidiarrheal medications following each loose stool; if not adequate, administer around-the-clock maximum dose.
2. Monitor for constipation to prevent impaction.
3. Monitor to avoid complications from intractable diarrhea.
   a. Nutritional depletion.
   b. Electrolyte imbalance.
4. Provide appropriate diet: bland, low-fiber, low-milk products.
5. Give client incontinence pads to prevent accidents.

J. Provide measures to reduce pain.

1. Administer analgesics to relieve pain (do not allow client to go for long periods without medication if pain is extensive).
2. Allow client to monitor own pain medication to increase effectiveness.
3. Provide alternate pain relief.
   a. Massage and touch help to relieve pain.
   b. Teach visualization techniques to reduce pain.
   c. Give client warm baths.
   d. Provide emotional support—talking, touching, etc.

K. Monitor client to prevent injuries.
1. Evaluate degree of weakness.
   a. Encourage use of call bell.
   b. Assist with ambulation.
   c. Use siderails if necessary.
   d. Keep belongings within reach.
2. Evaluate degree of mental confusion.
   a. Reorient frequently; remind client to call for assistance.
   b. Restrain as appropriate.
3. Provide bedpan or bedside commode and assistance.

Psychosocial Care for AIDS Client

✦ A. Identify problem area.
1. Fear of contagion.
   a. Family and friends fear contagion because of lack of knowledge about AIDS transmission.
   b. The person with AIDS is actually the most vulnerable to contagion.
2. Fear of rejection.
   a. Disclosing AIDS, especially if one is a homosexual, to family or friends leads to fear of rejection.
   b. Guilt and shame accompany a diagnosis of AIDS.
3. Planning for terminal care.
   a. Resources and funds may be depleted when terminal care is needed.
   b. Long-term total care is often needed for physical as well as mental debilitation.

B. Provide milieu of individual acceptance.
1. Use of nonjudgmental attitudes.
2. Encourage open, honest communication from staff to client.

✦ C. Assist client to clarify fears and concerns of rejection.
1. Encourage verbalization of fears and feelings but only if client is ready to verbalize.
2. Encourage honesty when telling others of diagnosis, concerns, and needs.

D. Mediate between client, parents, and loved ones.
   1. Clarify role client wishes friends, partner, and family to take during illness.
   2. Assist client to clarify decisions regarding treatment, finances, and caregiving.
E. Assist client to go through grieving process caused by loss (of self-image, independence, identity, and worthiness).
F. Support parents and loved ones who are bereaved at loss of partner or child.

Hepatitis

See Hepatitis A, B, C, D in Chapter 8.

Healthcare Workers' Exposure to HIV

A. In 1997, the Public Health Service updated recommendations for management of healthcare workers' exposure to HIV. The decision to recommend HIV postexposure prophylaxis (PEP) takes into account two factors:
   1. The nature of the exposure.
   2. The amount of blood or body fluid involved in the exposure.
✦ B. Healthcare facilities should have the protocols available and mandate prompt reporting and post-exposure care.
   1. Healthcare workers must be educated to report occupational exposures immediately after they occur.
   2. PEP is most likely to be effective if implemented as soon after the exposure as possible.
   3. Exposure is defined as a percutaneous injury, contact of mucous membrane or nonintact skin, or contact with intact skin when the duration of contact is prolonged.
   4. Risk assessment is performed on all healthcare workers who have been exposed to potentially HIV-infected blood or body fluids.
   5. The FDA has recently approved a point-of-care HIV test that provides results in 5 minutes. If positive, a follow-up confirmation test must be done.
   6. Goal is to balance risk for infection against potential toxicity of the PEP drugs.
C. Recommendations for PEP:
   1. A basic 4-week regimen of two drugs (zidovudine and lamivudine) is appropriate for most HIV exposures.
   2. Expanded regimen that includes the addition of a protease inhibitor (indinavir or nelfinavir) is recommended for increased risk for transmission of HIV exposures.
   3. There is now available a boosted protease inhibitor (Kaletra) that helps to reduce the viral load.

HIV–HBV Healthcare Worker Alert

A. Accidental contact with blood or body fluids.
✦ 1. Any percutaneous or mucocutaneous exposure should receive immediate first aid.
   a. Percutaneous exposure—a break in the skin caused by contaminated needle or sharp instrument, broken glass container holding blood or body fluids, or human bite.
   b. Mucocutaneous exposure—body fluid contact to open wounds, nonintact skin (eczema), or body fluid splash to mucous membranes (mouth, eyes).
✦ 2. Apply immediate first aid to site.
   a. Needlestick or puncture wound; scrub area vigorously with soap and water for 5 minutes.
   b. Oral mucous membrane exposure: rinse area several times with water.
   c. Ocular exposure: irrigate immediately with water or normal saline solution.
   d. Human bite: cleanse wound with povidone–iodine (Betadine) and sterile water.
   3. Report unusual occurrence to the charge nurse or supervisor.
   4. Complete an unusual occurrence form and follow reporting requirements mandated by OSHA.
B. Health Care Worker Protection Act.
   1. The Health Care Worker Protection Act was passed to reduce number of healthcare workers who are accidentally exposed to potentially contaminated, infected blood via a needlestick.
   a. More than 600,000–800,000 needlesticks and injuries are reported yearly.
   b. Most common cause of exposure to blood-borne pathogens is needlestick injuries with post risk for HIV exposure.
   2. This act makes the use of safe needle devices a requirement if facility receives Medicare funding.
✦ 3. More than 20 pathogens can be transmitted through small amounts of blood.
   a. Hepatitis B is the most common infectious disease transmitted through work-related exposure to blood and needlesticks.
   b. In addition to HIV and hepatitis B, syphilis, varicella-zoster, and hepatitis C can be transmitted via this route.

INFECTION CONTROL REVIEW QUESTIONS

1. A nurse is just exiting an isolation room. Considering infection control protocol, which actions, in order, would the nurse take _____ ?

   1. Bag equipment and double-bag it out at the door.
   2. Remove protective gear.
   3. Dispose of equipment appropriately inside the room.
   4. Wash hands.

2. The nurse is assigned to care for two clients. One client has just returned from surgery for an abdominal resection. The second client is hospitalized with an acute case of tuberculosis. Which special precautions should the nurse take when providing care for these two clients?

   1. Proper hand hygiene between clients and use of specific isolation garb.
   2. Provide care to the client with tuberculosis before the client with abdominal surgery.
   3. Strictly adhere to barrier nursing principles.
   4. Thorough hand hygiene and gloving is sufficient in this situation.

3. CDC guidelines are specific for clients with tuberculosis. The major differences in providing care for the client with TB versus other clients requiring barrier nursing are

   1. The staff must wear gowns, mask, and gloves.
   2. The client should be in a private room with a special ventilation system.
   3. The client may be placed in a room with other clients requiring barrier nursing protocol.
   4. The protocol of donning and removing isolation garb before entering or leaving the client's room is different.

4. A nurse is assigned to take two clients' vital signs, complete a focus assessment and provide hygienic care, administer meds, and complete a dressing change for a client with an abdominal wound. Which task will have priority with this assignment?

   1. Take vital signs and provide hygienic care on the first client.
   2. Administer medications to the clients.
   3. Complete the dressing change.
   4. Take vital signs on the two clients.

5. All staff must wear disposable particulate respirators (HEPA filter) when

   1. Working with a client in isolation.
   2. There is inadequate room ventilation.
   3. Working with a client with tuberculosis.
   4. There are suspected colonized microorganisms.

6. When removing an isolation gown, steps the nurse should take would be to

   1. Untie the neck strings, remove gloves, and untie waist strings.
   2. Untie front waist strings, remove gloves, and untie neck ties.
   3. Remove gloves, untie waist strings, and wash hands.
   4. Remove gloves, untie neck strings, and wash hands.

7. A nurse is assigned to provide care for an AIDS client. Infection control guidelines specify that a gown should be worn when the nurse

   1. Enters the room to provide client care.
   2. Administers IV medications.
   3. Completes a dressing change.
   4. Administers an IM injection.

8. Gloves are an important component of infection control protocol. Which of the following situations would require that gloves be worn? List all the numbers that apply _____ .

   1. When the nurse is in contact with urine.
   2. Suctioning a client who does not have an infectious disease.
   3. Changing an ostomy pouch.
   4. Delivering a food tray to a client with AIDS.

9. Protective eye wear should be worn at all times when the nurse is

   1. Giving personal care to an AIDS client.
   2. Bathing a neonate for the first time.
   3. Drawing cord blood.
   4. Taking a specimen to the laboratory.

10. The RN team leader will assign a healthcare worker to care for a client in isolation. Which team member would be appropriate for this assignment?

   1. LVN/LPN only.

2. LVN/LPN, CNA.
3. LVN/LPN, UAP.
4. LVN/LPN, CNA, UAP.

11. The nurse is assigned to draw blood from a suspected AIDS client. Standard Precautions dictate that she should use

1. Gown, clean gloves, and mask.
2. Gown, sterile gloves.
3. Hand hygiene and sterile gloves.
4. Hand hygiene, gown, clean gloves.

12. The rationale for isolating a newborn who was born to a mother who had rubella is that

1. The newborn may be actively shedding the virus.
2. The newborn is more susceptible to infections.
3. The child may develop encephalitis, a complication of rubella.
4. A newborn's autoimmune system is depressed.

13. The nurse is responsible to check that the nursing assistant (UAP) is aware of Standard Precautions/isolation techniques. If the nursing assistant understands these techniques, she will say that she must wear

1. Gloves at all times when in contact with any clients, regardless of the diagnosis.
2. Gloves and gown when in contact with blood or body fluids.
3. Sterile gloves, gown and mask at all times when caring for identified AIDS clients.
4. Mask and gloves at all times when caring for diagnosed AIDS clients.

14. Which of the following is a type of transmission-based precaution?

1. Droplet.
2. Respiratory.
3. Blood.
4. Body fluids.

15. Two major factors that influence whether an infection occurs in an individual are

1. Age and general health status.
2. Underlying disease status and exposure to infectious agent.
3. Inherent health and immunologic status.
4. Type of organism and age.

16. When an area becomes inflamed, the substance that is released around the injured site is labeled

1. Plasmin.
2. Histamine.

3. Kinin.
4. Leukocytes.

17. Which of the following statements is true when evaluating infection control practices?

1. Gloves should be worn for contact with blood and body fluids of all clients.
2. Gloves should be changed after contact with blood or body fluid; otherwise, it is not necessary to change them between client care.
3. Gowns should be worn at all times when caring for clients with drainage.
4. Healthcare workers with open lesions should wear special gloves when providing client care.

18. The census on the unit is 90 percent and there are no private rooms available. An elderly client with influenza is admitted. To which of the following rooms would it be appropriate to assign this client?

1. A double room with another client with the same diagnosis.
2. A four-bed room with three clients who have had orthopedic surgery.
3. A double room with an elderly client with a diagnosis of chickenpox.
4. A double room with a client admitted for impetigo.

19. For an infection to occur, six links or steps must be present. Which of the following is not considered a link?

1. Infectious agent.
2. Reservoir.
3. Portal of entry.
4. Droplet transmission.

20. The nurse has instituted contact precautions on a client with herpes infection. These precautions would *not* include

1. Special particulate (HEPA) filter mask.
2. Private room or double room with a client with the same illness.
3. Gloves when providing client care and changing gloves following contact procedures.
4. Gown if clothing will come in contact with the client, environmental surfaces, or items in the room.

21. The single major risk a client faces when entering a hospital in the United States for any reason is

1. Resistant strain of *Staphylococcus*.
2. Vancomycin-resistant enterococcus.
3. Nosocomial infection.
4. Death.

22. Considering the most basic infection control measures, which of the following statements is correct?

    1. Wearing gloves eliminates the need to wash hands between clients.
    2. Donning gloves, even with unclean hands, will protect the client.
    3. It is important to wash hands between clients and before and after using gloves.
    4. OSHA stipulates that gloves must be worn for all client contact.

23. The most common nosocomial infection is

    1. Urinary tract infection.
    2. Infectious diarrhea *(C. difficile)*.
    3. Pneumonia (gram-negative bacteria).
    4. Bloodstream infection.

24. A client returns to the unit following neurosurgery for removal of a meningioma. The client has been in intensive care for 2 days and now is assigned to a step-down unit. When completing an assessment, the nurse notes that the client has a fever of 102°F and is complaining of cramps and pain in the stomach. The appropriate intervention is to

    1. Repeat the assessment in 12 hours.
    2. Notify the physician.
    3. Do nothing—these symptoms are expected with this condition.
    4. Suggest a stool assay for toxin A or B.

25. A nurse accidentally has had a needlestick in her hand as she pulled an IM needle from the muscle. The first action is to

    1. Report the accident to the charge nurse.
    2. Scrub the area vigorously with soap and water for 5 minutes.
    3. Cleanse area with povidone–iodine (Betadine).
    4. Irrigate the wound with sterile water.

INFECTION CONTROL

Answers with Rationale

1. The answer is *3 2 1 4.* The first action would be to dispose of "dirty" equipment in a garbage bag before removing protective gear. Then, the nurse would remove gear beginning with the gown (2) and place in garbage bag (1). Finally, the nurse would wash hands (4) and dispose of all "double-bagged" equipment in the dirty utility room and wash hands again.

NP:P; CN:S; CA:M; CL:A

2. (3) There are no special precautions; however, the nurse must strictly adhere to barrier nursing principles and the two clients must be treated separately. Providing care to the abdominal surgery client before the TB client would be appropriate. Proper hand hygiene is essential, but isolation garb is needed only for the TB client.

NP:P; CN:S; CA:M; CL:A

3. (2) Clients with tuberculosis are placed in private rooms with directional air-flow, negative-pressure ventilation systems. Negative pressure pulls air away from the hallway and exhausts it out of the room to areas away from the intake vents. The other elements are the same for any client requiring barrier nursing precautions or isolation protocols.

NP:A; CN:S; CA:M; CL:C

4. (4) Taking vital signs on the two clients would be the priority nursing action to determine if there are any emergent problems. Even if one of the clients had TB, the nurse could don gloves and a HEPA filter mask to complete the assignment. Next, the nurse would give the meds (2) that need to be given within a certain time frame. Because changing the dressing (3) might also involve a pain assessment, this would take more time and should probably be done last.

NP:P; CN:S; CA:M; CL:AN

5. (2) Staff must wear disposable respirators when there is inadequate room ventilation. If the room has a directional negative-pressure ventilation system, the staff would not be required to wear a HEPA filter mask, even if the client had TB. These masks are required for droplet transmission–based conditions.

NP:P; CN:H; CA:M; CL:A

6. (2) Removing the waist strings first is appropriate because when they are tied in front, they are considered dirty. The nurse would remove gloves, untie the neck strings (which are considered clean), and then remove the gown. Only if there were no waist strings in front would the nurse remove the gloves first.

NP:P; CN:S; CA:M; CL:K

7. (3) Whenever a dressing is changed, the nurse could come in contact with body fluids; thus a gown should always be worn. Entering a room (1) and administering IV meds (2) or an IM injection (4) are interventions that do not necessarily require gowning.

NP:P; CN:S; CA:M; CL:C

8. The answer is *1 2 3.* Answer (4), delivering a food tray to an AIDS client, would not require the nurse to don gloves. However, correct protocol would require the nurse to wash hands before delivering another tray. The other interventions would absolutely require gloving because the nurse is in contact with body fluids.

NP:AN; CN:S; CA:M; CL:C

9. (3) Protective eyewear should be worn when drawing cord blood, because the blood could easily splash into the nurse's eyes. Gloves should be worn when giving personal care to an AIDS client or bathing a neonate for the first time, but eyewear is not required protocol.

NP:P; CN:S; CA:M; CL:C

Coding for Questions/Answers Abbreviations: **Nursing Process: NP,** Assessment: A, Analysis: AN, Planning: P, Implementation: I, Evaluation: E; **Client Needs: CN,** Safe, Effective Care Environment: S, Health Promotion and Maintenance: H, Psychosocial Integrity: PS, Physiological Integrity: PH; **Clinical Area: CA,** Medical Nursing: M, Surgical Nursing: S, Maternal/Newborn Nursing: MA, Pediatric Nursing: P, Psychiatric Nursing: PS; **Cognitive Level: CL,** Knowledge: K, Comprehension: C, Application: A, Analysis: AN.

10. (4) All members of the team, even unlicensed personnel, can perform some activities of care for a client in isolation.

    NP:P; CN:S; CA:M; CL:A

11. (4) The most important protection for the nurse is hand hygiene and clean gloves. She should wear a gown to protect herself, especially if the client is not alert. A mask is advised if the client is coughing.

    NP:P; CN:S; CA:M; CL:C

12. (1) These infants continue to shed the rubella virus for up to 18 months postdelivery. Mental retardation, congenital cataracts, and cardiac anomalies can occur as a result of exposure to the virus. The newborn examination should be thorough to check for these potential problems.

    NP:P; CN:S; CA:M; CL:A

13. (2) Standard (universal) Precautions, a code advocated by the CDC, include protecting oneself when there is any possibility of being in contact with contaminated body fluids or blood. The nurse manager is responsible for ensuring that those on the team understand these precautions.

    NP:E; CN:S; CA:M; CL:C

14. (1) Droplet is a type of transmission-based precaution. The other two types are contact and airborne. The remaining answers are not considered types of precautions.

    NP:A; CN:S; CA:M; CL:K

15. (3) Inherent health and the health of one's immune system are the two major factors that determine whether an infection will occur. Other factors that have an impact are general health status (1) and underlying disease status (2) (which would weaken the immune system). Neither age nor exposure time to the infectious agent is a major factor.

    NP:A; CN:S; CA:M; CL:C

16. (2) Histamine is released, which causes increased vascular permeability. When an area becomes inflamed, cells at the site activate the plasmin, clotting, and kinin systems, which cause the release of histamine around the injured site. Phagocytes are then summoned to the site to combat the infection by ingesting the harmful microorganisms.

    NP:A; CN:S; CA:M; CL:K

17. (1) The only completely true statement is that gloves should be worn for contact with blood and body fluids for all clients. It is always necessary to change gloves between clients for their protection (2). Gowns do not have to be worn (3) if the nurse will not be in direct contact with drainage. Double gloving, but not special gloves (4), may provide more protection if a healthcare worker has an open lesion.

    NP:P; CN:S; CA:M; CL:C

18. (1) If a private room is not available, the client should be placed with another client with the same diagnosis where droplet precautions would already be in place. The staff and visitors should be told to stay at least 3 feet away without a mask because large-particle droplets travel only about 3 feet before falling from the air. Orthopedic clients (2) should not be exposed to the flu or chickenpox (3) (which require airborne precautions). Impetigo (4) requires contact precautions, so this client should not be exposed to the flu, and vice versa.

    NP:P; CN:S; CA:M; CL:AN

19. (4) Droplet transmission is not considered a link in the six-step process of infection. Droplet is one of the three precautions (the other two are contact and airborne) based on the route of transmission. The additional three links needed for an infection to occur are route of transmission, portal of exit, and susceptible host.

    NP:A; CN:S; CA:M; CL:K

20. (1) A HEPA filter mask would work for droplet precautions for a client with tuberculosis or any disease that is spread via droplet (such as diphtheria or pertussis) rather than contact (skin to skin).

    NP:P; CN:S; CA:M; CL:C

21. (3) The major risk for any hospitalized client for any reason is developing a nosocomial infection. There are more than 2 million infections per year acquired in hospitals, with 90,000 deaths as a direct or indirect result of infections (CDC statistics).

    NP:A; CN:S; CA:M; CL:K

22. (3) The only totally correct statement is to perform hand hygiene between clients as well as before and after using gloves. Wearing gloves does *not* eliminate the need to wash hands (1) and microorganisms can be transmitted (when the hands are unclean) even if gloves are worn (2). Gloves are not necessary for all

client contact (4)—just contact that may result in blood or body fluid exposure to the hands.

23. (2) The most common cause of nosocomial infections is *C. difficile* diarrhea. Twenty to 40 percent of hospital clients become colonized within a few days. The second most common cause is pneumonia—gram-negative, gram-positive, and viral.

24. (4) The symptoms suggest infectious diarrhea. Up to 40 percent of hospitalized clients contract this infection within days of entering the hospital. A stool assay is indicated so that antibiotics or antimicrobial medication can be initiated immediately.

25. (2) Immediate first aid is to scrub the area vigorously. The nurse would then report and write up the accidental needlestick (1). Cleansing the area with Betadine (3) would be appropriate for a human bite. Irrigating with sterile water (4) is appropriate first aid for ocular exposure to blood or body fluid.

Disaster Nursing: Bioterrorism

✦ The icon denotes content of special importance for NCLEX.

INTRODUCTION TO DISASTER NURSING

A. Preparedness for a terrorist-caused disaster is critical for containment and protection of the population.

B. The Centers for Disease Control and Prevention (CDC) has developed a strategic plan based on five focus areas.
    1. Preparedness and prevention.
    2. Detection and surveillance.
    3. Diagnosis and characterization of biological and chemical agents.
    4. Response.
    5. Communication.

✦ C. Disaster is defined as an event of such magnitude that essential services are disrupted and current resources are overwhelmed.
    1. Disasters may be natural (caused by an earthquake, hurricane, tornado, blizzard, flood, etc.).
    2. Disasters may be caused by human actions such as civil disturbance, a hazardous material incident, or act of terrorism.
    3. Disasters have several characteristics in common.
        a. They are unexpected with little or no warning.
        b. Lives, public health, and the environment are endangered.
        c. Emergency services and personnel must be called to action.

D. Public policy in relation to mass casualties.
    1. Hospitals are the last link in community response to a mass-casualty incident and will receive most seriously injured and ill casualties.
    ✦ 2. Hospitals must follow federal legislation known as EMTALA (Emergency Medical Treatment and Labor Act).
        a. By federal law, a hospital is not allowed to turn away clients.
        b. EMTALA ensures that all individuals must be screened, evaluated, and stabilized before being transferred.
    3. The Public Health Security and Bioterrorism Response Act of 2002 authorizes $4.3 billion to combat terrorism through detection, treatment, and containment.

E. A disaster's impact on the infrastructure will affect transportation, electrical systems, telephone, water, and fuel supplies.

F. JCAHO has focused on security management and has a developed plan.
    1. Provides for designation of personnel to report and investigate security incidents.
    2. Provides identification for participants.
    3. Controls access and egress to sensitive areas.
    4. Provides an education program and performance standards for a mass-casualty event.

NATURAL DISASTERS

A. The type and timing of a disaster event will determine the types of injuries or illnesses that occur.
    1. Disasters may have a prior warning—hurricanes or floods.
    2. Disasters may occur with no warning—tsunamis or earthquakes.

B. Natural disasters include earthquakes, hurricanes, floods, tornadoes, tsunamis, typhoons, volcano eruptions, wildfires, landslides/mudslides, extreme heat, and snow or extreme cold.

C. Natural disasters affect public health.
    1. Access to medical care is limited.
    2. Resources (food, water, medicines) are limited or depleted.

D. Government agencies cannot always provide immediate relief (Hurricane Katrina was an example of this situation).

E. Develop a home disaster kit.
    1. Water—1 gallon/person/day for a minimum of 1–2 weeks.
    2. Food—selection of ready-to-eat foods, high in protein, for 1–2 weeks.
    3. First-aid kit with bandages, gloves, soap, H_2O_2. Over-the-counter medications for pain, stomach problems, etc.

Safety Issues in a Disaster	Disaster Preparation
No electricity	Flashlights, batteries, oil lamps
Gas lines broken	Turn off gas, anchor gas-powered water heater
Oil not available	Have wood available to burn
Structure may collapse	Have building inspected
	Have home bolted to foundation
	Plan safe areas in the home
	Carry a whistle to notify searchers
No communication available	Carry a cell phone—keep cell phone charged
	Have available battery radio for information
Food and water are contaminated	Keep 1 gallon of water/person/day for 15 days
	Have a portable water purifier available
	Have a safe food supply stored for 1 week
Lack of sanitation	Keep heavy plastic bags, buckets, and shovel available

4. Prescription drugs (with written prescriptions) essential for health (insulin, heart medications), 1-month supply.

5. Various supplies—radio, battery-operated flashlights or oil-burning lamps; wood for heat; personal maintenance items such as contact lens, denture needs, feminine products.

6. Appropriate clothing and bedding supplies, rain protection gear, sleeping bags.

7. Family documents—personal identification, passports, wills, trusts, insurance records.

8. Credit cards, ATM cards and cash.

F. Check and replenish supplies and kits once a year; update your disaster plan with the family and practice evacuation procedures.

✦ WEAPONS OF MASS DESTRUCTION

A. Biological agents.
1. Biological terrorism is the use of specific agents to cause harm or kill people, and includes the use of organisms such as bacteria, viruses and toxins.
2. Agents possess unique characteristics.
   a. Easily disseminated or transmitted via person-to-person contact and can be dispersed over a wide geographical area.
   b. Cause high mortality with the potential for major public health impact.
   c. Require specific actions so that public health preparedness is secured.

B. Chemical agents.
1. Chemical terrorism is the deployment of chemical weapons with the intention of causing death.
2. Chemical weapons can be pulmonary agents (phosgene, chlorine), cyanide agents (hydrogen cyanide), vesicant agents (mustard, oxime), nerve agents (tabun, sarin, VX), or incapacitating agents (agent 15, BZ).
   a. The most dangerous of these agents are nerve gases (sarin, tabun, VX), which are extremely toxic and easy to disseminate in the air.
   b. Nerve agents are designed to kill people by binding up a compound known as acetylcholinesterase, which is the body's "off" switch.

C. Radiation.
1. Radioactive substances emit radiation in the form of rays (waves) or extremely small particles.
   a. *Waveforms* are x-ray and gamma rays. *Particle forms* are alpha, beta, and neutron.
   b. Ionizing radiation is radiation that has enough energy to cause atoms to lose electrons and become ions.
   c. Charged particles are emitted from ionizing radiation, the most likely to be dispersed following a terrorist attack.
2. A cell that has been exposed to any type of radiation is damaged and may die.
3. A critical point of discrimination is whether a victim is exposed to, or contaminated by, radiation.
   a. If exposed, the victim is *not* a hazard to others. Radiation is absorbed by or passes through the body, but does not result in radioactive contamination.
   b. Radioactive contamination as radioactive particulate material is a major cause for concern. The source of contamination, resulting from spillage, leakage, deliberate dispersal, or attached to dust particles in the air, can be passed on to healthcare workers.

✦ 4. Measuring radiation.
   a. RAD (radiation absorbed dose) is a unit of measure for radiation exposure; 1 rad results in absorption of 100 ergs of energy/gram of tissue exposed.
   b. The international system now measures the unit of exposure by Gray (Gy). 1 Gy equals 100 rads.
   c. Radiation dose is a specific calculated measurement of the amount of energy deposited in the body.
   d. The unit of dose is called REM, which takes into account the type of radiation.
   e. A survey instrument measures radiation levels.
      (1) The readout is in units of R (either rad or rem), which is exposure or dose.
      (2) An instrument reading of 50 R/hr tells the healthcare worker that if he stays in the exposed area for 1 hour, he will receive a 50-rad exposure.
      (3) A radiation detection device (film badge) should be worn by personnel who come in contact with the exposed area or victims.

✦ 5. Health effects of radiation.
   a. A victim contaminated by radiation is at risk. How much risk depends on how much radiation is absorbed.
   b. Victims who absorb less than 0.75 Gy will not experience symptoms of exposure.
   c. Victims who absorb 8 Gy could die. Between 0.75 and 8 Gy, the victim could develop acute radiation syndrome (ARS).

    d. Background radiation is derived from natural sources such as radiation from outer space, industrial, academic, military or radiation used in medicine.

    e. All of these sources combine to give us a background radiation dose of 0.360 rem per person per year.

BIOLOGICAL AGENTS AND ANTIDOTES

Assessment

A. Identify epidemiologic features.
1. Rapidly increasing incidence of specific signs and symptoms.
2. An unusual number of clients seeking care, especially with flu-like symptoms, fever, or respiratory complaints.
3. An endemic disease that rapidly emerges.
4. Clusters of clients from one area.
5. Large numbers of fatalities.

B. Identify mode of dissemination and incubation period.

C. Assess the appropriate therapy/antidotes necessary to treat victims of a bioterrorist attack.

D. Assess need for collecting a clinical specimen to identify a specific bioterrorism agent.

Anthrax

Definition: An acute infectious disease caused by *Bacillus anthracis*, a spore forming gram-positive bacillus. Human anthrax occurs in three forms: cutaneous, gastrointestinal or inhalation, the form most dangerous.

Characteristics

✦ A. Clinical features.
1. Inhalation or pulmonary form.
    a. Early signs and symptoms: developing within days, nonspecific flu-like illness with malaise, dry cough, mild fever, and headache.
    b. Delayed signs and symptoms: severe respiratory distress, hemodynamic collapse—victim may die, even with antibiotic treatment.
2. Cutaneous form.
    a. Early signs and symptoms: local skin involvement with intense itching; painless, papular lesions (commonly seen on head, forearms or hands).
    b. Delayed signs and symptoms: papular lesion turned vesicular, developing into black eschar with edema.

3. Gastrointestinal form (from contaminated meat).
    a. Early signs and symptoms: abdominal pain, nausea and vomiting, severe diarrhea.
    b. Delayed signs and symptoms: gastrointestinal bleeding and fever; usually fatal after progression to toxemia and sepsis.

B. Mode of dissemination and incubation period.
1. Inhalation of spores: aerosol—no person-to-person transmission; incubation: 2–60 days (usually 48 hours).
2. Cutaneous: direct contact with skin lesions.
3. Gastrointestinal ingestion of contaminated food: no person-to-person transmission; incubation: 1–7 days.

Implementation

A. The first line of defense for an outbreak of anthrax is rapid identification.

✦ B. Manage decontamination.
1. Remove contaminated clothing.
2. Instruct clients to shower thoroughly with soap and water.
3. Instruct personnel to use Standard Precautions.*
4. Decontaminate environment with 0.5% bleach (1 part to 9 parts water), or EPA approved germicidal agent.

C. Institute isolation precautions.
1. Inhalation—Standard Precautions,* wash victim thoroughly (use 0.5% diluted bleach for visible contamination); store clothing in sealed plastic bag with biohazard label.
2. Cutaneous—contact precautions (gown and gloves).
3. Gastrointestinal—Standard Precautions.*

D. Assign client placement.
1. Private room placement *not* necessary.
2. Airborne transmission does *not* occur.
3. Skin lesions may be transmitted by direct skin contact only.

E. Implement therapy for anthrax infection.
1. Ciprofloxacin 400 mg IV q8–12 hrs; 500 mg PO q12 hrs; doxycycline 200 mg IV (1 dose); 100 mg IV q8–12 hrs; or 100 mg PO q12 hrs, or amoxicillin may also be ordered.
2. Continue treatment for 60 days.
3. Mass casualty—oral therapy with standard doses.

Plague

Definition: Acute, severe bacterial infection, caused by gram-negative bacillus. Seen in bubonic or pneumonic form; caused by *bacillus yersinia pestis*. A bioterrorism outbreak could be airborne, causing pneumonic plague.

*Standard Precautions: *See* p. 115

✦ A. Clinical features.
   1. Bubonic form.
      a. Swollen, tender lymph nodes (femoral or inguinal commonly most involved).
      b. High temp (39.5 to 41°C), chills.
      c. Pulse rapid, hypotension.
      d. Extreme exhaustion.
   2. Pneumonic form.
      a. High fever, chills, tachycardia, headache.
      b. Cough with foamy hemoptysis.
      c. Tachypnea and dyspnea.
B. Know mode of dissemination and incubation period.
   1. Transmitted from rodents to humans by infected fleas; incubation 2–8 days.
   2. Human-to-human transmission occurs by inhaling droplets through cough.
   3. Bioterrorism-related through dispersion of aerosol. Incubation: 1–3 days.

Implementation
✦ A. Manage decontamination—procedure should be done in a room designed for this purpose or at a special site outside the hospital.
   1. Instruct clients to remove clothing and store in closed plastic biohazard bags.
   2. Instruct clients to shower thoroughly with soap and water—include all crevices.
   3. Home decontamination: employ Standard Precautions (gloves, gown, face shield, when necessary).
   4. Use 0.5% diluted bleach or EPA-approved germicidal agent.
B. Institute isolation precautions.
   1. Bubonic form—routine aseptic (Standard) Precautions.
   2. Pneumonic form—add droplet precautions to Standard Precautions (eye protection and surgical mask when within 3 feet of client) until 72 hours of antimicrobial therapy.
C. Assign client placement.
   1. Bubonic form—private isolation room or cohort with clients with similar symptoms.
   2. Maintain at least 3 feet between clients when cohorting is not possible.
   3. Do not place client with immunosuppressed client.
D. Implement therapy.
   1. Doxycycline 100 mg 2 × daily.
   2. Ciprofloxacin 500 mg 2 × daily.

Botulism

Definition: A muscle-paralyzing disease caused by an anaerobic gram-positive bacillus that produces a potent neurotoxin. Food-borne botulism is the most common form; inhalational botulism is most likely to occur through a bioterrorist release of aerosol.

Characteristics
A. Recognize clinical features.
   1. Food-borne botulism.
      a. Gastrointestinal symptoms: nausea, vomiting, diarrhea.
      b. Leads to symptoms of inhalational botulism.
   2. Inhalational botulism.
      a. No fever—client is responsive.
      b. Symetric cranial nerve paralysis: drooping eyelids, blurred vision, diplopia, difficulty swallowing, dry mouth.
      c. Symptoms progress to paralysis of arms, respiratory muscles, and legs.
      d. Symptoms may be confused with Guillain-Barré syndrome.
B. Know mode of dissemination and incubation period.
   1. Food-borne botulism: generally transmitted through toxin-contaminated food; incubation is 12–36 hours after ingestion.
   2. Inhalational botulism: transmitted through aerosolization of the toxin. Incubation is 24–72 hours post-exposure.

Implementation
A. Manage decontamination.
   1. Client does not require decontamination.
   2. Contaminated clothing washed with commercial soap.
B. Institute isolation precautions.
   1. No evidence of person-to-person transmission.
   2. Standard Precautions for clients.
C. Assign client placement: implement client room selection and care according to facility policy. Client-to-client transmission does not occur.
D. Implement therapy.
   1. Early recognition of botulism is important for administration of antitoxin that may stop or reduce paralysis.
   2. Administer trivalent botulinum antitoxin (per CDC orders); requires skin testing due to 95% hypersensitivity reactions.
   3. Monitor client for respiratory failure and provide supportive care.

Typhoidal Tularemia

Definition: A disease caused by *firaneisella tularensis* bacterium. Extremely infectious and can be transmitted via aerosol or contaminated water or food.

Characteristics

A. Clinical features.
1. Early symptoms: headache, cough, fever, and chills, malaise.
2. Delayed symptoms: pharyngeal ulcers, pleuritic chest pain, pneumonia, pericarditis—may progress to respiratory failure.

B. Mode of dissemination and incubation period.
1. Bioterrorism mode is aerosol.
2. This disease may not be recognized unless a bioterrorism attack is suspected.
3. Incubation period: 2–12 days (average 3–5 days) after exposure.

Implementation

A. Manage decontamination: general decontamination measures for clothing of infected person—shower with soap or use 0.5% bleach. Because there is no person-to-person transmission, no other measures are necessary.

B. Institute isolation precautions.
1. This disease is not transmitted person-to-person, so isolation measures are not required.
2. Standard Precautions recommended.

C. Assign client placement: cohort clients and do not place with immunosuppressed clients.

D. Implement therapy: ciprofloxacin 250 mg PO q12 hrs × 14 days. Streptomycin 15 mg/kg BID IM × 10–14 days or gentamycin 1.5 mg/kg q8 hrs IV × 10–14 days.

Viral Hemorrhagic Fever (VHF)

Definition: An infection caused by agents such as Ebola, Marburg, Lassa, Argentine, Yellow and Dengue fevers. These viruses could be life-threatening (moderately high lethality) and could be delivered by aerosol in a biological attack.

Characteristics

A. Clinical features.
1. Each illness has unique clinical manifestations; however, some features are similar.
2. Characterized by abrupt onset of fever, myalgia, headache, prostration.
3. Other signs and symptoms are nausea and vomiting, diarrhea, pain in abdomen and chest, cough, and pharyngitis.
4. A maculopapular rash, prominent on the trunk, develops in most clients 5 days after onset of illness.
5. Bleeding manifestations may occur as the disease progresses. Even though it is rare for this life-threatening condition to occur, bleeding (intracranial hemorrhage) could result; hence, the term, hemorrhagic fever.

B. Mode of dissemination and incubation period.
1. Viruses are zoonotic (animal-borne), but can be spread person-to-person.
2. All viruses (except Dengue fever) could be spread by aerosol in a biological attack.
3. Incubation period: usually 5–10 days, with a range of 2–21 days.

Implementation

A. Manage decontamination: the virus is transmitted person-to-person; decontamination with overt attack: victim undresses, showers with soap or 0.5% diluted bleach.

B. Institute isolation procedures.
1. Communicable person-to-person; risk is highest after infection has progressed. Isolation precautions (including airborne and contact), including respirators, face shields, gowns, gloves, shoe and head covers.
2. Negative-pressure ventilated rooms with an anteroom.

C. Assign client placement.
1. Clients should be under strict isolation precautions, including a negative-pressure room with anteroom.
2. Only clients with the same form of hemorrhagic infection should be cohorted.

D. Implement therapy.
1. Primarily supportive.
2. Ribavirin, 30 mg/kg IV × 1 dose; 15 mg/kg IV q6 hrs × 4 days.

Q Fever

Definition: A rickettsial organism (*coxiella gurnetti*), naturally found in sheep, cattle, and goats. Bioterrorism mode of dissemination will be aerosol or food supply sabotage.

Characteristics

A. Clinical features.
1. Early signs and symptoms: headache, fever, chills, malaise, diaphoresis, anorexia; insidious onset with nonspecific flu-like symptoms.
2. Delayed signs and symptoms: double vision, sore throat, cough, chest pain, nuchal rigidity, encephalitis, hallucinations, weight loss.
3. Differential diagnosis: atypical pneumonias.

B. Mode of dissemination and incubation period.
1. Aerosol or food supply.
2. Incubation period: 10–40 days (average 10–14 days).

Implementation

A. Manage decontamination.
1. Have victim undress and shower thoroughly with soap. May use 0.5% diluted bleach.

2. Clean environment with 0.5% diluted bleach.
B. Institute isolation precautions: none required. Rarely transmitted person-to-person. Use Standard Precautions.
C. Assign client placement: transmissibility rare, so clients can be cohorted.
D. Implement therapy.
   1. Tetracycline 500 mg PO q6 hrs × 5–7 days; doxycycline 100 mg PO q12 hrs × 5–7 days.
   2. Continue treatment for 2 days post-febrile condition.

Ricin Toxin

Definition: Produced from the castor bean plant and secreted in castor seeds; *Ricinus communis* is a cytotoxin that blocks protein synthesis, killing the cell.

Characteristics
A. Clinical features.
   1. Signs and symptoms depend on route of exposure. Diagnosis is difficult. ELISA test of blood will identify ricin.
      a. Ingestion: nausea, vomiting, diarrhea, and severe abdominal cramps occur before vascular collapse (GI bleeding) leading to death on 3rd day.
      b. Aerosol—inhalation: cough, fever, hypothermia and hypotension (usually nonspecific symptoms); cardiovascular collapse leads to death in 36 to 48 hours.
   2. This biotoxin has been used by assassins to cause death; in 2003 ricin was found in a terrorist cell in England—potential use unknown.

B. Mode of dissemination and incubation period.
   1. Ricin can be delivered via the castor bean through a chemical process (ingested) or through inhalation method.
   2. Incubation period is within hours to days (ingestion: 3 days; inhalation 3–4 days).

Implementation
A. Manage decontamination.
   1. Ingested biotoxin does not require decontamination.
   2. Aerosol exposure—victim should shower with soap or use 0.5% diluted bleach.
B. Institute isolation precautions. This toxin is not transmitted to others, but Standard Precautions should be implemented.
C. Assign client placement. There is no communicability person-to-person or transport through the skin, so placement is planned to protect client's immune system.
D. Implement therapy. There is no approved antitoxin treatment or prophylaxis (vaccination) at this time.
   1. Therapy is supportive; give oxygen and hydration.
   2. If there is ingestion, GI decontamination would be implemented.

SMALLPOX: AGENT OF TERROR

Smallpox Disease

Definition: An acute viral disease caused by the *variola* virus. It was eradicated in 1977, and in the early 1980s routine vaccinations were discontinued. Because there is a large nonimmune population, authorities fear it could be a bioterrorism weapon, transmitted via the airborne route as aerosol.

Characteristics
A. Recognize clinical features.
   1. Initially, symptoms resemble an acute viral illness like influenza with fever, myalgia, headache, and backache.
   2. Rash appears, progressing from macules to papules (in 1 week) to vesicles, and then to scabs over in 1–2 weeks.
   3. Distinguishing rash from varicella (chickenpox): smallpox has a synchronous onset on face and extremities, rather than arising in "bunches," starting on the trunk.
B. Mode of dissemination and incubation period.
   1. Smallpox is transmitted by large and small respiratory droplets; thus, both respiratory and oral secretions spread the disease, as well as lesion drainage.

2. Clients are considered more infectious if they are coughing or have a hemorrhagic form of the disease.
3. Vaccination effective if given within 3 to 4 days.
4. Incubation: 7–17 days; average is 12 days.

Assessment

A. For those clients who have contracted smallpox, identify those in a high-risk group.
B. Assess need for smallpox vaccination.
C. Observe post-vaccination reactions and compare with adverse reactions.
D. Assess client's understanding of post-vaccination evaluation.

Implementation

A. Manage decontamination.
    1. Decontamination of clients is not indicated with smallpox.
    2. Careful management using contact precautions of potentially contaminated equipment and environmental surfaces—clean, disinfect, and sterilize when possible.
    3. Dedicated or disposable equipment for each client should be used.
◆ B. Institute strict isolation precautions *immediately*.
    1. Airborne and contact precautions in addition to Standard Precautions; includes gloves, gown, eye shields, shoe covers and correctly fitted masks (very important).
    2. Airborne precautions: microorganisms transmitted by airborne droplet nuclei (particles 5 microns or smaller).
        a. Respiratory protection when entering client's room (particulate respirators, N95); must meet N1OSH standards for particulate respirators.
        b. Isolate in room under negative pressure with high-efficiency particle air (HEPA) filtration.
    3. Contact precautions: clients known to be infected or colonized with organisms that can be transmitted by direct contact or indirect contact with contaminated surfaces.
        a. Perform hand hygiene using antimicrobial agent when entering and leaving room.
        b. Don gloves when entering room.
        c. Wear gown for all client contact or contact with client's environment.
        d. Wear gown when entering room and remove before leaving isolation area.
C. Assign client placement.
    1. Rooms must meet ventilation and engineering requirements for airborne precautions.

a. Monitored negative air pressure with 6–12 air exchanges/hour.
b. Appropriate discharge of air to outdoors, or high-efficiency filtration of air.

2. Door to room must remain closed; private room is preferred. Clients with same diagnosis may be cohorted.
3. Limit transport of clients; use appropriate mask if unavoidable.

D. Implement therapy.
    1. Post-exposure immunization (*vaccinea* virus) is available.
        a. Vaccination alone if given within 3 to 4 days of exposure.
        b. Passive immunization (VIG) if greater than 3 days post-exposure.
        c. VIG given at 0.6 mL/kg IM. Check with CDC for up-to-date recommendations.
    2. Prophylactic care with precautions.
E. Identify clients exposed to the smallpox virus.
    1. Persons who were exposed to initial release of the virus.
    2. Persons who had face-to-face, household or close-proximity contact (<2 meters = 6.5 feet) with a confirmed or suspected smallpox client after client developed fever and until all scabs have separated (no longer infectious).
F. Identify healthcare workers exposed to the virus— must be evaluated for possible vaccination.
    1. Personnel involved in evaluation, care, or transportation of confirmed, probable, or suspected smallpox clients.
    2. Laboratory personnel involved in collection or processing of clinical specimens.
    3. Other persons with increased likelihood of contact with infectious materials from a smallpox client (laundry or medical waste handlers).
    4. Other persons or staff who have a reasonable probability of contact with smallpox clients or infectious materials (e.g., selected law enforcement, emergency response, or military personnel).
    5. Because of potential for greater spread of smallpox in a hospital setting due to aerosolization of the virus from a severely ill client, all individuals in the hospital may be vaccinated.
G. Determine contraindications for vaccination of non-contacts.
    1. Certain medical conditions (heart disease) have a higher risk of developing severe complications following vaccination.
    2. Diseases or conditions which cause immunodeficiency (HIV, AIDS, leukemia, lymphoma, generalized malignancy, agammaglobulinemia).

3. Serious, life-threatening allergies to the antibiotics.
4. Persons who have ever been diagnosed with eczema or other acute or chronic skin conditions such as atopic dermatitis, burns, impetigo or varicella zoster (shingles).
5. Women who are pregnant.

Administering Smallpox Vaccine

Implementation

A. Prepare the vaccine.
   1. Identify client(s) to be vaccinated according to public health protocol.
   2. Reconstitute *vaccina* vaccine.
      a. Bring vaccine vial to room temperature.
      b. Don gloves.
      c. Use prefilled syringe of diluent and inject into vaccine vial.
      d. Allow vial to stand for 3–5 minutes.
      e. Record date and time of reconstitution.
      f. Dispose of equipment in biohazard bag.
   3. Gather equipment.
   4. Perform hand hygiene.

✦ B. Administer the smallpox vaccine.
   1. Remove aluminum seal and rubber stopper from vaccine vial and place in sterile container.
   2. Choose site of vaccination—one that is easily accessible for vaccination and later evaluation of site. (The outer aspect of the upper right arm over the insertion of the deltoid muscle is the standard vaccination site.)
   3. Clean vaccination site only if grossly contaminated. Let dry thoroughly.
   4. Dip point of a sterile bifurcated needle into vial of reconstituted vaccine and withdraw needle perpendicular to the floor.
   5. Do not redip needle into vaccine vial if needle has touched skin. This contaminates the vial.
   6. Hold needle at a 90° angle (perpendicular) to skin and apply 15 up-and-down (perpendicular) strokes rapidly within a 5mm diameter area. This number of strokes will deliver specified dose to client.
   7. Examine for a trace of blood at vaccination site which will indicate successful vaccine delivery.
   8. Cover vaccination site with gauze bandage and tape.
   9. Dispose of bifurcated needle in a puncture-resistant medical waste sharps container.
   10. Instruct client to keep site dry.
   11. Recap vial with sterile rubber stopper and store capped vial at 2 to 8°C.
   12. Remove gloves, dispose in appropriate receptacle, and wash hands.

C. Assess post-vaccination reactions.
   1. Identify persons who should be revaccinated. If the vaccination did not take, the individual will remain vulnerable to the smallpox virus.
      a. They will have delayed type of skin sensitivity consisting of *erythema only* within 24 to 48 hours.
      b. This represents a response to inert protein in a previously sensitized person and can occur in a highly immunized person or in individuals with little or no immunity; it is indistinguishable from the immediate or immune reaction.
   ✦ 2. Confirm successful vaccination.
      a. Presence of a pustular lesion in previously unvaccinated persons.
      b. Pustular lesion or an area of definite induration or congestion surrounding a central lesion 7 days following revaccination in a previously vaccinated person.
      c. Vaccinees who do not exhibit a "major" reaction at vaccination site on day 7 should be revaccinated.
   ✦ 3. Recognize adverse reactions.
      a. The overall risk of serious complications following vaccination with *vaccinia* vaccine is low.
      b. Complications occur more frequently in persons receiving their first dose of vaccine and among young children (< 5 years of age).
      c. The *most frequent* complications of vaccination are inadvertent inoculation, generalized vaccinia, eczema vaccination, progressive vaccinia, and postvaccination encephalitis.

D. Instruct client in post-vaccination evaluation.
   1. Successful vaccination is associated with tenderness, redness, swelling, and a lesion at the vaccination site.
   2. May also be associated with fever for a few days, malaise, and enlarged, tender lymph nodes in the axilla of the vaccinated arm.
   3. Inoculation site becomes reddened and pruritic 3–4 days after vaccination.
   4. A vesicle surrounded by a red areola enlarges, becomes umbilicated, and then pustular by the 7th to 11th day after vaccination.
   5. The pustule begins to dry, redness subsides, and lesion becomes crusted between 2nd and 3rd week.
   6. By the end of the 3rd week, scab falls off, leaving a permanent scar that at first is pink in color, but eventually becomes flesh-colored.

Table 7-1. BIOTERRORISM AGENTS

Disease	Signs and Symptoms	Incubation Period	Person-to-Person Transmission
Anthrax (inhalational)	Nonspecific flu-like, with fever, malaise, fatigue, cough. Delayed symptoms—severe respiratory distress.	1–7 days (usually 48 hours). Can be 6 weeks.	No.
Botulism (inhalational)	Increasing muscle weakness, drooping eyelids, blurred vision, difficulty speaking and swallowing; progresses down body to paralysis.	12–36 hours after exposure.	No.
Pneumonic plague	Sudden onset of high fever, chills, chest pain, headache, and cough with bloody sputum. Possibly vomiting and diarrhea. Advanced: skin lesions, respiratory failure.	2–3 days (1–6 days after exposure).	Yes; through droplet, aerosol.
Smallpox	Sudden onset of high fever, headache, and backache. Then, painful rash of small, red spots starts on face and spreads over entire skin surface. Progresses from macules to papules.	7–17 days after exposure (average is 12 days).	Yes; airborne, droplet, or direct contact with skin lesions (until scabs fall off, 3–4 weeks).
Typhoid tularemia	Sudden onset of high fever, weakness, weight loss, chest pain, and cough.	3–5 days after exposure.	No.
Viral hemorrhagic fevers (filo-viruses, such as Ebola and Marburg, and arenaviruses, such as Lassa and Junin)	Sudden onset of fever, muscle aches, and profound weakness, followed by circulatory compromise.	2–21 days after exposure.	Yes; risk higher during late stages of disease.
Ricin toxin	Depends on route of exposure: ingestion (nausea, vomiting, cramps); aerosol (cough, fever, cardiovascular collapse).	Hours to 3–4 days.	No.

Source: Adapted from Smith, S. & Duell, D. (2008). *Clinical nursing skills* (7th ed.). Upper Saddle River, NJ: Prentice Hall Health.

E. Identify indications for *vaccinia* immune globulin (VIG) administration.
   1. Identify post-vaccination complications for which VIG may be indicated.
      a. Eczema vaccinatum.
      b. Progressive vaccinia (vaccinia necrosum).
      c. Severe generalized vaccinia if client has a toxic condition or serious underlying illness.
      d. Inadvertent inoculation of eye or eyelid without vaccinial keratitis.
   2. Check physician's orders for VIG treatment of complications due to *vaccinia* vaccination.
   3. Administer VIG intramuscularly (IM) as early as possible after onset of symptoms.
   4. Give VIG in divided doses over a 24- to 36-hour period. Doses may be repeated at 2- to 3-day intervals until no new lesions appear.

Collecting and Transporting Specimens

Implementation

A. Acquire and follow specific recommendations for diagnostic sampling of the specific agent.
   1. Perform all sampling according to Standard Precautions.

   2. Check that laboratory has capacity and equipment to handle specific sample. There are 4 laboratory levels.
      a. Local clinical labs for minimal identification of an agent.
      b. County or state labs.
      c. State and other large labs with advanced capacity for testing.
      d. CDC or select Department of Defense labs with Bio Safety Level (BSL) testing capacity.
B. Wear protective gear when entering environment where potential for exposure exists.
C. Collect specimen and place in appropriate container (zip-closure plastic bag, sealed).
   1. Remove original gloves handling specimen, and place in biohazard container.
   2. Don new pair of gloves.
   3. Place specimen bag in second zip-closure bag and seal, or if specimen is large, in trash bag.
D. Remove protective gear and place in biohazard bags.
E. Perform hand hygiene.
F. Label specimen with appropriate label outside of bag: date, person collecting specimen, location, and contact person.

Treatment	Death Rate If Untreated	Death Rate If Treated	Isolation Precautions/ Standard Precautions
Antibiotics, including ciprofloxacin 500 mg PO q12 hrs. Doxycycline 100 mg PO q12 hrs; also, combined IV and PO.	High.	Improved chances for survival. Once symptoms appear, treatment is less effective.	Standard Precautions.
Antitoxim—requires skin testing. Supportive care and ventilate until victim can breathe on his own.	High.	Low, if breathing can be supported for duration of illness (weeks to months, in some cases).	Standard Precautions
Antibiotics, including ciprofloxacin 400 mg IV q12 hrs. Doxycycline 200 mg PO, then 100 mg PO q12 hrs.	Almost always fatal.	Treatment is highly effective if taken within 24 hours of first symptoms.	Bubonic form: Standard Precautions. Pneumonic form: Standard Precautions plus droplet precautions until 48–72 hours after antibiotic treatment.
Vaccination is effective if given within 3–4 days of exposure; passive immunization with VIG if 3 days post-exposure.	3–30%.	If vaccinated, less than 1%	Strict isolation precautions: airborne (includes N95 mask) and contact, in addition to Standard Precautions.
Antibiotics, including doxycycline and ciprofloxacin.	33%.	1–3% if treated within 24 exposure.	Standard Precautions.
Little is known. Antiviral agents, such as ribavirin, may be useful.	15–90%.	Unknown.	Strict isolation precautions, including negative-pressure room with anteroom.
No approved antitoxin; high O_2, supportive therapy.	Death is probable outcome.	High.	Isolation precautions.

G. Collect an acute phase serum sample, as well as a later convalescent serum sample for comparison.

H. Transport specimens.
   1. Coordinate with local and state health departments and the FBI.
   2. Include a chain of custody form with specimen information from moment of collection, completed each time specimen is transferred to another party.

CHEMICAL AGENT EXPOSURE

Assessment

◆ A. Pulmonary agents (chlorine, chloropicrin or phosgene): when inhaled produce pulmonary edema with little damage to other pulmonary tissues (with resulting hypoxemia) and hypovolemia.
   1. Immediate symptoms are irritation of eyes, nose and upper airways—often not distinctive enough to be recognized as chemical agent exposure.
   2. Two to 24 hours later, victim develops chest tightness, shortness of breath with exertion (later, at rest).
   3. Cough produces clear, frothy sputum, fluid that leaked into lungs.
   4. If symptoms begin soon after exposure, death may occur within hours.

B. Cyanide agents (gases or solids, such as hydrogen cyanide or cyanogens chloride): with high concentrations death occurs in 6 to 8 minutes.
   1. Initial symptoms are burning irritation of eyes, nose and airways, and smell of bitter almonds.
   2. Victim's skin may be acyanotic, cherry-red (oxygenated venous blood) or normal.
   3. Large amount of gas inhaled: hyperventilation, convulsions, cessation of breathing (3 to 5 minutes) and no heartbeat (6 to 10 minutes).

C. Vesicant agents: cause vesicles or blisters; common agents are sulfur mustard and lewisite. More lethal than pulmonary agents and cyanide.
   1. Mustard—initial symptoms not observable; effects begin hours after exposure: erythema, burning and itching with blisters; burning of eyes; airway pain, sore throat, nonproductive cough.
   2. Lewisite—oily liquid that results in topical damage; vapor causes immediate pain, burning and irritation of eyes, skin and upper airways.

TRIAGE IN THE HOT ZONE FOLLOWING A CHEMICAL AGENT TERRORIST ATTACK

- First responders will probably not be able to identify the exact agent.
- Early intervention is critical for nerve agents and cyanide.
- Pulmonary agent exposure will be treated later.
- Intervention in the hot zone generally has to do with airway, breathing and circulation (ABCs); add antidotes for nerve agents.

3. Cellular damage occurs that can result in hypovolemic shock.

D. Nerve agents (sarin, tabon, soman, GF and VX): liquids or vapors that are the most toxic of all chemical agents.

1. Nerve agents block the enzyme acetylcholinesterase, so activity in organs, glands, muscles, smooth muscles and central nervous system cannot turn off; body systems wear out.

2. Effects of nerve agent depends on route (vapor or droplet) of exposure and amount; it is felt within seconds.

   a. Felt first on face: eyes, nose, mouth and lower airways—watery eyes, runny nose, increased salivation and constriction of airways, shortness of breath.

   b. The most common sign of nerve vapor exposure is constricted pupils (miosis) with reddened, watery eyes.

   c. Large concentration of vapor: loss of consciousness, convulsions, no breathing.

Implementation

A. Pulmonary agents: client with pulmonary edema must be on immediate bedrest with no exertion and receive oxygen.

B. Cyanide agents: administer antidotes.

1. Client inhales amyl nitrite, or is given sodium nitrite IV (10 mL; 300 mg); frees bound cyanide from hemoglobin to allow O_2 transport.

2. Sulflur thiosulfate IV (50 mL; 12.5 g); sulfur converts cyanide to form a nontoxic substance.

3. Give antidotes sequentially and slowly, titrated to monitor effects; ventilate with oxygen, and correct acidosis.

C. Vesicant agents.

1. Mustard: immediate decontamination (within 1 minute) will minimize damage; longer will be too late. Irrigate affected skin areas and eyes frequently and apply antibiotics to skin 3 to 4 times/day.

2. Lewisite: similar to mustard; immediate decontamination is important. An antidote for systemic lewisite is British-Anti-Lewisite (BAL), a drug given IV for heavy metal poisoning.

D. Nerve agents.

1. Personal protection equipment is necessary when decontaminating victims. Decontamination must take place first, before management begins.

2. Antidotes.

   a. *Atropine* 2 to 6 mg (average dose 2 to 4 mg) IM. 2 mg more may be administered in 5 to 10 minutes if no improvement. A high initial dose is necessary to block excess neurotransmitter, especially if victim is unconscious.

   b. *Protopam*, an oxime, 600 mg given slowly IV to counteract nerve agent by removing agent from the enzyme.

   c. *Valium* might be used for prolonged convulsions.

3. The military has a device (Mark I Auto-Injection Kit) that holds 2 spring-powered injectors containing two antidotes, atropine and protopam, that can be used effectively and quickly to administer antidotes.

4. Chempacks, which include chemical weapon antidotes, are being shipped to all states from a federal stockpile. Within hours, they will be available following an emergency.

ACUTE RADIATION SYNDROME

Characteristics

A. An acute illness characterized by manifestations of cellular deficiencies caused by the body's reaction to ionizing radiation.

1. Prodromal period: loss of appetite, nausea, vomiting, fatigue, diarrhea.

2. Latent period: symptoms disappear for a period of time.

3. Overt illness follows the latent period—infection, electrolyte imbalance, diarrhea, bleeding.

4. The final phase is a period of recovery or death.

B. The higher the radiation dose, the greater the severity of early effects and possibility of late effects.

Assessment

A. Attempt to identify dose exposure of client. (Treatment is according to dose exposure.)

1. Dose less than 2 Gy (200 rads) is usually not severe; nausea and vomiting seldom experienced at 0.75 to 1 Gy (75–100 rads) of penetrating gamma rays.

   a. Hospitalization unnecessary at less than 2 Gy, thus outpatient care indicated.

   b. Closely monitor and administer frequent CBC with differential blood tests.

2. Dose greater than 2 Gy (200 rads). Signs and symptoms become increasingly severe with increased dose.

✦ B. Identify if radiation dose includes radioactive iodine—uptake of this isotope could destroy thyroid tissue.

C. Identify acute radiation syndromes.
   1. Hematopoietic syndrome.
      a. Characterized by deficiencies of RBC, lymphocytes and platelets, with immuno-deficiency.
      b. Increased infectious complications, including bleeding, anemia, and impaired wound healing.
   2. Gastrointestinal syndrome.
      a. Characterized by loss of cells lining intestine and alterations in intestinal motility.
      b. Fluid and electrolyte loss with vomiting and diarrhea.
      c. Loss of normal intestinal bacteria, sepsis, and damage to the intestinal microcirculation, along with the hematopoietic syndrome.
   3. Cerebrovascular–central nervous system.
      a. Primarily associated with effects on the vasculature and resultant fluid shifts.
      b. Signs and symptoms include vomiting and diarrhea within minutes of exposure, confusion, disorientation, cerebral edema, hypotension, and hyperpyrexia.
      c. Fatal in short time.
   4. Skin syndrome.
      a. Can occur with other syndrome.
      b. Characterized by loss of epidermis (and possibly dermis) with "radiation burns."

Implementation

A. Give supportive care—treat gastric distress with H_2 receptor antagonists (Tagamet, Pepcid, etc.).

B. Prevent and treat infections—monitor viral prophylaxis.

C. Consult with hematologist and radiation experts.

D. Observe for erythema, hair loss, skin injury, mucositis, weight loss and fever.

E. Administer potassium iodide before exposure, if possible, or as soon as available (within 4 hours).
   1. Blocks uptake of specific damaging isotope.
   2. Protects thyroid tissue.

PERSONAL PROTECTION EQUIPMENT

Assessment

A. Identify clients who present risk to healthcare professionals.

B. Assess need for special equipment (biohazard bags, specimen bags, etc.).

C. Determine type of protection equipment required according to biohazard that is identified (biological, chemical or radiological).

D. Assess need for decontaminating victims prior to triage.

E. Assess strategy for decontamination at site of incident.

F. Assess need for mass casualty decontamination.

Implementation

✦ A. Protective equipment for biological exposure.
   1. Respirators—type selected according to hazard identified and its airborne concentration.
      a. High level of protection: Self-contained breathing apparatus (SCBA) with full facepiece. Provides highest level of protection against airborne hazards when used correctly—reduces exposure to hazard by a factor of 10,000.
      b. Minimal level of protection: Half-mask or full facepiece air-purifying respirator with particulate filters like N95 (used for TB) or P100 (used for hantavirus).
   2. Protective clothing includes gloves and shoe covers—necessary for full protection.
      a. Level A Protective Suit used when a suspected biological incident occurs and type, dissemination method, and concentration is unknown.
      b. Level B Protective Suit used when biological aerosol is no longer present.
      c. Full facepiece respirator (P100 or HEPA filters) used if agent was *not* aerosoled or dissemination was by letter or package that could be bagged.

✦ B. Protective equipment for chemical exposure.
   1. Cover all skin surfaces with protective clothing impervious to chemicals—necessary for protection until exact chemical agent is identified.
      a. Use Mission Oriented Protective Posture (MOPP) suit, if available (chemical protection suit).
      b. Use fire department chemical suits as alternative.
   2. Don masks with filtered respirator. (HEPA filter respirator—N100 with full facepiece—and fit-tested N95 meet CDC performance criteria for chemical exposure.)
   3. Wear boots or boot covers to prevent tracking contaminant.
   4. Initiate decontamination procedures with trained personnel.
      a. Decontaminate at site, if possible.

b. Otherwise, decontaminate outside of facility.

5. Use chemical detection devices, if available, to validate presence or absence of agent.
   a. M8 Paper: sheet of chemically treated paper—if colored spots appear within 20 seconds, chemical agent is present.
   b. M9 Tape: affix adhesive backed paper to equipment or protective clothing—color changes when exposed to chemical agent.
   c. M2S6A1 Chemical Agent Detector Kit: can detect nerve, blister or blood agent vapors; a glass ampoule contains substance that, when placed on test spot, changes color.
   d. Chemical Agent Monitors (CAMs): contain a microprocessor chip that identifies presence of certain nerve and blister agents.

✦ C. Protective equipment for a radiological attack.
   1. Don protective clothing: basic gear will stop alpha and some beta particles, not gamma rays.
      a. Scrub suit.
      b. Gown and cap.
      c. Mask.
      d. Eye shield.
      e. Double gloves—one pair under cuff of gown and taped to close all entry; second pair can be removed and/or replaced.
      f. Masking tape, 2" wide.
      g. Shoe cover with all seams taped.
      h. Radiation detection device: able to detect energy emitted from a radiation source. Several detectors available: Geiger counters, dosimeters, etc.
      i. Film badge.
   2. If radiation incident is suspected, self-contained breathing apparatus (SCBA) and flash suits are indicated to reduce potential exposure of healthcare providers.
   3. If SCBA suits not available:
      a. Use surgical attire or disposable garments (such as those made of Tyvek).
      b. Use eye protection and double gloves.
      c. Use masks with respirators.
   4. Triage client's medical condition first, regardless of radiation exposure—first priority is delivery of emergency medical services, including transport.
      a. Administer emergency medical treatment to radiation-exposed clients.
      b. Decontaminate clients who have been contaminated on the scene before transport.
   5. Complete decontamination of victims.
      a. Remove client's clothing and have client do a total body wash, scrubbing skin with soap and soft brush.

b. Place contaminated clothing in bins or biohazard bag labeled "Radioactive."
c. Capture runoff of water; contain and label "Radioactive."
d. Wash area down between washing victims to prevent transfer of contaminated material.
e. Capture material with vacuum cleaner with HEPA filter, if appropriate, to prevent release of radioactive material into the air.
f. Open wounds or non-intact skin: irrigate with sterile water or normal saline (NS); cover with dry, sterile dressing.
g. Eyes: irrigate with sterile water or NS according to skill, "Irrigating the Eyes."
h. Intact skin: wash skin with soap and warm water. Bleach, 0.5%, may also be used.
i. Radiation burns: treat as other burns are treated.

6. Implement isolation techniques for contaminated victims to confine contamination and protect personnel.
7. Recheck radiation levels at each stage of treatment until reduced to background levels.
8. Dispose of used protective gear appropriately.

DECONTAMINATION: GENERAL PROTOCOL

✦ **Implementation**

A. Utilize Standard Precautions for all clients admitted to or arriving at the hospital.
B. Follow routing client placement for normal number of admissions.
   1. Isolate suspicious cases.
   2. Group similar cases.
C. Utilize alternative placement for large numbers of clients.
   1. Co-group clients with similar syndromes in a designated area.
   2. Establish designated unit, floor, or area in advance.
   3. Place clients based on pattern of airflow and ventilation with respirator problems, smallpox, or plague.
   4. Place clients after consultation with engineering staff.
D. Control entry to client designated areas.
E. Transport bioterrorism clients as little as possible—limit to essential movement.
F. Clean, disinfect, and sterilize equipment according to principles of Standard Precautions.
   1. Use procedures facility has in place for routine cleaning and disinfection.

SALVAGEABLE VICTIMS

SALVAGEABLE VICTIMS

- First priority: Decontaminate exposed victims with no symptoms.
- Second priority: Decontaminate exposed victims with minor injuries who require minimal resources.
- Third priority: Decontaminate exposed victims needing maximum medical care.
- Last: Decontaminate deceased victims.

SETTING UP A SITE FOR DECONTAMINATION

- Establish the decontamination site upwind from contamination area.
- Set up site on a downhill slope, if possible, or on flat ground (so that runoff can be captured).
- Have water source available and, if possible, decontamination solution.
- Have decontamination equipment available, if possible.
- Supply personal protection equipment for healthcare personnel.
- Notify healthcare facilities nearby to be available, if possible.
- Maintain security and privacy for site.
- Institute post-decontamination monitoring and checks.

2. Have available approved germicidal cleaning solutions.
3. Contaminated waste should be sorted and disposed of in accordance with biohazard waste regulations.
4. For clients with bioterrorism-related infections, use Standard Precautions for cleaning unless infecting organism indicated special cleaning.

Decontamination Procedures

Implementation

✦ A. Decontaminate at scene of incident (hot zone) to prevent hospital system from absorbing contaminated victims and protect healthcare providers and uncontaminated casualties.

✦ B. Familiarize emergency personnel with stages of decontamination.
   1. Gross decontamination.
      a. Decontaminate those who require assistance.
      b. Remove and dispose of exposed victim's clothing. (This will remove 70–80 percent of contaminant.)
      c. Perform a thorough head-to-toe tepid water rinse. (Cold water can cause hypothermia and hot water can result in vasodilation, speeding distribution of the contaminants.)
   2. Secondary decontamination.
      a. Perform a full-body rinse with clean tepid water. (Water is an effective decontaminant because of rapidity of application.)
      b. Wash rapidly from head to toe with cleaning solution (HTH chlorine is effective) and rinse with water. (HTH chlorine can decontaminate both chemical and biological contaminants.) *Note:* Undiluted household bleach is 5.0% sodium hypochlorite.
   3. Definitive decontamination.
      a. Perform thorough head-to-toe wash and rinse.
      b. Dry victim and don clean clothes.

C. Initial decontamination may be accomplished by the fire department with hoses spraying water at reduced pressure. (This will remove a high percentage of contaminant at an early stage.)

✦ D. Decontaminate salvageable clients first. (This allows those in need of medical intervention to be treated.)
   ✦ 1. Non-symptomatic and ambulatory victims have lowest priority for decontamination. (The goal is to decontaminate victims who have been exposed, yet are salvageable.)
   2. Clients who are dead or unsalvageable have lowest priority for decontamination.

✦ E. Reduce extent of contamination in facility by decontaminating clients prior to receiving in healthcare facility—to ensure safety of clients and staff.
   1. Establish decontamination site outside facility using a decontamination tent prior to needing it.
   2. Set up procedures for decontamination, depending on infectious agent.

F. Implement procedure for decontaminating client.
   1. Don appropriate personal protective gear before assisting clients to decontaminate.
   2. Remove decontaminated clothing and place in appropriate double biohazard bags.
   3. Instruct or assist client to shower with soap and water.
   4. Use clean water, normal saline, or ophthalmic solution for rinsing eyes.

Specific Decontamination Steps

✦ Implementation

A. Following a biological terrorist event.
   1. Identify dermal exposure, if possible.
   2. Remove victim's clothing as soon as possible and place in biohazard bags.
   3. Cleanse exposed areas using soap and tepid water (large amounts) or diluted sodium hypochlorite (0.5%).

4. Adhere strictly to Standard Precautions for emergency personnel to prevent secondary contamination of personnel.
5. Send victims home, if possible, to continue decontamination procedure.
   a. Instruct to wash thoroughly with soap and water.
   b. Instruct victims to monitor for signs and symptoms of agent.

B. Following a chemical terrorist event.
1. Know general principles to guide actions following a chemical agent incident.
   a. Expect a 5:1 ratio of unaffected to affected casualties.
   b. Decontaminate immediately (ASAP).
   c. Disrobing is decontamination, head-to-toe; the more removal, the better.
   d. Large volume water flush is best decontamination method.
   e. Following exposure, first-responders must decontaminate immediately to avoid serious effects.
2. Practice triage guidelines for Mass Casualty Decontamination. (Chemical exposure can be deadly, so early decontamination is critical.) Prioritize casualties by identifying those:
   a. Closest to point of release.
   b. Reporting exposure to vapor or aerosol.
   c. With liquid deposits on clothing or skin.
   d. With serious medical conditions.
   e. With conventional injuries.
3. Decontaminate victims as early as possible. (Requirements differ according to type of chemical agent used: Sarin dissipates quickly in the air; VX remains lethal for hours.)
   a. Nerve agents may be absorbed on all body surfaces—must be removed quickly to be effective.
   b. Vesicant (blister) agents are not always identified due to latent effects.
4. Treat eyes and mucous membranes with special protocol.
   a. Flush with copious amounts of water.
   b. If available, isotonic bicarbonate (1.26%) or saline (0.9%) may be used as a flushing agent.
5. Monitor victim for remains of agent or contaminate using chemical agent monitor (CAM) or M8 paper for chemical agents.

C. Following radiation exposure.
1. Determine cause of incident to identify radiation exposure or contamination. (Exposure does not necessarily indicate need for decontamination.)

   a. First responders may be told by those requesting assistance that there has been a radiation-exposure event.
   b. First responders may recognize radiation exposure from observation at incident site.
2. Understand difference between exposure and contamination.
   a. Exposed victim: presents no hazard; requires no special handling; and presents no radiological threat to personnel.
   b. Externally-contaminated victim: may mean individual has come in contact with unconfined radioactive material.
3. Decontaminate all victims; remove all clothing and complete a full body wash.
4. Institute isolation techniques to confine contamination and protect others.
5. Decontaminate equipment touched by client.
   a. Gurney used to transfer client.
   b. Equipment used in client care, e.g., BP cuff, stethoscope, etc.
   c. Ambulance.
6. Decontaminate care providers who touched or moved client (protective clothing may be contaminated).
7. Examine surrounding area (walls, floor that client may have touched).
8. Control victims' entry and exit to/from area. (Radioactive particles adhere to dust, may become airborne, and can contaminate other clients and personnel.)

TRIAGE

Characteristics

✦ A. Triage, a French word (*trier*) meaning "to sort," is a medical process of prioritizing treatment urgency.
1. The triage system can quickly assess large numbers of people with multiple problems.
2. Rapid identification determines which clients require immediate treatment and which can safely wait.

✦ B. The goal of triage is to do the greatest good for the greatest number.
C. From triage, victims are taken to a designated medical treatment area (Immediate Care, Delayed Care, or Morgue), and from there, transported out of the disaster area (*see* flow chart on the next page).
D. Three-level triage has been used for years to differentiate levels of emergency cases.
E. Now, a five-level system is preferred because it reduces ambiguity of middle level emergency care.

TWO WAYS TO CATEGORIZE THREE-LEVEL TRIAGE

Method One

- **Emergent** triage refers to a life-threatening or potentially life-threatening condition that requires immediate treatment.
- **Immediate,** or Urgent, triage is not life-threatening or acute, but refers to clients who need treatment as soon as possible (within 2 hours). These clients have stable vital signs and require no immediate intervention.
- **Nonemergent,** or Nonurgent, includes clients who have a condition that would not be affected by a delay in treatment.

Method Two

- **Immediate (I)** – the victim has a life-threatening injury (airway, bleeding or shock) that demands immediate attention (the same as Emergent);
- **Delayed (D)** – an injury that does not jeopardize the victim's life if definitive treatment is delayed; and finally,
- **Dead (DEAD)** – no respiration after 2 attempts to open airway. (CPR is not performed in a disaster environment because it demands extensive resources, including personnel time.)

EXAMPLE OF A FIVE-LEVEL TRIAGE SYSTEM: EMERGENCY SEVERITY INDEX (ESI)

Level

1.	Most acute	Life-threatening—potentially fatal
2.		Includes vital sign assessment
3.	Lower acuity	Some resources required from this level to 5
4.		
5.	Least acute	Not life-threatening—minimal resources

TRIAGE CATEGORIES

Field Triage

Red	=	Emergent (hyperacute–1st priority)
Yellow	=	Immediate (serious–2nd priority)
Green	=	Urgent (injured–3rd priority)
Blue	=	First Aid
Black	=	Dead or dying

Catastrophic Triage (First Option)

I	=	Immediate (life-threatening)
D	=	Delayed (may delay treatment without death)
Dead	=	Dead

Catastrophic Triage (Second Option)

Red Tag	=	Potential to survive
No other victims tagged.		

START Categories

Color Tag			Decontamination Priority
Red Tag	=	Immediate	1. Serious signs/symptoms Known agent contamination
Yellow Tag	=	Delayed	2. Moderate-to-minimal signs/symptoms Known agent or aerosol contamination Close to point of release
Green Tag	=	Minor	3. Minimal signs/symptoms No known exposure to agent
Black Tag	=	Deceased/ Expectant	4. Very serious signs/ symptoms Grossly contaminated Unresponsive

Assessment

A. Assess need to establish triage treatment areas.

B. Validate that public health parameters are established.

C. Observe that steps of triage are followed.

D. Assess that victim is not in immediate danger, or conversely, requires immediate intervention.

E. Assess vital signs of victims.

F. Assess the treatment steps necessary to treat life-threatening conditions.
  1. Observe for signs of respiratory distress.
  2. Assess need for establishing an airway.
  3. Observe for amount and source of bleeding and need for intervention.
  4. Recognize shock state and need for intervention.

G. Assess victims post-triage and observe for any signs or symptoms that indicate major injury.

H. Identify victims having a severe psychological reaction to bioterrorism event.

I. Assess possibility of post-traumatic stress syndrome developing.

✦ Implementation

A. Assign roles to personnel in treatment areas.

B. Select a site as soon as possible—advance planning is essential.
  1. Select safe area, free of hazards and debris.
  2. Position site upwind of hazard zone.
  3. Determine site is accessible to transportation vehicles (ambulances, trucks, helicopters).
  4. Be sure site is able to expand.
  5. Survey entire scene, including area above you, for threats to your safety before beginning triage or team work.

C. Protect treatment area and delineate area using tarps, covers, etc.

D. Set up signs to identify subdivisions of area.
  I = Immediate care.
  D = Delayed care.
  Dead = Dead for morgue.

1. Establish I and D areas close together in order to facilitate verbal communication between workers; this also allows them to share medical supplies and transfer victims quickly when status changes.
2. Position victims in head-to-toe configuration, with 2 to 3 feet between victims, facilitating effective use of space and personnel.
3. Establish a secure morgue site that is away (and not visible) from medical treatment areas.

✦ E. Establish public health parameters.
1. Assign personnel to monitor public health concerns where disaster victims are sheltered.
2. Have available search and rescue safety equipment.
3. Maintain proper hygiene by washing hands and using gloves.
    a. Wash hands with soap and water if dirty or antibacterial gel between victims.
    b. Wear gloves at all times.
    c. Change gloves between victims if possible. If not, clean them between victims in a bleach and water solution (1 part bleach to 10 parts water).
4. Wear a mask and goggles.
5. Avoid direct contact with body fluids.
6. Maintain sanitation.
    a. Mark and have available specific biohazard waste disposal containers where bacterial sources (gloves, dressings, etc.) are discarded.
    b. Place waste products in plastic bags and bury them in designated area.
    c. Bury human waste.
7. Purify water for drinking, cooking, medical use, if potable water is not available.
    a. Boil water at rolling boil for 10 minutes.
    b. Use water purification tablets.
    c. Use unscented liquid bleach (16 drops per gallon of water or 1 teaspoon per 5 gallons; mix and let stand for 30 minutes).

✦ F. Steps of trauma assessment applied to triage.
1. Perform a rapid systematic assessment. (Trauma is a multisystem condition so all systems must be assessed.)
2. Complete a primary trauma assessment. (To identify victim's primary and critical problem.)
    a. Airway.
    b. Breathing capability.
    c. Shock—circulation and bleeding.
    d. Neurological—level of consciousness, mental status.
    e. Exposure to contaminate.
    f. Disability.
    g. Evacuation necessity.
3. Complete a secondary assessment (post-triage) that includes a focus assessment.

DISASTER MANAGEMENT

Hospital Evacuation Plans

A. Every hospital must have an evacuation plan in place with a designated authority in charge.
B. Types of evacuation
1. Shelter in place—keeping everyone where they are may be the safest plan.
2. Moving occupants either up (flooding) or down (protection from air attack).
3. Removing all persons from building and relocating to a safe area.

Communication

Characteristics

A. Communication systems are likely to be overwhelmed in a disaster.
1. Establishing backup and redundant communication systems is essential.
2. Communication coordination is an important component in the infrastructure system.
B. There must be communication among the triage team (out-of-hospital) for establishing victim care priorities, the hospital or treatment staff (in-hospital), and state and federal agencies.
1. The local communication structure should appoint one community-identified person or small group to be in command and act as liaison agent.
2. The state and federal response teams will be integrated into the communication system.
3. The Incident Command System (ICS) is an example of a local system.
    a. Specific roles and positions carry specific duties and responsibilities.
    b. The ICS tells people how and with whom to communicate.
    c. Each position has a prioritized list of tasks that are checked off as they are completed.
    d. This system organizes emergency responses in five categories: command, planning, operations, logistics and administration.
✦ C. Hospitals must have an ongoing, open channel of communication with emergency response teams, who will have been notified first of a mass casualty incident.
1. A community-wide network, all using the same channel of communication, is necessary.

a. A single communication site for obtaining victim and locator information should be established.

b. A clear and open information system, using both telecommunication and a position-to-position cascade in the event of the primary system being overloaded, is necessary.

2. Adequate equipment, such as cell phones, walkie-talkies, even runners, must be available if current phone land lines are overwhelmed.

Assessment

A. Assess that lines of communication are established and activated.

B. Assess that internal, external, and collaborative communication networks are in place.

C. Assess that Federal Response Plan is activated.

Implementation

A. Understand lines of communication. (When lines of communication are compromised, effective triage and intervention cannot take place.)
1. Mass casualty incident occurs.
2. Local public health official notifies FBI—lead agency for crisis plan.
3. FBI notifies HHS and CDC and FEMA.
4. State health agency requests CDC to deploy response teams if needed.

B. Understand the network of communication that will be activated in response to a suspected or actual bioterrorism event.
1. Emergency response team.
   a. Local and state public health officials.
   b. Infection control personnel in notified facilities.
   c. FBI field offices.
   d. CDC.
   e. Local emergency medical services (EMS).
   f. Local police and fire departments.
2. In turn, the Federal Response Plan will be activated.

C. Activate Federal Response Plan. (When the local area cannot cope with the disaster, federal assistance is available.)
1. Department of Health and Human Services (HHS) is primary agency.
2. Office of Emergency Preparedness is action agency.
3. Emergency Support Function N8 coordinates federal assistance to supplement state and local resources (directed by HHS).
4. Implemented when state requests assistance and FEMA agrees.

◆ D. Establish a viable communication system.

1. Set up **external communication** system designated spokesperson.
   a. A viable system will minimize disruption.
   b. All communication goes through designated spokesperson—no staff will communicate with the public, press, or outside persons.
2. Report to appointed community-wide regional spokesperson or small group designated as being in command throughout the incident. Spokesperson will be in charge of coordination of all media relations.
3. Set up a single community site for family and friends to obtain victim-locator information.
   a. Provide clear, consistent and verifiable information to clients and general public.
   b. Plan in advance methods and channels of communication to be used to inform the public.
4. Establish **internal communication**.
   a. Determine position (not person) that will be in charge, i.e., emergency department supervisor, called "incident commander." Position, rather than person, will prevent confusion when staff turnover, multiple shifts, or reassignment of staff occur.
   b. Communicate only through established lines of communication with designated commander or liaisons.
5. Establish a **collaborative communication system**.
   a. Establish on-going, open channels of communication with emergency response teams. (Response teams may have first awareness of the disaster and will need to communicate with the hospital.)
   b. Appoint person (reporting to spokesperson) to collaborate with response team and link to community representative.
   c. Develop a community-wide communications network. (If different organizations cannot communicate with each other, precious time will be lost.)
   d. Test the communications network so overload does not occur in the event of a mass-casualty incident.
6. Develop clear communication systems that have access to telecommunications, as well as a person-to-person communication system. This position-to-position or person-to-person method is necessary if telecommunications are overwhelmed or unavailable.
   a. Use pagers, walkie-talkies, and the Internet via e-mail as substitutes for a communication network during a disaster.

b. Develop horizontal and vertical relationships between organizations, governmental and private, that will have to work together in a mass-casualty event.

TREATING LIFE-THREATENING CONDITIONS

Implementation

A. Implement Simple Triage and Rapid Treatment (START), the first step for treating multiple casualties in a disaster.

B. Gather all equipment needed for interventions.
   - 1. Check breathing immediately.
      a. Open airway. (If airway is obstructed, victim cannot get oxygen.)
      b. Move fast—time is critical. (Heart function will be affected within minutes, and brain damage is possible after 4 minutes.)
      c. Check if tongue is obstructing airway. (This is the most common airway obstruction, especially when victim is positioned on back).
   2. Use head-tilt/chin-lift method if victim is not breathing and airway is not obstructed.
      a. Touch victim and shout "CAN YOU HEAR ME?"
      b. If victim does not respond, place one hand on forehead, 2 fingers of other hand under chin, and tilt jaw upward and head back slightly.
      c. Look for chest to rise, listen for air exchange, and feel for abdominal movement.
      d. If no response (victim does not start breathing) repeat procedure. (If AED is available, may apply to victim.)
      e. If victim does not respond after 2nd attempt, move on to next victim. (Goal of disaster intervention is to do the greatest good for the greatest number of victims.)
      f. If the victim begins breathing, maintain airway (hopefully with a volunteer holding airway open) or place soft object under victim's shoulders to elevate them, keeping airway open.
   - 3. Control bleeding. (If bleeding is not controlled within a short period of time, victim will go into shock—loss of 1 liter of blood (out of a total of 5 in the human body) will present risk of death.
   4. Identify type of bleeding.
      a. Arterial bleeding (spurting blood).
      b. Venous bleeding (flowing blood).
      c. Capillary bleeding (oozing blood).

   - 5. Choose appropriate method to control bleeding.
      a. Direct local pressure—place direct pressure over wound (using clean or sterile pad) and press firmly. (95% of bleeding can be controlled by direct pressure with elevation.)
      b. Maintain compression by wrapping wound firmly with pressure bandage.
      c. Elevate wound above level of heart.
      d. Use pressure point to slow blood flow to wound, brachial point for arm, femoral point for leg.
   - 6. Use tourniquet if bleeding cannot be controlled by other methods (consider this a last resort, as tourniquets can pose serious risks to affected limbs).
      a. Incorrect material or application can cause more damage and bleeding; if the tourniquet is too tight, nerves, blood vessels or muscles may be damaged.
      b. If tourniquet is left in place too long, limb may be lost.
      c. If tourniquet is applied, leave in plain sight and affix label to victim's forehead, stating time tourniquet was applied.
      d. Notify physician to remove tourniquet.
   7. Recognize and treat shock.
      a. Body will initially compensate for blood loss, so signs of shock may not be observable.
      b. Continually evaluate victim's condition.
   8. Observe for signs/symptoms of shock.
      a. Rapid, shallow breathing (> 30/minute).
      b. Cold, pale skin (capillary refill > 2/second).
      c. Failure to respond to simple commands.
   - 9. Administer treatment for shock.
      a. Position victim supine with feet elevated 6–10 inches.
      b. Maintain open airway.
      c. Maintain body temperature (cover ground and victim).
      d. Avoid rough or excessive handling, and do not allow victim to eat or drink.

POST-TRIAGE INTERVENTIONS

Assessment

A. Perform head-to-toe assessment, always in the same order. This will enable you to complete it more quickly and accurately: head, neck, shoulders, chest, arms, abdomen, pelvis, legs, back.

B. Complete assessment before beginning any treatment—to prioritize treatment interventions, a complete assessment must be done.

C. Observe for any sign/symptom that indicates major injury.

1. Assess how person received injury (mechanism of injury).
2. Airway obstruction.
3. Signs of shock.
4. Labored or difficult breathing.
5. Excessive bleeding.
6. Swelling/bruising.
7. Severe pain.

Implementation

A. Provide immediate treatment. Reclassify victim during treatment, if necessary.

✦ B. Evaluate that victim is not in immediate danger.
1. If available staff, continue to assess for signs of head, neck, and spinal injury.
   a. Change in level of consciousness (unconscious, confused).
   b. Unable to move body part.
   c. Severe pain in head, neck, back.
   d. Tingling or numbness in extremities.
2. Continue to assess other signs and symptoms.
   a. Difficulty breathing or seeing.
   b. Heavy bleeding/blood in eyes or nose.
   c. Seizures.
   d. Nausea, vomiting.

C. Immobilize head, neck or spine by keeping spine in straight line, putting cervical collar on neck, or placing victim on board—if equipment is available.

D. Document person's identity and relevant medical information.

✦ E. Care for those who died.
1. Victims pronounced DOA (dead on arrival) must be tagged.
   a. Add special tag "not to remove personal effects."
   b. Incorporate special instructions for people performing autopsies, preparing bodies for burial or transportation.
2. Place bodies in cordoned off area for field triage. (Decontamination may have to be completed before transport.)
3. Notify those performing post-mortem care of victim's diagnosis to protect staff handling post-mortem care.
   a. Autopsies performed carefully using all personal protective equipment and Standard Precautions, including use of masks and eye protection.
   b. Incorporate any special instructions about biological–chemical–radiological agent present.
4. Complete a record for all bodies including identification, name of person declaring death,

diagnosis, if known, name of agency removing body, etc.

✦ F. Care for clients with psychological reactions.
1. Expect major psychological reactions of fear, panic, anger, horror, paranoia, etc., following a bioterrorism event.
2. Plan prior to such an event for professional and educated volunteers to be on site.
3. Minimize fear and panic in staff.
   a. Provide educational materials that include risks to healthcare workers, accurate information on bioterrorism facts, plans for protecting workers, and use of personal protection equipment.
   b. Encourage team participation in disaster drills, as experience in handling a disaster will build confidence and allay anxiety.
4. Cope with psychological reactions of fear and anxiety.
   a. Minimize panic by clearly explaining the care given.
   b. Offer rapid evaluation and treatment and avoid isolation, if possible.
✦ 5. Treat major anxiety reactions in unexposed persons with factual information, reassurance and medication, if indicated. (Anxiety is communicable; prompt intervention will allay group anxiety. "Worried well" persons could overwhelm hospitals if they leave area and go to closest healthcare facility.)
6. Prevent post-terrorism trauma.
   a. Gather victims into a group with a skilled therapist soon after event (within 24 hours) to prevent a major post-trauma reaction.
      (1) Early opportunity for catharsis will help prevent suppression of traumatic event emotions.
      (2) Group victims according to age and experience.
   b. Follow initial group meeting with subsequent meeting within one week to discuss feelings about event. (Research has found that group meetings following traumatic event has eliminated 80% post-traumatic stress disorder.)

G. Identifying post-traumatic stress disorder.
1. Recognize possibility of existing condition.
   a. Traumatic event occurs and is re-experienced as flashbacks, dreams, or memory state.
   b. Abreaction occurs: vivid recall of painful experience with original emotions.
   c. Individual cannot adjust to event.
2. Assess signs and symptoms of anxiety and depression.

a.   Emotional instability, withdrawal and isolation.

b.   Nightmares, difficulty sleeping.

c.   Feelings of detachment or guilt.

3.   Assess aggressive or acting-out behavior; may be explosive or impulsive behavior.

4.   Assist client to go through recovery process.

a.   Recovery—reassure client that he is safe following experience of the traumatic event.

b.   Avoidance—client will avoid thinking about traumatic event; support client.

c.   Reconsideration—client deals with event by confronting it, talking about it, and working through feelings.

d.   Adjustment—client rehabilitates and adjusts to environment following event; client functions well and is able to view future positively.

DISASTER NURSING: BIOTERRORISM REVIEW QUESTIONS

1. You are assigned to complete mass-casualty decontamination. Which group, according to triage guidelines, will be decontaminated *last*?

   1. Those closest to the point of release of the toxin.
   2. Those who have serious medical conditions.
   3. Those with liquid deposits on their skin.
   4. Those with conventional injuries.

2. If a disaster occurs, one example of how the disaster will impact the infrastructure of a city is by the effect it will have on the

   1. People who live in the city.
   2. Houses and land of the city.
   3. Water supply of a city.
   4. First responders.

3. A preparedness plan for a community-wide communication network includes the local emergency response system being activated. The individual person or agency who is notified *first* would be the

   1. Local health officer commander.
   2. FBI field office.
   3. Health and Human Services.
   4. Centers for Disease Control and Prevention (CDC).

4. Healthcare workers exposure to radiation is measured by an instrument readout in units of rads (R). 50 R tells the worker that if he stays in the exposed area 1 hour, he will receive a rad exposure of

   1. 50 rad.
   2. 5 rad.
   3. 0.75 rad.
   4. 100 rad.

5. You are assigned to decontaminate casualties. Which decontamination material will you use as a *first* step?

   1. Bleach.
   2. Hydrogen peroxide.
   3. Tepid water.
   4. Hot water.

6. Which piece of equipment is *not* necessary when implementing Standard Precautions?

   1. Soap or waterless antiseptic.
   2. Gloves.
   3. Gown.
   4. Shoe covers.

7. You are assigned to administer smallpox vaccinations to a group of people. Of the following groups, which group would be appropriate to receive the vaccination?

   1. Those with immunodeficiency, such as HIV infection or AIDS.
   2. Those who have life-threatening allergies to antibiotics.
   3. Those with flu, cold, or bronchitis.
   4. Those who have been diagnosed with eczema.

8. When establishing a triage site following a major disaster, the area that will *not* be included is

   1. Immediate care.
   2. Intermediate care.
   3. Delayed care.
   4. The morgue or other designated area for the deceased.

9. There is a suspected attack of anthrax. The precautions necessary to implement are

   1. Strict isolation.
   2. Isolation.
   3. Droplet precautions.
   4. Standard Precautions.

10. The precaution protocol necessary to implement for the biohazard of pneumonic plague is

   1. Standard Precautions plus droplet.
   2. Strict isolation with Standard Precautions.
   3. Droplet precautions.
   4. Contact precautions.

11. The best rationale for informing clients about the smallpox vaccination process is to

   1. Avoid a later lawsuit.
   2. Meet government expectations.
   3. Provide safety information.
   4. Make clients comfortable in signing the permission form.

12. The most toxic of all chemical agents is/are

    1. Cyanide.
    2. Vesicant.
    3. Pulmonary.
    4. Nerve.

13. The rationale for setting up a decontamination unit for radiological exposure prior to victims entering the hospital is

    1. That it is closer to medical care than a unit in the field.
    2. To prevent contamination of clients and healthcare workers.
    3. That it is preferable to decontamination at the site.
    4. Protection for healthcare workers is better closer to the hospital.

14. If a mass-casualty incident occurs and first responders do *not* know what type of personal protection gear is needed, the team should

    1. Wait until the type of equipment needed is known.
    2. Decontaminate victims before intervening.
    3. Choose the highest level of equipment available—full Level A protection.
    4. Wear a radiation and biological device before entering the area.

15. Place in order the steps for treating life-threatening conditions _____ .

    1. Control bleeding.
    2. Treat shock.
    3. Check breathing.
    4. Use head-tilt method if airway is obstructed.

DISASTER NURSING: BIOTERRORISM

Answers with Rationale

1. (4) When triaging casualties, you will first triage serious medical conditions, then those close to the point of release with liquid on their skin or those who report exposure to the agent; you will then treat those with conventional injuries. Last you would treat those who do not have a serious medical condition.

   NP:P; CN:S; CA:M; CL:AN

2. (3) The infrastructure of a city includes transportation, electrical equipment, telephone connections, fuel supplies, and water. People and housing are not part of the infrastructure. Water could be affected by disruption of service, inadequate supply to fight a fire, and increased risk to public health if the supply is not pure.

   NP:AN; CN:H; CA:M; CL:C

3. (1) Once the local emergency response system is activated, the local health officer commander (who has been pre-chosen) is notified first, and he/she in turn notifies the FBI field office, HHS, and the CDC.

   NP:A; CN:H; CA:M; CL:K

4. (1) One hour is equal to an exposure of 50 rad. Gray is also a unit of exposure; so the worker should know that if he receives less than 0.75 Gy (when 1 Gray equals 100 rad), his exposure will be in the safe range.

   NP:E; CN:S; CA:M; CL:C

5. (3) The primary decontamination material used is tepid water. Water is an effective decontaminant because of the rapidity of application. Water should be tepid because cold water can cause hypothermia and hot water will cause vasodilation, speeding distribution of the contaminants.

   NP:P; CN:H; CA:M; CL:A

6. (4) Shoe covers are not considered standard equipment for precautions, but a mask and eye or face shield are included.

   NP:P; CN:S; CA:M; CL:A

7. (3) Persons who have a cold, flu, or bronchitis could receive a smallpox vaccination. Other categories of conditions that are excluded (in addition to the ones mentioned in the question) are cardiac conditions, leukemia, lymphoma, pregnancy, or burns.

   NP:P; CN:H; CA:M; CL:AN

8. (2) Triage sites will be set up in three areas. The area that is not included is intermediate care. Following a disaster, the area sites are simple and straightforward—those who need immediate care, delayed care or no care (dead).

   NP:P; CN:H; CA:M; CL:C

9. (4) An attack of anthrax would require Standard Precautions. Isolation is not necessary because anthrax is not transmitted via droplet or person to person.

   NP:I; CN:S; CA:M; CL:A

10. (1) Precautions include Standard Precautions plus droplet precautions (eye protection and surgical mask) until 48–72 hours after antibiotic treatment.

    NP:I; CN:S; CA:M; CL:A

11. (3) The best rationale for providing information is the safety element, so the client will know how to recognize side effects, care for the blister, and not contaminate others. Regulations state that clients cannot sue following a vaccination. The government has specific regulations about vaccination being voluntary, rather than a government expectation. A permission form must be signed and adequate

---

Coding for Questions/Answers Abbreviations: **Nursing Process: NP,** Assessment: A, Analysis: AN, Planning: P, Implementation: I, Evaluation: E; **Client Needs: CN,** Safe, Effective Care Environment: S, Health Promotion and Maintenance: H, Psychosocial Integrity: PS, Physiological Integrity: PH; **Clinical Area: CA,** Medical Nursing: M, Surgical Nursing: S, Maternal/Newborn Nursing: MA, Pediatric Nursing: P, Psychiatric Nursing: PS; **Cognitive Level: CL,** Knowledge: K, Comprehension: C, Application: A, Analysis: AN.

information would make the client more comfortable, but it is not a safety issue.

NP:E; CN:S; CA:M; CL:C

12. (4) The most toxic chemical agents are nerve agents, such as Sarin, Tabon, Soman, GF and VX. These agents block acetylcholinesterase, which regulates activity in organs, glands, muscles, and the CNS. With no ability to "turn off," the body wears out and death occurs in a short time.

NP:AN; CN:S; CA:M; CL:C

13. (2) It is preferable to decontaminate at the site of radiological exposure, but if it cannot be done, the next choice is to decontaminate prior to entering the hospital to prevent contamination of clients and workers.

NP:P; CN:H; CA:M; CL:C

14. (3) Because it is critical that the response team be fully protected, they must wear the highest level of equipment; this includes SCBA full protection suit, shoe covers, double gloves and biological detection device, if available.

NP:P; CN:S; CA:M; CL:AN

15. The answer is 3 4 1 2. After gathering equipment, check breathing. If victim is not breathing or airway is obstructed, use head-tilt/chin-lift method. Next, you would control bleeding, followed by treating shock.

NP:I; CN:H; CA:M; CL:C

Medical–Surgical Nursing

✦ The icon denotes content of special importance for NCLEX.

NEUROLOGICAL SYSTEM

The nervous system (together with the endocrine system) provides the control functions for the body. Unique in its incredible ability to handle thousands of bits of information and stimuli from the sensory organs, this system of nerves and nerve centers coordinates and regulates all of this data and determines the responses of the body.

ANATOMY AND PHYSIOLOGY OF THE NERVOUS SYSTEM

Central Nervous System: Brain and Spinal Cord

A. Brain.
  1. Cerebrum (two hemispheres).
    a. Function.
      (1) Highest level of functioning.
      (2) Governs all sensory and motor activity, thought, and learning.
      (3) Analyzes, associates, integrates, and stores information.
    ✦ b. Cerebral cortex (outer gray layer)—divided into four major lobes.
      (1) Frontal.
        (a) Precentral gyrus—motor function.
        (b) Broca's area—motor speech area.
        (c) Prefrontal—controls morals, values, emotions, and judgment.
      (2) Parietal.
        (a) Postcentral gyrus—integrates general sensation.
        (b) Interprets pain, touch, temperature, and pressure.
        (c) Governs discrimination.
      (3) Temporal.
        (a) Auditory center.
        (b) Wernicke's area—sensory speech center.
      (4) Occipital—visual area.
    c. Basal ganglia.
      (1) Collections of cell bodies in white matter.
      (2) Controls motor movement.
      (3) Part of extrapyramidal tract.
  2. Diencephalon.
    a. Thalamus.
      (1) Screens and relays sensory impulses to cortex.
      (2) Lowest level of crude conscious awareness.
    ✦ b. Hypothalamus—regulates autonomic nervous system, stress response, sleep, appetite, body temperature, fluid balance, and emotions.
  3. Brain stem.
    a. Midbrain—motor coordination, conjugate eye movements.
    b. Pons.
      (1) Contains projection tracts between spinal cord, medulla, and brain.
      (2) Controls involuntary respiratory reflexes.
    c. Medulla oblongata.
      (1) Contains all afferent and efferent tracts.
      (2) Decussation of most upper motor neurons (pyramidal tracts).
      (3) Contains cardiac, respiratory, vomiting, and vasomotor centers.
  4. Cerebellum.
    a. Connected by afferent/efferent pathways to all other parts of CNS.
    b. Coordinates muscle movement, posture, equilibrium, and muscle tone.
B. Spinal cord.
  1. Structure.
    a. Conveys messages between brain and the rest of the body.
    b. Extends from foramen magnum to second lumbar vertebra.
    c. Inner column of H-shaped gray matter that contains two anterior and two posterior horns.
    d. Posterior horns—contain cell bodies that connect with afferent (sensory) nerve fibers from posterior root ganglia.
    e. Anterior horns—contain cell bodies giving rise to efferent (motor) nerve fibers.
    f. Lateral horns—present in thoracic segments; origin of autonomic fibers of sympathetic nervous system.
    g. White matter of cord contains nerve tracts.
      (1) Principal ascending tracts (sensory pathways).
        (a) Lateral spinothalamic—governs pain, temperature (contralateral).
        (b) Anterior spinothalamic—governs touch, pressure (contralateral).

(c) Posterior column to medial lemniscus—governs proprioception, vibration, touch, pressure (ipsilateral).

(d) Spinocerebellar—governs bilateral proprioception to posterior and anterior portions of the cerebellum.

(2) Principal descending tracts (motor pathways).

(a) Pyramidal, upper motor neuron, or corticospinal—from motor cortex to anterior horn cell. Tract crosses in medulla.

(b) Extrapyramidal tracts consist of corticorubrospinal, corticoreticulospinal and vestibulospinal. These tracts facilitate or inhibit flexor/extensor activity.

2. Protection for CNS.

a. Skull—rigid chamber with opening at the base (foramen magnum).

b. Meninges—three layers of protective membranes.

(1) Dura mater—tough, fibrous membrane—forms falx, tentorium.

(2) Arachnoid membrane—delicate membrane that contains subarachnoid fluid.

(3) Pia mater—vascular membrane.

c. Ventricles.

(1) Four ventricles.

(2) Communication between subarachnoid space.

(3) Subarachnoid space—formed by the arachnoid membrane and the pia mater.

(4) Produce and circulate cerebrospinal fluid.

✦ d. Cerebrospinal fluid.

(1) Secreted from choroid plexuses in lateral ventricles, third ventricle, and fourth ventricle.

(2) Circulates within interconnecting ventricles and subarachnoid space.

(3) Protective cushion; aids exchange of nutrients and wastes.

(4) Normal pressure: 60 to 180 mm H_2O.

(5) Volume: 80 to 200 mL, average 130 mL.

(6) Allows fluid shifts from cranial cavity to the spinal cavity.

e. Blood–brain barrier.

(1) Cerebrospinal fluid (CSF).

(2) Brain parenchyma.

(3) Structure of brain capillaries differs from other capillaries. Some substances that normally pass into most tissue are prevented from entering brain tissue. This barrier protects the brain from certain harmful agents and limits penetration of some drugs.

f. Blood supply—conductor of oxygen vitally needed by nervous system.

(1) Internal carotids branch to form anterior and middle cerebral arteries.

(2) Vertebral arteries arise from the subclavian arteries and merge to form the basilar arteries, which then subdivide into the two posterior cerebral arteries.

(3) Circle of Willis—formed as the anterior communicating artery bridges the anterior cerebral arteries, and as the posterior communicating artery bridges each posterior and middle cerebral artery.

Neuron Structure and Function

A. Structure.

1. Cell body (gray matter).

2. Processes (nerve fibers).

a. Axon conducts impulses from cell body.

b. Dendrites receive stimuli from the body and transmit them to the axon.

3. Synapse—chemical transmission of impulses from one neuron to another.

B. Myelin sheath (white matter).

1. Surrounds axon.

2. Insulates; correlates with function and speed of conduction.

3. Produced by neurolemmal cells in peripheral nerve fibers (sheath of Schwann).

4. Produced by neuroglial cells in CNS fibers.

✦ C. Classification by function.

1. Sensory (afferent)—conducts impulses from end of the organ to CNS.

2. Motor (efferent)—conducts impulses from CNS to muscles and glands.

3. Internuncial (connector)—conducts impulses from sensory to motor neurons.

4. Somatic—innervates body wall.

5. Visceral—innervates the viscera.

D. Reflex arc (basic unit of function).

1. Receptor—receives stimulus.

2. Afferent pathway—transmits impulses to spinal cord.

3. CNS—integration takes place at synapse between sensory and motor neurons.

4. Efferent pathway—motor neurons transmit impulses from CNS to effector.

CRANIAL NERVES

The following table correlates cranial nerves (CN) to areas of the brain stem, classification, and major function. The brain stem is responsible for vital functions. Disruption of this area can cause cranial nerve deficits, ataxia, coma, or brain death. CN evaluation can identify the level of the lesion in the brain stem. New onset cranial nerve deficits or changes in response to stimulation may indicate brain herniation.

Nerve	Brain Stem Area	Classification Sensory/Motor	Major Functions
Olfactory	Directly Above Midbrain	Sensory	Smell
Optic	Directly Above Midbrain	Sensory	Vision (acuity and field of vision); pupil reactivity to light and accommodation (afferent impulse)
Oculomotor	Midbrain	Motor	Most extraocular movements (EOMs): upward, downward and medial gaze, eyelid opening pupil size and reactivity (efferent impulse)
Trochlear	Midbrain	Motor	EOM (turns eye downward and laterally—inward gaze)
Trigeminal	Pons	Both	Movement of jaw, chewing; facial and mouth sensation; corneal reflex (sensory)
Abducens	Pons	Motor	EOM (turns eye laterally)
Facial	Pons	Both	Facial expression; taste; corneal (blink) reflex (motor); eyelid and lip closure
Accoustic	Pons	Sensory	Hearing; equilibrium—vestibular response
Glossopharyngeal	Medulla	Both	Gagging and swallowing (sensory); taste
Vagus	Medulla	Both	Gagging and swallowing (motor); speech (phonation), cough reflex
Spinal accessory	Medulla	Motor	Shoulder movement; head rotation, neck muscle
Hypoglossal	Medulla	Motor	Tongue movement; speech (articulation)

Sources: 1. Hickey, J. V. (2003). *The clinical practice of neurological and neurosurgical nursing.* Philadelphia: Lippincott Williams & Wilkins. 2. Marshall, R. S., & Mayer, S. A. (2001). *On call neurology* (2nd ed.). New York: W. B. Saunders. 3. Messner, R., & Wolfe, S. (1997). *RN's pocket assessment guide.* Montvale, NJ: Medical Economics. 4. Vos, H. (2002). The neurologic assessment. In E. Barker (Ed.), *Neuroscience nursing: Spectrum of care* (2nd ed.). St. Louis: Mosby. 5. Noah, P. (2004). *Neurological assessment: A refresher.* Retrieved February 28, 2008, from http://www.rnweb.com/rnweb/article/articleDetail.jsp?id=120796&searchString=cranial%20nerves

5. Effector—the organ or muscle that responds to the stimulus.

E. Regeneration of destroyed nerve fibers.
　1. Peripheral nerve—can regenerate, possibly due to neurolemma.
　2. CNS—cannot regenerate; lacks neurolemma.

Peripheral Nervous System

Nerves (Cranial and Spinal)

◆ A. Cranial nerves—12 pairs of parasympathetic nerves with their nuclei along the brain stem.

B. Spinal nerves (31 pairs).
　1. All mixed nerve fibers formed by joining the anterior motor and posterior sensory roots.
　2. Anterior root—efferent nerve fibers to glands and voluntary and involuntary muscles.
　3. Posterior root—afferent nerve fibers from sensory receptors. Contains posterior ganglion—the cell body of sensory neuron.

Dysfunction of Cranial Nerves

A. Eye deviation from midline or unusual movements.
　1. Unilateral pupil dilation: compression of the third cranial nerve (controls pupillary constriction).
　2. Fixed pupils, often unequal: midbrain injury.
　3. Pinpoint, fixed pupils, often unequal: pontine damage.

◆ B. Reflexes present with dysfunction.
　1. Plantar (called Babinski): dorsiflexion ankle and great toe with fanning of other toes; indicates disruption of pyramidal tract.
　　a. Paralyzed side in CVA.
　　b. Bilateral presence with spinal cord injury.
　2. Corneal (blink): loss of blink reflex indicates dysfunction of fifth cranial nerve (danger of corneal injuries).
　3. Gag: loss of gag reflex indicates dysfunction on the ninth and tenth cranial nerves (danger of aspiration).

Autonomic Nervous System (ANS)

A. Structure and function.
　1. The term "autonomic" means that this system operates independently of desires and intentions.
　2. Part of the peripheral nervous system controlling smooth muscle, cardiac muscle, and glands.
　3. The ANS is divided into two components.

a. Sympathetic.

b. Parasympathetic.

c. Two divisions make involuntary adjustments for integrated balance (homeostasis).

B. Diseases of sympathetic nerve trunks result in specific syndromes.

1. Dilation of pupils.

2. Bowel paralysis.

3. Variations in pulse rate and rhythm.

C. Structure of sympathetic nervous system—thoracolumbar division.

1. Long postganglionic (adrenergic) fibers.

2. Fibers arise in brain stem and descend to gray matter in spinal cord from C8 to L2.

D. Structure of parasympathetic nervous system—craniosacral division.

1. Short postganglionic (cholinergic) fibers.

2. Cells lie in brain stem and sacral region of spinal cord.

System Assessment

A. Evaluate client's history regarding common signs and symptoms.

1. Numbness, weakness.

2. Dizziness, fainting, loss of consciousness.

3. Headache, pain.

4. Speech disturbances.

5. Visual disturbances.

6. Disturbances in memory, thinking, personality.

7. Nausea, vomiting.

✦ B. Assess client's level of consciousness.

1. Evaluate cerebral function (most sensitive and reliable index of consciousness).

2. Evaluate level of consciousness.

3. Assess behavior to determine level of consciousness: clouding, confusion, delirium, stupor, coma.

✦ C. Evaluate pupillary signs.

1. Assess size: measure in millimeters; compare each eye.

2. Assess equality: equal, unequal, fluctuations.

3. Assess reactions to light: brisk, slow, fixed.

a. Light reflex is most important sign differentiating structural from metabolic coma.

b. Early warning of deterioriating condition or elevated ICP.

4. Evaluate unusual eye movements or deviations from midline.

✦ D. Evaluate motor function.

1. Assess face and upper and lower extremities for:

a. Muscle tone, strength, equality; normal is equal bilaterally.

b. Voluntary movement.

c. Involuntary movements.

SIGNS SUGGESTING INCREASED INTRACRANIAL PRESSURE (ICP)

Normal pressure is 10 to 15 mm Hg.

- Level of consciousness (LOC) is the most sensitive indication of increased ICP.
- Specific signs to assess for:

1. Observe for deteriorating LOC, restlessness, confusion, irritability to declining level of consciousness and coma.

2. Check for severe headache caused by tension and displacement of the brain.

3. Observe for vomiting—caused by irritation of the vagal nuclei floor of fourth ventricle.

4. Assess papillary changes—dilated or pinpoint, slow/no reaction to light; fixed dilated pupils is an ominous sign requiring immediate nursing intervention.

5. Assess deterioration in motor function—weakness, hemiplegia, positive Babinski, abnormal posturing (decorticate or decerebrate), flaccidity, seizure activity.

6. Assess vital signs:

a. Cushing reflex—a late sign characterized by severe hypertension with rise in blood pressure, widening pulse pressure (systolic–diastolic) and bradycardia.

b. Note abnormalities in respiration, especially periods of apnea; Cheyne–Stokes respirations, central neurogenic hyperventilation, temperature elevation.

---

d. Reflexes: Babinski, corneal, gag.

2. Evaluate patterns of motor function.

3. Inappropriate—nonpurposeful.

a. Involuntary.

(1) Choreiform (jerky, quick).

(2) Athetoid (twisting, slow).

(3) Tremors.

(4) Spasms.

(5) Convulsions.

E. Assess reflexes.

1. Evaluate for presence of reflexes.

2. Identify reflex response.

a. Scale is 0 to 4.

b. Absence of reflex is rated 0.

c. Weak response is rated 1.

d. Normal response is rated 2.

e. Exaggerated response is rated 3.

f. Hyperreflexia is rated 4.

g. Clonus is an abnormal response of continued rhythmic contraction of the muscle after the stimulus has been applied.

F. Evaluate sensory function.

G. Evaluate vital signs.

✦ 1. Increasing blood pressure with reflex slowing of pulse—compensatory stage with increasing intracranial pressure.

✦ 2. Fall in blood pressure with increasing or irregular pulse—decompensation.

3. Assess respiratory rate and rhythm.

✦ H. Evaluate intracranial pressure.
I. Evaluate autonomic nervous system.
✦   1. Assess for sympathetic function.
      a. Fight, flight, or freeze; diffuse response.
      b. Increases heart rate, blood pressure.
      c. Dilates pupils, bronchi.
      d. Decreases peristalsis.
      e. Increases perspiration.
      f. Increases blood sugar.
✦   2. Assess for parasympathetic function.
      a. Repair, repose; discrete response.
      b. Decreases heart rate, blood pressure.
      c. Constricts pupils, bronchi.
      d. Increases salivation and peristalsis.
      e. Dilates blood vessels.
      f. Bladder contraction.
J. Assess for pain.
  1. Assess for nonverbal signs of pain (i.e., facial grimaces, retracting from painful stimuli).
  2. Evaluate onset, location, intensity, duration, and aggravating factor.
  3. Observe for precipitating factors, associated manifestations, and alleviating factors.
  4. Assess ability to distinguish between sharp and dull sensation; use cotton-tip applicator and wooden end.

DIAGNOSTIC PROCEDURES

Skull Series

A. Procedure: x-rays of head from different angles.
B. Purpose: to visualize configuration, density, and vascular markings.
C. Tomograms: layered vertical or horizontal x-ray exposures.

Myelography

A. Injection of dye or air into lumbar or cisternal subarachnoid space followed by x-rays of the spinal column.
✦ B. Purpose: to visualize spinal subarachnoid space for distortions caused by lesions or tumors.
C. Potential complications.
  1. Same as for lumbar puncture.
  2. Cerebral meningeal irritation from dye.
D. Nursing implementation.
  1. If dye is used, elevate head and observe for meningeal irritation.
  2. If air is used, keep head lower than trunk.
  3. Frequently observe neurological signs and vital signs and compare to baseline.
  4. Check for adequate voiding.

Cerebral Angiography

A. Injection of radiopaque dye into carotid and/or vertebral arteries followed by serial x-rays.
B. Purpose: to visualize cerebral vessels and localize lesions such as aneurysms, occlusions, angiomas, tumors, or abscesses.
✦ C. Potential complications.
  1. Anaphylactic reaction to dye.
  2. Local hemorrhage.
  3. Vasospasm.
  4. Adverse intracranial pressure.
✦ D. Nursing implementation.
  1. Prior to procedure.
      a. Check for allergies.
      b. Take baseline assessment.
      c. Measure neck circumference.
  2. During procedure and postprocedure.
      a. Have emergency equipment available.
      b. Monitor neurological and vital signs for shock, level of consciousness, hemiparesis, hemiplegia, and aphasia.
      c. Monitor swelling of neck and difficulty in swallowing or breathing.
      d. Apply ice collar.

Magnetic Resonance Imaging (MRI)

A. Visualization of distribution of hydrogen molecules in the body in three dimensions.
B. Purpose: to differentiate types of tissues, including those in normal and abnormal states (includes brain, both tumors and vascular abnormalities, as well as cardiac, respiratory and renal conditions).
C. MRI yields greater contrast in the images of soft-tissue structures than CT scan.

SAFETY MEASURES AND NURSING INTERVENTIONS FOR THE MRI

- Review client history for contraindications: pins, plates, pacemakers, artificial heart valves, or other implants that may be dislodged by a magnetic field.
- Explain procedure.
- Obtain informed consent.
- Assess ability to withstand being in a confined area—client must remain in a cylindrical machine for up to 90 minutes. Open MRI may be required for those who cannot tolerate closed spaces.
- Have client use the bathroom before test.
- Have client remove all jewelry, hair clips, clothing with metal fasteners, dentures.
- Instruct client to remove hearing aids and glasses before entering the scanner.
- Closely monitor clients with potential respiratory or cardiac collapse.

Computerized Tomography Scan (CT Scan)

A. Procedure: a diagnostic imaging procedure that uses a combination of x-rays and computer technology to produce horizontally and vertically cross-sectional images of the body to analyze relative tissue density as an x-ray beam passes through.

B. Purpose: provides detailed three-dimensional images of any part of the body, including the bones, muscles, fat, and organs, to determine location and extent of tumors, infracted areas, vascular lesions/abnormalities, or tissue atrophy.

C. Nursing implementation.
   1. Explain procedure; advise client that he or she will have to lie still.
   2. Obtain informed consent.
   3. Assess for allergy to iodine, a component of the contrast material.
   4. Withhold food for approximately 2 hours; contrast may cause nausea and vomiting.
   5. Have client use the bathroom before the test.
   6. Have client remove all hair pieces, pins and clips prior to CT of head.
   7. Instruct client to remove hearing aids and glasses before the test.

Tomography

✦ A. Type of brain scan that relies on tissue density and shadows to reflect internal state of brain tissue.

B. EMI/scanner (CT scan).

C. Xenon computed tomography quantitative cerebral blood flow (Xe/CT/CBF).
   1. Precisely measures blood flow to various areas of the brain.
   2. Defines degree and extent of ischemia in an acute neurologic condition.
   3. Enables clinicians to identify irreversibly damaged brain tissue hours to days before changes become evident on standard CT or MRI tests.
   4. Most often used to select stroke clients for thrombolytic therapy.
   5. Identifies and manages vasospasm after subarachnoid hemorrhage.
   6. Diagnoses brain death by confirming the absence of cerebral blood flow.
   7. Determines the effect of hyperventilation when used with head trauma clients with increased intracranial pressure (ICP).
   8. Evaluates the effectiveness of interventions to increase cerebral perfusion (i.e., hypertensive therapies).
   9. Provides both quantitative and qualitative measurement of blood flow.
   10. Xenon gas eliminated from body within 20 minutes, test can be repeated quickly if needed.
   11. Client prep as for normal noncontrast CT.

Positron Emission Tomography (PET)

A. Procedure: a computerized image of regional metabolic activity of the body tissues used to determine the presence of disease. The test involves injecting a very small dose of a radioactive glucose, called a radiotracer, into a vein. A scanner is used to make detailed, computerized pictures of areas inside the body where the glucose is metabolized, blood flows, and oxygen is extracted.

B. Purpose: a PET scan differs from other imaging tests such as CT scan or MRI in that it reveals cellular-level metabolic changes occurring in an organ or tissue where disease processes begin.
   1. A PET scan can often detect these very early changes, whereas a CT or MRI detects changes a little later—as the disease causes changes in the structure of organs or tissues.
   2. PET scans can detect cancer, brain disorders (including brain tumors, memory disorders, and seizures), and other CNS problems.

C. Nursing implementation.
   1. Explain procedure. Advise client that he or she will have to lie still during procedure and may require sedation—if so, use carefully with head injury or surgery.
   2. Obtain informed consent.
   3. Withhold food for approximately 4–6 hours.
   4. Have client use the bathroom before the test.

Electroencephalography (EEG)

A. Procedure: graphic recording of brain's electrical activity by electrodes placed on the scalp.

B. Purpose: to detect intracranial lesion and characteristic abnormal electrical activity (seizures).

C. Nursing implementation.
   1. Wash hair.
   2. Withhold sedatives or stimulants.
   3. Administer fluids as ordered.

Electromyography (EMG)

A. Procedure: recording the potential of muscle action by surface or needle electrodes.

B. Purpose: to diagnose or localize neuromuscular disease.

Lumbar Puncture (LP)

✦ A. Procedure: insertion of spinal needle through L3–4 or L4–5 interspace into lumbar subarachnoid space.

B. Purpose.
 1. To obtain cerebrospinal fluid (CSF).
 2. To measure intracranial pressure and spinal fluid dynamics.
 3. To instill air, dye, or medications.
C. Potential complications: headache, backache and herniation with brain stem compression (especially if intracranial pressure is high).
D. Nursing implementation.
 1. Explain procedure. Advise client that he or she will have to lie or sit still during procedure.
 2. Obtain informed consent.
 3. Have client empty bowel and bladder before the test.
 4. Monitor vital signs.
 5. Position client in a position that will facilitate enlarging the opening of the vertebral space.
  a. Lying on side with feet drawn up, head to chest on edge of bed.
  b. Sitting on side of bed, leaning over bedside table, support feet on flat surface.
 6. Assist with specimen collection and spinal fluid dynamics.
 7. Post procedure.
  a. Maintain client in prone position for 2 hours or flat side-lying for 2–3 hours to avoid headache.
  b. Assess puncture site for CSF leakage—a complication of LP.
 8. Label specimens, send to lab; note color and amount of fluid.
 9. Assess for signs of shock.
 10. Maintain asepsis and administer fluids unless contraindicated.
E. Spinal fluid dynamics—Queckenstedt–Stookey test.
 1. Normal pressure is 60–150 mm H_2O when client is in lateral recumbent position. Pressure increases with jugular compression and drops to normal 10–30 seconds after release of compression.
 2. Partial block: slow rise and return to normal.
 3. Complete block: no rise.

✦ **System Implementation**

A. Observe for and treat seizure activity.
B. Monitor vital signs for signs of hyperthermia, increased intracranial pressure, and infection.
C. Observe motor and sensory function.
D. Observe pupillary signs for metabolic or structural complications.
E. Prevent muscle weakness and atrophy through range-of-motion exercises.
F. Promote bowel and bladder function.
G. Maintain nutritional status.

H. Prevent complications of immobility (i.e., skin breakdown).
I. Provide emotional support for client and family during hospitalization and upon discharge.
J. Monitor cardiac and respiratory function for identification of potential complications.
K. Provide appropriate preoperative and postoperative nursing interventions.
L. Establish an individualized rehabilitative program.
M. Administer drug therapy and monitor side effects.
N. Institute nursing implementation to assist in decreasing intracranial pressure.
O. Establish appropriate measures for pain relief.

NEUROLOGIC DYSFUNCTION

The Unconscious Client

Definition: Unconsciousness is a state of depressed cerebral functioning with altered sensory and motor function.

Assessment

A. Possible causes: vascular disorders, intracranial mass, head trauma, cerebral toxins, metabolic disorders, acute infection.
 1. Intracranial.
  a. Supratentorium mass/lesion compressing or displacing brain stem.
  b. Infratentorium destructive lesions.
 2. Extracranial.
  a. Metabolic encephalopathy (most common).
  b. Psychiatric conditions.
✦ B. Glasgow Coma Scale provides objective, consistent way to monitor client's neurological condition.
 1. Comatose state based on three areas associated with level of consciousness.
 ✦ 2. Scoring system.
  a. Based on a scale of 1 to 15 points.
  b. Any score below 8 indicates coma is present; the lowest score, 3, indicates severe impairment.
 ✦ 3. Eye opening is the most important indicator.
C. Respiratory function and airway patency.
D. Adequate circulation.
E. Fluid and electrolyte balance.

Implementation
✦ A. Maintain open airway and adequate ventilation.
 1. Check for airway obstruction.
  a. May result in retention of carbon dioxide (with cerebral vasodilation, edema, and increased intracranial pressure).
  b. Hypoxia (with potential irreversible brain damage).

(GLASGOW) COMA SCALE

A. Motor response. **Points**
  1. Obeys a simple command 6
  2. Localizes painful stimuli; attempts to remove offending stimulus; lack of obedience 5
  3. Withdrawn—moves purposelessly in response to pain 4
  4. Abnormal flexion—decorticate posturing 3
  5. Extensor response—decerebrate posturing 2
  6. No motor response to pain 1

B. Verbal response. **Points**
  1. Oriented—to time, place, and person 5
  2. Confused conversation; disorientation in *one* or more spheres 4
  3. Inappropriate or disorganized use of words (cursing); lack of sustained conversation 3
  4. Responds with incomprehensible sounds 2
  5. No verbal response (Record T if an endotracheal or tracheostomy tube is in place) 1

C. Eye opening. **Points**
  1. Spontaneous when a person approaches 4
  2. In response to speech 3
  3. Only in response to pain 2
  4. Do not open, even to painful stimuli (Record C if eyes are closed by swelling) 1

This scale is a tool for assessing a client's response to stimuli. Scores range from 3 (deep coma) to 15 (normal). Add numbers to determine a total score.

2. Monitor respiratory signs and symptoms continuously.
  a. Color, chest expansion, deformities.
  b. Rate, depth, and rhythm of respirations.
  c. Air movement at nose/mouth or through endotracheal tube.
  d. Breath sounds, adventitious sounds.
  e. Accumulation of secretions or blood in mouth.
  f. Signs of respiratory distress: hypoxemia, hypercapnia or atelectasis.
3. Provide airway.
  a. Head tilt; modified jaw thrust if cervical injury suspected.
  b. Cuffed endotracheal or tracheostomy tube (maintain airway, avenue for suctioning and/or mechanical ventilation).
  c. Assisted ventilation if necessary.
4. Position client to facilitate breathing.
  a. Side-lying or semiprone (to prevent tongue from occluding airway and secretions from pooling in pharynx).
  b. Frequent change of position.
5. Provide pulmonary toilet.

  a. Deep breathing and coughing if not contraindicated.
  b. Suctioning of secretions as necessary.
6. Have emergency equipment available.
B. Maintain adequate circulation.
  1. Blood pressure.
    a. Hypertension—result of increased intracranial pressure.
    b. Hypotension—result of immobility.
  2. Pulse.
    a. Check quality and presence of all pulses.
    b. Check rate and rhythm of apical and/or radial pulse.
  3. Heart sounds.
    a. Arrhythmias due to hypoxia.
    b. Usually premature ventricular contractions.
C. Monitor neurological status.
  1. Level of consciousness.
  2. Pupillary signs.
  3. Motor function.
  4. Sensory function.
D. Maintain nutrition, fluid and electrolyte balance.
  1. Keep client NPO while unconscious (check for gag and swallowing reflexes).
  2. Give intravenous fluids, hyperalimentation as required—check for dehydration.
  3. Use caution with IV rates in presence of increased intracranial pressure.
  4. Record intake, output and daily weight.
  5. Maintain oral and nasal hygiene.
  6. Resume oral intake carefully as consciousness returns.
    a. Check gag reflex.
    b. Use ice chips or water as first liquid.
    c. Keep suction equipment ready.
E. Promote elimination.
  1. Urinary: retention catheter.
    a. Maintain daily hygiene of meatus.
    b. Ensure patency to prevent bladder distention, urinary stasis, infection, and urinary calculi.
    c. Evaluate amount, color, consistency of output; check specific gravity.
  2. Bowel: suppositories and enemas.
    a. Establish routine elimination patterns.
    b. Observe for complications.
    c. Check for paralytic ileus.
      (1) Abdominal distention.
      (2) Constipation and/or impaction.
      (3) Diarrhea.
F. Maintain integrity of the skin.
  1. High risk of pressure ulcers due to:
    a. Loss of vasomotor tone.
    b. Impaired peripheral circulation.

      c.   Paralysis, immobility, and loss of muscle tone.

      d.   Hypoproteinemia.

  2.   Loss of sensation of pressure, pain, or temperature—decreased awareness of developing pressure ulcers or burns.

  3.   Monitor for edema: dependent areas.

  4.   Skin care.

      a.   Clean and dry skin; avoid powder because it may cake.

      b.   Massage with lotion around and toward bony prominences once a day if area is not red.

      c.   Alternate air fluidized therapy bed with eggcrate mattress.

      d.   Keep linen from wrinkling; avoid mechanical friction against linen.

      e.   Turn client every 2 hours; position with pillows to protect pressure on bony prominences.

G. Maintain personal hygiene.

  ✦ 1.   Eye: loss of corneal reflex may contribute to corneal irritation, keratitis, blindness.

      a.   Assess corneal reflex and signs of irritation.

      b.   Instill artificial tears or close eyelids and cover with moistened pads to protect cornea.

  2.   Nose: trauma or infection in nose or nasopharynx may cause meningitis.

      a.   Observe for drainage of CSF.

      b.   Clean and lubricate nares; do not clean inside nostrils.

      c.   Change nasogastric tube per policy and PRN.

  3.   Mouth: mouth breathing contributes to drying and crusting excoriation of mucous membranes, which may contribute to aspiration and respiratory tract infections.

      a.   Examine the mouth daily with a good light.

      b.   Clean teeth, gums, mucous membranes, tongue, and uvula to prevent crusting and infection; lubricate lips.

      c.   Inspect for retained food in the mouth of clients who have facial paralysis; follow with mouth care.

  ✦ 4.   Ear: drainage of CSF from the ear indicates damage to the base of the brain and a danger of meningitis.

      a.   Inspect ear for drainage of CSF; if clear drainage tests positive for glucose (using a Labstix), drainage is CSF.

      b.   Loosely cover ear with sterile, dry dressing.

✦ H. Maintain optimal positioning and movement.

  1.   Prevent further trauma.

      a.   Maintain body alignment, support head and limbs when turning, logroll.

      b.   Do not flex or twist spine or hyperextend neck if spinal cord injury is suspected.

  2.   Provide adequate positioning.

      a.   Disuse of muscle leads to contractures, osteoporosis, and compromised venous return.

      b.   Maintain and support joints and limbs in most functional anatomic position.

      c.   Avoid improper use of knee gatch or pillows under knee.

      d.   Use a footboard or high-top sneakers to prevent footdrop. If sneakers are used, be sure to remove daily and inspect feet.

  3.   Avoid complete immobility.

      a.   Perform range of motion (against resistance if possible), weight bearing, and/or tilt table.

      b.   Change position every 2 hours.

I. Provide psychosocial support for client and family.

  1.   Assume that an unconscious client can hear; frequently reassure and explain procedures to client.

  2.   Encourage family interaction.

✦ J. Institute safety precautions.

  1.   Use siderails at all times.

  2.   Remove dentures and dental bridges.

  3.   Remove contact lenses.

  4.   Avoid restraints.

  5.   Do not leave client who is unstable unattended for more than 15–30 minutes.

  6.   Keep tongue blade at bedside.

Increased Intracranial Pressure (ICP)

Definition: An increase in intracranial bulk due to blood, CSF, or brain tissue leading to an increase in pressure. Can be caused by trauma, hemorrhage, tumors, abscess, hydrocephalus, edema, or inflammation.

Assessment

✦ A. Level of consciousness (most sensitive indication of increasing intracranial pressure)—changes from restlessness to confusion to declining level of consciousness and coma.

  1.   Orientation to person, place, purpose, time.

  2.   Response to verbal/tactile stimuli or simple commands.

  3.   Response to painful stimuli: purposeful/nonpurposeful, decorticate, decerebrate, no response.

✦ B. Respiration: rate, depth, and rhythm are more sensitive indications of intracranial pressure than blood pressure and pulse—abnormal breathing patterns associated with ICP.

1. Cheyne–Stokes—rhythmically waxes and wanes, alternating with periods of apnea.
2. Neurogenic hyperventilation.
   a. Sustained regular, rapid, and deep.
   b. Low midbrain, middle pons.
3. Apneustic—irregular breathing with pauses at end of inspiration and expiration.
4. Ataxic (Biot's)—totally irregular, random rhythm and depth.
5. Apnea may occur.
✦ C. Headache—tension, displacement of brain.
✦ D. Vomiting—irritation of vagal nuclei in floor of fourth ventricle; may be projectile.
✦ E. Pupillary changes.
   1. Unilateral dilation of pupil; slow reaction to light (light reflex is most important sign differentiating structural from metabolic coma).
   2. Unilateral, fixed, dilated pupil is ominous sign requiring immediate action—may indicate transtentorial herniation of the brain.
✦ F. Motor function—weakness, hemiplegia, positive Babinski, seizure activity.
   1. Posturing in response to noxious stimuli.
      a. Decorticate—nonfunctioning cortex, internal capsule (upper-extremity flexion, and may stiffen and extend legs).
      b. Decerebrate—brain stem lesion (total stiff extension of one or both arms and legs).
✦ G. Pulse and blood pressure.
   1. Monitor for trends; changes are often unreliable and occur late with increasing intracranial pressure.
   2. Rise in blood pressure, widening pulse pressure; reflex slowing of pulse.
      a. Cushing reflex—when systolic pressure rises and pulse slows but is more forceful—tells you ICP is rising but body is coping.
      ✦ b. When systolic pressure drops (below 50 mm Hg) and pulse becomes irregular, thready, and rapid, body is no longer coping—danger.
   H. Hyperthermia—possible complication—can signal infection, hemorrhage, or traction on the hypothalamus or brain stem.

Implementation

A. Acute phase: medical management.
   ✦ 1. Elevate head of bed—30 or 40 degrees as ordered—this allows gravity to drain cerebral veins.
      a. Avoid Trendelenburg position.
      b. Avoid tilting client's head, which would impede venous flow through jugular veins.
   ✦ 2. Limit fluid intake; restricted to 1200 mL/day.

3. Maintain normal body temperature—administer Tylenol as ordered and temperature-regulating blanket. Prevent shivering, which can raise ICP (chlorpromazine will control shivering).
4. Administer medications: steroids, osmotic diuretics.
   ✦ a. Steroids (Decadron) decrease cerebral edema by their anti-inflammatory effect and decrease capillary permeability in inflammatory processes, thus decreasing leakage of fluid into tissue.
   ✦ b. Histamine blocker (Zantac) given concomitantly with steroids to counter excess gastric acid secretion.
   ✦ c. Mannitol decreases cerebral edema; provides diuretic action by carrying out large volume of water through nephrons. Sometimes combined with Lasix to increase excretion of water and sodium from kidneys.
   ✦ d. Hypertonic IV solution administered because it is impermeable to blood–brain barrier; reduces edema by rapid movement of water out of ventricles into bloodstream.
   e. Sedation may be ordered to counter effects of noxious stimuli of ICP and make client comfortable.
✦ 5. Maintain patent airway and administer mechanical ventilation. Maintain $PaCO_2$ at 25–30 mm Hg to cause vasoconstriction of cerebral blood vessels, decrease blood flow, and decrease ICP.
6. Prevent further complications.
   a. Monitor neurological dysfunction versus cardiovascular shock.
   b. Prevent hypoxia: avoid morphine—it masks signs of increased ICP.
   c. Monitor fluids: electrolytes for hypo- and hypernatremia, and acid–base balance. (If client is receiving a loop diuretic, electrolyte replacement is indicated.)
✦ 7. Decrease environmental stimuli—dim lights, speak softly, limit visitors, avoid routine procedures if client is resting, etc.
✦ B. Chronic phase: surgical management.
   1. Ventriculoperitoneal shunt systems (most common). Designed to shunt cerebrospinal fluid from the lateral ventricles into the peritoneum.
   2. Preoperative care.
      a. Follow care of client with increased intracranial pressure.
      b. Prepare client for craniotomy if necessary.
   3. Postoperative care.

✦ a. Monitor closely for signs and symptoms of increasing intracranial pressure due to shunt failure.
  b. Check for infection (a common and serious complication). If present, removal of the shunt system is indicated in addition to appropriate chemotherapy.
  c. Position client supine and turn from back to unoperative side.

Cerebral Edema

Definition: Swelling of the brain that disrupts the stable relationship of the three components housed in the skull: brain, cerebrospinal fluid, and blood.

Characteristics

✦ A. Cerebral edema causes the intracranial pressure to rise.
B. Characterized by accumulation of fluid in the extra-cellular space, intracellular space, or both.
C. Regardless of the cause, cerebral edema results in an increase in tissue volume, with the potential to cause ICP.
D. Three types.
  1. Vasogenic edema results from increased extra-cellular fluid—most common type.
  2. Cytotoxic edema—the result of local disruption of the functional and/or morphologic integrity of cell membrane. Develops from destructive le-sions or trauma to the brain resulting in cerebral hypoxia or anoxia, sodium depletion, syndrome of inappropriate antidiuretic hormone (SIADH) secretion.
  3. Interstitial edema, associated with movement of cerebrospinal fluid.

Assessment

✦ A. Earliest indicator is change in level of consciousness (LOC).
  1. Lethargic.
  2. Talkative or quiet.
  3. Restlessness.
  4. Irritability.
  5. Nausea and vomiting.
  6. Disorientation: first to time, then to place and person.
B. Altered respiratory pattern.
✦ C. Pupillary changes.
  1. Unequal pupils.
  2. Sluggish response to light.
  3. Fixed and dilated pupils.
  4. Pupillary dysfunction is first noted on the ipsi-lateral side.
  5. Oculomotor dysfunction—inability to move eyes upward, ptosis of the eyelid.

D. Decorticate or decerebrate posturing.
✦ E. Monitor for late signs of increased ICP.
  1. Cushing's triad: increased systolic blood pressure, widened pulse pressure, and slowed heart rate.
  2. Irregular respirations.
  3. Rise in temperature.

Implementation

See Nursing Management for Increased Intracranial Pressure, page 177.

Hyperthermia

✦ *Definition:* Temperature of 41°C (106°F); associated with increased cerebral metabolism, increasing risk of hy-poxia, dysfunction of thermoregulatory center—trauma, tumor, cerebral edema, CVA, intracranial surgery; pro-longed exposure to high environmental temperatures—heatstroke; infection.

Assessment

A. Shivering.
B. Respiratory function—ventilation and patent airway.
C. Cardiac function—pulse and rhythm; arrhythmias.
D. Urinary function—color, specific gravity, and amount.
E. Nausea and vomiting.
F. Increased temperature—when very high, seizures.
G. Peripheral pulses for systemic blood flow.
H. Skin and mucous membranes for signs of dehydration.

Implementation

✦ A. Maintain patent airway if temperature is very high.
✦ B. Provide safety measures for possible seizure activity.
C. Monitor fluid balance by observing skin condition, urine output, lung sounds, peripheral pulses.
✦ D. Provide methods for inducing hypothermia.
  1. External—cool bath, fans, ice bags, hypothermic blanket (most common).
  ✦ 2. Drugs.
    a. Chlorpromazine—reduces peripheral vaso-constriction, muscle tone, shivering; depresses thermoregulation in hypothala-mus.
    b. Meperidine—relaxes smooth muscle, reduces shivering.
    c. Promethazine—dilates coronary arteries, reduces laryngeal and bronchial irritation.
  3. Extracorporeal—usually reserved for surgery.
E. Monitor effects of hypothermia.
  1. Prevent shivering.
    a. Shivering increases CSF pressure and oxy-gen consumption.
    b. Treatment: chlorpromazine or meperidine.
  ✦ 2. Prevent trauma to skin and tissue.

a. Frostbite—crystallization of tissues with white or blue discoloration, hardening of tissue, burning, numbness.

b. Fat necrosis—solidification of subcutaneous fat, creating hard tissue masses.

c. Initially give complete bath and oil the skin; during procedure, massage skin frequently with lotion or oil to maintain integrity of the skin.

◆ 3. Monitor and prevent respiratory complications.

a. Hypothermia may mask infection, cause respiratory arrest.

b. Institute measures to maintain open airway and adequate ventilation.

4. Monitor and prevent cardiac complications.

a. Hypothermia can cause arrhythmias and cardiac arrest.

b. Monitor cardiac status and have emergency equipment available.

5. Monitor renal function.

a. Insert Foley catheter.

b. Monitor urinary output, BUN; may monitor specific gravity.

6. Prevent vomiting and possible aspiration; client may have loss of gag reflex and reduced peristalsis.

7. Monitor changes in neurological function during hypothermia.

SEIZURE DISORDERS

Convulsions/Seizures

Definition: Temporary alterations in brain function resulting in sudden episodes of altered consciousness or involuntary movement expressing themselves as a changed mental state, tonic or clonic movements, and various other symptoms. Seizures may occur as isolated events, possibly after head trauma, and do not persist once the underlying cause is eliminated.

Characteristics

A. Causes: cerebral trauma, congenital defects, epilepsy, infection, tumor, circulatory defect, anoxia, metabolic abnormalities, excessive hydration, idiopathic, acute alcohol withdrawal.

◆ B. Classification.

1. *Tonic convulsion:* sustained contraction of muscles.

2. *Clonic convulsion:* alternating contraction–relaxation of opposing muscle group.

3. *Epileptiform:* any convulsion with loss of consciousness.

◆ **Assessment**

A. Identify if aura present.

B. Observe type of motor activity.

C. Observe pattern of seizure activity.

D. Identify length of seizure activity.

E. Evaluate loss of bowel or bladder control.

F. Evaluate loss of consciousness.

G. Observe for signs of respiratory distress.

H. Identify characteristics during the postictal state.

Implementation

◆ A. Observe and record characteristics of seizure activity.

1. Level of consciousness.

2. Description of any aura.

3. Description of body position and initial activity.

4. Motor activity: initial body part involved, character of movements (tonic/clonic), progression of movement, duration, biting of the tongue.

5. Respiration, color.

6. Pupillary changes, eye movements.

7. Incontinence, vomiting.

8. Total duration, frequency, number of seizures, injuries.

9. Postictal state.

a. Loss of consciousness.

b. Sleepiness.

c. Impaired speech, motor or thinking.

d. Headache.

e. Neurological and vital signs.

◆ B. Protect client from trauma.

1. Ensure patent airway; may need to use a nasal airway.

2. Do not force any object between teeth if they are already clenched.

3. Avoid use of any restraints; loosen restrictive clothing.

4. Remove any objects from environment that may cause injury.

5. Stay with client.

6. If the client is standing, place client on the floor; protect head and body from hard surfaces.

7. Be prepared to suction.

8. Keep siderails up; pad siderails.

C. Provide nursing care after seizure.

1. Keep turned to side to prevent aspiration.

2. Reorient to environment when awakened.

Epilepsy

◆ *Definition:* A combination of several disorders characterized by chronic, recurrent seizure activity; a symptom of brain or CNS irritation. A seizure is an abnormal, sudden, excessive discharge of electrical activity within the brain.

Characteristics

A. Incidence in United States may be as low as 1 million or as high as 2.5 million—many clients hide their seizure disorder.

B. Major problems may be an electrical disturbance (dysrhythmia) in nerve cells in one section of the brain.

C. Seizures are associated with changes in behavior, mentation and motor or sensory activity.

D. Causes may be related to several factors.
  1. Genetic factors, trauma, brain tumor, circulatory or metabolic disorders, toxicity, or infection.
  2. May be symptoms of underlying brain pathology such as scar tissue, vascular disease, meningitis, or secondary to a birth injury.
  3. Heredity may play a part in absence, akinetic, or myoclonic seizures.

E. Diagnostic tests include CT to determine underlying CNS changes, EEG for a distinctive pattern, MRI, blood studies, lumbar puncture, etc.

Assessment

◆ A. Observe specific phases of seizure activity.
  1. Occurs without warning or following an aura (peculiar sensation that warns of an impending seizure—dizziness, visual or auditory sensation).
  2. Behavior at onset of seizure.
     a. Change in facial expression—fixation of gaze, flickering eyelids, etc.
     b. Sound or cry at time of seizure.

◆ B. Observe movements of body.
  1. *Tonic phase*—parts of body involved, length of time (usually 10–20 seconds).
  2. *Clonic phase*—parts of body that jerk, sequence of jerking movements, how long activity lasts (usually 30–40 seconds).

C. Observe behavior following seizure.
  1. State of consciousness, orientation.
  2. Motor ability, speech ability, activity.

D. Seizure history through client report or observation.
  1. Seizure onset, pattern or sequence of progression, precipitating events, frequency, description.
  2. Whether seizure is a simple staring spell or prolonged convulsive movements.
  3. Excess or loss of muscle tone or movement.
  4. Disturbance of behavior, mood, sensation, and/or perception.
  5. Prodromal signs or symptoms: mood changes, irritability, insomnia, etc.
  6. Effect of epilepsy on life and lifestyle (work limitations, social interaction, psychological adjustment).

Generalized Seizures: Four Types

◆ A. Tonic–clonic seizures, traditionally known as "grand mal."
  1. May begin with an aura, then a tonic phase—symmetrical stiffening or rigidity of muscles, particularly arms and legs, followed by loss of consciousness.
  2. Clonic phase follows—hyperventilation with rhythmic jerking of all extremities.
  3. May be incontinent of urine and feces.
  4. May bite tongue.
  5. May last 2–5 minutes.
  6. Full recovery may take several hours.

◆ B. Absence seizures, formerly "petit mal."
  1. Brief, often just seconds, loss of consciousness; almost no loss or change in muscle tone.
  2. May occur 100 times/day. More common in children; may appear to be "daydreaming."

◆ C. Myoclonic seizures.
  1. Characterized by a brief, generalized jerking or stiffening of the extremities; jerks may be single or multiple.
  2. May occur as single movement or in groups; seizure may throw person to the floor.

◆ D. Atonic or akinetic seizures, also called "drop attacks."
  1. Characterized by sudden, momentary loss of muscle tone.
  2. Usually causes person to fall to the ground (injuries from falling are common).

◆ Partial Seizures (Focal Seizures)

A. Simple partial seizure.
  1. Localized (confined to a specific area).
     a. *Motor symptoms:* abnormal unilateral movement of leg or arm.
     b. *Sensory symptoms:* abnormal smell or sensation.
     c. *Autonomic symptoms:* include tachycardia, bradycardia, increased respirations, skin flushing, epigastric distress.
     d. *Psychic symptoms:* may report déjà vu or fearful feelings.
  2. Client remains conscious throughout episode and may report an aura before seizure takes place.

B. Complex partial (psychomotor) seizure; may progress to generalized tonic–clonic.
  1. Area of brain most involved is temporal lobe (thus this type of seizure is called psychomotor).
  2. Characterized by a period of altered behavior and automatism (client is not aware of behavior); evidenced by such mannerisms as lip smacking, chewing, picking at clothes, focal

motor activity, such as posturing or jerking movements.

    3.   Client loses consciousness for a few seconds.

C. Idiopathic or unclassified seizures.

    1.   This type of seizure accounts for half of all seizure activity.

    2.   Occurs for no known reason and fits into no generalized or partial classification.

Implementation

✦ A. Prevent injury during seizure.

    1.   Remove objects that may cause harm.

    2.   Remain with client during seizure.

    3.   Do not force jaws open during seizure.

    4.   Do not restrict limbs or restrain.

    5.   Loosen restrictive clothing.

    6.   Turn head to side, if possible, to prevent aspiration and allow secretions to drain.

    7.   Check that airway is open. Do not initiate artificial ventilation during a tonic–clonic seizure.

✦ B. Observe and document seizure pattern.

    1.   Note time, level of consciousness, and presence of aura before seizure.

    2.   Record type, character, progression of movements.

    3.   Note duration of seizure and client's condition throughout.

    4.   Observe and record postictal state.

✦ C. Administer and monitor medications.

    1.   Seizure control may be achieved with one or a combination of drugs.

    2.   Dosage is adjusted to achieve seizure control with few side effects.

✦   3.   Medications must be given continuously and on time throughout life of client to maintain therapeutic blood levels.

✦   4.   Phenytoin (Dilantin).

       a.   Prevents seizures through depression of motor areas of the brain.

       b.   Side effects: GI disturbance, visual changes, rash, anemia, gingival hyperplasia.

       c.   Check CBC and calcium levels.

       d.   Give PO drug with milk or meals; supplemental vitamin D and folic acid.

    5.   Diazepam (Valium).

       a.   Give to stop motor activity associated with status epilepticus; for restlessness.

       b.   Side effects: if given IV, monitor for respiratory distress.

    6.   Phenobarbital (Luminal).

       a.   Reduces responsiveness of normal neurons to impulses arising in focal site.

       b.   Side effects: drowsiness, ataxia, nystagmus, respiratory depression.

> ### ✦ STATUS EPILEPTICUS
>
> • A seizure that lasts longer than 4 minutes, or successive seizures without regaining consciousness.
>
> • A potential complication with all seizures—a neurological emergency with generalized tonic–clonic seizures.
>
> • Cause may be sudden withdrawal from medication, infection, head trauma, metabolic disorders, alcohol withdrawal.
>
> • Management.
>
>   a. Maintain airway.
>
>   b. Notify physician.
>
>   c. Administer oxygen.
>
>   d. Monitor IV medication: Valium, Dilantin, phenobarbital.

✦   7.   Carbamazepine (Tegretol).

       a.   Inhibits nerve impulses by limiting influx of sodium ions across cell membranes.

       b.   Give with meals; monitor for side effects—diplopia, blurred vision, ataxia, vomiting, leukopenia.

    8.   Clonazepam (Klonopin).

       a.   Decreases frequency, duration, and spread of discharge in minor motor seizures (absence, akinetic, myoclonic seizures).

       b.   Side effects: lethargy, ataxia, vertigo, thrombocytopenia—monitor CBC.

    9.   Gabapentin (Neurontin).

       a.   Do not take 1 hour before or less than 2 hours after antacids.

       b.   Monitor liver function studies regularly (as ordered) to detect early signs of hepatitis or liver problems.

    10. Fosphenytoin (Cerebyx).

       a.   Thought to modulate sodium channels of neurons, modulate calcium flux across neuronal membranes, enhance sodium–potassium ATPase activity of neurons and glial cells.

       b.   Must be prescribed in PE units.

       c.   Side effects—nystagmus, dizziness, somnolence, drowsiness.

D. Promote physical and emotional health.

    1.   Establish regular routines for eating, sleeping and physical activity.

    2.   Avoid alcohol, stress and excessive fatigue.

    3.   Foster self-esteem and promote self-confidence.

    4.   Contact Epilepsy Foundation of America.

       a.   Recent studies suggest specially trained dogs can tell when a seizure is about to happen.

       b.   For clients with poorly controlled seizures, suggest referral to special programs.

E. Surgical treatment.

1. When attempts to control seizure fail, excision of tissue involved in the seizure activity may be a safe and effective treatment.
2. Goal: control—reduce client's uncontrolled seizures.
3. Postop care—general postop care for a client having intracranial surgery.

TRAUMA

Head Injury

Definition: A trauma to the skull resulting in varying degrees of injury to the brain by compression, tension and/or shearing force.

✦ Types of Injury

A. Concussion—violent jarring of brain within skull; temporary loss of consciousness.
  ✦ 1. Symptoms are worse at point of impact.
       a. Immediate loss of consciousness (usually no longer than 5 minutes).
       b. Amnesia for events surrounding injury.
       c. Headache.
       d. Drowsiness, confusion, dizziness.
       e. Visual disturbances.
       f. Possible brief seizure activity, with *transient* apnea, bradycardia, pallor, hypotension.
    2. Postconcussion syndrome.
       a. Persistent headache.
       b. Dizziness.
       c. Irritability, insomnia.
       d. Impaired memory and concentration, learning problems.
✦ B. Contusion—bruising, injury of brain.
    1. Acceleration—slower-moving contents of cranium strike bony prominences or dura (coup).
    2. Deceleration—moving head strikes fixed object and brain rebounds, striking opposite side of cranium (contrecoup).
C. Fracture—linear, depressed, compound, comminuted.
D. Hematoma.
  ✦ 1. Epidural—most serious; hematoma between dura and skull from tear in meningeal artery; forms rapidly.
  ✦ 2. Subdural—under dura due to tears in veins crossing subdural space; forms slowly.
    3. Intracerebral—usually in frontal and temporal lobes, usually caused by gunshot wounds, stabbing, depressed skull fractures, long history of systemic hypertension, contusion.
✦ E. Subarachnoid hemorrhage—bleeding directly into brain, ventricles, or subarachnoid space.
    1. Monitor symptoms suggestive of complications.

a. Keep BP within normal limits—administer drugs as ordered.
b. Administer phenobarbital to control seizures; codeine for pain; corticosteroids for edema; fibrinolytic inhibitor (Amicar) to minimize risk of rebleed.
    2. Maintain bedrest, prevent exertion, keep room quiet and dark.
    3. Prevent straining, administer laxatives and stool softeners.
    4. Avoid stimulants like caffeine (i.e., coffee).
F. Intracerebral hemorrhage—usually multiple hemorrhages around contused area.

Assessment

✦ A. Level of consciousness, unconsciousness, or confusion.
✦ B. Patent airway and breathing pattern.
C. Headache, nausea, vomiting.
✦ D. Pupillary changes—ipsilateral dilated pupil.
✦ E. Changes in vital signs, reflecting increased intracranial pressure or shock.
F. Vasomotor or sensory losses.
G. Rhinorrhea, otorrhea, nuchal rigidity.
H. Overt scalp or skull trauma.
I. Positive Babinski sign (dorsiflexion of toes when bottom of foot is stroked).

Implementation

✦ A. Primary nursing objective is to recognize, prevent, and treat complications; observe for signs of increased intracranial pressure.
✦ B. Maintain adequate respiratory exchange—increased CO_2 levels increase cerebral edema.
    1. Maintain patent airway.
    2. Encourage to avoid coughing (increases ICP); may require frequent suctioning.
✦ C. Complete neurological assessment, including Glasgow Coma Scale, every 15 minutes initially; then every hour until stable; then every 4 hours.
    1. Awaken client as completely as possible for assessment.
    2. Maintain slight head elevation to reduce venous pressure.
D. Monitor temperature—utilize hypothermia as ordered to reduce fever.
E. Control pain and restlessness.
  ✦ 1. Avoid morphine, a respiratory depressant that might increase ICP.
    2. Use codeine or other mild, safe analgesic.
F. Monitor and treat seizure activity—administer anticonvulsants as ordered.
✦ G. Observe for complications.
    1. Shock—significant cause of death.
    2. Cranial nerve paralysis.

3. Rhinorrhea (fracture ethmoid bone) and otor-rhea (temporal).
   a. Check discharge—bloody spot surrounded by pale ring; positive Tes-Tape reaction for sugar.
   b. Do not attempt to clean nose or ears.
      (1) Do not suction nose.
      (2) Instruct client not to blow nose.
✦ 4. Ear—drainage of CSF from the ear indicates damage to the base of the brain and a danger of meningitis.
   a. Inspect ear for drainage of CSF.
   b. Loosely cover ear with sterile, dry dressing.
5. Eye—loss of corneal reflex may contribute to corneal irritation, keratitis, blindness.
   a. Assess corneal reflex and signs of irritation.
   b. Instill artificial tears or close eyelids and cover with moistened pads to protect cornea.
6. Fluid and electrolyte imbalance—diabetes insipidus.
H. Prevent infection.
   1. High risk of meningitis, abscess, osteomyelitis, particularly in presence of rhinorrhea, otorrhea.
   2. Maintain strict asepsis.
I. Prevent complications of immobility.
   1. Continue range-of-motion activities.
   2. Prevent contractures.
J. Establish individualized rehabilitation program.

Spinal Cord Injury (SCI)

Definition: Partial or complete disruption of nerve tracts and neurons resulting in paralysis, sensory loss, altered re-flex activity, and autonomic nervous system dysfunction.

Characteristics

A. The mechanisms of trauma associated with SCI are usually related to vertebral fracture; resulting injuries include flexion, hyperflexion, hyperextension, flexion-rotation, rotation beyond normal range, axial-loading/compression, and penetrating injury.
✦ 1. Most common causes of abnormal spinal cord movements.
   a. Acceleration—when an external force is applied in rear-end collision, upper torso and head are forced backward and then forward.
   b. Deceleration—in a head-on collision, the external force is applied from the front.
2. Direction of motion.
   a. Hyperflexion.
   b. Hyperextension.
   c. Axial loading.
   d. Excessive rotation.

B. Common traumas.
   1. Automobile and motorcycle accidents.
   2. Sports and industrial injuries.
   3. Falls and crushing injuries, stab wounds, bullets.
C. Other conditions associated with spinal cord pathology.
   1. Infections, tumors.
   2. Disruption of blood supply to cord—thrombus.
   3. Degenerative diseases.
   4. Congenital or acquired anomalies—spina bifida, myelomeningocele.
D. Improper handling and transport may result in extension of cord damage.
E. Vascular disruption, biochemical changes, and direct tissue damage cause pathology associated with trauma.
   1. Inflammatory process leads to edema and neu-ronal dysfunction.
   2. Ischemia and hypoxia due to vasoconstriction, edema and hemorrhage.
   3. Hypoxia of gray matter stimulates release of catecholamines, which increases hemorrhage and necrosis.

Classification of Cord Involvement

✦ A. Functional deficiencies.
   1. Level of spinal cord involvement dictates conse-quences of the cord injury.
   2. Quadriplegia (tetraplegia)—all four extremities functionally involved—cervical injuries (C1 through C8).
   3. Paraplegia—both lower extremities functionally involved—thoracic–lumbar region (T1 through L4).
B. Transection of the cord.
   1. Complete cord transection.
      a. All voluntary motor activity below injury is permanently lost.
      b. All sensation dependent on ascending pathway of segment is lost.
      c. Reflexes may return if blood supply to cord below injury is intact.
   2. Incomplete injuries.
      a. Motor and sensory loss varies and is dependent on degree of incompleteness.
   ✦ b. Extent of reflex dysfunction dependent on location of neurological deficit.
✦ C. Types of injuries.
   1. Central cord syndrome—leg function returns, arm function does not, as damage has occurred to peripheral cord, which innervates arms.
      a. More common in older adults.
      b. Motor weakness in *both* upper and lower extremities—greater in upper extremities than lower.

(1) Sensory dysfunction varies according to site of injury.

(2) Bladder dysfunction is variable.

   c. Frequently a result of hyperextension of osteoarthritic spine.

2. Brown–Séquard's syndrome—one side of cord damaged, resulting in paralysis on one side of body and loss of sensation on the other side.

   a. Transection or lesion of half of spinal cord.

   b. Usually caused by penetrating injuries (i.e., gunshot, stabbing).

   c. Characteristics.

     (1) Loss of motor function (paralysis), position and vibratory sense, vasomotor paralysis on the same side (ipsilateral) and below the hemisection.

     (2) Loss of pain and temperature sensation on the opposite side—contralateral (below the level of the lesion or hemisection).

3. Anterior cord syndrome—paralysis below the level of injury, loss of temperature and pain sensation below the level of injury.

   a. Often caused by a flexion injury.

   b. Lesion on anterior two-thirds of cord.

   c. Compression caused by disk or bony fragment.

   d. May be caused by spinal artery occlusion.

   e. Characteristics.

     (1) Complete motor paralysis from site of injury and below.

     (2) Hyposthesia—decreased pain sensation and loss of temperature below the injury.

     (3) Because posterior cord tracts are not injured, sensation of touch, position, vibration and motion remains intact.

4. Posterior cord syndrome—weakness in isolated muscle groups, tingling, pain, decreased or absent reflexes in the involved area.

   a. Associated with hyperextension trauma.

   b. Results from compression or damage to the posterior part of the spinal cord.

   c. Loss of proprioception.

   d. Pain, temperature sensation and motor function below the level of the lesion remain intact.

5. Horner's syndrome—ipsilateral ptosis of the eyelid, constricted pupil, and facial anhidrosis (inability to perspire).

D. Upper and lower motor neuron damage.

1. Upper motor neuron originates in cerebral cortex and terminates at anterior horn cell in cord.

✦ AUTONOMIC HYPERREFLEXIA

- Also called autonomic dysreflexia—a massive, uncompensated cardiovascular reaction mediated by the sympathetic nervous system.
- Occurs in clients with lesions above T6, most often those with cervical injuries, after spinal shock has resolved.
- Acute emergency—result of exaggerated autonomic responses to stimuli (most often distended bladder or impacted rectum)—treat immediately to prevent stroke, status epilepticus, myocardial infarction, even death.
- Symptoms include severe headache, profuse diaphoresis, nausea, bradycardia, hypertension, piloerection, blurred vision, spots in the visual field, nasal congestion and anxiety.
- Interventions focused on reducing blood pressure and eliminating stimulus.
  - a. Immediately elevate head to decrease blood pressure and monitor vital signs every 15 minutes.
  - b. Eliminate stimulus—relieve bladder distention by catheterizing or remove fecal mass.
- If severe hypertension does not resolve with removal of stimulus, an antihypertensive drug will be ordered (Apresoline) IV.

---

   a. Postspinal shock reflexes return resulting in spastic paralysis. No reflex return if blood supply to cord is lost.

   b. Spasms and reflexes used to retrain activities of daily living—bowel evacuation and bladder control.

2. Lower motor neuron begins at anterior horn cell and becomes part of peripheral nerve to muscle, motor side of reflex arc.

   a. Areflexia continues, flaccid paralysis.

   b. Usually cauda equina injuries.

Assessment

✦ A. Level of injury. The last cord segment in which normal motor, sensory, and reflex activity can be demonstrated is labeled level of injury (e.g., "C5, level of injury" means neurofunction is intact for C5 but not C6).

B. Degree of sensory, motor and reflex loss depends upon severity of cord damage.

C. Respiratory insufficiency or failures occur in injuries above C4 due to lack of diaphragm innervation.

D. Assess general sensory function in all extremities: touch, pressure, pain.

E. Assess motor response to command.

1. Pattern of motor dysfunction yields information about anatomic location of lesions, independent of level of consciousness.

2. Appropriate response—spontaneous movement to stimulus or command.

3. Absent response—hemiplegia, paraplegia, quadriplegia.

<hr>

◆ SPINAL SHOCK

- Absence of reflexes slightly above and completely below level of lesion. (This is a *neurologic emergency* that requires immediate attention.)
- Temporary condition: lasts days to months.
- Initial flaccid paralysis, absent reflexes, loss of sensation, loss of urinary and bowel retention, hypotension (especially positional), bradycardia.
- Active rehabilitation may begin in the presence of spinal shock.

<hr>

4. Use minimal amount of stimulus necessary to evoke a response.

F. Assess for bladder control.
1. Reflex (autonomic or spastic) bladder occurs when reflexes are still present and, with stimulation, the bladder involuntarily empties.
2. Spastic bladder responds to minor stimulus and empties before it is full.

G. Evaluate bowel control.
1. Observe ability to evacuate stool.
2. Assess consistency and number of stools.
3. Identify need for bowel training program.

Implementation

A. Complete a head-to-toe neurological examination to determine motor, sensory, and reflex loss due to spinal cord injury.

◆ B. Provide emergency care—suspect spinal cord injury if neurological deficits present in extremities.
1. Immobilize entire body, especially head and neck; do not flex head; stabilize cervical spine.
2. Transport in log fashion with sufficient help.
3. Maintain open airway and adequate ventilation —high cervical injuries can cause complete paralysis of muscles for breathing; observe for signs of respiratory failure.

◆ C. Immobilize client, as ordered, to allow fracture healing and prevent further injury.
1. Special beds (Stryker frame) permit change of position between prone and supine.
   a. Maintain optimal body alignment.
   b. Place client in center of frame without flexing or twisting.
   c. Position arm boards, footboards, canvas.
   d. Turn; reassure client while turning.
   e. Free all tubings; secure bolts and straps.
2. Regular hospital beds used in many rehabilitation centers. (Some use Roto-Rest beds or Foster frame.)
◆ 3. Halo traction with body cast allows for early mobilization. (*See also* page 365.)

a. Consists of a circular headpiece with four pins: two anterior, two posterior. These are inserted into client's skull, and then halo jacket or cast is applied.
b. Once fracture is stable, the headpiece can be attached to halo vest.
c. Assess client's neurological status for decreased strength or changes in movement.
◆ d. **Never** turn or move the client by pulling on the halo traction.
e. Assess for tightness of the jacket. Be sure one finger can fit under the jacket.
f. Assess skin integrity to be sure there are no pressure areas from the cast or jacket; protect with fleece or foam.
g. Provide care to the pin sites.
◆ h. Keep correct-size wrench available at all times for any emergency situation that may occur and require removal of the device.
i. If client requires cardiopulmonary resuscitation, the anterior portion of the vest will be loosened and the posterior portion will remain in place to provide stability.
4. Soft and hard collars and back braces used about 6 weeks postinjury.
◆ 5. Maintain skeletal traction if part of treatment.
   a. Cervical tongs for hyperextension (Crutchfield, Gardner–Wells, Vinke).
      (1) Traction is applied to vertebral column by attaching weights to pair of tongs.
      (2) Tongs are inserted into outer layer of parietal area of skull.
   b. Facilitates moving and turning of client while maintaining spine immobilization.
   c. Observe site of insertion for redness or drainage, alignment and position of traction, and pressure areas.

D. Complete frequent neurological assessment: note changes in muscle tone, motor movement, sensation, bladder and bowel function, presence or absence of sweating, temperature and reflexes.
◆ E. Monitor for autonomic nervous system disturbances.
1. Heart, lung, and bowel sounds for complications, such as embolus, ileus.
2. Temperature fluctuations—unable to adapt to environmental changes or infection-related.
   a. Excessive perspiration causes dehydration.
   b. Absence of perspiration leads to hyperthermia.
◆ F. Prevent postural hypotension and syncope, which occur when head is elevated.
1. Apply Ace bandage or TED elastic hose.
2. Administer ephedrine PO 30 minutes before client is to get up.

✦ G.   Monitor for autonomic dysreflexia. (*See* page 184.)
  1.   Signs and symptoms: extreme hypertension, flushing, bradycardia, headache (usually occipital), sweating, diplopia, convulsions.
  2.   Provide immediate treatment.
    a.   Catheterize bladder; manually evacuate bowel.
    b.   May administer parasympatholytic (Banthine) or ganglionic blocking agent (Hyperstat, Apresoline).
    c.   If client is lying down and fracture status permits, immediately elevate the head of bed or elevate client to sitting position.
  3.   Control factors that precipitate episode to prevent recurrence.
    a.   Set up regular bowel and bladder programs.
    b.   Apply Nupercainal ointment prior to rectal stimulation.
    c.   Administer alpha-adrenergic blocking agents (phenoxybenzamine) BID.

H.   Prevent infections.
  1.   Administer prophylactic antibiotics while client is on catheterizations.
  2.   Evaluate client with elevated temperature for urinary or respiratory infection.

✦ I.   Prevent circulatory complications.
  1.   Turn entire body every 2 hours. Give range-of-motion exercises to extremities.
  2.   Apply Ace bandages and TED elastic hose to legs.
  3.   Monitor for edema, thrombus and emboli; provide prompt anticoagulant therapy if needed.
  4.   Do not overhydrate based on blood pressure (normal BP is 100/60 or below).

✦ J.   Maintain optimal positioning.
  1.   Logroll with firm support to head, neck, spine, and limbs; do not allow neck flexion.
  2.   Maintain good body alignment with 10-degree flexion of knees, heels off mattress or canvas, and feet in firm dorsiflexion.
  3.   During convalescence, provide cervical collar, tilt table, wheelchair, braces, parallel bars.

K.   Promote optimal physical activity.
  1.   Provide physical therapy, exercises, range of motion.
  2.   Encourage independent activity.
  3.   Provide extensive program of rehabilitation and self-care.

✦ L.   Maintain integrity of the skin.
  1.   Turn client every 2 hours and check skin.
  2.   Do not administer IM medication below the level of the lesion due to impaired circulation and potential skin breakdown.
  3.   Provide elastic stockings to improve circulation in legs.
  4.   Later, instruct client how to look for and prevent injury; reinforce the necessity for self-care.
  5.   Provide prompt treatment of pressure areas.

✦ M.   Promote adequate nutrition, fluid and electrolyte balance.
  1.   Provide diet adequate in protein, vitamins, calories, and bulk; limit milk.
  2.   Avoid citrus juices, which alkalize the urine; give cranberry juice and vitamin C tabs to acidify urine.
  3.   Avoid gas-forming foods.
  4.   Monitor calcium, electrolytes, and hemoglobin.
  5.   Restrict fluids if client is on intermittent catheterization; otherwise, encourage fluids—3000 mL+ per day.

✦ N.   Provide psychological support to client and family.
  1.   Support client and family through grief process.
  2.   Promote sustained therapeutic relationships.
  3.   Provide diversionary activities, socialization.
  4.   Promote independence; teach client to problem solve.
  5.   Give encouragement and reassurance but never false hope.
  6.   Encourage family involvement in care.
  7.   Provide sexual counseling if needed.
    a.   Client should be aware of his or her sexual abilities postinjury.
    b.   Role perception may need expansion.
  8.   During rehabilitation stage, provide employment counseling if needed.

O.   Establish individualized rehabilitation program for client.
  1.   Based on level of injury.
  2.   Determined by willingness of client to adapt to new body image.
  3.   Availability of family and community support services.

✦ P.   Optimal bladder function.
  1.   During spinal shock, bladder is atonic with urinary retention; danger of overdistention, stretching.
  2.   Possible reactions.
    a.   Hypertonic, retention with overflow—sacral reflex center injury (lower motor neuron).
    b.   Hypertonic, sudden reflex voiding—injury above sacral area (upper motor neuron).
  3.   Check for bladder distention, voiding, incontinence, and symptoms of infection.
  4.   Provide aseptic intermittent catheterizations—prophylactic antimicrobials (nitrofurantoin).
  5.   Prevent urinary tract infection, calculi.
    a.   Monitor urinary residuals.

    b.   May have periodic bladder and kidney function studies—IVP, cystogram.

6. Initiate bladder retraining.
   a. Hypertonic—sensation of full bladder, trigger areas, regulation of fluid intake.
   b. Hypotonic—manual expression of urine (Credé).
7. Administer medications to treat incontinence.
   a. Hypertonic—propantheline bromide, diazepam.
   b. Hypotonic—bethanechol chloride.

✦ Q. Optimal bowel function.
1. Incontinence and paralytic ileus occur with spinal shock; later, incontinence, constipation, impaction.
2. For severe distention, administer neostigmine methylsulfate and insert rectal tube, which decompresses intestinal tract.
3. Give enema only if necessary. Excessive amount of fluid distends bowel. Manual evacuation is preferred.
4. Initiate bowel retraining.
   a. Record bowel habits before and after injury.
   b. Provide well-balanced diet with high-fiber foods—fruits, vegetables, grains (bran), and legumes.
   c. Encourage fluid intake—2000 to 3000 mL per day.
   d. Provide stool softeners, bulk producers, mild laxative.
   e. Encourage the development of muscle tone.
   f. Administer suppository (glycerin or Dulcolax) as indicated.
   g. Most important is to establish a regular, consistent routine and time for elimination.

✦ R. Pharmacology.
1. Corticosteroids—high-dose steroid protocol using methylprednisolone (Medrol) must be given intravenously within 8 hours of injury to be effective. It is used to prevent secondary spinal cord damage from edema and ischemia. Initial loading dose given, followed by a maintenance dose over the next 23 hours.
   a. Criteria for selection.
      (1) Spinal cord injury less than 8 hours old.
      (2) Spinal lesion cannot be below L2 or be a cauda equina lesion.
   b. Special considerations.
      (1) Pregnant client.
      (2) Client less than 13 years old.
      (3) Client with penetrating spinal cord lesion.
      (4) Client with fulminating infection like TB, AIDS, or severe diabetes mellitus.

2. Vasopressors—used in the immediate critical care period to treat bradycardia or hypotension due to spinal shock.
3. Antispasmodics—used to treat spasms. They depress the central nervous system and inhibit transmission of impulse from spinal cord to skeletal muscle (not always effective).
   a. Baclofen (Lioresal).
   b. Chlorzoxazone (Paraflex).
   c. Cyclobenzaprine hydrochloride (Flexeril).
   d. Diazepam (Valium).
   e. Orphenadrine citrate (Norflex).
   f. Dantrolene sodium (Dantrium).
4. Analgesics.
   a. Nonsteroidal anti-inflammatory drugs (NSAIDs).
   b. Opioids, non-opioids.
   c. Tricyclic antidepressants (amitriptyline [Elavil], imipramine [Tofranil]).
   d. Anticoagulant—heparin or low-molecular-weight heparin for DVT prophylaxis.

INFECTIOUS PROCESSES

Brain Abscess

Definition: Infectious process resulting in an encapsulated collection of pus usually found in the temporal lobe, frontal lobe, or cerebellum. May result from local or systemic infection.

Assessment
A. Increased temperature unless abscess is walled off, in which case temperature can be subnormal.
B. Headache, anorexia, malaise, vomiting.
C. Neurological deficits relative to area involved (focal seizures, blurred vision, etc.).
D. Signs of increased intracranial pressure.
E. Weight loss.

Implementation
A. Observe neurological signs for alterations.
B. Decrease temperature.
   1. Sponge bath.
   2. Antipyretic drugs.
   3. Cooling blanket.
C. Administer appropriate antibiotics for causative agent.
D. Prepare client and family for surgical intervention.
E. Provide appropriate postoperative care.

Meningitis

✦ *Definition:* An acute infection of the pia–arachnoid membrane, usually as the result of another bacterial infection such as upper respiratory, otitis media, or pneumonia (may be viral). May result in a degeneration of nerve cells or congestion of adjacent brain tissue.

Assessment

✦ A. Inflammation, infection, and increased intracranial pressure cause the cardinal signs and symptoms.
1. Headache, high fever, nuchal rigidity, and changes in mental status are first indications.
2. Later symptoms include nausea, vomiting, disorientation, muscle aches, and positive Kernig's sign.
✦ B. Observe for signs of meningeal irritation.
1. Brudzinski's sign: flexion of head causes flexion of both thighs at hips and knee flexion.
2. Kernig's signs: supine position, thigh and knee flexed to right angles. Extension of leg causes spasm of hamstring, resistance, and pain.
3. Nuchal rigidity.
C. Other symptoms may be severe headache, stiff neck and back, photophobia.
D. As illness progresses, lethargy, irritability, stupor, coma, possible seizures.
E. Diagnosis made by testing CSF obtained by lumbar puncture.

Implementation

✦ A. Maintain patent airway—give oxygen as ordered.
✦ B. Treat the infective organism—antimicrobial therapy by intravenous route for 2 weeks, followed by oral antibiotics.
✦ C. Droplet isolation for 24 hours after antibiotic therapy is initiated.
1. Treat all secretions from nose and mouth as infectious.
2. Check nasal cultures for organism.
✦ D. Treat increased intracranial pressure or seizures (Mannitol may be ordered for cerebral edema).
E. Control body temperature.
F. Provide adequate fluid and electrolyte balance—be aware of fluid overload, which can cause cerebral edema.
G. Provide bedrest and a quiet environment; sedate if needed. Do not give narcotics or sedatives that would interfere with neurologic assessment.
✦ H. Prevent complications of immobility.
1. Raise head of bed 30 to 45 degrees—decreases ICP.
2. Reposition frequently and provide range-of-motion exercises.
I. Relieve headache and fever with acetaminophen.
J. Maintain restful environment with dim lights to decrease photophobia.

Encephalitis

Definition: Severe inflammation of the brain caused by arboviruses or enteroviruses. Can be fatal. Diagnosed by CT, MRI, PET scan, and spinal fluid culture. Polymerase chain reaction (PCR) test is a laboratory method for detecting the presence and/or level of antibodies to an infectious agent in serum. It allows for early detection of HSV and West Nile encephalitis antibodies, substances made by the body's immune system to fight a specific infection.

✦ Assessment

A. Fever, headache, vomiting.
B. Signs of meningeal irritation.
C. Neuronal damage, drowsiness, coma, paralysis, ataxia.
D. Symptoms vary and depend on organism and area of brain involved.
E. Symptoms resemble meningitis but have a more gradual onset.

Implementation

A. Monitor vital signs frequently.
✦ B. Monitor neurological signs for alterations in client's condition.
✦ C. Administer anticonvulsant medications such as phenytoin.
✦ D. Administer glucocorticoids to reduce cerebral edema.
E. Administer sedatives to relieve restlessness.
F. Administer antiviral medications as ordered.
G. Manage fluid and electrolyte balance to prevent fluid overload and dehydration.
H. Position client to maintain patent airway and prevent contractures. Provide range-of-motion exercises.
I. Promote adequate nutrition through tube feedings, and parenteral hyperalimentation if necessary.
J. Provide hygienic care (i.e., skin care, oral care, and perineal care).
K. Provide safety measures if client is confused.

Post-Polio Syndrome (PPS)

✦ *Definition:* A neurological condition caused by the polio virus that invaded the central nervous system decades earlier.

Characteristics

A. Risk of developing PPS.
✦ 1. Risk manifests as people reach age 45–60 (35 years from the original polio infection).
2. Progresses over time but becomes a major risk if acute health problem develops.
3. Clients who had nonparalytic or "mild" polio are also at risk for developing PPS.
B. For original polio infection, *see* Pediatrics chapter, page 619.

✦ C. Cause of PPS appears to be neuromuscular failure—chronic overuse of polio-damaged nerves and muscles together with normal aging process.

D. If no medical records are available, electromyographic testing will confirm diagnosis of PPS.

Assessment

✦ A. Clinical manifestations of PPS.
1. Excessive fatigue.
2. Muscle weakness (both in muscles involved in original infection and those that were not).
3. Joint pain.
4. Breathing problems.
5. Impaired swallowing.
6. Intolerance to cold.
7. Inability to carry out activities of daily living.

B. Onset usually insidious; but with any sudden change in health status (severe illness or general anesthesia for surgery), onset may be sudden.

Implementation

A. No specific treatment for PPS.

B. Management is targeted at controlling symptoms, especially fatigue, weakness and pain. Overexertion can worsen weakness, and fatigue.

C. Promote pacing of activities to avoid feelings of fatigue.

D. Planning includes rest periods as well as learning to use assistive devices such as canes, scooters and wheelchairs.

E. Adaptive equipment will help with self-care.

F. Physical therapy can support fitness and mobility in light of limitations.

G. Weight loss interventions are helpful if the client is overweight.

H. Management of client focuses on lifestyle modifications to conserve energy and to support maximal performance of ADLs.

I. Rigorous and aggressive therapy used after initial polio infection is contraindicated during the post-polio period.

J. An interdisciplinary team approach is essential to manage the client.

K. Monitor for respiratory function.
1. Position for maximum chest excursion.
2. Monitor oxygen—may present risk if breathing based on hypoxic drive, not CO_2.
3. Muscle-relaxing medications and narcotic analgesics may be life-threatening if respirations are depressed.
4. Assess for speech, swallowing or respiratory difficulties. Take nursing measures to prevent aspiration. These are similar to those described for clients with Guillain-Barré syndrome.

L. Effective pain management through pharmacologic and nonpharmacologic approaches will help the client to remain active and achieve a greater sense of well-being.

M. Protection from the cold will aid in pain relief.

N. Surgery presents special risks.
1. General anesthesia not tolerated well—regional anesthesia is a better option.
2. Clients should not have nonessential surgical procedures performed.

O. Maintain blood volume, fluid and electrolyte balance (especially important to replace potassium after surgery).

P. Cold intolerance may present a special challenge for client undergoing surgery.

Q. Results of experiencing reemergence of symptoms:
1. Can be devastating to the client.
2. May impact psychological well-being.
3. May evoke a sense of fear, anxiety, and/or depression.

R. Nurse can help the client by active listening, providing information about PPS, encouraging participating in support groups, helping client gain a sense of control through active participation in lifestyle modifications.

Creutzfeldt-Jakob Disease (CJD)

Definition: Rare and fatal brain disorder thought to be caused by prion protein. Prions are small infectious pathogens containing protein but lacking nucleic acid.

Characteristics

A. Causes
1. May be inherited (10 percent).
2. Clients who received human growth hormone prior to more stringent purification methods instituted after 1978.
3. Clients who receive corneal transplants or cadaver dural grafts.

B. Types:
1. Sporadic CJD.
2. Familial CJD.
3. Acquired CJD.
4. Variant CJD (vCJD)—from infected beef; also called mad cow disease; found in Great Britain.

C. Incubation ranges from 4 to 20 years.

Assessment

A. There are no diagnostic tests to detect CJD. It is definitively determined by autopsy and examination of brain tissue.

B. Onset is gradual, with memory loss as first symptom.
1. Assess for memory loss progressing to global dementia.
2. Death may occur after a few months.

Implementation

A. Nursing care emphasizes safety, skin and mouth care, nutrition and comfort.

B. Prevention focuses on both caution in handling body fluids (blood or tissue) from clients with this diagnosis and, for mad cow disease, not eating contaminated beef.

C. The U.S. Blood Bank implemented guidelines in 2000 that refuse blood from anyone who has lived in Great Britain for more than 6 months.

ALTERED BLOOD SUPPLY TO BRAIN

Brain Attack (Cerebrovascular Accident [CVA], Stroke)

✦ *Definition:* A sudden focal neurological deficit due to cerebrovascular disease; the most common cause of brain disturbances.

Characteristics

✦ A. Causes.
1. Thrombosis.
2. Embolism.
3. Hemorrhage (extradural, subdural, subarachnoid or intracerebral).

B. Risk factors.
1. Circulatory—atherosclerosis, hypertension, anticoagulation therapy, cardiac valvular disease, synthetic valve and organ replacement, atrial arrhythmias.
2. Diabetes.
3. Sickle cell disease.
4. Substance abuse.
5. Sedentary lifestyle.
6. Hyperlipidemia.

MEDICAL IMPLICATIONS

✦ **Transient ischemic attack (TIA):** a precursor symptom or warning of impending CVA.
A. Rapid onset and short duration (30 minutes to 24 hours); by definition, must be resolved within this time period. No permanent neurological deficit.
B. Most common symptoms: vision loss, diplopia, contralateral hemiparesis, aphasia, confusion, slurred speech, and vertigo.

✦ **Carotid endarterectomy:** surgical procedure for carotid stenosis—often done following TIA or in presence of bruit indicating stenosis.
A. Procedure removes atherosclerotic plaque from arterial wall.
B. Monitor closely first 24 hours for cerebral ischemia or thrombosis or intolerance from carotid clamping.

✦ BRAIN LESION MANIFESTATIONS

Left Hemisphere
Lesion manifestations
✦• Usually dominant, containing speech center; right hemiplegia; aphasia, expressive and/or receptive.
• Behavior is slow, cautious, disorganized.
• Impaired left/right discrimination.
• Slow performance.
• Aware of deficits: depression, anxiety.
• Impaired comprehension related to language and math.
Nursing guidelines
• Do not underestimate ability to learn.
• Assess ability to understand speech.
• Act out, pantomime communication; use client's terms to communicate; speak in normal tone of voice.
• Divide tasks into simple steps; give frequent feedback.

Right Hemisphere
Lesion manifestations
• Left hemiplegia; spatial–perceptual deficits.
✦• Behavior is impulsive, quick; unaware of deficits; poor judge of abilities, limitations; neglect of paralyzed side.
• Tends to deny or minimize problems.
• Rapid performance, short attention span.
• Impulsive, safety problems.
• Impaired judgment.
• Impaired time concept.
Nursing guidelines
• Do not overestimate abilities.
• Use verbal cues as demonstrations; pantomimes may confuse.
• Use slow, minimal movements and avoid clutter around client.
• Divide tasks into simple steps; elicit return demonstration of skills.
• Promote awareness of body and environment on affected side.

---

7. Polycythemia.
8. Use of oral contraceptives.

✦ C. Interruption of blood supply to brain via carotid and vertebral–basilar arteries—causes cerebral anoxia.

D. Cerebral anoxia longer than 10 minutes to a localized area of the brain—causes cerebral infarction (irreversible changes).

E. Surrounding edema and congestion causes further dysfunction.

✦ F. Lesion in cerebral hemisphere (motor cortex, internal capsule, basal ganglia)—results in manifestations on the contralateral side.

G. Permanent disability unknown until edema subsides. Order in which function may return: facial, swallowing, lower limbs, speech, arms.

✦ **Assessment**

A. *Generalized signs*—headache; hypertension; changes in level of consciousness, convulsions; vomiting, nuchal rigidity, slow bounding pulse; Cheyne–Stokes respirations.

B. *Focal signs*—upper motor lesion in motor cortex and pyramidal tracts: hemiparesis, hemiplegia, central facial paralysis, language disorders, cranial dysfunction, conjugate deviation of eyes toward lesion, flaccid hyperreflexia (later, spastic hyporeflexia).

C. Evaluate general residual manifestations.
   1. Memory deficits; reduced memory span; emotional lability.
   2. Visual deficits such as homonomous hemianopia (loss of half of each visual field).
   3. Apraxia (can move but unable to use body part for specific purpose).

D. Evaluate client for rehabilitative program.

Implementation

A. Initial nursing objective is to support life and prevent complications.

◆ B. Give oxygen as needed. Begin at 3 L/min unless client has COPD.

◆ C. Maintain patent airway and ventilation—elevate head of bed 20–30 degrees unless shock is present—encourage flat in bed if possible (except for ADLs).

◆ D. Monitor clinical status to prevent complications.
   1. Neurological.
      a. Assess for recurrent CVA, increased intracranial pressure, bulbar involvement, hyperthermia.
      b. Continued coma—negative prognostic sign.
   2. Cardiovascular—shock and arrhythmias, hypertension.
   3. Apply elastic stockings or pneumatic compression stockings as ordered to reduce risk of deep vein thrombosis.
   4. Lungs—pulmonary emboli.

◆ E. Maintain optimal positioning during bedrest period—prevent contractures.
   1. During acute stages, quiet environment and minimal handling to prevent further bleeding.
   2. Upper motor lesion—spastic paralysis, flexion deformities, external rotation of hip.
   3. Positioning schedule—2 hours on unaffected side; 20 minutes on affected side; 30 minutes prone, BID–TID.
   4. Begin passive–active range-of-motion exercises, 4 to 5 times daily.
   5. Complications common with hemiplegia—frozen shoulder (vulnerable to injury due to stroke-induced injury to muscles); footdrop, use footboard.

◆ F. Maintain skin integrity: provide skin care every 2 hours; special protocol for back, bony prominences, and skin.

COLLABORATIVE CARE FOR A STROKE

Prevention
1. Control of hypertension.
2. Control of diabetes mellitus.
3. Treatment of underlying cardiac problems.
4. Anticoagulation therapy with Coumadin (warfarin sodium) for clients with atrial fibrillation.
5. Smoking cessation.
6. Limit alcohol intake.
7. Surgical intervention if client has an aneurysm and is at risk for bleeding.
8. Carotid endarterectomy.
9. Carotid artery stent.
10. Transluminal angioplasty.
11. Extracranial–intracranial (EC–IC) bypass.

Acute Care
1. Maintain airway.
2. Maintain hydration—fluid therapy.
3. Treatment of cerebral edema.
4. Drug therapy.
   a. Antiplatelet drugs are usually chosen to prevent further strokes in clients who have had TIA related to atherosclerosis.
   b. Platelet inhibitors used: aspirin (acetylsalicylic acid), Plavix (clopidogrel), Ticlid (ticlopidine), Persantine (dipyridamole), Aggrenox [combined Persantine (dipyridamole) and aspirin (acetylsalicylic acid)], Coumadin (warfarin sodium) for clients with atrial fibrillation.
5. Surgical therapy.
   a. Carotid endarterectomy.
   b. Carotid artery stent.
   c. Transluminal angioplasty.
   d. Extracranial–intracranial (EC–IC) bypass.

G. Maintain personal hygiene: encourage self-help.

◆ H. Keep siderails up and safety straps on if required.

I. Promote adequate nutrition, fluid and electrolyte balance.
   1. Encourage self-feeding with swallowing and assess if gag reflexes present.
   2. Food should be placed in unparalyzed side of mouth.
   3. Enteral feeding or gastrostomy feeding may be necessary.

J. Promote elimination.
   1. Bladder control may be regained within 3–5 days.
   2. Offer urinal or bedpan every 2 hours, day and night.
   3. Diet should have roughage and fiber to encourage elimination and prevent fecal impaction.
   4. Activity and exercises will stimulate elimination.

K. Provide emotional support.

1. Behavior changes as consciousness is regained—loss of memory, emotional lability, confusion, language disorders.
2. Reorient, reassure and increase self-esteem by encouraging client. Establish means of communication.

✦ L. Promote rehabilitation to maximal functioning.

Types of Stroke

A. Ischemic stroke—thrombotic or embolitic.
  1. Drug therapy—Tissue plasminogen activator (tPA).
    a. Must be administered within 3 hours of the onset of clinical signs.
    b. Timing of the administration of the med is the most critical factor.
    c. Screening includes:
      (1) Non-contrast CT or MRI to rule out hemorrhagic stroke.
      (2) Coagulation studies.
      (3) Screen for a recent history of a GI bleed.
      (4) Head trauma within the past 3 months.
      (5) Major surgery within the past 14 days.
    d. During drug infusion.
      (1) Monitor neuro signs to assess for improvement or for potential deterioration related to intercerebral hemorrhage.
      (2) Control of BP is critical during treatment and for 24 hours following.
  2. Surgical therapy.
    a. MERCI Retriever—MERCI stands for mechanical embolus removal for cerebral ischemia.
    b. During this procedure, which is used for ischemic strokes, a catheter with a coiled tip is placed directly into the blood vessel, allowing the physician to pull the clot out.

B. Hemorrhagic stroke.
  1. Surgical decompression if needed.
  2. Clipping, wrapping or coiling of aneurysm.
  3. Medical therapy.
    a. Anticoagulants and platelet inhibitors are contraindicated.
    b. Calcium-channel blocker nimodipine (Nimotop) is given to clients with subarachnoid hemorrhage to decrease the effects of vasospasm and minimize cerebral damage.
      (1) Must assess BP and AP prior to administration.
      (2) Hold if AP ≤ 60 beats/min or systolic BP ≤ 90 mm Hg, contact physician.
    c. Hyperthermia is treated with aspirin or acetaminophen (Tylenol).

(1) Increase in body temp by 1°C can increase brain metabolism by 10 percent and cause further brain damage.
(2) Cooling blankets may also be used. Monitor client temperatures closely.
(3) Maintaining temperature during the first 24 hours after a stroke is most important in preventing detrimental outcomes.

d. Seizure prevention—5–7 percent of stroke victims have seizures.
  (1) Antiseizure drug such as Dilantin (phenytoin) is given if a seizure occurs.
  (2) Seizure prophylaxis is recommended in the acute period after intracerebral or subarachnoid hemorrhage. In other types of strokes, it is not recommended.

Cerebral Aneurysm

✦ *Definition:* A dilation of the walls of a weakened cerebral artery leading to rupture from arteriosclerosis or trauma.

Assessment

✦ A. Alteration in level of consciousness may be earliest sign—monitor for subtle changes indicating a change in condition.
B. Suggest pupillary reaction, diplopia.
C. Slurred speech, drowsiness may be early signs LOC is deteriorating.
D. Hemiparesis, nuchal rigidity, headache.

Implementation

✦ A. Establish and maintain a patent airway.
✦ B. Closely monitor client.
  ✦ 1. Check for deteriorating condition—pulse, blood pressure, level of responsiveness.
    2. Monitor respiratory status—reduced oxygen increases chances of cerebral infarction.
C. Place client on bedrest in semi-Fowler's or side-lying position (elevate bed 15–30 degrees to promote venous drainage).
D. Turn and deep-breathe client every 2 hours.
E. Suction only with specific order.
F. Provide darkened room without stimulation (i.e., limit visitors and lengthy discussions).
G. Avoid any exertion or strenuous activity; provide range-of-motion exercises.
H. Provide diet low in stimulants such as caffeine. Restrict fluid intake to prevent increased intracranial pressure.
I. Monitor intake and output.
✦ J. Monitor vital signs for hypertension or cardiac irregularities. *Do not take rectal temperature due to vagal stimulation leading to cardiac arrest.*

K. Observe for complications indicating rebleeding, deep vein thrombosis (DVT), or increased size of aneurysm.

L. Surgical therapy: aneurysm and hemorrhage.
1. Immediate evacuation of aneurysm induced hematomas greater than 3 cm.
2. Clipping, wrapping, or coiling of the aneurysm to prevent bleeding—Gugliemi detachable coils (GDCs) provide immediate protection against hemorrhage by decreasing pulsation within the aneurysm.
3. Over time, a thrombus forms within the aneurysm. Plugging the weak, bulging section of the artery or fistula stops blood flow to the affected area and markedly decreases the risk of rupture.
4. Coils are designed to remain anchored within the aneurysm or fistula and do not require eventual removal.

DEGENERATIVE DISORDERS

Multiple Sclerosis (MS)

✦ *Definition:* A chronic, slowly progressive, noncontagious, degenerative disease of the CNS. Characterized by demyelination of the neurons, this disease affects the brain and spinal cord.

Characteristics

A. Definite cause unknown; may be autoimmune, associated with a deficit in the T lymphocytes.
B. Precipitating factors: pregnancy, fatigue, stress, infection, and trauma.
C. Incidence is greater in colder climate, equal in the sexes, and usually occurs between 20 and 40 years of age. More than 300,000 in U.S. alone are affected.
D. Demyelination of nerve fibers occurs within long conducting pathways of spinal cord and brain.
E. Lesions (plaques) are irregularly scattered—disseminated in pyramidal tract, posterior column, and ventricle of brain.
F. Destruction of myelin sheath creates patches of sclerotic tissue, degeneration of the nerve fiber, and disturbance in conduction of sensory and motor impulses.
G. Initially, the disease is characterized by periods of remission with exacerbation and variable manifestations, followed by irreversible dysfunction.
H. Clinical course may extend over 10–20 years.
I. Diagnostic tests; abnormal EEG, lumbar puncture (LP) indicating increased gamma globulin but normal serum levels.

Assessment

A. Clinical manifestations—variable, depending on area of involvement: sensory fibers, motor fibers, brain stem, cerebellum, internal capsule. Often insidious and gradual.
✦ B. Initial signs and symptoms: ataxia, diplopia, blurred vision, impaired speech; ascending numbness, starting in the feet.
✦ C. Weakness, paralysis, uncoordinated, intention tremor, spasticity, numbness, tingling, analgesia, anesthesia, loss of position sense; heat intolerance and symptoms of overheating.
D. Lhermitte's sign is a transient sensory symptom described as an electric shock radiating down the spine or into the limbs with neck flexion.
E. Bladder/bowel retention or incontinence.
F. Impaired vision (nystagmus), dysphagia.
G. Emotional instability, impaired judgment.
H. Charcot's triad—nystagmus, intention tremor, scanning speech.

Implementation

✦ A. Avoid precipitation of exacerbations.
1. Avoid fatigue, stress, infection, overheating, chilling.
2. Establish regular program of exercise and rest.
3. Provide a balanced diet, low in fat, rich in linoleic acid.
✦ B. Administer and assess effects of medications.
1. Steroids hasten remission. Prednisone is used for short-term therapy.
2. Chlordiazepoxide for mood swings.
3. Baclofen or dantrolene for spasticity.
4. Bethanechol to relieve urinary retention, or oxybutynin to increase bladder capacity.
5. Tegretol to treat paresthesia.

CHARCOT'S TRIADS

There are two sets of **Charcot's triads,** both of which are sets of clinical signs relating to quite separate diseases. One pertains to multiple sclerosis; the other refers to ascending cholangitis. Charcot's triads are named for Jean-Martin Charcot (1825–1893), the French neurologist who first described these combinations of signs in relation to these diseases.

Charcot's triad 1: the combination of nystagmus, intention tremor, and scanning or staccato speech. This triad is sometimes associated with multiple sclerosis but is not, as previously considered by some authors, pathognominic for multiple sclerosis.

Charcot's triad 2: the combination of jaundice; fever, usually with rigors; and right upper quadrant abdominal pain. Occurs as a result of ascending cholangitis. When the presentation also includes hypotension and mental status changes, it is known as Reynolds' pentad.

6. Symmetrel or Cylert to treat fatigue.
7. Inderal or an anticonvulsant (Neurontin) to treat ataxia.
8. Interferons (Betaseron and Avonex) used in relapsing–remitting MS.

C. Promote optimal activity.
   1. Moderation in activity with rest periods.
   2. Physical and speech therapy.
   3. Diversionary activities, hobbies.
   4. During exacerbation, client is usually put on bedrest.

D. Promote safety.
   1. Sensory loss—regulate bath water; caution with heating pads; inspect skin for lesions.
   2. Motor loss—avoid waxed floors, throw rugs; provide rails and walker.
   3. Diplopia—eye patch.

E. Promote regular elimination—bladder/bowel training programs.

F. Alternative treatments: hyperbaric oxygen, nutrition supplements (omega 3 and 6).

G. Provide education and emotional support to client and family.
   1. Encourage independence and realistic goals; assess personality and behavior changes; observe for signs of depression.
   2. Provide instruction and assistive devices; provide information about services of the National Multiple Sclerosis Society.

H. Assess and prevent potential complications.
   1. Most common: urinary tract infection, calculi, pressure ulcers.
   2. Common cause of death: respiratory tract infection, urinary tract infection.
   3. Contractures, pain due to spasticity, metabolic or nutritional disorders, regurgitation, depression.

Myasthenia Gravis

◆ *Definition:* A neuromuscular disease characterized by marked weakness and abnormal fatigue of voluntary muscles. Cause is unknown; question autoimmune reaction.

Characteristics

A. Clients with myasthenia have a high incidence of thymus abnormalities and frequently have systemic lupus erythematosus.

B. Basic pathology is a defect in transmission of nerve impulses at the myoneural junction, the junction of motor neuron with muscle.

◆ C. Normally, acetylcholine is stored in synaptic vesicle of motor neurons to skeletal muscles. Defect may be due to
   1. Deficiency in acetylcholine/excess acetylcholinesterase.

2. Defective motor-end plate and/or nerve terminals.
3. Decreased sensitivity to acetylcholine.

D. Muscles supplied by bulbar nuclei (cranial nerves) are commonly involved.

◆ E. Muscle involvement usually progresses from ocular to oropharyngeal, facial, proximal muscles, respiratory muscles.

F. Generally, there is no muscle atrophy or degeneration; there may be periods of exacerbations and remissions.

G. Symptoms are related to progressive weakness and fatigue of muscles when used; muscles generally strongest in the morning.

Assessment

A. Changes in eyes (affected first): ptosis, diplopia, and eye squint.

B. Impaired speech; dysphagia; drooping facies; difficulty chewing, closing mouth, or smiling; breathing difficulty and hoarse voice.

C. Respiratory paralysis and failure.

D. Severe weakness during Tensilon test.

Implementation

A. Assist with disease diagnosis.
   ◆ 1. Have Tensilon available for physician to inject—rapid, brief-acting anticholinesterase for testing purposes.
   2. Assess results of Tensilon injections.
      a. Positive for myasthenia—improvement in muscle strength.
      b. Negative—no improvement or even deterioration.

B. Administer medications as ordered.
   ◆ 1. Anticholinesterase drugs increase levels of acetylcholine at myoneural junction.
      ◆ a. Neostigmine, pyridostigmine, ambenonium —main difference is duration of effect.
      ◆ b. Edrophonium (Tensilon).
      c. Monitor side effects.
         (1) Related to effects of increased acetylcholine in parasympathetic nervous system: sweating, excessive salivation, nausea, diarrhea, abdominal cramps; possibly bradycardia or hypotension.
         (2) Excessive doses lead to cholinergic crisis —atropine given as cholinergic blocker.
      d. Nursing measures.
         (1) Give medication exactly on time, 30 minutes before meals.
         (2) Give medication with milk and crackers to reduce gastrointestinal upset.
         (3) Observe therapeutic or any toxic effects; monitor and record muscle strength and vital capacity.

2. Steroids.
   a. Suppress immune response.
   b. Usually the last resort after anticholinesterase and thymectomy.
✦ 3. The following drugs must be avoided:
   a. Streptomycin, kanamycin, neomycin, gentamicin—block neuromuscular transmission.
   b. Ether, quinidine, morphine, curare, procainamide, beta-adrenergic blockers, Innovar (opioid analgesic), sedatives—aggravate weakness of myasthenia.
4. Psychotropic drugs (e.g., lithium carbonate, phenothiazines, benzodiazepines, tricyclic antidepressants) have been associated with worsening of MG.

✦ C. Monitor client's condition for complications.
   1. Vital signs.
   2. Respirations: depth, rate, vital capacity, ability to deep-breathe and cough.
   3. Swallowing: ability to eat and handle secretions.
   4. Muscle strength.
   5. Speech: provide method of communication if client is unable to talk.
   6. Bowel and bladder function.
   7. Psychological status.

D. Promote optimal activity.
   1. Plan short periods of activity and long periods of rest.
   2. Time activity to coincide with maximum muscle strength.
   3. Encourage normal activities of daily living.
   4. Encourage diversionary activities.

E. Provide education and emotional support for client and family.
   1. Give reassurance and facts about the disease, medications and treatment regimen, importance of adhering to medication schedule, difference between myasthenic/cholinergic crisis, and emergency care.
   2. Instruct client to avoid infection, stress, fatigue and over-the-counter drugs.
   3. Instruct client to wear identification medal and carry emergency card.
   4. Provide information about services of Myasthenia Gravis Foundation.

F. Provide appropriate nursing measures in the event of thymectomy surgery.

✦ G. Use of Tensilon.
   1. Tensilon test differentiates crises, as symptoms are similar.
   2. Give Tensilon; if strength improves, it is symptomatic of myasthenic crisis and the client needs more medication; if weakness is more

---

CRISIS CONDITIONS

- **Myasthenic crisis**
  a. Acute exacerbation of disease may be due to rapid, unrecognized progression of disease; failure of medication; infection; or fatigue or stress.
  b. Myasthenic symptoms—weakness, dyspnea, dysphagia, restlessness, difficulty speaking.
- **Cholinergic crisis**
  a. Cholinergic paralysis with sustained depolarization of motor-end plates is due to overmedication with anticholinesterase.
  b. Symptoms similar to myasthenic state—restlessness, weakness, dysphagia, dyspnea.
  c. Cholinergic symptoms—fasciculation, abdominal cramps, diarrhea, nausea, vomiting, salivation, sweating, increased bronchial secretion.

---

severe, it is symptomatic of cholinergic crisis and overdose has occurred.

3. Be prepared for emergency with atropine, suction and other emergency equipment for respiratory arrest.
4. Crisis with respiratory insufficiency—client cannot swallow secretions and may aspirate.
   a. Maintain bedrest.
   b. May require endotracheal or tracheostomy tube to assist with ventilation.
   c. Monitor vital capacity, blood gases.
   d. Give atropine and may hold anticholinesterase (cholinergic).
   e. Begin anticholinesterase (myasthenic).

Parkinson's Disease

Definition: A degenerative disease resulting in dysfunction of the extrapyramidal system.

Characteristics

A. Possible causes: atherosclerosis, drug induced, post-encephalitic, idiopathic.
B. Degeneration of basal ganglia due to depleted concentration of dopamine.
C. Depletion of dopamine correlated with degeneration of substantia nigra (midbrain structures that are closely related functionally to basal ganglia).
D. Loss of inhibitory modulation of dopamine to counterbalance cholinergic system and interruption of balance-coordinating extrapyramidal system.
E. Slowly progressive disease with high incidence of crippling disability; mental deterioration occurs very late.

Assessment

✦ A. Assess stage of disease—five stages: unilateral, bilateral, impaired balance, fully developed severe disease, confinement to bed or wheelchair.

B. Identify presence of initial symptoms.
   1. Slowing of all movements.
   2. Aching shoulders and arms.
   3. Monotonous and indistinct speech.
   4. Writing becomes progressively smaller.
C. Evaluate major symptoms.
   ✦ 1. Tremor at rest, especially in hands and fingers (pill rolling).
       a. Increases when stressed or fatigued.
       b. May decrease with purposeful activity or sleep.
   2. Rigid or blank facial expression (masklike).
       a. Drooling, difficulty swallowing or speaking.
       b. Short, shuffling steps with stooped posture.
       c. Propulsive gait.
       d. Immobility of muscles in flexed position, creating jerky cogwheel motions.
       e. Loss of coordinated and associated automatic movement and balance.
   3. Bradykinesia—abnormal slowness and reduction in automatic movement; sluggishness of responses.
   4. Increased muscle tone rigidity.

Implementation

✦ A. Administer and monitor drugs—drug therapy is aimed at correcting an imbalance of neurotransmitters within the CNS.
   1. Amantadine (Symmetrel): used to treat clients with mild symptoms but no disability; side effects uncommon with usual dose.
   ✦ 2. Anticholinergic drugs: most effective is ethopropazine (Parsidol); used to treat tremors and rigidity, and inhibit action of acetylcholine; side effects include dry mouth, dry skin, blurring vision, urinary retention, and tachycardia.
   ✦ 3. Levodopa (Larodopa, Dopar) (converted in body to dopamine).
       a. Reduces akinesia, tremor, and rigidity.
       b. Passes through blood–brain barrier.
       c. Effectiveness may decline after 2–3 years.
       d. Side effects.
           (1) Anorexia, nausea and vomiting (administer drug with meals or snack; avoid coffee, which seems to increase nausea).
           (2) Postural hypotension, dizziness, tachycardia, and arrhythmias (monitor vital signs; caution client to sit up or stand up slowly; have client wear support stockings).
       e. Contraindicated in clients with closed-angle glaucoma, psychotic illness, and peptic ulcer disease.

✦ 4. Sinemet—combination of carbidopa and levodopa; has fewer side effects than levodopa.
   5. Antihistamines: reduce tremor and anxiety; side effect is drowsiness.
   6. Antispasmodics (Artane, Kemadrin): improve rigidity but not tremor.
   7. Bromocriptine (Parlodel): drug often used to replace levodopa when it loses effectiveness.
       a. Acts on dopamine receptors.
       b. Side effects: anorexia, nausea, vomiting, constipation, postural hypotension, cardiac arrhythmias, headache.
       c. Contraindicated in clients with mental illness, myocardial infarction, peptic ulcers, peripheral vascular disease.
✦ B. Avoid the following drugs:
   1. Phenothiazines, reserpine, pyridoxine, vitamin B_6: blocks desired action of levodopa.
   2. Monamine oxidase inhibitors: precipitate hypertensive crisis.
   3. Methyldopa: potentiates effects of the primary drug.
C. Maintain regular patterns of elimination.
   1. Constipation is often a problem due to side effects of medications, reduced physical activity, muscle weakness, and excessive drooling.
   2. Provide stool softeners, suppositories, mild cathartics.
✦ D. Promote physical therapy and rehabilitation.
   1. Provide preventive, corrective, and postural exercises.
   2. Institute massage and stretching exercises, stressing extension of limbs.
   3. Encourage daily ambulation—have client lift feet up when walking and avoid prolonged sitting.
   4. Facilitate adaptation for activities of daily living and self-care; encourage rhythmic patterns to attain timing; foster independence; utilize special aids and devices.
   5. Remove hazards that might cause falls.
E. Provide education and emotional support to client and family.
   1. Remember—intellect is usually not impaired.
   2. Assess changes in self-consciousness, body image, sexuality, moods.
   3. Instruct client to avoid emotional stress and fatigue, which aggravate symptoms.
   4. Instruct client to avoid foods high in vitamin B_6 and monamine oxidase.
F. Complete preoperative teaching for specific surgical intervention.
   1. Stereotactic surgery to reduce tremor.
       a. Pallidotomy—lesion in globus pallidus.

b. Thalamotomy—lesion in ventrolateral portion of thalamus.
2. Implantation of electrodes through burr holes into target area of brain; creation of lesion with high-frequency coagulation probe.
G. Provide appropriate nursing care following surgery.

CRANIAL AND PERIPHERAL NERVE DISORDERS

Trigeminal Neuralgia (Tic Douloureux)

◆ *Definition:* A sensory disorder of the fifth cranial nerve, resulting in severe, recurrent paroxysms of sharp, facial pain along the distribution of the trigeminal nerve. Etiology and pathology are unknown; incidence is rare, more common in women in fifth or sixth decade of life.

Assessment

A. Assess for trigger points on the lips, gums, nose, or cheek.
B. Conditions that stimulate symptoms: cold breeze, washing, chewing, food/fluids of extreme temperatures.
C. Assess pain—limited to those areas innervated by the three branches of the fifth nerve.
D. Diagnostic tests.
1. History and physical exam.
2. Brain or CT scan.
3. Audiologic evaluation.
4. EMG.
5. CSF analysis to rule out MS.
6. MRI to rule out MS.

Implementation

A. Observe and record characteristics of the attack.
B. Record method client uses to protect face.
C. Avoid extremes of heat or cold.
D. Provide small feedings of semiliquid or soft food.
E. Administer medication and record effects.
◆ F. Complete postoperative care.
1. Ophthalmic nerve—client needs protective eye care.
2. Maxillary and mandibular nerves.
a. Avoid hot food and liquids, which might burn.
b. Instruct client to chew on unaffected side to prevent biting denervated portion.
c. Encourage client to visit dentist within 6 months.
d. Provide frequent oral hygiene to keep the mouth free of debris.

MEDICAL IMPLICATIONS

Medical—Pharmacologic
1. Massive doses of vitamin B_{12}.
2. Carbamazepine (Tegretol, Carbatrol) remains criterion standard of treatment for this condition.
3. Phenytoin (Dilantin) has a lower rate of success; the dose varies greatly among clients.
4. Gabapentin (Neurontin) seems to be effective in some cases.
5. Lamotrigine (Lamictal) has proven effective. Dosage should be increased slowly for better tolerance (e.g., 25 mg daily dose each week; up to 250 mg twice a day).

Surgical Care
1. Surgical therapy can be divided into external or percutaneous procedures.
2. Microvascular decompression (MVD).
3. Alcohol injection of the trigeminus.
4. Glycerol injection of the gasserian ganglion to selectively destroy the pain-transmitting fibers.
5. Percutaneous radiofrequency rhizotomy.
6. Percutaneous microcompression with balloon inflation.

Radiation
1. Gamma-knife treatment.

Alternative Options
1. Acupuncture has proven to be successful.

Bell's Palsy (Facial Paralysis)

◆ *Definition:* A lower motor neuron lesion of the seventh cranial nerve, resulting in paralysis of one side of the face. May occur secondary to intracranial hemorrhage, tumor, meningitis, trauma. Diagnosis made by exclusion. No definitive tests.

Assessment

A. Flaccid muscles.
B. Shallow nasolabial fold.
C. Ability to raise eyebrows, frown, smile, close eyelids, or puff out cheeks.
D. Upward movement of eye when attempting to close eyelid.
E. Loss of taste in anterior tongue.

Implementation

◆ A. Majority of clients recover in a few weeks without residual effects.
B. Palliative measures account for majority of interventions; acupuncture; moist heat, massage.
C. Monitor use of analgesics and steroids.
D. Protect facial muscles.
1. Provide face sling to prevent stretching of weakened muscles and loss of tone.
2. Promote active facial exercises to prevent loss of muscle tone and support of facial muscles.

E. Monitor diet.
1. Instruct client to chew food on unaffected side.
2. Provide attractive, easy-to-eat foods to prevent anorexia and weight loss.
F. Provide special eye care to protect cornea and prevent keratitis, dark glasses, artificial tears.
G. Reassure and support.

Ménière's Disease

✦ *Definition:* Dilatation of the endolymphatic system causing degeneration of the vestibular and cochlear hair cells.

Characteristics
A. Etiology is unknown.
B. Possible causes may include allergies, toxicity, localized ischemia, hemorrhage, viral infection, and edema.
C. Surgical procedures.
1. Surgical division of vestibular portion of nerve or destruction of labyrinth may be necessary for severe cases.
2. Endolymphatic shunt.
3. Vestibular nerve section.
4. Labyrinthotomy.
5. Labyrinthectomy.

Assessment
A. Chronic recurrent process.
✦ B. Severe vertigo, nausea, vomiting, nystagmus, and loss of equilibrium.
C. Impaired hearing and tinnitus.
D. Nutritional needs, which will depend on amount of nausea and vomiting.

Implementation
✦ A. Maintain bedrest during acute attack.
1. Prevent injury during attack.
2. Provide siderails if necessary.
3. Keep room dark when photophobia is present.
✦ B. Provide drug therapy.
1. Vasodilators (nicotinic acid).
2. Diuretics, antihistamines (Benadryl), anticholinergics.
3. Sedatives.
C. Monitor diet therapy.
1. Low sodium.
2. Lipoflavonoid vitamin supplement.
3. Restricted fluid intake.
D. Assist with ambulation if necessary.

Bulbar Palsy

✦ *Definition:* A dysfunction of the ninth and tenth cranial nerves. The disease is secondary to tumors, infections, vascular or degenerative diseases.

Assessment
✦ A. Glossopharyngeal paralysis: absent gag reflex; difficulty swallowing, increased salivation; anesthesia of posterior palate and base of tongue.
✦ B. Vagal paralysis: difficulty with speech, breathing, and regurgitation.
C. Possible aspiration.
D. Breathing capability.
E. Difficulty in swallowing.
F. State of depression and fear.

✦ ### Implementation
A. Medical/surgical treatment is directed toward underlying cause.
B. Nursing care is directed toward prevention of complications.
C. Keep suction equipment at bedside.
D. Elevate head of bed.
E. Provide oral care.
F. Maintain open airway.
G. Keep emergency equipment available.
H. Avoid milk products and sticky carbohydrates.
I. Use small cup instead of straw for liquids.
J. Provide relationship therapy.
1. Give client time to express fears and concerns.
2. Provide consultation for depression if present.

Guillain–Barré Syndrome

✦ *Definition:* An acute, rapidly progressing and potentially fatal form of polyneuritis. Immune system overreacts to an infection, destroying the myelin sheath.

Characteristics
A. Etiology is unknown.
B. Occurs at any age but increased incidence between 30 and 50 years of age.
C. Both sexes equally affected.
D. Presyndrome clients may report a mild upper respiratory infection or gastroenteritis.
E. Recovery is a slow process, taking 2 months to 2 years.
F. Diagnostic test results: cerebrospinal fluid (CSF) contains high protein, abnormal EMG and nerve conduction.

Assessment
✦ A. Initial symptom of weakness of lower extremities with ascending paralysis/paresthesia.
B. Gradual progressive weakness of upper extremities and facial muscles (24–72 hours); paresthesias may precede weakness.
C. Respiratory failure occurs in some clients.
D. Cardiac arrhythmias, tachycardia.
E. Sensory changes—usually minor, but in some cases severe impairment of sensory information occurs.

Implementation

+ A. No specific treatment available; supportive treatment includes monitoring for complications (respiratory, circulatory).
  B. Carefully observe for respiratory paralysis and inability to handle secretions.
  C. Provide chest physiotherapy and pulmonary toilet.
  D. Maintain cardiovascular function.
    1. Monitor vital signs and cardiac rhythm.
    2. Vasopressors and volume replacement.
+ E. Prevent complications of immobility.
    1. Turn frequently.
    2. Provide skin care.
  F. Provide appropriate diversion.
  G. Reassure client, especially during paralysis period.
  H. Previous treatment included corticosteroids; this is now considered controversial.

Amyotrophic Lateral Sclerosis (Lou Gehrig's Disease)

+ *Definition:* The most common motor neuron disease of muscular atrophy. It is a rapidly fatal, upper and lower motor neuron deficit affecting the limbs.

Characteristics

+ A. May result from several causes.
    1. Nutritional deficiency related to disturbance in enzyme metabolism.
    2. Vitamin E deficiency resulting in damage to cell membranes.
    3. Metabolic interference in nucleic acid production by nerve fibers.
    4. Autoimmune disorder.
  B. Inherited as an autosomal dominant trait in 10 percent of cases.
  C. Occurs after age 40; most common in men.
  D. Is fatal within 2–6 years after onset. Riluzole slows progression of the disease.
  E. Diagnostic tests: EMG and muscle biopsy; increased protein in CSF.

Assessment

  A. Atrophy and weakness of upper extremities.
+ B. Difficulty swallowing and chewing.
  C. Respiratory excursion and breathing patterns.
  D. Impaired speech.
  E. Secondary depression.

Implementation

  A. Assist with rehabilitation program to promote independence.
+ B. Monitor for complications.
    1. Prevent skin breakdown: reposition regularly, provide back care, and utilize pressure-relieving devices.
    2. Prevent aspiration of food or fluids: offer soft foods and keep client in upright position during meals.
    3. Promote bowel and bladder function.
  C. Provide emotional support.

SURGICAL INTERVENTION

General Preoperative Care

Assessment

  A. Follow general assessment modalities for preoperative care.
  B. Observe and record neurological symptoms relative to site of problem (clot, lesion, aneurysm, etc.); for example:
    1. Paralysis.
    2. Seizure foci.
    3. Pupillary response.

Implementation

  A. Provide psychological support to client and family.
  B. Prep and shave cranial hair (save hair).
  C. Apply scrub solution to scalp, as ordered.
  D. Avoid using enemas unless specifically ordered; the strain of defecation may lead to increased intracranial pressure.
  E. Explain postoperative routine orders such as neurological checks and headaches.
  F. Administer steroids or mercurial diuretics as ordered, to decrease cerebral edema.
  G. Insert NG tube and/or Foley catheter, as ordered.

General Postoperative Care

Assessment

  A. Follow general assessment modalities for postoperative clients.
+ B. Observe neurological signs.
    1. Evaluate level of consciousness.
       a. Orientation to time and place.
       b. Response to painful stimuli: pinch Achilles tendon or test with safety pin.
       c. Ability to follow verbal command.
    2. Evaluate pupil size and reactions to light.
       a. Are pupils equal, not constricted or dilated?
       b. Do pupils react to light?
       c. Do pupils react sluggishly or are they fixed?
    3. Evaluate strength and motion of extremities.
       a. Are handgrasps present and equal?
       b. Are handgrasps strong or weak?
       c. Can client move all extremities on command?
       d. Are movements purposeful or involuntary?
       e. Do the extremities have twitching, flaccid, or spastic movements (indicative of a neurological problem)?

C. Observe vital signs.
1. Keep client normothermic to decrease metabolic needs of the brain.
2. Observe respirations for depth and rate to prevent respiratory acidosis from anoxia.
3. Observe blood pressure and pulse for signs of shock or increased intracranial pressure.
D. Evaluate reflexes.
1. Babinski—positive Babinski is elicited by stroking the lateral aspect of the sole of the foot, backward flexion of the great toe, or spreading of other toes.
   a. Most important pathological reflex in neurology.
   b. If positive, indicative of pyramidal tract involvement (usually upper motor neuron lesion).
2. Romberg—when client stands with feet close together, he or she falls off balance. If positive, may have cerebellar, proprioceptive, or vestibular difficulties.
3. Kernig—client is lying down with thigh flexed at a right angle; extension of the leg upward results in spasm of hamstring muscle, pain, and resistance to additional extension of leg at the knee (indicative of meningitis).
E. Observe for headache, double vision, nausea, or vomiting.

Implementation

A. Maintain patent airway.
1. Oxygen deprivation and an increase of carbon dioxide may produce cerebral hypoxia and cause cerebral edema.
2. Intubate if values indicate to be necessary:
   a. PO_2 below 80 mm Hg.
   b. PCO_2 above 50 mm Hg.
B. Suction if necessary, but not through nose without specific order.
C. Maintain adequate oxygenation and humidification.
D. Place client in semi-prone or semi-Fowler's position (or totally on side). Turn every 2 hours, side to side (unless contraindicated by surgical procedure).
E. Maintain fluid and electrolyte balance.
1. Do not give fluid by mouth to semiconscious or unconscious client.
2. Weigh to determine fluid loss.
3. Administer IV fluids slowly; overhydration leads to cerebral edema.
F. Record accurate intake and output.
G. Watch serial blood and urine samples; sodium regulation disturbances accompany head injuries.
H. Keep temperature down with cooling blanket if necessary. If temperature is down, the metabolic requirements of brain as well as oxygen requirements are less.

✦ PRECAUTIONS FOR CARE OF NEUROSURGICAL CLIENT

A. Do not lower head in Trendelenburg position or place in supine position.
B. Do not suction through nose without specific order.
C. Be careful when administering sedation and narcotics.
   1. Cannot evaluate neurological status.
   2. May cause respiratory embarrassment.
D. Do not give oral fluids unless client is fully awake.
E. Do not administer enemas or cathartics (may cause straining, which then increases intracranial pressure).
F. Do not place on operative side if large tumor or bone is removed.

I. Take vital and neurological signs every 15–30 minutes until stable.
J. Use seizure precautions. Administer anticonvulsants as ordered.
K. Provide hygienic care, including oral hygiene.
L. Observe dressing for unusual drainage (bleeding, cerebrospinal fluid).
M. Prevent straining with bowel movements.
N. Administer steroids and osmotic diuretics to decrease cerebral edema.
O. Observe for and treat postoperative complications.
1. Increased intracranial pressure.
2. Seizures.
3. Hemorrhage.
4. Wound infection.
5. Brain abscess.
6. Meningitis.

EYE AND EAR

Glaucoma

Definition: An eye disorder in which intraocular pressure is too high for the health of the eye—causes atrophy of the optic nerve and peripheral visual field loss.

Characteristics

A. Glaucoma classified into two main types: open-angle and angle-closure.
B. Also classified by cause: primary, cause is not known; secondary, cause is known.
C. Primary open-angle (chronic) glaucoma.
1. Results from an overproduction or obstruction to the outflow of aqueous humor. Aqueous humor flows from the trabecular network, Schlemm's canal, or aqueous veins.
2. 60% to 70% of all glaucoma cases are of this type.
D. Primary angle-closure (narrow angle—acute) glaucoma follows an untreated attack of acute angle-closure glaucoma.

1. Results from an obstruction to the outflow of aqueous humor.
2. Causes of obstruction.
   a. A narrow angle between the anterior iris and the posterior corneal surface.
   b. Shallow anterior chambers.
   c. A thickened iris that causes angle closure upon pupil dilation.
   d. A bulging iris that presses on the trabecula to close the angle.
3. Caused by trauma, drugs, or inflammation.

Assessment
✦ A. Type of glaucoma.
   1. Primary open-angle—slow, progressive course.
   2. Angle-closure.
   3. Other glaucomas (associated with inflammation, trauma, surgery, etc.).
✦ B. Risk conditions: over 40 years of age, diabetes, African American, hypertensive, familial history of glaucoma, and history of eye injury.
✦ C. Results of Schiotz or Goldman's Applanation Tonometer Test (7 to 21 mm Hg is normal) and optic-disc cupping.
✦ D. Primary open-angle manifestations.
   1. Slow loss of peripheral vision.
   2. Eventual loss of central vision; tunnel vision.
✦ E. Primary angle-closure glaucoma manifestations (accounts for 10 percent of all glaucomas).
   1. Unilateral inflammation.
   2. Pain; pressure over eye.
   3. Increased intraocular pressure (24–32 mm Hg to much higher). One-sixth of clients have pressure within normal range.
   4. Moderate pupil dilation, nonreactive to light.
   5. Cloudy cornea.
   6. Blurring and decreased visual acuity.
   7. Photophobia.
   8. Halos around light.
   9. Nausea and vomiting.

Implementation
A. Chronic or primary open-angle glaucoma.
   1. Decrease aqueous humor production through beta blockers or prostaglandins.
   2. Treated first with medication. New drugs include topical α_2-selective adrenergic agonists, carbonic anhydrase inhibitors and prostaglandin analogs.
   ✦ 3. When medication no longer controls intraocular pressure and peripheral vision is lost, prepare client for argon laser treatments.
      a. Trabeculoplasty—laser alters trabecular meshwork and facilitates aqueous humor drainage.

   b. Trabeculectomy—creates a new opening at limbus to allow drainage of aqueous humor.
   c. Seton implants (Moltemo).
   d. Photocoagulation—uses argon laser heat to destroy portions of the ciliary body.
   e. Cyclocryotherapy—freezes tissue and destroys portions of the ciliary body.
B. Acute or primary angle-closure glaucoma.
   1. Treat as a medical emergency problem.
   ✦ 2. Administer drugs to lower intraocular pressure—beta blockers, IV or oral carbonic anhydrase inhibitors, or topical adrenergic agonists.
   3. Prepare client for laser peripheral iridotomy (definitive treatment).
      a. Allows aqueous humor to flow from posterior to anterior chamber.
      b. Administer ordered drugs: pilocarpine, acetazolamide, Mannitol, etc.
C. Provide postoperative care.
   ✦ 1. Administer cycloplegic eyedrops to affected eye to relax the ciliary muscle and decrease inflammation.
   2. Observe unaffected eye for symptoms of acute angle-closure glaucoma if cycloplegic drops are given by mistake.
✦ D. Instruct client to limit activities that increase intraocular pressure—straining, coughing, stooping, or lifting.

Cataracts

Definition: Clouding or opacity of the lens that leads to blurred vision.

Characteristics
✦ A. Opacity is due to physical changes of the fibers or chemical changes in protein of the lens—most often caused by the slow, degenerative changes of age.
B. The goal of cataract surgery is to restore functional vision.
C. Surgical procedure is usually based on individual needs.
   1. If any inflammation is present, surgery is not performed.
   2. Cataracts are usually removed under local or topical anesthesia.
   3. Some simple cataracts are removed by use of alphachymotrypsin, which weakens the zonular fibers that hold the lens in position.
   4. Surgery is performed on one eye at a time.
✦ D. Types of surgical extraction.
   1. *Extracapsular*—the lens is lifted out without removing the posterior lens capsule.
   2. *Phacoemulsification (ultrasonic)*—the lens is broken up by ultrasonic vibrations and extracted via extracapsular route.

3. *Intracapsular* (rarely done today)—the lens is removed within its capsule through a small incision.

E. Intraocular lens implant at time of surgery is a common alternative to sight correction with glasses.
   1. Cataracts are now removed through smaller incisions to promote rapid visual rehabilitation.
   2. New intraocular lens designs have helped to prevent lens epithelial cell migration.

Implementation

A. Check that client understands preoperative instructions.
   1. Client must be transported to and from hospital.
   2. Client must have someone at home for assistance following surgery.
   3. Client should be NPO, and shampoo hair before surgery.
   4. Review instructions to decrease intraocular pressure (do not bend, cough, strain, or lift).

B. Administer prescribed preoperative medications.
   1. Mydriatics and cycloplegics (Cyclogyl) to paralyze ciliary muscle—note whether pupil dilates following drug instillation.
   2. Topical antibiotics—prevention of infection.

C. Provide postoperative care. Most procedures are done on outpatient basis.
   1. Instruct client in postoperative drugs.
      a. Mydriatics are occasionally used.
      b. Steroids (prednisolone suspension) and antibiotic drops.
      c. Analgesics.
   2. Instruct in ways to alleviate symptoms that could result in complications.
      a. Increased intraocular pressure may occur with nausea and vomiting; restlessness; coughing or sneezing; lifting more than 15 pounds; constipation.
      b. Observe for signs of infection: increasing redness, tearing, green drainage, or photophobia.
   3. Instruct client to notify physician of sudden pain in operative eye—may be due to ruptured vessel or suture.
   4. Apply dressing and shield at night to prevent injury to operative eye. Unoperative eye is usually left uncovered.
   5. Instruct client to maintain low-Fowler's position the day of surgery and to turn only to unoperative side (as ordered).
   6. Instruct client to avoid rapid movements and not to bend over—may be ambulatory first postoperative day.

7. Reinforce instructions on dressing changes and eye drops. (Client returns to physician's office first postoperative day for change of dressing.)
8. Inform client that temporary glasses are prescribed 1–4 weeks postoperatively if lens is not implanted.

D. Assist client with specific adjustment problems.
   1. Intraocular lens implant at time of surgery is very common.
      a. This lens provides means of focusing light on the retina—approximates human lens.
      b. If no implant, the eye cannot accommodate and glasses must be worn at all times.
      c. Mydriatic drops frequently used to prevent lens displacement.
   2. Cataract glasses magnify—objects appear closer. Teach client to accommodate, judge distance, and climb stairs carefully.

Ophthalmic Drugs

A. Miotics: pilocarpine HCl 1–4 percent solution; carbachol; cholinergic agonists.
   1. Action is contraction of ciliary muscle, which increases flow of aqueous humor.
   2. Treatment for glaucoma and certain types of lens implants.
   3. Side effects: headache, conjunctiva irritation, and inflammation.

B. Beta blockers: timolol; betaxolol, levobunolol.
   1. Action is to reduce intraocular pressure by decreasing formation of aqueous humor or may facilitate outflow of aqueous humor.
   2. Treatment for glaucoma.
   3. Side effects: eye irritation.

C. Carbonic anhydrase inhibitors: acetazolamide, dichlorphenamide.
   1. Action is to restrict action of the enzyme necessary to produce aqueous humor—thus, decrease aqueous production.
   2. Treatment for glaucoma.
   3. Side effects: CNS disturbance, GI irritation, acidosis, hypokalemia.

D. Hyperosmotic agents: glycerin (oral) or Mannitol (IV).
   1. Action is to draw fluid from the eye (increase blood osmolarity)—reduce intraocular pressure.
   2. Treatment for cataract surgery as preoperative medication.
   3. Side effects: CNS—headache, confusion, blurred vision, GI irritability, nausea, dehydration.

E. Nonselective adrenergic agonists: epinephrine, dipivefrin.
   1. Action is to increase aqueous outflow and decrease aqueous production.

2. Topical treatment for glaucoma.

F. Topical antibiotics are used to prevent infection.

Retinal Detachment

Characteristics

✦ A. The retina is the part of the eye that perceives light; it coordinates and transmits impulses from its seeing nerve cells to the optic nerve.

B. There are two primitive retinal layers: the outer pigment epithelium and an inner sensory layer.

C. Retinal detachment occurs when
   1. The two primitive layers of the retina separate, due to the accumulation of fluid between them.
   2. Both retinal layers elevate away from the choroid, due to a tumor.

D. As the detachment extends and becomes complete, blindness occurs.

✦ Assessment

A. Opacities before the eyes.

B. Flashes of light.

C. Floating spots—blood and retinal cells freed at the time of the tear cast shadows on the retina as they drift about the eye.

D. Progressive constriction of vision in one area.
   1. The area of visual loss depends on the location of detachment.
   2. When the detachment is extensive and rapid, the client feels as if a curtain has been pulled over his or her eyes.
   3. Painless.

Implementation

✦ A. Provide preoperative care.
   1. Keep client on bedrest.
   2. Cover both eyes with patches to prevent further detachment.
   ✦ 3. Position client's head so the retinal hole is in the lowest part of the eye.
   4. Immediate surgery with drainage of fluid from subretinal space so that retina returns to normal position.
   5. Retinal breaks are sealed by various methods that produce inflammatory reactions (chorioretinitis).
      a. Cryosurgery—cold probe applied to sclera causes a chorioretinal scar. Most common procedure.
      b. Diathermy—causes retina to adhere to choroid.
      c. Laser—seals small retinal tears before detachment occurs.

✦ B. Provide postoperative care.
   1. Maintain safe environment.
      a. Keep siderails up.
      b. Feed client.
      c. Maintain bedrest for 1 or 2 days.
      d. Give client call bell and answer immediately.
   ✦ 2. Prevent complications.
      a. Observe for hemorrhage, which is a common complication. Notify physician immediately of any sudden, sharp eye pain, restlessness.
      b. Cover both eyes; keep lights dim.
      c. Position so area of detachment is in dependent position. (If air bubble is present, position on abdomen.)
      d. Prevent clinical manifestations that can cause hemorrhage.
         (1) Nausea and vomiting.
         (2) Restlessness.
      e. Encourage client to do deep breathing but to avoid coughing (increases intraocular pressure).
      f. Administer good skin care to prevent breakdown.
   3. Provide emotional support.
      a. Provide audible stimulation.
      b. Warn client as you enter the room and always speak before touching.
      c. Orient to surroundings.

C. Provide client instruction.
   1. Convalescent period.
      a. Wear patch at night to prevent rubbing of eyes.
      b. Wear dark glasses; avoid squinting.
      c. No reading for 3 weeks.
   2. Postconvalescent period.
      a. Avoid straining and constipation.
      b. Avoid lifting heavy objects for 6–8 weeks.
      c. Avoid bending from the waist.
      d. May return to more active life in 6–8 weeks.

Age-Related Macular Degeneration (ARMD)

✦ *Definition:* Macula cells fail to function and cell regeneration lessens, which causes loss of central vision.

Characteristics

✦ A. The leading cause of new cases of uncorrectable vision loss in adults over 60 years of age.
   1. Most cases are age-related.
   2. Much more common in Caucasians than in African Americans.

B. There are two types.
   1. Dry (atrophic)—photo receptors in the macula of the retina fail to function and are not replaced due to age.

2. Wet (exudative)—less common form in which retinal tissue degenerates, allowing fluid to leak into the subretinal space.

Assessment

✦ A. Painless loss of central vision in one or both eyes.
1. Blurred vision.
2. Distortion of straight lines.
3. Dark spot in the central vision area.
B. Decreased ability to distinguish colors.
C. Check if client has difficulty with everyday activities—reading, driving, watching television, recognizing faces.

✦ ### Implementation

A. Assist client to learn to compensate for visual deficit in the home.
B. Discuss client's fear of blindness.
C. Discuss optical aids available, closed-circuit television, telescopic lenses.
D. Refer client to a low-vision support group.
E. If client is hospitalized with this condition, orient to room, remove clutter, assist with meals, and always identify self when entering room.
F. Alternative therapy and prevention: vitamin and nutrient supplements (lutein, leucopene, zinc, and beta-carotene, vitamin C, vitamin E).

✦ ### Removal of Foreign Body from Eye

A. Have client look upward.
B. Expose and evert lower lid to expose conjunctival sac.
C. Wet cotton applicator with sterile normal saline, and gently twist swab over particle and remove it.
D. If particle cannot be found, have client look downward. Place cotton applicator horizontally on outer surface of upper lid.
E. Grasp eyelashes with fingers, and pull upper lid outward and upward over cotton stick.
F. With twisting motion upward, loosen particle and remove.
G. If penetrating object—do not remove. Cover with cup, do not bend, and notify physician STAT.

Stapedectomy

Characteristics
A. Surgery is performed when the client has otosclerosis.
✦ B. Otosclerosis is a condition in which the stapes is replaced.
✦ 1. A graft is placed over the oval window and a prosthesis is positioned between the incus and covered oval window.

2. Stapes replacement surgery has a high success rate, with the client experiencing improved hearing.
C. Surgical procedure.
✦ 1. An incision is made deep in the ear canal, close to the eardrum, so that the drum can be turned back and the middle ear exposed.
2. The surgeon frees and removes the stapes and the attached footplate, leaving an opening in the oval window.
3. The client can usually hear as soon as this procedure has been completed.
✦ 4. The opening in the oval window is closed with a plug of fat or Gelfoam, which the body will eventually replace with mucous membrane cells.
✦ 5. A steel wire or a Teflon piston is inserted to replace the stapes.
   a. It is attached to the incus at one end and to the graft or plug at the other end.
   b. The wire transmits sound to the inner ear.
6. External canal is packed, covered with "eye patch" dressing over auricle.

Implementation

✦ A. Position client in low-Fowler's, on unoperated side, or as ordered.
B. Do not turn the client.
✦ C. Put siderails up.
D. Have client deep-breathe every 2 hours until ambulatory, but do not allow client to cough.
✦ E. Check for drainage; report excessive bleeding.
F. Prevent vomiting.
G. Give antibiotics as ordered.
H. Client may have vertigo when ambulatory; stay with the client and avoid quick movements.
I. Advise client not to smoke.

Irrigation of External Auditory Canal

A. Remove any discharge on outer ear.
B. Place emesis basin under ear.
✦ C. Gently pull outer ear upward and backward for adult, or downward and backward for child.
D. Place tip of syringe or irrigating catheter at opening of ear.
✦ E. Gently irrigate with solution at 95°F to 105°F, directing flow toward the sides of the canal.
F. Dry external ear.
G. If irrigation does not dislodge wax, instillation of drops will need to be carried out.

NEUROLOGICAL SYSTEM REVIEW QUESTIONS

1. Following a car accident, a newly admitted client seems concerned about his sudden loss of memory. He seeks out the nurse for an explanation. Before responding to the client, the nurse needs to consider that

   1. Her answer should be reassuring and brief because the client is still very anxious.
   2. She needs to wait until all the test results are in before responding.
   3. The client's amnesia is a result of his guilt.
   4. The client's anxious behavior would be best dealt with by having the physician order a tranquilizer.

2. The nurse has orders to administer phenytoin (Dilantin) 100 mg IV as an anticonvulsant. The priority action while administering this drug is to

   1. Administer the drug as quickly as possible to prevent a seizure.
   2. Assess for infiltration of the drug.
   3. Assess for effects of the drug.
   4. Check pupil dilation of the client to assess for overdose.

3. A 42-year-old client has been diagnosed with a right-sided acoustic neuroma. The tumor is large and has impaired the function of the seventh and eighth cranial nerves. Which of the following nursing actions will be carried out to prevent complications?

   1. Keeping a suction machine available.
   2. Use of an eyepatch or eyeshield on the right eye.
   3. Use of only cool water to wash the face.
   4. Advising the client to use only the left eye.

4. A client admitted to a surgical unit for possible bleeding in the cerebrum has vital signs taken every hour to monitor the neurological status. Which of the following neurological checks will give the nurse the best information about the extent of bleeding?

   1. Pupillary checks.
   2. Spinal tap.
   3. Deep tendon reflexes.
   4. Evaluation of extrapyramidal motor system.

5. A client with an admitting diagnosis of head injury has a Glasgow Coma Scale score of 3–5–4. The nurse's understanding of this test is that the client

   1. Can follow simple commands.
   2. Will make no attempt to vocalize.
   3. Is unconscious.
   4. Is able to open his eyes when spoken to.

6. The nursing diagnosis that would have the highest priority in the care of a client who has become comatose following a cerebral hemorrhage is

   1. Impaired physical mobility.
   2. Altered nutrition: less than body requirements.
   3. Ineffective airway clearance.
   4. Constipation.

7. A 28-year-old male client is admitted to the hospital for a suspected brain tumor. While assessing this client, the nurse would keep in mind that the most reliable index of cerebral status is

   1. Pupil response.
   2. Deep tendon reflexes.
   3. Muscle strength.
   4. Level of consciousness.

8. If a client with increased intracranial pressure (ICP) demonstrates decorticate posturing, the nurse will observe

   1. Flexion of both upper and lower extremities.
   2. Extension of elbows and knees, plantar flexion of feet, and flexion of the wrists.
   3. Flexion of elbows, extension of the knees, and plantar flexion of the feet.
   4. Extension of upper extremities and flexion of lower extremities.

9. A client was in an automobile accident and sustained a head injury. Following admission to the hospital, a diagnosis of increasing intracranial pressure was made. The nursing intervention appropriate in the care of this client is to

   1. Teach controlled coughing and deep breathing.
   2. Provide a quiet and brightly lit environment.
   3. Elevate the head 15 to 30 degrees.
   4. Encourage the intake of clear fluids.

10. The nurse enters the room of a client who is in the clonic phase of a tonic–clonic seizure. The initial nursing action should be to

1. Insert a padded mouth gag.
2. Place some padding under the head.
3. Gently restrain the limbs.
4. Obtain equipment for orotracheal suctioning.

11. A client, admitted to the emergency room following a car accident, complains of a severe headache and demonstrates nuchal rigidity and Kernig's sign. The nurse will assess for which complication?

1. Subdural hemorrhage.
2. Increased intracranial pressure.
3. Shock.
4. Subarachnoid hemorrhage.

12. A 16-year-old girl has a known arteriovenous malformation of the middle cerebral artery. In talking to the school nurse, she complains of a headache and stiff neck. The nurse would take which of the following actions?

1. Call her mother and have her picked up from school to see the physician.
2. Send her home right away to rest.
3. Make preparations for emergency transfer to an acute care setting.
4. Have the client rest for 2 hours, then reevaluate the situation.

13. A client is admitted following an automobile accident in which he sustained a contusion. The nurse knows that the significance of a contusion is that

1. It is reversible.
2. Amnesia will occur.
3. Loss of consciousness may be transient.
4. Laceration of the brain may occur.

14. A client is admitted to the trauma unit with a suspected arterial bleed in his head following an injury. He is experiencing periods of confusion and lucidity. As the nurse assesses his status, she will further assess for

1. Subdural hematoma.
2. Increased intracranial pressure.
3. Epidural hematoma.
4. Increased blood pressure.

15. A 24-year-old client is admitted to the hospital following an automobile accident. She was brought in unconscious with the following vital signs: BP 130/76, P 100, R 16, T 98°F. The nurse observes bleeding from the client's nose. Which of the following inter-

ventions will assist in determining the presence of cerebrospinal fluid?

1. Obtaining a culture of the specimen using sterile swabs and sending to the laboratory.
2. Allowing the drainage to drip on a sterile gauze and observing for a halo or ring around the blood.
3. Suctioning the nose gently with a bulb syringe and sending specimen to the laboratory.
4. Inserting sterile packing into the nares and removing in 24 hours.

16. A young client who was hit by a car was fortunate because the level of his injury did not interrupt his respiratory function. The cord segments involved with maintaining respiratory function are

1. Thoracic level 5 and 6.
2. Thoracic level 2 and 3.
3. Cervical level 7 and 8.
4. Cervical level 3 and 4.

17. Following an accident, a client is admitted with a head injury and concurrent cervical spine injury. The physician will use Crutchfield tongs. The purpose of these tongs is to

1. Hypoextend the vertebral column.
2. Hyperextend the vertebral column.
3. Decompress the spinal nerves.
4. Allow the client to sit up and move without twisting his spine.

18. A quadriplegic client tells the nurse that he believes he is experiencing an episode of autonomic hyperreflexia (dysreflexia). The first nursing intervention is to

1. Ask him what he thinks has precipitated this episode.
2. Assess his blood pressure and pulse.
3. Elevate his head as high as possible.
4. Assist him in emptying his bladder.

19. In developing a nursing care plan for a client with multiple sclerosis, the nurse would *not* include

1. Preventive measures for falls.
2. Interventions to promote bowel elimination.
3. Instructions on doing only moderate activities.
4. Techniques to promote safe swallowing.

20. Myasthenic crisis and cholinergic crisis are the major complications of myasthenia gravis. Which of the following is essential nursing knowledge when caring for a client in crisis?

1. Weakness and paralysis of the muscles for swallowing and breathing occur in either crisis.
2. Cholinergic drugs should be administered to prevent further complications associated with the crisis.
3. The clinical condition of the client usually improves after several days of treatment.
4. Loss of body function creates high levels of anxiety and fear.

21. A 21-year-old male has a confirmed diagnosis of a brain tumor. Following surgery for a tumor near the hypothalamus, the nursing assessment should include observing for

   1. Inability to regulate body temperature.
   2. Bradycardia.
   3. Visual disturbances.
   4. Inability to perceive sound.

22. For a client who has ataxia, which of the following tests would be performed to assess the ability to ambulate?

   1. Kernig's.
   2. Romberg's.
   3. Riley–Day's.
   4. Hoffmann's.

23. The nurse is counseling a client with the diagnosis of glaucoma. She explains that if left untreated, this condition leads to

   1. Blindness.
   2. Myopia.
   3. Retrolental fibroplasia.
   4. Uveitis.

24. A male client has just had a cataract operation without a lens implant. In discharge teaching, the nurse will instruct the client's wife to

   1. Feed him soft foods for several days to prevent facial movement.
   2. Keep the eye dressing on for 1 week.
   3. Have her husband remain in bed for 3 days.
   4. Allow him to walk upstairs only with assistance.

25. A client has just been admitted with a diagnosis of detached retina and surgery is scheduled. The preoperative ophthalmic medication that will most likely be ordered for this client will be

   1. Atropine sulfate.
   2. Carbamylcholine.
   3. Pilocarpine.
   4. Timolol maleate.

NEUROLOGICAL SYSTEM

Answers with Rationale

1. (1) The client is very anxious, and his ability to comprehend and process information is extremely limited. A quiet, reassuring manner with a brief, concrete response will be most helpful at this point. Interventions to decrease the client's anxiety are the priority here, whether or not the cause is guilt feelings.

   NP:P; CN:PS; CL:C

2. (2) It is important to assess for infiltration because it can cause erosion of the tissue and even loss of a limb. Injecting the drug at a faster rate may induce severe hypotension. Assessing for effects of the drug is too general an answer (3) and pupil dilation will not reveal overdose (4).

   NP:P; CN:PH; CL:A

3. (2) The seventh nerve closes the eyelid. Without a patch, the cornea is subject to damage. The temperature of the water (3) does not matter. A suction machine (1) is not necessary.

   NP:I; CN:PH; CL:AN

4. (1) Pupillary checks reflect function of the third cranial nerve, which stretches as it becomes displaced by blood, tumor, etc.

   NP:E; CN:PH; CL:A

5. (4) A Glasgow Coma Scale score of 3–5–4 means that the client is able to open his eyes when spoken to and can localize pain, attempting to remove noxious stimuli when motor function is tested. He is not able to follow commands. He is able to vocalize but is confused. Verbal response is usually tested by asking the client to state who he is, where he is, or what day it is.

   NP:E; CN:PH; CL:C

6. (3) An unconscious person is unable to independently maintain a clear airway; therefore, the highest priority should be given to planning and providing nursing interventions that promote effective airway clearance. The other nursing diagnoses are of lower priority.

   NP:AN; CN:PH; CL:AN

7. (4) The state or level of consciousness is the most reliable index of cerebral status.

   NP:A; CN:PH; CL:C

8. (3) Decorticate posturing results from lesions of the corticospinal tracts within or near to the cerebral hemispheres. When assessing decortication, the nurse observes adduction of the upper arms with the elbows, wrists, and fingers flexed. The legs are extended and internally rotated. Plantar flexion of the feet is also noted.

   NP:A; CN:PH; CL:C

9. (3) Elevating the head promotes reduction of cerebral edema through gravity drainage. Coughing increases intracranial pressure. The environment should be nonstimulating (dim lights and quiet) to limit the risk of seizures. Fluids are restricted to avoid increasing the cerebral edema.

   NP:I; CN:PH; CL:A

10. (2) Preventing cerebral trauma during the convulsion is a priority activity. Placing some form of padding under the head will protect the skull and brain from injury. Inserting a mouth gag (1) and restraining the limbs (3) are unsafe interventions. The nurse would not leave a seizing person to go and obtain equipment (4).

    NP:I; CN:PH; CL:A

11. (4) Hemorrhage or blood in the CSF, within the brain, ventricles, or subarachnoid space, is irritating to the meninges and causes headache and nuchal rigidity.

    NP:A; CN:PH; CL:AN

Coding for Questions/Answers Abbreviations: **Nursing Process: NP,** Assessment: A, Analysis: AN, Planning: P, Implementation: I, Evaluation: E; **Client Needs: CN,** Safe, Effective Care Environment: S, Health Promotion and Maintenance: H, Psychosocial Integrity: PS, Physiological Integrity: PH; **Clinical Area: CA,** Medical Nursing: M, Surgical Nursing: S, Maternal/Newborn Nursing: MA, Pediatric Nursing: P, Psychiatric Nursing: PS; **Cognitive Level: CL,** Knowledge: K, Comprehension: C, Application: A, Analysis: AN.

12. (3) The client's complaints are consistent with meningeal irritation from bleeding into the subarachnoid space; therefore, she needs immediate transfer to an acute care setting.

NP:I; CN:H; CL:AN

13. (4) Laceration, a more severe consequence of closed head injury, occurs as the brain tissue moves across the uneven base of the skull in a contusion. Contusion causes cerebral dysfunction, which results in bruising of the brain. A concussion causes transient loss of consciousness and retrograde amnesia, and is generally reversible.

NP:AN; CN:PH; CL:C

14. (3) Epidural hematomas usually form quickly within 6 hours after injury, as a result of an arterial bleed. They usually cause periods of confusion and lucidity, and may or may not cause loss of consciousness. Epidural hematomas are fatal if left untreated; subdural hematomas—not epidural hematomas—have the highest mortality of all head injuries.

NP:A; CN:PH; CL:AN

15. (2) The halo or "bull's-eye" sign seen when drainage from the nose or ear of a head-injured client is collected on a sterile gauze is indicative of CSF in the drainage. The collection of a culture specimen (1) using any type of swab or suction would be contraindicated because brain tissue may be inadvertently removed at the same time or other tissue damage may result.

NP:I; CN:PH; CL:AN

16. (4) Nervous control for the diaphragm (phrenic nerve) exists at C3 or C4. Quadriplegia involves cervical injuries at C1–C8.

NP:AN; CN:PH; CL:C

17. (2) The purpose of the tongs is to decompress the vertebral column through hyperextending it. Both (1) and (3) are incorrect because they might cause further damage. (4) is incorrect because the client cannot sit up with the tongs in place; only the head of the bed can be elevated.

NP:AN; CN:PH; CL:K

18. (3) Blood pressure can become dangerously elevated during an episode of dysreflexia and can cause cerebral and retinal hemorrhages. Elevating the head will help prevent these complications and should be the nurse's first action. Identifying the precipitant (1) is useful in terminating the episode by removing the noxious stimulus that provoked the exaggerated autonomic response. A full bladder may precipitate dysreflexia, and emptying the bladder (4) would be appropriate if it was the precipitant. The blood pressure and pulse (2) should be monitored throughout the episode of dysreflexia.

NP:I; CN:PH; CL:AN

19. (4) Clients with MS do not usually have difficulty swallowing; therefore, techniques to promote safe swallowing would not be included on a care plan. The three other responses are important aspects in client care and should be included in the care plan.

NP:P; CN:PH; CL:C

20. (1) The client cannot handle his own secretions, and respiratory arrest may be imminent. Atropine may be administered to prevent crisis. Anticholinergic drugs are administered to increase the levels of acetylcholine at the myoneural junction. Cholinergic drugs (2) mimic the actions of the parasympathetic nervous system and would not be used.

NP:P; CN:PH; CL:A

21. (1) The hypothalamus controls body temperature, fluid balance, particular emotions (such as pleasure and fear), sleep, and appetite. The visual area (3) is controlled by the occipital lobe. The temporal lobe contains the auditory center (4). Bradycardia (2) can be caused by a problem in the medulla oblongata.

NP:A; CN:PH; CL:A

22. (2) Romberg's test is the ability to maintain an upright position without swaying when standing with feet close together and eyes closed. Kernig's sign (1), a reflex contraction, is pain in the hamstring muscle when attempting to extend the leg after flexing the thigh.

NP:P; CN:PH; CL:C

23. (1) The increase in intraocular pressure causes atrophy of the retinal ganglion cells and the optic nerve, and leads eventually to blindness.

NP:I; CN:PH; CL:C

24. (4) Without a lens, the eye cannot accommodate. It is difficult to judge distance and climb stairs when the eyes cannot accommodate. Therefore, the client should walk up and down stairs only with assistance.

NP:I; CN:PH; CL:A

25. (1) Mydriatic drugs are used preoperatively so that the pupil is widely dilated. Either atropine sulfate or epinephrine HCl is commonly used. Pilocarpine (3) and carbamylcholine (2) are miotics used for glaucoma and certain types of lens implants. Timolol maleate (4) is a beta blocker used for glaucoma.

NP:P; CN:PH; CL:C

CARDIOVASCULAR SYSTEM

The heart and the circulatory system, both systemic and pulmonary, constitute one of the most essential parts of the body; failure to function results in death of the organism. The heart is a hollow muscular organ that, by contracting rhythmically, effectively pumps the blood through the circulatory system to nourish all of the body tissues.

ANATOMY

Gross Structure of the Heart

Layers

A. Pericardium—protective covering.
   1. Fibrous pericardium—fibrous sac.
   2. Serous pericardium—allows for free cardiac motion.
B. Epicardium—covers surface of heart, extends onto great vessels, and becomes continuous with inner lining of pericardium.
C. Myocardium—muscular portion of heart that pumps blood and is responsible for the contractile force of the heart.
D. Endocardium—thin, delicate layer of tissue that lines cardiac chambers and covers surface of heart valves.

Chambers of the Heart

Definition: The heart is a four-chambered muscular organ. It is divided by a thick, muscular wall into right and left halves. Each half is divided into upper and lower chambers; upper chambers are called atria and lower chambers are called ventricles.

✦ A. Right atrium (RA)—(receiving chamber) is a thin-walled, distensible, low-pressure collecting chamber that receives deoxygenated bood from the systemic venous system and sends most blood to right ventricle during ventricular diastole or filling. The venous blood remaining in right atrium is propelled forward into right ventricle during atrial systole or contraction.
   1. Inlets: superior vena cava, inferior vena cava, coronary sinus, thebesian veins.
   2. Outlet: tricuspid valve.
B. Right ventricle (RV)—(ejecting chamber) is a thin-walled, low-pressure crescent-shaped pump for propelling blood into the low-resistance pulmonary circuit.

   1. Normal thickness: 0.5 cm.
   2. Inlet: right atrium, tricuspid valve.
   3. Outlet: pulmonic valve into pulmonary artery.
   4. Generates pressure of 25 mm Hg, which is enough to close tricuspid valve and open pulmonic valve—propelling blood into pulmonary artery and lungs.
   5. Work load of right ventricle is less than that of left ventricle because pulmonary system is normally low pressure; therefore there is less resistance to blood flow.
C. Left atrium (LA)—(receiving chamber) is a thin-walled, medium-pressure collecting chamber that receives oxygenated blood from the pulmonary venous system.
   1. Inlets: four pulmonary veins.
   2. Outlet: mitral valve.
D. Left ventricle (LV)—(ejecting chamber) is a thick-walled, high-pressure, cone-shaped pump for propelling blood into the high-resistance systemic circuit.
   1. Normal thickness: 1.5 cm (about 2–3 times the thickness of the right ventricle).
   2. Inlet: left atrium, mitral valve.
   3. Outlet: aortic valve into aorta.
   4. Must generate a higher pressure than right ventricle because it is contracting against the high-pressure systemic circulation where there is a much greater resistance to blood flow.

Valves

Definition: Valves are strong membranous openings responsible for maintaining the forward flow of blood through the chamber. These valves open and close passively in response to pressure and volume changes within chambers of the heart.

✦ A. Atrioventricular valves prevent backflow of blood from the ventricles to the atria during systole.
   1. Tricuspid—right heart valve; between right atrium and right ventricle.
      a. Three cusps or leaflets.
      b. Open during ventricular diastole.
      c. Free edges anchored to papillary muscles in right ventricle by chordae tendineae, which contract when the ventricular walls contract (systole).
   2. Mitral—left heart valve; between left atrium and left ventricle.
      a. Two cusps or leaflets.
      b. Open during ventricular diastole.
      c. Free edges anchored to papillary muscles in left ventricle by chordae tendineae, which contract when the ventricular walls contract (systole).

✦ B. Semilunar valves prevent backflow from the aorta and pulmonary artery into the ventricles during diastole.
  1. Pulmonic—three cusps or leaflets; opens from the right ventricle into the pulmonary artery.
  2. Aortic—three cusps or leaflets; opens from the left ventricle into the aorta; orifices for coronary arteries arise from wall of aorta above two of the three cusps.
C. Valves function passively.
  1. Close when backward pressure pushes blood backward.
  2. Open when forward pressure forces blood in a forward direction.

Conduction System

Definition: Conduction system is composed of specialized tissue that allows rapid transmission of electrical impulses through the myocardium.

✦ A. Sinoatrial (SA) node—main pacemaker of heart in which normal rhythmic self-excitatory impulse is generated.
  1. Located at the junction of right atrium and superior vena cava.
  2. Activates myocardial cells, initiates process of depolarization.
  3. 60–100 electrical impulses/min.
  4. External control is through autonomic nervous system.
    a. Sympathetic—increases rate.
    b. Parasympathetic—slows rate.
  5. Nerves affect cardiac pumping in two ways.
    a. Change heart rate.
    b. Change strength of contraction of the heart.
  6. Intrinsic automaticity—initiates electrical impulses automatically.
B. Internodal tracts—transmission of electrical impulses through atria from sinoatrial node to atrioventricular node.
C. Atrioventricular (AV) node—contains delay tissue that delays impulse transmission, allowing atrial contraction to eject blood into ventricle before ventricular contraction ("atrial kick").
D. Bundle of His.
  1. Conducts electrical impulse from AV node into ventricles.
  2. Divides into right bundle branch and left bundle branch.
E. Purkinji fibers—conduct electrical impulse from right and left bundle branches to all parts of the ventricles.

Coronary Blood Supply

Definition: Oxygen and other nutrients are supplied to cells of heart by vessels of the coronary circulation. Coro-

nary circulation consists of coronary arteries and coronary veins. Coronary artery blood flow to the myocardium occurs primarily during diastole, when coronary vascular resistance is lower. To maintain adequate blood supply through coronary arteries to nourish the myocardium, mean arterial pressure (MAP) must be at least 60 mm Hg. A MAP between 60 and 70 mm Hg is necessary to maintain vital body organs (i.e., brain and kidneys).

A. Coronary arteries—transport oxygen-rich blood from the heart, under high pressure, to the body tissues.
  1. Right coronary artery (RCA)—in most people supplies
    a. Atrioventricular (AV) node.
    b. Right ventricle.
    c. Inferior and posterior walls of left ventricle.
  2. Posterior descending coronary artery (PDA) supplies posterior wall of left ventricle.
  3. Left coronary artery—left main (LM) and left anterior descending (LAD) supply
    a. Intraventricular septum.
    b. Bundle branches.
    c. Anterior wall and apex of left ventricle.
  4. Left circumflex coronary artery (LCX) supplies
    a. Left atrium.
    b. Lateral and posterior surfaces of left ventricle.
    c. Sometimes portions of intraventricular septum.
    d. SA node in about 45 percent of people.
    e. AV node in about 10 percent of people.
    f. Peripheral branches arise from both LCX and LAD and form a network of vessels throughout myocardium.
✦ B. Veins—generally parallel arterial system.
  1. Coronary sinus veins empty into right atrium.
  2. Thebesian veins empty into right atrium.

Gross Structure of Vasculature

Arteries

A. The function of the arteries is to transport blood under high pressure to the body tissues.
  1. Arteries have thick, elastic walls.
  2. Move blood forward through the circulatory system.
B. Arterioles.
  1. Small arteries with little elastic tissue and more smooth muscle.
  2. Serve as major control of blood pressure and flow.
  3. Respond to O_2 and CO_2 levels by constricting or dilating.

Capillaries

Definition: Microcirculation between arterioles and venules. The exchange of fluid, cellular nutrients, and metabolic waste products takes place through thin-walled vessels.

A. Capillary walls are thin and permeable to fluid and small substances.

B. Blood flow is slowest in capillaries.

Veins

✦ *Definition:* Primary function is to act as conduits for transport of the blood from tissues back to the heart.

A. Venous system.
   1. Low-pressure, high-volume system.
   2. Walls are thin but muscular.
   3. Walls are able to contract or expand, thereby storing a small or large amount of blood.
   4. Larger veins have valves to maintain forward blood flow and prevent backflow.

✦ B. Factors influencing venous return.
   1. Muscle contraction (e.g., walking, leg exercises).
   2. Gravity (e.g., elevating legs).
   3. Competent valves.
   4. Respiration.
      a. Inspiration increases venous return.
      b. Expiration decreases venous return.
   5. Compliancy of right heart (CVP).

C. Venules: small vessels made up of muscle and connective tissue. Collect blood from capillary beds and direct it to larger veins.

PHYSIOLOGY

Regulation of Cardiac Function

Contraction

✦ *Definition:* The heart muscle utilizes chemical energy to do the work of contraction—a shortening or increase in tension.

A. The sarcomere is the unit of contraction and contains the proteins actin and myosin.

B. Sliding theory of contraction.
   1. Actin slides inward on myosin causing shortening of sarcomere, resulting in systole.
   2. When calcium is used up, actin and myosin slide apart, resulting in systole.

C. Each cardiac cell is composed of many sarcomeres.

Cardiac Muscle Principles

✦ A. Frank–Starling law: the greater the heart is filled during diastole, within physiological limits, the greater the quantity of blood pumped into the aorta and pulmonary artery.
   1. The heart can pump a large amount of blood or a small amount depending on the amount that flows into it from the veins.
   2. It automatically adapts to whatever the load or volume may be (within physiological limits of the total amount the heart can pump).

B. All-or-none principle: cardiac muscle either contracts or does not contract when stimulated.

C. Two phases of contractility.
   1. Isometric—increasing tension while maintaining length of muscle fiber.
   2. Isotonic—shortening muscle fiber while tension remains constant.

D. Cardiac output—the amount of blood pumped out by the heart in one minute.
   1. Calculation: CO = SV (stroke volume) × HR (heart rate).
      a. Cardiac output is 4–7 L/min.
      b. Varies according to body size; cardiac index is used to adjust for differences in body size.
   2. Stroke volume—amount of blood ejected from the ventricle with each contraction.
   3. Factors affecting cardiac output.
      a. Heart rate.
      b. Stroke volume.
         (1) Preload—volume of blood in the ventricles before contraction.
         (2) Afterload—peripheral vascular resistance that the left ventricle must pump against.
         (3) Contractility.

E. Cardiac reserve—ability of heart to respond to increased demands by increasing cardiac output. CO is increased by increasing heart rate or increasing stroke volume, by increasing either preload or contractility. Increased demands on cardiovascular system may be due to many conditions, such as exercise, stress, hypovolemia, etc.

Properties of Cardiac Cells

✦ A. Automaticity: ability to initiate an electrical impulse without external stimuli; spontaneously and repetitively.
   1. Although all cells of the heart can initiate an electrical impulse, certain areas of the heart will initiate impulses within the following ranges:
      a. SA node: 60–100.
      b. Junctional node: 40–60.
      c. Bundle branch Purkinje system: 20–40.
   2. Causes depolarization and repolarization.

✦ B. Conductivity: ability to transmit electrical impulse.

✦ C. Contractility: ability of muscle to shorten in response to electrical impulse.

✦ D. Excitability: ability to be stimulated by an impulse (depolarization).

✦ E. Refractoriness: inability to respond to a stimulus until the cells return to a resting state (repolarized).

1. Absolute refractory period—no amount of electrical stimulation will cause contraction.
2. Relative refractory period—strong enough electrical stimulation will cause contraction.

F. Electrical and mechanical properties determine system function.

Pulse

Definition: The rhythmic dilation of an artery caused by the contraction of the heart.

A. Number of times the "ventricles" contract.
B. Rate—extrinsically controlled by the ANS, which adjusts rapidly to regulate CO.
C. Increased heart rate = increased myocardial O_2 demand.
D. Pulse deficit—difference between apical and radial pulse, due to weakened or ineffective contraction of heart.
E. Pulse pressure—difference between systolic and diastolic pressure.

Blood Pressure

A. A measure of pressure exerted on walls of arterial systems.
   1. Systolic BP is the maximum amount of pressure exerted on walls of arterial system when heart contracts.
   2. Diastolic BP is pressure within arterial system following contraction during "relaxation" phase.
B. Factors influencing blood pressure.
   1. CO (cardiac output).
   2. SVR (systemic vascular resistance—resistance created in the small arteries and arterioles).
   3. Volume of fluid: hypovolemia (decreased blood pressure) such as hemorrhage.
   4. Diameter and elasticity of blood vessels; for example, arteriosclerosis (increased blood pressure).

Autonomic Nervous System Influence

Cardiac Muscle

A. Sympathetic nervous system (adrenergic)—innervates all cardiac muscle.
   1. Secretes epinephrine and norepinephrine.
   2. Response stimulates beta$_1$ receptors.
      a. Increases SA node rate of discharge.
      b. Increases conductivity.
      c. Increases contractility of cardiac muscle.
      d. Increases cell irritability.
B. Parasympathetic nervous system (cholinergic)—innervates primarily atrial tissue.
   1. Mediated via vagus nerve.
   2. Secretes acetylcholine.
   3. Maintenance of homeostasis—"brake of heart."
      a. Decreases SA node rate of discharge.

   b. Decreases conductivity, especially of AV node.
   c. Decreases atrial contractility.

Systemic Blood Vessels

A. Sympathetic nervous system.
   1. Vasoconstriction of blood vessels through action mainly on alpha$_1$ receptors of precapillary sphincter (one exception: vasodilation of coronary arteries).
   2. Causes vasodilation of selected blood vessels via beta$_2$ receptor stimulation.
B. Parasympathetic nervous system.
   1. Usually predominates so that blood vessels are not vasoconstricted.
   2. Effect is vasodilation in certain areas such as cerebrum, salivary glands, and lower colon.

Baroreceptor Reflex

A. Most important circulatory reflex is called baroreceptor reflex.
   1. Initiated by baroreceptors (also called pressoreceptors) located in arch of the aorta and at beginning of internal carotid arteries.
   2. Rise in pressure results in baroreceptors transmitting signals to CNS to inhibit sympathetic action.
   3. Other signals, in turn, sent to circulatory system reduce pressure back toward normal.
   4. Result is decreased heart rate, vasodilation and decreased blood pressure.
B. Effect of decreased pressure on baroreceptors.
   1. Sympathetic stimulation overrides vagal response.
   2. Result is increased heart rate, vasoconstriction and increased blood pressure.

Other Chemical Controls of Blood Pressure

A. Kidney.
   1. Juxtaglomerular apparatus releases renin, which causes vasoconstriction to increase blood pressure.
   2. Adrenal cortex releases aldosterone, causing sodium and water to be reabsorbed. This increases blood volume and blood pressure.
B. Antidiuretic hormone (vasopressin)—acts on kidney tubules to reabsorb water, thereby increasing blood volume and blood pressure.
C. Histamine release from mast cells' response to antigen.
   1. Arterioles dilate.
   2. Venules constrict.
D. Capillary fluid shift mechanisms (balance of hydrostatic/oncotic forces); for example, decreased blood pressure or an increase in oncotic pressure allows capillaries to reabsorb interstitial fluid.

System Assessment

✦ A. Assess client's cardiac history.
  ✦ 1. Pain—onset, character, location, radiation, duration, intensity, precipitating or aggravating factors, relieving factors, and intensity/severity on a scale of 0–10.
    a. Ischemic pain of angina.
      (1) Substernal, neck, jaw, arms/shoulders; vague pressure, radiates; confused with "indigestion."
      (2) Precipitated by emotional or physical activity, relieved by rest or nitroglycerin.
    b. Pain of myocardial infarction.
      (1) Similar location of angina, more intense.
      (2) Accompanied by dyspnea, diaphoresis, nausea/vomiting; not precipitated.
      (3) Not relieved by rest or nitroglycerin.
  ✦ 2. Dyspnea—subjective feeling of inability to get enough air.
    a. Exertional dyspnea (DOE) occurs with activity.
    b. Orthopnea occurs while in a reclining position—client sits up or uses several pillows to sleep.
    c. Paroxysmal nocturnal dyspnea (PND) interrupts client's sleep—gets up to relieve.
  ✦ 3. Respiratory rate and depth.
    a. Tachypnea: increase in rate of breathing.
    b. Hyperpnea: increase in depth of breathing (causes decrease in PCO_2).
  4. Cough—dry or productive of mucoid foamy sputum with heart failure; pink tinged with acute pulmonary edema.
  5. Cyanosis—bluish mucous membranes or skin color due to significant deficiency of oxygen in the blood (O_2 saturation less than 85 percent).
  6. Fatigue—result of decreased cardiac output.
  7. Palpitations—awareness of rapid or irregular heartbeat.
  8. Syncope—transient loss of consciousness due to inadequate cerebral blood flow (e.g., bradycardia).
  ✦ 9. Edema.
    a. Bilateral, dependent (ankles or sacrum) due to accumulation of interstitial fluid secondary to increased venous pressure (e.g., volume overload)—accompanied by weight gain.
    b. Unilateral due to venous insufficiency.
  10. Skin—color, temperature, dry or moist, hair growth, nails, capillary refill.
B. Evaluate pressure through inspection and palpation of venous and arterial systems.

CONSIDER GERIATRIC STATUS

- Valves: thicker and stiffer.
- SA node: decreased number of pacemaker cells.
- Sympathetic nerve system.
  a. Decreased response to physical stress (e.g., exercise).
  b. Decreased response to psychological stress.
  c. Less sensitive to beta-adrenergic agonist drugs.
- Arterial bood vessels: thicker, with decreased elasticity, resulting in elevated blood pressure.

---

1. Internal jugular veins—located deep in sternocleidomastoid muscle.
2. Venous pulsations.
   a. Observe venous pulsation in neck to assess central venous pressure (CVP) and adequacy of circulating blood volume.
   b. Assessment of jugular venous pressure (JVP) done to estimate volume and pressure on right side of heart. Increased JVP causes increased jugular vein distention.
   c. Normal JVP 3–10 cm H_2O. Increase caused by
      (1) Right ventricular failure.
      (2) Tricuspid stenosis or regurgitation.
      (3) Pulmonary hypertension.
      (4) Cardiac tamponade.
      (5) Constrictive pericarditis.
      (6) Hypervolemia.
      (7) Superior vena cava obstruction.
3. Arterial system.
   a. Neck—carotid artery.
   b. Upper extremities—radial, brachial, and ulnar.
   c. Lower extremities—femoral, popliteal, posterior tibial, dorsalis pedis, pedal.
4. Grading peripheral pulses.
   a. 0 = absent.
   b. 1+ = weak.
   c. 2+ = diminished.
   d. 3+ = strong.
   e. 4+ = full/bounding.
5. Pulsus paradoxus: systolic blood pressure drop greater than 10 mm Hg during inspiration (cardiac tamponade).
✦ C. Assess heart sounds by auscultation.
   1. Auscultatory areas.
      a. Aortic: second intercostal space right of sternum.
      b. Pulmonic: second intercostal space left of sternum.
      c. Tricuspid: fifth intercostal space left, close to sternum.

d. Mitral: fifth intercostal space mid-clavicular line at the apex of the heart.

e. PMI: point of maximal impulse.

✦ 2. Heart sounds—frequency, pitch, intensity, duration.

a. S_1—("lub") closure of mitral and tricuspid valve.

b. S_2—("dub") closure of aortic and pulmonic valve.

c. S_3 and S_4—diastolic filling sounds.

(1) S_3—rapid filling of ventricle in early diastole; heard after S_2; sign of heart failure in client over age 40.

(2) S_4—coincides with atrial contraction due to poorly compliant ventricle; prior to S_1; normal in older adult.

✦ 3. Murmurs: turbulence of blood flow through valve; classified by their timing and heard between heart sounds.

a. Systolic: occurring between S_1 and S_2.

(1) Mitral and tricuspid insufficiency.

(2) Aortic and pulmonic stenosis.

(3) Patent foramen ovale.

(4) Ventricular septal defect.

b. Diastolic: occurring between S_2 and S_1.

(1) Mitral and tricuspid stenosis.

(2) Aortic and pulmonic insufficiency.

c. Location: point where murmur is loudest.

d. Radiation: transmission from point of maximal intensity to surrounding areas.

e. Quality: blowing, harsh, musical, or rumbling.

f. Pitch: high, medium, or low.

g. Pattern: determined by intensity over time.

(1) Crescendo: soft to loud.

(2) Decrescendo: loud to soft.

(3) Crescendo–decrescendo: soft to loud to soft.

(4) Plateau: same throughout.

h. Intensity (loudness): Grade 1–6.

(1) Grade 1 = barely audible through stethoscope.

(2) Grade 6 = audible with the stethoscope just off the client's skin.

4. Pericardial friction rub due to inflammation—"squeak" timed with heart sounds.

D. Evaluate arterial pressure.

✦ 1. Measurement of blood pressure—indirect via cuff.

a. Both arms.

b. Lying, standing.

2. Presence of bruits (sound of abnormal turbulence of blood flow usually around obstruction).

E. Evaluate chest x-ray to determine abnormalities of lung fluids and cardiac silhouette.

F. Assess lungs for adventitious sounds.

1. Rales: fine, medium, coarse.

2. Rhonchi: sibilant, sonorous.

G. Assess client's readiness for a cardiac rehabilitation program.

DIAGNOSTIC PROCEDURES

Chest X-ray

A. Silhouette of heart, chambers and great vessels observed on routine chest x-ray.

B. Pulmonary vascular congestion seen when there is increased left heart pressure.

C. Enlarged heart seen with dilation/hypertrophy.

12-Lead Electrocardiography

A. An electrocardiogram (ECG or EKG) is a surface record of the electrical activity of the heart.

B. Purpose: to determine areas of myocardial ischemia, injury or necrosis, cardiac irregularities, and electrolyte imbalances. (*See* Figures 8-1 through 8-9.)

1. Noninvasive.

2. Limited to resting state of heart function.

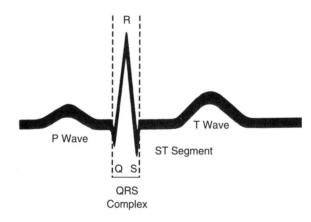

FIGURE 8-1. ECG pattern.

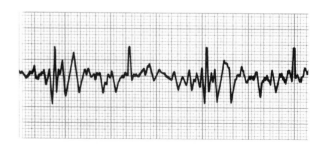

✦ FIGURE 8-2. ECG pattern showing artifact.

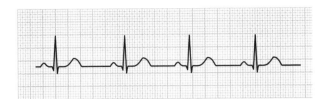

✦ **FIGURE 8-3.** Sinus bradycardia.

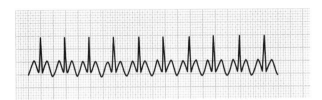

✦ **FIGURE 8-4.** Atrial flutter.

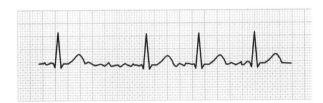

✦ **FIGURE 8-5.** Atrial fibrillation.

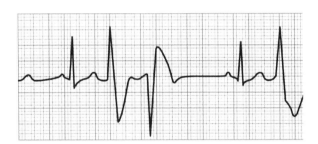

✦ **FIGURE 8-6.** Multifocal PVCs.

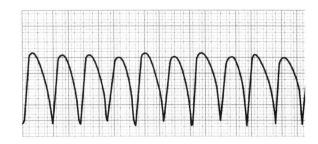

✦ **FIGURE 8-7.** Ventricular tachycardia.

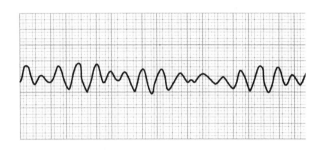

✦ **FIGURE 8-8.** Ventricular fibrillation.

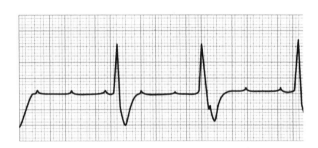

✦ **FIGURE 8-9.** Third-degree heart block.

C. ECG components.
   ✦ 1. Normal cardiac cycle.
      a. P wave—atrial depolarization.
      b. P-R interval—conduction through the electrical system, SA node, AV node, and His–Purkinje system.
      c. QRS wave—ventricular depolarization.
      d. ST segment—early ventricular repolarization.
      e. T wave—rapid ventricular repolarization.
   ✦ 2. Interpretation of ECG.
      a. Determine heart rate by calculating atrial rate (P-P interval) and ventricular rate (R-R interval). Normal 60 to 100—one P wave for each QRS complex.
      b. Determine regularity of rhythm (atrial and ventricular).
      c. Measure P-R interval to determine conduction time through electrical system (0.12 to 0.20 second).
      d. Measure QRS duration to determine ventricular conduction time (0.04 to 0.10 second).
      e. Measure Q-T interval—represents ventricular systole. Duration varies with heart rate.
      f. Note configuration and relation of P waves to QRS. Note for ST-segment depression or elevation, T-wave inversion.
   ✦ 3. Etiology of arrhythmias.
      a. Ischemia, electrolyte imbalance, acid–base imbalance, hypoxia, myocardial stretch, sympathetic stimulation, antiarrhythmic agents.

b. Precipitating or contributing disease states—heart failure, coronary artery disease, myocardial infarction, congenital or acquired heart disease, hyperthyroidism.

Echocardiography

A. Noninvasive cardiac procedure that records sound vibrations and reflects mechanical cardiac activity.
B. Used to detect valvular/structural anomalies, ventricular wall thickness, decreased (hypokinesis) or absent (akinesis) wall movement, ventricular ejection fraction, intramural thromboses.
C. May demonstrate exercise-induced ventricular wall motion abnormalities when performed during exercise (or pharmacologic-induced stress).
D. Transesophageal (TEE): as probe passes through esophagus, strictures can be viewed without interference from lungs or ribs.

Exercise Electrocardiography (Treadmill)

A. Noninvasive electrocardiography procedure for evaluating myocardial response to increased demands (exercise).
B. Treadmill or bicycle used.
C. Monitor vital signs and ECG for ischemic changes.
D. Clients with positive test may be referred for cardiac catheterization and/or coronary arteriography.
E. Test often combined with scintigraphic studies or echocardiography.

Ambulatory Electrocardiographic Monitoring

A. Records ECG for 24–48 hours.
B. Identifies episodes of ischemic ST-segment depression, rhythm changes, and/or correlation with symptoms.
C. Silent (asymptomatic) episodes recorded.

Scintigraphic (Nuclear Medicine) Studies

A. Involves IV injection of radioactive isotopes; thallium-201 or technetium-99 sestamibi; myocardial uptake is proportionate to blood flow.

B. Special camera scans heart to identify areas of diminished uptake reflecting region of hypoperfusion.
C. When combined with exercise, or pharmacologic vasodilation, region of hypoperfusion may represent ischemia or scar, and may then perfuse at rest indicating reversible ischemia.
D. Technetium-99m pyrophosphate is taken up by an area of myocardial infarction and produces a "hot spot."
E. Positron emission tomography (PET)—two radionuclides are used: one evaluates myocardial perfusion; second shows myocardial metabolic function. In a normal heart, scans match; differences indicate ischemic or myocardial injury.

Cardiac Magnetic Resonance Imaging (MRI)

A. Provides high-resolution images of heart and great vessels without radiation exposure or use of iodinated contrast media.
B. Demonstrates pericardial disease, myocardial thickness, chamber size/defects, aneurysms.

Cardiac Catheterization/Coronary Angiography

A. Invasive angiography procedure in which a catheter is passed into the heart and its major vessels for examination of blood flow, pressures in chambers and vessels, and oxygen content and saturation. The catheter may be passed through the arterial system into the left side of the heart or through the venous system into the right side of the heart.
B. Radiopaque compound is injected into heart chambers and coronary vessels for selective arteriography.
   1. Evaluates blood flow through chambers.
   2. Demonstrates anatomy of coronary circulation.
   3. Reveals coronary occlusive disease.
C. Obtain baseline data prior to test.
   1. History of allergy, especially shellfish, iodine, or drugs.
   2. Serum BUN and creatinine for renal function.
   3. Obtain baseline vital signs.
   4. Check coagulation studies.
   5. Mark peripheral pulses bilaterally.

IMPORTANT CARDIAC EFFECTS OF ELECTROLYTES			
Electrolytes	Normal Value	Decreased (Hypo)	Increased (Hyper)
K (potassium)	3.5–5.0	Flat T waves, ST depression U wave, ventricular dysrhythmia	Peaked T waves, wide QRS ↑ PR interval, asytole
Mg (magnesium)	1.3–2.1	↑Ventricular dysrhythmia	
Ca (calcium)	9.0–10.3	↑ QT interval ↓ Inotropic effect	↓ QT interval ↑ Inotropic effect

D. Nursing responsibilities prior to procedure.
1. Be sure consent form is signed.
2. Assess client/family understanding of the procedure.
3. Reinforce physician's explanation.
4. Describe cath lab and equipment or show video.
5. Provide techniques to decrease anxiety and fear.
6. Keep NPO 8 hours or as ordered.
7. Administer pretest medications.

E. Post-procedure responsibilities.
1. Compare data with baseline data obtained prior to procedure.
2. Notify physician if blood pressure (taken every 15 minutes for 1 hour, then every 30 minutes for 2 hours) is decreased by 10 percent from baseline.
3. Take apical pulse for 1 full minute to determine if arrhythmia is present.
4. Monitor urine output.
5. Encourage increased PO fluid intake to flush system (contrast dye is nephrotoxic).
6. Keep on bedrest in supine position with leg straight for prescribed time.
7. Maintain hemostasis at access site by pressure (e.g., sandbag) for several hours.
8. Check puncture site frequently for bleeding, swelling, hematoma.
9. Observe for allergy to dye.
   a. Tachycardia.
   b Nausea and vomiting.
   c. Shortness of breath.
   d. Rash
10. Palpate pulses distal to catheter insertion site to assess for perfusion.
   a. Palpable pulses—bilateral and strong (grade 0, 1+, 2+, 3+, 4+).
   b. Color—no cyanosis or pallor.
   c. Temperature of skin—warm.
   d. No pain.

F. Observe for complications.
1. Respiratory complications—hypoventilation, hypoxia, pulmonary edema.
2. Hypolemia due to osmotic diuresis.
3. Notify physician if peripheral pulse is lost or if pain, tingling or coolness occurs.
4. Arrhythmias or alterations of heart rate.
5. Cardiac tamponade—notify physician immediately.
6. Decreased urine production (< 30 mL/hr).

G. Discharge teaching.
1. Instruct client to
   a. Avoid strenuous activity as directed.
   b. Immediately report bleeding at insertion site, chest pain, shortness of breath, diffi-

culty breathing, tingling, numbness or change in color/temperature of extremities.
   c. Restrict lifting to < 10 lb for prescribed time.
2. Clients with stent placement will require anti-coagulation therapy for 6–8 weeks. Instruct client to
   a. Take medication at the same time each day.
   b. Follow up with laboratory tests as ordered to maintain therapeutic blood levels.
   c. Avoid activities that could cause bleeding.
   d. Follow lifestyle guidelines recommended: smoking cessation; weight management; low-fat, low-cholesterol diet; limit alcohol intake; exercise.

Hemodynamic Monitoring

A. Pulmonary artery catheter measures several parameters.
1. CVP 5–10 cm H_2O (same as right atrial pressure—RAP normal is 5 mm Hg).
2. Pulmonary artery pressure (PAP): normal is 20/10 mm Hg with mean of 15 mm Hg.
3. Pulmonary artery wedge pressure (PAWP): mean pressure 10 mm Hg.

B. Pulmonary artery catheter has 4–5 lumens.
1. Proximal lumen used to measure CVP and inject selected solutions.
2. Distal lumen used to measure PAWP.
3. Third lumen used for balloon inflation.
4. Fourth lumen used to measure cardiac output.

C. Prepare for insertion.
1. Prepare pressure (300 mm Hg) solution bag with heparin.
2. Balance zero transducer.
   a. Transducer must be at level of client's right atrium (fourth intercostal space).
   b. Continuously monitor client's ECG.
3. Assist physician to insert catheter.

D. Obtain PCWP pressure readings.
1 Expose distal port for PAWP.
2. Inject air into balloon port and leave in no longer than required to obtain wedge.
3. Observe waveform change—wedge pressure "A" depicts left atrial contraction and left ventricular relaxation, and "V" depicts left atrial relaxation and left ventricular contraction.

Central Venous Pressure (CVP) Monitoring

A. CVP is pressure within right atrium and reflects right ventricular function—indicates the right side of the heart's ability to manage fluid load.
1. CVP is a guide for fluid replacement.
2. It is a measure of circulating blood volume.

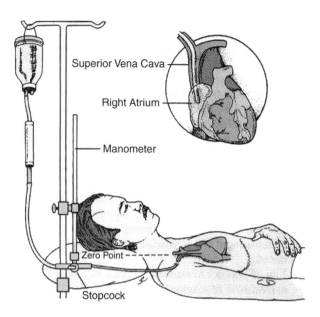

FIGURE 8-10. CVP reading: Manometer zero must be level with client's right atrium.

+ B. Changes in CVP correlate with client's clinical status.
    1. Elevated CVP can be late sign of left ventricular failure or hypervolemia.
    2. Lowered CVP indicates hypovolemia.
+ C. CVP measured by height of column of water in a manometer (*see* Figure 8-10).
    1. Measuring CVP is done by using zero mark on manometer as standard reference point.
    2. Transducer placed at phlebostatic axis.
    + 3. Normal CVP is 5–10 cm H_2O.

+ **System Implementation**

A. Monitor apical pulse for alterations in cardiac rhythm and rate.
B. Monitor for alterations in blood pressure.
C. Assess peripheral pulses to determine adequacy of circulation.
D. Monitor laboratory values for alterations in electrolytes, coagulation and cardiac enzymes to prevent complications.
E. Provide diet appropriate for client's need.
F. Provide emotional support for client and family when alterations in lifestyle are indicated.
G. Administer and instruct client on medications and their side effects.
H. Instruct client on preoperative and postoperative care modalities.
I. Monitor for complications following surgical intervention.
J. Plan an acceptable rehabilitation program with client and family.
K. Administer life support measures when client's condition is compromised.

CORONARY ARTERY DISEASE (CAD)

Coronary Atherosclerosis

+ *Definition:* The most common type of cardiovascular disease—occurs as the result of accumulation of fatty materials (lipids and, the primary one, cholesterol) and fibrous tissue, which narrow the lumen of coronary arteries. Clinical manifestations of disease reflect ischemia to the myocardium, resulting from inadequate blood supply to meet metabolic demands.

Characteristics
A. This form of heart disease originates from an abnormal accumulation of fatty substances and fibrous tissue.
B. Continued development of CAD involves an inflammatory response.
C. Deposits are formed on vessel walls called atheromas or plaque, which narrows vessel and obstructs blood flow.
D. Fibrous cap of plaque may be thick and stable or thin; if thin, it may rupture and form a thrombus.
E. The thrombus may obstruct blood flow and lead to sudden cardiac death or MI.

Assessment
+ A. Assess for presence of risk factors.
+ B. Evaluate chest pain.
    1. Angina, burning, squeezing, crushing tightness substernally or in precordal area. Pain may radiate to neck, jaw, shoulder, arms.
    2. Associated with nausea, vomiting, increased perspiration, and cool extremities.
+ C. Assess heart sounds for presence of arrhythmias and/or murmurs.

Implementation
+ A. Risk reduction (lifestyle modification).
    1. Engage in regular aerobic exercise.
    2. Reduce caloric intake if overweight.
    3. Refrain from smoking.
    4. Control hypertension, diabetes.
    5. Nutritional therapy: adhere to a diet that emphasizes a decrease in saturated fat and cholesterol.
        a. American Heart Association (AHA) Step 1 diet.
        b. For further restrictions of saturated fats and cholesterol, an AHA Step 2 diet is recommended.
        c. For elevated triglycerides, eliminate or reduce simple sugars and alcohol.
    6. Stress reduction.
B. Lipid-lowering agents.

C. Revascularization.
  1. Percutaneous transluminal coronary angioplasty (PTCA).
  2. Stent placement.
  3. Atherectomy.
  4. Laser angioplasty.
  5. Coronary artery bypass grafting (CABG).
D. In-hospital care.
  1. Monitor vital signs, particularly blood pressure and pulse.
  2. Evaluate ECG findings for changes of ischemia, injury, or necrosis.
  3. Administer nitrates if chest pain present.
  4. Evaluate chest pain—type, duration, radiation, relieved with medication.
  5. Monitor breath sounds and signs of peripheral edema to detect early complications.

Types of Angina

Stable Angina Pectoris

✦ *Definition:* Intermittent chest pain or discomfort due to the inability of coronary arteries to meet oxygen needs of myocardium. Angina is the result of ischemia caused by reversible cell injury.

Assessment

✦ A. Precipitating factors:
  1. Physical exertion.
  2. Emotional upset.
  3. Tachyarrhythmias.
  4. Extremes of temperature, especially cold.
  5. Smoking.
  6. Consumption of heavy meal.
  7. Sexual activity.
✦ B. Evaluate pain.
  1. Location: precordial, substernal.
  2. Character: compressing, choking, burning, squeezing, crushing heaviness.

  3. Radiation: arm or jaw, neck, back.
  4. Duration: usually 5–15 minutes, relieved by rest or nitroglycerin.
✦ C. Observe for signs of dyspnea, diaphoresis, unrelieved discomfort.
D. Assess ECG changes (may not be present at rest); ST-segment depression or elevation during pain.

Implementation

✦ A. Current approach to therapy is to decrease oxygen demand of myocardium—restrict activity.
B. Understand medication usage for stable angina.
  1. Action of nitroglycerin medication.
    a. Dilates coronary arteries that are not atherosclerotic to increase blood flow to myocardium.
    b. Lessens cardiac work by decreasing venous return—decreases peripheral vascular resistance.
  2. Beta blocker—reduces cardiac response to exertion and stress.
  3. ASA inhibits platelet activity.
  4. Morphine sulfate for relief of pain from myocardial ischemia.
  5. Side effects: hypotension, headache, bradycardia.
✦ 6. Instruct in use of sublingual nitroglycerin (tablets or metered-dose mouth spray).
    a. Usual recommended dosage: one tablet, may be repeated at 5-minute intervals until pain is relieved, up to 3 doses.
    b. If pain persists after 15 minutes, instruct client to seek immediate medical attention (call 911 where available).
    c. May be used prophylactically before engaging in activity known to precipitate angina.
    d. Take precautions for postural hypotension.
    e. Keep tablets in tightly closed, dark-glass bottle.
    f. Do not allow tablets to age—drug potency is 3–6 months.
    g. Wear Medic-Alert band and keep medication on person at all times.
✦ 7. Alternative: instruct client in use of nitroglycerin ointment/transdermal patch.
    a. Apply directly to skin.
    b. Remove patch and wash off remaining ointment before new application.
    c. Change skin placement with each application.
    d. Wear patch as directed by physician.
C. Provide client instruction.
  1. Learn to live in moderation; physical activity should be sufficient to maintain general physical state, but short of causing angina.
  2. Change in lifestyle.
    a. Avoid stress and emotional upset.

b. Engage in regular exercise.

c. Reduce caloric intake if overweight.

d. Refrain from smoking.

e. Avoid saturated fats and cholesterol.

f. Instruct client in use of medication.

✦ D. Other antianginal agents.

1. Beta blockers (propranolol, atenolol) reduce myocardial oxygen requirements during exertion and stress.

2. Calcium-entry blocking agents (verapamil, diltiazem) dilate coronary arteries, lower blood pressure, reduce heart rate—effective for vasospastic angina.

3. Platelet-inhibiting agents (low-dose aspirin or clopidogrel).

E. Myocardial revascularization (if medical management ineffective).

1. Percutaneous transluminal coronary angioplasty (PTCA).

2. Stent placement.

3. Atherectomy.

4. Laser angioplasty.

5. Coronary artery bypass grafting (CABG).

✦ **Unstable Angina**

Definition: Also called preinfarction angina—previously stable angina has new onset while at rest, lasts longer, is less responsive to medication. Signifies dynamic change in the vessel (a *supply* problem). Most clients have complex coronary stenoses with plaque rupture, ulceration, or hemorrhage with subsequent thrombus formation; may occur due to vasospasm.

Assessment

A. Unstable angina leads to myocardial infarction (MI).

1. ST-elevated MI (STEMI).

2. Non-ST-elevated MI (non-STEMI).

✦ B. ECG changes—transient ST-segment depression or T-wave flattening or inversion, or ST-segment elevation (vasospastic angina).

C. Serial ECG recordings ordered.

D. Presence of S_3 diastolic filling sound.

E. Serial cardiac enzyme determinations (troponin elevation may indicate small amount of myocardial damage).

✦ F. Unstable status may progress to complete occlusion and MI or may resolve and return to stable angina.

G. Noninvasive and invasive cardiac diagnostic procedures to identify diseased coronary artery.

✦ **Implementation**

A. Immediate medical intervention; bedrest, with cardiac and hemodynamic monitoring.

B. Heparin infusion (weight-based bolus, then infusion titrated to achieve activated partial thromboplastin time [APTT] ratio 1.5–2.3).

C. Platelet-inhibiting agents (ASA, clopidogrel).

D. Narcotic pain management (morphine sulfate).

E. Oxygen administration (2–4 L/min).

F. Nitroglycerine infusion (Tridil) titrated for pain relief (requires continuous blood pressure monitoring for hypotension).

1. Potent, concentrated drug; must be diluted in glass bottle of D_5W or sodium chloride 0.9 percent.

2. Given as a continuous infusion. Begin at 5 μg/min.

3. Increase by increments every 3–5 minutes, until the desired response occurs.

4. IV infusion pump is used to deliver continuous flow rate.

5. Closely monitor BP, PA, PCWP, HR, CO (cardiac output).

G. Administration of beta blockers.

H. Antiembolytic therapy.

I. Revascularization management (PTCA, CABG).

Myocardial Infarction

✦ *Definition:* The process by which cardiac muscle cells die due to insufficient blood supply (oxygen deprivation). Caused by vessel occlusion due to thrombus formation on ruptured or eroded coronary artery atheroma; coronary artery embolism or vasospasm; decreased blood volume with shock and/or hemorrhage; direct trauma.

Assessment

✦ A. Assess pain (history very important)—precipitating factors, interventions leading to relief, associated symptoms.

✦ B. Identify anxiety, feeling of doom.

✦ C. Note dyspnea, nausea, vomiting, and diaphoresis.

D. Low-grade temperature elevation after 24 hours.

E. Diagnostic findings.

1. History of ischemic type chest discomfort (very important).

✦ 2. Serial 12-lead ECGs to note evolutionary changes that reflect areas of involvement.

a. ST elevated (STEMI, acute injury).

b. ST-segment depression (subendocardial infarction).

c. Evolving abnormal Q waves (transmural infarction).

✦ 3. Serial cardiac enzymes lab tests. (*See* Chapter 11, Laboratory Tests.)

a. Elevated creatine kinase MB (CK-MB)—rises in 3–6 hours after onset of myocardial damage, peaks in 12–24 hours, returns to normal in 48–72 hours.

b. Myoglobin—protein found in cardiac and skeletal muscle. Sensitive and early indicator of myocardial infarction, occurring 1–2 hours following injury. Declines rapidly after approximately 7 hours.

c. Troponin—myocardial muscle protein released after injury.
(1) Troponin T—peaks in 12 hours; high specificity at 3–6 hours following onset of injury.
(2) Troponin I—rises in 4–6 hours (remains elevated 6 days).

4. Elevated WBCs and sedimentation rate.
5. Isotope scanning of myocardium.
6. Echocardiogram.

F. Infarction sites.
1. Transmural—entire thickness of myocardium involved—produces Q wave on reflecting ECG leads.
2. Subendocardial—death confined to inner layer of myocardium—produces non–Q wave MI.
3. Location: depends on which coronary artery is occluded.
a. Most MIs occur in left ventricle, with damage limited to area supplied by blocked vessel.
b. Left ventricular infarcts may be localized to anterior, septal, inferior, posterior, or lateral walls.
(1) RCA blockage = inferior wall infarcts.
(2) LAD blockage = anterior or antero-septal infarcts.

DIAGNOSTIC STUDIES FOR CARDIAC DISEASE*

Cardiac Enzymes	Rises	Peaks	Returns to Normal
CK-MB	4–6°	12–24°	48–72°
Troponin T	3–6°	12°	> 9 days
Troponin I	3–6°	12°	> 9 days
Myoglobin	30–60 min	6–10°	12–24°

	Normal	Moderate Risk	High Risk
C-reactive protein (CRP)	< 1 mg/L	< 1–3 mg/L	> 3 mg/L

	Optimal	Moderate Risk	High Risk
Homocystine	< 12 μmol/L	12–15 μmol/L	> 15 μmol/L

Congestive Heart Failure Marker	Normal
B-type natriuretic peptide (BNP)	< 100 pg/mL

*See cardiac enzymes tests in Chapter 11, Laboratory Tests.

Implementation

A. Immediate hospitalization for early diagnosis of acute myocardial injury by ECG, serial enzymes.

B. Pain management with sublingual nitroglycerine or intravenous narcotics (morphine sulfate).

C. Early reperfusion therapy by PTCA or thrombolysis (streptokinase, TPA, APSAC) to reduce infarction size.

D. Antiplatelet therapy.

E. Anticoagulant continuation therapy following reperfusion (heparin weight-based bolus, then infusion titrated to keep APTT ratio 1.5–2.3).

F. Coronary care unit continuous monitoring.
1. Physical and emotional rest.
2. Bedrest with bedside commode.
3. Liquid diet for 24 hours, then advanced.
4. Stool softeners to prevent constipation/Valsalva maneuver.
5. Beta blocker therapy (reduces reinfarction rate and sudden death).
6. ACE inhibitor if low ejection fraction (reduces mortality).
7. Lidocaine for frequent and complex PVCs, ventricular tachycardia.
8. Lipid-lowering agents (if appropriate).

G. Monitor for complications.
1. Arrhythmias.
2. Heart failure.
3. Cardiogenic shock.
4. Papillary muscle dysfunction (new murmur).
5. Pericarditis (friction rub).
6. Ventricular aneurysm/cardiac rupture.

H. Step down care with telemetry cardiac monitoring progressive ambulation.

I. Rehabilitation with progressive ambulation and client teaching about lifestyle modification, prudent (AHA) Step 2 diet, medications, etc.

VALVULAR DISEASE (MURMURS)

Mitral Stenosis

Definition: A progressive fibrous thickening and calcification of the valve cusps that results in the leaflets fusing and becoming stiff, causing narrowing of lumen of mitral valve.

Assessment

A. Evaluate history for congenital heart disease or rheumatic heart disease.

B. Assess for signs of decreased cardiac output. Asymptomatic until valve area is less than 1.5 cm² and tachycardia or atrial fibrillation occurs.

C. Assess for symptoms and signs of left, and then right, ventricular failure.

D. Auscultate heart sounds for diastolic murmur and opening snap crescendo and loud S_1 at apex.
E. Assess for complications.
  1. Atrial fibrillation.
  2. Subacute infective (bacterial) endocarditis.
  3. Thrombi formation.

Implementation

A. Treat heart failure and arrhythmias.
B. Decrease cardiac workload.
✦ C. Prevent and/or treat infections—prophylactic antibiotic therapy used to prevent recurrence of infection.
✦ D. Monitor administration of anticoagulants for treatment and/or prevention of thrombi/emboli in clients with atrial fibillation.
E. Provide emotional support to client.
F. Prepare client for plan if there is no calcification of valve or for surgical replacement of the mitral valve.

Mitral Insufficiency

✦ *Definition:* Congenital or acquired abnormality of the valve that prevents the mitral valve from closing completely during systole, allowing regurgitation (backflow) of blood from left ventricle to atrium.

Assessment

A. Assess for presence of cardiac disease associated with mitral insufficiency.
  1. Rheumatic heart disease.
  2. Congenital disease.
  3. Infective (bacterial) endocarditis.
  4. Rupture of chordae tendineae supporting structures.
  5. Rupture or dysfunction of papillary muscle.
  6. Dilatation of left ventricle.
  7. Decreased cardiac output (fatigue, weakness).
  8. Dyspnea on exertion.
  9. Orthopnea.
  10. Atrial fibillation.
B. Observe for evidence of heart failure.
✦ C. Auscultate at apex for decreased intensity of S_1; pansystolic murmur; S_3.
✦ D. Assess for palpable thrill.
✦ E. Evaluate for systemic emboli.

Implementation

Same as for *mitral stenosis.*

Mitral Valve Prolapse

Definition: Leaflets of the mitral valve enlarge and prolapse into left atrium during systole.

Assessment

A. Asymptomatic.

B. May experience chest pain, palpations, exercise intolerance.

Implementation

A. Benign abnormality.
B. Can progress to mitral regurgitation.

Aortic Valve Stenosis

✦ *Definition:* The narrowing of the aortic valve opening due to fibrosis and calcification. This results in increased afterload to the left ventricle.

Assessment

A. Assess history for predisposing conditions.
  1. Rheumatic heart disease. (Mitral valve commonly affected as well.)
  2. Arteriosclerosis.
  3. Congenital defect.
✦ B. Observe for dizziness and syncope with exertion.
C. Observe for symptoms of heart failure.
D. Auscultate for systolic murmur; faint S_2 at aortic area.
E. Assess for dyspnea, angina.

Implementation

A. Follow nursing care protocols for clients with heart failure.
B. Prepare client psychologically and physiologically for prosthetic valve replacement.

Aortic Insufficiency

✦ *Definition:* Allows blood to regurgitate (backflow) into left ventricle from the aorta. The left ventricle compensates and dilates to accommodate increased blood volume; leads to left ventricular hypertrophy.

Assessment

A. Assess for presence of the following conditions:
  1. Rheumatic heart disease.
  2. Marfan syndrome.
  3. Arteriosclerotic and hypertensive dilatation of aortic root.
  4. Dissecting aortic aneurysm.
  5. Prosthetic valve leakage.
B. Observe for signs of heart failure.
✦ C. Assess for pounding arterial pulse (Corrigan-type arterial pulse) in the neck.
✦ D. Observe if widened pulse pressure present (difference between systolic and diastolic pressure).
E. Auscultate for early diastolic murmur.
F. Assess for weakness, severe dyspnea, hypotension.

Implementation

Same as for *aortic valve stenosis.*

Tricuspid Stenosis

✦ *Definition:* Narrowing of the valve lumen, usually associated with mitral valve defect. (Extremely uncommon.)

Assessment

A. Assess for presence of the following conditions:
1. Rheumatic heart disease with mitral valve involvement.
2. Congenital disease.
3. Infective (bacterial) endocarditis.
✦ B. Observe for evidence of heart failure.
✦ C. Auscultate for late diastolic murmur—use bell over tricuspid area.

Implementation

A. Follow nursing protocols for clients with heart failure.
B. Prepare client psychologically and physiologically for valvotomy or tricuspid valve replacement.

Tricuspid Insufficiency

✦ *Definition:* Allows regurgitant blood flow back into the right atrium from the ventricle—usually due to right ventricular dilation. (Extremely uncommon.)

Assessment

A. Note chest x-ray for heart dilatation and failure.
B. Auscultate for holosystolic murmur over tricuspid area.
C. Observe for symptoms of heart failure.

Implementation

Same as for *tricuspid stenosis.*

Heart Failure

Definition: Insufficient cardiac output to meet metabolic needs of the body. Regardless of type, it results in decreased cardiac output (forward failure) and venous congestion (backward failure) secondary to pump failure.

Characteristics

A. Differentiate heart failure types: left-sided or right-sided, systolic or diastolic, high output failure and acute or chronic.
✦ B. Heart failure may be due to left-sided cardiac failure or right-sided failure.
1. One side of the heart may fail separately from the other side because the heart is two separate pumping systems.
2. Impaired pumping ability results in heart's inability to maintain adequate circulation.
✦ C. Either the left or right ventricle may be affected; while most heart failure begins on the left side when the left ventricle cannot pump blood out of the chamber, failure usually then progresses to both ventricles.
1. Coronary artery disease and hypertension are the usual causes of left-sided failure.
2. Pulmonary congestion occurs and pressure is increased in the left ventricle, causing dyspnea and shortness of breath.
3. Pressure in the left atrium increases, which increases pressure in the pulmonary circulation.
4. Venous congestion occurs due to decreased compliance (decreased relaxation) of the left ventricle (decreased preload).
5. Acute pulmonary edema may result from left ventricular failure.
✦ D. Right ventricular failure—congestion occurs when blood is not pumped adequately from the systemic circulation into the lungs, resulting in systemic congestion.
1. The right side of the heart cannot eject blood and, therefore, cannot handle all of the blood that flows into it from venous circulation.
2. Congestion of the viscera (liver congestion) and peripheral tissues occurs.
3. Signs of right-sided failure will be edema of the extremities; congestion of GI tract causes nausea and vomiting.
E. Differentiating systolic from diastolic dysfunction—heart failure is manifested as systolic and diastolic dysfunction, or both.
✦ 1. Systolic dysfunction.
   a. Inadequate ventricular emptying leads to increased preload, diastolic volume and pressure (the tissues do not receive adequate circulatory output).
   b. Most common causes are coronary artery disease, hypertension, and cardiomyopathy, with viruses and toxic substances such as alcohol and medications being a possible cause.
   c. Conventional therapy includes diuretics (loop diuretics preferred), digitalis, ACE inhibitors, and beta blockers to improve performance of left ventricle.
   d. The above regimens may be inappropriate for diastolic dysfunction; avoid digitalis and vasodilators.
✦ 2. Diastolic dysfunction.
   a. Resistance to ventricular filling as a consequence of reduced ventricular compliance—results in prolonged ventricular relaxation time.
   b. Ejection fraction may be normal or increased.
   c. Clients cannot tolerate reduced blood pressure or plasma volume so diuretics, ACE

inhibitors and vasodilators are usually contraindicated. Digoxin is also contraindicated.

d. May respond to calcium-channel blockers and beta blockers (to slow the heart rate).

e. Nitrates may be used to decrease preload.

f. High output failure occurs with hypermetabolic states (infection, hyperthyroidism) and requires increased blood flow to meet oxygen demands.

g. Acute vs. chronic: acute is abrupt onset (MI); chronic is progressive deterioration.

Assessment: Left-Sided Failure

◆ A. Evaluate for presence of pulmonary symptoms.
1. Dyspnea, labored breathing (early symptoms).
2. Orthopnea (difficulty breathing when lying flat).
3. Moist, hacking cough.
4. Bibasilar crackles.
5. Cyanosis or pallor; cool extremities.
6. Increased pulmonary artery and/or pulmonary wedge pressure.

◆ B. Assess for anxiety, weakness and fatigue (after activities that usually are not tiring).

C. Identify behavior changes.

D. Check for palpitations and diaphoresis.

E. Assess for gallop rhythm—presence of S_3.

F. Evaluate for tachycardia, arrhythmias and cardiomegaly.

G. Assess for reduced pulse pressure.

◆ **Assessment: Right-Sided Failure**

A. Assess client for presence of conditions that could lead to right ventricular failure.
1. Any disease resulting in left ventricular failure.
2. Pulmonary embolism.
3. Fluid overload.
4. COPD.
   a. Pulmonary hypertension.
   b. Cor pulmonale.
5. Cirrhosis, portal hypertension.

◆ B. Evaluate symptoms primarily related to systemic congestion.
1. Peripheral edema (pitting type) in dependent parts: feet, legs, sacrum, back, buttocks.
   a. Results from elevation in venous pressure.
   b. Necessitates good skin care and positioning.
2. Ascites, which can result in pulmonary distress.
3. Anorexia and nausea due to congestion in liver and gut.
4. Weight gain.
5. Oliguria during day and polyuria at night.
6. Hepatomegaly and tenderness in right upper quadrant of abdomen.
7. Fatigue from poor tissue perfusion.
8. Difficulty concentrating.

Implementation

◆ A. Goal is to reduce workload on the heart, increase efficiency of contractions, and reduce fluid.

◆ B. Provide physical rest and emotional support.

◆ C. Optimize oxygenation—bedrest with Fowler's position.
1. Oxygen therapy based on degree of pulmonary congestion.
2. May require oxygen (cannula better than mask) or intubation.

D. Reduce preload (volume of blood heart receives) and afterload (resistance to pump).

◆ E. Monitor medications.
1. ACE inhibitors (decrease renin angiotensin–aldosterone response).
   a. Monitor for hypotension, hypovolemia, and hyponatremia (if receiving diuretics).
   b. Dosage according to BP, fluid and renal status, and degree of cardiac failure.
   c. Avoid NSAIDs (counteract action of ACE inhibitors, diuretics).
2. Diuretics to improve urine output to reduce preload (Lasix, Aldactone).
3. Beta blockers to decrease effects of catecholamines.
4. Digitalis if ejection fraction is < 40 percent (for systolic dysfunction).
   a. Increases contractility and improves cardiac output.
   b. Not used in diastolic failure.
5. Administer nitrates (ischemia) for vasodilation.
6. Administer beta blocker.
7. Administer potassium chloride for electrolyte replacement.

◆ F. Monitor diet—sodium restriction, as ordered to reduce fluid retention; and monitor and maintain fluid restriction as ordered.

G. Monitor brain natriuretic peptide (BNP) assay to detect abnormal hormone levels produced by failing ventricles.

H. Monitor daily weights.

I. Monitor for complications of treatment.
◆ 1. Digitalis toxicity.
   a. Most common predisposing factor for toxicity is hypokalemia, which potentiates effect of digitalis.
   b. Low potassium levels (from diuretics) lead to excitable heart and dysrhythmias.
◆ 2. Electrolyte imbalance from diuretics, especially decreased potassium.
3. Oxygen toxicity, especially with COPD clients.
4. Myocardial failure.
5. Cardiac dysrhythmia.

6. Pulmonary infarction; emboli, pneumonia from bedrest—circulatory stasis.

Cardiomyopathy

Definition: Heart muscle disease that primarily affects structural or functional ability of myocardium. It is classified as primary or secondary, and manifests as three types: dilated, hypertrophic, and restrictive cardiomyopathy.

Characteristics
A. Types.
    1. Dilated: most common type. Diffuse inflammation and rapid degeneration of myocardial fibers, which leads to decreased contractile function and dilation of both ventricles. This results in impaired systolic function and decreased cardiac output.
    2. Hypertrophic: asymmetrical ventricular hypertrophy, leading to hypercontractility of the left ventricle, obstruction of the left ventricle outflow, and stiffness of the ventricular walls. This results in impaired ventricular filling and decreased cardiac output.
    3. Restrictive: least common and impairs diastolic volume and stretch, resulting in decreased cardiac output.
✦ B. Regardless of the type manifested or cause, result is impaired pumping of the heart and decreased cardiac output.
C. Decreased stroke volume stimulates sympathetic nervous system resulting in increased vascular resistance with eventual left ventricular failure.

Assessment
✦ A. Effort dyspnea and fatigue due to elevated left ventricular diastolic pressure and low cardiac output.
✦ B. Physical signs include pitting edema, sinus tachycardia, basal rales, low blood pressure, and possible enlarged liver.
C. Chest x-ray reveals cardiomegaly.

Implementation
✦ A. Treatment begins with finding any specific cause (most often there is none) and treating it.
    1. Therapy for heart failure and low cardiac output is implemented.
    2. Combined afterload and preload reduction with ACE inhibitors, hydralazine plus nitrate, is the mainstay of treatment.
    3. Digitalis, diuretics are also used in the treatment protocol.
B. Nursing focus is aimed at improving cardiac output.
    ✦ 1. Bedrest and increased oxygenation.
        a. Gradually increase activity alternating with rest.

b. Identify activities that cause shortness of breath and teach client how to plan.
✦ 2. Monitor medications—compliance is vital.
3. Plan with client how to reduce anxiety—stress exacerbates condition.

Acute Pulmonary Edema

✦ *Definition:* A medical emergency characterized by excessive fluid in the pulmonary interstitial spaces or alveoli, usually due to severe, acute left ventricular decompensation.

Characteristics
✦ A. Most common cause is greatly elevated capillary pressure resulting from acute failure of left heart pump and pooling of blood in lungs.
B. Fluid fills alveoli and causes bronchospasm.
C. May also be associated with barbiturate/opiate poisoning or other noncardiac condition.

✦ ### Assessment
A. Observe initially for anxiety, feelings of impending doom, and restlessness.
B. Observe for marked dyspnea.
C. Assess for pink, frothy sputum.
D. Evaluate for marked cyanosis.
E. Observe for profuse diaphoresis—cold and clammy.
F. Evaluate for tachyarrhythmias.
G. Evaluate for (S_3) diastolic sound.
H. Evaluate for marked increase in pulmonary artery and/or pulmonary capillary wedge pressure.
I. Evaluate for hypoxemia and low PCO_2 (hyperventilation).

Implementation
✦ A. Place in high-sitting position—feet over side of bed.
✦ B. Administer oxygen at 6 L/min.
✦ C. Administer drugs (diuretics, digitalis, morphine, nitroglycerin) to improve myocardial contractility and reduce preload (volume of blood in ventricle after diastole).
D. Instruct client in deep breathing.
E. Monitor fluid intake and output; weigh daily.
F. Monitor vital signs and hemodynamic parameters (PCWP).
G. Provide sedation with ordered medication. Observe respiratory rate and depth.
H. Monitor drug therapy used for preload or afterload (nitroglycerin, nitroprusside, hydralazine).
✦ I. Rotating tourniquets on client's extremities used in emergency situation to reduce venous return to heart and pool blood temporarily in extremeties, thus reducing preload. Not commonly used—may be used in emergencies.

CARDIAC PROCEDURES

Angioplasty

A. Percutaneous transluminal coronary angioplasty procedure that can be balloon stent or laser to open narrowed or blocked arteries.
B. Preparation of client.
1. NPO after midnight.
2. In cath lab, catheter is inserted through groin or arm and contrast dye is injected.
3. Procedure takes 30–60 minutes.
4. Vital signs checked frequently following procedure.

Atherectomy

A. Procedure used to cut away blockage (plaque responsible for narrowing of the artery).
B. There are several atherectomy techniques.
1. Rotational extraction, using a high-speed rotational burr, a cutting device that removes plaque through a vacuum suction system.
2. Rheolytic thrombectomy, a system designed for clot removal via a special pump to deliver a saline "jet" to break away the clot, transform it into fragments, and vacuum it out.

Coronary Stents

A. A stainless steel structure placed in a coronary vessel to expand and help keep the artery open.
B. Stents are metabolic wires implanted at the site of a narrowed coronary artery.
C. Treatment of choice for lesions in diseased bypass grafts.

Pacemaker Insertion

Definition: A temporary or permanent device to initiate and maintain heart rate when client's intrinsic pacemaker is unreliable.

Assessment

A. Assess client for conditions requiring pacemaker insertion.
1. Conduction defect following heart surgery.
2. Heart block [usually third-degree (complete) heart block] due to anterior MI.
3. Tachyarrhythmias (overdrive pacing).
4. Bradyarrhythmias ("sick sinus syndrome").
B. Assess vital signs for baseline data.
C. Obtain and assess monitor rhythm strips for baseline.
D. Determine type of pacemaker inserted.

✦ 1. Temporary pacemaker—external generator used in emergency situations.
a. Pacing lead wire threaded transvenously to right ventricle and attached to external power source.
b. Right atrial and ventricular epicardial wires placed during heart surgery, exist transthoracically and connected to external pulse generator.
c. Transcutaneous—gelled electrode patches placed anteriorly and posteriorly.
d. Used for heart block, bradycardia, or tachyarrhythmias.
e. Client at risk for microshock if transvenous or transthoracic.
✦ 2. Permanent pacemaker.
a. Pacing lead wire with electrodes inserted through central vein and advanced into apex of right ventricle.
b. Pulse generator implanted into subcutaneous tissue below clavicle.
c. Demand—mode functions only if client's own heart rate is inadequate (most common type).
(1) Pacemaker is set at a specific rate and is inhibited if client's heart rate is adequate.
(2) May be dual-chamber or AV synchronous.
(3) Used mainly in bradyarrhythmias or heart block.
(4) Programmable pacemaker allows noninvasive adjustment of pacemaker.

Implementation

A. Observe for hematoma at site of insertion.
B. Immobilize extremity on side of pacemaker generator.
C. Do not lift client under arm on side of pacemaker.
✦ D. Evaluate pacemaker function/malfunction.
1. Absence of pacemaker artifact when client's rate is inadequate (failure to sense or discharge).
2. Failure of pacemaker inhibition (failure to sense)—leads to inappropriate pacing.
3. Pacing without depolarization response (failure to capture).
4. Assess for cardiac tamponade (decreased BP).
5. Monitor for hiccoughs—indicates dislodged pacing wire.
E. Monitor vital signs.
F. Provide client teaching.
1. Purpose of pacemaker.
2. Medication dose and side effects.
3. Monitoring pulse.

4. Signs and symptoms of infection.
5. No ROM on affected side for 2 days.
6. Wear medical alert bracelet and carry pacemaker ID card.
7. Follow up with pacemaker evaluation (e.g., clinic).
8. Avoid large electromagnetic fields.

✦ G. Counsel client to observe for pacemaker malfunction.
1. Dizziness or fatigue.
2. Shortness of breath.
3. Slowed pulse rate (5 beats less than pacemaker rate).
4. Chest pain.
5. Edema or weight gain.

Surgical Procedures

Definition: Surgical procedures on the cardiac vessels, valves, or myocardium.

Assessment

A. Assess type of heart surgery to be done.
✦ 1. *Percutaneous transluminal coronary angioplasty* (PTCA)—less invasive than bypass surgery and preferred as initial procedure.
   a. A catheter with a deflated balloon is threaded into artery at site of blockage.
   b. Balloon is inflated and opens artery by breaking up and compressing plaque against artery wall.
   c. Stent often placed to maintain patency.
✦ 2. *Coronary bypass surgery*—healthy sections of a leg or chest blood vessel are grafted distal to blocked area of coronary artery.
✦ 3. *Commissurotomy of stenosed valve.*
   a. Closed commissurotomy—finger inserted to dilate valvular opening.
   b. Open commissurotomy—dissection of scarred area by means of a scalpel.
✦ 4. *Valve replacement:* artificial, or prosthetic, valves; heterografts (porcine or bovine).
5. *Transplantation*—therapeutic option for severe heart disease.
   a. Immunosuppressant drugs decrease body's rejection of foreign protein (another's human heart).
   b. Clients must balance risk of rejection with risk of infection.
B. Evaluate client's knowledge of operative procedure to prepare for preoperative teaching.
C. Assess vital signs, heart and lung sounds, other vital parameters for baseline data.

Implementation

✦ A. Observe for fluid and electrolyte imbalance.
1. Obtain lab specimens for hypokalemia and hyperkalemia.
2. Measure CVP for hypovolemia and volume overload.
3. Measure blood gases for acidosis and alkalosis.
4. Monitor hematocrit and hemoglobin.
5. Weigh daily after voiding and before breakfast.

✦ B. Observe respiratory function.
1. Client receives mechanical ventilation for varying length of time postoperatively.
   a. Endotracheal intubation with cuffed tube.
   b. Suction airway PRN.
   c. Auscultate for bilateral breath sounds.
   d. Monitor pulmonary volumes; pulse oximetry.
2. Auscultate for abnormal lung sounds.

✦ C. Observe for circulatory complications.
1. Decreased blood pressure.
2. Tachycardia, thready pulse.
3. Weak peripheral pulses.
4. Decreased urine output.
5. Skin—cool, clammy, cyanotic.
6. Restlessness.
7. Elevated cardiac and central venous pressures.
8. Electrolyte imbalance.

✦ D. Observe for signs of cardiac tamponade (mediastinal/chest tubes output over 100 mL/hr).

✦ E. Place in semi-Fowler's position to facilitate cardiac and respiratory function.

✦ F. Administer pain medication such as morphine sulfate IV.

✦ G. Monitor IV fluid and blood requirements by use of intracardiac pressures, blood pressure, urine output, hemoglobin and hematocrit.
1. Keep CVP between 5 and 12 cm water pressure (or 0–6 mm Hg) or as directed by physician.
2. Keep urine above 30 mL/hr.
3. Hematocrit maintained at 30–35.

H. Maintain circulation.
1. Inotropic medications.
2. Vasoactive medications.
3. IV fluids.
4. Antibiotics.

✦ I. Maintain kidney function.
1. Keep urine output above 30 mL/hr with IV fluids or plasma expanders.
2. Maintain blood pressure above 90 mm Hg systolic.
3. Diuresis is common.
4. Report cloudy or pink urine.

✦ J. Maintain patent chest tubes.
1. Used to remove fluid and air from mediastinum/pleural space.
2. Maintain 20 cm H_2O suction.

✦ K. Maintain body temperature. (Clients are usually hypothermic following cardiac surgery.)
   1. Raise body temperature gradually.
      a. Blankets used cautiously following hypothermic surgical procedure.
      b. Monitor core temperature with PA catheter.
   2. Client at risk for developing fever caused by infection or postpericardiotomy syndrome.
      a. Bedrest and anti-inflammatory agents primary treatment.
      b. Keeping temperature below 100°F prevents increased metabolic rate, which increases cardiac workload.
✦ L. Assess level of consciousness, pupil response, motor response.
   1. Neurologic complications may result from extra corporeal perfusion or aorta clamping.
   2. Orient client frequently.
✦ M. Administer anticoagulant therapy for valve replacements.
✦ N. Monitor laboratory values for anticoagulation.
   1. Partial thromboplastin time for heparin administration based on weight and sliding scale protocol.
   2. Prothrombin time/INR for Coumadin therapy.
✦ O. Monitor for complications associated with valve replacement.
   1. Conduction defects (may require temporary pacing).
   2. Cardiac tamponade.
   3. Supraventricular tachyarrhythmias (may use pacemaker overdrive).
   4. Malfunction of prosthetic valve (murmur).
P. Monitor for complications associated with use of cardiopulmonary bypass.
   1. Fluid and electrolyte imbalance.
   2. Decreased cardiac output.
   3. Coagulation defects.
   4. Atelectasis (hypoventilation).
   5. Thromboembolic disorders.
   6. Alterations of BP.
   7. Cardiac tamponade.
   8. Arrhythmias.
   9. Renal failure.
   10. Neurologic dysfunction.
   11. Pain.
Q. Progressive care.
   1. Progressive ambulation.
   2. Lifestyle modification teaching (smoking cessation, AHA diet, exercise).
   3. Medications (antithrombotics/anticoagulants, inotropic agents, beta blockers, antihypertensives, antiarrhythmics).
   4. Sternal incision protection/wound care.

INFLAMMATORY HEART DISEASE

Infective (Bacterial) Endocarditis

Definition: An infection of the lining of the heart and valves caused by pathogenic microorganisms.

Characteristics
✦ A. Acute—fulminating disease due to organisms engrafted on a preexisting heart lesion.
   1. Occurs following open heart surgery or with IV drug use.
   2. Causative agents—gram-positive, gram-negative bacilli, yeasts; more rapid serious infection with *Staphylococcus aureus.*
B. Subacute—slowly progressive disease of rheumatic or congenital lesions or prosthetic valve.
   1. Occurs following dental, genitourinary, gynecological procedures, bacteremia or surgery.
   2. *Streptococcus* most common organism.

✦ ### Assessment
A. Observe for chills, diaphoresis, lassitude, anorexia, weight loss, arthralgia.
B. Check for fever and night sweats that recur for several weeks.
C. Assess for regurgitant heart murmur.
D. Identify history of recent infection, dental work, cystoscopy, IV drug use.
E. Evaluate for systemic emboli.
   1. Assess for petechiae on skin or mucous membranes: tender, red nodules on fingers, palms, or toes (arterial emboli).
   2. Splenic infarction—pain, upper left quadrant, radiating to left shoulder.
   3. Renal infarction—hematuria, pyuria, flank pain.
   4. Cerebral infarction—hemiparesis or neurological deficits.
   5. Pulmonary infarction—cough, pleuritic pain, dyspnea, hemoptysis.
F. Evaluate lab tests—increased WBC, erythrocyte sedimentation rate (ESR), blood culture, echocardiogram.

Implementation
✦ A. Maintain intensive chemotherapy with antibiotic drugs for several weeks.
B. Follow general nursing measures.
   1. Decrease cardiac workload—bedrest.
   2. Ensure physical and emotional rest.
C. Encourage fluids.
D. Anticoagulant therapy contraindicated because of danger of cerebral hemorrhage.
E. Monitor for signs of CHF.
F. Prophylactic antibiotics for high-risk client with existing cardiac lesion or prosthetic valve.

Pericarditis

Definition: Inflammation of the pericardium.

Assessment

A. Assess for possible cause of inflammation.
1. Transmural infarction—frequent cause.
2. Inflammation of heart or lungs.
3. Radiation.
4. Trauma/cardiac surgery.
5. Neoplasms.
◆ B. Evaluate type of pain—stabbing and knifelike; starts at sternum and radiates to neck and shoulder or back; aggravated by deep inspiration, supine position, and turning from side to side; relieved by sitting.
C. Identify if pericardial friction rub is present.
D. Assess vital signs for indication of infection.
◆ E. Evaluate lab tests—increased WBC, ESR, slightly elevated cardiac enzymes, and ECG changes (elevated ST segment, inverted T waves).

Implementation

◆ A. Maintain client on bedrest in semi-Fowler's position.
B. Administer and observe for side effects of salicylates and indomethacin.
C. Monitor vital signs.
◆ D. Monitor for pericardial friction rub on forced expiration with client in forward leaning position.
E. Relieve pain with analgesics.
F. Prepare client for pericardiocentesis if required.
G. Observe for complications following pericardiocentesis.
1. Monitor vital signs and CVP for possible cardiac tamponade recurrence.
2. Auscultate heart sounds to determine if decrease in intensity of heart sound is present.
◆ H. Monitor for pericarditis complications.
1. Pericardial effusion leading to tamponade.
2. Constrictive pericarditis—prevents adequate diastolic filling of ventricles, leading to decreased cardiac output.

PERIPHERAL VASCULAR DISORDERS

Hypertension

◆ *Definition:* Defined as blood pressure that is greater than either 140 mm Hg systolic or 90 mm Hg diastolic.

Characteristics

A. Approximately 50 million people have hypertension in United States—only 25 percent are controlled to normotensive.
B. More frequent in African Americans. Higher incidence in white men than women before age 50; after age 50, this is reversed.
C. Risk factors.
1. Obesity.
2. Family history.
3. Age > 60 years.
4. Race.
5. Diabetes.
6. Smoking.
7. Dyslipidemia.
8. Gender—male.
D. Types of hypertension.
◆ 1. Primary or essential—no known etiology (accounts for 90 percent of clients).
◆ 2. Secondary—directly related to another condition.
a. Renal disease.
b. Endocrine disorders.
(1) Pheochromocytoma.
(2) Adrenal cortex lesions—hyperaldosteronism, Cushing's syndrome.
c. High-dose estrogen use.
d. Pregnancy.
e. Acute autonomic dysreflexia.
f. Increased intracranial pressure.

Assessment

A. Assess for risk factors by evaluating history.
◆ B. Assess for common manifestations.
1. Headache in early AM.
2. Loud S_2 heart sound.
3. Epistaxis.
C. Identify if target organ complications are present.
1. Brain—mental and neurologic abnormalities.
2. Kidneys—renal insufficiency (especially if diabetic).
3. Cardiovascular system—left ventricular hypertrophy, heart failure, atherosclerosis, PVD.
4. Eyes—narrowing of arteries, papilledema, visual disturbances.

Implementation

◆ A. Lifestyle modifications.
1. Weight loss.
2. Reduce sodium intake.
3. Maintain adequate intake of dietary potassium and magnesium.
4. Decrease stress.
5. Engage in regular aerobic exercise.
6. Limit alcohol intake.
7. Stop smoking.
◆ B. Drug therapy (combination frequently used).
◆ 1. Diuretics.
a. Act on kidneys to increase urine output.

b. Thiazides (Diuril).

c. Loop (potent) diuretics (Lasix, Bumex).

d. Potassium-sparing (Aldactone)—weak diuretic effect, often used in combination with other diuretic.

◆ 2. Beta blockers (Inderal).

a. Decrease response to sympathetic stimulation; decrease contractility and myocardial workload.

b. Can cause bradycardia, conduction blocks.

3. ACE inhibitors (Captopril): inhibit the conversion of angiotensin I to angiotensin II.

a. Allow blood vessels to dilate.

b. Help prevent target organ damage.

c. May cause dry cough, due to increased bradykinin levels.

d. Used cautiously with renal insufficiency.

e. May cause hyperkalemia if potassium supplements also used.

4. Angiotensin II receptor blockers (Losartan).

a. Dilate vessels without increasing bradykinin levels.

b. Used for those who cannot tolerate ACE inhibitor.

c. May cause hyperkalemia if potassium supplements also used.

5. Calcium-channel blockers (nifedipine).

a. Relax smooth muscles.

b. Block calcium flow into the cell.

6. Central alpha agonists (Clonidine)—centrally acting agents that cause vasodilation.

a. Available in transdermal patch changed weekly.

b. May cause sedation, dry mouth.

7. Alpha$_1$ blockers (Prazosin)—peripherally acting antiadrenergic.

a. Risk for postural hypotension.

b. Also used for prostatic urinary obstruction.

8. Arterial vasodilators (Hydralazine)—direct acting.

a. May cause tachycardia—often used with beta blocker.

b. May cause fluid retention—monitor weight.

C. Client education.

1. Importance of regimen compliance.

2. Not to discontinue medication abruptly.

3. Avoid concurrent use of alcohol.

4. Check with physician before taking over-the-counter (OTC) medications (e.g., NSAIDs counteract the effect of many antihypertensive agents).

Hypertensive Crisis

Definition: Critical ("accelerated/malignant") elevation of blood pressure that becomes acute and life-threatening.

Assessment

◆ A. Assess for signs/symptoms.

1. Diastolic blood pressure usually over 120 mm Hg.

2. Known history of hypertensive disease or diseases that cause hypertension (e.g., renal vascular disease, head injury).

3. Medical therapy (medications and compliance) or use of sympathomimetic drug.

B. Monitor for potential end-organ complications.

1. Depressed level of consciousness.

2. Focal neurologic signs.

3. Chest pain.

4. Pulmonary edema.

5. Signs of renal failure (azotemia—increased BUN and creatinine).

Implementation

◆ A. Monitor vital signs, ECG, and neurological signs closely.

1. Assess blood pressure every 5 minutes with antihypertensive drug therapy.

2. Avoid too-rapid reduction in blood pressure.

3. Note for end-organ signs/symptoms worsening with rapid pressure reduction.

4. Note for side effects of antihypertensive agents (tachycardia).

◆ B. Administer antihypertensive medications (and particular agents relative to cause of crisis) as prescribed.

1. Drug most frequently used is nitroprusside (Nipride) because of its rapid onset of action (increased intracranial pressure). Possible cyanide poisoning with high doses.

2. Drugs such as hydralazine hydrochloride (Apresoline), nicardipine hydrochloride (Cardene), or esmolol hydrochloride (Brevibloc) take longer to act than Nipride.

◆ C. Monitor urinary output closely.

1. Indwelling urinary catheter may be indicated.

2. Oliguria or anuria should be reported immediately.

◆ D. Maintain client on strict bedrest.

1. Elevate head of bed 45 degrees.

2. Keep room quiet.

E. Support client and assist to remain calm.

1. Do not leave the client unattended.

2. Use anxiety-reducing measures; client may sense impending doom and be frightened.

◆ F. Provide safety interventions.

1. Keep siderails up if client is not fully alert.

2. Employ seizure precautions if indicated.

3. Place client on side if level of consciousness is diminished to prevent aspiration.

4. Keep suction equipment readily available.

Thromboangiitis Obliterans (Buerger's Disease)

Definition: Inflammatory occlusions of distal arteries and veins. Most often affects males under 40 years of age who smoke.

Assessment

◆ A. Observe for signs of arterial insufficiency: impaired pulse, intermittent claudication, pain, postural color changes in foot.

B. Disease may involve upper and lower extremities.

C. Observe for signs of neuropathy; decreased sensation, paresthesia.

Implementation

◆ A. Urge client to stop smoking.

◆ B. Administer vasodilator drugs to increase blood supply to lower extremities (Trental).

◆ C. Administer low-dose aspirin.

D. Instruct client in foot care.

E. Instruct client to prevent chemical, mechanical, and thermal trauma to feet.

F. Monitor peripheral pulses frequently.

G. May require arterial bypass surgery or amputation.

Raynaud's Disease and Phenomenon

Definition: Episodic vasospasms of the small cutaneous arteries, usually involving the fingers and toes. Primarily seen in young women.

Assessment

◆ A. Raynaud's disease.
   1. Primary idiopathic paroxysmal arteriolar vasospasm due to abnormality of the sympathetic nervous system.
   2. Precipitated by cold or emotional stimuli; relieved by warmth.
   3. Bilateral or symmetric pallor and cyanosis followed by redness of the digits (usually fingers).
   4. May have throbbing and paresthesia during recovery.
   5. Ulcers near fingertips.

◆ B. Raynaud's phenomenon.
   1. Often related to underlying collagen or connective tissue disease (rheumatoid arthritis, lupus).
   2. May be unilateral and involve few digits, but usually symmetric.
   3. Pallor, cyanosis, redness, and changes in skin temperature in response to cold or strong emotion.

Implementation

◆ A. Encourage client to stop smoking.

◆ B. Encourage client to avoid precipitating factors such as cold temperature and emotional stress—keep warm.

◆ C. Wear warm clothing when in cold weather: boots, gloves, etc.

D. Protect hands from injury—wounds heal slowly.

E. Keep skin soft with emollients—avoid dry skin.

F. Administer vasodilator drugs.
   1. Calcium-channel blocker—nifedipine.
   2. Nitrates (transdermal or oral).

G. May require sympathectomy.

Deep Vein Thrombophlebitis (DVT)

◆ *Definition:* Formation of clot in a vein with inflammatory changes in the vein wall. Most prevalent sites: deep veins of lower extremities and pelvis. Usually begins in calf and propagates proximally.

Characteristics

A. Persons most vulnerable are from 45–65 years of age.

◆ B. Causes of DVT (Virchow's triad).
   1. Impaired venous flow—stasis. Associated with periods of inactivity (bedrest, surgery, long plane trips, or car rides).
   2. Endothelial injury exposes platelets in bloodstream to collagen, promoting thrombosis.
   ◆ 3. Hypercoagulopathy (increased tendency to clot).
      a. Dehydration.
      b. Malignancy (breast, prostate, ovary, pancreas).
      c. Polycythemia and sickle-cell disease.
      d. Use of oral contraceptive agents and smoking.
      e. Inherited disorders (antithrombin III deficiency).

Assessment

A. Symptoms closely related to size and location of clot—may have no signs or symptoms.

◆ B. Assess leg.
   1. Unilateral edema.
   2. Calf pain—dull ache.
   3. Changes in color and temperature; may be warm with red color, but may also be pale "milk leg."
   4. Affected area may also feel firm and hard.
   5. Distended superficial veins.
   6. Homan's sign (not recommended or reliable and may mobilize clot).

C. Doppler flow studies, phlebography, and impedance plethysmography confirm diagnosis.

Implementation

◆ A. Administer anticoagulant therapy.
   1. Heparin therapy for 7–10 days.
   2. Coumadin prescribed for 3 months; dose adjusted to keep INR between 2.0 and 3.0.

3. Observe for signs of bleeding (urine, stool occult blood, ecchymosis).
+ B. Maintain strict bedrest for minimum 3–4 days.
   1. Do not use knee gatch or pillows under knees.
   2. Elevate foot of bed 20 degrees.
   3. Handle affected limb with care to prevent compression of tissue.
+ C. Monitor for pulmonary embolism (PE).
   1. Assess subtle changes; report immediately (confusion, anxiety, restlessness).
   2. Cough; rapid, shallow respirations; dyspnea.
   3. Chest pain that is worse with deep breath.
   4. Tachycardia.
D. Position client to avoid venous stasis and turn every 2 hours.
E. Take vital signs at least every 4 hours.
+ F. Promote venous return.
   1. Use ROM exercises on unaffected limbs only.
   2. Do not massage or exercise affected leg.
   3. Apply antiembolic stocking to unaffected leg or use pneumatic compression device.
+ G. Provide client education.
   1. Avoid standing in one position or sitting for long periods (either walk or lie flat; avoid crossing legs at knees; elevate legs while sitting).
   2. Avoid wearing constrictive clothing.
   3. Wear support hose.
   4. Understand correct use of anticoagulants and the necessity for follow-up lab tests.
      a. Include measures to reduce risk of bleeding (soft toothbrush, electric razor).
      b. Avoid contact sports; notify physician if injury occurs.
   + 5. Teach prevention.
      a. Elevate foot of bed.
      b. Avoid sitting in chair for long periods.
      c. Leg and ankle exercises.
      d. Pneumatic compression device/TEDs.
      e. Low-dose heparin or low-molecular-weight heparin.

Varicose Veins

Definition: A condition in which the veins are dilated and tortuous caused by incompetent venous valves.

Characteristics
A. Causes.
   1. Pregnancy.
   2. Standing for long periods of time.
   3. History of DVT.
   4. Prolonged and heavy lifting.
B. Pathology.
   1. Most commonly affects superficial saphenous veins.
   2. Possible inherited defect of valves or vein wall.

Assessment
+ A. Visible dilated, tortuous veins.
+ B. Assess for dull aching, heaviness in legs after standing.
C. Observe for edematous ankles with itching.
D. Skin brown above ankles from blood that has escaped due to increased venous pressure.
E. Secondary ulceration (medial ankle).

Implementation
+ A. Encourage client to use antiembolic stockings, support hose.
+ B. Elevate legs when possible.
+ C. Educate client to see need for cessation of smoking (makes blood hypercoagulable).
D. Prevent constrictive clothing and positions; protect legs from pressure/trauma.
E. Prepare client for vein stripping or sclerosing injections.

SURGICAL INTERVENTIONS FOR VASCULAR DISORDERS

Femoral Popliteal Bypass Graft

Definition: Prosthetic or autologous vein graft is anastomosed to the artery proximal and distal to the atherosclerotic obstruction.

Assessment
+ A. Observe peripheral circulation pre- and postoperatively.
   1. Check for presence of distal pulses—use Doppler if necessary.
   2. Check that extremities are warm and pink postoperatively.
   3. Compare both extremities.
+ B. Check vital signs, particularly blood pressure.
C. Check for comorbidity (heart or renal disease).

Implementation
+ A. Mark on skin where pulses are palpated or heard.
+ B. Keep leg flat postoperatively initially—avoid wound strain.
+ C. Monitor edema in operative leg—usual but may require compression hosiery and diuretic; resolves in 4–8 weeks.
+ D. Administer perioperative antibiotics, postoperative anticoagulants and antithrombotics as prescribed and monitor drug lab effects.
E. Report bleeding from wound.
F. Encourage ambulation/exercise post discharge.

Aortic Aneurysms

Definition: A localized abnormal dilatation of the vascular wall occurring most often in the abdominal aorta and less commonly in the thoracic aorta.

Characteristics

✦ A. Caused by weakening of arterial wall due to athero-sclerosis; thoracic aneurysm due to trauma, Marfan syndrome.

B. Risk factors include dyslipidemia, diabetes mellitus, smoking, hypertension, family history.

C. Highest incidence in older men—25 percent also have peripheral vascular occlusive disease.

Assessment

A. Evaluate symptoms to determine area involved. (*See* p. 215.)

✦ 1. Abdominal aneurysm.
   a. Pulsating mass in abdomen may be palpated.
   b. Bruit over aorta.
   c. Lumbar pain radiating to flank and groin indicates impending rupture.
   d. Detected by abdominal CT scan or sonog-raphy.

✦ 2. Thoracic aneurysm.
   a. Pain—most are asymptomatic—substernal, back or neck.
   b. Symptoms due to pressure—dysphagia, hoarseness, dyspnea.
   c. Most accurate means for imaging are CT scan and MRI.

B. Assess vital signs to obtain baseline data.

C. Evaluate peripheral pulses.

Implementation

✦ A. Control hypertension—with antihypertensives (e.g., beta blocker).

B. Prepare asymptomatic client for surgery if aneurysm exceeds 5 cm in diameter.

C. Monitor fluid balance. Administer whole blood when needed.

D. Prepare symptomatic client for immediate surgery.

✦ E. Provide postoperative nursing management.

1. Follow same procedures as for open heart surgery if client has thoracic aneurysm; monitor vital signs and hemodynamic variables.
2. Observe circulatory status distal to graft site.
3. Observe all peripheral pulses and temperature of extremities.
4. Monitor renal function with accurate intake and output (cross clamp of aorta during surgery).
5. Observe for emboli to brain or lung.
6. Monitor neurological signs.
7. Monitor for complications.
   a. Hypertensive preoperatively, but can easily become hypotensive due to excessive bleeding.
   b. Acute renal failure. (Monitor I&O.)
   c. Hemorrhage from graft site. (Assess for back bruising.)

d. Cerebral vascular accident.
e. Paraplegia.
f. Infection.

COMMONLY USED DRUGS FOR THE CARDIOVASCULAR SYSTEM

Summary of Cardiac Drug Categories

ACE Inhibitors: use to treat high blood pressure, post heart attack and kidney disease. Also useful in management of heart failure by decreasing stress on heart muscle.

Antiarrhythmics: help heart to beat in a regular rhythm.

Anticoagulants: slow down blood-clotting process. Prescribed for blocked arteries or blood clot in an artery.

Antioxidants: prevent chemical reaction in blood causing oxidation, which leads to plaque formation.

Antiplatelets: prevent platelets from clumping or forming clots. They lower the risk of heart attack.

Beta Blockers: lower heart rate and blood pressure, thus reducing work of the heart.

Calcium-Channel Blockers: used for high blood pressure to prevent artery spasm or angina, or to control rapid heartbeat.

Cardiac Glycosides: help to maintain normal heart rhythm and rate. Also strengthen heart muscle.

Cholesterol-Lowering Agents: lower blood cholesterol levels, reducing risk of developing coronary heart disease.

Diuretics: lower blood pressure by allowing kidneys to rid body of excess fluid.

Nitrates: dilate blood vessels, which decrease workload of the heart. Primary indication is to prevent or stop angina.

Specific Drug Categories

Diuretics

A. Action: most diuretics block sodium reabsorption in tubules of kidney, thereby eliminating water.

B. Agents.

✦ 1. Thiazide and thiazide-like diuretics.
   a. Common preparations: chlorothiazide (Diuril), hydrochlorothiazide (Hydrodiuril), chlorthalidone (Hygroton), Exna, Enduran, etc.
   b. Thiazide-like: chlorthalidone (Thalitone), indapamide (Lozol), Zaroxolyn, Mykrox.
   c. Administration: oral and parenteral.
   d. Advantages: potent by mouth; effective antihypertensives.

      e.   Disadvantages: electrolyte imbalances; loss of potassium, metabolic alkalosis, hypotension, hyperlipidemia.

      f.   Nursing implementation.
        (1) GI upset, gout, hyperglycemia.
        (2) Allergic reaction.
        (3) Monitor kidney function (BUN, serum creatinine), signs of hypokalemia.

✦ 2. Potassium-sparing agents.
      a.   Common preparations: spironolactone (Aldactone), triamterene (Dyrenium).
      b.   Administration: oral only.
      c.   Advantages: conserve potassium.
      d.   Disadvantages: weak diuresis; usually not effective when used alone.
      e.   Nursing implementation.
        (1) Electrolyte imbalance; hyperkalemia.
        (2) Gynecomastia and nitrogen retention.
        (3) If diarrhea or GI problems occur, give after meals.
        (4) If drowsy, headache, or lethargy, decrease dose as ordered.

✦ 3. Loop diuretics: moderate to severe volume overload.
      a.   Common preparations: furosemide (Lasix), bumetanide (Bumex), Edecrin, Demadex.
      b.   Administration: oral and parenteral.
      c.   Advantages: rapid, potent action useful in cases of severe pulmonary edema and refractory edema.
      d.   Nursing implementation/evaluation.
        (1) Note weight loss with diuresis.
        (2) Monitor/watch for signs of electrolyte imbalance (potassium and chloride loss); dehydration.
        (3) Thirst, nausea, skin rash; monitor blood pressure.
        (4) Hyperuricemia, secondary aldosteronism, hyperglycemia.
        (5) Give oral doses with food to decrease GI side effects.
      e.   Advese reactions: hypotension, electrolyte imbalance, rash, azotemia.

Nitrates

A. Action.
  1. Promotes vasodilation by reducing vascular tone in arteries and veins.
  2. Decreases venous blood return to heart (preload)—primary action.
  3. Decreases peripheral arterial vascular resistance (afterload)—in larger doses.
  4. Reduces myocardial oxygen consumption and pulmonary congestion.

B. Uses.
  1. First-line therapy for acute angina.
  2. Heart failure related to ischemic heart disease.
✦ C. Agents.
  1. Short acting—for acute attack or prophylactically.
    a.   Sublingual—nitroglycerin for acute attack (repeat in 3- to 5-minute intervals).
    b.   Buccal spray.
    c.   IV sodium nitroprusside—for heart failure decompensation combined with dopamine or dobutamine.
  2. Long acting.
    a.   Oral—Imdur, Ismo.
    b.   Nitro-Dur, Transdermal.
  3. Extended release—buccal tablets; capsules.
✦ D. Major side effects.
  1. Headache is a common side effect.
  2. Postural hypotension.
  3. Cyanide poisoning with sodium nitroprusside use.
✦ E. Nursing implementation.
  1. Development of tolerance minimized with intermittent therapy.
  2. Advise client to take drug, in short-acting doses, while sitting or lying down to prevent hypotension.
  3. Drug should be replaced in 3 months after opening bottle.
  4. Instruct client to notify physician if severe headache, weakness, blurry vision, irregular heartbeat, or dry mouth is experienced.

ACE Inhibitors

Captopril (Capoten), Lotensin, Vasotec, Zestril, Univase, etc.

✦ A. Action.
  1. Angiotensin-converting enzyme (ACE) inhibitor.
  2. Inhibits renin–angiotensin–aldosterone activity.
  3. Effective for heart failure (reduces mortality and improves cardiac function).
  4. Used as initial therapy for early CHF.
  5. Stimulates synthesis of nitric oxide and prostaglandin.
  6. Used post-infarction to reduce ventricular remodeling.
✦ B. Adverse side effects.
  1. Hypotension—especially with first dose.
  2. Dry, irritating cough is often present.
  3. Swelling of lips, tongue or glottis may occur.
  4. Renal insufficiency.
✦ C. Nursing implementation.
  1. Instruct client to take medication at same time every day.

2. Instruct client to move from lying to sitting to standing position slowly.
3. Avoid salt substitutes that could lead to hyperkalemia.
4. Notify physician if cough, fatigue, or nausea develop.

Beta-Adrenergic Blockers

Propanolol (Inderal), Lopressor, Tenormin, Sectral, Zebeta, Coref, etc.

◆ A. Action.
  1. Blocks cardiac response to sympathetic stimulation—slows heart, decreases blood pressure, slows AV conduction.
  2. Pure beta or beta$_1$-specific action.
  3. Carvedilal (alpha and beta blocker for heart failure).
◆ B. Uses.
  1. Prevent chronic angina; used in unstable angina.
  2. Slow heart rate, slow AV conduction, lower blood pressure.
  3. Prolong life in postinfarction clients.
  4. Prevent sudden death.
  5. Improve left ventricular function.
C. Contraindications/major side effects.
  1. Bronchospasm (COPD), wheezing.
  2. Bradyarrhythmias.

Angiotensin Receptor Blockers

A. Action: appropriate alternative for vasodilation if clients are intolerant to ACE inhibitors due to cough, edema or rash.
B. Example: Iosartan-Cozzar, Losartan.

Cardiac Glycosides

Digitalis (Digoxin, Lanoxin), Digitoxin (Crystodigin)

◆ A. Action.
  1. Increases contractile force (pumping ability) of heart positive inotropism), which increases cardiac output in systolic heart failure (ejection fraction < 40%).
  2. Slows heart rate.
    a. Direct effect.
    b. Increases vagal tone and decreases sympathetic tone.
  3. Slows conduction through AV node.
  4. Increases nonpacemaker cell automaticity that may cause arrhythmias.
◆ B. Uses.
  1. Systolic heart failure—increases contractility, reduces oxygen needs, increases cardiac efficiency, and reduces heart size.

2. Supraventricular tachyarrhythmias—slows ventricular rate by slowing conduction of impulses through AV node.
◆ C. Dosage.
  1. Individualized to client and clinical situation; loading dose, then maintenance dose (usually 0.25 mg QD).
  2. Monitor blood level with Digoxin (normal is 0.9–2.0 mg/mL).
◆ D. Major side effects—signs of toxicity.
  1. Cardiac.
    a. Bradycardia.
    b. Conduction disturbances (advanced AV block).
    c. Arrhythmias, due to increased automaticity (premature ventricular beats).
  2. Gastrointestinal.
    a. Anorexia.
    b. Nausea and vomiting.
    c. Diarrhea.
◆ E. Nursing implementation.
  ◆ 1. Monitor for toxic effects—incidence high.
    a. Signs and symptoms: anorexia, nausea, vomiting, bradycardia.
    b. Elderly are more sensitive to digitalis, so monitor carefully for toxicity.
  ◆ 2. Check apical pulse before administering digitalis drugs.
    a. If below 60, hold dose and notify physician.
    b. If above 120, check for toxicity/arrhythmias.
  3. Client teaching.
    a. Ensure that client understands drug action and dosage.
    b. Monitor pulse before taking medication.
    c. Report unusual effects (toxic symptoms).
    d. Store in tightly covered, light-resistant containers.
  ◆ 4. Precautions.
    a. Hypokalemia—predisposes client to toxicity.
    b. Renal failure—predisposition to digitalis toxicity.
    c. Should not be given with advanced AV block.
    d. Increased risk of toxicity when given with antiarrhythmics.

Calcium-Channel Blockers (Ion Antagonists)

Verapamil, Diltiazem, Nifedipine, Amlodipine, Isoptin

◆ A. Action.
  1. Inhibits the influx of calcium ions across cell membrane.
  2. Decreases heart rate as conduction is slowed through SA and AV nodes.

3. Reduces extension of non-Q MI. Increases myocardial oxygenation by causing coronary vasodilation (verapamil, diltiazem).
4. Decreases peripheral vascular resistance (especially nifedipine)—dilates blood vessels.

✦ B. Uses.
1. Prescribed for angina especially vasospastic-angina.
2. Slows ventricular response to atrial tachy-arrhythmias.
3. Antihypertensive agents.

✦ C. Major side effects.
1. Cardizem (diltiazem hydrochloride)—nausea, edema, bradycardia.
2. Calan, Isoptin (verapamil hydrochloride)—hypotension, peripheral edema, vertigo, bradycardia.
3. Procardia (nifedipine)—nausea, peripheral edema, headache, flushing, dyspnea, reflex tachycardia.

✦ D. Nursing implementation.
1. Cardizem: observe for hypotension; report irregular heartbeats, or bradycardia; do not discontinue suddenly.
2. Calan, Isoptin: give on empty stomach; do not discontinue suddenly; monitor for bradycardia, constipation.
3. Procardia: give on empty stomach.

Antiarrhythmic Drugs

Quinidine, Pronestyl, Lidocaine, Amiodarone

✦ A. Action.
1. Increases recovery time of atrial and ventricular muscle; prolongs repolarization.
2. Decreases myocardial excitability.
3. Increases conduction in cardiac muscle, Purkinje fibers, and AV junction (exception: lidocaine).
4. Decreases contractility (exception: lidocaine).
5. Decreases automaticity.

✦ B. Uses.
1. Quinidine used for atrial fibrillation, atrial flutter, supraventricular tachycardia, premature systoles.
2. Procainamide hydrochloride (Pronestyl) used for premature ventricular systoles.
3. Xylocaine (lidocaine), drug of choice for short-term management of ventricular tachyarrhythmias associated with MI.
4. Amiodarone for life-threatening arrhythmias unresponsive to other agents.

✦ C. Major side effects.
1. Quinidine.

a. Cinchonism—nausea, vomiting, diarrhea, tinnitus, vertigo, visual disturbances.
b. Hypersensitivity, thrombocytopenia.
c. Conduction disturbances.
d. Potentiates digitalis toxicity.
2. Pronestyl.
a. Anorexia, nausea, vomiting, diarrhea.
b. Systemic lupus erythematosus.
c. Agranulocytosis.
d. AV block.
3. Lidocaine.
a. CNS disturbances—drowsiness, slurred speech, blurred vision, seizures, coma.
b. Cautious use in clients with liver disease or low cardiac output (metabolism of drug slowed).
4. Amiodarone.
a. Visual disturbances.
b. Bradycardia, hypotension.
c. Liver function abnormality.
d. Potentiates digitalis toxicity.

✦ D. Nursing implementation.
1. Monitor ECG and assess vital signs.
2. Client teaching.
a. Observe for individual drug side effects. (*See* Major side effects.)
b. Notify physician if arrhythmia develops.
3. Monitor blood levels as indicated.

Sympathomimetic Agents

✦ A. Action.
1. Epinephrine HCl (Adrenalin): beta and alpha stimulation—increases heart rate, contractility, and peripheral vascular resistance; bronchodilation.
2. Norepinephrine (Levophed).
a. Alpha-adrenegic stimulation—peripheral vasoconstriction.
b. Beta stimulation mild.
3. Isoproterenol HCl (Isuprel): beta stimulation.
a. Increases heart rate, contractility, and oxygen consumption.
b. Decreases vascular resistance.
c. Bronchodilation.
4. Dopamine (Depostat)—precursor of norepinephrine.
a. Raises blood pressure.
b. Increases myocardial contractility.
c. Increases cardiac output and perfusion.
d. Dilates renal vessels; improves urine output.
5. Dobutrex (dobutamine hydrochloride).
a. Cardiac stimulation, but no significant increase in heart rate.
b. Increases cardiac output.

✦ B. Uses.

1. Epinephrine (Adrenalin): allergic states, anaphylactic shock.
2. Norepinephrine (Levophed).
   a. Elevates blood pressure.
   b. Used for hypotension, cardiac arrest.
3. Isoproterenol (Isuprel).
   a. Cardiogenic shock with high peripheral vascular resistance.
   b. AV block—increases pacemaker automaticity and improves AV conduction.
4. Dopamine (Intropin)—precursor of norepinephrine.
   a. Cardiogenic shock (hypotension).
   b. Heart failure.
5. Dobutrex (dobutamine hydrochloride).
   a. Short term for heart failure.
   b. Cardiac surgical procedures.
✦ C. Major side effects.
1. Epinephrine (Adrenalin).
   a. Chest pain, arrhythmias, tachycardia, hypertension.
   b. Hyperglycemia.
2. Norpinephrine (Levophed).
   a. Anxiety (mimics physiological reaction to stress), headache.
   b. Hypertension.
   c. Arrhythmias.
3. Isoproterenol (Isuprel).
   a. Tachyarrhythmias, especially ventricular tachycardia.
   b. Hypotension.
   c. Headache, skin flushing, angina, dizziness, weakness.
4. Dopamine (Intropin).
   a. Renal vasoconstriction with high dose.
   b. Hypertension.
   c. Tachycardia, arrhythmias.
5. Dobutrex (dobutamine hydrochloride).
   a. Arrhythmias, palpitations.
   b. Angina, chest pain, shortness of breath.
✦ D. Nursing implementation.
1. Carefully monitor ECG and vital signs.
2. Prevent IV infiltration of vasoconstricting agents —could cause tissue necrosis. (Central vein preferred.)
3. Client teaching.
   a. Recognition of side effects.
   b. Diet—high fiber to reduce constipation.

Antihyperlipidemic Agents

✦ A. Action.
1. Lowers low-density lipoprotein (LDL) cholesterol levels and triglycerides. Raises high-density lipoprotein (HDL) cholesterol.

   a. Binds with bile acids in the intestine and excreted in feces, resulting in removal of LDL and cholesterol.
   b. May interfere with absorption of digoxin, thiazides, beta-adrengic blockers, fat-soluble vitamins, folic acid and vancomycin.
✦ B. Uses and side effects.
1. Bile acid sequestrants (Questram).
   a. Causes liver to produce bile acid from cholesterol.
   b. Lowers LDL and total cholesterol.
   c. May raise serum triglyceride level.
   d. GI side effects (constipation, flatulence, nausea).
2. HMG-CoA reductase inhibitors [lovastatin (Mevacor) or simvastatin (Zocor)].
   a. Blocks synthesis of cholesterol.
   b. Lowers LDL cholesterol and triglycerides; raises HDL cholesterol.
   c. May cause constipation, diarrhea, liver enzymes elevation, muscle aches.
3. Fibric acid derivatives [clofibrate (Atromids), tricor (Lopid)].
   a. Inhibits liver synthesis of triglycerides and very-low-density lipoprotein (VLDL).
   b. Used for hypertriglyceridemia and type III hyperlipidemia.
   c. GI side effects common; gallstones.
   d. May increase effects of anticoagulants and hypoglycemics.
4. Nicotinic acid (niacin); Nicobid, Niacor.
   a. Inhibits VLDL production in liver.
   b. Decreases LDL level; raises HDL level.
   c. Used in mixed dyslipidemias.
   d. Used in combination with other antihyperlipidemics.
   e. May cause cutaneous flushing, pruritus, hepatitis.
✦ C. Nursing implementation.
1. Review dietary restrictions (AHA diet).
2. Encourage regular exercise program.
3. Vitamin supplementation may be indicated.
4. HMG-CoA reductase inhibitors taken in evening.
5. Encourage smoking cessation.

Platelet Inhibitors

Aspirin, Persantine, Ticlid

✦ A. Action.
1. Agents interfere with platelet adhesion or aggregation.
2. Used to prevent venous thromboembolism and arterial thrombosis (CVA, MI).
✦ B. Uses and side effects.

1. Acetylsalicylic acid (aspirin).
   a. Inhibits platelet formation of thromboxane A (reduces adhesiveness).
   b. Low dose used in angina, acute coronary syndromes, MI, TIA, post cardiac surgery, post coronary artery interventional therapy.
   c. Prolongs bleeding time; interacts with Coumadin to prolong PT.
   d. Monitor for GI bleeding; tinnitus.
2. Dipyridamole (Persantine).
   a. Increases platelet cyclic adenosine monophosphate (AMP) levels.
   b. Used for peripheral vascular disease, prosthetic heart valves, TIA.
   c. May cause hypotension.
3. Ticlopidine (Ticlid).
   a. Blocks platelet recruitment by binding to adenosine diphosphate (ADP) receptor on platelet.
   b. Same indications as aspirin.
   c. Used if unable to tolerate aspirin.
   d. May cause bleeding, neutropenia, thrombocytopenia; may increase serum lipids.
4. GPIIb/IIIa antiagonists (Plavix—oral, abciximab—IV).
   a. Inhibit platelet aggregation.
   b. Used as adjunct to interventional coronary procedures (angioplasty, stent placement).
   c. Used in unstable angina.
   d. May cause hypotension, bradycardia, serious bleeding.
+ C. Nursing implementation.
   1. Recommend appropriate safety precautions for bleeding.
   2. Discuss possible drug interactions (consult physician before taking OTC medications).
   3. Reinforce teaching of early signs of stroke, heart attack, DVT.
   4. Monitor closely for bleeding (especially following interventional therapies).

Anticoagulant Therapy

+ A. Action.
   + 1. Medications used to prevent intravascular thrombosis by decreasing blood coagulability.
      a. Heparin (IV, sub q).
      b. Warfarin sodium (Coumadin, PO).
      c. Lovenox (sub q).
   + 2. Pharmacological action.
      a. Prevents fibrin deposits.
      b. Prevents extension of a thrombus.
      c. Prevents thromboembolic complications.

B. Contraindications for use of drug.
   1. Blood dyscrasia.
   2. Liver and kidney disease.
   3. Peptic ulcer.
   4. Chronic ulcerative colitis.
   5. Active bleeding (except DIC).
   6. Spinal cord or brain injuries.
+ C. Drugs and foods to avoid when on anticoagulant therapy.
   1. Leafy green vegetables (foods high in vitamin K) more than usual—antagonist.
   2. Salicylates/NSAIDs, acetaminophen, and steroids potentiate.
+ D. Nursing implementation—safety precautions.
   + 1. Keep antagonist nearby; *see* Antagonist, below.
   + 2. Observe for signs of bleeding (gums, ecchymosis, hematuria, melena).
   3. Avoid/prevent bleeding.
   4. Carry identification card (Coumadin).
   5. Keep appointments for blood work (PT).
   6. Teach first aid for bleeding.

Intravenous Anticoagulants

Heparin Sodium, Enoxaparin (Lovenox)

+ A. Mode of administration: IV or sub q (inactivated orally).
+ B. Action.
   1. Interferes with formation of thrombin from prothrombin.
   2. Prevents thrombin from converting fibrinogen to fibrin.
   3. Therapeutic dose by continuous infusion (e.g., 1000 U/hr) prolonged PTT.
   4. Dose lasts 3–4 hours if given IV intermittently (3500–5000 U q 8–12 hr) for prophylaxis.
+ C. Lab findings.
   1. Prophylactic dose not monitored by PTT.
   2. Therapeutic dose—weight-based dose adjusted to achieve desired PTT; values 1.5 to 2 times normal values.
+ D. Antagonist.
   1. Discontinue infusion (short half-life).
   + 2. Protamine sulfate: 1 mg protamine sulfate for each 100 U of heparin in last dose if necessary.
E. Used for treatment of various conditions.
   1. Quickly stops development of clots.
   2. Serious unstable angina.
   3. Certain strokes.
   4. Severe thrombophlebitis.
   5. Acute pulmonary edema.
+ F. Nursing implementation.
   + 1. Check PTT or clotting time routinely for weight-based dosing per IV titration.

2. Check patency of IV.
3. Assess client for bleeding.
4. Avoid aspirin during anticoagulant therapy.
5. Instruct client to carry medical alert card.
✦ 6. Take following precautions when administering drug sub q into abdomen:
   a. Use small needle (27 gauge).
   b. Form pouch of skin on abdomen no closer than 5 cm around umbilicus—avoid extremities.
   c. Administer injection at 90-degree angle sub q.
   d. Do not aspirate needle or massage skin around injection site to prevent ecchymosis.

Oral Anticoagulants

Dicumarol, Coumadin, Miradon

✦ A. Mode of administration: oral.
✦ B. Action.
  1. Prevents utilization of vitamin K by liver.
  2. Depresses hepatic synthesis of several clotting factors.
  3. Decreases prothrombin formation.
  4. Takes 24–72 hours for action to develop and continues for 24–72 hours after last dose.
✦ C. Antagonist.
  ✦ 1. Vitamin K—AquaMEPHYTON IM or IV.
  2. Returns to hemostasis within 6 hours.
  3. Blocks action of Coumadin for 1 week.
✦ D. Nursing implementation.
  1. Check prothrombin or INR time before giving.
    ✦ a. Keep prothrombin time at 18–30 seconds (normal is 12–14 seconds).
    ✦ b. Keep INR between 2 and 3.5.
  2. Give at same time each day.
  ✦ 3. Teach client to avoid usual intake of foods high in vitamin K (cabbage, cauliflower, spinach, and other dark leafy vegetables), alcohol, ASA, NSAIDs, Tylenol.
  4. Encourage client to wear Med-Alert bracelet.
  5. Avoid invasive procedures (IM injection) and injury.
  6. Check with physician before taking any OTC medications.

Thrombolytic Agents

✦ A. Action.
  1. Activates formation of plasmin, which digests fibrin and dissolves formed blood clots—limits infarct size.
  2. Stimulates conversion of plasminogen to plasmin (fibrinolysin).
  3. Prescribed for acute pulmonary emboli, deep vein thrombosis, arterial thrombosis, and coronary thrombosis.
  4. Greatest benefit if initiated in 1–3 hours.
✦ B. Agents infused.
  1. Streptokinase (Streptase); urokinase.
  2. Tissue plasminogen activator (Activase).
  3. Antistreplase, APSAC, Eminase.
  4. Reteplase (Retavase).
  5. Tenecteplace (TNKase) was FDA approved in 2000.
    a. Can be administered in one single injection to dissolve clots rather than 90-minute infusion.
    b. Advantage over Activase is that TNKase is more specific for a clot in coronary artery.
C. Major side effects.
  ✦ 1. Serious bleeding (increased fibrinolytic activity).
  2. Fever up to 100°F.
  3. Allergic reactions; rash (streptokinase).
  4. Reperfusion arrhythmias when used for coronary clots.
D. Contraindications for use.
  1. Recent major surgery, GI bleed.
  2. History of CVA.
  3. Bleeding tendency.
  4. Uncontrolled hypertension.
  5. Pregnancy.
✦ E. Nursing implementation.
  1. Obtain PTT, PT, fibrinogen level, and platelet count.
  2. Monitor infusion of IV (use controller or pump).
  3. Monitor closely for signs of bleeding, blood pressure.
    a. 24 hours for pulmonary embolism.
    b. 24–72 hours for deep vein or arterial thrombosis.
  4. Avoid invasive procedures.

CARDIOVASCULAR SYSTEM REVIEW QUESTIONS

1. In assessing a client's history for a cardiac work-up, which of the following is the most important parameter to question?

   1. Amount of weight loss.
   2. Character of pain experienced.
   3. Respiratory rate and depth.
   4. Amount of coughing.

2. A 54-year-old client was put on quinidine (a drug that decreases myocardial excitability) to prevent atrial fibrillation. He also has kidney disease. The nurse is aware that this drug, when given to a client with kidney disease, may

   1. Cause cardiac arrest.
   2. Cause hypotension.
   3. Produce mild bradycardia.
   4. Be very toxic even in small doses.

3. Thrombolytic therapy would be appropriate for which of the following conditions?

   1. Continual blood pressure above 200/120.
   2. History of diabetic retinopathy.
   3. History of significant kidney disease.
   4. Myocardial infarction.

4. When assessing an ECG, the nurse knows that the P-R interval represents the time it takes for the

   1. Impulse to begin atrial contraction.
   2. Impulse to traverse the atria to the AV node.
   3. SA node to discharge the impulse to begin atrial depolarization.
   4. Impulse to travel to the ventricles.

5. Monitoring a central venous pressure (CVP), the nurse understands that a normal reading is between

   1. 5 cm and 15 cm.
   2. 10 cm and 15 cm.
   3. 5 cm and 10 cm.
   4. 10 cm and 20 cm.

6. Following a treadmill test and cardiac catheterization, the client is found to have coronary artery disease. After discharge from coronary care unit with a significant MI, the client is referred to the cardiac rehabilitation unit. During his first visit to the unit, he says that he doesn't understand why he needs to be there because there is nothing that can be done—and the damage is done. The best nursing response is

   1. "Cardiac rehabilitation is not a cure but can help restore you to many of your former activities."
   2. "Here we teach you to gradually change your lifestyle to accommodate your heart disease."
   3. "You are probably right but we can gradually increase your activities so that you can live a more active life."
   4. "Do you feel that you will have to make some changes in your life now?"

7. A client admitted with the diagnosis of cardiac disease tells the nurse he is afraid of dying from a heart attack. The most therapeutic response is

   1. "Perhaps you should discuss this with your physician."
   2. "Of course you aren't going to die."
   3. "What makes you think you will die?"
   4. "Tell me more about these fears of dying from a heart attack."

8. To evaluate a client's condition following cardiac catheterization, the priority intervention is to palpate the pulse

   1. In all extremities.
   2. At the insertion site.
   3. Distal to the catheter insertion.
   4. Above the catheter insertion.

9. While admitting a client scheduled for a cardiac catheterization the client states to the nurse, "I always get a rash when I eat shellfish." Following safety protocol, the most appropriate initial nursing intervention is to

   1. Notify the physician.
   2. Place a note on the chart regarding this reaction.
   3. Ask the client if there are any other foods that cause such a reaction.
   4. Notify the dietitian of the reaction and request a "no shellfish" diet.

10. A client's physician orders nuclear cardiography and makes an appointment for a thallium scan. The pur-

pose of injecting a radioisotope into the blood stream is to detect

1. Normal versus abnormal tissue.
2. Damage in areas of the heart.
3. Ventricular function.
4. Myocardial scarring and perfusion.

11. For a client who presents with a heart murmur, the nurse can best explain how a murmur manifests in the body by saying

1. "The systolic occurs between S_1 and S_2."
2. "The diastolic occurs between S_2 and S_1."
3. "It is determined by intensity over time."
4. "It is a measure of turbulence of blood flow through the valve."

12. When auscultating the apical pulse of a client who has atrial fibrillation, the nurse would expect to hear a rhythm that is characterized by

1. The presence of occasional coupled beats.
2. Long pauses in an otherwise regular rhythm.
3. A continuous and totally unpredictable irregularity.
4. Slow but strong and regular beats.

13. A client is experiencing tachycardia. The nurse's understanding of the physiological basis for this symptom is explained by which of the following statements?

1. The demand for oxygen is decreased because of pleural involvement.
2. The inflammatory process causes the body to demand more oxygen to meet its needs.
3. The heart has to pump faster to meet the demand for oxygen when there is lowered arterial oxygen tension.
4. Respirations are labored.

14. A client has the diagnosis of left ventricular failure and a high pulmonary capillary wedge pressure (PCWP). The physician orders dopamine to improve ventricular function. The nurse will know the medication is working if the client's

1. Blood pressure rises.
2. Blood pressure decreases.
3. Cardiac index falls.
4. PCWP rises.

15. A client is admitted with stable sinus tachycardia. The initial intervention will be based on

1. Elimination of the cause.
2. Availability of cardioversion.

3. Analysis of the P waves.
4. Whether this is a defect or a physiological variant.

16. A client is admitted, and the monitor shows an abnormal rhythm. A major sign of hemodynamic instability would be

1. Mild chest pain.
2. Client complaining of anxiety.
3. Shortness of breath.
4. Heart rate of 80.

17. A client has been admitted to the hospital with a diagnosis of suspected bacterial endocarditis. The complication that the nurse will constantly observe for is

1. Presence of a heart murmur.
2. Systemic emboli.
3. Fever.
4. Congestive heart failure.

18. For morning shift, you are assigned two clients, both on cardiac monitoring. Client 1, a 60-year-old, is on Lasix and digoxin, has clear lungs, and has lost 4 pounds. Client 2 is a 70-year-old, with an MI 2 days ago; he requires close monitoring. The first nursing action is to

1. Assess Client 2 first because he is older and unstable.
2. Obtain a rhythm strip for both clients and interpret them before intervening.
3. Cleck the amount of fluid Client 1 is losing.
4. Assess Client 1 first because of fluid loss.

19. Thrombophlebitis is a common complication following vascular surgery. Which of the following signs indicates that a possible thrombus has occurred?

1. Kernig's sign.
2. Homan's sign.
3. Dull, aching calf pain.
4. Soft, pliable calf muscle.

20. In preparation for discharge of a client with arterial insufficiency and Raynaud's disease, client teaching instructions should include

1. Walking several times each day as part of an exercise routine.
2. Keeping the heat up so that the environment is warm.
3. Wearing TED hose during the day.
4. Using hydrotherapy for increasing oxygenation.

21. A 45-year-old male client with leg ulcers and arterial insufficiency is admitted to the hospital. The nurse understands that leg ulcers of this nature are usually caused by

    1. Decreased arterial blood flow secondary to vaso-constriction.
    2. Decreased arterial blood flow leading to hyper-emia.
    3. Atherosclerotic obstruction of arteries.
    4. Trauma to the lower extremities.

22. A client comes into the outpatient clinic and tells the nurse that he has leg pains that begin when he walks but cease when he stops walking. Which of the following conditions would the nurse assess for?

    1. An acute obstruction in the vessels of the legs.
    2. Peripheral vascular problems in both legs.
    3. Diabetes.
    4. Calcium deficiency.

23. A client who recently started taking a daily dose of the drug methyldopa (Aldomet) for hypertension complains of drowsiness and lethargy when the nurse makes a home visit. The nursing intervention would be to

    1. Notify the physician of the negative side effects so the dose can be reduced.

    2. Ask the physician to prescribe another antihypertensive.
    3. Suggest that the client take the medication in the evening and reevaluate on the next visit.
    4. Explain that these are expected side effects and he will have to live with them.

24. Dyspnea associated with congestive heart failure is primarily due to

    1. Blockage of a pulmonary artery by an embolus.
    2. Accumulation of fluid in the interstitial spaces and alveoli of the lungs.
    3. Blockage of bronchi by mucous secretions.
    4. Compression of lungs by the dilated heart.

25. The client returns to the clinic a week after discharge following a leg fracture. The fracture was complicated by a clot in the left leg. The orders were to remain on Coumadin. The client has a prothrombin time drawn. The results indicate that it is 24 seconds. The follow-up care plan for the client is based on the knowledge that these results are

    1. Above normal and in the therapeutic range.
    2. Below normal and in the therapeutic range.
    3. Normal, within acceptable limits.
    4. Abnormal and test should be repeated.

CARDIOVASCULAR SYSTEM

Answers with Rationale

1. (2) The character of pain, including its location, duration, and intensity, is the most important for accurate diagnosis. Answers (3) and (4) should be included in the client's history, but are not as critical. Weight loss (1) is not relevant.

   NP:A; CN:S; CA:M; CL:A

2. (1) Kidney disease interferes with metabolism and excretion of quinidine, resulting in higher drug concentrations in the body. Quinidine can depress myocardial excitability enough to cause cardiac arrest.

   NP:E; CN:PH; CL:A

3. (4) For clients with an MI, thrombolytic therapy minimizes the infarct size through lysis of the clot in the occluded coronary artery. The patent artery then promotes perfusion of the heart muscle. The other three responses are all contraindications for the use of thrombolytic agents.

   NP:AN; CN:PH; CL:C

4. (4) The P-R interval is measured on the ECG strip from the beginning of the P wave to the beginning of the QRS complex. It is the time it takes for the impulse to travel to the ventricle.

   NP:AN; CN:PH; CL:K

5. (3) The normal CVP reading is between 5 cm and 10 cm. The rise and fall of CVP readings are more important than are pressure level readings, so it is necessary to observe a series of pressure readings.

   NP:A; CN:PH; CL:C

6. (1) Such a response does not give false hope to the client but is positive and realistic. This answer tells the client what cardiac rehabilitation is and does not dwell upon his negativity about it.

   NP:I; CN:H; CL:A

7. (4) This response opens up communication to allow the client to discuss his fears of dying. Referring to his physician (1) is nontherapeutic, as is answer (2), which is giving him false reassurance. Answer (3) questions his feelings and does not encourage him to express them.

   NP:I; CN:PS; CL:A

8. (3) Palpating pulses distal to the insertion site is important to evaluate for thrombophlebitis and vessel occlusion. They should be bilateral and strong.

   NP:E; CN:PH; CL:A

9. (1) Because the dye used during a cardiac catheterization contains iodine, the physician must be aware of this client's reaction to iodine (shellfish). The other interventions should be carried out, but they should follow notifying the physician.

   NP:I; CN:PH; CL:A

10. (4) This scan detects myocardial damage and perfusion, an acute or chronic MI. It is a more specific answer than (1) or (2). Specific ventricular function is tested by a gated cardiac blood pool scan.

    NP:AN; CN:PH; CL:K

11. (4) A murmur is heard as turbulence of blood flow through the valve. It is classified by timing, so answers (1) and (2) are correct, but they have to do with timing. Answer (3) has to do with pattern of flow.

    NP:P; CN:PH; CA:M; CL:C

12. (3) In atrial fibrillation, multiple ectopic foci stimulate the atria to contract. The AV node is unable to transmit all of these impulses to the ventricles, resulting in a pattern of highly irregular ventricular contractions.

    NP:AN; CN:PH; CL:C

Coding for Questions/Answers Abbreviations: **Nursing Process: NP,** Assessment: A, Analysis: AN, Planning: P, Implementation: I, Evaluation: E; **Client Needs: CN,** Safe, Effective Care Environment: S, Health Promotion and Maintenance: H, Psychosocial Integrity: PS, Physiological Integrity: PH; **Clinical Area: CA,** Medical Nursing: M, Surgical Nursing: S, Maternal/Newborn Nursing: MA, Pediatric Nursing: P, Psychiatric Nursing: PS; **Cognitive Level: CL,** Knowledge: K, Comprehension: C, Application: A, Analysis: AN.

13. (3) The arterial oxygen supply is lowered and the demand for oxygen is increased, which results in the heart's having to beat faster to meet body needs for oxygen.

    NP:AN; CN:PH; CL:C

14. (1) If dopamine has a positive effect, it will cause vasoconstriction peripherally, but increase renal perfusion and the blood pressure will rise. The cardiac index will also rise and the PCWP should decrease.

    NP:E; CN:PH; CL:AN

15. (1) With sinus tachycardia, determining the cause is critical, because the treatment depends on it. For example, if the client is in pain, pain relief will affect sinus tachycardia. If this condition is unstable, cardioversion would be the treatment of choice. Answers (3) and (4) are incorrect; P waves are normal, and a moderately fast heart rate may be a normal variant.

    NP:I; CN:PH; CA: M; CL:A

16. (3) A major sign of hemodynamic instability is shortness of breath, in addition to ongoing chest pain and a heart rate over 150 per minute. Anxiety would be present, but is not a determining factor.

    NP:A; CN:PH; CA:M; CL:C

17. (2) Emboli are the major problem; those arising in right heart chambers will terminate in the lungs, and left chamber emboli may travel anywhere in the arteries. Heart murmurs, fever, and night sweats may be present, but do not indicate a complication of emboli. Congestive heart failure may be a result, but this is not as dangerous an outcome as emboli. Emboli may occur in the spleen, kidneys, brain, lungs, and in the extremities.

    NP:A; CN:PH; CL:AN

18. (2) The first nursing action is to interpret the two rhythm strips to identify any unanticipated complications. Answer (1) is incorrect because the nurse will need to assess the degree of instability and current status by interpreting the rhythm strip first. Fluid loss is expected with Lasix and is a positive sign of status change.

    NP:I; CN:S; CA:M; CL:AN

19. (3) Dull, aching calf pain is a major sign of DVT. Homan's sign is now considered unreliable and may even mobilize the clot, so it is not used (2). Kernig's sign (1) indicates the presence of meningeal irritation. Rigidity in the muscle is found with DVT, not a soft and pliable muscle.

    NP:A; CN:PH; CL:A

20. (2) The client's instructions should include keeping the environment warm to prevent vasoconstriction. Wearing gloves, warm clothes, and socks will also be useful in preventing vasoconstriction, but TED hose would not be therapeutic. Walking (1) will most likely increase pain.

    NP:I; CN:H; CL:C

21. (1) Decreased arterial flow is a result of vasospasm. The etiology is unknown. It is more problematic in colder climates or when the person is under stress. Hyperemia occurs when the vasospasm is relieved.

    NP:AN; CN:PH; CL:C

22. (2) Intermittent claudication is a condition that indicates vascular deficiencies in the peripheral vascular system. If an obstruction were present, the leg pain would persist when the client stops walking. Low calcium level may cause leg cramps but would not necessarily be related to walking.

    NP:A; CN:PH; CL:A

23. (3) These side effects may be present with this medication, but may be alleviated by taking the drug in the evening. Often, taking one dose in the evening will minimize the sedation. The nurse needs to follow up with this client and report to the physician.

    NP:I; CN:H; CL:AN

24. (2) Failure of the left ventricle to pump effectively causes damming of blood back into the pulmonary circuit, increasing pressure, and causing extravasation of fluid into interstitial spaces and alveoli.

    NP:AN; CN:PH; CL:C

25. (1) Normal prothrombin time is 12 to 14 seconds, but for Coumadin therapy, the PT should be maintained between 18 and 28 seconds.

    NP:P; CN:PH; CL:AN

RESPIRATORY SYSTEM

The respiratory system is the body process that accomplishes pulmonary ventilation. The act of breathing involves an osmotic and chemical process by which the body takes in oxygen from the atmosphere and gives off end products, mainly carbon dioxide, formed by oxidation in the alveolar tissues. The respiratory system also works in conjunction with the kidneys in regulating acid–base balance.

ANATOMY OF RESPIRATORY SYSTEM

Upper Airway

A. Nasal passages.
   1. Filter the air.
   2. Warm the air.
   3. Humidify the air.
B. Nasopharynx.
   1. Tonsils: filter and destroy microorganisms.
   2. Eustachian tube: opens during swallowing to equalize pressure in the middle ear.
C. Oropharynx.
   1. Part of both the respiratory tract and the digestive tract.
   2. Swallowing reflex initiated here.
   3. Epiglottis closes entry to trachea as foodstuff passes en route to the stomach.

Lower Airway

A. Larynx.
   1. Protects the tracheobronchial tree from aspiration of foreign materials.
   2. Cough reflex initiated here, whether voluntary or involuntary.
   3. Houses the vocal cords, which are considered to be the dividing point between the upper and lower airways.
B. Trachea.
   1. Flexible cartilaginous tubular structure.
   2. Extends from the cricoid cartilage into the thorax, branching into the right and left mainstem bronchi.
C. Right lung.
   1. Contains three distinct lobes: upper, middle, and lower.
   2. Lobes are divided by interlobar fissures.
D. Left lung.
   1. Contains two lobes—upper and lower.
   2. Lingula is part of the upper lobe but is sometimes referred to as the middle lobe of the left lung.
   3. Lobes are divided by one interlobar fissure.
E. Bronchi.
   1. Right mainstem bronchus (RMSB): shorter and wider than left bronchus; nearly vertical to trachea.
      a. Most frequent route for aspirated materials.
      b. Endotracheal tube might enter the RMSB if tube is passed too far.
   2. Left mainstem bronchus (LMSB): branches off the trachea at a 45-degree angle.
   3. The bronchi subdivide into bronchioles, terminal bronchioles, respiratory bronchioles, and alveoli.
F. Alveoli.
   1. Air cells surrounded by pulmonary capillaries in which gas exchange takes place: oxygen, carbon dioxide.
   2. Contain a substance known as surfactant, which keeps the alveoli expanded. Without surfactant, the alveoli would collapse.
G. Pleura.
   1. Each lung enclosed in double-walled membrane sac. Parietal pleura lines the chest cavity. Visceral pleura lines the lungs. Space between the pleural layers is the intrapleural space and is filled with pleural fluid.
   2. The pleural fluid is a thin film of fluid, encasing each lung, which allows for a smooth, gliding motion between the lung and the chest wall and facilitates expansion of lung during inspiration.

PRINCIPLES OF VENTILATION

Respiration

Definition: A process in which oxygen is transported from the atmosphere to the cells and carbon dioxide is carried from the cells to the atmosphere.
A. Respiration is divided into four phases.
   1. Pulmonary ventilation—air movement caused by intrathoracic pressure changes in relation to the pressure at the airway opening.
   2. Diffusion of oxygen and carbon dioxide between alveoli and blood.
   3. Transportation of oxygen and carbon dioxide in blood to and from cells.
   4. Regulation of ventilation via respiratory center in medulla.

B. Respiratory cycle.
   1. Inspiration (active process)—diaphragm descends and external intercostal muscles contract; alveolar pressure decreases, allowing air to flow into the lungs.
   2. Expiration (normally a passive process)—muscles relax, alveolar pressure increases, allowing air to flow from the lungs.

Respiratory Pressures

A. At inspiration the intra-alveolar pressure is more negative than the atmospheric pressure.
B. At expiration the intra-alveolar pressure is more positive, thereby pressing the air out of the lungs.
C. A negative pressure exists in the intrapleural space and aids in keeping the visceral pleura of the lungs against the parietal pleura of the chest wall. Lung space enlarges as the chest wall expands.
D. Recoil tendency of the lungs is due to the elastic fibers in the lungs and the surfactant.

Surfactant

A. Surface-active material that lines the alveoli and changes the surface tension, depending on the area over which it is spread.
✦ B. Surfactant in the lungs allows the smaller alveoli to have lower surface tension than the larger alveoli.
   1. Results in equal pressures within both and prevents collapse.
   2. Production of surfactant depends on adequate blood supply.
C. Conditions that decrease surfactant.
   1. Hypoxia.
   2. Oxygen toxicity.
   3. Aspiration.
   4. Atelectasis.
   5. Pulmonary edema.
   6. Pulmonary embolus.
   7. Mucolytic agents.
   8. Hyaline membrane disease.

Compliance

A. Relationship between pressure and volume: elastic resistance.
   1. Measure of elasticity of lungs and thorax.
   2. When compliance is decreased, lungs are more difficult to inflate.
✦ B. Conditions that decrease chest wall compliance.
   1. Obesity—excess fatty tissue over chest wall and abdomen.
   2. Kyphoscoliosis—marked resistance to expansion of the chest wall.
   3. Scleroderma—expansion of the chest wall limited when the involved skin over the chest wall becomes stiff.

   4. Chest wall injury—as in crushing chest wall injuries.
   5. Diaphragmatic paralysis—as a result of surgical damage to the phrenic nerve, or disease process involving the diaphragm itself.
C. Conditions that decrease lung compliance.
   1. Atelectasis—collapse of the alveoli as a result of obstruction or hypoventilation.
   2. Pneumonia—inflammatory process involving the lung tissue.
   3. Pulmonary edema—accumulation of fluid in the alveoli.
   4. Pleural effusion—accumulation of pleural fluid in the pleural space, compressing lung on the affected side.
   5. Pulmonary fibrosis—scar tissue replacing necrosed lung tissue as a result of infection.
   6. Pneumothorax—air present in the pleural cavity; lung is collapsed as volume of air increases.

Airway Resistance

A. Opposition or counterforce. Resistance depends on the diameter and length of a given tube (respiratory tract).
   1. Flow may be laminar (smooth) or turbulent.
   2. Resistance equals pressure divided by flow (Poiseuille's law).
B. Conditions that increase airway resistance.
   1. Secretions.
   2. Bronchial constriction.

✦ ### Lung Volumes

A. Total lung capacity (TLC)—total volume of air that is present in the lungs after maximum inspiration.
B. Vital capacity (VC)—volume of air that can be expelled following a maximum inspiration.
C. Tidal volume (TV)—volume of air with each inspiration.
D. Inspiratory reserve volume (IRV)—volume of air that can be inspired above the tidal volume.
E. Inspiratory capacity (IC)—volume of air with maximum inspiration; comprises tidal volume and inspiratory reserve volume.
F. Expiratory reserve volume (ERV)—volume of air that can be expelled following a resting expiration.
G. Reserve volume (RV)—volume of air remaining in the lungs at the end of maximum expiration.
H. Functional reserve capacity (FRC)—volume of air remaining in the lungs at the end of resting expiration; comprises ERV and RV.
I. Forced expiratory volume (FEV_1)—volume of air of the vital capacity that is expelled within the first second.

Alveolar Ventilation

Definition: The rate at which the alveolar air is renewed each minute by atmospheric air—the most important factor of the entire pulmonary ventilatory process.

A. Rate of alveolar ventilation.

✦ 1. Alveolar ventilation is one of the major factors determining the concentrations of oxygen and carbon dioxide in the alveoli.

2. Alveolar ventilation per minute is the total volume of new air entering the alveoli each minute; equal to the respiratory rate times the amount of new air that enters the alveoli with each breath.

B. Anatomic dead space.

1. Dead space air is the air that fills the respiratory passages with each breath (nose to bronchioles).

2. The volume of air that enters the alveoli with each breath is equal to the tidal volume minus the dead space volume; usually 150 mL in adults. Air is not available for gas exchange.

3. Anatomical dead space refers to the volume of all spaces of the respiratory system besides the gas exchange areas (the alveoli and terminal ducts).

4. Physiological dead space refers to alveolar dead space (occurring because of nonfunctioning or partially functioning alveoli); included in the total measurement of dead space.

5. In the normal person, anatomical and physiological dead space are equal because all alveoli are functional.

Oxygen and Carbon Dioxide Diffusion and Transportation of Respiratory Gases

Ventilation

A. The first phase in respiration is ventilation, which is the constant replenishment of air in the lungs.

B. Composition of alveolar air.

✦ 1. Alveolar air is only partially replenished by atmospheric air each inspiratory phase.

a. Approximately 350 mL of new air (tidal volume minus dead space) is exchanged with the functional residual capacity volume each respiratory cycle (FRC = 2300 mL).

b. Sudden changes in gaseous concentrations are prevented when alveolar air is replaced slowly.

2. Alveolar air contains more carbon dioxide and water vapor than atmospheric air.

3. Alveolar oxygen concentration depends on the rate of oxygen absorbed into the blood and the ability of the lungs to take in carbon dioxide.

4. Carbon dioxide content is likewise affected by the rate at which carbon dioxide is passed into the alveoli from the blood and the ability of the lungs to expire it.

Diffusion of Gases

A. The next phase is movement of oxygen from the alveolar air to the blood and movement of carbon dioxide in the opposite direction.

B. Movement of gases through the respiratory membrane depends on the following factors:

1. Thickness of membrane.

2. Permeability of membrane (diffusion coefficient).

3. Surface area of the membrane.

4. Differences in gas pressures in the alveolar and blood spaces.

5. Rate of pulmonary circulation.

C. Blood low in carbon dioxide and high in oxygen leaves lungs.

D. Throughout the body there again is exchange of respiratory gases in the capillary beds.

1. Oxygen out of the blood and into the cells.

2. Carbon dioxide from cells into the blood.

✦ **Oxygen Transport in the Blood**

A. About 3 percent of the oxygen is carried in a dissolved state in the water of plasma and cells.

B. About 97 percent is carried in chemical combination with hemoglobin in red blood cells.

1. The percentage of oxygen combined with each hemoglobin molecule depends on the partial pressure of oxygen (PO_2).

2. The relationship is expressed as the oxygen–hemoglobin dissociation curve.

a. It shows the progressive increase in the percentage of hemoglobin that is bound with oxygen as the PO_2 increases.

b. When the PO_2 is high, oxygen binds with hemoglobin; when PO_2 is low (tissue capillaries), oxygen is released from hemoglobin.

c. This is the basis for oxygen transport from the lungs to the tissues.

3. Febrile states and acidosis permit less oxygen to bind with Hgb, thereby limiting the amount of oxygen available for the tissues.

4. The amount of oxygen that is available to the tissues depends on the oxygen content of the blood and the cardiac output.

C. Inadequate oxygen transport to the tissues—hypoxia.

1. Hypoxic hypoxia: low arterial PO_2.

a. Alveolar hypoventilation.

b. Ventilation–perfusion inequalities.

c. Diffusion defects.

d. Fraction of inspired oxygen (FIO_2) is less than atmosphere, such as in high altitudes.

2. Anemic hypoxia: decreased oxygen-carrying capacity to the blood.

a. Anemia—less Hgb; therefore, less oxygen is able to combine with it.

b. Carbon monoxide poisoning—carbon monoxide combines with Hgb, preventing oxygen from combining with Hgb.

3. Circulatory hypoxia: circulatory insufficiency.
   a. Shock—decreased cardiac output.
   b. Congestive heart failure.
   c. Arterial vascular disease—localized obstruction to arterial blood flow.
   d. Tissue need for oxygen surpasses supply available.

4. Histotoxic hypoxia: prevents tissues from utilizing oxygen.

✦ **Carbon Dioxide Transport in the Blood**

A. A small amount of carbon dioxide is dissolved in plasma and red blood cells in the form of bicarbonate.

B. Inside the red blood cells, carbon dioxide combines with water to form carbonic acid.
   1. It is catalyzed by the enzyme called carbonic anhydrase.
   2. The enzyme accelerates the rate to a fraction of a second.

C. In another fraction of a second, carbonic acid dissociates to form hydrogen ions and bicarbonate in the red cells.

D. Carbon dioxide combines with the hemoglobin molecule.
   1. The hemoglobin molecule has given off its oxygen to the tissues, and carbon dioxide attaches itself.
   2. The venous system carries the combined carbon dioxide back to the lungs, where it is expired.

Regulation of Respiration

A. Respiratory centers.
   1. Pons—two respiration areas: pneumotaxic and apneustic.
   2. Medulla oblongata—major brain area controlling rhythmicity of respiration.
   3. Spinal cord—facilitory role in maintaining respiratory center.
   4. Hering Breuer reflexes—stretch receptors located in lung tissue that assist in maintaining respiratory rhythm and prevent overstretch of the lung. Afferent fibers are carried in the vagus nerve.

B. Humoral regulation of respiration (chemical).
   1. Central chemoreceptors.
      a. Directly stimulated by an increase in hydrogen ion concentration (acidity) in the cerebrospinal fluid.
      b. An increase in arterial PCO_2 causes a rapid change in pH of the cerebrospinal fluid, increases the depth and rate of respiration, and decreases the PCO_2 level.
      c. Changes in hydrogen ion and bicarbonate ion concentrations are not as quickly recognized as changes in the PCO_2 by the central chemoreceptors; therefore, responses to metabolic imbalances are slower.
      d. Receptors are located in the medulla oblongata and adjacent structures.
   2. Peripheral chemoreceptors.
      a. Receptor cells are located in the carotid body at the bifurcation of the common carotid arteries and at the aortic arch.
      b. Impulses from the aortic arch are transmitted to the brain via the vagus nerve.
      c. Impulses from the carotid body are transmitted to the brain via the glossopharyngeal nerve.
      d. The peripheral chemoreceptors primarily respond quickly to a decreased PO_2 (below 50 mm Hg) and, to some extent, to alteration of the PCO_2 and hydrogen ion concentration in the arterial blood.

System Assessment

✦ A. Check for airway patency.
   1. Clear out secretions.
   2. Insert oral airway if necessary.
   3. Position client on side if there is no cervical spine injury.
   4. Place hand or cheek over nose and mouth of client to feel if client is ventilating.

✦ B. Listen to lung sounds.
   1. Absence of breath sounds: indicates lungs not expanding, due to either obstruction or deflation.
   2. Crackles (rales): indicate vibrations of fluid in lungs.
   3. Rhonchi (coarse sounds): indicate partial (fluid) obstruction of airway.
   4. Decreased breath sounds: indicate poorly ventilated lungs.
   5. Detection of bronchial sounds that are deviated from normal position: indicates mediastinal shift due to collapse of lung.
   ✦ 6. Where breath sounds are heard.
      a. Bronchovesicular—heard over mainstem bronchi.
      b. Vesicular (normal)—heard over lung parenchyma.
      c. Bronchial—heard over trachea above sternal notch.

C. Determine level of consciousness; decreased sensorium can indicate hypoxia.

D. Observe sputum or tracheal secretions; bloody sputum can indicate contusions of lung or injury to trachea and other anatomical structures.

E. Evaluate vital signs for temperature, respiratory rate, pulse, and changes in skin color.

F. Evaluate for tightness or fullness in chest.

G. Determine degree of pain client is experiencing.

H. Observe for PVCs if client is on monitor.

I. Assess for respiratory complications.
   1. Breathing patterns.
   2. Evaluate cough.
      a. Normally a protective mechanism utilized to keep the tracheobronchial tree free of secretions.
      b. Common symptom of respiratory disease.
   3. Assess for bronchospasm.
      a. Bronchi narrow and secretions may be retained.
      b. Condition may lead to infection.
   4. Observe for hemoptysis—expectoration of blood or blood-tinged sputum.
   5. Assess for cyanosis—late sign of hypoxia, due to large amounts of reduced hemoglobin in the blood (PaO_2 of about 50 mm Hg).
   6. Observe for hypoxia (anoxia)—a deficiency of oxygen in the body tissues.
   7. Evaluate for hypercapnia.
      a. Occurs when carbon dioxide is retained.
      b. High levels of oxygen depress and/or paralyze the medullary respiratory center.
      c. Peripheral chemoreceptors (sensitive to oxygen) become the stimuli for breathing.
   8. Assess for presence of respiratory alkalosis or acidosis.

J. Assess for other system complications.
   1. Evaluate for polycythemia—increase in RBCs as a compensatory response to hypoxemia.
   2. Observe for clubbing of fingers. Pathogenesis is not well understood.
   3. Evaluate for cor pulmonale—enlargement of the right ventricle as a result of pulmonary arterial hypertension following respiratory pathology.

✦ ABNORMAL BREATHING PATTERNS

- Dyspnea—labored or difficult breathing.
- Hyperpnea—abnormal deep breathing.
- Hypopnea—reduced depth of breathing.
- Orthopnea—difficulty breathing in other than upright position.
- Tachypnea—rapid breathing.
- Stridor—noisy respirations as air is forced through a partially obstructed airway.

---

   4. Evaluate for chest pain.
   5. Assess for atelectasis.
   6. Check for abdominal distention.
   7. Assess for hypertension.
   8. Evaluate cardiac status: CHF, cerebral edema, arrhythmias.
   9. Assess for trauma to thorax.

K. Assess oxygen concentration with noninvasive pulse oximetry.
   1. Sensor probe on earlobe, finger, or toe registers light passing through vascular bed.
   2. Allows continual monitoring of arterial oxygen saturation.

L. Assess for conditions associated with respiratory failure.
   1. Infectious diseases: tuberculosis, pneumonia.
   2. Obstruction of airway: pulmonary embolism, chronic bronchitis, bronchiectasis, emphysema, asthma, cardiac disorders leading to pulmonary congestion.
   3. Restrictive lung disease: pleural effusion, pneumothorax, atelectasis, pulmonary tumors, obesity.
   4. CNS depression: drugs, head injury, CNS infection.
   5. Chest wall trauma: flail chest, neuromuscular disease, congenital deformities.

Diagnostic Procedures

Radiologic Studies

A. Chest x-ray.

B. Lung scintigraphy: measures concentration of gamma rays from lung after intake of isotope.

C. Perfusion studies: outline pulmonary vascular structures after intake of radioactive isotopes IV. (Check for dye allergy.)

D. Computed tomography (CT).

E. Magnetic resonance imaging (MRI)—have client remove any metal before tests.

Bronchoscopy

A. A flexible fiberoptic scope to visualize the interior of the tracheobronchial tree.

B. Used as a therapeutic tool to remove foreign materials, diagnosis, biopsy, specimen collection.

C. Nursing care.
   1. Keep client NPO 6–8 hours before procedure.
   2. Explain sedation and local anesthesia of nasal and oral pharynx.
   3. Postprocedure: check client's ability to control secretions. Keep NPO until gag reflex returns.
   4. Observe for potential complications of laryngospasm, laryngeal edema, anesthesia complications, subcutaneous emphysema.
   5. Client may expect hoarseness and sore throat.

Biopsy of Respiratory Tissue

A. May be done by needle, via bronchoscope, or an open lung procedure biopsy.

B. Nursing care: observe for hemothorax and/or pneumothorax.

Thoracentesis

A. A needle puncture through the chest wall to remove air or fluid.

B. Used for diagnostic and/or therapeutic purposes.

✦ C. Nursing care: observe for possible pneumothorax postprocedure (↑ pulse, pallor, chest pain, dyspnea, tachycardia).

Pulmonary Function Tests

A. Measure of body's ability to mechanically ventilate and to effect gaseous exchange.

B. Tests include spirometry, measurement of gas volume and airway resistance, diffusing capacity, and arterial blood gases. (*See* Lung Volumes under Principles of Ventilation, page 248.)

C. Nursing care.
   1. Avoid scheduling immediately after meals.
   2. Hold bronchodilators (inhaled) for 6 hours prior to tests.

Skin Tests

✦ A. Mantoux test for tuberculosis.
   1. The most reliable test to confirm infection.
   2. 0.1 mL tuberculin injected intradermally—PPD is standard-strength purified protein derivative.
   3. Test read 48–72 hours postintradermal wheal production.
   4. Erythema not important.
   5. Area of induration is more than 10 mm: indicates positive reaction (client has had contact with the tubercle bacillus). For HIV or severely immune suppressed, test is positive if induration is 5 mm or greater.
   6. When skin test is positive, chest x-ray and sputum cultures important to rule out active TB or old, resolved TB lesions.
   7. Reactions of 5–9 mm require retest.

B. Tine test (not recommended for diagnosis).
   1. Test read on third day.
   2. Mantoux test required if induration is more than 2 mm.

Arterial Blood Studies

A. Arterial blood gases.
   ✦ 1. Indicate respiratory function by measuring:
      a. Oxygen (PO_2).
      b. Carbon dioxide (PCO_2).
      c. pH.
      d. Oxygen saturation.
      e. Bicarbonate (HCO_3).
   2. Determine state of acid–base balance.
   3. Reveal the adequacy of the lungs to provide oxygen and to remove carbon dioxide.
   4. Assess degree to which kidneys can maintain a normal pH.

✦ B. Normal arterial values.
   1. Oxygen saturation: 93–98 percent.
   2. PaO_2: 95 mm Hg.
   3. Arterial pH: 7.35–7.45 (7.4).
   4. PCO_2: 35–45 mm Hg (40).
   5. HCO_3 content: 24–30 mEq (25).
   6. Base excess: −3 to +3 (0).

System Implementation

✦ A. Maintain patent airway.
   1. Suction.
   2. Intubation.
      a. Oral airway.
      b. Endotracheal intubation.

B. Maintain adequate ventilation.
   1. Place in Fowler's position to facilitate lung expansion.
   2. Encourage coughing and breathing exercises.
   3. If client needs help breathing, a ventilator may be used.
      a. Ventilator simulates breathing action usually provided by diaphragm and thoracic cage.
      b. Type of ventilator depends on specific needs of client.

C. Administer oxygen therapy using specific oxygen equipment according to the percentage of oxygen required by client with humidity therapy.

D. Monitor blood gases to determine how well client's oxygen needs are being met.

E. Maintain fluid and electrolyte balance.
   ✦ 1. When blood and fluid loss are replaced, watch carefully for fluid overload, which can lead to pulmonary edema.
   2. Record intake and output.

F. Maintain acid–base balance; make frequent blood gas determination as acid–base imbalances occur readily with compromised respirations or with mechanical ventilation.

G. Provide for relief of pain.
   ✦ 1. Analgesics should be used with caution as they depress respirations. (Demerol is the drug of choice.)
   2. Atropine, morphine sulfate, and barbiturates should be avoided.
   3. Nerve block may be used.

H. Administer electrocardiogram to establish associated cardiac damage.

I. Provide for incentive spirometry and chest physio-therapy.

J. Maintain hydration status.
    1. Necessary to liquefy secretions or prevent formation of thick, tenacious secretions.
    2. Monitor oral intake of fluids, IV administration of fluids, or humidification to tracheobronchial tree.

K. Administer appropriate drug therapy for respiratory condition.

Hypoxic Condition

✦ *Definition:* Oxygen deficiency—the primary indication for initiation of oxygen therapy.

✦ **Assessment**

A. Check to see if client has a patent airway.
B. Assess client's vital signs.
C. Observe existence of PVCs if client is on monitor.
D. Observe client for any of the following signs. If these signs are evident, you may need to administer oxygen.
    1. Tachycardia.
    2. Gasping and/or irregular respirations (dyspnea).
    3. Restlessness.
    4. Flaring nostrils.
    5. Cyanosis.
    6. Substernal or intercostal retractions.
    7. Increased blood pressure followed by decreased blood pressure.
    8. Abnormal ABGs.
✦ E. Assess for side effects of oxygen therapy.
    ✦ 1. Atelectasis.
        a. Nitrogen is washed out of the lungs when a high FIO_2 is delivered to client.
        b. In alveoli free of nitrogen, oxygen diffuses out of the alveoli into the blood faster than ventilation brings oxygen into the alveoli.
        c. This results in a collapse (atelectasis) of the affected alveoli.
    ✦ 2. Pulmonary oxygen toxicity.
        a. High FIO_2 delivered over a long period of time (48 hours) results in destruction of the pulmonary capillaries and lung tissue.
        b. The clinical picture resembles that of pulmonary edema.
    ✦ 3. Retrolental fibroplasia.
        a. Blindness resulting from high FIO_2 delivered to premature infants.
        b. This condition is seen in prolonged FIO_2 of 100 percent when high levels of oxygen are not needed.
    ✦ 4. Carbon dioxide narcosis.

✦ STAGES OF HYPOXIA

Early symptoms
Restlessness
Headache, visual disturbances
Slight confusion
Hyperventilation
Tachycardia
Hypertension (mild)
Dyspnea
Decreased pulse oximetry
Late symptoms
Hypotension
Bradycardia
Metabolic acidosis (production of lactic acid)
Cyanosis
Chronic oxygen lack
Polycythemia
Clubbing of fingers and toes
Thrombosis

---

        a. Carbon dioxide narcosis can develop if hypoxic drive is removed by administering FIO_2 to return the arterial PO_2 to normal range.
        b. Symptoms of carbon dioxide narcosis.
            (1) Decreased mentation.
            (2) Flushed, pink skin.
            (3) Flaccid (sometimes twitching) extremities.
            (4) Shallow breathing.
            (5) Respiration arrest.
F. Evaluate client for clinical manifestations of COPD.
    1. Ventilatory drive is hypoxemic.
    2. Oxygen administration requires critical observation. Start at 2 L/min.

Implementation

A. Monitor lung sounds for adequate ventilation.
B. Monitor client for signs of oxygen toxicity.
C. Provide skin care for areas surrounding oxygen equipment.
✦ D. Administer oxygen at appropriate flow with specified equipment.
    1. Nasal prongs and cannula.
        a. Easily tolerated by clients.
        b. The FIO_2 will vary depending on the flow.
            (1) FIO_2: 24–28 percent.   Flow: 1–2 L.
            (2) FIO_2: 30–35 percent.   Flow: 3–4 L.
            (3) FIO_2: 38–44 percent.   Flow: 5–6 L.
    2. Simple face mask.
        a. Requires fairly high flows to prevent rebreathing of carbon dioxide.
        b. Accurate FIO_2 difficult to estimate.
        c. FIO_2: 35–65 percent.   Flow: 8–12 L.

3. Mask with reservoir bag.
   a. Higher FIO_2 is delivered because of the reservoir.
   b. At flows less than 6 L/min, risk of rebreathing carbon dioxide increases.
      (1) Partial rebreathing mask: FIO_2: 40–60 percent.   Flow: 6–10 L.
      (2) Nonrebreather: FIO_2: 60–100 percent. Flow: 6–15 L.
4. Venturi mask.
   a. Delivers fixed or predicted FIO_2.
   b. Utilized effectively in clients with COPD when accurate FIO_2 is necessary for proper treatment.
   c. FIO_2: 24–50 percent.
5. Face tent.
   a. Well tolerated by clients but sometimes difficult to keep in place.
   b. Convenient for providing humidification with compressed air in conjunction with nasal prongs.
   c. FIO_2: 28–100 percent.   Flow: 8–12 L.
6. Oxygen hood.
   a. Hood fits over child's head.
   b. Provides warm, humidified oxygen at high concentrations.
   c. FIO_2: 28–85 percent.   Flow: 5–12 L.
7. Intratracheal oxygen device for long-term therapy.

INFECTIOUS DISEASES

Pulmonary Tuberculosis

✦ *Definition:* Airborne, infectious, communicable disease thought to be caused by *Mycobacterium tuberculosis*. May affect any part of the body, but is most common in the lungs. Disease may be acute or chronic.

✦ A. Tubercle bacilli is rod-shaped and gram-positive, acid fast.
B. Diagnostic findings.
   1. Early AM sputum for smear and culture: positive acid-fast bacillus.
   2. Fiberoptic bronchoscopy and chest x-ray (to determine presence and extent of TB).
   3. Increased WBC and ESR.
   4. Positive Mantoux skin test.
C. Most people infected do not develop clinical illness because the immune system brings infection under control.
D. Persons at risk: persons with HIV, immunosuppressed, the elderly, certain minority groups, persons in close contact with infectious TB, persons who have live dormant bacilli from an initial infection

---

✦ MANTOUX SKIN TEST

- Purified protein derivative (PPD) tuberculin antigen.
- PPD tuberculin injected intradermally to form wheal 5–10 mm.
- Test read 48–72 hours: positive induration is 10-mm diameter or more.
- Results mean client has had contact recently or in the past—does not signify active disease is present, or has recently been vaccinated with BCG.
- BCG (bacille Calmette–Guérin) vaccine produces a greater resistance to developing TB—more commonly used in Europe than in United States.
- If false positive for Mantoux is suspected, chest x-ray and AFB (acid-fast bacilli) sputum done.

---

acquired years before. Also, those with lowered resistance from alcoholism, those who take steroids, or those who are poorly nourished.
E. Pathophysiology.
   1. Inhaled airborne droplets containing the bacteria infect the alveoli, which become the focus of infection—transmission requires close frequent or prolonged exposure.
   2. After entrance of tubercle bacilli, the body attempts to wall off the organism by phagocytosis and lymphocytosis.
   3. Macrophages surround the bacilli and form tubercles.
   4. Tubercles go through the process of caseation— a necrotic process. (Cells become an amorphous cheese-like mass and may be encapsulated to form a nodule.)
   5. Caseous nodule erodes and sputum is released, leaving an air-filled cavity.
   6. Initial lesion may disseminate by extension, via bloodstream or lymph system, and through bronchi.

Assessment
A. Evaluate pulmonary symptoms.
   1. Cough (at cavitation stage).
   2. Sputum production—initially dry, then purulent.
   3. Dyspnea.
   4. Hemoptysis.
   5. Pleuritic pain (with pleural involvement).
   6. Rales.
B. Evaluate systemic symptoms.
   1. Fatigue, malaise.
   2. Night sweats, low-grade fever in afternoon.
   3. Weight loss.
   4. Anorexia.
   5. Irritability, lassitude.
   6. Tachycardia.

C. Complete physical examination.

D. Complete social and medical history.

E. Examine sputum—takes 3–8 weeks for results.

F. Check tuberculin test.

Implementation

✦ A. Maintain respiratory precautions.
  1. Client is not considered infectious 2–3 weeks after initiation of chemotherapy.
  2. Teach client methods to prevent spread of droplets when coughing.

✦ B. Monitor administration of medications—a combination of drugs are used to destroy variable microbial organisms.

✦ C. Sputum smears obtained every 2–4 weeks until negative (sputum cultures become negative in 3–5 months).

✦ D. Chemoprophylaxis.
  ✦ 1. Isoniazid and vitamin B_6 therapy for 6 months given to those infected with tubercle bacillus without the disease, or to those at high risk for development of the disease.
  ✦ 2. Evaluate for potential complications of INH therapy: check for hepatitis (rare), excessive tiredness, weakness, loss of appetite, nausea, vomiting, dark yellow or brown urine, jaundice, diarrhea, vision problems, eye pain, numbness or tingling in hands and feet, rash, fever, swollen glands, joint pain, sore throat, stomach pains or RUQ tenderness.
  3. Evaluate for potential complications of RIF therapy: hepatitis (rare), headache, muscle pain, bone pain, heartburn, nausea, vomiting, stomach cramps, chills, diarrhea, rash, sores on skin or in mouth, fever, jaundice. Urine, stools, saliva, sputum, sweat, and tears may turn red–orange.
  4. Evaluate for potential complications of PZA therapy: hepatitis (rare), upset stomach, fatigue, rash, fever, vomiting, loss of appetite, jaundice, darkened urine, pain and swelling in joints, unusual bleeding or bruising, difficulty urinating.
  5. Evaluate for potential complications of EMB therapy: blurred vision, sudden changes in vision, inability to see colors red and green, loss of appetite, upset stomach, vomiting, numbness and tingling in hands or feet, rash, itching.
  6. Encourage client to report for frequent prescribed liver function studies.

✦ E. Work with client to maintain compliance—the major problem in eliminating TB.
  1. Strict compliance to drug regimen.
  2. Monthly follow-up visits for sputum smear until conversion.

F. Directly observed therapy (DOT).

TB MEDICATIONS

Drugs Used to Treat TB

The following drugs are recommended as initial treatment regimen for active TB. Treatment almost always consists of four antibiotics: Isoniazid—INH (Laniazid, Nydrazid), rifampin—RIF (Rifadin, Rimactane), pyrazinamide—PZA, ethambutol—EMB (Myambutol).

First-line TB drugs: 2 months of isoniazid (INH), rifampin (RIF), and pyrazinamide (PZA); followed by 4 months of INH and RIF.

✦• Streptomycin or ethambutol will be added for 1–3 weeks until sensitivity results and then discontinued if organisms are sensitive to other drugs in the regimen.
  a. Daily alcohol intake and antacids containing aluminum interfere with metabolism and absorption, respectively.
  b. Monitor kidney function if client is taking streptomycin.
• Rifapentine (Priftin) was a new drug approved in 1998—first new TB drug in 10 years.
  a. As effective as rifampin, but with a longer half-life.
  b. Clients need to take it less often, so compliance is increased.
• Drug regimen varies with age, number of bacilli in client's smear, and susceptibility to drug therapy and compliance.
• **Adverse Effects:** Relatively common, especially during the first few weeks of therapy, but clients should not discontinue treatment because of minor side effects. If more serious side effects—particularly drug-induced hepatitis—develop, isoniazid, rifampin, and pyrazinamide should be stopped immediately and then restarted one-by-one to determine which drug was causing the problem. (Ethambutol does not damage the liver.)

Second-line drugs: used for resistant clients: capreomycin, kanamycin, para-aminosalicylic acid, cycloserine and lerofloxacin, ofloxacin, ciprofloxacin.
• Drugs are more effective when administered in single daily dose.
• Drug resistance is a problem, especially in certain populations: poor compliance, previously treated for TB.
• Corticosteroids may be used in severe cases, together with antituberculosis agents, to reduce symptoms.
• Clients with latent TB are sometimes prescribed drug therapy—typically isoniazid once daily for 6 months to a year—to prevent the disease from progressing to active TB.

---

1. This therapy involves observing the ingestion of every dose of medicine the TB client is supposed to take.
  a. This observation continues for the entire course of treatment.
  b. Completing the course of therapy is essential; incomplete treatment can lead to reactivation of TB.
2. The decision to implement DOT is based on risk factors evaluated by the nurse.

✦ G. Instruct client in ways to prevent spread of disease.

1. Cover nose and mouth with a few layers of disposable tissue when sneezing or coughing.
2. Expectorate into a disposable sputum container.
3. Maintain adequate air ventilation.

H. Decontaminate infected air by nonrecirculated air or ultraviolet rays.
I. Provide well-balanced diet: high carbohydrate, high protein, high vitamin B_6.
J. Provide frequent oral hygiene.
K. Drug resistent TB is beginning to appear in the United States.

Pneumonia

Definition: An acute inflammatory process of the lung parenchyma, resulting in lung consolidation as the alveoli and bronchioles fill with exudate. Can be caused by bacteria, viruses, fungi, chemicals.

Assessment

A. Assess for type of pneumonia (classification).
1. Community-acquired pneumonia (CAP)—acquired outside the hospital; lower respiratory tract infection.
   a. Typical.
      (1) *Streptococcus pneumoniae* is the most common bacterial organism, followed by *Haemophilus influenzae.*
      (2) Communicable disease.
      (3) Young males most affected.
      (4) Clinical manifestations.
         (a) Rapid onset, severe chills, high temperature (103–106°F).
         (b) Tachypnea, rapid pulse.
         (c) Productive cough with purulent sputum.
         (d) Pleuritic pain.
         (e) Anxiety.
         (f) Dyspnea.
         (g) Bronchial breath sounds, crackles.
   b. Atypical.
      (1) *Legionella, Mycoplasma,* and *Chlamydia* are the common organisms causing infections.
      (2) More gradual onset.
      (3) Dry cough.
      (4) Headache, fatigue, sore throat.
      (5) Nausea, vomiting.
      (6) Crackles.
2. Hospital-acquired pneumonia (HAP)—leading cause of mortality stemming from nosocomial infections. Occurs 48 hours after hospitalization.
   a. Common organisms include *Pseudomonas, Enterobacter, Staphylococcus aureus,* and

Streptococcus pneumoniae, which enter lungs after aspiration of particles from client's own pharynx.
   b. Risk factors.
      (1) Aspiration.
      (2) Abdominal surgery.
      (3) Immunosuppressant therapy.
      (4) Prolonged mechanical ventilation.
      (5) Structural lung disease.
   c. Clinical manifestations—may represent other disease processes like tuberculosis, heart failure.
      (1) Fever, chills, diaphoresis.
      (2) Wheezing, inspiratory rales.
      (3) Productive cough, increased pulmonary secretions.
      (4) Fatigue, pallor, malaise.
      (5) Tachypnea, tachycardia.
3. Aspiration pneumonia—aspiration of material in mouth into trachea and lungs. Dependent areas of lung most often affected. Aspirate can be food, water, vomitus, chemicals.
   a. Secondary to other conditions such as age, debilitation, stasis, loss of consciousness.
   b. Onset insidious—initial manifestation may be airway obstruction.
4. Opportunistic pneumonia—clients with altered immune response very susceptible to respiratory infections.
   a. At-risk individuals include those with malnutrition, HIV/AIDS, transplants, cancer, immune deficiencies.
   b. Most common organisms involved are *Pneumocystis carinii,* cytomegalovirus and fungi.
   c. Clinical manifestations: fever, chills, dry nonproductive cough, malaise, fatigue.

B. Assess for excerbation of chronic obstructive pulmonary disease as respiratory infections precipitate this condition.
C. Observe for an increase in the amount of sputum.
1. Change in the character of sputum (particularly color—yellow to green).
2. Onset of malaise or fever may indicate infection.

Implementation

◆ A. If possible, keep client ambulatory or change position frequently.
B. Elevate head of bed 30 degrees.
C. Encourage fluids to 3000 mL or more to provide hydration.
D. Observe and record type and amount of sputum.
E. Administer antibiotics as ordered.
1. Given for a period of 10–14 days.

2. Antibiotics most commonly used are penicillin G IV, ampicillin, Bactrim, vancomycin (staph pneumonia) and cephalosporins.
F. Provide physiotherapy as ordered (cough, deep-breathe, incentive spirometry).
G. Obtain throat sputum and blood cultures for specific organisms.
H. Determine O_2 need according to O_2 saturation and ABGs. Administer O_2 as indicated.
I. Administer antipyretic drugs and analgesics as needed.

Legionnaires' Disease

✦ *Definition:* An acute respiratory infection caused by gram-negative bacteria. The name was derived from an outbreak of the disease in Philadelphia in 1973 when members of the American Legion were attending a convention.

Assessment

✦ A. Assess the lungs, the organs most targeted by the bacteria.
1. Primary entry into the body is through the lungs.
2. The organisms are in infected water, usually transmitted via air conditioners and cooling towers.
3. Disease is not transmitted person to person.
B. Early symptoms.
1. Malaise.
2. Mild headache.
3. Dry cough.
C. Later symptoms.
1. Fever and chills—unremitting until therapy.
2. Other symptoms may be pleuritic pain, confusion, and impaired renal function.

Implementation

A. Diagnosis made from specific serum antibodies or by culture.
B. Monitor antibiotic therapy—erythromycin is drug of choice.
C. Nursing care is the same as for pneumonia.

Emerging Viruses

See Infection Control chapter, Chapter 6.

CHRONIC OBSTRUCTIVE PULMONARY DISEASE (COPD)

Definition: A functional category applied to respiratory disorders that obstruct the pathway of normal alveolar ventilation either by spasm of the airways, mucus secretions, or changes in the airway and/or alveoli.

COPD PRECAUTIONS

- Oxygen must be given via a low-flow controlled system.
- The Venturi mask provides O_2 at 24–40 percent.
- ABG measurements—important to maintain PaO_2 of 60–90 mm Hg. (If less than 55 mm Hg, client may require oxygen.)

Chronic Bronchitis

✦ *Definition:* A long-term inflammation of the mucous membranes of the bronchial tubes with recurrent cough and sputum production for 3 months or more in 2 consecutive years.

Characteristics

A. Cigarette smoking is probably the biggest culprit, inhibiting the ciliary activity of the bronchi, and resulting in increased stimulation of the mucous glands to secrete mucus.
B. Immunological factors and familial predisposition may also be implicated for those individuals who do not smoke.

Assessment

A. Assess for bronchoconstriction.
B. Evaluate malaise.
C. Check for exertional dyspnea.
D. Assess for hemoptysis.
E. Evaluate cough—may not be productive but may be purulent.
F. Assess for hypoxia.
G. Evaluate lung fields for the following: atelectasis, percussion—hyperresonant, tactile fremitus decreased, prolonged expiratory phase, expansion decreased, trachea midline, wheezes, rales.

✦ **Implementation**

A. Administer antibiotics when infection occurs.
B. Administer bronchodilators (drug of choice) to relieve bronchospasm and facilitate mucus expectoration.
C. Steroid therapy may be used, but it is still controversial.
D. Encourage fluids to 3000 mL daily to dilute secretions.
E. Provide chest physiotherapy.
✦ F. Monitor oxygen therapy.
✦ G. Teaching principles.
1. Stop smoking—this is the major irritant to the lungs and the major cause of death from cancer.
2. Avoid irritants or allergens and pollutants when possible.
3. Avoid high altitudes (where there is less oxygen).

4. Teach pursed-lip breathing (helps to open airway and stretching exercises).
5. Monitor edema in legs and ankles, which may signify right-sided heart failure.
6. Yearly flu and pneumococcal vaccines.

Bronchiectasis

✦ *Definition:* Thought to develop following airway obstruction or atelectasis. Characterized by permanent, abnormal dilation of one or more large bronchi, leading to destruction of elastic and muscular structures of bronchial wall. Most often associated with bacterial infections such as pneumonia or TB.

Assessment

A. Evaluate for frequent, severe paroxysms of coughing.
B. Assess for hemoptysis.
C. Check for fetid breath.
D. Assess for thick, profuse sputum.
E. Observe for breathlessness, fatigue.
F. Assess for profuse night sweats.
G. Assess for weight loss, anorexia.
✦ H. Evaluate lung fields and chest for the following:
   1. Trachea deviates to the affected side.
   2. Decreased expansion.
   3. Percussion—dull.
   4. Vocal fremitus and breath sounds absent if bronchus occluded.
   5. Vocal fremitus increased; bronchovesicular/bronchial breath sounds if bronchus open.
   6. Rales, rhonchi.

✦ Implementation

A. Administer antibiotics as ordered. Usually given for 7–10 days—may be long term.
B. Provide chest physiotherapy—postural drainage.
C. Administer bronchodilators and aerosolized nebulizer treatments to assist in removal of secretions.
D. Monitor oxygen therapy if hypoxia occurs.
E. Prepare client for surgery if severe hemoptysis occurs.
F. Encourage client to rest by providing quiet environment.
G. Provide high-protein diet with increased fluid intake.
H. Provide frequent mouth care.

Emphysema

Definition: The permanent overdistention of the alveoli with resulting destruction of the alveolar walls. (*Emphysema* is a Greek word meaning "overinflated.")

✦ Assessment

A. Alpha-antitrypsin deficiency causes condition to develop at a younger age.

B. Individual usually has a history of smoking, chronic cough, wheezing, and shortness of breath.
C. Observe for dyspnea—chief complaint.
D. Assess sputum production.
E. Observe for weight loss.
F. Assess for hypoxia, hypercapnia.
G. Observe physical characteristics of chest.
   1. Barrel chest.
   2. Expansion decreased.
   3. Flat diaphragm.
   4. Accessory muscles of respiration used.
H. Assess for decreased tactile fremitus.
I. Percuss for hyperresonance.
J. Auscultate for distant breath sounds.
K. Assess for prolonged expiratory phase.
L. Assess for wheezes, forced expiratory rhonchi.
M. Assess for complications.
   1. Pulmonary hypertension.
   2. Right-sided heart failure.
   3. Spontaneous pneumothorax.
   4. Acute respiratory failure.
   5. Peptic ulcer disease, GERD.

Implementation

A. Monitor for signs of impending hypoxia.
B. Monitor for alterations in lung sounds.
C. Instruct on pursed lip breathing exercises.
✦ D. Administer low concentration oxygen.
   1. Usually 2 L/min.
   2. Raise PaO_2 to 65–80 mm Hg.
E. Monitor for signs of carbon dioxide narcosis.
✦ F. Monitor medications.
   1. Inhaled bronchodilators (beta agonists: Proventil, Ventolin, Alupent)—to improve gas exchange by stimulating beta receptors in the lungs.
   2. Systemic corticosteroids—controversial: used when bronchodilators are unsuccessful or during an acute attack.
   3. Inhaled corticosteroids (Azmacort, Beclovent, AeroBid)—affect lungs with no systemic effects.
   4. Antibiotics—to combat infection.
G. Provide hydration.
   1. Necessary to liquefy secretions present, or to prevent formation of thick, tenacious secretions in clients with pulmonary disease.
   2. Modalities.
      a. Oral intake of fluids.
      b. IV administration of fluids.
      c. Humidification to tracheobronchial tree.
✦ H. Monitor humidification and aerosol therapy—important part of treatment plan.
   1. Humidity.
      a. Water content of a gas at a given temperature.

    b. Humidification can be delivered through humidifier or nebulizer.

2. Metered-dose inhaler therapy, nebulizer.
   a. Corticosteroids, beta$_2$-adrenergic agonists (isoproterenol), and anticholinergic agents may be administered alone or in combination.
   b. Nebulizers deliver aerosols.
3. Clinical implications.
   a. Relief of bronchospasm and mucosal edema.
   b. Mobilization of secretions.
   c. Humidification of the tracheobronchial tree.

✦ I. Provide for chest physiotherapy.
1. Postural drainage.
   a. Positions are utilized to promote gravitational drainage and mobilization of secretions of affected lung segments.
   b. Allows the client to expectorate secretions.
   c. Secretions may be aspirated through a sterile suctioning procedure.
✦ 2. Percussion and vibration.
   a. Valuable and necessary adjunct to postural drainage. Cupped-hand position used in percussion.
   b. Vibration of the chest is performed only during the expiratory phase of respiration.
✦ 3. Deep breathing and coughing.
   a. Should be encouraged often.
   b. Clients with COPD should be taught the mechanics of an effective cough.
      (1) Contract intercostal muscles.
      (2) Contract diaphragm.
      (3) Fill lungs with air.
✦ 4. Breathing exercises or exercise regimen—an integral part in the management of clients with coronary disease.
   ✦ a. Diaphragmatic breathing.
      (1) Breathe in via nose.
      (2) Exhale through slightly pursed lips.
      (3) Contract abdominal muscles while exhaling.
      (4) Chest should not move, but abdomen should do the moving. (Abdomen contracts at expiration.)
      (5) Exercises can be learned with client flat on back and then done in other positions.
   b. Accelerated diaphragmatic breathing.
   c. Chest expansion—apical, lateral (unilateral, bilateral), basal.
   d. Controlled breathing with daily activities and graded exercises to improve general physical fitness.
   e. Relaxation and stretching.
   f. General relaxation.
5. Pressure ventilation options.
   a. PEP (positive expiratory pressure).
   b. NIPPV (noninvasive positive-pressure ventilation).
   c. IPV (intrapulmonary percussive ventilation).
   d. IPPB use is very controversial and is not treament of choice.

J. Monitor carefully for complications of right-sided (cor pulmonale) and left-sided heart failure.

Asthma

Definition: An obstructive chronic inflammatory disorder of the airways manifested by narrowing of the airways and characterized by generalized bronchoconstriction, excess mucus secretion, and mucosal edema. More than 14.6 million people have asthma in the United States.

Assessment

✦ A. Assess classification of asthma.
1. Mild intermittent.
2. Mild persistent.
3. Moderate persistent.
4. Severe persistent.

B. Evaluate for precipitating factors and triggers, which may include emotions, infection, seasonal changes, occupational exposure to dusts or chemical irritants, certain drugs, exercise.

C. Evaluate for respiratory problems.
1. Cough may be nonproductive or very purulent.
2. Air hunger, dyspnea.
3. Wheezing.
4. Tachypnea.
5. Prolonged expiratory phase.
6. Tachycardia.
7. Hypoxia, cyanosis, hypercapnia.
✦ 8. Assess physical signs.
   a. Retraction of intercostal and sternal muscles.
   b. Percussion—hyperresonant.
   c. Distant breath sounds.
   d. Rhonchi, wheezes, rales.

✦ 9. Ominous signs.
    a. Diminished breath sounds.
    b. No wheezing (quiet chest).
    c. Increased respiratory rate.

Implementation

A. Provide supportive respiratory care.
B. Identify and avoid known triggers for asthma.
C. Avoid aspirin, NSAIDS.
D. Teach peak-flow monitoring.
E. Administer drug therapy.
✦ 1. Beta agonists (epinephrine, albuterol, terbutaline, isoetharine–Bronkosol).
    2. Methylxanthines (aminophylline and derivatives).
    3. Corticosteroids.
    4. Anticholinergics (atropine).
    5. Mast cell inhibitors (cromolyn sodium).
✦ F. Current treatment approach for asthma attack.
    1. During attack, bronchial mucosa releases histamine and slow-reacting substances of anaphylaxis (SRS-A) bronchoconstrictors.
    2. SRS-A are leukotrienes that cause airway inflammation, edema, and mucus secretion.
    3. New drugs are available that antagonize leukotrienes and reduce symptoms.
    4. Anti-inflammatory drugs taken orally are Accolate, Zyflo, and Singulair.
G. Sedatives and narcotics should be used with caution.
H. Administer oxygen via nasal cannula.
✦ I. Encourage fluids to 3000 mL daily.
J. Breathing exercises, postural drainage.
✦ K. Metered-dose inhaler (MDI) therapy has advantages over nebulized medications.
    1. Teach client to coordinate puff of drug with breath, hold for 10 seconds, one puff at a time.
    2. Use of holding chambers attached to MDI mouthpiece (spacers) enhance effectiveness.

RESTRICTIVE RESPIRATORY DISORDERS

Pleural Effusion

✦ *Definition:* A collection of nonpurulent fluid in the pleural space. Many pathological processes can irritate the pleurae and cause effusion, but in older clients cancer is a common cause. Empyema is a pleural effusion that contains pus.

✦ **Assessment**

A. Assess for dyspnea.
B. Check fatigue level, malaise.
C. Assess for elevated temperature.

TYPES OF PNEUMOTHORAX CONDITIONS

• **Tension pneumothorax—a medical emergency**
    a. The mediastinum shifts away from the side of the pneumothorax, compressing the unaffected lung.
    b. A large-bore needle introduced into the pleural cavity to release the pressure will change a tension pneumothorax into a simple pneumothorax.
    c. A tube thoracostomy is then performed.
• **Spontaneous (or closed) pneumothorax**
    a. Occurs suddenly when lung is weakened—air moves from lung to intrapleural space, causing collapse.
    b. If the pneumothorax is large or increasing in size, closed tube thoracostomy is performed.
    c. Chest tubes attached to water seal are utilized to reexpand the lung.
    d. A small pneumothorax may reabsorb on its own.
• **Hemothorax (blood in the thoracic cavity)**
    a. Hemothorax occurs with pneumothorax, especially if trauma is the causative factor.
    b. Treatment: evacuate the blood through chest tube insertion.

D. Assess for dry cough.
E. Assess for pleural pain.
F. Check for tachycardia.
G. Assess physical signs.
    1. Absence of movement on side of effusion.
    2. Percussion—dull.
    3. Decreased breath sounds.
    4. Pleural friction rub occurs in dry pleurisy; as effusion develops, friction rub disappears.
    5. Collapse of lung—when fluid increases in amount.
    6. Mediastinal structures shift position.
    7. Cardiac tamponade.

Implementation

✦ A. Assist with thoracentesis, which is used to aid in diagnosis and to relieve pressure by draining excess fluid.
    1. Explain procedure to client.
    2. Instruct client to tell you any compromising symptoms such as difficulty in breathing or discomfort.
    3. Give client reassurance during procedure.
B. Monitor vital signs.
C. Following removal of fluid, observe for bradycardia, hypotension, pain, pulmonary edema or pneumothorax.
D. Monitor administration of drugs if ordered for empyema.
E. Administer oxygen as ordered; high-Fowler's position.
F. Teach deep-breathing exercises to increase lung expansion and coughing.

G. Monitor chest tubes and drainage.

H. Encourage intake of fluids.

Pneumothorax

✦ *Definition:* A collection of air in the pleural cavity. As the air collects in the pleural space, the lung collapses and respiratory distress ensues. This condition occurs as a result of chest wall penetration by surgery or injury or when a disease process interrupts the internal structure of the lung.

✦ **Assessment**

A. Assess for sharp, sudden chest pain.

B. Assess for gasping respirations, dyspnea.

C. Check anxiety, vertigo.

D. Assess for hypotension.

E. Look for pallor.

F. Evaluate cough.

G. Check tachycardia.

H. Evaluate elevated temperature, diaphoresis.

I. Assess for hypoxia, hypercapnia.

J. Assess for physical signs.

    1. Paradoxical or diminished movement on the affected side.

    2. Percussion—hyperresonant.

    3. Absent breath sounds.

    4. Tactile fremitus decreased.

Implementation

A. Monitor vital signs frequently for impending shock.

B. Auscultate lungs frequently.

C. Monitor for respiratory distress.

D. Assist client to semi- or high-Fowler's position—maintain bedrest initially.

E. Reassure client, who will be anxious.

F. Prepare for possible thoracentesis and/or chest tube placement.

Acute Respiratory Distress Syndrome (ARDS)

Definition: Inflammatory syndrome marked by disruption of the alveolar-capillary membrane. Sudden, progressive form of acute respiratory failure from damaged alveolar-capillary membranes, with increased permeability to intravascular fluid. Mortality rate approximately 50%.

Characteristics

A. Conditions predisposing to ARDS.

    1. Aspiration.

    2. Pneumonia.

    3. Chest trauma.

    4. Oxygen toxicity.

    5. Embolism.

B. Manifestations.

    1. Dyspnea, cough, restlessness, scattered crackles (early).

    2. Severe dyspnea, retractions.

    3. Hypoxemia, hypercapnia.

    4. Crackles, rhonchi, pulmonary edema.

    5. Decreased lung compliance.

    6. Mental status changes.

Assessment

A. Assess for cyanosis.

B. Assess for shallow, increased respirations, restlessness.

C. Evaluate use of accessory muscles for breathing.

D. Assess for decreased breath sounds.

Implementation

A. Monitor oxygen therapy—leading to intubation and ventilation.

B. Use prone positioning to increase PaO_2.

C. Monitor ABGs.

D. Monitor pulmonary artery catheter for pressure monitoring.

E. Maintain fluid balance.

Cancer of the Lung

Definition: Pulmonary tumors are either primary or metastatic and interrupt the normal physiological internal structures of the lung.

Characteristics

✦ A. Classification of lung cancer is designated by anatomic location or by histological pattern.

    1. Anatomic classification.

        a. Central lesions involve the tracheobronchial tube up to the distal bronchi.

        b. Peripheral lesions extend from the distal bronchi and include the bronchioles.

    2. Four histologic types.

        a. Squamous cell (epidermoid).

            (1) Most frequent lung lesions.

            (2) Affects more men than women.

            (3) Associated with cigarette smoking.

            (4) Lesion usually starts in bronchial area and extends.

            (5) Metastasis not usually a rapid process.

        b. Adenocarcinoma.

            (1) Usually develops in peripheral tissue (smaller bronchi).

            (2) Metastasizes by blood route.

            (3) May be associated with focal lung scars.

            (4) Affects more women than men.

            (5) Bronchiole—alveolar cell and bronchogenic are two types.

  c. Small-cell anaplastic or oat cell carcinoma.
      (1) Aggressive and spreads bilaterally.
      (2) Considered metastatic because usually spreads to distant sites.
  d. Large-cell (undifferentiated) carcinoma—usually spreads through the bloodstream; high correlation with smoking.
B. Detection—pulmonary lesions are not usually detected by physical exam, and symptoms do not occur until process is extensive. Chest x-ray is very helpful in diagnosis; also CT scan and MRI.

✦ **Assessment**

A. Assess for pulmonary symptoms.
    1. Persistent cough that changes in character (most common sign).
    2. Dyspnea.
    3. Bloody sputum.
    4. Long-term pulmonary infection.
    5. Atelectasis.
    6. Bronchiectasis.
    7. Chest pain.
    8. Chills, fever.
B. Assess for systemic symptoms.
    1. Weakness.
    2. Weight loss.
    3. Anemia.
    4. Anorexia.
    5. Metabolic syndromes.
        a. Hypercalcemia.
        b. Inappropriate ADH.
        c. Cushing's syndrome.
        d. Gynecomastia.
    6. Neuromuscular changes.
        a. Peripheral neuropathy.
        b. Corticocerebellar degeneration.
    7. Connective tissue abnormalities.
        a. Clubbing.
        b. Arthralgias.
    8. Dermatologic abnormalities.
    9. Vascular changes.

Implementation

A. Comprehensive supportive care of client in the preoperative and postoperative state. (*See* section on care of the operative client.)
✦ B. Nursing care for common lung cancer symptoms.
    1. Cough.
        a. Encourage fluid intake.
        b. Monitor amount, type, and change of color of sputum.
        c. Avoid lung irritants.
        d. Give antitussives as ordered.

MEDICAL IMPLICATIONS

Diagnostic Evaluation
- Chest x-ray—a negative film does not rule out cancer.
- Cytologic examination of sputum—to detect malignant cells.
- Bronchoscopy—view of tracheobronchial tree; to stage cancer.
- Percutaneous fine-needle aspiration—tissue for diagnosis.
- Bone scan or bone marrow for metastasis; computed tomography may show primary tumor and metastasis.
- Mediastinoscopy—examination of lymph nodes through a small incision over sternal notch.

Management
- Surgery for localized tumors (Stage I and II)
- Radiation therapy
- Chemotherapy with multiple drugs (cisplatin and topoisomerase inhibitors)

✦ 2. Dyspnea.
      a. Teach coughing, deep breathing, and pursed-lip breathing.
      b. Administer humidified oxygen as ordered.
      c. Suction to remove secretions as needed.
      d. Position for comfort—high-Fowler's leaning over a cushion may help.
      e. Administer medications: bronchodilators, anxiolytic agents.
  3. Hemoptysis.
      a. Administer antibiotics as needed.
      b. Mild symptoms may resolve; instruct client to notify physician if bleeding continues or worsens.
  4. Fatigue.
      a. Monitor blood count.
      b. Teach client to pace activities, rest frequently, and ask for help.
  5. Pain.
      a. Develop a plan for analgesia administration.
      b. Teach alternative techniques for managing pain: relaxation, biofeedback.
  6. Weight loss.
      a. Consult with nutritionist for planning—use nutritional supplements.
      b. Request appetite stimulant from physician.
      c. Encourage client to rest before and after meals.
C. Give appropriate information to client to allay anxiety and clarify expectations.
D. Instruct client in postoperative procedures to minimize complications.
E. Give psychological support.
See Chapter 9, Oncology Nursing.

THORACIC TRAUMA

Trauma Assessment

✦ A. Check for airway patency.
  1. Clear out secretions.
  2. Insert oral airway if necessary.
  3. Position client on side if there is no cervical spine injury.
  4. Place hand or cheek over nose and mouth of client to feel if client is breathing.
✦ B. Inspect thoracic cage for injury.
  1. Inspect for contusions, abrasions, and symmetry of chest movement.
  2. If open wound of chest, cover with a nonporous dressing, taped on three sides to allow vent and prevent tension pneumothorax.
  3. Watch for symmetrical movement of chest. Asymmetrical movement indicates
    a. Flail chest.
    b. Tension pneumothorax.
    c. Hemothorax.
    d. Fractured ribs.
  4. Observe color; cyanosis indicates decreased oxygenation.
  5. Observe type of breathing; stertorous breathing usually indicates obstructed respiration.
✦ C. Auscultate lung sounds.
  1. Absence of breath sounds: indicates lungs not expanding, due to either obstruction or deflation.
  2. Rales or crackles (crackling sounds): indicate vibrations of fluid in lungs.
  3. Rhonchi (coarse sounds): indicate partial obstruction of airway.
  4. Decreased breath sounds: indicate poorly ventilated lungs.
  5. Detection of bronchial sounds that are deviated from normal position: indicates mediastinal shift due to collapse of lung.
D. Determine level of consciousness; decreased sensorium can indicate hypoxia.
E. Observe sputum or tracheal secretions; bloody sputum can indicate contusions of lung or injury to trachea and other anatomical structures.

Trauma Implementation

A. Take history from client if feasible or family member, witness to trauma or emergency personnel to aid in total evaluation of client's condition.
B. Administer electrocardiogram to establish if there is associated cardiac damage.
✦ C. Maintain patent airway.
  1. Suction.

  2. Intubation.
    a. Oral airway.
    b. Endotracheal intubation.
D. Maintain adequate ventilation.
E. Maintain fluid and electrolyte balance.
  1. When blood and fluid loss is replaced, watch carefully for fluid overload, which can lead to pulmonary edema.
  2. Record intake and output.
F. Maintain acid–base balance; make frequent blood gas determinations, as acid–base imbalances occur readily with compromised respirations or with mechanical ventilation.
G. Provide relief of pain.
  1. Analgesics should be used with caution because they depress respirations. (Demerol is rarely used now due to its CNS neurotoxic effects.)
  2. Morphine sulfate and other opioids can be used with careful monitoring.
  3. Nerve block may be used.

THORACIC INJURIES

Definition: Thoracic injuries involve trauma to the chest wall, lungs, heart, great vessels and esophagus. Injuries occur as a result of blunt trauma (i.e., crush injury) or penetrating trauma (i.e., gunshot wound).

✦ ### Hemothorax or Pneumothorax

✦ *Definition:* Hemothorax refers to blood in pleural space. Pneumothorax refers to air in pleural space. As air or fluid accumulates in pleural space, positive pressure builds up, collapsing the lung.

Assessment

A. Evaluate pain.
B. Auscultate for decreased breath sounds.
C. Observe for tracheal shift to unaffected side.
D. Observe for dyspnea and respiratory embarrassment.
E. Observe for hypovolemic shock, hypotension.
F. Inspect chest for asymmetrical expansion.

Implementation

✦ A. Assist with the insertion of a large-bore needle into the second intercostal space, midclavicular line, followed by aspiration of the fluid or air by means of thoracentesis.
B. Assist with insertion of chest tubes and connection to closed-chest drainage.
C. Continuously observe vital signs for complications such as shock and cardiac failure.
D. *See* Restrictive Respiratory Disorders: Pneumothorax.

✦ Open Wounds of the Chest

✦ **Assessment**

A. Assess for air entering and leaving the wound during inspiration and expiration.

B. Evaluate if intrapleural negative pressure is lost, thereby embarrassing respirations, leading to hypoxia. Death can occur if not corrected promptly.

✦ **Implementation**

A. Cover with occlusive dressing taped on three sides and vented to allow air to escape and decrease risk of tension pneumothorax.

B. Place client on assisted ventilation if necessary.

C. Prepare for insertion of chest tubes.

D. Place client in high-Fowler's position (unless contraindicated) to assist in adequate ventilation.

Fractured Ribs

Assessment

A. Evaluate pain and tenderness over fracture area, especially on inspiration.

B. Observe for bruising at injury site.

C. Evaluate respiratory embarrassment occurring from splinters puncturing lung and causing pneumothorax.

D. Observe client for splinting of chest causing shallow respirations. Splinting causes a reduction in lung compliance as well as respiratory acidosis.

Implementation

✦ A. Decrease pain to promote good chest expansion. Narcotics drug therapy used with caution due to respiratory depression.

B. Encourage deep breathing and coughing to prevent respiratory complications such as atelectasis and pneumonia.

C. Observe for signs of hemorrhage and shock.

D. Assist with intercostal nerve block if necessary to decrease pain.

Flail Chest

Definition: Multiple rib fractures that result in an unstable chest wall, with subsequent respiratory impairment causing flail area to move paradoxically to intact portion of chest during respiration.

Assessment

A. Evaluate for severe chest pain.

B. Observe for dyspnea leading to cyanosis.

C. Assess for tachypnea with shallow respirations.

✦ D. Assess if detached portion of flail chest is moving in opposition to other areas of chest cage and lung.

   1. On inspiration, the affected chest area is depressed; on expiration, it is bulging outward.

   2. This causes poor expansion of lungs, which results in carbon dioxide retention and respiratory acidosis.

✦ E. Evaluate ability to cough effectively. Inability leads to accumulation of fluids and respiratory complications such as pneumonia and atelectasis.

F. Assess for signs of cardiac failure due to impaired filling of right side of heart. This condition results from high venous pressure caused by paradoxical breathing.

G. Observe for rapid, shallow, and noisy respirations and accessory muscle breathing.

✦ **Implementation**

A. Progressive respiratory failure is treated with intubation and mechanical ventilation.

B. Positive end-expiratory pressure (PEEP) used to improve oxygenation.

C. Suction as needed to maintain airway patency.

D. Pain medications as ordered.

E. Observe for signs of shock and hemorrhage.

F. For client on ventilator, use nasogastric tube to prevent abdominal distention and emesis, which can lead to aspiration.

G. For client with mild to moderate chest injuries when client is not on mechanical ventilator:

   1. Encourage turning, coughing, and hyperventilating every hour.

   2. Administer oxygen.

   3. Incentive spirometry.

   4. Suction as needed.

Cardiac Tamponade

✦ *Definition:* Acute accumulation of blood or fluid in the pericardial sac (interferes with diastolic filling, which causes decreased cardiac output, myocardial hypoxia and cardiac failure). Can occur from blunt or penetrating wounds.

✦ **Assessment**

A. Assess for Beck's triad: increased CVP with neck vein distention, muffled heart sounds, and pulsus paradoxus.

B. Assess for decreased blood pressure.

C. Assess for narrowed pulse pressure.

✦ D. Evaluate paradoxical pulse (pulse disappears on inspiration and is weak on expiration because of changed intrathoracic pressure).

   1. Paradoxical pulse is an exaggeration of the normal fall in arterial BP on inspiration.

   2. Defined as a fall in systolic arterial BP of 10–20 mm Hg or more on inspiration.

E. Observe for agitation.

F. Observe for cyanosis.

G. Chest pain.

Implementation

A. Assist with pericardiocentesis. Large-bore needle (16–18 gauge) is inserted by physician into pericardium, and blood is withdrawn.

B. Maintain cardiac monitoring to observe for arrhythmias due to myocardial irritability.

C. Have cardiac defibrillator and emergency drugs available to treat cardiac arrhythmias.

D. Monitor vital signs and watch for shock.

TREATMENT FOR TRAUMATIC INJURY

Chest Tube

Definition: Chest tubes remove air and fluid from lungs and restore normal intrapleural pressure so lungs can reexpand.

Assessment

A. Before insertion.
   1. Complete client procedure verification.
   2. Obtain consent after physician explains procedure.
   3. Perform baseline cardiopulmonary assessment.
   4. Monitor VS and pulse oximetry.
   5. Observe chest excursion.
   6. Assess changes in LOC.
   7. Obtain a preprocedure chest x-ray if ordered.
   8. Assess anxiety and medicate 30 minutes prior to insertion.
   9. Prepare necessary equipment and supplies, including two rubber-tipped hemostats for each chest tube at bedside and to travel with client should he or she leave the unit.
   10. Position client according to physician's specifications.

B. During insertion.
   1. Evaluate client's safety while tubes inserted.
   2. Assess patency of chest tubes.
   3. Observe for mediastinal shift.
   4. Auscultate breath sounds for air flow.
   5. Observe for bilateral chest expansion.
   6. Evaluate chest drainage, color and amount.

✦ Implementation

A. Purpose: To reestablish negative pressure in pleural space by the evacuation of air and fluid.
   1. Uses: Used for pleural effusions, pneumothorax and hemothorax.
   ✦ 2. Safety measure: Always keep rubber-tipped Kelly clamps and Vaseline gauze at bedside. There should be two Kelly clamps per chest tube.

B. Assist physician in placement of tubes.
   1. Tubes placed in pleural cavity following thoracic surgery.
   2. Provides for removal of air and serosanguineous fluid from pleural space.

C. Attach to water-seal suction—maintains closed system.
   1. Tape all connectors.
   2. Ensure that all stoppers in bottles are tight fitting.

D. Apply suction.
   1. Keep unit below level of bed.
   2. Keep suction level where ordered (be sure that bubbling is not excessive in the pressure-regulating chamber).
   3. Maintain water level in chamber.

E. Nursing care immediately following procedure.
   1. Obtain repeat chest x-ray.
   2. Assess respirations.
   3. Assess integrity of the system.
   4. Assess drainage.
   5. Assess for fluctuation in tubing during respirations.

F. Follow-up nursing care (hourly initially, once stabilized q 2 hours).
   1. Respiratory rate and effort.
   2. Bilateral lung sounds.
   3. Symmetrical chest excursion.
   4. Assess and medicate for pain.
   5. Check integrity of dressing.
   6. Subcutaneous emphysema (should ↓ unless air leak).
   7. Tidaling with inspiration.
   8. Water seal—no bubbling unless leak (client or system).

G. Facilitating drainage.
   1. Keep tubing looped on bed—avoid dependent drainage.
   2. Reposition every 2 hours or as ordered.
   3. Encourage client to cough and deep-breathe.
   4. Use gentle wall suction if ordered.
   5. Monitor drainage (color, amount), initially every hour, when < 100 mL/hr, monitor q 2 hours. Document every 4 hours.
   6. Drainage should be no more than 100 mL/hr or 500 mL in 8 hours.

H. Maintain integrity of system.
   1. Keep water seal filled to the 2-cm level.
   2. Keep suction control chamber to ordered level (usually 20 cm and check for evaporation of water q shift) or dry suction to ordered level.
   3. Keep system below level of chest.
   4. Tape all connections.
   5. Secure drainage system to bed or floor.
   6. If transporting, secure drainage system to stretcher or W/C.

7. Position system for safety prior to raising or lowering bed.
8. Never clamp unless ordered.
✦ 9. Milking of chest tubes is not done unless specifically ordered by physician.
   a. With specific physician's orders, milk every 30–60 minutes.
   b. Milk away from client toward the drainage receptacle (Pleur-evac or bottles).
   c. Pinch tubing close to the chest with one hand as the other hand milks the tube. Continue going down the tube in this method until drainage receptacle is reached.
   d. Milking may be ordered—stripping should be avoided unless specifically ordered.

I. Change drainage system.
   1. Prepare new drainage system.
   2. Fill under water seal.
   3. Fill suction control to desired level (if ordered).
   4. Clamp and disconnect chest tube.
   5. Attach to new drainage system.
   6. Retape all tubing connections.
   7. Open clamp.

J. Nursing care following removal of chest tubes.
   1. Explain procedure to client.
   2. Medicate 30 minutes prior to removal.
   3. Prepare necessary equipment and supplies.
   4. Post-procedure chest x-ray as ordered.
   5. Perform baseline cardiopulmonary assessment.
   6. Monitor VS and pulse oximetry.
   7. Observe chest excursion.
   8. Monitor insertion site.
   9. Encourage cough, deep breathing, position change.

Chest Drainage Systems

Characteristics

A. The disposable water-seal drainage system is most commonly used.
✦ B. General principles.
   1. Used after some intrathoracic procedures.
   2. Chest tubes placed intrapleurally.
   3. Breathing mechanism operates on principle of negative pressure (pressure in chest cavity is lower than pressure of atmosphere, causing air to rush into chest cavity when injury such as stab wound occurs).
   4. When chest has been opened, vacuum must be applied to chest to reestablish negative pressure.
   5. Closed water-seal drainage is method of reestablishing negative pressure.

   a. Water acts as a seal and keeps the air from being drawn back into pleural space.
   b. Open drainage system would allow air to be sucked back into chest cavity and collapse lung.
6. Closed drainage is established by placing catheter into pleural space and allowing it to drain under water.
   a. The end of the drainage tube is always kept under water.
   b. Air will not be drawn up through catheter into pleural space when tube is under water.

Assessment

A. Assess client's respiratory rate, rhythm, and breath sounds for signs of respiratory distress.
B. Check that all connections on tubing are airtight and suction control is connected.
C. Examine system to see if it is set up and functioning properly.
D. Identify any malfunctions in system (i.e., air leaks, negative pressure, or obstructions).

Implementation

A. Maintain chest drainage system.
B. Most pleural drainage systems have 3 basic compartments (*see* Figures 8-11 and 8-12).
   1. Collection chamber (1). Fluid and air from chest cavity drain into chamber. Air in this chamber is vented to the second chamber.
   2. Water-seal chamber (2). Acts as one-way valve so air drains from the chest cavity, but can't return to the client. Air bubbles out into water. Water level fluctuates as intrapleural pressure changes.
   3. Suction-control chamber (3). Amount of suction applied regulated by amount of water in chamber or depth of tubing in water, not by the amount of suction applied.

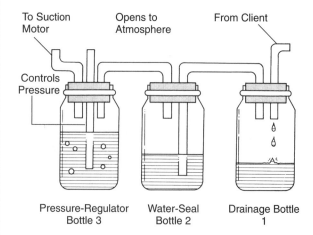

FIGURE 8-11. Three-bottle suction system—use illustration to understand mechanics of system.

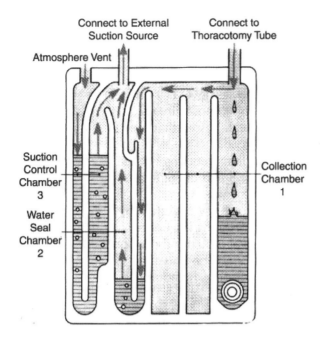

FIGURE 8-12. Disposable water-seal system.

4. When drainage system pressure becomes too low, outside air is sucked into the system. Results in constant bubbling in the pressure regulator bottle.
5. Whenever suction is off, drainage system must be open (vented) to the atmosphere.
   a. Intrapleural air can escape from the system.
   b. Detach the third chamber tubing from the suction motor to provide the air vent.

Mechanical Ventilation

Assessment

A. Assess respiratory status for need to use mechanical ventilation.
B. Identify type of mechanical ventilation needed.
   1. Negative-pressure ventilator.
      a. Helpful in problems of a neuromuscular nature, spinal cord injuries.
      b. Not effective in the treatment of increased airway resistance.
   ✦ c. Types—full body, chest, and chest–abdomen. Employs intermittent negative pressure around chest wall to pull wall out and decrease intrathoracic pressure.
   2. Positive-pressure ventilator.
      a. Uses positive pressure (pressure greater than atmospheric) to inflate lungs. Primary use in acutely ill clients.
      b. Types.
         (1) Pressure cycle.
            (a) Pressure ranges from 10 to 30 cm of water pressure.

         (b) Air is actively forced into lungs.
         (c) Expiration is passive.
      (2) Volume cycle.
         (a) Uses physiological limits.
         (b) Predetermined total volume is delivered irrespective of airway pressure.
         (c) Positive end-expiratory pressure (PEEP) utilized to maintain positive pressure between expiration and beginning of inspiration.
C. Assess for complications of positive-pressure therapy.
   1. Respiratory alkalosis.
   2. Gastric distention and paralytic ileus.
   3. Gastrointestinal bleeding.
   4. Diffuse atelectasis.
   5. Infection.
   6. Circulatory collapse.
   7. Pneumothorax.
   8. Sudden ventricular fibrillation.

Implementation

A. Monitor ventilator for complications.
B. Suction client or check for kinks in tubing when pressure alarm sounds.
C. Monitor blood gas values frequently.
D. Maintain fluid therapy.
   1. IV route.
   2. Oral route if client able to swallow.
E. Monitor intake and output.

Thoracic Surgical Procedures

Assessment

✦ A. Identify type of procedure done.
   1. Exploratory thoracotomy: incision of the thoracic wall; performed to locate bleeding, injuries, tumors.

2. Thoracoplasty: removal of ribs or portions of ribs to reduce the size of the thoracic space.
3. Pneumonectomy: removal of entire lung.
4. Lobectomy: removal of a lobe of the lung (three lobes on right side, two on the left).
5. Segmented resection: removal of one or more segments of the lung (right lung has ten segments and left lung has eight).
6. Wedge resection: removal of a small, localized area of disease near the surface of the lung.

B. Assess for postoperative client care needs.

Implementation

◆ A. Provide postoperative nursing management.
   1. Closed chest drainage is employed in all but pneumonectomy. In pneumonectomy, there is no lung to reexpand, so it is desirable that the fluid accumulate in empty thoracic space. Eventually the thoracic space fills with serous exudate, which consolidates to prevent extensive mediastinal shifts.
   2. Maintain patent chest tube drainage by chest tube milking—milk away from client toward drainage bottle, *only* with physician's orders.
   ◆ 3. Maintain respiratory function.
      a. Have client turn, cough, and deep-breathe.
      b. Suction if necessary.
      c. Provide oxygen therapy.
      d. Provide incentive spirometry.
      e. Ventilate mechanically if necessary.
      f. Auscultate lungs.
      g. Observe for complications.
   ◆ 4. Ambulate early to encourage adequate ventilation and prevent postoperative complications. (Ambulate clients with pneumonectomies in two or three days to facilitate cardiopulmonary adjustment.)
   5. Provide range-of-motion exercises to all extremities to promote adequate circulation.
   6. Monitor central venous pressure with vital signs—watch for indications of impaired venous return to heart.
   ◆ 7. Position client correctly to maximize ventilation.
      a. Use semi-Fowler's position when vital signs are stable to facilitate lung expansion.
      b. Turn every 1–2 hours.
      c. Pneumonectomy.
         (1) No chest tubes inserted. Fluid left in space to consolidate.
         (2) Position on operative side to maximize ventilation.
         (3) Some physicians will allow positioning on either side after 24 hours.
      d. Segmental resection or wedge resection: position on back or unoperative side (aids in expanding remaining pulmonary tissue).
      e. Lobectomy: turn to either side (can expand lung tissue on both sides).
8. Maintain fluid intake as tolerated. Watch for overload in pneumonectomy clients.
9. Provide arm and shoulder postoperative exercises—prevent adhesion formation.
   a. Put affected arm through both active and passive range of motion every four hours.
   b. Start exercises within four hours after client has returned to room following surgery.

B. Monitor postoperative complications.
   ◆ 1. Respiratory complications.
      a. Causes of inadequate ventilation.
         (1) Airway obstruction due to secretion accumulation.
         (2) Atelectasis due to underexpansion of lungs and anesthetic agents during surgery.
         (3) Hypoventilation and carbon dioxide buildup due to incisional splinting because of pain.
         (4) Depression of CNS from overuse of medications.
      b. Tension pneumothorax.
         (1) Caused by air leak through pleural incision lines.
         (2) Can cause mediastinal shift.
      c. Pulmonary embolism.
      d. Bronchopulmonary fistula.
         (1) Air escapes into pleural space and is forced into subcutaneous tissue around incision, causing subcutaneous emphysema.
         (2) Caused by inadequate closure of bronchus when resection is done.
         (3) Another cause is alveolar or bronchiolar tears in surface of lung (particularly following pneumonectomy).
      e. Atelectasis and/or pneumonia: caused by airway obstruction or as result of anesthesia.
      f. Respiratory arrest can occur.
   ◆ 2. Circulatory complications.
      a. Hypovolemia: due to fluid or blood loss.
      b. Arrhythmias: due to underlying myocardial disease.
      c. Cardiac arrest: can occur from either of these conditions.
      d. Pulmonary edema: can occur due to fluid overload of circulatory system.

Tracheostomy

Characteristics

A. Bypasses upper airway obstruction.
B. Facilitates removal of secretions.
C. Permits long-term mechanical ventilation.

Assessment

A. Determine need for tracheostomy as compared to less intrusive methods of providing patent airway.
B. Assess client's level of consciousness to determine client's ability to understand explanation and instructions.
C. Observe client's respiratory status: shortness of breath, severe dyspnea, tachypnea, or tachycardia.
D. Auscultate for presence and forced expiration of rhonchi, rales, or wheezes.
E. Observe for dried or moist secretions surrounding cannula or on tracheal dressing.
F. Observe for excessive expectoration of secretions.
G. Assess result of routine tracheal care to determine if routine care is adequate for this client.
H. Observe client's ability to sustain respiratory function by ability to breathe through normal airway.
I. Assess respiratory status: breath sounds, respiratory rate, use of accessory muscles for breathing while tracheal tube is plugged (must be a fenestrated tube).
J. Assess for labored breathing, flaring of nares, retractions, and color of nailbeds.

Implementation

A. Provide tracheal suction as ordered or PRN. (*See* Tracheostomy Suctioning.)
  ✦ 1. Always wear sterile gloves for these procedures.
  2. Always apply oral or nasal suction first so that when cuff is deflated, secretions will not fall into lung from area above cuff.
  3. Catheter must be changed before doing tracheal suctioning as a sterile technique.
B. Provide humidity by using trach mist mask, if client is not on ventilator.
C. Monitor for hemorrhage around tracheostomy site.
D. Change dressings (nonraveling type) and cleanse surrounding area with hydrogen peroxide at least every four hours.
E. Provide care for cuffed tracheostomy tube.
  ✦ 1. Hyperoxygenate client before and after cuff is deflated with ambu bag.
  2. Deflate tracheal cuff (no longer a routine procedure).
    a. Suction airway before deflating cuff.
    b. Attach 10-mL syringe to distal end of inflatable cuff, making sure seal is tight.
    c. Slowly withdraw 5 mL of air. Amount of air withdrawn is determined by type of cuff used and whether air leak is utilized.
    d. Keep syringe attached to end of cuff.
    e. Suction if cough reflex stimulated.
    f. Assess respirations; if labored, reinflate cuff.
    ✦ g. If high-volume/low-pressure cuff is used, cuff is not routinely deflated. (In fact, deflating cuff does not help tracheal lining. The pooled secretions above the tracheal cuff are the problem.)
  ✦ 3. Inflate cuff.
    a. Suction airway before inflating cuff.
    ✦ b. Inflate prescribed amount of air to create leak-free system. *Cuff is inflated correctly when you cannot hear the client's voice or any air movement from nose or mouth.*
    c. Remove syringe and apply rubber-tipped forceps to maintain air in cuff if there is no self-sealing.
    d. If high-volume/low-pressure cuff is used, cuff is not routinely deflated .
✦ F. Administer inner cannula tracheal cleaning.
  1. Suction before cleaning tracheal tube.
  2. Unlock the inner cannula by turning the lock to the right about 90 degrees and secure the outer cannula of the neck plate with your left index finger and thumb.
  3. Gently pull the inner cannula slightly upward and out toward you.
  4. Wash cannula thoroughly with cool, sterile water, saline, or hydrogen peroxide to remove secretions. (Tap water may be used if hospital policy allows.) Soak the cannula in a hydrogen peroxide–filled sterile bowl to further remove dried secretions.
  5. Rinse cannula thoroughly with sterile water or saline, and gently shake to dry.
  6. Replace the inner cannula carefully by grasping the outer flange of the cannula with your left hand as you insert the cannula. Lock the inner cannula by turning the lock to the left so that it is in an upright position.
  7. Cleanse around the incision site with applicator sticks soaked in normal saline and/or hydrogen peroxide (one-half strength).
  8. Apply trach dressing around insertion site, and change trach ties if needed.
  9. If trach ties are to be changed, ask another person to hold the tracheal tube in place while you change the ties. This procedure prevents accidental extubation if the client coughs.
  10. Repeat care TID and as needed.

11. Keep obturator at bedside for emergency use if tube is dislodged.
✦ G. Current research advises against instilling saline into airway—increases chance of infection and causes hypoxemia.
✦ H. Provide tracheostomy plugging.
1. Suction nasopharynx if cuffed tube is in place using clean technique.
2. Deflate tracheal cuff; if tracheostomy tube is plugged and cuff is *not* deflated, client has no airway.
3. Place tracheal plug in either the inner cannula or the outer cannula with inner cannula removed.
4. Observe client for respiratory distress.

Suctioning

Assessment
A. Determine need for suctioning.
1. Ineffective cough.
2. Thick, tenacious mucus.
3. Impaired pulmonary function.
4. Repressed level of consciousness.
5. Restlessness.
B. Observe vital signs for increases in pulse and respirations, and for changes in skin color.
C. Auscultate sounds to evaluate lung field.
D. Determine level of consciousness to assess hypoxia.

Implementation
A. Provide nasotracheal suction.
1. Gather equipment.
   a. Sterile suction catheter, usually no. 14 or no. 16 French.
   b. Sterile saline.
   c. Suction machine.
   d. Gloves.
✦ 2. Complete suctioning procedure.
   a. Hyperoxygenate (100 percent oxygen) before suctioning.
   b. Lubricate catheter with normal saline.
   c. Insert catheter into nose for 15–20 cm (clean technique is used when catheter does not extend to lower airway).
   d. Do not apply suction while introducing catheter.
   e. When advanced as far as possible, begin suctioning by withdrawing catheter slowly; if single-eyed catheter, rotate it with pressure applied. (Usually, a whistle-tip catheter or Y connector tube is used to apply pressure.)
   f. Withdraw catheter slightly if cough reflex is stimulated.

✦ g. Remember that hypoxia can occur if suctioning is done incorrectly.
   (1) More than 10 seconds of suctioning—oxygen will be decreased in respiratory tree.
   (2) Causes chemoreceptors to respond by increasing ventilation rate.
   h. Postoxygenate after suctioning.
✦ B. Closed suction system.
1. Suction catheter attached directly to ventilator tubing presents advantages over open system.
2. More effective—no need to disconnect client from ventilator; thus, oxygenation is better.
3. Safer—catheter is enclosed in plastic sheath (a closed system) so risk of infection is decreased for both client and nurse.

PULMONARY MEDICATIONS

✦ Sympathomimetic (Adrenergic) Bronchodilators

Definition: Relax smooth muscle and increase respirations by effect on beta-adrenergic receptor in bronchus.
A. Epinephrine (Adrenalin).
1. Beta and alpha stimulant; relaxes bronchial smooth muscle.
2. Routes: sub q, IV, MDI (metered-dose inhaler).
3. Used to treat severe bronchial attacks and for anaphylaxis.
4. May cause arrhythmias, increased BP, urinary retention, increased blood sugar, headache.
B. Ephedrine sulfate.
1. Relaxes smooth muscle of the tracheobronchial tree.
2. Route: PO.
3. Used for mild bronchospasm.
4. Similar side effects as epinephrine.
C. Isoproterenol (Isuprel).
1. Pure beta agonist; relaxes smooth muscle of tracheobronchial tree; relieves bronchospasms.
2. Routes: IV, MDI.
3. May cause marked tachycardia, arrhythmias, angina, palpitations.
D. Albuterol (Proventil, Ventolin).
1. Very selective $beta_2$ agonist with rapid onset of action.
2. Routes: PO, MDI (2–3 puffs every 4–6 hours).
3. Minimal cardiovascular side effects.
E. Isoetharine (Bronkosol, Bronkometer).
1. More $beta_2$ specific than Isuprel; relaxes smooth muscle of the tracheobronchial tree; less potent.
2. Route: Nebulized solution or MDI.

3. Side effects similar to Isuprel, but appear less frequently; may cause tachycardia.
4. Tolerance to bronchodilating effect may develop with too-frequent use of medication.

F. Metaproterenol (Alupent).
   1. Relieves bronchospasm, has rapid onset.
   2. Routes: PO, MDI (2–3 puffs every 4–6 hours).
   3. Side effects same as isoetharine.

G. Terbutaline (Bricanyl, Brethine).
   1. Beta-adrenergic receptor agonist; bronchodilator; relieves bronchospasms associated with COPD, asthma. Slow onset with PO, MDI.
   2. Routes: sub q, PO, Brethaire by MDI (2–3 puffs every 4–6 hours).
   3. May cause nervousness, palpitations; nausea if taken on an empty stomach.

✦ Anticholinergic Bronchodilators

Definition: Prevents bronchospasm caused by acetylcholine.

A. Ipratropium bromide (Atrovent).
   1. Greater bronchodilating effect than conventional beta agonists. Primarily local and site specific; more potent than sympathomimetics in COPD. Also used for severe acute asthma.
   2. Route: MDI (2–3 puffs every 4–6 hours).
   3. Minimal side effects, dry mouth, cough.

B. Atropine.
   1. Prevents bronchospasm associated with asthma, bronchitis and COPD.
   2. Routes: nebulizer 3–4 times/day.
   3. Monitor for tachycardia and hypertension.

✦ Methylxanthine Bronchodilators

Definition: Relaxes smooth muscle of tracheobronchial tree. Less effective than inhaled beta agonists. Used later in treatment regimen, as an additional bronchodilator.

A. Aminophylline.
   1. Relaxes smooth muscle of the tracheobronchial tree; bronchodilator.
   2. Routes: PO, IV, rectal suppository.
   3. Therapeutic serum level 8–20 μg/mL.
   4. May cause tachycardia, hypotension, arrhythmias, GI distress, tremors, anxiety, headache.
   5. Toxic levels cause arrhythmias, seizures.

B. Theophylline (Theo-Dur, Slo-Bid, Uni-Dur).
   1. Long-acting bronchodilator—relaxes smooth muscle of the bronchi and pulmonary vessels.
   2. Routes: PO, rectally.
   3. Therapeutic serum level 10–20 μg/mL.
   4. Side effects similar to aminophylline.

C. Oxtriphylline (Choledyl).
   1. Similar to other bronchodilators.
   2. Route: PO.
   3. Less GI irritation than aminophylline.

✦ Leukotriene Inhibitors/Receptor Antagonists

Definition: Inhibit formation of leukotrienes, which cause airway inflammation, edema, bronchoconstriction, and mucus secretion.

A. Zafirlukast (Accolate), Zileuton (Zyflo), and montelukast sodium (Singulair).
   1. Basic action is anti-inflammatory.
   2. Taken orally (not through MDI) so compliance is improved for long-term control, not for acute asthma episode.

B. Side effects: headache, nausea, diarrhea, dizziness, fever, and myalgia.

✦ Antimediators (Mast Cell Stabilizers)/ Anti-inflammatory Agents

Definition: Mast cell stabilizers inhibit release of histamine; glucocorticoids reduce inflammation and act as bronchodilators.

A. Cromolyn sodium (Intal, Nalcrom).
   1. Decreases airway inflammation and irritation—used for younger clients with asthma.
   2. Route: MDI, nebulizer, nasal spray.
   3. Prevents bronchospasm when used before exercise or exposure to cold air.
   4. Can cause throat irritation.

B. Glucocorticoids (Beclovent, Vanceril, Beconase).
   1. Used in conjunction with bronchodilators for treatment of bronchospasms; anti-inflammatory effects, decrease mucus secretion. Aerosol use prevents systemic side effects of steroids.
   2. Routes.
      a. Prednisone PO.
      b. Methylprednisolone PO, IV, hydrocortisone IV.
      c. Beclomethasone diproprionate (Beclovent, Vanceril) MDI.
      d. Triamcinolone (Azmacort) MDI.
   3. Instruct client to rinse mouth after MDI use to prevent oral candidiasis.
   4. Side effects include increased appetite, sore throat, cough, thrush, Cushing-like appearance.

✦ Mucokinetic Agents

Definition: Reduces the viscosity of respiratory secretions by breaking down mucoproteins.

A. Acetylcysteine (Mucomyst).
   1. Used to loosen secretions; reduces viscosity.
   2. Routes: inhaled or instilled.

3. May cause bronchospasm, nausea.
4. Instruct client to rinse mouth after use.
B. Guaifenesin.
   1. Commonly used expectorant.
   2. Route: PO.
C. Iodide preparations (SSKI, Organidin).
   1. Expectorant liquefies tenacious bronchial secretions.
   2. Route PO; bitter taste, give with juice or milk.
   3. Do not administer if allergic to iodine or hyperthyroid.

✦ Antiprotozoal Drugs

Definition: Interferes with biosynthesis of deoxyribonucleic acid, ribonucleic acid, phospholipids, and proteins in susceptible organisms.
A. Pentamidine (NebuPent, Pentam 300) for prevention.
   1. Prevention of *Pneumocystis carinii* pneumonia.
   2. Routes: nebulizer (300 mg every 4 weeks).
   3. If client experiences fatigue, dizziness or anxiety during inhalation, stop treatment and allow client to rest. Well tolerated, expensive. No systemic protection. Least effective form of prophylaxis.
B. Pentamidine for treatment.
   1. Treatment of *Pneumocystis carinii*.
   2. Route: IV or IM (4 mg/kg daily for 14 days). IV used for those clients who do not tolerate Bactrim, Septa (trimethoprim-sulfamethoxazole).
   3. Closely monitor for hypotension—place client in supine position for IV administration.
   4. Nephrotoxic; can cause hyperglycemia, pancreatitis.
   5. Screen for active TB before treating moderate to severe PCP.

RESPIRATORY SYSTEM REVIEW QUESTIONS

1. A client is on a disposable water-seal system with chest tubes in place. The RN assigns the LVN to milk the chest tubes to maintain patency. The RN monitors that the first LVN action is to

   1. Milk the tubes toward the client.
   2. Check that the physician has written orders to milk the chest tubes.
   3. Tell the charge nurse that this assignment is not appropriate for LVNs.
   4. Complete the assignment and chart the intervention in the client's record.

2. A female client comes to the emergency department complaining of shortness of breath and pain in the lung area. She states that she started taking birth control pills 3 weeks ago and that she smokes. Her vital signs are as follows: BP 140/80, P 110, R 40. The physician orders ABGs; results are as follows:

pH	7.50
$PaCO_2$	29 mm Hg
PaO_2	60 mm Hg
HCO_3	24 mEq/L
SaO_2	86%

   Considering these results, the first intervention is to

   1. Begin mechanical ventilation.
   2. Place the client on oxygen.
   3. Give the client sodium bicarbonate.
   4. Monitor for pulmonary embolism.

3. Basilar crackles are present in a client's lungs on auscultation. The nurse knows that these discrete, non-continuous sounds are

   1. Caused by the sudden opening of alveoli.
   2. Usually more prominent during expiration.
   3. Produced by air flow across passages narrowed by secretions.
   4. Found primarily in the pleura.

4. A client's condition requires that a bronchoscopy procedure be done. Due to his physical condition, he will be awake during the procedure. As part of the pretest teaching, the nurse will instruct him that before the scope insertion, his neck will be positioned so that it is

   1. In a flexed position.
   2. In an extended position.
   3. In a neutral position.
   4. Hyperextended.

5. A cyanotic client with an unknown diagnosis is admitted to the emergency room. In relation to oxygen, the first nursing action would be to

   1. Wait until the client's lab work is done.
   2. Not administer oxygen unless ordered by the physician.
   3. Administer oxygen at 2 L flow per minute.
   4. Administer oxygen at 10 L flow per minute and check the client's nailbeds.

6. A client with tuberculosis is given the drug pyrazinamide (Tebrazid). Which one of these diagnostic tests should be monitored while the client is receiving the drug?

   1. Liver function tests.
   2. Gallbladder studies.
   3. Thyroid function studies.
   4. Blood glucose.

7. Care for a client following a bronchoscopy will include

   1. Withholding food and liquids until the gag reflex returns.
   2. Providing throat irrigations every 4 hours.
   3. Having the client refrain from talking for several days.
   4. Suctioning frequently, as ordered.

8. Immediately following a thoracentesis, which clinical manifestations indicate that a complication has occurred and the physician should be notified?

   1. Serosanguineous drainage from the puncture site.
   2. Increased temperature and blood pressure.
   3. Increased pulse and pallor.
   4. Hypotension and hypothermia.

9. If a client continues to hypoventilate, the nurse will continually assess for a complication of

   1. Respiratory acidosis.
   2. Respiratory alkalosis.
   3. Metabolic acidosis.
   4. Metabolic alkalosis.

10. A client is admitted to the hospital for acute bronchitis. While taking the client's vital signs, the nurse notices he has an irregular pulse. The nurse understands that cardiac arrhythmias in chronic respiratory diseases are usually the result of

    1. Respiratory acidosis.
    2. A buildup of carbon dioxide.
    3. A buildup of oxygen without adequate expelling of carbon dioxide.
    4. An acute respiratory infection.

11. Select the most effective nursing intervention for a client experiencing adult respiratory distress syndrome (ARDS).

    1. Maintain low-flow oxygen via nasal cannula.
    2. Encourage oral intake of at least 3000 mL fluids per day.
    3. Ask open-ended questions to promote expression of anxiety.
    4. Position in semi- to high-Fowler's with support to the back.

12. Which one of the following principles is *incorrect* when discussing the water-seal chest drainage system?

    1. When the chest has been opened, a vacuum must be applied to reestablish positive pressure.
    2. Water acts as a seal to prevent air from being drawn into the pleural space.
    3. Air drawn into the chest cavity collapses the lung.
    4. Water-seal mechanisms operate on a negative-pressure principle.

13. Your client is unable to use the incentive spirometer device. In counseling the client, the first advice would be to

    1. Start slowly and gradually increase volume over several sessions.
    2. Give up and do regular deep breathing.
    3. Obtain another device because this one is obviously faulty.
    4. Be much more vigorous in increasing increments.

14. Auscultation of a client's lungs reveals rales (crackles) in the left posterior base. The nursing intervention is to

    1. Repeat auscultation after asking the client to deep-breathe and cough.
    2. Instruct the client to limit fluid intake to less than 2000 mL/day.
    3. Inspect the client's ankles and sacrum for the presence of edema.

    4. Place the client on bedrest in a semi-Fowler's position.

15. The exercise that would be most beneficial for a client with COPD is

    1. Controlled coughing.
    2. Whistling while exhaling.
    3. Deep breathing.
    4. Use of the incentive spirometer.

16. The most reliable index to determine the respiratory status of a client is to

    1. Observe the chest rising and falling.
    2. Observe the skin and mucous membrane color.
    3. Listen to and feel the air movement.
    4. Determine the presence of a femoral pulse.

17. A client with COPD has developed secondary polycythemia. Which nursing diagnosis would be included in the care plan because of the polycythemia?

    1. Fluid volume deficit related to blood loss.
    2. Impaired tissue perfusion related to thrombosis.
    3. Activity intolerance related to dyspnea.
    4. Risk for infection related to suppressed immune response.

18. The nurse is assigned to care for a 20-year-old client who has just had chest tubes inserted. The priority nursing action is to

    1. Place a hemostat nearby in case of an air leak.
    2. Check the chest tubes every 2 hours for air leaks.
    3. Coil the tubes carefully to prevent kinking, which could result in an air leak.
    4. Keep the client flat to avoid leaks in the tubing.

19. The physician has scheduled a client for a left pneumonectomy. The position that will most likely be ordered postoperatively for him is the

    1. Unoperative side or back.
    2. Operative side or back.
    3. Back only.
    4. Back or either side.

20. Assessing a client who has developed atelectasis postoperatively, the nurse will most likely find

    1. A flushed face.
    2. Dyspnea and pain.
    3. Decreased temperature.
    4. Severe cough with no pain.

21. A client who has had a lobectomy for cancer of the left lower lobe of the lung is complaining of severe pain on inspiration. The drug the nurse expects the physician to order to relieve the pain is

1. Codeine sulfate.
2. Demerol.
3. Morphine sulfate.
4. Tylenol with codeine.

22. A 50-year-old client has a tracheostomy and requires tracheal suctioning. The first intervention in completing this procedure would be to

1. Change the tracheostomy dressing.
2. Provide humidity with a trach mask.
3. Apply oral or nasal suction.
4. Deflate the tracheal cuff.

23. A client has been diagnosed with a pulmonary embolism. The nurse would anticipate medical orders for the immediate administration of

1. Warfarin (Coumadin).
2. Dexamethasone (Decadron).
3. Heparin.
4. Protamine sulfate.

24. When a client asks the nurse why the physician says he "thinks" he has tuberculosis, the nurse explains to him that diagnosis of tuberculosis can take several weeks to confirm. Which of the following statements supports this answer?

1. A positive reaction to a tuberculosis skin test indicates that the client has active tuberculosis, even if one negative sputum is obtained.
2. A positive sputum culture takes at least 3 weeks, due to the slow reproduction of the bacillus.
3. Because small lesions are hard to detect on chest x-rays, x-rays usually need to be repeated during several consecutive weeks.
4. A client with a positive smear must have a positive culture to confirm the diagnosis.

25. The nurse would assess that a client is experiencing Cheyne–Stokes respiration when he has

1. Periods of hyperpnea alternating with periods of apnea.
2. Periods of tachypnea alternating with periods of apnea.
3. An increase in both rate and depth of respirations.
4. Deep, regular, sighing respirations.

RESPIRATORY SYSTEM

Answers with Rationale

1. (2) This is a management question and the RN must be sure that the LVN checked that the physician has written orders. Stripping and milking chest tubes is allowed only with a physician's order because it can cause excessive negative pressure, which could damage the lung tissue. Chest tubes are milked away from the client toward the drainage receptacle. LVNs are legally allowed to do this intervention.

   NP:I; CN:S; CL:AN

2. (2) The pH (7.50) reflects alkalosis, and the low $PaCO_2$ indicates that the lungs are involved. The client should immediately be placed on oxygen via mask, so that the SaO_2 is brought up to 95 percent. Encourage slow, regular breathing to decrease the amount of CO_2 she is losing. This client may have pulmonary embolism, so she should be monitored for this condition (4), but it is not the first intervention. Sodium bicarbonate (3) would be given to reverse acidosis; mechanical ventilation (1) may be ordered for acute respiratory acidosis.

   NP:I; CN:PH; CL:AN

3. (1) Basilar crackles are usually heard during inspiration and are caused by sudden opening of alveoli.

   NP:AN; CN:PH; CL:K

4. (4) Hyperextension brings the pharynx into alignment with the trachea and allows the scope to be inserted without trauma.

   NP:I; CN:PH; CL:A

5. (3) Administer oxygen at 2 L/min and no more. If the client is emphysemic and receives too high a level of oxygen, he will develop CO_2 narcosis and the respiratory system will cease to function.

   NP:I; CN:PH; CL:A

6. (1) Liver function tests can be elevated in clients taking pyrazinamide. This drug is used when primary and secondary antitubercular drugs are not effective. Urate levels may be increased, and there is a chemical interference with urine ketone levels if these tests are done while the client is on the drug.

   NP:E; CN:PH; CL:A

7. (1) Until the gag reflex returns, the client cannot handle foods or liquids, and may aspirate. Suctioning (4) is not usually ordered. The client does not require throat irrigations (2) and can talk (3) whenever he or she is ready.

   NP:E; CN:PH; CL:A

8. (3) Increased pulse and pallor are symptoms associated with shock. A compromised venous return may occur if there is a mediastinal shift as a result of excessive fluid removal. Usually no more than 1 L of fluid is removed at one time to prevent this from occurring.

   NP:E; CN:PH; CL:AN

9. (1) Respiratory acidosis represents an increase in the acid component, carbon dioxide, and an increase in the hydrogen ion concentration (decreased pH) of the arterial blood. It differs from metabolic acidosis (3) in that it is caused by defective functioning of the lungs.

   NP:A; CN:PH; CL:A

10. (2) The arrhythmias are caused by a buildup of carbon dioxide and not enough oxygen so that the heart is in a constant state of hypoxia.

    NP:AN; CN:PH; CL:C

11. (4) ARDS produces severe dyspnea and life-threatening abnormalities of blood gases; therefore, main-

---

Coding for Questions/Answers Abbreviations: **Nursing Process: NP,** Assessment: A, Analysis: AN, Planning: P, Implementation: I, Evaluation: E; **Client Needs: CN,** Safe, Effective Care Environment: S, Health Promotion and Maintenance: H, Psychosocial Integrity: PS, Physiological Integrity: PH; **Clinical Area: CA,** Medical Nursing: M, Surgical Nursing: S, Maternal/Newborn Nursing: MA, Pediatric Nursing: P, Psychiatric Nursing: PS; **Cognitive Level: CL,** Knowledge: K, Comprehension: C, Application: A, Analysis: AN.

taining an upright position will promote gas exchange and help relieve dyspnea. The client with ARDS requires high concentrations of oxygen, usually by mask or ventilator. Diuretics and fluid restrictions are used to combat the pulmonary edema, which is part of ARDS. Closed questions are used because of the client's dyspnea; the expected anxiety needs to be addressed through interventions other than verbalization.

NP:P; CN:PH; CL:A

12. (1) A seal must be established to prevent atmospheric air from entering the pleural space and to reestablish negative, not positive, pressure. The other options are correct.

NP:E; CN:PH; CL:A

13. (1) The best advice is to have the client start very slowly and gradually increase the volume. The device is not at fault; it is usually the inability of the client to expand the lungs. Deep breathing is an alternative *only* if the client is totally unable to use the device.

NP:I; CN:PH; CL:A

14. (1) Although crackles often indicate fluid in the alveoli, they may also be related to hypoventilation and will clear after a deep breath or a cough. It is, therefore, premature to impose fluid (2) or activity (4) restrictions. Inspection for edema (3) would be appropriate after reauscultation.

NP:I; CN:PH; CL:A

15. (2) Whistling while exhaling or pursed-lip breathing prevents the bronchi from collapsing, thereby permitting more effective exhalation of trapped carbon dioxide. The other exercises do not foster exhalation of carbon dioxide.

NP:P; CN:PH; CL:A

16. (3) To check for breathing, the nurse places her ear and cheek next to client's mouth and nose to listen and feel for air movement. The chest rising and falling (1) is not conclusive of a patent airway. Observing skin color (2) is not an accurate assessment of respiratory status, nor is checking the femoral pulse (4).

NP:A; CN:PH; CL:C

17. (2) Chronic hypoxia associated with COPD may stimulate excessive RBC production (polycythemia). This results in increased blood viscosity and the risk of thrombosis. The other nursing diagnoses are not applicable in this situation.

NP:AN; CN:PH; CL:A

18. (1) The most important safety measure is to tape a hemostat nearby to use in case of an air leak. Chest tubes should be checked periodically, but not necessarily every 2 hours (2). The client should be in semi-Fowler's position to increase lung expansion.

NP:I; CN:PH; CL:A

19. (2) Positioning the client on the operative side facilitates the accumulation of serosanguineous fluid. The fluid forms a solid mass, which prevents the remaining lung from being drawn into the space.

NP:P; CN:PH; CL:C

20. (2) Atelectasis is a collapse of the alveoli due to obstruction or hypoventilation. Clients become short of breath, have a high temperature, and usually experience severe pain but do not have a severe cough (4). The shortness of breath is a result of decreased oxygen–carbon dioxide exchange at the alveolar level.

NP:A; CN:PH; CL:C

21. (3) Morphine sulfate (3) is the drug of choice, but due to its depressing action on respirations, clients need to be closely monitored. Codeine (1) and Tylenol (4) are usually not sufficient pain relievers; therefore, the use of these drugs could interfere with other nursing interventions, such as deep breathing and coughing. Demerol is not commonly used today.

NP:P; CN:PH; CL:C

22. (3) Before deflating the tracheal cuff (4), the nurse will apply oral or nasal suction to the airway to prevent secretions from falling into the lung. Dressing change (1) and humidity (2) do not relate to suctioning.

NP:I; CN:PH; CL:A

23. (3) Heparin acts rapidly to prevent extension of emboli and the formation of thrombi. Warfarin (1) is a slow-acting anticoagulant. Protamine sulfate (4) inactivates heparin. Dexamethasone (2), a corticosteroid, is not indicated for the immediate treatment of pulmonary embolism.

NP:P; CN:PH; CL:C

24. (2) The culture takes 3 weeks to grow. Usually, even very small lesions can be seen on x-rays due to the natural contrast of the air in the lungs; therefore, chest x-rays do not need to be repeated frequently (3). Clients may have positive smears but negative cultures if they have been on medication (4). A positive skin test indicates the person has been infected with tuberculosis but may not necessarily have active disease (1).

NP:AN; CN:H; CL:K

25. (1) Periods of hyperpnea alternating with apnea is a breathing pattern that is easily missed if the client's respirations are not observed for a few minutes. It may indicate disorders of cerebral circulation, increased cerebral pressure, and/or injury to the brain tissue.

NP:A; CN:PH; CL:C

GASTROINTESTINAL SYSTEM

The alimentary tract's primary function is to provide the body with a continual supply of nutrients, fluids, and electrolytes for tissue nourishment. This system has three components: a tract for ingestion and movement of food and fluids; secretion of digestive juices for breaking down the nutrients; and absorption mechanisms for the utilization of foods, water, and electrolytes for continued growth and repair of body tissues.

ANATOMY AND PHYSIOLOGY

Main Organs

Description: The main organs of the gastrointestinal system include the mouth, pharynx, esophagus, stomach, small intestine, and large intestine.

Functions
A. Normally, the GI system is the only source of intake for the body.
B. Provides the body with fluids, nutrients, and electrolytes.
C. Provides means of disposal for waste residues.

Activities
A. Secretion of enzymes and electrolytes are used to break down the raw materials ingested.
B. Movement of ingested products through the system.
C. Complete digestion of ingested nutrients.
D. Absorption of the end products of digestion into the blood.

Coats of Tissue Walls
A. Mucous lining.
   1. Rugae and microscopic gastric and hydrochloric acid glands in the stomach.
   2. Villi, intestinal gland Peyer's patches, and lymph nodes.
   3. Intestinal glands.
B. Submucous coat of connective tissue, in which the main blood vessels are located.
C. Muscular coat.
   1. Digestive organs have circular and longitudinal muscle fibers.
   2. The stomach has oblique fibers in addition to circular and longitudinal fibers.
D. Fibroserous coat, the outer coat.

   1. In the stomach, the omentum hangs from the lower edge of the stomach, over the intestines.
   2. In the intestines, it forms the visceral peritoneum.

The Mouth, Pharynx, and Esophagus
A. The buccal cavity.
   1. Cheeks.
   2. Hard and soft palates.
   3. Muscles.
   4. Maxillary bones.
   5. Tongue.
B. The pharynx.
   1. Tubelike structure that extends from the base of the skull to the esophagus.
   2. Compound of muscle lined with mucous membrane, composed of the nasopharynx, the oropharynx, and the laryngopharynx.
   3. Functions include serving as a pathway for the respiratory and digestive tracts, and playing an important role in phonation.
C. The esophagus begins at the lower end of the pharynx and is a collapsible muscular tube about 10 inches (25 cm) long.
   1. It leads to the abdominal portion of the digestive tract.
   2. The main portion is lined with many simple mucous glands; complex mucous glands are located at the esophagastric juncture.

The Stomach
A. Elongated pouch lying in the epigastric and left hypochondriac portions of the abdominal cavity (approximately 10 inches [25 cm]).
B. Divisions are the fundus, the body, and the pylorus (the constricted lower portion).
C. Curvatures are the lesser curvature and the greater curvature.
D. Sphincters.
   1. Cardiac sphincter—at the opening of the esophagus into the stomach.
   2. Pyloric sphincter—guards the opening of the pylorus into the duodenum.
E. Regions.
   1. Cardiac.
   2. Fundus.
   3. Body.
   4. Pyloris.
F. Coats.
   1. The mucous coat allows for distention and contains microscopic glands: gastric, hydrochloric acid, and mucous.
   2. The muscle coat contains three layers.
      a. Circular—forms the two sphincters.
      b. Longitudinal.

c.   Oblique.
3.   The fibroserous coat forms the visceral peritoneum; the omentum hangs in a double fold over the intestines.
G.   Glands.
1.   Mucous glands—secrete mucus to provide protection from gastric juice.
2.   Goblet cells—secrete viscid mucus.
3.   Gastric glands.
a.   Parietal—secrete hydrochloric acid and intrinsic factor.
b.   Chief cells—secrete pepsin, lipase, amylase, and renin.
✦ H.   Function: mechanical and chemical digestion.
1.   Mechanical.
a.   A storage reservoir for food.
b.   Churning provides for forward and backward movement.
c.   Peristalsis moves material through the stomach and, at intervals with relaxation of the pyloric sphincter, squirts chyme into the duodenum.
2.   Chemical.
a.   Hydrochloric acid provides the proper medium for action of pepsin and aids in the coagulation of milk in adults.
b.   Pepsin splits protein into proteoses and peptones.
c.   Lipase is a fat-splitting enzyme with limited action.
d.   Renin coagulates or curdles the protein of milk.
e.   Intrinsic factor acts on certain components of food to form the antianemic factor.
f.   Mixes food with gastric juices into a thick fluid called chyme.

The Small Intestine
A.   Approximately 21 feet (6 m).
✦ B.   Divisions.
1.   The duodenum [about 10 inches (25 cm)] includes the Brunner's glands (the duodenal mucous digestive glands) and the openings for the bile and pancreatic ducts.
2.   The jejunum is approximately 8 feet (2.4 m) long; the ileum is approximately 12 feet (3.6 m) long. Both have deep circular folds that increase their absorptive surfaces.
a.   The mucous lining has numerous villi, each of which has an arteriole, venule and lymph vessel that serve as structures for the absorption of digested food.
b.   The small intestine terminates by opening into the cecum (the opening is guarded by the ileocecal valve).

C.   Intestinal digestion.
1.   Intestinal juice has an alkaline reaction and contains a large number of enzymes.
2.   Enzymes.
a.   Peptidase splits fragments of proteins into free amino acids.
b.   Amylase digests starch to maltose.
c.   Maltase reduces maltose to monosaccharide glucose.
d.   Lactase splits lactose into galactose and glucose.
e.   Sucrase reduces sucrose to fructose and glucose.
f.   Nucleoses split nucleic acids into nucleotides.
g.   Enterokinase activates trypsinogen to trypsin.

The Large Intestine (Colon)
A.   Approximately 5 feet (1.5 m) long, with a relatively smooth mucous membrane surface. The only secretion is mucus.
B.   Muscle coats pucker the wall of the colon into a series of pouches (haustra) and contain the internal and the external anal sphincters.
✦ C.   Divisions.
1.   The cecum (the first part of the large intestine) is guarded by the ileocecal valve.
a.   Prevents regurgitation of the cecal contents into the ileum.
b.   3 L of fluid passes through the small bowel but only 500 mL passes through the ileocecal valve.
2.   The appendix is attached to its surface as an extension. The appendix is a twisted structure that may accumulate bacteria and become inflamed.
3.   Colon.
a.   Ascending—the portion of the colon on the right side of the abdomen that extends from the ileocecal valve to the right hepatic flexure.
b.   Transverse—the largest, most mobile section extending from the right hepatic flexure to the left splenic flexure.
c.   Descending—the narrowest portion of the large intestine, extending from the left splenic flexure to the brim of the pelvis.
d.   Sigmoid—S-shaped portion of the colon, beginning at the brim of the pelvis and extending to the rectum.
e.   Rectum—12-cm mucosa-lined tube. It has three transverse folds (valves of Houston) that serve to retain feces while allowing flatus to pass through the anus.
f.   Anus—a hairless, darker-skinned area at the end of the digestive tract. It has an

internal involuntary sphincter and an external voluntary sphincter.
D. Functions.
   1. Absorption and elimination of wastes.
   ✦ 2. Formation of vitamins: K, B_{12}, riboflavin, and thiamine.
   3. Mechanical digestion: churning, peristalsis and defecation.
   4. Absorption of water from fecal mass.

Accessory Organs

Description: The accessory organs of the gastrointestinal system include the teeth, tongue, salivary glands, pancreas, liver, gallbladder, and appendix.

Tongue
A. A skeletal muscle covered with a mucous membrane that aids in chewing, swallowing and speaking.
B. Papillae on the surface of the tongue contain taste buds.
C. The frenulum is a fold of mucous membrane that helps to anchor the tongue to the floor of the mouth.
D. The tongue mixes food with saliva to form a mass called a bolus.

Salivary Glands
A. Three pairs—the submaxillary, the sublingual, and the parotid glands.
B. Secretion.
   1. Saliva is secreted by the glands when sensory nerve endings are stimulated mechanically, thermally, or chemically.
   2. pH ranges: 6.0–7.9. Between 1000 and 1500 mL is secreted in a 24-hour period in adults.
   3. Contains amylase, an enzyme that hydrolyzes starch.

Teeth
A. Deciduous teeth (20 in the set) and permanent teeth (32 in the set).
B. The functions are mastication and mixing saliva with food.

Liver
A. Location and size.
   1. Located in the right hypochondrium and part of the epigastrium.
   2. It is the largest gland in the body, weighing about 3 pounds.
   3. It is protected by the lower ribs and is in contact with the undersurface of the dome of the diaphragm.
B. Lobes—right lobes (include the right lobe proper, the caudate, and the quadrate) and left lobe.
   1. Lobes are divided into lobules by blood vessels and fibrous partitions.

   2. The lobule is the basic structure of the liver and contains hepatic cells and capillaries.
C. Ducts include the hepatic duct from the liver, the cystic duct from the gallbladder, and the common bile duct (the union of the hepatic and cystic ducts).

✦ **Functions of the Liver**
A. Metabolism of carbohydrates.
   1. Converts glucose to glycogen and stores glycogen.
   2. Converts glycogen to glucose.
   3. Glycogenolysis—the supply of carbohydrates released into bloodstream.
B. Metabolism of fats.
   1. Oxidation of fatty acids and formation of aceto-acetic acid.
   2. Formation of lipoproteins, cholesterol, and phospholipids.
   3. Conversion of carbohydrates and protein into fat.
C. Metabolism of proteins.
   1. Deamination of amino acids.
   2. Formation of urea.
   3. Formation of plasma proteins.
   4. Interconversions among amino acid and other compounds.
D. Vascular functions for storage and filtration of blood.
   1. Blood (200–400 mL) can be stored by the liver.
   2. Fat-soluble vitamins (A, D, E, and K), B_{12}, copper, and iron are stored in the liver.
   3. Detoxifies harmful substances in the blood.
   4. Breaks down worn-out blood cells.
   5. Filters blood as it comes through the portal system.
   6. Synthesizes prothrombin, fibrinogen, and factors I, II, VII, IX, and X, which are necessary for blood clotting.
E. Secretory functions.
   1. Constant secretion (500–1000 mL in 24 hours) of bile, which is stored in the gallbladder.
   2. Bile is a yellow–brown viscous fluid, alkaline in reaction, and consists of bile salts, bile pigments, cholesterol, and inorganic salts.
   3. Bile emulsifies fats.
   4. Red blood cell destruction releases hemoglobin, which changes to bilirubin; bilirubin unites with plasma proteins and is removed by the liver and excreted in the bile.
   5. The bile pigment bilirubin is converted by bacterial action into urobilin and to urobilinogen (appears in urine and gives feces brown color).
F. Hepatic reticuloendothelial functions.
   1. Inner surface of the liver sinusoids contains Kupffer cells.

2. Kupffer cells are phagocytic and are capable of removing bacteria in the portal venous blood.

G. Sex hormone and aldosterone metabolism.

The Gallbladder

✦ A. Small sac of smooth muscle located in a depression at the edge of the visceral surface of the liver, which functions as a reservoir for bile.
  1. Cystic duct—the duct of the gallbladder joins the hepatic duct, which descends from the liver, to form the common bile duct.
  2. The common bile duct is joined by the duct of the pancreas (Wirsung's duct) as it enters the duodenum.
  3. The sphincter of Oddi guards the common entrance.

B. Secretion—the presence of fatty materials in the duodenum stimulates the liberation of cholecystokinin, which causes contraction of the gallbladder and relaxation of the sphincter of Oddi.

The Pancreas

A. A soft, pink–white organ, 15 cm long and 2.5 cm wide, which adheres to the middle portion of the duodenum.

B. Divided into lobes and lobules.
  1. Exocrine portion secretes digestive enzymes, which are carried to the duodenum by Wirsung's duct.
  2. Endocrine secretion is produced by the islets of Langerhans; insulin is secreted into the bloodstream and plays an important role in carbohydrate metabolism.

✦ C. Pancreatic juices contain enzymes for digesting proteins, carbohydrates, and fats.
  1. Enzymes are secreted as inactive precursors, which do not become active until secreted into the intestine (otherwise they would digest the gland).
  2. Actions.
     a. Converts trypsinogen to trypsin to act on proteins, producing peptones, peptides and amino acids.
     b. Pancreatic amylase acts on carbohydrates, producing disaccharides.
     c. Pancreatic lipase acts on fats, producing glycerol and fatty acids.

D. Two regulatory mechanisms of pancreatic secretion.
  1. Nervous regulation—distention of the intestine.
  2. Hormonal regulation.
     a. Chyme in the intestinal mucosa causes the release of secretin (which stimulates the pancreas to secrete large quantities of fluid) and pancreozymin.

     b. Pancreozymin passes by way of the blood to the pancreas and causes secretion of large quantities of digestive enzymes.

See Chapter 4, Nutritional Management, Assimilation of Nutrients in the Gastrointestinal Tract section.

System Assessment

A. Evaluate client's history regarding reported signs and symptoms.

B. Assess overall condition of client, including vital signs and level of consciousness.

C. Evaluate condition of mouth, teeth, gums, and tongue.
  1. Foul odor to breath may indicate diseased teeth, gums, or poor assimilation along gastrointestinal tract.
  2. Coated tongue may indicate chemical imbalance in system.
  3. Check voice for hoarseness.

D. Check for presence of gag reflex.

E. Assess general contour of abdomen with client lying flat. Look for concave or protuberant abdomen.

F. Assess for bowel sounds: hyperactive or hypoactive.
  1. Hypoactive bowel sounds may be due to peritonitis, paralytic ileus or no obvious cause.
  2. Absent bowel sounds may be due to bowel obstruction or systemic illness.

G. Check bowel habits and/or alterations in bowel elimination.

H. Palpate abdominal muscles for tenderness or rigidity; evaluate all quadrants of abdomen.

I. Assess bowel motility.
  1. Hypermotility may be result of irritation of autonomic nervous system or inflammatory process.
  2. Hypomotility may be result of blockage, intestinal muscle weakness, or chemical agents.

J. Check for amount of flatulence client reports, which indicates malfunction of system or dietary indiscretion.

K. Assess stool specimen.
  1. Check for presence of blood.
  2. Check for presence of mucus.
  3. Evaluate consistency, color, and odor of stool.

L. Assess for parasites.

M. Assess fluid intake per day.

N. Evaluate dietary program (e.g., type of foods, amount).

O. Evaluate laboratory tests.

P. Note presence or absence of hemorrhoids.

Q. Assess the degree of sphincter control by the client's reports of his or her ability to control and regulate bowel movements.

R. Assess for presence of pain along gastrointestinal tract and in accessory organs.

1. Assess nonverbal signs, such as flinching, grimacing, etc.
2. Evaluate onset, location, intensity, duration, and aggravating factors.
S. Palpate for rebound tenderness of spleen.
T. Check skin color for yellow tinge, pallor, or heavy flushing.
U. Assess for signs of shock following trauma to abdomen.
V. Assess client's knowledge of diagnostic tests or surgical interventions.
W. Assess sclerae for jaundice.

Diagnostic Procedures

Roentgenography of the Gastrointestinal Tract

A. The gastrointestinal tract cannot be visualized unless a contrast medium is ingested or instilled into it.
B. Barium sulfate—a white, chalky radiopaque substance that can be flavored—is normally used as a contrast medium.
C. For an upper GI tract study, the client ingests an aqueous suspension of barium. The progression of barium is followed by the fluoroscope.
D. Roentgenography of the upper tract reveals
1. Structure and function of the esophagus.
2. Size and shape of the right atrium.
3. Esophageal varices.
4. Thickness of gastric wall.
5. Motility of the stomach.
6. Ulcerations, tumor formations, and anatomic abnormalities of the stomach.
7. Pyloric valve patency.
8. Emptying time of the stomach.
9. Structural abnormalities of the small intestine.
E. X-rays are taken for permanent records.
F. Preparation of client for an upper GI roentgenograph.
1. Maintain NPO after midnight, prior to the test.
2. Withhold medication.
3. Explain procedure.
G. The lower GI roentgenograph involves rectal instillation of barium, which is viewed with the fluoroscope. Then, permanent x-rays are taken.
H. The lower GI roentgenograph reveals the following information:
1. Abnormalities in the structure of the colon.
2. Contour and motility of the cecum and appendix.
✦ I. Preparation of client for a lower GI roentgenograph.
1. Empty intestinal tract by giving an enema, laxatives or suppositories as ordered.
2. Maintain NPO after midnight, prior to the examination.

3. Explain procedure to client.
4. Increase fluid intake and administer laxative, if needed, following procedure.

Endoscopy

A. Visualization of the inside of a body cavity by means of a lighted tube.
B. Flexible scopes are used for these examinations; scopes may be equipped with a camera.
C. Purposes.
1. Direct visualization of mucosa to detect pathologic lesions.
2. Obtaining biopsy specimens.
3. Securing washings for cytologic examination.
D. Organs capable of being scoped: esophagus, stomach, duodenum, rectum, sigmoid colon, transverse colon, and right colon.
✦ E. Nursing implementation.
1. Explain procedure to client.
2. Ensure that a signed consent for the procedure is present in the chart. Endoscopy is an invasive procedure and requires an informed consent.
3. Have client fast, prior to the examination.
4. Prepare the lower bowel with laxatives, enemas or suppositories as ordered.
5. Remove dentures and check for loose teeth prior to the procedure.
6. Prior to gastroscopy, conscious sedation and a local anesthetic may be used in the posterior pharynx. Withhold fluids and food after the procedure until the gag reflex has returned.
7. Support client during the procedure. The muscles of the GI tract tend to go into spasm with the passage of the scope, causing pain.
✦ 8. Following the endoscopy.
   a. Observe for hemorrhage, swelling or dysfunction of the involved area.
   b. Monitor vital signs.
   c. Evaluate client for evidence of complications (bleeding, dyspnea, fever, abdominal pain).
   d. For upper GI, withhold all food and fluids until gag and swallow reflexes have returned.
   e. Inform client that a sore throat, hoarseness, abdominal bloating, belching, and flatulence are common.
   f. Ensure that client is not discharged alone until sedation is completely worn off.
   g. Instruct client to inform physician immediately if the following occur: persistent difficulty swallowing; epigastric, substernal, or shoulder pain; vomiting blood; black, tarry stools; or fever.

Analysis of Secretions

A. Contents of the GI tract may be examined for the presence or absence of digestive juices, bacteria, parasites, and malignant cells.

B. Stomach contents may be aspirated and analyzed for volume and free and total acid.

✦ C. *Gastric analysis,* performed by means of a nasogastric tube.
1. Maintain NPO 6–8 hours prior to the test.
2. Pass nasogastric tube; verify its presence in the stomach; tape to client's nose.
3. Collect fasting specimens.
4. Administer agents, such as alcohol, caffeine, histamine (0.2 mg subcutaneous), as ordered, to stimulate the flow of gastric acid.
   a. Watch for side effects of histamine, including flushing, headache and hypotension.
   b. Do not give drug to clients with a history of asthma or other allergic conditions.
5. Collect specimens as ordered, usually at 10- to 20-minute intervals.
6. Label specimens and send to laboratory.
7. Withdraw nasogastric tube; offer oral hygiene; make client comfortable.
8. Gastric acid is high in the presence of duodenal ulcers and low in pernicious anemia.

✦ D. *Tubeless gastric analysis.*
1. Determines acidity or its absence.
2. Have client fast for 6–8 hours prior to the examination.
3. Administer gastric stimulant, followed by Azuresin or Diagnex Blue, as ordered.
4. Acid in the stomach displaces the dye, which is then released, absorbed by the bowel mucosa, and excreted in the urine.
5. The bladder is emptied; the specimen saved. One hour after taking dye resin, client is instructed to void again. Urine is analyzed, and an estimation is made of the amount of free acid in the stomach.

E. *Gastric washings for acid-fast bacilli.*
1. Have client fast 6–8 hours prior to the procedure.
2. Insert nasogastric tube and secure to client's nose.
3. Send specimens to the laboratory to determine the presence of acid-fast bacilli.
4. Wash your hands carefully, wear gloves, and protect yourself from direct contact with specimens.
5. This procedure is performed on suspected cases of active pulmonary tuberculosis when it is difficult to secure sputum for analysis.

F. *Analysis of stools.*
1. Stool specimens are examined for amount, consistency, color, shape, blood, fecal urobilinogen, fat, nitrogen, parasites, food residue, and other substances.
2. Stool cultures are also done for bacteria and viruses.
3. Some foods and medicines can affect stool color: spinach, green; cocoa, dark red; senna, yellow; iron, black; upper GI bleeding, tarry black; lower GI bleeding, bright red.
✦ 4. Stool abnormalities.
   a. Steatorrhea: bulky, greasy and foamy, foul odor.
   b. Biliary obstruction: light gray or clay-colored.
   c. Ulcerative colitis: loose stools, with copious amounts of mucus or pus.
   d. Constipation or obstruction: small, hard masses.
✦ 5. Specimen collection.
   a. Specimens for detection of ova and parasites should be sent to the laboratory while the stool is still warm and fresh.
   b. Examination for guaiac (occult blood) is performed on a small sample that is sent to the lab; or, a sample is placed on a commercially prepared card. A positive result indicates blood in the stool.
   c. Stools for chemical analysis are usually examined for the total quantity expelled, so the complete stool is sent to the laboratory.

Biopsy and Cytology

A. Specimens for microscopic examination are secured by endoscopy examination, cell scrapings, and needle aspiration.

B. Specimens are examined, and the laboratory then determines their origin, structure, and functions, and the presence of malignant cells.

Radionuclide Uptake

A. Radionuclides are used for diagnosis by measuring the localization of the substance, such as radioiodine in the thyroid, and the excretion of the material.

B. Various substances are studied, such as vitamin B_{12}, iron, and fat, and major organs can be scanned.

C. Substances are tagged with radioactive isotopes to assess the degree of absorption.

Blood Examinations

A. Hematologic studies and electrolyte determinations reveal information about the general status of the client.

B. Results of these examinations in conjunction with other assessment procedures and clinical symptoms help to localize the disorder.

System Implementation

A. Monitor vital signs.
B. Check for signs of dehydration.
   1. Dry mucous membranes.
   2. Poor skin turgor.
   3. Decreased urination.
   4. Increased pulse.
C. Monitor fluid intake or IV administration if ordered.
D. Monitor dietary intake or NPO status as ordered.
E. Check and record stool pattern, consistency, color, odor, presence of blood or pus, etc.
F. Evaluate laboratory results of stool culture.
G. Observe skin tone, color, and changes.
H. Administer enema if ordered.
I. Promote bowel regulation through client teaching of dietary information.
J. Perform and teach colostomy or ileostomy care to client.
K. Place or assist physician in placing Miller–Abbott tube for relief of distention if ordered.
L. Instruct client on diagnostic tests.
M. Instruct client in preoperative and postoperative care.

GENERAL GASTROINTESTINAL CONDITIONS

Definition: General symptoms of the gastrointestinal tract that may occur singly or concurrently and may be due to a wide variety of causes.

Anorexia

Definition: Loss of appetite.

Assessment

A. Assess for physiological basis for anorexia.
   1. Most illnesses, especially active stages of infections and disorders of the digestive organs, cause anorexia.
   2. Physical discomfort.
   3. Constipation.
   4. Fluid and electrolyte imbalances.
   5. Oral sepsis.
   6. Intestinal obstruction.
B. Assess for psychological source of anorexia.
   1. Fear and anxiety.
   2. Depression.
   3. Anorexia nervosa.
C. Assess for mechanical problems resulting in anorexia.
   1. Improperly fitting dentures.
   2. Excessive amounts of food.

Implementation

A. Be aware of client's eating habits, food likes and dislikes, and cultural and religious beliefs regarding food.
B. Permit choices of food when possible.
C. Show interest, but do not force client to eat.
D. Provide a pleasant environment.
E. Serve small, attractive portions of food.

Nausea and Vomiting

Definitions: Nausea is a feeling of revulsion for food, accompanied by salivation, sweating, and tachycardia. Vomiting is the contraction of the expiratory muscles of the chest, spasm of the diaphragm with contraction of the abdominal muscles, and subsequent relaxation of the stomach, allowing the gastric contents to be forced out through the mouth.

Characteristics

A. Accompanying symptoms: decreased blood pressure, increased salivation, sweating, weakness, faintness, paleness, vertigo, headache, and tachycardia.
B. Vomiting centers.
   1. Chemoreceptor emetic trigger zone.
   2. Vomiting center in the medulla.
C. Stimulation of vomiting centers.
   1. Impulses arising in the gastrointestinal tract.
   2. Impulses from cerebral centers.
   3. Chemicals via the bloodstream to the centers.
   4. Increased intracranial pressure.

Assessment

A. Assess for cerebromedullary causes.
   1. Stress, fear and depression.
   2. Neuroses and psychoses.
   3. Shock.
   4. Pain.
   5. Hypoxemia.
   6. Increased intracranial pressure.
   7. Anesthesia.
◆ B. Assess for toxic causes.
   1. Drugs ingested.
      a. Direct action on the brain.
      b. Irritant effects on the stomach or the small bowel.
   2. Food poisoning—ask about foods recently ingested.
   3. Acute febrile disease—evaluate temperature.
C. Evaluate possible visceral causes.
   1. Allergy.
   2. Intestinal obstruction—evaluate bowel sounds.
   3. Constipation.
   4. Diseases of the stomach.
   5. Acute inflammatory disease of the abdominal and pelvic organs.

6. Pregnancy.
7. Cardiovascular diseases.
8. Visceral disease.
9. Motion sickness.

D. Check for severe hypovitaminosis, especially B vitamins.
E. Assess for eating patterns: fasting or starvation.
F. Check for endocrine disorders, such as hypothyroidism and Addison's disease.
G. Observe character and quantity of emesis.
H. Evaluate hydration status and fluid and electrolyte balance.
I. Check daily weights.
J. Assess for complications: alkalosis, convulsions or tetany, atelectasis, or pneumonitis.

Implementation

A. Administer drugs: antiemetics, antihistamines, phenothiazines.
B. Monitor parenteral fluid and electrolyte replacements.
C. Perform gastric decompression.
D. Closely monitor prolonged vomiting, as hemorrhage could result.
E. Monitor hydration status, as dehydration will result in electrolyte imbalance leading to alkalosis.
F. Monitor for aspiration of vomitus, which may cause asphyxia, atelectasis, or pneumonitis.
G. Protect the client from unpleasant sights, sounds, and smells.
H. Promptly remove used emesis basin and equipment.
I. Promptly change soiled linens and dressings.
J. Ventilate room and use unscented air fresheners.

Constipation and Diarrhea

Definitions: Diarrhea is a condition characterized by loose, watery stools resulting from hypermotility of the bowel (not determined by frequency). Constipation is the undue delay in the evacuation of feces, with passage of hard and dry fecal material.

Assessment

A. Assess all other systems of the body to determine causal factors.
✦ B. Assess for constipation.
1. Lack of regularity.
2. Psychogenic causes.
3. Drugs such as narcotics.
4. Inadequate fluid and bulk intake.
5. Mechanical obstruction.
✦ C. Assess for diarrhea.
1. Fecal impaction.
2. Ulcerative colitis.
3. Intestinal infections.

4. Drugs such as antibiotics.
5. Neuroses.
✦ D. Evaluate hydration status.
E. Assess for presence of metabolic acidosis.
F. Assess for fecal impaction—pain.
G. Observe the condition of the stool, such as color, odor, shape, consistency, amount, and any unusual features, such as mucus, blood, or pus.

Implementation

A. Administer drugs—laxatives and cathartics.
✦ 1. Laxative may be used temporarily to relieve constipation, but regular use will cause loss of bowel tone.
   a. Bulk-forming/fiber (Metamucil, psyllium seed, bran) stimulates peristalsis.
   b. Milk of magnesia alters stool consistency to stimulate peristalsis.
   c. Lubricants, such as mineral oil, soften stool.
   d. Dulcolax stimulates colon; cascara, castor oil.
   e. Stool softener; Colace, Surfak.
✦ 2. Antidiarrheals, such as absorbents, astringents, and antispasmodics, may relieve symptoms.
   a. Mild diarrhea: oral fluids replace lost fluids.
   b. Moderate diarrhea: drugs that decrease motility (Lomotil and Imodium).
   c. Severe diarrhea caused by infectious agent: antimicrobials and fluid replacement.
   d. Anticholinergics (Atropine) reduce bowel spasticity. Used to treat irritable bowel and diarrhea caused by peptic ulcer disease.
✦ B. Provide fluid and electrolyte replacement therapy to correct imbalances—IV therapy may be necessary to replace fluids.
C. Diet high in nutrients and calories—give supplements of vitamins (especially fat-soluble A, D, E and K).
D. Prevent skin excoriation with emollients, powder, and cleanliness.
E. Change soiled linens and dressings.
F. Ventilate room.

DISORDERS OF THE UPPER GASTROINTESTINAL TRACT

Oral Infections

Definition: Stomatitis is an inflammation of the mouth; glossitis, an inflammation of the tongue; and gingivitis, an inflammation of the gums.

Characteristics

A. Causes may be mechanical, chemical, or infectious.

B. Types.
  ✦ 1. Herpes simplex—a group of vesicles on an ery-thematous base.
      a. Usually located at the mucocutaneous junc-tion of the lips and face.
      b. Caused by a virus that may be activated by sunlight, heat, fever, digestive disturbances, and menses.
    ✦ c. Antimicrobial treatment is not effective unless there is secondary bacterial infection. Treated with acyclovir.
      d. Treated symptomatically.
    2. Vincent's angina (trench mouth)—purplish-red gums covered by pseudomembrane.
      a. Caused by fusiform bacteria and spirochetes.
      b. Symptoms include fever, anorexia, enlarged cervical glands, and foul breath.
      c. May be acute, subacute, or chronic.
    3. Aphthous ulcers (canker sores).
      a. Unknown etiology.
      b. Usually less than 1 cm in diameter.
      c. Duration—lasts weeks to months.
      d. Very painful, shallow erosions of the mucous membranes.
      e. Well circumscribed with a white or yellow center, encircled by a red ring.

Assessment

A. Assess for anorexia.
B. Evaluate excessive salivation.
C. Check for foul breath.
D. Evaluate condition of gums and tongue.
E. Assess for jagged teeth or mouth breathing.
F. Check for foods or drinks that result in allergies.
G. Assess for presence of infection.

Implementation

A. Remove cause.
B. Provide frequent, soothing oral hygiene.
C. Administer topical medications or systemic anti-biotics.
D. Provide a soft, bland diet.
E. Administer pain medications as needed.
F. Avoid alcohol-based mouthwashes.

Disorder of the Salivary Glands

✦ *Definition:* Salivary gland infection is an inflammation (parotitis or surgical mumps) usually caused by *Staphylococcus aureus.*

Assessment

A. Assess for pain.
B. Check temperature.

C. Assess for enlargement of glands.
D. Assess for dysphagia.

Implementation

A. Administer preventive measures.
    1. Keep the glands active; calculus or calculi (stones) form when the gland is inactive.
    2. Provide adequate fluids.
    3. Give oral hygiene.
B. Provide warm packs.
C. Administer antibiotics.
D. Monitor hydration.
E. Care for incision.
F. Observe for drainage.

Malignant Tumors of the Mouth

Definition: Cancer of the mouth is a malignant tumor (squamous cell carcinoma) and usually affects the lips, the lateral border of the tongue, or the floor of the mouth.

Assessment

✦ A. Assess for lesions that tend to be painless and hard and ulcerate easily.
B. Assess for poor oral hygiene.
C. Check for chronic irritation.
D. Evaluate for chemical and thermal trauma (tobacco, alcohol, and hot, spicy foods).
E. Assess for metastasis by local extension.
    1. Cause symptoms by occupying space and exert-ing pressure.
    2. Usually fibromas, lipomas, or neurofibromas.

Implementation

A. Provide postsurgical interventions.
B. Monitor for complications.

Radical Neck Dissection

Definition: Removal of lateral lymph nodes and tissue, submandibular gland, jugular vein, sternocleidomastoid muscle, spinal accessory nerve and surrounding tissue of neck.

✦ Assessment

A. Assess for patent airway.
    1. Observe for airway obstruction (wheezing, stri-dor, retraction).
    2. Observe for respiratory distress, stertorous, labored breathing, increased respirations, and cyanosis.
B. Observe for edema that could constrict trachea.
C. Watch for difficulty in swallowing if allowed oral fluids. Difficulty may indicate nerve damage. If radi-cal procedure, client will probably be fed through either nasogastric tube, gastrostomy, or IV therapy.

D. Observe dressings for hemorrhage, which could lead to respiratory embarrassment.

E. Assess vital signs for indications of bleeding and infection.

F. Assess for infection; increase in temperature, foul odor to dressings.

G. Observe for carotid rupture or chylous fistula—milky drainage.

H. Assess catheter drainage and suture lines.

I. Evaluate wound healing.

J. Observe for lower facial paralysis indicating facial nerve injury.

K. Assess mental state for depression, damage to self-image, feelings of loss, etc.

Implementation

✦ A. Maintain adequate respiratory function.
   1. Place in high-Fowler's position.
   2. Monitor for respiratory distress.

✦ B. Suction to prevent aspiration and pneumonia.

C. Administer oxygen as needed.

D. Encourage intake of fluids, which is necessary to thin secretions.

E. Provide care for laryngectomy (frequently performed with radical neck dissection).
   1. Use mist mask.
   2. Clean laryngectomy tube as you would tracheostomy tube.

F. Change dressings frequently to prevent infection.
   1. Drains are frequently placed in surgical site; Hemovac is the drain most commonly used.
   2. Observe for drainage (amount, type, odor, color).

G. Give oral hygiene every 2–4 hours.

✦ H. Develop means to communicate, as client will not be able to talk postoperatively if laryngectomy was also performed.
   1. Provide method of writing for the first few days.
   2. Explain to client that hoarseness is usual for the first few weeks.
   3. Provide bell or readily accessible means of communication for client to decrease anxiety following surgery.

I. Provide privacy for client.

J. Develop nurse–client relationship, as client may be depressed, may suffer feelings of loss, and may need to verbalize concerns about self-image.

K. Teach or follow through with rehabilitation exercises for head and shoulder.
   1. Rotate neck, tilt head to both sides, and drop chin to chest.
   2. Swing arm on operated side in arc to extend range of motion.

L. Provide general postoperative care.

MEDICAL IMPLICATIONS

Diagnosis
- Laryngoscopic exam reveals nodes on or near the vocal cords.
- Biopsy reveals cancer cells.
- Assess involvement of the vocal cords.

Radiation
- Excellent result when only one cord is affected.
- Usually retains normal voice.
- May be used preoperatively to reduce tumor size.
- May not be a lasting cure.

Surgery

Cancer of the Larnyx

Definition: Cancer of the voice box and other surrounding structures.

Characteristics

A. Factors that increase risk.
   1. Age—occurs most often in people older than age 55.
   2. Gender—men are four times more likely than women.
   3. Race—increased in African Americans.
   4. Smoking.
   5. Alcohol.
   6. Personal history of head and neck cancer.
   7. Occupational—workers exposed to sulfuric acid mist, nickel, or asbestos have increased risk of disease.

B. Clinical manifestations.
   1. Hoarseness.
   2. Burning while drinking hot or acidic food.
   3. Dysphagia.
   4. Foul breath.
   5. Enlarged cervical nodes.
   6. Weight loss.
   7. Malaise.
   8. Pain radiating to the ear.

Laryngectomy

Definition: Removal of the voice box and other surrounding structures. May be partial or complete, which depends on the location and involvement of the tumor.

Characteristics

A. Total laryngectomy and radical neck dissection—procedure of choice for cancer under following circumstances:
   1. If tumor does not extend more than 5 mm up base of tongue or below upper edge of cricoarytenoid muscle.

2. If there is no evidence of distant metastasis.

B. Epiglottis, thyroid cartilage, hyoid bone, cricoid cartilage, and part of trachea are removed.

C. Stump of trachea is brought out to neck and sutured to skin. The pharyngeal portion is closed, and breathing through nose is eliminated.

D. Accompanied by radical neck dissection if neck tissue and lymph nodes are involved.

Assessment

A. Assess drainage from wound suction for amount, type, color, and odor.

B. Assess for carotid artery hemorrhage.

C. Evaluate lung fluids for atelectasis and pneumonia.

D. Monitor for complications.
1. Mucus plug.
2. Bleeding from stoma or incision.
3. Infection at incision site.
4. Respiratory infection.

✦ Implementation

A. Observe for hypoxia.

B. Position in semi-Fowler's position or higher.

C. Suction frequently using sterile technique until area has healed; then use clean technique.

D. Place pressure on neck wound for hemorrhage around site.

E. Instruct client regarding means for communication, as he or she will not be able to speak immediately postoperatively.

F. Speech rehabilitation is utilized after surgical area has healed.

G. Nutrition.
1. NPO 10–14 days.
2. NG tube and TPN for nutrition.
3. Thick fluids introduced first.
4. Avoid sweet foods.
5. Rinse mouth or brush teeth after eating.

H. Teaching.
1. Teach ways to handle increased mucus production.
2. Keep stoma clear of excess mucus.
3. Wear a bib to conceal mucus.
4. Cleanse peristomal skin BID.
5. Use nebulizer or humidifier.
6. Assure that taste and smell will adapt over time.
7. Cover stoma while showering.
8. Avoid swimming.
9. Avoid powders and and aerosols.
10. Carry medical alert information.

Gastroesophageal Reflux Disease (GERD)

Definition: Backward flow (reflux) of gastric contents into the esophagus; suffered by 15–20% of adults.

Assessment

A. Assess for heartburn after meals.

B. Check for regurgitation of material into the mouth.

C. Assess for difficulty or pain in swallowing—pain may be severe.

✦ Implementation

A. Monitor antacids (Maalox) for mild or moderate conditions.

B. Explain use of histamine$_2$ receptor blockers (cimetidine, ranitidine) to reduce acid production.

C. Monitor use of proton-pump inhibitors (PPIs) such as Prilosec or Prevacid to reduce gastric secretions and relieve symptoms.

D. Suggest dietary changes such as reduction in fat, coffee, spicy foods and cessation in smoking (which increases acidity).

Esophageal Varices

✦ *Definition:* Tortuous, dilated veins in the submucosa of the lower esophagus, possibly extending into the fundus of the stomach or upward into the esophagus; caused by portal hypertension and often associated with cirrhosis of the liver.

Assessment

A. Assess for bleeding.

B. Check for hypotension.

C. Evaluate neck veins for distention.

D. Assess for nutritional status.

E. Evaluate indications that lead to suspected varices.
1. Hematemesis.
2. Hematochezia.
3. History of alcoholism.

F. Observe for strain of coughing or vomiting, which could result in esophageal rupture.

✦ Implementation

✦ A. Carefully observe vital signs, watching for hemorrhage and shock. (Goal is to restore hemodynamic status.)

B. Maintain prescribed pressure levels in balloon tamponade.
1. Provide frequent oral hygiene and aspiration of the mouth and throat because the client cannot swallow saliva with the balloons in place.
2. Prevent esophageal erosion by deflating the balloons (only with physician's order).
✦ 3. Safety measure: keep scissors at bedside. If tube dislodges and causes obstruction, cut tube to deflate balloons.
4. Prevent nasal breakdown.
   a. Keep nostrils lubricated and clean.

MEDICAL IMPLICATIONS

✦A. Upper endoscopy evaluates and treats condition.
  1. Gastric lavage with normal saline to visualize varices.
  2. Varices may be banded or sclerosed.
    a. Varices are ligated with small rubber bands that occlude blood flow.
    b. Sclerosing agent injected into varices to induce inflammation and thrombosis.
✦B. Balloon tamponade—Sengstaken–Blakemore triple-lumen tube for pressure application against varices.
  1. May be used if endoscopy is unavailable or if vaso-constriction cannot control bleeding.
  2. Tube has three openings.
    a. One opening to gastric balloon.
    b. Second opening to esophageal balloon.
    c. Pressure in both balloons is 25–30 mm Hg.
    d. Third opening for aspiration of gastric contents.
  3. Traction with a 0.75- to 1.5-lb weight used to prevent downward movement.
  4. Iced saline irrigations may be used to vasoconstrict the small collaterals.
✦C. Transjugular intrahepatic portosystemic shunt (TIPS)—used for portal hypertension and varices.
  1. A needle inserted transcutaneously in which a stent is inserted that carries blood into hepatic vein, bypassing the damaged liver.
  2. Shunt relieves pressure in varices and increases perfusion of the liver and impaired ammonia metabolism.
✦D. Restoration of clotting factors.
  1. Vitamin K replacement.
  2. Platelet replacement (destroyed by damaged spleen).
  3. Fresh frozen plasma.
✦E. Surgical repairs.
  1. Direct ligation of varices.
  2. Portasystemic shunts.
    a. Portacaval.
      (1) End to side.
      (2) Side to side.
    b. Splenorenal.
      (1) End to side.
      (2) Side to side.
    c. Mesocaval.
      (1) End to side.
      (2) Use of synthetic graft.
  3. Esophageal transection and devascularization.

    b. Provide foam rubber padding to reduce pressure at nares.
  5. Observe for sudden respiratory crisis, which may occur with aspiration or upward displacement of the balloons.

C. Maintain fluid and nutritional balance.
✦D. Observe for complications of active bleeding varices.
  1. Hypovolemia.
  2. Hepatic encephalopathy due to increased ammonia production as blood protein is metabolized.
  3. Metabolic imbalances due to acid–base and electrolyte disturbances.
E. Comfort family and client.
  1. Explain procedures and utilize nursing comfort measures.
  2. Use sedatives and narcotics judiciously because the liver is usually impaired in its ability to detoxify.

Esophageal Hernia (Hiatal Hernia)

Definition: In esophageal hernia, a portion of the stomach herniates through the diaphragm and into the thorax (also called diaphragmatic hernia).

Characteristics

A. Congenital weakness.
B. Trauma.
C. Relaxation of muscles.
D. Increased intra-abdominal pressure.
E. Manifestations range from none to acutely severe manifestations.

Assessment

A. Assess for heartburn and substernal discomfort or pain.
B. Assess for dysphagia.
C. Check for vomiting pattern.
D. Reflux.
E. Indigestion or feeling of fullness.
F. Assess for complications.
  1. Ulceration.
  2. Hemorrhage.
  3. Regurgitation and aspiration of gastric contents.
  4. Incarceration of stomach in the chest, with possible necrosis, peritonitis and mediastinitis.
G. Diagnostic tests.
  1. Esophagogastroduodenoscopy (EGD).
  2. Barium swallow.

Implementation

✦A. Provide small, frequent meals, avoiding highly seasoned foods.
✦B. Maintain upright position during and after meals.
C. Give antacids after meals and at bedtime.
D. Elevate head of bed to avoid regurgitation while eating and for 30 minutes after meal.
E. Avoid anticholinergic drugs, which delay emptying of the stomach.

F. Prevent constricting clothing around the waist and sharp, forward bending.

G. Monitor medical treatment.
   1. Reduction of stomach distention.
   2. Reduction of stomach acidity.
   3. Reduction of increased levels of intra-abdominal pressure.

✦ H. Give postoperative care for surgical reduction of hernia, via a thoracic or abdominal approach.
   1. Surgery is indicated when the risk of complications or reflux is severe.
   2. Surgical approach reinforces the lower esophageal sphincter (LES) to restore sphincter competence and prevent reflux. A portion of the stomach fundus is wrapped around the distal esophagus to anchor it and reinforce the LES.

Esophageal Lesions

Characteristics

A. Benign lesions.
   1. Leiomyoma most common type.
   2. Asymptomatic.
B. Malignant lesions.
   1. Usually occur in lower two-thirds of esophagus.
   2. Mainly affect men over age 50.
   ✦ 3. Smoking and alcohol are risk factors.
      a. Poor prognosis (< 5 years survival) due to early lymphatic spread and late development of symptoms.
      b. Dysphagia is the most common symptom.
      c. Diagnosis made by barium swallow, esophagoscopy, biopsy.
C. Treatment.
   1. Surgical excision.
   2. Radiation therapy (fistulas may be a complication).

Assessment

A. Assess for extent of lesions.
B. Evaluate vital signs.
C. Observe for poor dietary status.
D. Observe for complications of ulceration and hemorrhage, fistula formation, and pneumothorax in end-stage disease.

Implementation

A. Maintain fluid and electrolyte balance.
B. Manage nutrition needs (hyperalimentation therapy may be used).
C. Administer gastrostomy tube feedings, if needed.
D. Monitor client's ability to handle secretions.
E. Provide emotional support.

GASTRIC DISORDERS

Dyspepsia Indigestion

Definition: Indigestion is caused by diseases of the gastrointestinal system, eating too rapidly, emotional problems, inadequate chewing, eating improperly cooked foods, systemic diseases, food allergies, and altered gastric secretion or motility.

Assessment

A. Assess for heartburn.
B. Assess for flatulence.
C. Observe for nausea.
D. Observe for eructations.
E. Identify feeling of fullness.

Implementation

A. Based on the cause of the disorder.
B. Antacids and bland diets.
C. Antispasmodics and tranquilizers.
D. Altered eating habits.

Anorexia Nervosa

✦ *Definition:* Underlying emotional disorders cause psychogenic aversion to food, with resulting emaciation. Usually occurs in females during the late teens or early twenties. Onset is often associated with a stressful life event. Client often has fear of obesity, body-image distortion, and disturbed self-concept. This eating disorder may be life-threatening. Death can occur from starvation or electrolyte imbalance.

Assessment

✦ A. Assess weight—loss of one-fourth to one-half or more of the body weight occurs with this disorder.
✦ B. Check for amenorrhea for at least 3 consecutive periods.
C. Observe for vomiting when food is forced.
D. Assess for hypotension, decreased temperature and pulse.
E. Evaluate for anemia.
F. Assess for hypoproteinemia.
G. Compulsive exercising.
H. Loss of appetite or refusal to eat.
I. Perfectionism and overachievement.
J. Self-administered enemas or self-induced vomiting.
K. Dry and scaly skin.
L. Sleep disturbances.
M. Gastrointestinal upsets.
N. Deterioration of gums and teeth.
O. Degeneration of bone.

Implementation

A. Give supportive care.

B. Administer tube feedings if necessary.
✦ C. Monitor psychiatric treatment. (*See* Chapter 14, Psychiatric Nursing, for more detailed information.)
   1. Set firm limits.
   2. Monitor eating patterns.

Acute Gastritis

Definition: An inflammation of the stomach by a local irritant.

Characteristics
A. Ingestion of an infectious, corrosive, or erosive substance (such as alcohol, aspirin, or food poisoning).
B. Acute systemic infections.
C. Radiotherapy or chemotherapy.

✦ Assessment
A. Assess for pain.
B. Evaluate nausea and vomiting pattern.
C. Check for malaise.
D. Observe for hemorrhage.
E. Assess for anorexia.
F. Check for headache.
G. Assess for dehydration.

Implementation
A. Remove cause and treat symptomatically.
B. Monitor drugs that include antacids and phenothiazines.
✦ C. Correct fluid and electrolyte balance; NPO during acute phase, then graduate to bland diet with fluid replacement.

Chronic Gastritis

Definition: Unrelated to acute gastritis, a nondescript, upper abdominal distress with vague symptoms. Other causes should be explored.

✦ Characteristics
A. Type A: autoimmune component affecting people of Northern European heritage.
   1. Antibodies destroy gastric mucosal cells—results in tissue atrophy, loss of HCl and pepsin.
   2. Intrinsic factor not present, so low absorption of B_{12} leads to pernicious anemia.
B. Type B: more common, with incidence increasing with age.
   1. Caused by chronic infection of gastric mucosa by *H. pylori*.
   2. Infection is associated with increased risk of peptic ulcer disease.

Assessment
A. Assess for dyspepsia, anorexia, and eructations.

B. Check for foul taste in mouth.
C. Assess for nausea and vomiting.
D. Assess for pain and mild epigastric tenderness.
E. Observe for complications.
   1. Hemorrhage.
   2. Scarring of mucosa.
   3. Ulcer formation.
   4. Malnutrition.

Implementation
The same as for peptic ulcer disease (PUD).

Peptic Ulcer Disease (PUD)

✦ *Definition:* An ulceration in the mucosal wall of the stomach, pylorus, or duodenum, occurring in portions that are accessible to gastric secretions. Erosion may extend through the muscle to the peritoneum.

Characteristics
✦ A. Pathophysiology.
   1. Any condition that upsets the balance between digestion and protection.
      a. No longer thought to be only caused by excess stomach acid. It can contribute to ulcer formation if too much acid is secreted.
   ✦ b. Bacterial invasion of mucosa caused by *Helicobacter pylori* bacterium.
      (1) Found in more than 70 percent of gastric ulcer clients.
      (2) Found in 95 percent of duodenal ulcers.
      (3) *H. pylori* is found in 50 percent of ulcers worldwide.
      c. Ingestion of certain drugs such as steroids, ASA, and NSAIDs.
      d. Smoking is a risk factor.
   ✦ 2. Ulcers tend to occur in lesser curvature of stomach near the pylorus (15%).
   ✦ 3. Duodenal ulcers account for 80 percent of peptic ulcers. (*See* Table 8-1.)
B. Diagnostic evaluation.
   1. Medical history and symptoms.
   2. Key test is endoscopy to locate ulcer.
   3. Gastric biopsy to detect *Helicobacter pylori*.

Assessment
✦ A. Assess pain.
   1. Location and intensity—duodenal ulcer symptoms usually occur 2–3 hours after eating and during the night.
   2. Duration.
   3. Aggravating factors.
B. Evaluate vital signs to establish a baseline to monitor for bleeding.
C. Evaluate laboratory results.

✦ Table 8-1. COMPARISON OF DUODENAL AND GASTRIC ULCER

	Chronic Duodenal Ulcer	Chronic Gastric Ulcer
Age	Usually 30 to 55	Usually 55 and older
Sex	Male:female—2–3:1	Male:female—1:1
Blood group	Most frequently type O	Blood group A
Social class	Executives, competitive leaders	Lower socioeconomic class
Incidence	80%	20%
General nourishment	Well nourished	Malnourished
Acid production in stomach	Hypersecretion	Normal to hyposecretion
Location	Within 3 cm of pylorus	Lesser curvature
Pain	2–3 hours after meals and at night Usually absent before breakfast—worsens as day progresses Ingestion of food, antacids or vomiting relieves pain	On an empty stomach or shortly after the meal Rarely is there pain at night Relieved by antacids or vomiting
Vomiting	Uncommon	Common
Hemorrhage	Melena more common than hematemesis	Hematemesis more common than melena
Malignancy possibility	None	Usually less than 10%

D. Check stool for blood.

✦ E. Observe for hemorrhage.
1. Dark, granular (coffee ground) emesis is a result of acid digestion of blood in the stomach.
2. Tarry, black stools result when blood is completely digested.
3. Hematemesis (vomiting of bright red blood).
4. Bright red blood from rectum. Occurs when bleeding originates from high in the gastrointestinal tract and there is concurrent rapid gastrointestinal motility.

Implementation

A. Administer and monitor medications.
✦ 1. Antimicrobial therapy—antibiotics (Amoxil), tetracycline.
   a. One course of therapy treats ulcers caused by *Helicobacter pylori* infection.
   b. Combined with proton-pump inhibitor, bismuth preparations, traditional antacids, H$_2$ antagonists, and Flagyl results in a full cure with fewer complications.
   c. Levofloxacin-based triple therapy is treatment of choice for persistent *H. pylori* infection.
✦ 2. Antacids.
   a. Action: reduces gastric acidity; given for pain.
   b. Taken 1 hour after meals; effects last longer.
   c. Side effects: diarrhea and constipation.
   d. Types of nonabsorbable antacids.

   (1) Calcium carbonate is most effective but may cause hypercalcemia, hypercalciuria (high urine calcium), and constipation.
   (2) Magnesium oxide is more potent than either magnesium trisilicate or magnesium carbonate.
   (3) Aluminum hydroxide—high sodium content and constipation are disadvantages.
   (4) Sodium bicarbonate is absorbed and should be avoided to prevent systemic alkalosis.
✦ 3. Histamine H$_2$-receptor antagonists.
   a. Cimetidine (Tagamet), ranitidine (Zantac), famotidine (Pepcid), and nizatidine (Axid), PO or IV.
   b. Action: blocking action reduces production of gastric acid and allows ulcers to heal.
   c. Drugs were 90 percent effective when taken PO for 8 weeks; now often replaced by antibiotics.
   d. Minimal side effects: headache and skin rash.
✦ 4. Sucralfate (Carafate).
   a. Action: adheres to ulcer surface, stimulates release of prostaglandins; reinforces mucosal barrier.
   b. Duration is 5 hours; administer 1 hour before or after meals and at bedtime on an empty stomach.

c. Prescribed when drug interactions or side effects negate use of H$_2$ antagonists.

d. Side effects: constipation, nausea and vomiting.

5. Anticholingeric drugs.

a. Used only for clients with severe pain in the early morning.

b. Drug action increases risk of gastric outlet syndrome.

✦ 6. Proton-pump inhibitors block release of HCl from parietal cells—very effective result with over 90 percent healing in 4 weeks.

a. Omeprazole (Prilosec).

b. Lansoprazole (Prevacid).

7. Synthetic prostaglandin.

a. Misoprostol (Cytotec).

b. Particularly useful for persons using long-term NSAIDs.

c. Protects stomach lining from erosive action of gastric acid. (This drug may induce abortions.)

✦ B. Provide dietary control of symptoms until ulcer is cured.

1. Ensure three nutritious meals.

2. Avoid black pepper, foods that cause distress until ulcer is cured (e.g., highly seasoned, rough, greasy, gas-forming, or fried).

3. Avoid prolonged use of milk and cream, as they stimulate acid production.

4. Avoid alcohol, as it releases gastrin, stimulates the parietal cells, and may damage the mucosa.

5. Avoid tea, coffee, and cola, because caffeine stimulates gastric secretion.

6. Do not provide any snacks, even at bedtime (stimulates acid secretion).

7. Provide iron and ascorbic acid to promote healing.

✦ C. Reduce stressful situations if client is hospitalized.

1. Allow client to care for important business obligations.

2. Eliminate visitors or duties that increase stress.

3. Teach autogenic methods of stress reduction, relaxation, tension-releasing activities.

D. Promote rest.

1. Adequate sleep is strongly advised.

2. Business and social responsibilities should be curtailed during acute phase.

3. Hospitalization may be required if therapy is not effective in 1 week.

4. Sedatives and tranquilizers may be helpful for the anxious, tense client.

✦ E. Provide client and family teaching regarding diet, activity level, medications, risk factors (smoking), and potential complications.

✦ F. Observe for complications.

1. Hemorrhage, ranging from slight blood loss (revealed by occult blood in stool) to massive blood loss, which may lead to shock.

a. Promote bedrest.

b. Observe vital signs.

c. Observe consistency, color, and volume of vomitus and stools.

d. Provide nasogastric suction to empty the stomach of clots and blood, and to watch the rate of bleeding.

e. Monitor blood, plasma, or IV fluids to support blood volume.

f. Administer narcotics and/or tranquilizers to reduce restlessness and to relieve pain.

g. Gavage with ice water to increase vaso-constriction.

2. Perforation: occurs almost exclusively in males 25–40 years of age.

a. Monitor acute onset of severe, persistent pain that increases in intensity and can be referred to the shoulder.

b. Examine for tender, boardlike rigidity of the abdomen.

3. Pyloric obstruction caused by scarring, edema, or inflammation at the pylorus.

a. Monitor for the following signs: nausea and vomiting, pain, weight loss, and constipation.

b. Be aware that persistent vomiting can lead to alkalosis.

G. For surgical interventions, *see* Surgical Implications under Gastric Cancer.

SURGICAL INTERVENTION

Gastric Cancer

Definition: Carcinoma of the stomach is a common cancer of the digestive tract.

Characteristics

A. Responsible for 20,000 deaths annually in the United States.

B. Has decreased in incidence during the last 20 years, but is a significant cause of death because of low cure rate.

C. Occurs twice as often in males as in females, and more often in African Americans than in other races.

D. Found frequently in conjunction with pernicious anemia and atrophic gastritis.

E. Worldwide incidence varies.

F. Early carcinoma causes no symptoms.

Assessment

A. Assess for weight loss and anorexia.

✦ SURGICAL IMPLICATIONS

A. Vagotomy and gastroenterostomy or pyloroplasty.
1. Vagus nerve is cut.
2. Drainage of stomach.
   a. Drainage operation necessary because vagotomy is often followed by gastric retention.
   b. Vagus nerve provides the motor impulses to the gastric musculature, whose division is often followed by gastric atony.
3. The pyloroplasty or gastroenterostomy also reduces the stimulation of gastric acid by reducing the formation of gastrin produced in the antral area of the stomach.
B. Vagotomy and antrectomy.
1. Decrease production of acid to point where ulcers will not recur.
2. Remove acid-stimulating mechanism of stomach (i.e., divide vagus nerve and remove antral portion of stomach).
C. Partial gastrectomy and possible vagotomy.
1. Billroth I—partial gastrectomy with remaining segment of stomach anastomosed to duodenum.
2. Billroth II—remaining segment of stomach is anastomosed to jejunum (usually for duodenal ulcer).

B. Check for feeling of vague fullness and sensation of pressure.
C. Assess for anemia from blood loss.
D. Examine stools for occult blood.
E. Assess vomiting if pylorus becomes obstructed.
F. Observe for late symptoms: ascites, palpable mass, and pain from metastasis.
G. Evaluate for metastasis.
1. Occurs by direct extension into surrounding tissue.
2. Spreads through lymphatic and hematogenous systems.

Implementation
A. Provide postoperative care for surgical resection.
1. Surgical mortality is 5–12 percent.
2. Five-year survival rate is 5–15 percent.
B. Monitor chemotherapy—response has not been consistent; may shorten life span if toxic effects occur.

Postoperative Period

Assessment
A. Observe color, amount, and consistency of nasogastric drainage.
B. Evaluate patency of nasogastric tube.
C. Evaluate type and severity of pain.
D. Evaluate client's ability to deep-breathe and cough.
E. Assess intravenous site for possible complications.

✦ DUMPING SYNDROME

- Rapid emptying of gastric contents into small intestine, which has been anastomosed to the gastric stump.
- Mechanical result of surgery in which a small gastric remnant remains after surgery.
- From this, there is a large opening from the gastric stump into the jejunum.
- Foods that are high in carbohydrates and electrolytes must be diluted in the jejunum before absorption can take place.
- The ingestion of fluid at mealtime is another factor in the rapid emptying of the stomach into the jejunum.
- Symptoms are caused by rapid distention of jejunal loop anastomosed to stomach.
  1. There is a withdrawal of water from the circulating blood volume into the jejunum to dilute the high concentration of electrolytes and sugars.
  2. A rapid movement of extracellular fluids into the bowel occurs and converts the hypertonic material to an isotonic mixture.
  3. This rapid shift decreases the circulatory blood volume, similar to hypovolemic shock.
- Foods high in sugars and salt produce the following symptoms: palpitation, perspiration, faintness, weakness that lasts from a few minutes to as long as 30 minutes and causes the client to lie down.
- Teach client how to prevent dumping syndrome.
  1. Avoid sugar and salt; maintain a high-protein, high-fat, low-carbohydrate diet.
  2. Avoid drinking fluids with meals, thereby delaying gastric emptying.
  3. Lie down after meals.
  4. Physicians can prevent symptoms by forming smaller stomas and larger gastric stump.
  5. Syndrome usually subsides in 6 months.

F. Listen for bowel sounds.
G. Assess all systems for possible complications.

Implementation
✦ A. After anesthesia recovery, place in modified Fowler's position for comfort and easy stomach drainage.
✦ B. Prevent pulmonary complications—medicate before turning, coughing, or hyperventilating.
✦ C. Institute nasogastric suction; drainage contains some blood for the first 12 hours.
1. Physician inserts tube.
2. Keep patent by irrigating with sodium chloride.
✦ D. See that client is NPO (no peristalsis).
E. Give intravenous fluids with potassium chloride.
✦ F. After nasogastric tube is out, give small sips of water. (Do not use a straw.)
1. Do not give cold fluids (cause distress); give warm, weak tea.
2. Offer bland foods so that client eats six small meals a day and drinks 120 mL fluid between meals.

G. Promote ambulation on first postoperative day unless contraindicated by physician.

H. Check drainage tubes if inserted. (Serosanguineous drainage is normal.)

✦ I. Observe for postoperative complications.
1. Shock (from hypovolemia).
2. Vomiting—usually due to blood left in stomach. (Nasogastric tube prevents vomiting.)
3. Hemorrhage.
4. Pulmonary complications.
5. Large fluid and electrolyte losses.
6. Dumping syndrome.
7. Diarrhea—complication of vagotomy (use Kaopectate).
✦ 8. Vitamin B_{12} deficiency.
   a. Production of "intrinsic factor" is halted. (The gastric secretion is required for the absorption of vitamin B_{12} from the gastrointestinal tract.)
   b. Unless supplied by parenteral injection throughout life, client suffers vitamin B_{12} deficiency.

INFLAMMATORY BOWEL DISEASE

Regional Enteritis (Regional Ileitis, Crohn's Disease)

✦ *Definition:* An inflammatory disease of the small intestine that is chronic and relapsing. It results in thickening, scarring, and granulomas of intestinal tissues, which causes narrow lumen, fistulas, ulcerations, and abscesses. The etiology is unknown, but may be related to altered immunologic reactivity.

Characteristics
A. Occurs at all ages.
B. Usually observed in second and third decades of life.
C. High incidence of familial occurrence.
D. High incidence in Jewish population; low incidence in African Americans.

✦ ### Assessment
A. Continuous or episodic diarrhea and cramp-like pain after meals.
B. Evaluate for weight loss.
C. Check for malnutrition.
D. Assess for secondary anemia.
E. Check for abdominal pain and tenderness.
F. Evaluate temperature.
G. Assess for complications: acute perforation, generalized peritonitis, and massive melena, which are sometimes present at onset.
H. Fever.
I. Electrolyte imbalance.

Implementation
✦ A. Provide appropriate diet: high calorie, high protein, low residue, bland, with iron and vitamin supplements (including B_{12}); elimination of all milk and milk products.
✦ B. Administer medications.
1. Anti-inflammatory drugs to reduce swollen membranes [corticosteroids, sulfasalazine (Azulfidine)].
2. Antidiarrheal agents to control diarrhea.
3. Sedatives and narcotics to reduce apprehension and pain.
4. Antibiotics such as Flagyl may be given to control infection.
5. Oral aminosalicylates (Asacol).
6. Immunosuppressives to prevent relapses.
7. Total parenteral nutrition (TPN) to maintain nutritional status is often prescribed.
C. Provide postoperative care for surgical intervention (ileostomy).

Ulcerative Colitis

✦ *Definition:* A chronic ulcerative and inflammatory disease that affects the mucosa and submucosa of the colon and rectum; commonly begins in the rectum and sigmoid colon and spreads upward. The disease is characterized by periods of exacerbations and remissions.

Characteristics
A. Cause unknown, but theories include autoimmune factor, allergic reaction, specific vulnerability of the colon, emotional instability, and bacterial infection.
B. Most common in young adulthood and middle life. More prevalent among the Jewish population; less common in African Americans than in Caucasians.

✦ ### Assessment
A. Assess for gradual onset.
1. Malaise.
2. Early—vague abdominal discomfort.
3. Later—cramp-like abdominal pain.
4. Bowel evacuation—pus, mucus, and blood.
5. Stools scanty and hard.
6. Painful straining with defecation.
B. Assess for abrupt onset.
1. Severe diarrhea (15–20 watery stools a day that may contain blood and mucus).
2. Fever.
3. Anorexia.
4. Weight loss.
5. Abdominal tenderness.
6. Rectal and anal spasticity.
7. Consistency of stools vary with areas of colon involved.

✦ C. Assess for complications.
1. Dehydration.
2. Magnesium and calcium imbalances.
3. Anemia and malnutrition—malabsorption and iron and vitamin K deficiency.
4. Perforation, peritonitis and hemorrhage.
5. Abscesses and strictures.
6. Carcinomatous degeneration (if more than 10 years' duration).
7. Toxic megacolon and colon perforation.
8. Bleeding tendency.
D. Evaluate results of client's history and diagnostic tests.
1. Medical history.
2. Clinical manifestations.
3. Lower GI series.
4. Stool and blood examinations.
5. Sigmoidoscopy.

Implementation

A. Major objective—prevent acute episodes and/or manage complications.
✦ B. Maintain nutritional status.
1. High-protein, high-calorie, high-fiber diet.
2. Avoid certain spices (pepper), gas-forming foods, and milk products (client may be lactose intolerant).
3. All foods should be cooked to reduce cramping and diarrhea.
4. Vitamins (A and E), minerals (zinc, calcium, and magnesium), and iron supplements.
5. Eating may increase diarrhea and anorexia.
6. Total parenteral nutrition (TPN) may be indicated.
✦ C. Replace fluid and electrolytes lost due to diarrhea.
1. 3–4 L/day.
2. Potassium chloride may need to be added.
D. Manage psychological disturbances.
1. Allow client to ventilate feelings; accept client as he or she is.
2. Help client live with chronic disease (a change in lifestyle may be necessary).
3. Avoid emotional probing during periods of acute illness.
4. Provide client and family with instructions about pathology of the disease and rationale for treatment.
✦ E. Administer drugs as ordered.
1. Steroid therapy for inflammation, toxicity, and emotional symptoms.
a. Induces remissions.
b. Given IV in acute episode.
c. Given rectally for long term.
2. Anti-infectives.
a. Routine sulfonamides to reduce severity of attack.

b. Antibiotic therapy for secondary bowel inflammation and systemic infections.
3. Immunosuppressives to prevent relapses.
4. Oral aminosalicylates have proven very effective (used with caution in clients with renal dysfunction).
5. Tranquilizers (e.g., phenobarbital) to relieve anxiety and decrease peristalsis.
6. Anticholinergics.
a. Relieve abdominal cramps.
b. Assist in controlling diarrhea.
7. In acute stages cathartics contraindicated, as they may lead to megacolon or perforation.
F. Maintain bedrest during acute phase.
G. Prepare client for surgery, if necessary. (*See* Table 8-2.)

INTESTINAL DISORDERS

Intestinal Malignant Tumors

Characteristics
✦ A. Adenocarcinoma of the duodenum is the most common lesion of the small intestines.
1. In the United States, less than 1 percent of gastrointestinal tract cancers arise in the small bowel.
2. Occurs in younger age group; twice as common in men.
✦ B. Malignant tumors of large intestine are second most frequent cause of death from cancer.
1. Men and women equally affected.
2. CA colon more common in women; CA rectum more common in men.
3. Metastasis is by direct extension, usually to stomach from transverse colon, bladder, and bowel.

Assessment
A. Assess for abnormal stools, malabsorption, intestinal bleeding.
B. Assess for weight loss, malaise, anemia.
C. Check for anorexia.
D. Check for vomiting.
E. Evaluate cramp-like pain.
F. Assess for intestinal obstruction or biliary obstruction.

Implementation
✦ A. Provide postoperative care for surgical intervention.
1. Large intestine tumors may result in a colostomy.
2. Instruct client in colostomy procedure and care.
3. Refer client to ostomy club.
B. Monitor cytotoxic drug therapy following surgery.

✦ Table 8-2. SURGICAL CORRECTIONS FOR THE COLON

Colostomy

A. Causes.
   1. Cancer of colon—permanent colostomy.
   2. Traumatic or congenital disruption of intestinal tract (permanent or temporary).
   3. Diverticulitis (double barrel)—can be reversed after inflammatory process is healed.
B. Procedure—portion of colon brought through abdominal wall.
C. Preoperative care.
   1. Provide high-calorie, low-residue diet for several days.
   2. Administer intestinal antibiotics, Kantrex, erythromycin, and neomycin (PO) to decrease bacterial content of colon and to soften and decrease bulk of contents of colon.
   3. Cleanse bowel by administering laxatives and enemas.
   4. Provide adequate fluids and electrolytes.
D. Postoperative care.
   1. Depends on which part of colon involved; contents are liquid to formed.
   2. Client has no voluntary control of bowel evacuation.
   3. Ascending colostomy is hard to train for evacuation.
   4. Evacuate bowel every 24–48 hours.
      a. May irrigate with 200–500 mL at first, but irrigation not commonly done today.
      b. Empty colostomy bag when $1/3$–$1/2$ full.
   5. Control with diet.
   6. Maintain skin care around stoma; use skin barrier.
   7. Assure proper fit and placement of appliance—$1/8$ inch from stoma.
   8. Normal fluid intake.
   9. Instruct client in colostomy self-care.
   10. Suppositories may be given via colostomy.

Ileostomy

A. Causes.
   1. Ulcerative colitis.
   2. Crohn's disease (regional ileitis).
   3. Distal obstruction.
B. Procedure.
   1. Total colectomy and ileostomy (anything less gives only temporary relief).
   2. Portion of ileum brought through abdominal wall.
C. Preoperative care.
   1. Provide intensified fluid, blood and protein replacement.
   2. Administer chemotherapy and antibiotics.
   3. If on steroids, maintain therapy after surgery and then gradually decrease.
   4. Provide low-residue diet in small, frequent feedings.
   5. Administer neomycin enemas.
D. Postoperative care.
   1. Contents always liquid (from small intestine).
   2. More chance of excoriation of skin around stoma.
   3. Provide increased fluids because of excessive fluid loss through stoma.
   4. Provide a low-residue, high-calorie diet until client is accustomed to new arrangement for bowel evacuation; give vitamin B_{12}.
   5. Do not give suppositories via ileostomy.

Continent Ileostomy

A. Internal reservoir created by short segment of small intestines.
B. Nipple valve is formed from terminal ileum.
C. As reservoir fills, fecal pressure closes valve.
D. Client catheterizes stoma 2–4 times a day.
E. Appliance may be needed if leaking occurs.

C. Provide psychological support.
D. Maintain low-residue or liquid diet.
E. Administer antibiotics if ordered.

Appendicitis

Definition: An inflammation of the appendix due to infection; can be classified as simple, gangrenous or perforated.

✦ **Assessment**
✦ A. Assess for generalized, severe upper abdominal or periumbilical pain that localizes in the right lower quadrant.
✦ B. Check for rebound tenderness or flatus.
C. Check for anorexia.
D. Evaluate slightly increased temperature.
E. Assess for nausea and vomiting.

F. Assess for abdominal distention and, if ruptured, paralytic ileus.
G. Check diagnostic tests: elevated WBC, urinalysis, abdominal x-rays and ultrasound.

Implementation

✦ A. Place in semi-Fowler's position to relieve abdominal strain.
✦ B. Give nothing by mouth until bowel sounds present. IV fluids may be given to maintain vascular volume.
C. Give antibiotics (third-generation cephalosporin) as ordered.
D. Insert nasogastric tube as required; rectal tube for flatus.
E. Client should *not* receive laxatives or enemas because these may perforate the appendix.

F. Follow routine postoperative nursing care for any abdominal surgery (return of bowel sounds).

G. Surgery may be laparoscopic.

Intestinal Obstruction

Definition: An impairment of the forward flow of intestinal contents caused by partial or complete stoppage.

Characteristics

◆ A. Mechanical type of obstruction.
   1. Adhesions—fibrous bands of scar tissue, following abdominal surgery, may become looped over a portion of the bowel.
   2. Hernias—incarcerated or strangulated.
   3. Volvulus—twisting of the bowel.
   4. Intussusception—telescoping of the bowel upon itself.
   5. Tumors.
   6. Hematoma.
   7. Fecal impaction.
   8. Intraluminal obstruction.

◆ B. Neurogenic type of obstruction.
   1. Paralytic, adynamic ileus.
   2. Ineffective peristalsis due to toxic or traumatic disturbance of the autonomic nervous system.

C. Vascular type of obstruction.
   1. Occlusion of the arterial blood supply to the bowel.
   2. Mesenteric thrombosis.
   3. Abdominal angina.

D. Pathophysiology.
   1. Fluids and air collect proximal to the obstruction.
      a. Peristalsis increases as the bowel attempts to force material through.
      b. Peristalsis ends and the bowel becomes blocked.
   2. Pressure increases in the bowel and decreases the absorptive ability.
   3. Circulating blood volume is reduced and shock may develop.
   4. Location of the obstruction determines the symptoms and progression of the clinical course.

Assessment

◆ A. Assess for small bowel obstruction (mortality is 10 percent) by evaluating following symptoms:
   1. Cramp-like, colicky pain in midabdomen may be intermittent.
   2. Nausea and early severe vomiting.
   3. Reverse peristalsis.
   4. Dehydration; signs of fluid and electrolyte imbalance.
   5. Abdominal distention.
   6. Shock and death.

◆ B. Assess for large bowel obstruction by evaluating following symptoms:
   1. Progression of symptoms is slower than with small bowel obstruction.
   2. Constipation.
   3. Abdominal distention.
   4. Cramp-like pain in lower abdomen.
   5. If ileocecal valve is incompetent, relief of colonic pressure occurs by reflux into the ileum.

◆ C. Assess for paralytic ileus by evaluating following symptoms:
   1. Dull, diffused pain.
   2. Gaseous distention.
   3. Bowel sounds diminished or absent.
   4. Vomiting after eating.

D. Observe and report the nature, duration, and character of pain.

E. Assess the presence and progression of distention and the absence of flatus and stool.

F. Observe for signs and symptoms of fluid and electrolyte imbalance.

G. Note lab test results: elevated hematocrit, BUN and blood glucose, and low potassium.

Implementation

A. Assist in placement of a long intestinal tube with weighted or balloon tip for intestinal decompression to remove gas and fluid.

B. Monitor parenteral fluids to replace fluids and electrolytes.
   1. Sodium, potassium, and chloride.
   2. Dextrose and water.

C. Administer antibiotics to prevent secondary infections (especially peritonitis).

D. Measure and record vital signs, intake and output (urinary output hourly—keep at 30 mL/hr or more), and emesis.

E. Save stool for testing.

F. Prepare client for surgery, if indicated.

Herniorrhaphy

Definition: A hernia is a protrusion of the intestine through an opening in the abdominal wall.

◆ ### Characteristics

A. Femoral—below groin.

B. Umbilical—around umbilicus, due to failure of orifice to close after birth.

C. Incisional—due to weakness in incisional area from infection or poor healing.

D. Inguinal—weakness in abdominal wall where round ligament is located in female and where spermatic cord emerges in male.

Assessment

A. Assess for possible wound healing at incision site.
B. Assess for edematous scrotum for inguinal hernia.
C. Check for constipation.
D. Assess for abdominal distention.

Implementation

✦ A. Treatment.
    1. Reducing hernia—place an appliance over hernia area to prevent abdominal contents from entering hernia area and strangulating.
    2. Surgical intervention.
B. Postoperative care.
    1. Maintain routine postoperative care.
    2. Ambulate day of surgery or next morning.
    3. Provide ice pack or scrotal support if inguinal hernia in male.
    4. Prevent urine retention.
    5. Report any abdominal distention.

Diverticulosis and Diverticulitis

✦ *Definition:* Diverticulum is the outpouching of intestinal mucosa, which may occur at any point in the gastrointestinal tract but more commonly in the sigmoid colon. It is caused by congenital weakness and increased pressure in the lumen. Diverticulosis is the presence of multiple diverticula. Diverticulitis is inflammation of diverticula.

Characteristics

A. No symptoms unless complications develop.
B. Large bowel diverticula are more apt to develop complications.
C. Complications are perforation, hemorrhage, inflammation, fistulas, and abscess.

Assessment

A. Assess for cramp-like pain (usually left-sided).
B. Check for flatulence.
C. Assess for nausea and vomiting.
D. Evaluate patterns of irregularity, irritability, and spasticity of the intestine.
E. Assess for fever.
F. Examine for dysuria associated with bladder involvement.

Implementation

✦ A. Provide care during acute phase.
    1. Intravenous fluids with electrolytes.
    2. Bedrest.
    3. Nothing by mouth (NPO).
    4. Nasogastric decompression.
    5. Drugs: antibiotics, analgesics, antispasmodics, and bulk former (Metamucil).

✦ B. Monitor appropriate diet.
    ✦ 1. Current studies indicate a high-fiber diet to increase stool bulk and reduce spasms. (Use bran fiber for diverticulosis.)
    ✦ 2. Bowel rest and low-fiber regimen for severe inflammatory phase of diverticulitis.
    3. Provide vitamin and iron supplements.
C. Instruct client and family in pathology and rationale for treatment.
D. Provide pain medication (Talwin) rather than MS or Demerol, which increase colonic pressure.
E. Monitor stool normalization: bowel lubricant nightly, stool softener, bulk preparation daily, evacuant suppository, vegetable oil, unprocessed bran, and fruit juice daily.
F. Prepare client for surgery if indicated. (*See* Table 8-2.)

Hemorrhoids

Definition: Dilated varicose veins of the anal canal that may be internal or external.

Characteristic

A. Types.
    1. Internal hemorrhoids (occur above the internal sphincter)—are covered by mucous membrane.
    2. External hemorrhoids (occur outside the external sphincter)—are covered by anal skin.
    3. Thrombosed hemorrhoids are infected and clotted.
✦ B. Causes.
    1. Portal hypertension.
    2. Straining from constipation.
    3. Irritation and diarrhea.
    4. Increased venous pressure from congestive heart failure.
    5. Increased abdominal pressure as from pregnancy.

Assessment

A. Assess for itching.
B. Assess for pain.
C. Check for bleeding.
D. Assess for complications: hemorrhage, strangulation, thrombosis, and prolapse.

Implementation

✦ A. Treat constipation with diet, stool softeners, and laxatives.
✦ B. Maintain diet low in roughage and high in fiber.
C. Provide suppositories, ointments and systemic analgesics.
D. Administer hot sitz baths.
✦ E. Surgical treatment.

1. Internal hemorrhoids ligated with rubber bands—tissue becomes necrotic and drops off.
2. Cryosurgical hemorrhoidectomy may be done.

F. Nonsurgical treatment.
   1. Infrared photocoagulation and laser therapy.
   2. Methods affix mucosa to underlying muscle.

Anorectal Surgery

Characteristics

A. Hemorrhoids or varicose veins of anal canal.
   1. External—outside rectal sphincter.
   2. Internal—above internal sphincter.
B. Pilonidal cyst—cyst located on lower sacrum with hair protruding from sinus opening.
C. Anal fissure—crack in the anal canal.
D. Anal fistula—abnormal opening near the anus and continuing into the anal canal.

✦ Implementation

A. Give routine postoperative care.
B. Keep perineal and rectal area clean by providing sitz baths 3 to 4 times/day (after first day) or irrigations.
C. Apply spray analgesics when needed to ease pain.
D. Medicate for pain but avoid codeine preparations as they are constipating.
E. Place in prone position or side-lying position for at least 4 hours postop to prevent hemorrhage.
F. Prevent urinary retention.
   1. Keep accurate intake and output.
   2. Observe for frequent, small voidings.
G. Clients usually have packing inserted with pressure dressing applied.
   1. Reinforce dressing as needed to apply pressure.
   2. Keep area clean.
H. Apply ice packs over rectal dressing immediately postoperatively.
   1. Prevents edema formation.
   2. Provides vasoconstriction.
I. When client is able to ambulate, encourage small steps; increase activity gradually.
J. When client is sitting in chair, use flotation pads, not rubber rings; limit sitting to short periods of time.
K. Force fluids to aid in keeping bowel movements soft.
L. Administer stool softeners and laxatives every day.
M. On second day, before first bowel movement, enemas are sometimes ordered.
   1. Medicate for pain.
   2. Administer an enema with a pliable, soft, well-lubricated tube.
   3. Place in sitz bath after expelling enema (will relieve excessive pain by relaxing anal area).

DISORDERS OF LIVER, BILIARY, AND PANCREATIC FUNCTION

Diagnostic Evaluation Studies

Physical Examination

A. Palpation of the abdomen to determine tenderness, size, and shape of liver and spleen.
B. Visual inspection for ascites, venous networks, and jaundice.

✦ Radiologic Techniques

A. Cholecystogram—to visualize the gallbladder for detection of gallstones, and to determine the ability of the gallbladder to fill, concentrate, contract, and empty normally.
   1. Organic radiopaque dye may be given by mouth 10–12 hours before x-ray, or intravenously 10 minutes before x-ray.
   2. Dyes taken orally (e.g., Telepaque, Priodax, Oragrafin) are given one at a time at 3- to 5-minute intervals with at least 240 mL of water. A low-fat evening meal precedes the dye ingestion. Clients are NPO until after examination. An enema is given before test.
B. Cholangiography—radiopaque dye (iodipamide methylglucamine) is injected directly into the biliary tree.
   1. May be injected into the common duct drain during surgery or postoperatively.
   2. Gallbladder disease is indicated by poor or absent visualization of the gallbladder.
   3. Stones will appear as shadows within the opaque medium.
C. Scanning of the liver—131-iodine or other like substances are administered intravenously; then a scintillation detector is passed over the area.
   1. Lesions appear as filling defects.
   2. The isotopes are concentrated in functioning tissue.
D. Other procedures with contrast media: celiac angiography, hepatoportography, splenoportography, and pancreatic angiography.
   1. With all of these procedures, organic iodine dye is injected into the vessel, flowing to and outlining the desired area.
   2. Reveals the patency of the vessels and the lesions that distort the vasculature.

✦ Liver Biopsy

A. Sampling of liver tissues by needle aspiration through abdominal wall to determine anatomic tissue changes and to facilitate diagnosis.
B. Nursing implementation prior to procedure.

Table 8-3. LABORATORY/RADIOGRAPHIC/DIAGNOSTIC ASSESSMENT FOR LIVER DISEASE

Test	Comments
Serum enzymes	Elevated during hepatic inflammation. As the liver deteriorates, hepatocytes may be unable to create an inflammatory response. AST and ALT may be normal.
↑ ALP	Enzyme found in the liver, bones, placenta, obstructive jaundice, hepatic metastasis.
↑ ALT/SGPT	Enzyme found primarily in liver cells, hepatitis, or hepatic cell destruction.
↑ AST/SGOT	Enzyme found in liver and other areas of the body; most specific indicator of hepatitis or hepatic cell destruction.
↑ LDH	Enzyme found in the liver.
GGTP/GGT	Enzyme found in the liver, pancreas, and kidneys.
Bilirubin	A waste product formed by the breakdown of RBCs.
↑ Total bilirubin	Hepatic cell disease.
↑ Serum direct conjugated bilirubin	Hepatitis, liver metastasis.
↑ Serum indirect conjugated bilirubin	Cirrhosis.
↑ Urine bilirubin	Hepatocellular obstruction, viral or toxic liver disease.
↑ Urine urobilinogen	Hepatic dysfunction.
↓ Fecal urobilinogen	Obstructive liver disease.
Serum proteins	Nutrients normally broken by the liver and its enzymes.
↑ Serum total protein	Acute liver disease.
↓ Serum total protein	Chronic liver disease, ↓ synthesis in the liver.
↓ Albumin	A protein synthesized by the liver, ↓ synthesis in the liver.
↑ Serum globulin	Immune response to liver disease.
Other Tests	
Total cholesterol	A substance stored in the liver.
↑ (Prolonged) Prothrombin time or INR	Hepatic cell damage, ↓ synthesis of prothrombin.
↑ Serum ammonia	Advanced liver disease or portal-systemic encephalopathy (PSE).
↓ Platelet count	Results in thrombocytopenia.
↑ Serum creatinine	Deteriorating kidney function.
X-ray	Show hepatomegaly, splenomegaly, or massive ascites.
Liver biopsy	Percutaneous—risk of bleeding, may thread through jugular to hepatic artery.
MRI	Reveals masses or lesions, helps to determine if condition is benign or malignant.
Arteriography	Portal vein thrombosis.
Ultrasound	Show hepatomegaly, splenomegaly, massive ascites, biliary stones, duct obstructions, portal vein thrombosis. Evaluation of portal blow flow—normal is from portal vein into liver, reverse blood flow is abnormal.

✦ 1. Verify test results of prothrombin times and blood typing; high PT may indicate deficiency in prothrombin, fibrinogen, or factor V, VII, or X. Administer vitamin K as ordered.
2. Obtain baseline vital signs and consent form.
3. Keep NPO and provide sedation as ordered.
4. Assemble equipment, have client empty bladder, place client in supine position on right side of bed.
5. Support client; let client verbalize fears.
C. Nursing implementation following procedure.
✦ 1. Position client on right side over biopsy site to prevent hemorrhage.
2. Measure and record vital signs.
3. Watch for shock.
4. Observe for complications: hemorrhage, puncture of the bile duct, peritonitis, and pneumothorax.

See Chapter 11, Laboratory Tests, Liver Function Tests.

Jaundice

Definition: A symptom of a disease that results in yellow pigmentation of the skin due to accumulation of bilirubin pigment. Jaundice is usually first observed in the sclera of the eye.

✦ Characteristics
A. Hemolytic.
1. Results from the rapid rate of red blood cell destruction, which releases excessive amounts of unconjugated bilirubin.
2. Caused by hemolytic transfusion reactions, erythroblastosis fetalis, and other hemolytic disorders.
B. Hepatocellular.

1. Results from the inability of the diseased liver cells to clear the normal amount of bilirubin from the blood.
2. Caused by viral liver cell necrosis or cirrhosis of the liver.

C. Obstructive.
   1. Caused by intrahepatic obstruction due to inflammation, tumors, or cholestatic agents.
   2. Bile is dammed into the liver substance and reabsorbed into the blood.
   3. Deep-orange, foamy urine; white- or clay-colored stools; and severe itching (pruritus).

Assessment

A. Evaluate laboratory findings indicating hemolytic jaundice.
   1. Increased indirect (unconjugated) serum bilirubin.
   2. Absence of bilirubin in urine.
   3. Increased urobilinogen levels.
◆ B. Evaluate laboratory findings indicating hepatocellular jaundice.
   1. Increased bilirubin.
   2. Increased SGOT.
   3. Increased SGPT.
   4. Increased alkaline phosphatase.
   5. Urobilinogen in urine.
   6. Increased PT.
   7. Decreased albumin.
C. Evaluate laboratory findings indicating obstructive jaundice.
   1. Increased bilirubin.
   2. Increased alkaline phosphatase.
   3. Decreased stool urobilinogen.

Implementation

◆ A. Control pruritus.
   1. Starch or baking soda baths.
   2. Soothing lotions, such as calamine.
   3. Antihistamines, tranquilizers, and sedatives.
   4. Cholestyramine—binds bile salt.
B. Provide emotional support.
   1. Allow client to ventilate feelings of altered body image.
   2. Notify family and visitors of client's appearance.
C. Provide dietary plan for anorexia and liver involvement.

Viral Hepatitis

Definition: An inflammation of the liver; the most common infection of the liver, often becoming a major health problem in crowded living conditions. Through vaccination, types A (2 vaccines—Havrix and Vaqta) and B can be prevented.

Characteristics

◆ A. Hepatitis A (formerly infectious hepatitis); HAV.
   1. Transmission.
      a. Oral–anal route, especially in conditions of poor hygiene.
      b. Blood transfusion with infected serum or plasma.
      c. Contaminated equipment, such as syringes and needles.
      d. Contaminated milk, water and food (uncooked clams and oysters).
      e. Respiratory route is possible, but not yet established.
      f. Antibodies persist in serum.
      g. Intimate contact with carriers of the virus.
   2. Prevention.
      a. Good handwashing and good personal hygiene.
      b. Do not eat uncooked shellfish (clams, oysters).
      c. Control and screening of food handlers.
      d. Passive immunization.
         (1) ISG to exposed individuals.
         (2) ISG for prophylaxis for travelers to developing countries.
   3. Incubation period: 20–50 days (short incubation period).
   4. Incidence.
      a. More common in fall and winter months.
      b. Usually found in children and young adults.
      c. Client is infectious 3 weeks prior to and 1 week after developing jaundice.
   5. Clinical recovery: 3–16 weeks.
◆ B. Hepatitis B (formerly serum hepatitis, SH virus); HBV.
   1. Transmission.
      a. Oral or parenteral route with infusion, ingestion or inhalation of the blood of an infected person.
      b. Contaminated equipment such as needles, syringes and dental instruments.
      c. Oral or sexual contact.
      d. Infected people can become carriers.
      e. Infected by filterable virus—Australian antigen.
      f. High-risk individuals include homosexuals, IV drug abusers, medical workers.
   2. Prevention.
      a. Screen blood donors for HB_3Ag.
      b. Use disposable needles and syringes.
      c. Registration of all carriers.
      d. Passive immunization: ISG for exposure and HBIG for finger stick, contact with mucous membrane secretions.

e. Active immunization: Hepatavax B vaccine and formalin-treated hepatitis B vaccine—purified antigen given in three doses (initial dose, 1 month, then 6 months).

3. Incubation: 45–180 days.

◆ C. Hepatitis C (formerly non-A, non-B); HCV.
 1. Transmission.
   a. Transmitted primarily by contact with contaminated blood.
   b. Incidence noted following injection of prophylactic gamma globulin.
   c. Increased incidence in population using drugs.
 2. Usual incubation period 14–180 days.
 3. May not show clinical jaundice—only 30–40 percent of clients have symptoms.

◆ D. Hepatitis D (delta agent).
 1. Transmission.
   a. Same as hepatitis B.
   b. Only clients with hepatitis B are at risk for hepatitis D because it requires B surface antigen for replication.
 2. Infections occur as coinfection with HBV or superinfection in HBV carrier.
 3. Incubation period: 45–180 days.

E. Hepatitis E.
 ◆ 1. Rare in United States but epidemic in areas of India.
 2. Transmitted through oral–fecal route by contaminated foods or water.
 3. Course of illness resembles hepatitis A.
 4. Incubation period: 15–60 days.

F. Hepatitis G—newly discovered, believed to be transmitted by infected blood. May exist only as a co-infection with HCV.

Assessment

A. Perform general assessment; keep in mind that client is not immediately sick after being infected; onset depends on incubation period and degree of infection.

◆ B. Assess preicteric phase.
 1. Signs are generally systemic.
   a. Lethargy and malaise.
   b. Anorexia, nausea and vomiting.
   c. Headache.
   d. Abdominal tenderness and pain.
   e. Diarrhea or constipation.
   f. Low-grade fever.
   g. Myalgia and polyarthritis.
 2. Above symptoms may precede jaundice or it may never appear.

◆ C. In anicteric hepatitis, client has symptoms of disease and altered lab tests, but no jaundice.

◆ D. Assess icteric phase.
 1. Dark urine and clay-colored stools generally occur a few days prior to jaundice.
 2. Jaundice is first observable in the eyes.
 3. Pruritus—usually transient and mild.
 4. Enlarged liver with tenderness.
 5. Nausea may continue with dyspepsia and flatulence.

E. Assess posticteric phase.
 1. Jaundice disappears.
 2. The absence of clay-colored stools is an indication of resolution.
 3. Fatigue and malaise continue.
 4. Enlarged liver continues for several weeks.

Implementation

◆ A. Type A.
 ◆ 1. Wash your hands carefully, always wear gloves, and take precautions during stool and needle procedures.
 2. Use disposable equipment or sterilized reusable equipment.
 ◆ 3. Provide diet.
   a. High-calorie, well-balanced diet; modified servings according to client response.
   b. Protein decreased if signs of coma.
   c. 10% glucose IV if not taking oral foods.
   d. Vitamin K supplements if prothrombin time is abnormally long.
   e. Promote adequate fluid intake.
 4. Instruct client and family.
   a. Stress the importance of follow-up care.
   b. Stress the restricted use of alcohol.
   c. Stress that client never offer to be a blood donor.
   d. Encourage gamma globulin for close contacts.
   e. Advise correction if any unsanitary condition exists in the home.
 ◆ 5. Bedrest during acute phase with bathroom privileges; reasonable activity level during subsequent phases.

◆ B. Type B.
 ◆ 1. Maintain bedrest until symptoms have decreased.
   a. Activities restricted while liver is enlarged.
   b. Activities discouraged until serum bilirubin is normal.
 ◆ 2. Alpha-interferon daily injections for 4 months induce remission in one-third of clients.
 ◆ 3. Provide well-balanced diet supplemented with vitamins. Protein may be restricted.
 4. Administer antacids for gastric acidity and soporifics for rest and relaxation.

5. Instruct client and family in pathology of the disease and rationale for treatment.
6. Counsel client to abstain from sexual activity during communicable period.
C. Other types of hepatitis follow the treatment principles for HAV and HBV.

Cirrhosis

Definition: Cirrhosis is a progressive disease of the liver characterized by diffuse damage to the cells with fibrosis and nodular regeneration.

Characteristics

✦ A. Types.
  1. Alcoholic or Laënnec's cirrhosis.
     a. Most common in the United States.
     b. Scar tissue surrounds the portal areas.
     c. Characterized by destruction of hepatic tissue, increased fibrous tissue, and disorganized regeneration.
  2. Posthepatic cirrhosis—a sequela to viral hepatitis in which there are broad bands of scar tissue. Results from chronic hepatitis B or C or unknown cause.
  3. Biliary cirrhosis.
     a. Pericholangitic scarring as a result of chronic biliary obstruction and infection.
     b. Least encountered of the three types.
B. Causes.
  1. Repeated destruction of hepatic cells, replacement with scar tissue, and regeneration of liver cells.
  2. Insidious onset with progression over a period of years.
  3. Occurs twice as often in males; primarily affects 40- to 60-year-old age group.
✦ C. Clinical progression.
  1. Early in the disease process, the liver becomes enlarged due to fat accumulation in the cells; accompanying this are gastrointestinal problems and fever.
  2. Subsequent symptoms are usually anorexia, weight loss, fatigue, and jaundice. (Jaundice is not always present in the active stage.)
  3. Continued structural changes in the liver result in obstruction of portal circulation. Collateral circulation increases to compensate for increased portal pressure.
     a. Obstruction of portal circulation results in portal hypertension, which in turn leads to esophageal varices and changes in bowel functioning with chronic dyspepsia.
     b. Liver function deteriorates; leads to peripheral edema and ascites, accompanied by

hormone imbalance, weakness, depression, and potential bleeding.
  4. As the liver is unable to synthesize protein, plasma albumin is reduced; leads to edema and contributes to ascites.
     a. Ascites, accumulation of serous fluid in the peritoneal cavity, increases as pressure in the liver increases.
     b. In addition, estrogen–androgen imbalance causes increased sodium and water to be retained.
  5. Hepatic coma results from the incomplete metabolism of nitrogenous compounds, particularly ammonia, by the incompetent liver.
  6. When the liver cannot detoxify this product, it remains in the systemic circulation and hepatic encephalopathy ensues.

Assessment

A. Evaluate client's history of failing health, weakness, gastrointestinal distress, fatigue, weight loss, and low resistance to infections.
✦ B. Assess for emaciation and ascites due to malnutrition, portal hypertension, and hypoalbuminemia.
C. Check for hematemesis.
✦ D. Assess for lower leg edema from ascites obstructing venous return from legs.
E. Palpate liver.
F. Assess for prominent abdominal wall veins from collateral vessel bypass.
G. Assess for esophageal varices and hemorrhoids from portal hypertension.
H. Evaluate skin manifestations: spider angiomas, telangiectasia, vitamin deficiency, and alterations.
✦ I. Evaluate laboratory tests.
  1. Impaired hepatocellular function; elevated bilirubin, AST (SGOT), ALT (SGPT), and LDH; reduced BSP; reduced albumin; elevated PT.
  2. Increased WBC, decreased RBC, coagulation abnormalities, increased gamma globulin, and proteinuria.
J. Assess for precoma state: tremor, delirium, and dysarthria.

Implementation

✦ A. Assist in maximizing liver function.
  1. Diet: ample protein to build tissue; carbohydrates to sustain weight and provide energy.
  2. With edema, restrict salt and fluids. With low Na, unrestricted fluids could lead to low serum Na and electrolyte imbalance.
  3. Multivitamin supplement (especially B complex).
  4. Diuretics (spironolactones) potassium-sparing to decrease ascites.

5. Antacids decrease gastric distress and minimize possibility of bleeding.

✦ B. Eliminate hepatotoxin intake (aldosterone antagonist).
   ✦ 1. Completely restrict use of alcohol.
   2. Lower the dosage of drugs metabolized by the liver.
   3. Avoid sedatives and opiates.
   4. Avoid all known hepatotoxic drugs (Thorazine, Halothane).
   5. Colchicine (anti-inflammatory drug to treat gout) has been shown to increase survival time.

C. Prevent infection by adequate rest, diet and environmental control.

D. Administer plasma proteins as ordered.

E. Maintain adequate rest during acute phase to reduce demand on the liver.

F. Monitor intake and output due to fluid restriction.

G. Provide good skin care and control pruritus.

H. Evaluate client's response to diet therapy.

I. Measure, record and compare vital signs.
   1. Character of pain.
   2. Progression of edema.
   3. Character of emesis and stools.

J. Evaluate level of consciousness, personality changes, and signs of increasing stupor.

K. Instruct client and family in disease process and rationale for treatment.

L. Prevent and control complications: ascites, bleeding esophageal varices, hepatic encephalopathy, and anemia.

M. Provide postoperative care if LeVeen peritoneovenous shunt is placed for intractable or circulatory failure.

COMPLICATIONS

Portal Hypertension

Definition: The result of altered liver structure that impedes normal hepatic blood flow and increases portal pressure.

✦ **Characteristics**
A. Obstruction of portal circulation causes portal hypertension and congestion of the spleen, pancreas, and gastrointestinal tract.
B. As the body compensates for increased pressure in the hepatic system, collateral circulation increases.

Assessment
A. Two major conditions result from portal hypertension.
   1. Evidence of increased collateral circulation: hemorrhoids, veins observable on abdomen, esophageal varices that bleed easily.

2. Weight gain and abdominal distention from ascites.
B. Assess for respiratory complications due to severe ascites.
C. Assess for abdominal pain (may be indication of infection or bleeding).

Implementation
A. Provide general nursing care for cirrhosis.
✦ B. Provide specific care for management of edema.
   1. Skin care to prevent breakdown.
      a. Use lanolin-based products to soften skin.
      b. Guard against cutting or scratching skin.
   2. Dietary control: negative sodium balance to reduce fluid retention, diuretics (Lasix, Edecrin) with potassium supplements, vitamin supplements of B complex, C, folate, and K.
   3. Monitor intake and output; weigh daily.
C. Provide care for ascites.
   1. Prevent complications associated with ascites (i.e., respiratory impairment, infection).
   2. Restrict fluids and sodium intake.
   ✦ 3. Position client in high-Fowler's to maximize respiratory capability.
   4. Weigh daily and measure abdominal girth to estimate status of fluid accumulation.
   5. Monitor use of diuretics (used with sodium restriction); is successful in 90 percent of clients with ascites.
   ✦ 6. Assist with paracentesis (will be avoided as long as possible due to the danger of precipitating shock, hypovolemia, or hepatic coma).
      a. Removal of fluid will relieve pressure on the diaphragm, stomach, or umbilical hernia.
      b. Because of high protein concentration in the ascitic fluid, IV infusion of salt-poor albumin may be administered over 24 hours.

Esophageal Varices

See page 289.

Hepatic Encephalopathy

Definition: Results from brain cell alterations caused by buildup of ammonia levels.

Characteristics
✦ A. Increased blood ammonia levels.
   1. Normally, ammonia is formed in the intestines from the breakdown of protein and is converted by the liver to urea.
   2. In liver failure, ammonia is not converted into urea, and blood ammonia concentrations increase.

Table 8-4. MEDICATIONS FOR LIVER DISEASE	
Medication	**Purpose**
Antacids: Mylanta, Maalox	Relief of dyspepsia
Vitamins: B_1, B_6, B_{12}, folic acid	Correct the deficiency seen in cirrhosis
Diuretics: Lasix, spirolactone	Treat ascites, reduce fluid accumulation, prevent cardiac and respiratory impairment
Laxatives: Dulcolax, milk of magnesia	Treat constipation
Colchicine	An inhibitor of collagen synthesis, for primary biliary cirrhosis—anti-inflammatory
Propranolol	↓ BP and help control bleeding
Steroids: prednisone	For autoimmune causes
Recombinant factor (Recombinate)	Bleeding problems, adjusts for coagulation problems
Milkweed thistle	Protects the liver from damage caused by viruses, toxins, alcohol, and certain drugs such as acetaminophen
Lactulose	To reduce ammonia levels in encephalopathy
Immunizations	Immunize for hepatitis A and B, pneumonia, yearly flu
Hepatitis C	C-PEG-alpha interferon and ribavirin
Hepatitis B	Lamivudine of PEG-alpha-interferon

◆ B. Any process that increases protein in the intestine, such as gastrointestinal hemorrhage and high protein intake, will cause elevated blood ammonia.

◆ C. Other factors involved in high ammonia levels.
   1. Electrolyte and acid–base imbalances. Alkalosis increases toxicity of NH_3.
   2. Constipation.
   3. Infectious diseases.
   4. Medications: sedatives, narcotic analgesics, central nervous system depressants.
   5. Shunting of blood into systemic circulation without passing through the hepatic sinusoids.

Assessment

◆ A. Assess for mental changes as blood ammonia level increases.
   1. Impaired memory, attention, concentration, and rate of response.
   2. Personality changes: untidiness, confusion, and inappropriate behavior.

◆ B. Assess for depressed level of consciousness and flapping tremor (liver flap) upon dorsiflexion of hand.

C. Evaluate disorientation and eventual coma.

Implementation

◆ A. Temporarily decrease protein from diet because ammonia cannot be converted to urea for excretion.
   1. Protein is restricted to 60–80 g/day.
   2. Sodium intake may be restricted to less than 2 g/day.
   3. High-calorie, moderate-fat diet recommended.

◆ B. Give client bile salts to assist with the absorption of vitamin A. Vitamin K may be given to reduce risk of bleeding.

◆ C. Give folic acid and ferrous sulfate (iron) to treat anemia.

◆ D. Administer antibiotics (Neomycin) to destroy intestinal bacteria and to reduce the amount of ammonia.

◆ E. Administer Lactulose to reduce blood ammonia—acidifies colon contents, resulting in retention of ammonium ion and decreased ammonia absorption.
   ◆ 1. Two or three stools/day indicate Lactulose is working.
   2. Watery diarrhea indicates drug overdose.

◆ F. Give enemas and/or cathartics to empty bowel and to reduce ammonia absorption.

G. Give salt-poor albumin to maintain osmotic pressure.

H. Use cation-exchange resins to remove toxic substances from the bowel.

I. Correct fluid and electrolyte imbalances.

J. Weigh daily to monitor for ascites and edema.

K. Measure and record intake and output.

L. Observe, measure, and record neurologic status daily.
   1. Test ability to perform mental tasks.
   2. Keep samples of handwriting.

M. Avoid depressants, which must be detoxified by the liver. Use agents, such as a benzodiazepine, that are excreted through the kidneys.

N. Prevent complications—pressure ulcers, thrombophlebitis, or pneumonia.

O. With coma, utilize same nursing skills as with the unconscious client.

Cholecystitis and Cholelithiasis

◆ *Definition: Cholecystitis,* either acute or chronic, is an inflammation of the gallbladder; *cholelithiasis* refers to stones in the gallbladder, formed of cholesterol (the most common) or pigment; *choledocholithiasis* refers to stones in the common bile duct.

Characteristics

A. Estimated 25 million in United States have gallstones.

B. Four times more common in women. Commonly occurs at ages 40–50.

C. Risk factors: cholesterol gallstones—age, race or ethnicity, obesity, estrogen, rapid weight loss, genetic predisposition, cholesterol-lowering drugs, and bile acid malabsorption; pigment gallstones—chronic liver disease, obstruction, or biliary infection.

D. Diagnostic procedures.
1. Serum bilirubin is elevated.
2. Gallbladder x-ray test.
3. IV cholangiogram.
4. Ultrasound determines gallstones.
5. Complete blood count (CBC); if WBC elevated, indicates infection or inflammation.

Assessment

A. Laboratory values.
1. Serum amylase elevated—may indicate pancreatic involvement of stones in common bile duct; alkaline phosphatase, bilirubin increased.
2. White blood cell count elevated—indicates inflammation and/or infection.

B. Differentiate between cholecystitis and cholelithiasis.

C. Assess for cholecystitis.
1. Epigastric distress—eructation after eating.
2. Pain—localized in right upper quadrant because of somatic sensory nerves.
   a. Murphy's sign: client cannot take a deep inspiration when assessor's fingers are pressed below hepatic margin.
   b. Pain begins 2–4 hours after eating fried or fatty foods and persists 12–18 hours.
3. Nausea, vomiting, and anorexia.
4. Low-grade fever.
5. Jaundice due to hepatocellular damage (seen in 25 percent of clients).
6. Weight loss.
7. Elevated serum bilirubin and alkaline phosphatase.

D. Assess for cholelithiasis.
1. Pain—excruciating, upper right quadrant—radiates to right shoulder (biliary colic).
2. Pain is sudden, intense, paroxysmal—occurs with contraction of gallbladder. Lasts 30 minutes to 5 hours.
3. Nausea and vomiting.
4. Jaundice due to obstruction and/or hepatocellular damage.
5. Intolerance to fat-containing foods.

E. Observe for biliary obstruction.
1. Jaundice—yellow sclera.
2. Urine—dark orange and foamy.
3. Feces—clay-colored.
4. Pruritus.

Implementation

A. Provide relief from vomiting.
1. Position nasogastric tube and attach to low suction. Tube reduces distention and eliminates gastric juices that stimulate cholecystokinin.
2. Provide good oral and nasal care; assure patency and flow of gastric secretions.

B. Maintain fluid and electrolyte balance.
1. Monitor intravenous fluids; record I&O.
2. Observe serum electrolyte levels; watch for signs of imbalance.

C. Monitor drug therapy.
1. Administer broad-spectrum antibiotics (Keflin) in presence of positive culture.
2. Chenodeoxycholic acid—bile acid dissolves cholesterol calculi (60 percent of stones).
3. Ursodiol (Actigal) and chenodiol (Chenix) reduce cholesterol content of stones, so they gradually dissolve; disadvantages are cost and long duration.
4. Nitroglycerin or papaverine to reduce spasms of duct.
5. Synthetic narcotics (Demerol, methadone) to relieve pain. Morphine sulfate may cause spasm of sphincter of Oddi and increase pain.
6. Questran/Benadryl to relieve pruritus.

D. Provide low-fat diet to decrease gallbladder stimulation; avoid alcohol and gas-forming foods.

E. Maintain bedrest.

Nonsurgical Management

A. Extracorporeal shock-wave lithotripsy: shock waves that disintegrate stones in the biliary system.
1. Ultrasound is used for stone localization before the lithotriptor sends waves through a water bag upon which the client is lying.
2. Analgesics and sedatives are given to reduce pain during procedure.
3. Oral-dissolution medication follows to dissolve stone fragments.
4. Postprocedure—monitor for biliary colic, results from gallbladder contractions.

B. Cholesterol stones removed through dissolution therapy. For high-risk clients—oral medications to decrease size or dissolve stones.

C. Stone removal by instrumentation.

Surgical Management

A. Laparoscopic cholecystectomy is treatment of choice: removal of gallbladder through small puncture hole in abdomen.
1. Laser dissects gallbladder.

2. Discharged day of surgery—normal activities resumed in 2–3 days.

✦ B. Cholecystectomy: removal of gallbladder after ligation of the cystic duct and vessels.
   1. Common bile duct may be explored.
   2. A Penrose drain is usually inserted for drainage following procedure.

✦ C. Choledochostomy: opening into the common bile duct for removal of stones.
   1. T-tube inserted to maintain patency of the duct; connected to drainage bottle to collect excess bile.
   2. Purpose is to decompress biliary tree and allow for postoperative cholangiogram.

Implementation

✦ A. Position client in low- to semi-Fowler's to facilitate bile drainage.

✦ B. Maintain skin integrity following surgery.
   1. Change position frequently; relieve pressure points.
   2. Protect skin around incision site from bile seepage.
      a. Change dressings frequently.
      b. Use protective skin paste or drainage pouches to prevent bile drainage from skin contact.

✦ C. Prevent respiratory complications (the most common postoperative complication).
   1. Turn, cough, and deep-breathe every 2 hours.
   2. Use IPPB or TRIFLO every 2 hours.
   3. Auscultate for abnormal breath sounds.
   4. Observe for signs of respiratory distress.
   5. Ambulate and activate as early as allowed.

✦ D. If nasogastric tube was inserted to relieve distention and increase peristalsis, irrigate tube every 4 hours and PRN.

✦ E. If T-tube inserted.
   1. Place client in Fowler's position to facilitate drainage.
   2. Keep tube below level of wound to promote bile flow and prevent backflow.
   3. Measure amount, and record character and color of drainage (may be up to 500 mL for first 24 hours).
   4. Clamp tube before eating.
   5. Protect skin around incision and cleanse surrounding area.

F. Prevent wound infections; clients tend to be obese—healing is often delayed.

G. Prevent thrombophlebitis.
   1. Encourage range of motion.
   2. Ambulate early.
   3. Provide antiembolic stockings.

H. Provide diet: low fat, high carbohydrate, and high protein.
   1. Instruct client to maintain diet for at least 2 or 3 months postoperatively.
   2. May require continued use of vitamin K as dietary supplement.

I. Prepare client for T-tube removal.
   1. As T-tube is clamped, observe for
      a. Abdominal discomfort and distention.
      b. Chills and fever; nausea.
   2. Unclamp tube if any nausea or vomiting.

Acute Pancreatitis

Definition: An inflammation of the pancreas with associated escape of pancreatic enzymes into surrounding tissue.

Characteristics

A. Etiology.
   ✦ 1. Inflammation is caused by the digestion of the organ from the very enzymes it produces—trypsin, elastase, and lipase.
   ✦ 2. The most common precipitating factor in United States is alcoholic indulgence.
   ✦ 3. Eighty percent of clients with pancreatitis have biliary tract disease with blocking of ampulla of Vater by gallstones.
   4. May be caused as a result of prednisone or thiazide therapy.
   5. May be a complication of viral or bacterial disease, peptic ulcer, trauma, etc.

B. Pathology.
   1. Cholecystitis with reflux of bile components into the pancreatic duct.
   2. Spasm and edema of ampulla of Vater following inflammation of the duodenum.

Assessment

✦ A. Assess for acute interstitial pancreatitis.
   1. Constant epigastric abdominal pain radiating to the back and flank. More intense in supine position. Aggravated by fatty meal, alcohol, or lying in the recumbent position.
   2. Nausea, vomiting, abdominal distention, paralytic ileus, and weight loss.
   3. Low-grade fever.
   4. Severe perspiration; anxiety.
   5. Possible jaundice.

✦ B. Laboratory values.
   1. Elevation of WBC—20,000 to 50,000.
   2. Elevated serum lipase (rises within 2–12 hours) and amylase (5–40 times); bilirubin and alkaline phosphatase elevated (due to compression of common duct) and transient elevation in glucose.
   3. Urine amylase elevated.

4. Abnormal low serum levels in calcium, sodium and magnesium—due to dehydration, binding of calcium in areas of fat necrosis.

✦ C. Assess for acute hemorrhagic pancreatitis.
   1. Pancreatic enzymes erode major blood vessels, causing hemorrhage into the pancreas and retroperitoneal tissues.
      a. Cullen's sign—gray–blue discoloration of the abdominal area may be seen in intra-abdominal hemorrhage.
      b. Turner's sign—bruising of the skin of the loin.
   2. Enzymatic digestion of the pancreas.
   3. Severe abdominal, back, and flank pain.
   4. Ascites.
   5. Shock.

Implementation

✦ A. Assess pain (using a standard pain scale) and take actions to alleviate pain.
   1. Give analgesic medication as ordered (pain and anxiety increase pancreatic secretions).
   2. Avoid opiates (morphine), which may cause spasms of sphincter of Oddi.
   3. Give anticholinergic medication—atropine, to decrease vagal stimulation.

✦ B. Reduce pancreatic stimulus.
   ✦ 1. Client is NPO to eliminate chief stimulus to enzyme release. TNA may be initiated.
   2. Nasogastric tube to low suction to remove gastric secretions and air if nausea, vomiting or ileus present.
   ✦ 3. Drugs to reduce pancreatic secretion.
      a. Sodium bicarbonate to reverse metabolic acidosis. Histamine H_2 antagonists may be used to neutralize hydrochloric acid secretion.
      b. Diamox to prevent carbonic anhydrase from catalyzing secretion of bicarbonate into pancreatic juice.
      c. Regular insulin to treat hyperglycemia.
   ✦ 4. Diet to avoid pancreatic secretion: low fat, low protein, high carbohydrate; no spicy foods, alcohol or caffeine; parenteral feedings if NPO.

C. Take vital signs every 15–30 minutes during acute phase; assess cardiovascular status.

D. Prevent or treat infection (and possible sepsis) with broad-spectrum antibiotics.

✦ E. Replace and maintain fluids and electrolytes.
   ✦ 1. Treat hypocalcemia with neuromuscular irritability with calcium gluconate IV. (Signs—nausea, vomiting; tetany; abdominal pain; positive Chvostek's sign.)

   ✦ 2. Treat hypokalemia—potassium is a major component in pancreatic juice. (Signs—muscle weakness; hyporeflexia; hypotension; apathy or irritability; arrhythmias.)
   ✦ 3. Treat hypomagnesemia (less than 1.4 mg/dL)—can be life-threatening.
   4. Blood and plasma administration may be necessary to maintain circulatory volume.

F. Aggressive respiratory care to prevent acute respiratory distress syndrome (ARDS).
   1. Atelectasis, effusion may be caused by elevation of the diaphragm.
   2. Hypoxemia may occur.
   3. Monitor arterial blood gases or ventilator if ordered.

G. Reduce body metabolism.
   ✦ 1. Oxygen for labored breathing.
   ✦ 2. Bedrest; Fowler's position for maximum chest expansion.
   3. Cool, quiet environment.

H. Provide client and family instruction.
   1. Discuss pathology of disease.
   2. Give rationale for treatment.
   3. Instruct client to avoid alcohol, coffee, heavy meals, and spicy foods.
   4. Stress importance of follow-up with physician.

Chronic Pancreatitis

Definition: Chronic fibrosis of the pancreatic gland—irreversible process of obstruction of ducts and destruction of secreting cells, following repeated attacks of acute pancreatitis.

Etiology

A. Alcohol abuse most common.
B. Other causes: hyperparathyroidism, malnutrition, and trauma.

Assessment

✦ A. Assess for pain—persistent epigastric and left upper quadrant pain radiating to upper left lumbar region.
✦ B. Check for anorexia, nausea, vomiting, constipation, and flatulence.
C. Evaluate disturbances of protein and fat digestion.
   1. Malnutrition.
   2. Weight loss from decreased intake due to fear of pain.
   3. Abdominal distention with flatus and paralytic ileus.
   4. Foul, fatty stools (steatorrhea) caused by a decrease in pancreatic enzyme secretion.
✦ D. Laboratory values.

1. Elevated serum amylase and lipase (indicates decreased pancreatic enzyme excretion).
2. Increased glucose and lipids.
3. Decreased calcium, potassium.

E. Assess for hyperglycemia with symptoms of diabetes.

F. Evaluate fecal fat in stool specimens; x-ray often shows pancreatolithiasis and mild ileus, indicating fibrous tissue and calcification.

Implementation

✦ A. Provide low-protein, low-fat, high-carbohydrate diet. Suggest bland and low-gas-forming foods in small, frequent feedings.

✦ B. Administer drug therapy.
   1. Antacids (Maalox) to neutralize acid secretions.
   2. Histamine antagonists (ranitidine [Zantac] and cimetidine [Tagamet]) to decrease hydrochloric acid production so pancreatic enzymes are not activated.
   3. Proton-pump inhibitors (Prilosec) may be given to neutralize or decrease gastric secretions.
   4. Anticholinergics (atropine, Pro-Banthine) to decrease vagal stimulation, GI motility, and inhibit pancreatic enzymes.
   5. Administer pancreatic enzyme replacements, such as pancreatin (Viokase) and pancrelipase (Cotazym), with meals or snacks to aid digestion. Dose depends on degree of malabsorption or maldigestion. Monitor for side effects.
   6. Narcotic analgesics (such as morphine sulfate) are used to control pain.

✦ C. Report diabetic symptoms—insulin or oral hypoglycemic agents will be administered; monitor blood glucose levels to control hyperglycemia and prevent insulin shock.

D. Monitor for potential complications: pseudocyst, ascites or pleural effusion, GI hemorrhage, biliary tract obstruction. Surgical treatment is done for specific complications and to relieve constant pain.

GASTROINTESTINAL SYSTEM REVIEW QUESTIONS

1. The nurse is completing the initial morning assessment on the client. Which physical examination technique would be used first when assessing the abdomen?

   1. Inspection.
   2. Light palpation.
   3. Auscultation.
   4. Percussion.

2. The client has orders for a nasogastric (NG) tube insertion. During the procedure, instructions that will assist in insertion would be

   1. Instruct the client to tilt his head back for insertion into the nostril, then flex his neck forward and swallow for final insertion.
   2. After insertion into the nostril, instruct the client to extend his neck.
   3. Introduce the tube with the client's head tilted back, then instruct him to keep his head upright for final insertion.
   4. Instruct the client to hold his chin down, then back for insertion of the tube.

3. The most important pathophysiologic factor contributing to the formation of esophageal varices is

   1. Decreased prothrombin formation.
   2. Decreased albumin formation by the liver.
   3. Portal hypertension.
   4. Increased central venous pressure.

4. The nurse analyzes the results of the blood chemistry tests done on a client with acute pancreatitis. Which of the following results would the nurse expect to find?

   1. Low glucose.
   2. Low alkaline phosphatase.
   3. Elevated amylase.
   4. Elevated creatinine.

5. A client being treated for esophageal varices has a Sengstaken–Blakemore tube inserted to control the bleeding. The most important assessment is for the nurse to

   1. Check that a hemostat is at the bedside.
   2. Monitor IV fluids for the shift.

   3. Regularly assess respiratory status.
   4. Check that the balloon is deflated on a regular basis.

6. A female client complains of gnawing midepigastric pain for a few hours after meals. At times, when the pain is severe, vomiting occurs. Specific tests are indicated to rule out

   1. Cancer of the stomach.
   2. Peptic ulcer disease.
   3. Chronic gastritis.
   4. Pylorospasm.

7. When a client has peptic ulcer disease, the nurse would expect a priority intervention to be

   1. Assisting in inserting a Miller–Abbott tube.
   2. Assisting in inserting an arterial pressure line.
   3. Inserting a nasogastric tube.
   4. Inserting an IV.

8. A 40-year-old male client has been hospitalized with peptic ulcer disease. He is being treated with a histamine-receptor antagonist (cimetidine), antacids, and diet. The nurse doing discharge planning will teach him that the action of cimetidine is to

   1. Reduce gastric acid output.
   2. Protect the ulcer surface.
   3. Inhibit the production of hydrochloric acid (HCl).
   4. Inhibit vagus nerve stimulation.

9. The nurse is admitting a client with Crohn's disease who is scheduled for intestinal surgery. Which surgical procedure would the nurse anticipate for the treatment of this condition?

   1. Ileostomy with total colectomy.
   2. Sigmoid colostomy with mucous fistula.
   3. Intestinal resection with end-to-end anastomosis.
   4. Colonoscopy with biopsy and polypectomy.

10. A client who has just returned home following ileostomy surgery will need a diet that is supplemented with

   1. Potassium.
   2. Vitamin B_{12}.
   3. Sodium.
   4. Fiber.

11. A client is scheduled for colostomy surgery. An appropriate preoperative diet will include which of the following foods? List all that apply _____ .

    1. Ground hamburger.
    2. Baked potato.
    3. Broiled fish.
    4. Rice.
    5. Salad.
    6. Winter squash or apple sauce.

12. As the nurse is completing evening care for a client, he observes that the client is upset, quiet, and withdrawn. The nurse knows that the client is scheduled for diagnostic tests the following day. An important assessment question to ask the client is

    1. "Would you like to go to the dayroom to watch TV?"
    2. "Are you prepared for the test tomorrow?"
    3. "Have you talked with anyone about the test tomorrow?"
    4. "Have you asked your physician to give you a sleeping pill tonight?"

13. Following abdominal surgery, a client complaining of "gas pains" will have a rectal tube inserted. The client should be positioned on his

    1. Left side, recumbent.
    2. Left side, Sims'.
    3. Right side, semi-Fowler's.
    4. Left side, semi-Fowler's.

14. If a colostomy irrigation was ordered, the appropriate instruction a homecare nurse would give a client would be to use

    1. The solution temperature at 100°F.
    2. 1000 mL of solution for the irrigation.
    3. The solution container placed 10 inches above the stoma.
    4. The irrigation cone in an upward direction in relation to the stoma.

15. The nurse is teaching a client with a new colostomy how to apply an appliance to a colostomy. The client leaves ½ inch of skin exposed between the stoma and the ring of the appliance. What teaching is indicated here?

    1. Telling the client this is too much skin exposed to fecal drainage.
    2. No teaching—this is a correct procedure.
    3. Telling the client that exposed skin should be between ¾ and 1 inch.

    4. Asking the client how much skin should be exposed before teaching.

16. Following a liver biopsy, the highest-priority assessment of the client's condition is to check for

    1. Pulmonary edema.
    2. Uneven respiratory pattern.
    3. Hemorrhage.
    4. Pain.

17. A client has a bile duct obstruction and is jaundiced. Which intervention will be most effective in controlling the itching associated with his jaundice?

    1. Keep the client's nails clean and short.
    2. Maintain the client's room temperature at 72 to 75°F.
    3. Provide tepid water for bathing.
    4. Use alcohol for back rubs.

18. When a client is in liver failure, which of the following behavioral changes is the most important assessment to report?

    1. Shortness of breath.
    2. Lethargy.
    3. Fatigue.
    4. Nausea.

19. A client with a history of cholecystitis is now being admitted to the hospital for possible surgical intervention. The orders include NPO, IV therapy, and bedrest. In addition to assessing for nausea, vomiting, and anorexia, the nurse should observe for pain

    1. In the right lower quadrant.
    2. After ingesting food.
    3. Radiating to the left shoulder.
    4. In the right upper quadrant.

20. The nurse taking a nursing history from a newly admitted client learns that he has a Denver shunt. This suggests that he has a history of

    1. Hydrocephalus.
    2. Renal failure.
    3. Peripheral occlusive disease.
    4. Cirrhosis.

21. A female client had a laparoscopic cholecystectomy this morning. She is now complaining of right shoulder pain. The nurse would explain to the client this symptom is

    1. Common following this operation.
    2. Expected after general anesthesia.

3. Unusual and will be reported to the surgeon.
4. Indicative of a need to use the incentive spirometer.

22. For a client with the diagnosis of acute pancreatitis, the nurse would plan for which critical component of his care?

    1. Testing for Homan's sign.
    2. Measuring the abdominal girth.
    3. Performing a glucometer test.
    4. Straining the urine.

23. After removing a fecal impaction, the client complains of feeling lightheaded and the pulse rate is 44. The priority intervention is to

    1. Monitor vital signs.
    2. Place in shock position.

3. Call the physician.
4. Begin CPR.

24. Peritoneal reaction to acute pancreatitis results in a shift of fluid from the vascular space into the peritoneal cavity. If this occurs, the nurse would evaluate for

    1. Decreased serum albumin.
    2. Abdominal pain.
    3. Oliguria.
    4. Peritonitis.

25. The assessment finding that should be reported immediately should it develop in the client with acute pancreatitis is

    1. Nausea and vomiting.
    2. Abdominal pain.
    3. Decreased bowel sounds.
    4. Shortness of breath.

GASTROINTESTINAL SYSTEM

Answers with Rationale

1. (1) Visual inspection is the first step in assessing the abdomen. Auscultation (3) is next because palpation (2) or percussion (4) can alter bowel motility, thereby producing inaccurate findings.

   NP:A; CN:PH; CL:C

2. (1) NG insertion technique is to have the client first tilt his head back for insertion into the nostril, then to flex his neck forward and swallow. Extension of the neck (2) will impede NG tube insertion.

   NP:I; CN:PH; CL:C

3. (3) As the liver cells become fatty and degenerate, they are no longer able to accommodate the large amount of blood necessary for homeostasis. The pressure in the liver increases and causes increased pressure in the venous system. As the portal pressure increases, fluid exudes into the abdominal cavity. This is called ascites.

   NP:AN; CN:PH; CL:K

4. (3) Amylase is produced by the pancreas. An inflamed pancreas is unable to adequately secrete the amylase into the intestinal tract producing elevated levels of amylase in the blood. Glucose (1) and alkaline phosphatase (2) are also likely to be elevated in acute pancreatitis. Creatinine (4) is unaffected by acute pancreatitis.

   NP:AN; CN:PH; CL:C

5. (3) The respiratory system can become occluded if the balloon slips and moves up the esophagus, putting pressure on the trachea. This would result in respiratory distress and should be assessed frequently. Scissors should be kept at the bedside to cut the tube if distress occurs. This is a safety intervention.

   NP:A; CN:PH; CL:A

6. (2) Peptic ulcer disease is characteristically gnawing epigastric pain that may radiate to the back. Vomiting usually reflects pyloric spasm from muscular spasm or obstruction. Cancer (1) would not evidence pain or vomiting unless the pylorus was obstructed.

   NP:AN; CN:PH; CL:C

7. (3) An NG tube insertion is the most appropriate intervention because it will determine the presence of active gastrointestinal bleeding. A Miller–Abbott tube (1) is a weighted, mercury-filled ballooned tube used to resolve bowel obstructions. There is no evidence of shock or fluid overload in the client; therefore, an arterial line (2) is not appropriate at this time and an IV (4) is optional.

   NP:I; CN:PH; CL:C

8. (1) These drugs inhibit action of histamine on the H_2 receptors of the parietal cells, thus reducing gastric acid output. Answer (2) refers to a cytoprotective drug; (3) to an antisecretory drug; and (4) to an anticholinergic drug.

   NP:P; CN:H; CL:C

9. (3) Crohn's disease is characterized by inflammation of the small and/or large intestine in a segmental pattern with diseased areas separated by areas of normal intestine. If surgery becomes necessary to treat the condition, a diseased area can be resected with a reanastomosis of the intestine. Ileostomy with colectomy (1) may be needed by clients with ulcerative colitis.

   NP:P; CN:PH; CL:K

10. (1) Potassium is lost through the liquid effluent, so it must be taken as a supplement. This surgery requires a low-residue diet that reduces fiber and fecal material. Vitamin B_{12} (2) is supplemented when the intrinsic factor is missing.

   NP:P; CN:PH; CL:C

Coding for Questions/Answers Abbreviations: **Nursing Process: NP,** Assessment: A, Analysis: AN, Planning: P, Implementation: I, Evaluation: E; **Client Needs: CN,** Safe, Effective Care Environment: S, Health Promotion and Maintenance: H, Psychosocial Integrity: PS, Physiological Integrity: PH; **Clinical Area: CA,** Medical Nursing: M, Surgical Nursing: S, Maternal/Newborn Nursing: MA, Pediatric Nursing: P, Psychiatric Nursing: PS; **Cognitive Level: CL,** Knowledge: K, Comprehension: C, Application: A, Analysis: AN.

11. The answer is *2 3 4 6*. The client's diet should be low residue and high calorie. Foods high in carbohydrates are usually low residue; chicken is acceptable without skin. Any salad, fresh vegetables, or grains would be considered high residue.

    NP:P; CN:H; CL:C

12. (3) An important assessment question is to find out how the client feels about the tests to be performed. Learning if he has talked with anyone about his concerns or fears will help the nurse assess the client's resources for emotional support and whether the client needs to talk about his fears or feelings.

    NP:A; CN:PS; CL:A

13. (1) The left-side position facilitates easy insertion of the rectal tube due to the anatomical position of the rectum. A recumbent position will be more comfortable for the client.

    NP:I; CN:PH; CL:C

14. (2) With the exception of the first irrigation, which is 500 mL, the amount of irrigating solution for a colostomy irrigation is 1000 mL. The temperature should be between 105° and 110°F. When the client is sitting up, the container is at shoulder level.

    NP:P; CN:PH; CL:K

15. (1) A colostomy appliance should be cut to fit the stoma so that there is a minimum amount of skin exposed to fecal drainage. Leaving ⅛ inch of skin exposed conforms to these criteria. Asking the client first is not necessary because he needs exact information, then clarification.

    NP:P; CN:PH; CL:K

16. (3) It is important to evaluate the client's condition for hemorrhage every hour for 12 hours, because this is a danger following a liver biopsy. Pulmonary edema (1) and respiratory problems (2) are not usually a concern.

    NP:A; CN:PH; CL:A

17. (3) Itching is made worse by vasodilation. Tepid water prevents excessive vasodilation. Warm environmental temperatures promote vasodilation. Alcohol not only produces vasodilation but also is drying to the skin, which further compounds the problem of itching. Keeping the nails clean and short will help prevent skin irritation and infection if the client scratches, but will not prevent the itching from occurring.

    NP:P; CN:PH; CL:C

18. (2) Lethargy may indicate impending encephalopathy and dictate the need for client safety measures. Fatigue is expected due to anemia, shortness of breath due to ascites, and nausea due to GI vascular congestion, but these are not as grave as lethargy.

    NP:A; CN:PH; CL:A

19. (4) Pain occurs 2–4 hours after eating fatty foods and is located either in the epigastric region or in the upper right quadrant of the abdomen.

    NP:A; CN:PH; CL:C

20. (4) The Denver shunt is a type of peritoneovascular shunt used in the treatment of clients who have cirrhosis with ascites. The shunt diverts ascitic fluid from the abdomen into the jugular vein or the vena cava.

    NP:AN; CN:PH; CL:C

21. (1) Carbon dioxide is insufflated into the abdomen during a laparoscopic cholecystectomy. It may irritate the diaphragm and cause referred shoulder pain. This client's complaint is a common response to this operation, so telling the client will be reassuring.

    NP:I; CN:PH; CL:C

22. (3) Hyperglycemia is a common finding in acute pancreatitis because the islet cells may not be able to produce adequate amounts of insulin. An important component of the treatment is to administer regular insulin to treat the hyperglycemia.

    NP:P; CN:PH; CL:AN

23. (2) The client requires treatment for shock. Vital signs are monitored (1) after placing the client in shock position. The physician is then called (3) for further orders.

    NP:I; CN:PH; CL:A

24. (3) Oliguria, with accompanying hypovolemic shock, is a dangerous complication of acute pancreatitis. This condition may necessitate large volumes of parenteral fluids to maintain vascular volume; a CVP catheter is often inserted for monitoring fluid needs.

    NP:E; CN:PH; CL:A

25. (4) Adult respiratory distress syndrome is a grave complication of pancreatitis. Pulmonary edema due to administration of large volumes of IV fluids and direct extension of inflammation resulting in pleural effusion are also seen. Pulmonary complications are associated with a poor prognosis. The other distractors are the more common presenting symptoms of pancreatitis.

    NP:A; CN:PH; CL:A

GENITOURINARY SYSTEM

The urinary system—the kidneys and their drainage channels—is essential for the maintenance of life. This system is responsible for excreting the end products of metabolism as well as regulating water and electrolyte concentrations of body fluids. The genitalia are the organs of reproduction.

ANATOMY AND PHYSIOLOGY

Kidney Structure

A. Paired organs located to the right and left of midline lateral to lower thoracic vertebrae.
B. Kidneys perform two major functions.
   1. Excrete most of the end products of body metabolism.
   2. Control the concentrations of most of the constituents of body fluids.
C. Composed of structural units, each of which functions the same as the total kidney and is capable of forming urine by itself.
D. The functional renal unit is called the nephron. Each nephron is composed of
   1. A glomerulus (a network of many capillaries) that filters fluid out of the blood. It is encased by Bowman's capsule.
   2. Tubules (proximal, Henle's loop, distal) in which fluid is converted to urine as it goes to the pelvis of the kidneys.
E. Fluid from Bowman's capsule moves through the proximal tubule located in the cortex.
F. Fluid then flows through Henle's loop and collecting duct located in medulla of kidney.
G. Fluid flows from loop to the collecting tubule.
H. After flowing through many convolutions, the fluid goes into a collecting sac called the pelvis of the kidney.
I. From the pelvis, fluid flows through the ureter and empties into the bladder.

Kidney Function

A. Urine production.
   1. As the fluid filtrate flows through the proximal tubules, 80 percent of the water and solutes are reabsorbed into tubular capillaries.
   2. The water and solutes that are not reabsorbed become urine.
   3. The amount of fluid and solutes excreted is determined through selective reabsorption.
B. Nephron function.
   1. The basic function is to rid the body of unwanted substances, the end products of metabolism (fluid and electrolytes).
   2. The nephron filters much of the plasma through the glomerular membrane into the tubules.
   3. The tubules filter the wanted elements of the blood (e.g., water and electrolytes) from the unwanted elements and reabsorb them into the plasma through the peritubular capillaries.
   4. Reabsorption and secretion take place by both active and passive transport.
C. Tubular reabsorption and secretion.
   1. Tubular secretion—passage of a substance by capillary action through tubular cells into tubular lumen.
   2. Three substances filtered at glomerulus.
      a. Electrolytes: Na^+, K^+, Ca^{++}, Mg^{++}, HCO_3^-, Cl^-, and HPO_4^{--}.
      b. Nonelectrolytes: glucose, amino acids, urea, uric acid, creatinine.
      c. Water.
   3. Proximal tubule reabsorption.
      a. Eighty percent of filtrate reabsorbed actively through obligatory reabsorption.
      b. H_2O, Na^+, and Cl^- continue through loop of Henle, where Cl^- is actively transported out of ascending loop, followed passively by Na^+.
D. Glomerular filtration.
   1. Glomerular membrane is semipermeable (proteins and glucose do not cross the membrane).
   2. Amount of filtration is determined by hydrostatic pressure. Normal glomerular filtration rate is 120–125 mL/min in adults.
   3. A decrease in blood pressure leads to a decrease in glomerular filtration rate (GFR) and, therefore, a decrease in urine output.
   4. Approximately 1000–2000 mL blood flows through kidneys each minute to produce 60 mL urine output per hour.
E. Concentrating and diluting mechanisms.
   1. Countercurrent flow of blood and tubular fluid increase concentration of NaCl and, therefore, H_2O reabsorption.
   2. ADH (antidiuretic hormone) released by posterior pituitary gland controls H_2O reabsorption at distal tubule.
      a. Concentrated urine leads to increased ADH secretion.

   b.   Dilute urine leads to decreased ADH secretion.
3.   Distal tubule and collecting duct.
   a.   Secretion and reabsorption completed—reabsorption of Na^+ and H_2O takes place.
   b.   Distal tubule—final regulation of H_2O and acid–base balance.
   c.   Uric acid and K^+ secreted into distal tubules and excreted in urine.
4.   Hormonal regulation.
   a. H_2O reabsorption depends on ADH.
   b. Na^+ and K^+ reabsorption influenced by aldosterone.
      (1)   Increased aldosterone causes increased Na^+ reabsorption and increased K^+ secretion.
      (2)   Decreased aldosterone exhibits opposite effect.
   c. Ca^{++} and HPO_4^{--} reabsorption regulated by parathyroid hormone.
      (1)   Increased parathyroid hormone leads to increased Ca^{++} reabsorption and increased HPO_4^{--} excretion.
      (2)   Decreased parathyroid hormone exhibits opposite effect.
5.   Water balance maintained through homeostasis—all functions of kidney must be maintained.
6.   Acid–base regulation.
   a.   Distal tubule maintains pH of ECF within 7.35–7.45.
   b.   Other actions: reabsorption, conservation of most of the bicarbonate and secretion of excess H^+ ions.

✦ F.   Blood pressure regulation.
1.   Regulation occurs through release of renin from juxtaglomerular cells in response to low blood volume or ischemia.
2.   Renin stimulates conversion of angiotensinogen to angiotensin I in liver.
3.   Angiotensin I changed to angiotensin II in pulmonary capillary bed.
4.   Angiotensin II increases blood pressure by vasoconstriction of peripheral arterioles and secretion of aldosterone.
5.   Increased aldosterone stimulates Na^+ reabsorption.
6.   Increased Na^+ reabsorption causes increased H_2O retention and plasma volume, which leads to increased blood pressure.

G.   Additional functions.
1.   Production of erythropoietin in response to hypoxia and decreased blood flow; stimulates production of RBCs in bone marrow.

2.   Renal failure leads to vitamin D deficiency, which leads to altered calcium and phosphate balance.

✦ Characteristics of Urine
A.   Components of urine include organic and inorganic materials in urine solution.
B.   Cloudy urine is of little significance and is usually the result of urates or phosphates that precipitate out.
C.   Red blood cells in the urine or hematuria are significant and indicate the presence of some disease or disorder in the body.
1.   Acute nephritis or exacerbation of chronic nephritis.
2.   Neoplasms, vascular accidents, or infections.
3.   Renal stones.
4.   Renal tuberculosis.
5.   Trauma to the urinary tract.
6.   A manifestation of thrombocytopenia.
7.   May be the result of problems along the genitourinary tract, such as the ureter, the bladder, or the prostate gland.
D.   The source of blood cells in urine must be determined.
1.   Blood during the initial period of voiding may be from the anterior urethra or prostate.
2.   Blood mixed with the total volume of urine may be from kidneys, ureters or bladder.

RENAL REGULATION OF FLUID AND ELECTROLYTES

Composition of the Body

Body Fluids
Definition: Total body water represents the largest constituent (45–80 percent) of the total body weight, depending on the amount of fat present.
✦ A.   Intracellular—represents 40 percent of total body fluid; contained inside the cell; includes the red blood cells.
✦ B.   Extracellular—represents 20 percent of total body fluid; includes remaining fluid not contained within the cell.
1.   Intravascular (plasma)—liquid in which the blood cells are suspended (5 percent).
2.   Interstitial—liquid surrounding tissue cells (15 percent).
3.   Percent varies with age and amount of fat.
   a.   Infant—70–80 percent of baby's weight is water.
   b.   Elderly clients—45–55 percent of body weight is water.
   c.   Thin person has more water.

d. Men—greater percentage of body weight is water, more lean body mass than women.

Electrolytes

Definition: Electrolytes are compounds that dissolve in a solution to form ions; each particle then carries either a positive or negative electrical charge.

✦ A. Types.
1. Cations—positive charge (Na^+, K^+, Ca^{++}, Mg^{++}).
2. Anions—negative charge (Cl^-, HCO_3^-, HPO_4^{--}, SO_4^{--}).
3. Equal number of cations and anions (154 each).

✦ B. Concentration in solution is expressed in mEq/L. Total number of cations (mEq) plus total number of anions (mEq) will be the same in both intracellular fluid and extracellular fluid, thereby rendering the body's fluid composition electrically neutral.

✦ C. Compartment composition.
1. Extracellular—large quantities of sodium, chloride and bicarbonate ions.
2. Intracellular—large quantities of potassium, phosphate and proteins.

Dynamics of Intercompartmental Fluid Transfer

✦ **Transport of Fluids and Electrolytes**
A. Diffusion—movement of solutes (substances that are dissolved in a solution) or gases from an area of higher concentration to an area of lower concentration; a passive transport system.
B. Filtration—passage of fluids through a semipermeable membrane as a result of a difference in hydrostatic pressures (pressure exerted by a fluid within a closed system). The semipermeable membrane prevents movement of solute particles.
C. Osmosis—passage of water or solvent through a semipermeable membrane from an area of lesser concentration to an area of greater concentration of solute; a passive transport system.
D. Facilitated diffusion—transport of molecules that are too large or insoluble across the membrane by means of a carrier molecule, creating a complex that is soluble in the membrane.
E. Active transport—transport (requiring external energy—ATP) of substances across a membrane from an area of low concentration to an area of high concentration.
1. Molecules move from an area of high concentration to one of low concentration. Glucose transport into cell is an example.
2. Active transport is used for sodium moving out of the cell and potassium moving into the cell.

F. Oncotic pressure—osmotic pressure that results from dispersed colloid particles (the largest being proteins) in the blood capillaries; the pressure draws water back into the vascular system, thereby maintaining blood volume.
G. Lymphatics—vessels responsible for returning the large molecules that have escaped from the blood capillaries (including protein molecules) to the bloodstream, returning them from the interstitial fluid and the gastrointestinal tract.

Balance of Body Fluid

A. Intake.
1. Ingestion of foodstuff and water. Usual intake of fluid is 2000–3000 mL/day.
2. Oxidation of foodstuff.
B. Output.
1. Skin and lungs.
a. Water is lost through vaporization from the skin surface and through expired air from the lungs.
b. The amount lost increases as metabolism increases.
c. About 900 mL loss/day.
2. Gastrointestinal tract.
a. Routes include saliva, gastric secretions, bile, pancreatic juices, and intestinal mucosa.
b. A volume in excess of 7 L is transferred from the extracellular fluid (ECF) into the gastrointestinal tract, only to be reabsorbed, excepting some 200 mL that is passed with feces.
✦ 3. Kidneys.
a. Carry the heaviest load.
b. Through glomerular filtration and tubular reabsorption, the kidneys maintain homeostasis.
c. Hormones influence the kidneys in terms of fluid balance.
(1) Antidiuretic.
(2) Aldosterone.

Fluid Imbalances

Assessment

✦ A. Assess for dehydration (extracellular fluid volume deficit).
1. Evaluate possible causes.
a. Vomiting, diarrhea.
b. Increased urine output.
c. Diuretics.
d. Excessive loss through respiration.
e. Insufficient IV replacement.
f. GI loss.

g. Hemorrhage.

h. Excessive perspiration.

2. Assess skin.

a. Loss of skin turgor (after being pinched and lightly pulled upward, skin returns to normal very slowly).

b. Dry, warm skin.

3. Assess febrile state (usually means there is fluid loss through perspiration).

4. Observe cracked lips, dry mucous membranes.

5. Assess decreased urinary output (normal output is > 30 mL/hr).

6. Concentrated urine—dark amber color and odorous.

7. Weight loss.

8. Low central venous pressure.

9. Increased respiration.

✦ B. Assess for circulatory overload (extracellular fluid volume excess).

1. Evaluate possible causes.

a. Excessive IV fluids.

b. Inadequate kidney function.

c. Cushing's syndrome.

d. Chronic liver disease.

2. Assess for headache.

3. Observe flushed skin.

4. Assess tachycardia.

5. Assess for venous distention, particularly neck veins.

6. Evaluate increased blood pressure and CVP.

7. Assess tachypnea (increased respiratory rate), coughing, dyspnea (shortness of breath), cyanosis, and pulmonary edema.

Implementation

✦ A. Take central venous pressure to determine fluid balance if CVP catheter is in place. The CVP reflects the competency of the heart (particularly the right side) to handle the volume of blood returning to it.

1. CVP indicates the comparison of the pumping capacity of the heart and the volume of the circulating blood.

✦ 2. Normal CVP reading: 5–10 cm H_2O.

3. Increased CVP (above 15 cm H_2O) can be indicative of congestive heart failure or circulatory overload.

4. Decreased CVP (below 5 cm H_2O) is indicative of hypovolemia (decreased fluid volume) whether from blood loss or other fluid losses.

B. Monitor client's condition.

1. Check condition of skin.

a. Dry, warm, cracked lips.

b. Elasticity.

2. Check body temperature—fever suggests loss of body fluids.

3. Check for venous distention, increased pulse rate and increasing blood pressure.

4. Ask client about unusual related symptoms, if possible, such as headache, shortness of breath.

5. Monitor fluid intake.

6. Check urine output at least every 8 hours for maintenance IV therapy, or as often as every hour for replacement fluid administration.

7. Check specific gravity (over 1.025 indicates dehydration; less than 1.010 indicates overhydration).

8. Check for symptoms of electrolyte disturbances at least every 4 hours.

9. Weigh client daily and watch for weight gain.

ELECTROLYTE IMBALANCES

Potassium Imbalance

See also Serum Electrolyte Levels in Chapter 11.

✦ A. Normal serum level is 3.5–5.0 mEq/L.

B. Potassium deficiency and excess is a common problem in fluid and electrolyte imbalance.

C. Major cell cation.

✦ D. General nursing management related to potassium imbalances.

1. Observe ECG tracings for change in T wave, ST segment, or QRS complex.

2. Measure intake and output accurately.

3. Draw frequent blood specimens for potassium level.

4. Observe for signs of metabolic acidosis and alkalosis.

Hypokalemia

Definition: Hypokalemia is a very low concentration of potassium ions in extracellular fluid (serum level below 3.5 mEq/L).

✦ A. Signs and symptoms of hypokalemia.

1. Muscle weakness, muscle pain, leg cramps, hyporeflexia, fatigue.

2. Hypotension, shallow respiration.

3. Arrhythmias—PVCs particularly.

4. Nausea, vomiting, diarrhea.

5. Apathy, drowsiness leading to coma.

6. ECG changes include peaked P wave, flat T wave, depressed ST segment, and elevated U waves.

7. Paralytic ileus.

✦ B. Causes of hypokalemia.

1. Renal loss most common (usually caused by use of diuretics).

2. Insufficient potassium intake.

3. Loss from gastrointestinal tract via NG tube placement without replacement electrolyte solution, or from vomiting or diarrhea.

✦ C. Nursing management of hypokalemia.
1. Maintain IVs with KCl added.
2. Replace K$^+$ when excess loss occurs (NG tubes, diarrhea, etc.).
3. Replace no more than 20 mEq of KCl in 1 hour; observe ECG monitor if possible.
4. Dilute KCl in 30–50 mL IV fluid and administer with an IV pump.
5. Observe for adequate urine output.

Hyperkalemia

Definition: Hyperkalemia is an excess of potassium in extracellular fluid (serum level greater than 5.0 mEq/L).

✦ A. Signs and symptoms of hyperkalemia.
1. Weakness, muscle cramp, flaccid paralysis, irritability.
2. Hyperreflexia proceeding to paralysis.
3. Bradycardia, arrhythmias.
4. Ventricular fibrillation.
5. ECG changes depict elevated or tented T wave, widened QRS complex, prolonged P-R interval, and flattened P wave with depressed ST segment.
6. Oliguria.
7. Diarrhea, nausea.

✦ B. Causes of hyperkalemia.
1. Usually renal disease (cannot excrete potassium).
2. Burns (due to cellular destruction releasing potassium from cells into extracellular space).
3. Crushing injuries (due to cellular breakage releasing potassium from cells).
4. Adrenal insufficiency.
5. Respiratory or metabolic acidosis.
6. Excess potassium administration.

✦ C. Nursing management of hyperkalemia.
1. Administer diuretics if kidney function is adequate.
2. Administer hypertonic IV glucose with insulin.
3. Provide exchange resins through NG or enema (Kayexalate).
4. Provide calcium IV to stimulate heart if depressed action.
5. Administer sodium bicarbonate if client is acidotic.
6. Withold food and medications with high potassium levels.

Sodium Imbalance

✦ A. Normal serum level is 135–145 mEq/L.
B. Sodium deficiency and excess are common problems in fluid and electrolyte imbalance.
C. General nursing management.
1. Observe skin condition.
2. Measure intake and output.
3. Auscultate lung sounds.
4. Observe urine for specific gravity and color.

Hyponatremia

Definition: Hyponatremia is caused by a very low concentration of sodium in extracellular fluid (serum level below 135 mEq/L).

✦ A. Signs and symptoms of hyponatremia.
1. Signs and symptoms are the same as those for extracellular fluid deficiency.
a. Weakness.
b. Restlessness.
c. Delirium, irritability, confusion.
d. Hyperpnea.
e. Oliguria.
f. Increased temperature and pulse.
g. Flushed skin, dry mucous membranes.
h. Abdominal cramps.
i. Convulsions.
j. Nausea, anorexia.
2. If sodium is lost but fluid is not, the following signs and symptoms will be present (similar to those of water excess):
a. Mental confusion, restlessness.
b. Headache.
c. Muscle twitching and weakness.
d. Coma.
e. Convulsions.
f. Oliguria.

✦ B. Causes of hyponatremia.
1. Excessive perspiration.
2. Use of diuretics.
3. Gastrointestinal losses—severe diarrhea, vomiting, pancreatic and biliary fistulas.
4. Lack of sodium in diet.
5. Burns, fibrocystic disease.
6. Excessive IV administration without NaCl.
7. Diabetic acidosis.
8. Adrenal insufficiency.

C. Nursing management of hyponatremia.
1. Administer IV fluids with sodium.
2. Maintain accurate intake and output.

Hypernatremia

Definition: Hypernatremia is caused by a very high concentration of sodium in extracellular fluid (serum level above 145 mEq/L).

✦ A. Signs and symptoms of hypernatremia.
1. Signs and symptoms are the same as for extracellular fluid excesses.
a. Pitting edema.
b. Excessive weight gain.
c. Increased blood pressure.
d. Dyspnea.

2. If hypernatremia is due to dehydration, in which a loss of fluid increases the number of ions, the signs and symptoms include
    a. Concentrated urine and oliguria.
    b. Dry mucous membranes, dry swollen tongue.
    c. Thirst.
    d. Flushed skin.
    e. Increased temperature.
    f. Tachycardia, hypertension.
    g. Seizures, coma.
+ B. Causes of hypernatremia.
    1. Severe diarrhea.
    2. Decreased water intake.
    3. Febrile states.
    4. Ingestion of sodium chloride.
    5. Excessive loss of water through rapid and deep respiration.
    6. Renal failure.
    7. Diabetes insipidus.
+ C. Nursing management of hypernatremia.
    1. Record intake and output.
    2. Restrict sodium in diet.
    3. Weigh daily.
    4. Observe vital signs.
    5. Administer fluids orally or IV.

Calcium Imbalance

+ A. Normal serum level is 4.3–5.3 mEq/L; 9–11 mg/dL.
  B. Mineral plays major role in blood coagulation, cardiac muscle function, and muscle and nerve function.

Hypocalcemia

Definition: Hypocalcemia results from a deficit of calcium in the extracellular fluid (serum level below 8.5 mg/dL).
+ A. Signs and symptoms of hypocalcemia.
    1. Abdominal cramps, muscle cramps, spasms of larynx and bronchus.
    2. Tetany, carpopedal spasms.
    3. Circumoral tingling, especially in fingers.
    4. Convulsions.
    5. Confusion, anxiety, and moodiness.
    6. ECG changes, prolonged QT interval, ventricular tachycardia.
+ B. Causes of hypocalcemia.
    1. Acute pancreatitis.
    2. Chronic renal insufficiency.
    3. Burns.
    4. Removal of parathyroid glands.
    5. Massive transfusion (over 2000 mL of blood) requires calcium supplement.
    6. Malabsorption syndrome.
    7. Vitamin D deficiency.

+ C. Nursing management of hypocalcemia.
    + 1. Calcium gluconate IV, followed by oral calcium supplements.
    2. Serum albumin if condition is due to low serum albumin concentration.
    3. Monitor for hypocalcemia.
        a. Trousseau's test positive.
        b. Chvostek's test positive.
    4. Monitor for signs of hypercalcemia and dysrhythmias.

Hypercalcemia

Definition: Hypercalcemia results from an excess of calcium in the extracellular fluid (serum level above 5.3 mEq/L).
+ A. Signs and symptoms of hypercalcemia.
    1. Anorexia, nausea, vomiting.
    2. Lethargy, weight loss, polydipsia, polyuria, dehydration.
    3. Flank pain, bone pain, decreased muscle tone, pathologic fractures.
    4. Stupor, coma.
    5. ECG changes, shortened QT segment, ventricular arrhythmia.
+ B. Causes of hypercalcemia.
    1. Excessive intake of vitamin D (milk) or calcium supplements.
    2. Hyperparathyroidism, neoplasm of parathyroids.
    3. Thyrotoxicosis.
    4. Immobilization.
    5. Paget's disease.
+ C. Nursing management of hypercalcemia.
    1. Treat the underlying cause of the high serum calcium level.
    2. Immediate reversal—sodium salts IV and diuretics (Lasix).

Magnesium Imbalance

+ A. Normal serum magnesium level is 1.3–2.1 mEq/L.
  B. Fifty percent of magnesium is in the bones and remaining 45 percent in intracellular compartment.

Hypomagnesemia

Definition: Deficit of magnesium due to chronic alcoholism, starvation, malabsorption, or vigorous diuresis (serum level below 1.3 mEq/L).
+ A. Signs and symptoms of hypomagnesemia.
    1. Neuromuscular irritability.
        a. Jerks, twitches.
        b. Hyperactive reflexes.
        c. Convulsions, hallucinations, coma.
        + d. Tetany.
    2. Cardiovascular changes.
        a. Tachycardia, ventricular dysrhythmias.

b. Hypotension.
c. ECG changes: prolonged PR and QT segments.
✦ B. Causes of hypomagnesemia.
1. Low intake.
2. Abnormal loss—chronic diarrhea.
3. Chronic nephritis.
4. Diuretic phase of renal failure.
5. Alcoholism.
6. Pancreatitis.
7. Toxemia of pregnancy.
8. Cancer chemotherapy.
✦ C. Nursing management of hypomagnesemia.
1. Magnesium sulfate.
a. Administer IV or IM slowly.
b. Observe for adequate urine output.
✦ c. Antidote: calcium gluconate.
2. Monitor cardiac rhythm.
3. Institute seizure precautions.

Hypermagnesemia

Definition: An excess of magnesium as a result of renal insufficiency or inability to excrete magnesium absorbed from food (serum level above 2.1 mEq/L).
✦ A. Causes of hypermagnesemia.
1. Renal insufficiency.
2. Overdose of magnesium.
3. Severe dehydration, oliguria.
4. Overuse of antacids with magnesium (Gelusil).
✦ B. Signs and symptoms of hypermagnesemia.
1. Hypotension, decreased respirations.
2. Curare-like paralysis.
3. Sedation.
4. Hypoactive deep tendon reflex.
5. Cardiac arrhythmias, bradycardia.
6. Warm sensation in body.
✦ C. Nursing management of hypermagnesemia.
1. Administer calcium gluconate IV slowly.
2. Give in peripheral veins (not CVP line).
3. Monitor vital signs and neurological status.

ACID–BASE REGULATION

Principles of Acid–Base Balance

✦ A. Acid–base balance is the ratio of acids and bases in the body necessary to maintain a chemical balance conducive to life.
B. Acid–base ratio is 20 parts base to 1 part acid.
✦ C. Acid–base balance is measured by arterial blood samples and recorded as blood pH. Range is 7.35–7.45.
D. Acids are hydrogen ion donors. They release hydrogen ions to neutralize or decrease the strength of the base.

E. Bases are hydrogen ion acceptors. They accept hydrogen ions to convert strong acids to weak acids (for example, hydrochloric acid is converted to carbonic acid).

Regulatory Mechanisms

A. The body controls the pH balance by use of
1. Chemical buffers.
2. Lungs.
3. Cells.
4. Kidneys.
✦ B. The chemical buffer system works fastest, but other regulatory mechanisms provide more reliable protection against acid–base imbalance.
1. A buffer is a substance that reacts to keep pH within normal limits. It functions only when excessive base or acid is present.
2. Chemical buffers are paired (for example, weakly ionized acid or base is balanced with a fully ionized salt).
a. Pairing prevents excessive changes in normal acid–base balance.
b. The buffers release or absorb hydrogen ions when needed.
3. The buffer systems in the extracellular fluid react quickly with acids and bases to minimize changes in pH.
a. Once they react, they are used up.
b. If further stress occurs, the body is less able to cope.
✦ 4. There are four primary buffer systems.
a. Carbonic acid–bicarbonate—maintains blood pH at 7.4 with ratio of 20 parts bicarbonate to 1 part carbonic acid.
b. Intracellular and plasma proteins—vary the amounts of hydrogen ions in the chemical structure of the protein (along with liver). They can both attract and release hydrogen ions.
c. Hemoglobin—maintains the balance by the chloride shift. Chloride shifts in and out of red blood cells according to the level of oxygen in the blood plasma. Each chloride ion that leaves the cell is replaced by a bicarbonate ion.
d. Phosphate buffer system—composed of sodium and other cations in association with HPO_4^{--} and $H_2PO_4^-$; acts like bicarbonate system.
✦ C. Lungs.
1. Next to react are the lungs.
2. It takes 10–30 minutes for lungs to inactivate hydrogen molecules by converting them to water molecules.

3. The carbonic acid that was formed by neutralizing bicarbonate is taken to lungs.
   a. There it is reduced to carbon dioxide and water and exhaled.
   b. When there is excessive acid in the body, the respiratory rate increases to blow off the excessive carbon dioxide and water.
4. When there is too much bicarbonate or base in the body, respirations become deeper and slower.
   a. This process builds up the level of carbonic acid.
   b. The result is that the strength of the excessive bicarbonate is neutralized.
5. Lungs can inactivate only the hydrogen ions carried by carbonic acid. The other ions must be excreted by the kidneys.

◆ D. Cells.
   1. They absorb or release extra hydrogen ions.
   2. They react in 2–4 hours.
◆ E. Kidneys.
   1. Most efficient regulatory mechanism.
   2. Begin to function within hours to days as integral part of buffering system.
   3. Blood pH is maintained by balance of 20 parts bicarbonate to 1 part carbonic acid.
   4. Four processes are involved in acid–base regulation.
      a. Dissociation of H^+ from H_2CO_3 (H^+ and HCO_3^-).
      b. Reabsorption of Na^+ from urine filtrate (Na^+ and H^+ change places).
      c. Formation and conservation of $NaHCO_3$ (Na^+ and HCO_3^-).
      d. NH_3 from metabolic process (Krebs cycle) enters kidney's tubular cell and adds an H^+ ion and then exchanges as ammonium with Na^+ (Na^+ and NH_4).
   5. Hydrogen and potassium compete with each other in exchange for Na^+ in the tubular urine.
      a. In acidosis, the H^+ ion concentration is increased and K^+ ion must wait to be excreted because hydrogen has preference.
      b. In alkalosis, the H^+ ion is low and K^+ is excreted in larger amounts.

ACID–BASE IMBALANCES

Metabolic Acidosis

◆ *Definition:* Metabolic acidosis occurs when there is a deficit of bases or an accumulation of fixed acids.
A. Changes in pH and serum HCO_3.
   1. The pH will become acidotic as a result of insufficient base.

> **NORMAL BLOOD GASES**
> - pH: 7.35–7.45
> - PCO_2: 35–45 mm Hg
> - HCO_3: 22–26 mEq/L
> - CO_2 content: 26–28 mEq/L
> - CO_2 combining power: 58 volume percent
> - PO_2: 80–100 mm Hg

   a. It falls below 7.35.
   b. There are either more hydrogen ions or fewer bicarbonate ions present in the blood.
2. The serum CO_2 level will be below 22 mEq/L (normal range of CO_2 is 26–28 mEq/L).
   a. Serum CO_2 measures the amount of circulating bicarbonate.
   b. Serum CO_2 acts as a bicarbonate (HCO_3) determinant. When serum CO_2 is low, HCO_3 is lost and acidosis results.
   c. In lab reports, the CO_2 may be reported as HCO_3, CO_2 content, or CO_2 combining power, depending on the laboratory.
   d. Laboratory values will vary depending on the methods used for analysis.
B. Compensatory mechanisms.
   1. When compensating for metabolic acidosis, the one clinical manifestation usually observed is the "blowing off" of excessive acids. This can be noted by a respiratory rate increase.
   2. The lungs are the fastest mechanism used to compensate for metabolic acidosis.
      a. If the lungs are involved, as in respiratory acidosis, they cannot function as a compensatory mechanism.
      b. Therefore, the kidneys must take over and the process is much slower.
   3. Renal excretion of acid occurs.
◆ C. Laboratory values.
   1. The partial pressure of the blood gas carbon dioxide (PCO_2) decreases below 35 mm of pressure when the client is compensating. (Normal values: 35–45 mm Hg.)
   2. The partial pressure of oxygen (PO_2) is usually increased due to increased respiratory rate. (Normal values PO_2: 80–100 mm Hg.)
   3. The serum potassium level is increased with acidosis, due primarily to the cause of the acidosis.
      a. For example, clients can go into metabolic acidosis from severe diarrhea.
      b. When this condition is present, the potassium moves out of the cell and into the extravascular space due to the dehydration process.

4. Sodium and chloride levels may be decreased. Again, this is usually due to excessive loss through urine or gastrointestinal disorders.
5. Laboratory values when a client is in metabolic acidosis and in the compensatory state.
   a. Metabolic acidosis.
      (1) pH: < 7.35 (decreased).
      (2) HCO_3: < 22 mEq/L (decreased).
      (3) PCO_2: 38–40 mm Hg (normal).
      (4) PO_2: 95 mm Hg.
      (5) Cl: 120 mEq/L.
      (6) K: 5.5 mEq/L.
   b. Compensated metabolic acidosis.
      (1) pH: 7.40.
      (2) HCO_3: 16 mEq/L.
      (3) PCO_2: < 35 mm Hg.

✦ D. Causes of metabolic acidosis (seen particularly in the surgical client).
   1. Diabetes—diabetic ketoacidosis.
      a. When insufficient insulin is produced or administered to metabolize carbohydrates, increased fat metabolism results, thus producing excess accumulations of ketones and other acids.
      b. This is the most common problem associated with metabolic acidosis in the surgical client.
   2. Renal insufficiency—kidneys lose their ability to reabsorb bicarbonate and secrete hydrogen ions.
   3. Diarrhea—excessive amounts of base are lost from the intestines and pancreas, resulting in acidosis.

E. Clinical manifestations.
   1. Headache, mental dullness.
   2. Drowsiness, confusion.
   3. Nausea, vomiting, diarrhea.
   4. Coma, twitching, convulsions (late changes).
   5. Kussmaul's respiration (increased respiratory rate due to compensation).
   6. Fruity breath (as evidenced in diabetic ketoacidosis as a result of improper fat metabolism).

F. Nursing management.
   ✦ 1. Administer sodium bicarbonate intravenously to alkalize the client and return client to normal acid–base balance as quickly as possible.
      a. Usual dosage: 1–3 ampules of 50 mEq bicarbonate/ampule.
      b. This is usually the immediate treatment rendered for metabolic acidosis.
   ✦ 2. Administer sodium lactate solution to increase the base level.
      a. Sodium lactate is converted to bicarbonate by the liver.

      b. Lactated Ringer's IV solution may be used.
   3. Administer insulin in ketoacidosis. Insulin moves glucose out of the blood serum and into the cell, thereby decreasing ketosis. Insulin decreases ketones by decreasing the release of fatty acids from fat cells.
   4. Monitor laboratory values closely while managing metabolic acidosis.
   5. Watch for signs of hyperkalemia and dehydration in the client (oliguria, vital sign changes, etc.).
   6. Record intake and output.

Metabolic Alkalosis

✦ *Definition:* Metabolic alkalosis is a malfunction of metabolism, causing an increase in blood base or a reduction of available acids in the serum.

A. Changes in pH and serum bicarbonate (HCO_3).
   1. The pH will become more alkaline; therefore, it will be above 7.45.
   2. Bicarbonate will increase above 26 mEq/L. CO_2 measures the amount of circulating bicarbonate or the base portion of the plasma. [A good way to remember these acid–base values is to recall that as the pH increases, so does the HCO_3 (and CO_2). The reverse is true for acidosis.]
   3. The PCO_2 will not change unless the lungs attempt to compensate.
   4. Serum potassium and chloride levels decrease, due to the basic cause of the alkalosis, whether it be excessive vomiting or the use of diuretics.

B. Compensatory mechanisms.
   1. The lungs attempt to hold on to the carbonic acid in an effort to neutralize the base state; therefore, the rate of respiration decreases.
   2. When the lungs are compensating for the alkalotic state, the PCO_2 will increase above 45 mEq/L.
   3. Renal excretion of bicarbonate occurs.

✦ C. Laboratory values when client is in metabolic alkalosis and compensatory states.
   1. Metabolic alkalosis.
      a. pH: > 7.45 (increased).
      b. HCO_3: > 26 mEq/L (increased).
      c. PCO_2: 38–40 mm Hg (normal).
      d. PO_2: 95 mm Hg.
      e. K: 3.0 mEq/L.
      f. Cl: 88 mEq/L.
   2. Compensated metabolic alkalosis.
      a. pH: 7.45.
      b. HCO_3: 38 mEq/L.
      c. PCO_2: > 45 mm Hg.
      d. PO_2: 95 mm Hg.

D. Causes of metabolic alkalosis.
   1. Ingestion of excessive soda bicarbonate (used by individuals for acid indigestion).
   2. Excessive vomiting, which results in the loss of hydrochloric acid and potassium.
   3. Placement of NG tubes that causes a depletion of both hydrochloric acid and potassium.
   4. Use of potent diuretics, particularly by cardiac clients. They tend to lose not only potassium but also hydrogen and chloride ions, causing an increase in the bicarbonate level of the serum.
   5. Excessive intake of mineralocorticoids.
E. Clinical manifestations.
   1. Confusion, dizziness.
   2. Nausea, vomiting, diarrhea.
   3. Restlessness, irritability, agitation, nervousness.
   4. Twitching of extremities, coma, convulsions (late signs).
   5. Numbness or tingling of fingers and toes.
   6. ECG changes indicate tachycardia, with the T wave running into the P wave.
✦ F. Nursing management.
   1. Give acetazolamide (Diamox) to promote kidney excretion of bicarbonate.
   2. Administer IV solution of added electrolytes.
      a. Estimate the potassium loss from gastric fluid at 5–10 mEq for each liter lost.
      b. In many institutions, the gastric fluid loss is replaced mL for mL every 2–4 hours.
      c. In other institutions, the approximate electrolyte loss is calculated and this amount is added to the 24-hour IV solution.
      d. Chloride replacement enables renal absorption of NA^+ with Cl^- and renal excretion of excessive HCO_3.
✦ 3. Maintain diet of foods high in potassium and chloride (bananas, apricots, dried peaches, Brazil nuts, dried figs, oranges).
   4. Administer potassium chloride maintenance doses to clients on long-term diuretics.
   5. Give ammonium chloride to increase the amount of available hydrogen ions, thereby increasing the availability of acids in the blood.
   6. Check laboratory values frequently to watch for electrolyte imbalance.
   7. Watch client for physical signs indicative of hypokalemia or metabolic alkalosis.
   8. Keep accurate records of intake and output and vital signs.

Respiratory Acidosis

✦ *Definition:* Respiratory acidosis refers to increased carbonic acid concentration (accumulated CO_2 that has combined with water) caused by retention of carbon dioxide through hypoventilation. Differs from metabolic acidosis in that it results from altered alveolar ventilation.

A. Changes in pH, PCO_2, and PO_2.
   1. With an increased acidic state, the pH will fall below 7.35.
   2. The PCO_2 will be increased above 45–50 mm Hg.
   3. The PO_2 will be normal (80–100 mm Hg) or it can be decreased as hypoxia increases.
   4. The HCO_3 will be normal if respiratory acidosis is uncompensated.
B. Compensatory mechanisms.
   1. Because the basic problem in respiratory acidosis is a defect in the lungs, the kidneys must be the major compensatory mechanism.
      a. The kidneys work more slowly than the lungs.
      b. Therefore, it will take from hours to days for the compensation to take place.
   2. The kidneys will retain bicarbonate and return it to the extracellular fluid compartment.
   3. The bicarbonate level will be elevated with partial or complete compensation.
✦ C. Laboratory values when client is in respiratory acidosis and compensated acidosis.
   1. Respiratory acidosis.
      a. pH: < 7.35 (decreased).
      b. PCO_2: < 45 mm Hg (increased).
      c. PO_2: 90 mm Hg.
      d. HCO_3: 24 mEq/L (normal or increased).
   2. Compensated acidosis.
      a. pH: 7.35.
      b. PCO_2: 50 mm Hg.
      c. PO_2: 90 mm Hg.
      d. HCO_3: > 26 mEq/L.
D. Causes of respiratory acidosis.
   1. Sedatives.
   2. Oversedation with narcotics in postoperative period.
   3. A chronic pulmonary disorder such as emphysema, asthma, bronchitis, or pneumonia, leading to
      a. Difficulty in the expiratory phase of respiration, leading to retention of carbon dioxide.
      b. Airway obstruction.
   4. Poor gaseous exchange during surgery.
E. Clinical manifestations.
   1. Dyspnea after exertion, tachycardia.
   2. Visual disturbances.
   3. Hyperventilation when at rest.
   4. Headache, vetigo, tremors, confusion.

5. Sensorium changes—drowsiness leading to coma (late changes).
6. Carbon dioxide narcosis.
   a. When body has adjusted to higher carbon dioxide levels, the respiratory center loses its sensitivity to elevated carbon dioxide.
   b. Medulla fails to respond to high levels of carbon dioxide.
   c. Client is forced to depend on anoxia for respiratory stimulus.
   ✦ d. If a high level of oxygen is administered, client will cease breathing.
✦ F. Nursing management.
1. Turn, cough and deep-breathe client at least every 2–4 hours as part of general postoperative care. Use oropharyngeal suction if necessary. Maintain semi-Fowler's position.
2. Encourage the use of the incentive spirometer.
3. When pulmonary complications present a threat, do postural drainage, percussion and vibration, followed by suctioning.
4. Keep client well hydrated (2–3 L) to facilitate removal of secretions. If client is dehydrated, secretions become thick and more difficult to expectorate.
5. Monitor vital signs carefully, particularly rate and depth of respirations.
6. Monitor ABGs for changes in pH and CO_2.
7. Teach pursed-lip breathing to chronic respiratory clients.
8. If oxygen is administered, watch carefully for signs of carbon dioxide narcosis. Usually O_2 at 2 L is started.
9. Place client on mechanical ventilation if necessary.
10. Administer aerosol medications through nebulizer treatment.
    a. Bronchodilators (aminophylline)—relieve bronchospasms.
    b. Detergents (Tergemist)—liquefy tenacious mucus.
    c. Antibiotics specific to causative agent.
11. Administer drug therapy.
    a. Sodium bicarbonate IV (0.25 g/kg body weight).
    b. Sodium lactate IV.
    c. Ringer's lactate IV to replace electrolyte loss.
    d. Potassium to maintain serum levels.

Respiratory Alkalosis

✦ *Definition:* Respiratory alkalosis occurs when an excessive amount of carbon dioxide is exhaled, usually caused by hyperventilation. The loss of carbon dioxide results in a decrease in H^+ concentration along with a decrease in PCO_2 and an increase in the ratio of bicarbonate to carbonic acid. The result is an increase in the pH level.

A. Changes in pH, PCO_2 and PO_2.
1. With an increased alkalotic state, the pH will increase above 7.45, indicating there is a decreased amount of carbonic acid in the serum.
2. The PCO_2 will be normal to low, as this measures the acid portion of the acid–base system (30–45 mm Hg).
3. The PO_2 should be unchanged.
4. The bicarbonate level (HCO_3 or CO_2 content) should be normal unless the client is compensating.
B. Compensatory mechanisms.
1. Because the basic problem is related to the respiratory system, the kidneys compensate by excreting more bicarbonate ions and retaining hydrogen ions.
2. This process returns the acid–base balance to a normal ratio.
✦ C. Laboratory values when client is in respiratory alkalosis and compensated alkalosis.
1. Respiratory alkalosis.
   a. pH: > 7.45 (increased).
   b. PCO_2: 35 mm Hg (decreased).
   c. PO_2: 95 mm Hg.
   d. HCO_3: < 22 mEq/L.
2. Compensated alkalosis.
   a. pH: 7.45.
   b. PCO_2: 30 mm Hg.
   c. PO_2: 95 mm Hg.
   d. HCO_3: < 22 mEq/L.
D. Causes of respiratory alkalosis.
1. Hysteria or acute anxiety: client hyperventilates and exhales excessive amounts of carbon dioxide.
2. Hypoxia: stimulates client to breathe more vigorously.
3. Following head injuries or intracranial surgery.
4. Increased temperature.
5. Overventilation with mechanical ventilator.
6. Salicylate poisoning.
   a. Stimulation of respiration causes alkalosis through hyperventilation.
   b. Acidosis may occur from excessive salicylates in the blood.
E. Clinical manifestations—increased neuromuscular irritability.
1. Lightheadedness, vertigo, tinnitus, palpatations.
2. Hyperreflexia.
3. Numbness of fingers and toes, tetany.
4. Muscular twitching, convulsions (late changes).
✦ 5. Gasping for breath, rapid, deep respirations.

Table 8-5. ACID–BASE BALANCE COMPARISON

	Respiratory Acidosis	Respiratory Alkalosis
How it happens	Client hypoventilates CO_2 builds up in the bloodstream pH drops (respiratory acidosis) Kidneys try to compensate by conserving bicarbonate ions or generating bicarbonate ions (base)	Client hyperventilates (increase in rate or depth) This causes the lungs to eliminate or blow off CO_2 Most common causes: • Anxiety • Pain • Hypermetabolic state (fever, liver failure, sepsis)
Signs and symptoms	Apprehension Confusion ↓ deep tendon reflexes Diaphoresis Dyspnea with rapid shallow respirations Nausea or vomiting Restlessness Tachycardia Tremors Warm flushed skin	Anxiety Diaphoresis Dyspnea ECG changes Hyperreflexia Paresthesia Restlessness Tachycardia Tetany
What tests show	ABG analysis: pH < 7.35 and $PaCO_2$ > 45 Chest x-ray—COPD, pneumonia, pulmonary edema, pneumothorax Serum potassium > 5 = hyperkalemia Drug screening may confirm suspected OD	ABG analysis: pH > 7.45 and $PaCO_2$ < 3; HCO_3 may be normal (22–26 mEq/L) when alkalosis is acute, but usually falls below 22 mEq/L when chronic Serum electrolytes may point to a metabolic disorder that could be causing compensated respiratory alkalosis Hypokalemia may be evident (↓ LOC) ECG may indicate arrhythmias Toxicology screening may reveal salicylate poisoning
How it is treated	Goal: improving ventilation and lowering $PaCO_2$ level If respiratory acidosis stems from nonpulmonary conditions such as neuromuscular disease or drug OD, correct the underlying cause Bronchodilator to open constricted airways Supplemental oxygen as needed Treat hyperkalemia Antibiotic to treat infection Chest PT to remove secretions from lungs	Correct the underlying disorder—which may require removing the causative agent such as salicylate If acute hypoxemia is the cause—O_2 therapy is initiated; if anxiety—sedative Hyperventilations can be counteracted by having the patient breathe into a paper bag, which forces the patient to rebreathe exhaled CO_2, thereby raising CO_2. If the cause is iatrogenic, may need mechanical ventilation
Role of nurse	Maintain patent airway Provide humidification Administer O_2 as ordered Suction, incentive spirometry, C&DB Be prepared for artificial ventilation Remove foreign bodies in airway, establish artificial airway Monitor VS, cardiac rate, rhythm, respiratory pattern, neurologic status, pulse ox, ABGs, electrolytes Encourage fluids	Monitor clients at risk for developing respiratory alkalosis Allay anxiety to prevent hyperventilation Promote relaxation, maintain calm quiet environment Monitor VS, cardiac rate, rhythm, respiratory pattern, neurologic status If client is on a ventilator, monitor settings (do not adjust) Monitor pulse ox, ABGs, electrolytes Stay with client during periods of extreme anxiety
What to document	VS, cardiac rate and rhythm, I&O, assessment, interventions chosen and client's response, notification of physician, client teaching, meds given, O_2 therapy, % of O_2, character of pulmonary secretions, serum electrolyte levels, ABG results	VS, IV therapy, assessment, interventions chosen and client's response, notification of physician, client teaching, meds given, O_2 therapy, % of O_2, character of pulmonary secretions, serum electrolyte levels, ABG results, safety measures

Metabolic Acidosis	Metabolic Alkalosis
Loss of HCO_3^- from extracellular fluid, an accumulation of metabolic acids (or a combination of both) Overproduction of ketones ↓ ability of kidneys to excrete acids Excessive GI loss from diarrhea Hyperaldosteronism Use of potassium-sparing diuretics Poisoning or toxic drug reaction	Client loses hydrogen ions (acid) and gains HCO_3^- or both. Excessive loss of acid from the GI tract: • Vomiting • Nasogastric tube drainage Diuretic use Kidney disease Cushing's disease
Confusion ↓ deep tendon reflexes Dull headache Hyperkalemic signs Hypotension Kussmaul's respirations Lethargy Warm, dry skin	Anorexia Apathy Confusion Cyanosis Hypotension Loss of reflexes Muscle twitching Nausea Paresthesia Polyuria Vomiting Weakness
ABG analysis: pH < 7.35 and $PaCO_2$ < 35 Serum potassium > 5 Blood glucose and serum ketones ↑ in client with diabetic ketoacidosis (DKA) Plasma lactase ↑	ABG analysis: pH > 7.45 and HCO_3 > 26 mEq/L Serum electrolytes usually show low potassium, calcium, and chloride ECG may show low T wave that merges with the P wave
Correct the underlying disorder Mechanical ventilation Adjust potassium Rapid-acting insulin for DKA Replace bicarbonate Antibiotic to treat infection	IV administration of ammonium chloride is rarely done in severe cases D/C nasogastric suctioning and thiazide diuretics Diamox may be given to increase renal excretion of HCO_3^-
Monitor VS, cardiac rate, rhythm, respiratory pattern, neurologic status Administer O_2 as ordered Administer sodium bicarbonate as ordered Institute seizure precautions Maintain patent IV access as ordered Administer meds as ordered Monitor I&O	Monitor VS, cardiac rate, rhythm, respiratory pattern, neurologic status Administer O_2 as ordered Institute seizure precautions Maintain patent IV access as ordered Administer meds as ordered Monitor I&O
VS, IV therapy, assessment, interventions chosen and client's response, notification of physician, client teaching, meds given, O_2 therapy, % of O_2, character of pulmonary secretions, serum electrolyte levels, ABG results, ventilator or dialysis data, safety measures	VS, IV therapy, assessment, interventions chosen and client's response, notification of physician, client teaching, meds given, O_2 therapy, % of O_2, character of pulmonary secretions, serum electrolyte levels, ABG results, safety measures

ACID–BASE IMBALANCES

Metabolic Alkalosis			Compensation
pH:	↑	> 7.40	7.40
HCO_3^-:	↑	> 24	
PCO_2:	normal	40	↑ > 40

Metabolic Acidosis			Compensation
pH:	↓	< 7.40	7.40
HCO_3^-:	↓	< 24	
PCO_2:	normal	40	↓ < 40

Respiratory Alkalosis			Compensation
pH:	↑	> 7.40	7.40
PCO_2:	↓	< 40	
HCO_2:	normal	24	↓ < 24

Respiratory Acidosis			Compensation
pH:	↓	< 7.40	7.40
PCO_2:	↑	> 40	
HCO_3^-:	normal	24	↑ > 24

SOLVING THE PUZZLE: IS IT RESPIRATORY OR METABOLIC ACIDOSIS OR ALKALOSIS?

When pH is in same column as
- PCO_2 = a respiratory problem
- HCO_3 = a metabolic problem

If third component is in *opposite* column = partial compensation.
If third component is in *normal* column = no compensation.
If pH is normal (7.40) = full compensation.

	Acidosis	Normal	Alkalosis
pH	< 7.35	7.35–7.45	> 7.45
PCO_2	> 45	35–45	< 35
HCO_3	< 22	22–26	> 26

F. Nursing management.
1. Eliminate cause of hyperventilation, instruct client to breathe slowly to decrease CO_2 loss.
2. Remain with client and be supportive to reduce anxiety.
3. Use rebreathing bag to return client's carbon dioxide to self (paper bag works just as well).
4. Provide sedation as ordered.
5. Monitor lab values, especially K^+ and HCO_3^-.

System Assessment

A. Take history to determine presence of renal or urologic problems.
B. Determine use of prescriptions, over-the-counter drugs and herbs. Many drugs are nephrotoxic.
C. Evaluate urinalysis findings to determine presence of infection, bleeding, or signs of renal failure.
D. Assess (palpate) for kidney pain between last thoracic and third lumbar vertebrae.
1. Severe pain or discomfort may indicate kidney infection, stone or kidney disease.
2. Kidney enlargement may indicate neoplasm or polycystic disease.
✦ E. Assess pain for location, intensity and precipitating factors.
1. Arterial pain is related to obstruction and is usually an acute manifestation.

a. Site of obstruction may be found by tracing the location of radiation of pain.
b. Pain may be severe and usually radiates down ureter into scrotum or vulva and to the inner thigh.
2. Bladder pain is due to infection and overdistention of the bladder in urinary retention.
3. Testicular pain is caused by inflammation or trauma, and is acute and severe.
4. Pain in the lower back and leg may be caused by prostate cancer with metastasis to pelvic bones.
5. Pain caused by renal disease.
a. Dull ache in flank, radiating to lower abdomen and upper thigh.
b. Pain may be absent if there is no sudden distention of kidney capsules.
✦ F. Assess bladder for distention.
G. Examine the urinary catheter for abnormal findings.
H. Evaluate intake and output values; dehydration leads to infection, calculi formation and renal failure.
I. Measure vital signs to determine presence of complications.
J. Assess patency of shunts.
K. Assess all body systems for potential alterations as a result of kidney problems.
1. Peripheral edema.
2. Hypertension.
3. Eye disorders.
4. Anemia.
5. Lethargic or irritable condition.
6. Congestive heart failure.
L. Observe for signs and symptoms of fluid and electrolyte imbalances.
M. Evaluate urinary test results for signs of renal abnormalities.
N. Assess client's feelings about body image.
O. Assess for type of imbalance.

DIAGNOSTIC PROCEDURES

Renal Function Tests

✦ A. Renal concentration tests.
1. Underlying principles.
    a. Evaluate the ability of the kidney to concentrate urine.
    b. As kidney disease progresses, renal function decreases. Concentration tests evaluate this process.
    c. Renal concentration is measured by specific gravity readings (normal range 1.010–1.030).
    d. If specific gravity is 1.018 or greater, it may be assumed that the kidney is functioning within normal limits.
    e. Specific gravity that stabilizes at 1.010 indicates kidney has lost ability to concentrate or dilute.
2. Common tests.
    a. Urine osmolality—used to evaluate clients with renal disease (i.e., SIADH and diabetes insipidus).
    b. Urinary sodium—24-hour test that determines amount of sodium excretion in urine. Used to determine clients with fluid volume deficits, acute renal failure and acid–base imbalances.
3. Concentration and dilution tests.
    a. Fishberg concentration test—high-protein dinner with 200 mL fluid is ordered. Next AM on arising, client voids q 1/hr. One specimen should have specific gravity more than 1.025.
    b. Dilution test—NPO after dinner. Morning voiding discarded. Client drinks 1000 mL in 30–45 minutes. Four specimens at 1-hour intervals are collected. One specimen will fall below 1.003.
    c. Specific gravity—urine 1.010–1.030. Increased solutes cause increased specific gravity.
B. Glomerular filtration test (endogenous creatinine clearance).
1. Kidney function is assessed by clearing a substance from the blood (filtration in the glomerulus).
2. Common test is the amount of blood cleared of urea per minute.
3. Test done on 12-hour or 24-hour urine specimen.
4. Normal range is approximately 100–120 mL/min (1.67–2.0 mL/sec).
5. Blood urea nitrogen (BUN).
    a. Normal 10:1 ratio for BUN to creatinine.
    b. High BUN indicates severe catabolic state, GI bleeding or use of corticosteroids.
C. Electrolyte tests.
1. Kidney function is essential to maintain fluid and electrolyte balance.
2. Tests for electrolytes (sodium, potassium, chloride, and bicarbonate) measure the ability of the kidney to filter, reabsorb, or excrete these substances.
3. Impaired filtration leads to retention, and impaired reabsorption leads to loss of electrolytes.
4. Tests are performed on blood serum, so venous blood is required.

Analysis of Urine

A. Urinalysis is a critical test for total evaluation of the renal system and for indication of renal disease.
B. Specific gravity shows the degree of concentration in urine.
1. Indicates the ability of the kidney to concentrate or dilute urine.
2. Change from normal range indicates diabetes mellitus (> 1.030) or kidney damage (< 1.010).
3. Renal failure—specific gravity constant at 1.010.
C. Analysis of the pH of urine—normal urine pH is 6–7. Lower than 6 is acidic urine, and higher than 7 is alkaline urine.
D. Urinary sodium—random sample used to identify renal failure.

See also Urine Analysis in Chapter 11, Laboratory Tests.

Renal Imaging

A. Flat plate of abdomen without contrast dye.
1. Outlines size of kidney.
2. Outlines stone formation.
B. Intravenous pyelogram (IVP).
1. Contrast dye identifies changes in kidney structure.
2. Identifies presence of stones.
3. Outlines ureteral obstructions.
C. Voiding cystourethrogram (VCUG)-XR.
1. Contrast dye inserted through catheter into bladder.
2. Determines reflux, cancer on wall of bladder, and increased residual volume.
D. Retrograde pyelogram (XR).
1. Contrast inserted into ureters retrograde from bladder.
2. Visualizes collecting system.
E. Renal ultrasound.
1. Noninvasive and useful in identifying kidney size, hydronephrosis and obstructions.
2. Used to guide percutaneous needle biopsies of kidneys.

GU Examination

Male Examination

✦ A. Testicular self-exam (TSE).
   1. Instruct client to perform monthly following warm bath or shower. (Between ages 15 and 25, third highest cause of cancer deaths in men.)
   2. Stand before mirror and check for swelling on skin and scrotum.
   3. Rotate each testicle between thumb and forefinger, feeling for a firm surface.
   4. If painless lump is felt (*not* the epididymis), notify physician immediately.
✦ B. Prostate evaluation.
   1. Rectal exam annually beginning at age 40.
   2. Blood chemistry for cancer.
      a. Prostatic acid phosphate (PAP)—elevated.
      b. Prostate-specific antigen (PSA)—elevated. Most sensitive tumor marker.
      c. May be false-positive readings.
      d. Second most common cause of death in men over 55.
   3. Ultrasound with biopsy if indicated.

Female Examination

A. Pelvic examination.
   1. Inspection of external genitalia for signs of inflammation, bleeding, discharge, and epithelial cell changes.
   2. Visualization of vagina and cervix.
   3. Bimanual examination.
   4. Rectal examination.
✦ B. Papanicolaou smear.
   1. Diagnosis for cervical cancer.
   2. Vaginal secretions and secretions from posterior fornix are smeared on a glass slide.
   ✦ 3. Pathological classifications.
      a. Class I: no abnormal or atypical cells present.
      b. Class II: abnormal or atypical cells present but no malignancy found; repeat Pap smear and followup if necessary.
      c. Class III: cytology suggests malignancy; additional procedures: biopsy, D&C.
      d. Class IV: cytology strongly suggests malignancy; additional procedures: biopsy, D&C.
      e. Class V: cytology conclusive of malignancy.
✦ C. Breast self-examination (BSE).
   1. Perform 5–7 days after menses, counting first day of menses as day 1. Less fluid is retained.
   2. Instruct female client to place pillow under the shoulder and, using three fingers, compress breast tissue in a circular motion, beginning at outer edge and moving toward nipple.
      a. Examine entire breast including nipple area.
      b. Move pillow to other shoulder and repeat examination.
   3. Remind client to immediately report any lump, irregularity, edema, skin changes, discharge, nipple changes, changes in contour of breasts.
D. Mammography.
   1. X-ray of soft tissue to detect nonpalpable mass.
   2. Baseline (one time) age 35–39; yearly after age 40.

Cystoscopy

Definition: The direct visualization of the bladder and urethra by means of a cystoscope.

Purpose

A. Inspect bladder and urethra for stones, etc.
B. Evaluate results of tissue examination obtained from biopsy.

Implementation

A. Measure vital signs.
B. Observe for urethral bleeding.
C. Chart intake and output, and consistency of urine.
D. Monitor for signs of infection.
   1. Frequency.
   2. Urgency.
   3. Burning during urination.
E. Monitor for perforation of bladder.
   1. Sharp abdominal pain.
   2. Anuria.
   3. Boardlike abdomen.
F. Maintain client on bedrest for 4–6 hours; then ambulate if no complications. (Many procedures are outpatient and the client is released 1–2 hours after test if no complications.)
G. Monitor vital signs for shock and infection.

System Implementation

✦ A. Monitor fluid intake at least every shift for clients with renal dysfunction.
   1. Encourage fluids.
      a. Urinary tract infection.
      b. Cystitis.
      c. Pyelonephritis.
      d. Urolithiasis.
   2. Restrict fluids.
      a. Glomerulonephritis.
      b. Renal failure.
      c. Nephrotic syndrome.
✦ B. Provide appropriate diet for renal dysfunction.
   1. Pyelonephritis—high calorie, vitamins, and protein; if oliguria is present, change diet to low protein.
   2. Glomerulonephritis—low saturated fat, 0.8 g/kg/day protein, low sodium.

3. Nephrotic syndrome—0.8 g/kg/day protein, high calorie, low sodium, liberal potassium.
4. Renal failure—restricted protein to 40–60 mEq/day; low in nitrogen, potassium; 2 g/day sodium, phosphate, and sulfate.

C. Monitor client for complications associated with renal dysfunction, especially congestive heart failure, pulmonary edema, and hypertension.
D. Provide good skin care; edematous areas are easily broken down.
E. Encourage bedrest for clients in an acute stage of the disease.
F. Administer medications on time to keep blood levels stable and in therapeutic range.
G. Monitor vital signs for early detection of changes in client status.
H. Provide shunt care to maintain patency and prevent infection.
I. Instruct client on diet, fluid alteration, and shunt care as needed.
J. Encourage client to express feelings and concerns with altered body image.

RENAL DISORDERS

Injuries to the Kidney

Definition: Injury to the kidney includes any trauma that bruises, lacerates, or ruptures any part of the kidney organ.

Assessment

A. Assess for hematuria.
B. Assess for shock, if hemorrhage has occurred.
C. Evaluate pain over costovertebral area.
D. Observe for gastrointestinal symptoms of nausea and vomiting.

Implementation

A. Promote bedrest.
B. Monitor vital signs frequently for possible hemorrhage.
C. Monitor blood work and laboratory examination of urine to assess for hematuria.
D. Prevent infection.
E. Frequently monitor the total status of the client following injury.
    1. Observe for pain and tenderness.
    2. Observe any sudden change in status.
F. Prepare for surgery (nephrectomy) if health status deteriorates (shock indicating severe hemorrhage).

Urinary Tract Infections

✦ *Definition:* A term that refers to a wide variety of conditions affecting the urinary tract in which the common denominator is the presence of microorganisms. Classified as infections involving the upper or lower urinary tract. Most common healthcare problem in United States. More common in women.

✦ **Characteristics**

A. Urine is sterile until it reaches the distal urethra.
B. Any bacteria can be introduced into the urinary tract, resulting in infection, which may then spread to any other part of the tract. *Escherichia coli* is most frequent organism causing about 80 percent of all cases; 5–15 percent are caused by *Staphylococcus.*
C. The most important factor influencing ascending infection is obstruction of free urine flow.
    1. Free flow, large urine output, and pH are antibacterial defenses.
    2. If defenses break down, the result may be an invasion of the tract by bacteria.
D. Microscopic examination is completed for an accurate identification of the organism (especially important in chronic infections).

Assessment

A. Determine location of infection.
    1. Lower UTI—cystitis, urethritis or prostatitis.
    2. Upper UTI—pyelonephritis, interstitial nephritis.
B. Evaluate urine cultures and chemical tests to determine presence and number of bacteria.
C. Evaluate urine colony count. Colony count over 100,000/mL indicates urinary tract infection.
D. Assess for location, type and precipitating factors leading to pain.
E. Observe urine for color, consistency, specific gravity.
F. Assess for frequency, urgency, nocturia, incontinence and suprapubic or pelvic pain.
G. Blood or urine test to rule out STDs, which produce similar symptoms.

Implementation

✦ A. Encourage fluids to 3000 mL.
✦ B. Administer urinary antimicrobials as ordered.
    1. Standard treatment—therapy for lower tract infection.
        a. Single-dose therapy effective in 80 percent of cases.
        b. Trimethoprim (Primsol), sulfamethoxazole (Gantanol), or quinolones (Cipro or Noroxin) may be used.
        c. Fosfomycin antibiotics (Monurol).
            (1) Acts by inhibiting bacterial cell-wall synthesis and reducing adherence of bacteria to epithelial cells of urinary tract.
            (2) First drug approved as single-dose treatment.

(3) Single-dose treatment—one packet of granules dissolved into 90–120 mL of water (not hot). May be taken with or without meals.

(4) Adverse reactions include dysuria and burning.

2. Short-course therapy—3 or 4 days, more commonly prescribed.

3. Longer course—10–14 days, for upper tract infections.

    a. Antibacterial may be prescribed with single-dose therapy.

    b. Urinary antiseptics may be used with antimicrobials.

4. Action of antimicrobials—inhibits cell-wall mucopeptide synthesis; interferes with enzyme needed for bacterial metabolism.

5. Adverse effects—hypersensitivity, nausea, vomiting, diarrhea, rash.

◆ C. Administer antiseptics—interfere with vital processes of the bacteria.

    1. Medications: nitrofurantoin (Furadantin); methenamine salts (Hipres, Urised).

    2. Adverse effects—anorexia, nausea, vomiting.

    3. Avoid foods that increase urinary pH.

D. Antispasmodics and analgesics may be used to relieve pain, frequency, urgency, and burning.

◆ E. Encourage client to void every 2 to 3 hours and to empty bladder—reduces urinary stasis and risk of reinfection.

F. Avoid beverages that irritate bladder—alcohol, coffee, carbonated beverages.

◆ G. Teach women hygiene measures to prevent reoccurrence (wipe front to back, keep perineum clean and dry, do not douche, and avoid tight-fitting pants; also, voiding after sexual intercourse helps).

Cystitis

◆ *Definition:* Inflammation of the bladder from infection or obstruction of the urethra is the most common cause.

Assessment

◆ A. Observe for frequency, urgency, and burning sensation on urination.

B. Evaluate lower abdominal discomfort.

C. Observe for dark and odorous urine (often a manifestation), hematuria.

D. Assess laboratory findings for presence of bacteria and hematuria.

E. Bacterial counts exceeding 10^5 colonies/mL of urine indicate infection using clean catch technique for urine sample.

Implementation

A. Assist physician in identifying and removing the cause of the condition (infection, obstruction, etc.).

◆ B. Administer antibiotics on time. Drugs usually administered—sulfamethoxazole with trimethoprim is drug of choice (Bactrim, Septra). May use Macrodantin (nitrofurantoin macrocrystals).

C. Instruct client on how to prevent infection. Empty bladder completely and frequently.

D. Instruct client on measures for symptomatic relief of chronic conditions. Antispasmodics are used for pain and bladder irritability.

E. Collect an uncontaminated urine specimen (midstream specimen) for laboratory test.

◆ F. Maintain adequate fluid intake.

    1. Force fluids only if specifically ordered.

    2. Check and record intake and output.

G. Encourage bedrest or a decrease in activity during the acute stage.

H. Maintain acid urine (pH 5.5).

I. Avoid urinary tract irritants—coffee, tea, citrus.

J. Instruct client in follow-up urinary tests for pH.

Pyelonephritis

◆ *Definition:* An acute or chronic infection and inflammation of one or both kidneys that usually begins in the renal pelvis. Women are more commonly affected. Gram-negative organisms are most often responsible, especially *E. coli*.

Assessment

◆ A. Observe for attacks of chills, fever, malaise, gastrointestinal upsets.

◆ B. Evaluate for tenderness and dull, aching pain in back.

C. Assess for fatigue, headache, poor appetite, excessive thirst, and weight loss.

◆ D. Identify frequent and burning urination (more common in lower tract involvement).

E. Evaluate pus and bacteria in urine.

F. Evaluate renal function. May have normal renal function except for inability to concentrate urine.

G. Evaluate for renal insufficiency.

    1. Progressive destruction of renal tubules and glomeruli.

    2. Inability of kidneys to excrete large amounts of electrolytes.

    3. Ultrasound or CT scan is used to locate any obstruction in urinary tract.

H. Assess for hypertension in presence of bacterial pyelonephritis.

I. Identify if overt symptoms disappear in a few days but urine is still infected.

Implementation

✦ A. Administer and monitor drug therapy.
   1. Antibiotic therapy usually for two weeks (organism-specific for infection).
   2. Usual drugs—trimethoprim and sulfamethoxazole, ciprofloxacin, gentamicin, or a third-generation cephalosporin.
   3. Analgesics and sedatives as needed.
   4. May be on antibiotics up to six months.
B. Maintain bedrest until asymptomatic.
✦ C. Force fluids to maintain urine output of 1500 mL/day (3–4 L/day).
D. Continue monitoring for presence of bacteria.
E. Instruct client in methods to prevent chronic renal insufficiency.
F. Monitor urinalysis.
   1. Check urine concentration.
   2. Check electrolytes.
G. Provide diet high in calories and vitamins, and low in protein if oliguria is present.
H. Monitor temperature every 4 hours.
I. Observe for edema and signs of renal failure.
J. Instruct client in good hygiene to prevent further infections.
K. Instruct to empty bladder regularly.

Glomerulonephritis

✦ *Definition:* A group of kidney diseases caused by inflammation of the capillary loops in the glomeruli of the kidney.

Characteristics

A. The kidney's glomeruli are affected by an immunological disorder.
✦ B. Most frequently follows infections with group A beta-hemolytic *Streptococcus.*
C. Upper respiratory infections, skin infections, other autoimmune processes (systemic lupus), and acute infections predispose to glomerulonephritis.
D. Glomerulonephritis symptoms appear 2–3 weeks after original infection.

✦ Assessment

A. Initially, symptoms may be mild—assess for pharyngitis, fever, malaise.
B. Assess urine.
   1. Evaluate for hematuria—first symptom.
   2. Urine may be dark, smoky, cola-colored.
   3. Assess urine for persistent and excessive foam caused by protein.
   4. Assess specific gravity for high values.
   5. Observe for oliguria, anuria.
   6. Observe for hypoalbuminemia due to increased loss via urine. (Proteinuria 2–8 g daily.)
C. Observe for weakness, anorexia, mild anemia.
D. Evaluate edema—leg, face, or generalized.
E. Assess abdominal pain, nausea, vomiting.
F. Flank pain.
G. Identify if hypertension, headache, or convulsions are present.
H. Assess for congestive heart failure.
I. Evaluate presence of increased BUN and creatinine.
J. Reduced visual acuity.
K. Observe for signs of encephalopathy.

✦ Implementation

✦ A. Administer penicillin for residual infection.
B. Administer loop diuretics and antihypertensives if necessary.
C. Administer corticosteroids and immunosuppressive agents if disease is progressing rapidly.
✦ D. Provide appropriate diet.
   ✦ 1. Protein restriction if oliguria is severe; otherwise, protein allowed at low normal range (normal 40–60 g/day).
   2. BUN level watched for protein determination.
   3. Protein should be of the complete type (milk, eggs, meat, fish, poultry).
   ✦ 4. High carbohydrate to provide energy and spare protein.
   ✦ 5. Potassium usually restricted.
   6. Sodium restriction for hypertension, edema, and CHF. If diuresis is great, sodium replacement may be necessary.
   7. Fluid restriction: replacement is based on insensible loss plus measured sensible loss of previous day or hour.
   8. Vitamin replacement.
✦ E. Prolonged bedrest is of little value and does not improve long-term outcomes.
F. Monitor vital signs continuously.
G. Allow client to verbalize feelings on body image changes (due to edema), loss of health, fear of death.
H. Monitor fluid intake.
   1. Measure fluids according to urinary output.
   2. Record intake and output.
   3. Weigh daily.
I. Monitor for signs of overhydration.
J. Take blood pressure frequently and observe for hypertension, signs of congestive failure and pulmonary edema.
K. Evaluate for symptoms of renal failure.
   1. Oliguria.
   2. Azotemia.
   3. Acidosis.

Nephrotic Syndrome

Definition: A term that refers to renal disease characterized by massive edema and albuminuria, high cholesterol and low-density lipoproteins. Considered a disease of childhood.

Characteristics

◆ A. The syndrome is seen in any renal condition that has damaged glomerular capillary membrane: glomerulonephritis, lipoid nephrosis, syphilitic nephritis, amyloidosis, or systemic lupus erythematosus.

B. There is a loss of plasma proteins, especially albumin, in the urine.

C. A specific form of intercapillary glomerulosclerosis is associated with diabetes mellitus (Kimmelstiel–Wilson syndrome).

D. Occurrence thought to be related to thyroid function.

Assessment

◆ A. Evaluate edema (at first, dependent; later, generalized).

◆ B. Identify if proteinuria (3–3.5 g/day) is present.

◆ C. Identify if decreased serum albumin is present.

D. Identify if elevated serum cholesterol, triglycerides, hyperlipemia are present.

E. Assess hypertension (related to function of renin–angiotensin system).

F. Evaluate decreased cardiac output (secondary to fluid loss).

G. Observe for pallor.

H. Observe for malaise, anorexia, lethargy.

Implementation

◆ A. Provide nursing care directed toward control of edema.
   1. Sodium restriction in diet.
   2. Avoidance of sodium-containing drugs.
   3. Diuretics (Lasix and Edecrin) that block aldosterone formation.
   4. Salt-poor albumin.

◆ B. Provide dietary instruction.
   1. High protein (100 g or 0.8 g/kg/day) to restore body proteins.
   2. High calorie, low saturated fat.
   3. 500 mg sodium if edema present.

◆ C. Administer drug therapy.
   1. Adrenocortical therapy (prednisone) to reduce proteinuria.
   2. Immunosuppressives (Imuran) or antineoplastic agents (Cytoxan).
   3. Angiotensin-converting enzyme (ACE) inhibitors with diuretics to reduce proteinuria (4–6 weeks).

◆ D. Client education for home care is necessary.

E. Instruct client in the maintenance of general health status, as the disorder may persist for months or years.

1. Avoiding infections.
2. Nutritious diet (low sodium, high protein).
3. Activity as tolerated.

F. Maintain fluid balance.
   1. Daily weights.
   2. Intake and output.

Tuberculosis of the Kidney

◆ *Definition:* Tuberculosis of the kidney is an infection caused by *Mycobacterium tuberculosis,* which is usually blood-borne from other foci such as the lungs, lymph nodes, or bone.

Assessment

A. Identify frequency and pain on urination.

B. Evaluate burning, spasm, and hematuria.

C. Assess for slight afternoon fever, weight loss, night sweats, loss of appetite and general malaise.

D. Evaluate findings of physical examination. Tuberculosis nodules may be present in the prostate.

E. Evaluate outcome of diagnostic studies.
   1. Urine cultures to isolate the tubercle bacilli.
   2. X-ray to reveal lesions.
   3. Cystoscopic examination.
   4. ESR elevation.

Implementation

◆ A. Administer medications on time.
   1. Drug therapy aimed at treating the original focus of infection as well as the genitourinary involvement.
   2. Combinations of isoniazid, ethambutol or rifampin are used for 4 months.
   3. Usually given together in a single daily dose.
   4. Observe for side effects.

B. Instruct client on methods to improve general health status.
   1. Good dietary habits.
   2. Adequate rest.

C. Prepare the client for possible nephrectomy if kidney is extensively diseased.

SURGICAL INTERVENTIONS FOR THE RENAL SYSTEM

Cystostomy

Definition: An opening into the bladder for suprapubic drainage.

Characteristics

A. Diverts urine flow from urethra.

◆ B. Empties bladder (similar for Foley catheter, but catheter is inserted in suprapubic area rather than through urinary meatus).

C. Provides less risk of infection for client.

D. Used for
1. Urethral stricture.
2. Following vaginal surgery.
3. Neurogenic bladder.
4. Following surgery on prostate and bladder.

Implementation

A. Provide care the same as for any client with indwelling catheter.

◆ B. Clamp catheter and then client is allowed to void on his or her own (through urinary meatus).

C. Remove when able to void on own.

Urolithiasis

◆ *Definition:* The presence of stones in any portion of the urinary system.

Characteristics

A. Causes: dehydration; immobilization; hypercalcemia; excessive uric acid excretion; obstruction; deficiency of citrate, magnesium, nephrocalcin, and uropontin (prevent crystallization in urine); and urinary stasis.

◆ B. Diagnostic tests.
1. Retrograde pyelography.
2. Renal ultrasound.
3. KUB x-ray.
4. CT scan.
5. MRI.
6. Blood chemistries.
7. 24-hour urine.

◆ C. Surgical interventions.
1. Ureterolithotomy: removal of stone from ureter.
2. Pyelolithotomy: removal of stone from kidney pelvis.
3. Lithotripsy.
   a. Extracorporeal shock-wave lithotripsy (ESWL): under general anesthesia, client is immersed in water and shock waves disintegrate stones that are then excreted in urine.
   b. Percutaneous ultrasonic.
   c. Laser therapy.

D. Chemolysis.
1. Dissolves stones using infusion of chemicals: alkylating agents, acidifying agents.
2. Used for "at risk" clients who could have complications with other procedures.
3. Use percutaneous nephrostomy to inject warm solution continuously into stone.

Assessment

A. Evaluate pain (starts low in back and radiates around front and down the ureter).

B. Observe for nausea, vomiting and diarrhea.

C. Observe for hematuria.

D. Assess for chills and fever.

E. Observe for pyuria.

Implementation

A. Manage pain with opioids or NSAIDs.

B. Apply moist heat or provide warm bath if not vomiting.

◆ C. Force fluids to at least 3000 mL/24 hr.

D. Record intake and output.

◆ E. Strain all urine for stones.

F. Send stones to laboratory for chemical analysis.

G. Administer appropriate antibiotics (infections occur especially when stones block off a portion of kidney).

H. Place heating pad on affected area.

I. Watch vital signs for indication of infection.

J. Instruct client in methods to prevent urolithiasis.
1. Provide adequate fluid intake (8 glasses of 8 oz H_2O/day).
2. Immediately treat urinary tract infection with appropriate antibiotics.
3. Ambulate clients to prevent urinary stasis (or reposition in bed frequently).
4. Dietary restrictions related to type of stone.

Urinary Diversion

◆ *Definition:* Procedure that diverts urine from bladder to a new exit site, through an opening in the skin termed a stoma. Most common type is the ileal loop.

Characteristics

A. Cancer of neck of bladder or ureters.

B. Cancer of pelvic area.

C. Neurogenic bladder.

Assessment

A. Assess type of urinary diversion.
1. Cutaneous—urine drains through an opening created in abdominal wall and skin.
2. Continent—a portion of intestine is used to create a new reservoir for urine.

B. Assess client's fluid balance.
1. Ensure output is 30 mL/hr.
2. Intake and output.
3. Daily weights.

C. Observe characteristics of urine. (Hematuria common in first 48 hours.)

D. Observe for complications related to surgical intervention.
1. Urinary fistula (urine around incision).
2. Bowel fistula (feces from incision).
3. Wound complications (dehiscence or evisceration).

E. Assess skin.

Implementation

A. If nasogastric tube is inserted, irrigate when necessary.
B. Provide routine abdominal postoperative care.
C. Provide stoma and skin care.
D. Provide psychological support for altered body image, change in lifestyle, chronic disease.
E. Refer to enterostomal therapist or cancer society for help with ostomy care.
F. Provide range-of-motion exercise.
G. Ensure tight-fitting ostomy bag around opening to prevent skin irritation.
H. Provide home care teaching regarding appliance change, odor control and skin care.

Nephrectomy

Definition: Surgical removal of a kidney.

Assessment

A. Evaluate possible cause.
   1. Polycystic kidneys.
   2. Stones.
   3. Preparation for transplantation.
   4. Injury.
   5. Infection that has destroyed kidney function.
B. Assess urine output for hematuria, cells, pus.
C. Observe for signs of hemorrhage and shock.
D. Evaluate intake and output (anuria can result if remaining kidney is damaged).
✦ E. Check for bowel sounds and abdominal distention (paralytic ileus may be a complication).
F. Assess nasogastric tube drainage, both amount and consistency, if inserted.

Implementation

✦ A. Obtain urine specimens as ordered to detect renal function of remaining kidney.
✦ B. Force fluids after bowel sounds return.
C. Monitor intake and output frequently.
D. Monitor blood replacement therapy as needed.
✦ E. Turn, cough, and deep-breathe every 2 hours (turn to operative side and back).
F. Encourage use of incentive spirometer.

G. Begin range-of-motion exercises immediately.
H. Encourage early ambulation.
✦ I. Observe that Foley or suprapubic catheter is draining adequately.
   1. Tape catheter to leg or abdomen to prevent trauma to bladder.
   2. Position catheter bag below bed level to facilitate drainage.
J. If nephrostomy tube is inserted, measure drainage and record characteristics of drainage (drains kidney after surgery).
   1. Do not clamp tubes unless ordered.
   2. Do not irrigate tubes unless ordered.
K. Administer antibiotics as ordered.
L. Administer low-dose heparin to reduce risk of thrombophlebitis.

RENAL FAILURE

Acute Renal Failure

✦ *Definition:* The sudden loss of kidney function caused by failure of renal circulation or damage to the tubules or glomerulus. Condition reversible with spontaneous recovery in a few days to several weeks.

Categories of Acute Renal Failure

A. Prerenal—condition decreasing blood flow.
   1. Decreased glomerular filtration rate (GFR).
   2. Severe dehydration; diuretic therapy.
   3. Circulatory collapse: hypovolemia, shock.
B. Intrarenal—disease process, ischemic or toxic conditions.
   1. Acute glomerulonephritis.
   2. Vascular disorders.
   3. Toxic agents (e.g., carbon tetrachloride, sulfonamides, arsenic).
   4. Severe infection.
   5. Burns, crushing injuries.
C. Postrenal obstruction to urine flow.

Assessment

✦ A. Clinical phases—an initial period of oliguria followed by period of diuresis, and a period of recovery.
   1. Evaluate urine output often. If less than 20 mL/hr, measure at least every 2–4 hours.
   2. Observe lab reports for increased BUN and creatinine.
✦ B. Evaluate serum levels of potassium, sodium, pH, PCO_2, and HCO_3—indication of complications.
C. Observe urinalysis for proteinuria, hematuria, casts.
D. Note if specific gravity fixed at 1.010–1.016 (normal is 1.025).
E. Evaluate for potassium intoxication; hyperkalemia.

F. Assess for signs of infection—client may not demonstrate fever or increased WBC.

Implementation

◆ A. Monitor urinary output.
   1. Record intake and output (oliguria followed by diuresis).
   2. Weigh daily; lack of weight loss (½–1 pound daily) indicates retention of too much fluid.
◆ B. Monitor fluid intake (observe for signs of CHF).
◆ C. Monitor for complications of electrolyte imbalances.
   1. Acidosis (treated with sodium bicarbonate).
   2. Serum potassium levels (above 6 mEq/L together with peaking T waves and shortening QT interval) for hyperkalemia.
D. Allow client to verbalize concerns and effect of altered body image.
◆ E. Encourage the prescribed diet: moderate protein restriction (1 g/kg/day); high carbohydrate; restrict foods high in K⁺ and phosphorus (coffee, bananas, juices).
   1. Elevated potassium reduced by exchange resins (Kayexalate).
   2. High level of serum potassium may require dialysis.
   3. Restrict sodium to 2 g daily.
F. Be cautious when using antibiotics and other drugs.
G. Continually assess status of client for potential complications: dyspnea, tachycardia, increased blood pressure.
H. Evaluate slow return of decreased serum BUN, creatinine, phosphorus, and potassium to normal after diuresis phase begins.
I. Maintain bedrest to decrease exertion and metabolic state.

Chronic Renal Failure

Definition: The progressive loss of kidney function that occurs in three stages and, without intervention, ends fatally in uremia.

◆ Characteristics
A. First stage: diminished renal reserve.
   1. 40–75% loss of nephron function.
   2. Abnormal renal function tests.
   3. No accumulation of metabolic waste.
B. Second stage: renal insufficiency.
   1. 75–90% loss of nephron function.
   2. Metabolic waste begins to accumulate.
   3. Increase in BUN and creatinine (10:1 ratio).
   4. Polyuria and nocturia occur.
   5. Stress poorly tolerated (e.g., infection).
   6. Chemical abnormalities resolve slowly.
   7. Anemia occurs.

C. Third stage: end-stage renal failure or uremia.
   1. Less than 10% functioning nephrons.
   2. Normal regulatory, excretory, and hormonal functions of kidneys are impaired severely.
   3. Hypertension; edema.
   4. Poor urine output.
   5. Severe alterations of electrolytes.
   6. Moderately increased BUN and creatinine.
   7. Anemia common with this condition.
   8. Metabolic acidosis.

◆ Assessment

A. Assess for weakness, fatigue, and headaches.
B. Assess for anorexia, nausea, vomiting, and hiccups.
C. Evaluate for hypertension, heart failure, and pulmonary edema.
D. Evaluate for anemia, azotemia (nitrogen retention in the blood), and acidosis.
E. Observe for personality changes (e.g., anxiety, irritability, hallucinations, convulsions, and coma).
F. Evaluate for low and fixed specific gravity of urine of 1.010.
G. Respirations may become Kussmaul, with deep coma following.
H. Observe for severe skin itching.

Implementation

◆ A. Provide diet (low protein with supplemented vitamins and amino acids) and fluids (500–600 mL/day) for acute renal failure.
◆ B. Provide electrolyte replacement.
   1. Sodium supplements provided.
   2. Potassium and phosphorus restricted.
   3. Acidosis replacement of bicarbonate stores.
C. Monitor and plan nursing care for hypertension and heart failure.
D. Prepare client for dialysis or kidney transplant.
E. Administer medications with caution—impaired renal function may require adjustment.
   1. Administer antihypertensives, Epogen, iron supplements, phosphate-binding agents, and calcium supplements.
   2. Antacids are used to treat hyperphosphatemia and hypocalcemia.

Uremic Syndrome (Uremia)

◆ *Definition:* The accumulation of nitrogenous waste products in blood due to inability of kidneys to filter out waste products.

Characteristics

A. May occur after acute or chronic renal failure.
B. Increased urea, creatinine, uric acid.

C. Extensive electrolyte imbalances (increased K⁺, increased Na⁺, decreased Cl⁻, decreased Ca⁺⁺, increased phosphorus).

D. Acidosis—bicarbonate cannot be maintained at adequate level.

E. Urine concentration ability lost.

F. Anemia caused by decreased rate of production of RBCs.

G. Metabolic acidosis accumulation affects all body systems.

H. Disorders of calcium metabolism with secondary bone changes.

Assessment

✦ A. Observe for signs of oliguria for 1–2 weeks (produces less urine than 400 mL/day).

✦ B. Assess changes in urine characteristics.
   1. Urine contains protein, red blood cells, casts.
   2. Specific gravity of 1.010.
   3. Rise in urine solutes (e.g., urea, uric acid, potassium, magnesium).

C. Assess for metabolic acidosis.

D. Observe for hypotension or hypertension.

E. Assess for gastrointestinal problems: stomatitis, nausea, vomiting, and diarrhea or constipation.

F. Assess for respiratory complications.

G. Evaluate coma—with alterations of blood chemistry and acid load.

Implementation

A. Monitor restoration of blood volume.

B. Monitor fluid and electrolyte balance.

✦ C. Provide dietary regulation.
   1. Limit protein (0.8 g/kg) unless on peritoneal dialysis.
   2. Reduce nitrogen, potassium, phosphate, and sulfate.
   3. Limit sodium intake.
   4. Provide glucose to prevent ketosis.
   5. Control potassium balance to prevent hyperkalemia.
   6. Carbohydrate intake 100 g daily.

DIALYSIS

Peritoneal Dialysis

Definition: A method of separating substances by interposing a semipermeable membrane. The peritoneum is used as the dialyzing membrane and substitutes for kidney function during failure.

✦ **Principles of Peritoneal Dialysis**

A. Usually temporary; can be used for clients in acute, reversible renal failure.

   1. Treatment of choice for clients who are unable or unwilling to undergo hemodialysis or transplantation.
   2. Used for clients with diabetes and cardiovascular disease who are at risk for fluid shifts, cannot use heparin, or are not responsive to other treatments.

B. Basic goals of dialysis therapy.
   1. Removal of end products of protein metabolism, such as creatinine and urea.
   2. Maintenance of safe concentration of serum electrolytes.
   3. Correction of acidosis and blood's bicarbonate buffer system.
   4. Removal of excess fluid.

C. Renal perfusion is compromised when increased size of the intravascular compartment and redistribution of blood volume result from
   1. Gram-negative sepsis.
   2. Overdoses of some drugs.
   3. Anaphylactic shock.
   4. Electrolyte disturbances, such as acidosis.

D. Drugs may be used to check for renal failure before client is placed on dialysis.
   ✦ 1. In most cases, Mannitol is tried before dialysis.
      a. Not reabsorbed by kidney.
      b. Has great osmotic effect and increases urinary flow.
      c. Administration.
         (1) Given quickly to get higher blood level, which initiates diuresis and may prevent or minimize renal failure.
         (2) If infusion is too slow, changes in the urinary flow rate are delayed, as urine flow depends on the amount of Mannitol filtered.
         (3) Give 12.5 g of a 25% solution in 3 minutes; if flow rate can be increased to 40 mL/hr, the client is in reversible renal failure.
         (4) Keep urine at 100 mL/hr with Mannitol.
   2. Drugs such as Lasix (furosemide) and Edecrin (ethacrynic acid) may be used if Mannitol is not effective.
      a. If the client does not respond to Lasix or Edecrin, diagnosis of acute tubular necrosis is made.
      b. If the client has increased urine output with drugs, be sure to check electrolytes, as sodium and potassium depletion occurs along with water loss.
      c. In renal disease, make sure that drugs that depend on kidneys for excretion are not given.

Peritoneal Dialysis Function

✦ A. Works on principles of diffusion and osmosis, similar to hemodialysis; however, in this instance, the peritoneum is the semipermeable membrane.

✦ B. Peritoneum is impermeable to large molecules (proteins).

✦ C. Peritoneum is permeable to low-molecular-weight molecules (urea, glucose, electrolytes).

D. Cannot be used with clients who have the following conditions:
1. Peritonitis.
2. Recent abdominal surgery.
3. Abdominal adhesions.
4. Impending renal transplant.

E. Dialysate.
1. Contains electrolytes but no urea, creatinine.
   a. Common electrolytes in dialysate in mEq/L.
      Na^+ 140–145
      Cl^- 101–110
      Ca^{++} 3.5–4.0
      Mg^{++} 1.5
      Lactate/acetate (base) 43–45
   b. Osmolarity.
      1.51% = 365 mOsm
      4.25% = 504 mOsm
   c. Amount: 1500–2000 mL infused over 5–10 minutes.
2. Sterile.
3. Solutions vary in dextrose concentration.
   a. Solution of 1.5 percent: used for drug intoxication and acute renal failure if large amounts of fluid are not required to be removed.
   b. Solutions of 2.5 percent: used for clients requiring moderate amount of fluid removal.
   c. Solution of 4.25 percent: used for removal of excessive fluid.
4. If hyperkalemia is not a problem, 4 mEq of potassium chloride is added to each solution.
5. Heparin is added to bottles to prevent clotting of the catheter.
6. Antibiotics may be added to prevent peritonitis.

F. Exchange process.
1. A series of exchanges or cycles that includes an infusion, dwell and drainage of dialysate.
2. Cycles are repeated according to client need and MD orders.
3. Dialysate is infused by gravity through catheter into peritoneal cavity over 5–10 minutes; catheter is clamped.
4. Usual dialysate is 2 L per cycle and dwell time (time dialysate stays in peritoneal cavity) allows for process of diffusion and osmosis. Time varies from 30 minutes to 4 hours.
5. Catheter is unclamped and dialysate is drained by gravity for 10–30 minutes.

G. Observe dialysate solution during exchange.
1. Bloody drainage may be seen in first few exchanges after insertion of catheter.
2. Usual dialysate is straw-colored or colorless and clear.
3. Cloudy effluent indicates infection.

✦ H. Monitor electrolyte balance throughout cycle.
1. Check muscle weakness, nausea, diarrhea as signs of hyperkalemia.
2. Monitor ECG for tall, peaked T waves and widening QRS as evidence of hyperkalemia.
3. Observe for hypokalemia—frequently decreased with dialysis: muscle weakness, hypotension, arrhythmias, anorexia, nausea, and vomiting.
4. Check for positive Chvostek's and Trousseau's signs as indications of low calcium levels.

Continuous Ambulatory Peritoneal Dialysis (CAPD)

✦ A. A variation of peritoneal dialysis developed to allow the client to be dialyzed while ambulatory.

✦ B. Procedure for CAPD.
1. Peritoneal catheter is inserted.
2. 500–2000 mL of dialysate infused through catheter by gravity (10–20 minutes).
3. The catheter is clamped, bag folded and placed in waistband of client's clothes.
4. Every 4–6 hours client drains fluid from peritoneal cavity.
   a. Unclamp catheter.
   b. Place pouch to allow drainage by gravity—below level of abdomen.
   c. Drain for approximately 20 minutes.
   d. Reclamp catheter and remove bag with drainage.
   e. Examine drainage—a change in color may indicate infection (glucose in dialysate predisposes client to infection).
5. Aseptically attach a new bag of dialysate and repeat procedure.
6. Repeat procedure 4–5 times daily.
7. Instruct client to change tubing every 24 hours using strict aseptic technique.

C. Be alert for possible complications: peritonitis, fluid and electrolyte imbalances, dehydration, catheter infection, abdominal pain and tenderness, and hemorrhage.

D. Body image is altered when fluid fills abdomen.

E. Altered sexuality and sexual dysfunction may occur.

Dialysis Procedure

A. Preparation for hospitalized clients.

1. Client voids before catheter insertion to prevent bladder damage.
2. Abdominal skin is prepped.
3. The area between the umbilicus and the pubic bone near the midline is most often used for catheter insertion.
4. Client is weighed before procedure.
5. Baseline vital signs (including weight).

B. Dialysis process.
   1. Dialysis fluid instilled in abdominal cavity.
   2. Occurrence of osmosis, diffusion and filtration via peritoneal membrane (called equilibration).
   3. Fluid drained from abdominal cavity.
   4. Process repeated with a time sequence allowed for each step. Period of time and number of cycles will vary according to client problem, tolerance, response, and type of solution.

C. Duration of dialysis depends on the following factors:
   1. Client's height and weight.
   2. Severity of uremia.
   3. Physical state of client.
   4. Usual time period for dialysis is 24–72 exchanges or runs.

D. Monitoring the procedure.
   1. Client's electrolyte status is monitored during the process.
   2. Periodic samples of the return dialysate are sent for culture.
   3. Compare client's weight before and after procedure to assess effectiveness.
   4. Vital signs must be monitored closely.

E. Care of equipment during procedure.
   1. Tubing should be changed every 8 hours using sterile technique when the procedure continues for days.
   2. Warming the dialysate not only improves urea clearance but also maintains client's body temperature and comfort.
   3. Avoid getting air into tubing as this is uncomfortable for the client and impedes smooth and easy return of flow.

F. Quality and quantity of return.
   1. Initial few outflows may be slightly bloody due to insertion process.
   2. Cloudy fluid is usually an indication of peritonitis.
   3. Bowel perforation should be suspected if flow is brown.
   4. Record amount and type of solution for each inflow. This includes the medications added (e.g., potassium chloride, heparin, antibiotics).
   5. Record outflow amount and characteristics.
   6. Duration of each phase of the process should be recorded.

7. Keep a total net balance (difference between input and output for each exchange) and cumulative net balance.
8. Inform physician if client loses or retains large volumes of fluid.
   a. Periodically test urine for presence of sugar, which may be absorbed from dialysate.
   b. Heparin helps prevent drainage problems.

G. Procedures to check when drainage slows.
   1. Check proper position of clamps.
   2. Look for kinking in tubes.
   3. Milk the drainage tube.
   4. Observe air vent in drainage bottle for patency.
   5. Flush catheter.
   6. Reposition direction of catheter within means.
   7. Have client change positions.
   8. Have physician change catheter.

Implementation

A. Each morning, send culture on returning dialysate solution to observe for signs of infection.
B. Each day at the same time, weigh client with abdomen empty of solution.
C. Monitor vital signs to observe for complications.
D. Monitor dialysis exchange.
   1. Keep exchange on time.
   2. Maintain aseptic technique when changing bottles and tubing.
   3. Record accurate intake and output on flow sheet.
E. Try the following interventions to assist in returning dialysate from peritoneal cavity:
   1. Turn client on side and prop with pillows.
   2. Place in Fowler's position after solution is infused into abdomen.
   3. Ambulate and/or have client sit in chair if client is able.
   4. Palpate abdomen.
   5. Place pillow or bath blanket under small of back (this also assists in relieving hiccoughs).
F. Test urine for sugar.
G. Monitor for complications of peritoneal dialysis.
   1. Peritonitis.
      a. Diffuse abdominal pain.
      b. Abdomen tender on palpation.
      c. Abdominal wall rigidity.
      d. Cloudy outflow.
   2. Hypertension.
   3. Pulmonary edema.
   4. Hyperglycemia (insulin may be needed).
   5. Hyperosmolar coma.
   6. Protein loss (0.5–1.0 g/L of drainage).
   7. Intestinal perforation.

Other Types of Peritoneal Dialysis

✦ A. Continuous cycling peritoneal dialysis (CCPD).
1. Requires a peritoneal cycling machine.
2. Consists of having 3 cycles done at night and 1 cycle with an 8-hour dwell time in morning.
3. Peritoneal cavity opened only for the *on* and *off* procedures, thereby reducing risk of infection.
4. Client does not need to do exchanges during the day.

✦ B. Intermittent peritoneal dialysis (IPD).
1. Requires peritoneal cycling machine.
2. Performed for 10–14 hours three to four times a week.

C. Nightly peritoneal dialysis (NPD).
1. Performed 8–12 hours each night.
2. No daytime dwells.

Hemodialysis

✦ *Definition:* The diffusion of dissolved particles from one fluid compartment into another across a semipermeable membrane. In hemodialysis, the blood is one fluid compartment and the dialysate is the other.

✦ Principles of Hemodialysis

A. The semipermeable membrane is a thin, porous, hollow, fiber (cellophane) system or flat-plate dialyzer.
B. The pore size of the membrane permits the passage of low-molecular-weight substances such as urea, creatinine, and uric acid to diffuse through the pores of the membrane.
C. Water molecules are also very small and move freely through the membrane.
D. Most plasma proteins, bacteria, and blood cells are too large to pass through the pores of the membrane.
E. The difference in the concentrations of the substances in the two compartments is called the concentration gradient.
F. The blood, which contains the waste products, flows into the dialyzer, where it comes in contact with the dialysate.
G. A maximum gradient is established so that movement of these substances occurs from the blood to the dialysate.
H. Dialysate (bath).
1. Composed of water and major electrolytes.
2. Tap water can be used (need not be sterile because bacteria are too large to pass through membrane).

✦ Hemodialysis Function

A. Removes by-products of protein metabolism: urea, creatinine, and uric acid.

B. Removes excessive fluid by
1. Changing osmotic pressure (by adding more dextrose to dialysate).
2. Negative or positive hydrostatic pressure.
C. Maintains or restores body buffer system.
D. Maintains or restores level of electrolytes in the body.

Dialysis Management

Implementation

A. Take vital signs to observe for shock and hypovolemia.
1. Hypotension is caused by
   a. Fluid loss initially.
   b. Decreased blood volume, especially if hematocrit is low.
   c. Use of antihypertensive drugs between dialysis procedures.
2. Plasma or volume expanders can be used to increase blood pressure; sometimes blood is used while the client is on dialysis.
B. Check serum electrolytes frequently (pre-, mid-, and post-dialysis).
C. Observe for painful cramping near end of dialysis as a result of rapid fluid and electrolyte loss.
D. Weigh client before and after dialysis to determine fluid loss.
E. Monitor for dysrhythmias resulting from electrolyte and pH changes.
F. Watch for leakage around shunt site.
G. Observe for dialysis disequilibrium syndrome.
1. Cerebral dysfunction symptoms.
   a. Nausea and vomiting.
   b. Headache.
   c. Hypertension leading to agitation.
   d. Twitching, mental confusion, and convulsions.
2. Syndrome is caused by rapid, efficient dialysis, resulting in shifts in water, pH and osmolarity between fluid and blood.
3. In acutely uremic clients, avoid this syndrome by dialyzing slowly, for short periods of time over 2–3 days.
4. Use Dilantin to prevent this syndrome in new clients.
H. If client is heparinized while on dialysis machine, do the following:
1. Take clotting time about 1 hour before client comes off the machine. If less than 30 minutes, do not give protamine sulfate (heparin antagonist)—not usually given, as there is usually no need to counteract effect of heparin.
2. Keep clotting time at 30–90 minutes while on dialysis (normal 6–10 minutes).

◆ I. Shunt care.
1. Temporary vascular access.
   a. Percutaneous cannulation of subclavian, internal jugular and femoral veins.
   b. Catheters are double or multilumen.
   c. Internal jugular and subclavian vein catheters in place 3–12 weeks, femoral catheter 2–3 days.
   d. Assess for signs of infection, thrombosis with pulmonary emboli, and hematoma.
   e. Maintain patency with intermittent heparin injection.
2. Arterial–venous fistula.
   a. Anastomosis of an artery and vein creates a fistula.
   b. Arterial blood flow into the venous system results in marked dilation of veins, which are then easily punctured with a 14-gauge needle.
   c. Two venipunctures are made at the time of dialysis.
      (1) One for blood source.
      (2) One for return.
      (3) Arterial needle is inserted to within 2.5–3.8 cm (1–1½ inches) from fistula, and venous needle is directed away from fistula.
   d. Observe for patency of graft site.
      (1) Check for bruit with stethoscope.
      (2) Observe for signs of infection.
      (3) Palpate pulses distal to shunt for circulation.
   e. No BPs, tourniquet, or blood drawing on shunt arm.
3. Arteriovenous graft.
   a. Graft is implanted subcutaneously between an artery and a vein.
   b. Performed when client's own vessels are not adequate for shunt.
   c. Venipuncture same as for AV fistula.

◆ **Guidelines for Dialysis Management**

A. Limit fluid intake (500 mL over previous day's output); provide accurate intake and output. (Goal is to keep client's weight gain under 1.5 kg between dialyses.)
B. Provide diet low in sodium (2–3 g), 1 g/kg protein, high carbohydrate, high fat, and foods low in potassium.
   1. Dietary protein should be of animal source.
   2. Include meat, eggs, milk, poultry, fish in diet.
C. Check vital signs for indication of hypovolemia; check temperature elevation for indication of possible infection.

D. Auscultate lungs for signs of pulmonary edema.
E. Provide shunt care for clients on hemodialysis.
F. Observe level of consciousness—indicative of electrolyte imbalance or thrombus.
G. Administer antihypertensive drugs between dialysis if ordered.
H. Administer diuretics if ordered.
I. Administer blood if ordered (cellular portion only is needed because of low hematocrit).
J. Weigh daily to assess fluid accumulation.
K. Prevent use of soap (urea causes dryness and itching, and soap adds to this problem).
L. Provide continued emotional support.
   1. Allow for expression of feelings about change in body image.
   2. Encourage expression of fears of death, especially during dialysis.
   3. Encourage family cooperation.
   4. Support required change in lifestyle.

Renal Transplant*

Definition: Implantation of a human kidney from a compatable donor to the recipient.

Characteristics

A. Irreversible kidney failure.
B. Recipient must take immunosuppressive medications for life.

Donors

A. Living related.
   1. Most desirable source.
   2. Screened for ABO blood type, human leukocyte antigen (HLA) suitability, tissue-specific antigen and histocompatibility.
   3. Must be in excellent health.
   4. Must have two fully functioning kidneys.
   5. Emotional well-being determined early in screening process.
   6. Must be able to comprehend the donation process and outcomes.
B. Cadaver.
   1. Must be < 60 years of age.
   2. Must meet criteria for "brain death," cannot have cardiac death.
   3. Renal function must be normal.
   4. Cannot have metastatic disease, HIV-positive status, or hepatitis B–positive status.
   ◆ 5. Donor cannot have the following:
      a. Abdominal or renal trauma.
      b. Hypotension.
      c. Generalized infection.

*See Legal Aspects of Organ Transplant, Chapter 2.

6. Must have cardiopulmonary support maintained until the kidneys are surgically removed.
7. Once brain death has occurred, restore intravascular volume, wean from vasopressors, and maintain diuresis.

C. Warm ischemic time—time elapsed between cessation of perfusion and cooling of the kidney and the time required to anastomose the kidney.
   1. Maximum time—30–60 minutes.
   2. Kidney can be cooled; this increases transplant time to between 24 and 48 hours.

Implementation

◆ A. Preoperative.
   1. Verify histocompatibility tests (per hospital policy).
   2. Administer medications.
   3. Keep client free from infection (follow protective isolation as indicated).
   4. Follow hospital policy for dialysis prior to transplant.
   5. Provide emotional support to donor and recipient.

◆ B. Postoperative.
   1. Assess kidney function—may occur immediately or be delayed a few days; monitor every hour.
   2. Maintain hemodialysis until adequate kidney function is maintained.
   3. Monitor VS, I&O, daily blood work, urine tests.
   4. Keep client in semi-Fowler's position.
   5. Maintain patency of Foley—urine will be pink to bloody initially, returns to clear yellow within days to weeks. If clots occur, notify physician immediately.
   6. Remove Foley as soon as indicated to prevent infection.
   7. Maintain protective isolation with strict aseptic technique.
   8. Monitor for possible complications.
      a. Hemorrhage from anastomosis.
      b. Failure of ureteral anastomosis—causing leakage of urine into peritoneal cavity.
      c. Renal artery thrombosis.
      d. Infection.
      e. Resection.
   9. Provide teaching to client and family.
      a. Use and side effects of prescribed medications.
      b. Vital signs and weight.
      c. Signs and symptoms of organ rejection.
      d. Dietary changes.
   10. Provide psychological support to client and family.

MALE GENITOURINARY DISORDERS

Prostatitis

◆ *Definition:* Inflammation of the prostate gland caused by an infectious agent (bacteria, mycoplasma) or structure, hyperplasia.

Assessment

A. Assess for peritoneal discomfort, burning, urgency, or frequency.
B. Assess for generalized pain or pain associated with ejaculation or voiding.
C. If acute, client may have sudden onset of fever, chills, and pain.
D. Evaluate clients with chronic conditions, even with absence of pain.

Implementation

◆ A. Monitor broad-spectrum antimicrobials (sensitive to causative agent)—may be tetracycline, doxycycline. Treatment is 10–14 days.
B. Maintain client on bedrest until symptoms are alleviated.
C. Promote comfort with analgesics, antispasmodics, sedatives, sitz baths, stool softeners.

Benign Prostatic Hypertrophy (BPH)

◆ *Definition:* Enlargement of prostate gland from normal tissue, usually in males over 50 years of age.

Assessment

A. Causes narrowing of urethra, which may result in obstruction.
◆ B. Clinical manifestations.
   1. Recurring infection and urinary stasis.
   2. Nocturia, frequency, dysuria, urgency, dribbling, retention, and hematuria.
   3. Hesitancy in starting urination, abdominal straining with urination.

Implementation

A. Treatment.
   1. Drug—finasteride (Proscar) reduces hypertrophy through inhibition of enzyme that blocks uptake of androgens; has severe side effects (impotence).
   2. Alpha-adrenergic receptor blockers (terazosin) relax smooth muscles of bladder neck and prostate.
   3. Herbs (saw palmetto) and nutrients: magnesium, calcium, and zinc reduce hypertrophy.
   4. Monitor drug therapy if indicated.
B. Encourage fluids—2000–3000 mL/day.

C. Suggest diet high in minerals: calcium, magnesium, zinc, manganese.

D. Avoid drugs that could cause urinary retention (anticholinergics).

E. Provide postoperative care for removal of the hypertrophied fibroadenomatous portion of the prostate. (*See* Prostatectomy.)

Cancer of the Prostate

Characteristics

A. Type: androgen-dependent adenocarcinoma.

B. Clinical manifestations.
   1. Early symptoms similar to BPH.
   2. Urinary obstruction late in disease.
   3. Pain radiating from lumbosacral area down legs strongly indicative of cancer.

C. Many cancers so slow-growing the client will die of other diseases before the cancer spreads significantly.

✦ D. Prostate-specific antigen (PSA) test shows concentration is proportional to total prostatic mass.
   1. Does not necessarily indicate malignancy.
   2. Used routinely to monitor client's response to cancer therapy.
   3. Only biopsy determines malignancy.

Prostatectomy

Definition: Removal of the prostate gland.

✦ **Assessment**

A. Observe for signs of hemorrhage and shock.

B. Assess for fluid and electrolyte balance.
   1. Observe for water intoxication (after TURP).
   2. Symptoms are confusion; warm, moist skin; nausea; vomiting.

C. Observe for complications.
   1. Epididymitis (most frequent).
   2. Gram-negative sepsis.
   3. Overdistended bladder.

Implementation

A. Maintain adequate bladder drainage via catheter.
   1. Suprapubic catheter used following suprapubic prostatectomy.
   ✦ 2. Continuous bladder irrigation (or triple-lumen catheter) is used following transurethral resection.
      a. One lumen is used for inflating balloon (usually 30 mL), one for outflow of urine, and one for instillation of irrigating solution.
      b. Function.
         (1) Continuous antibacterial irrigation of solution to prevent infection.
         (2) Continuous saline irrigation to rid the bladder of tissue and clots following surgery.

✦ A. Medical regimen.
   1. Estrogen therapy or luteinizing-hormone antagonist (Lupron or another antiandrogen agent) may be given to slow rate of growth and extension of tumor.
   2. Orchiectomy decreases androgen production.
   3. Radiation to local lesion to reduce tumor: external beam radiation or implant.
   4. Do no procedure—monitor annually.

B. Surgical options.
   ✦ 1. Transurethral resection (TUR) most common intervention—removal of prostatic tissue by instrumentation through urethra.
   2. Suprapubic prostatectomy—removal of prostate by abdominal incision with bladder incision.
   3. Retropubic prostatectomy—low abdominal incision without opening bladder.
   4. Perineal prostatectomy (may be radical resection)—perineal incision between scrotum and anus for gland removal.
   5. Transurethral incision (TUIP)—instrument passed through urethra, one or two incisions made in prostate to reduce pressure and obstruction. Effective for treatment of BPH.
   6. Homium laser (Coherent Co.) may replace TUR for prostate surgery—advantages are less bleeding, fewer complications, and shorter hospital stay.

   ✦ c. Nursing management.
      (1) Run solution in rapidly if bright red drainage or clots are present; when drainage clears, decrease to about 40 drops/min. Urine should be red to light pink in 24 hours, amber in 3 days.
      (2) If clots cannot be rinsed out with irrigating solution, irrigate with syringe as ordered, usually 50 mL.
      (3) Maintain accurate I&O. Observe color and consistency of fluid.
   3. After catheter removal, monitor for urinary retention and continence.
   4. Instruct client in perineal exercises to regain urinary control.
      a. Tense perineal muscles by pressing buttocks together; hold for as long as possible.
      b. Repeat this process 10 times every hour.

B. Provide fluids to prevent dehydration (2–3 L).

C. Provide high-protein, high-vitamin diet.

D. Ambulate early (after urine has returned to nearly normal color)—avoid strenuous activity.

E. Administer analgesics; urinary antiseptics or antibiotics to prevent infection; antispasmodics (spasms decrease within 24–48 hours).

F. Provide wound care for suprapubic and retropubic prostatectomies (similar to that for abdominal surgery)—change dressing frequently.

G. Provide sitz bath and heat lamp treatments to promote healing.

CONDITIONS OF THE FEMALE REPRODUCTIVE TRACT

Menstruation

Definition: The sloughing off of the endometrium, which occurs at regular monthly intervals if conception fails to take place. The discharge consists of blood, mucus, and cells, and it usually lasts for 4–5 days.

✦ Characteristics

A. Menarche—onset of menstruation—usually occurs between the ages of 11 and 14.

B. Abnormalities of menstruation.
   1. Dysmenorrhea (painful menstruation).
      a. May be caused by psychological factors: tension, anxiety, preconditioning.
      b. Physical examination is usually done to rule out organic causes.
      c. May subside after childbearing.
      d. Treatment.
         (1) Oral contraceptives: produce anovulatory cycle.
         (2) Mild analgesics such as aspirin.
         (3) Client urged to carry on normal activities.
   2. Amenorrhea (absence of menstrual flow).
      a. Primary: over the age of 17 and menstruation has not begun.
         (1) Complete physical necessary to rule out abnormalities.
         (2) Treatment aimed at correction of underlying condition.
      b. Secondary: occurs after menarche; does not include pregnancy and lactation.
         (1) Causes include psychological upsets or endocrine conditions.
         (2) Evaluation and treatment by physician is necessary.
   3. Menorrhagia (excessive menstrual bleeding). May be due to endocrine disturbance, tumors or inflammatory conditions of the uterus.
   4. Metrorrhagia (bleeding between periods). Symptom of disease process, benign tumors, or cancer.

Assessment

A. Assess characteristics of the menstrual cycle.

B. Evaluate cycle pattern.

C. Evaluate discomforts associated with menstruation.
   1. Breast tenderness and feeling of fullness.
   2. Temperament and mood changes because of hormonal influence. Levels of estrogen and progesterone drop sharply.
   3. Discomfort in pelvic area, lower back, and legs.
   4. Retained fluids and weight gain.

Implementation

A. Educate client about the physiology of normal menstruation. Answer questions about the myths and cultural beliefs associated with menstruation.

B. Educate client about abnormal conditions associated with menstruation: absence of bleeding, bleeding between periods, etc.

C. Educate client about normal hygiene during menstruation.
   1. Importance of cleanliness.
   2. Use of perineal pads and tampons.
   3. Continuing normal activities.

Menopause

Definition: The cessation of menstruation caused by physiologic factors; ovulation no longer occurs. Menopause usually occurs between the ages of 45 and 52.

Characteristics

A. Ovaries lose the ability to respond to pituitary stimulation and normal ovarian function ceases.
   ✦ 1. Gradual change due to alteration in hormone production.
      a. Failure to ovulate.
      b. Monthly flow becomes smaller, irregular, and gradually ceases.
   2. Menopause is accompanied by changes in reproductive organs: vagina gradually becomes smaller; uterus, bladder, rectum, and supporting structures lose tone, leading to uterine prolapse, rectocele, and cystocele.

B. Atherosclerosis and osteoporosis are more likely to develop at this time.

Assessment

A. Clinical manifestations vary from mild to severe.

B. May be accompanied by psychological symptoms (i.e., feelings of loss, children grown, aging process occurring).

C. May be accompanied by hot flashes and nervous symptoms, such as headache, depression, insomnia, weakness, and dizziness.

Implementation

✦ A. Instruct client in use of hormone replacement therapy (HRT) as alternative way to cope with menopause.

1. Postmenopausal estrogen/progestin intervention (PEPI) appears to improve lipoproteins and lowers fibrinogen levels.
2. Estrogen alone is not recommended for women who have not had a hysterectomy. It is associated with endometrial hyperplasia.
3. Hormone replacement therapy (HRT) is contraindicated for women who have a history of breast cancer, vascular thrombosis, active liver disease.
4. Methods of treatment vary from daily doses of both estrogen and progestin (now very controversial and not recommended) to 25 days of estrogen and natural progesterone taken 10–14 days during the cycle.
5. Estrogen patches must have accompanying oral progestin or natural progesterone.

B. Answer questions, clarify and/or counsel client on menopausal issues and alternatives to HRT.
C. Alternatives to HRT.
   1. Selective estrogen receptor modulators (SERMs) such as roloxifene (Evista).
      a. Acts like estrogen in some tissues but not in others.
      b. Significantly reduces risk of breast cancer.
      c. Used in treatment of osteoporosis.
   2. Studies done in 2003 indicate HRT (especially estrogen–progesterone combination) may present major cancer risk to women.
   3. Herbal combination used to decrease symptoms of menopause. (*See* Herbal Chart, Pharmacology, Chapter 5.)
   4. Other alternative is to use natural estrogen (estriol) and natural progesterone.

Vulvitis/Vaginal Infections

✦ *Definition:* An inflammation of the vulva or vagina, which usually occurs in conjunction with other conditions such as vaginal infections and venereal disease.

Characteristics

A. Vagina normally protected from infection by acidic environment.
B. Leukorrhea (whitish vaginal discharge) normal in small amounts at ovulation and prior to menstruation.

Assessment

A. Evaluate burning pain during urination.
B. Assess for itching.
C. Observe for red and inflamed genitalia.
D. Observe for discharge and odor.
✦ E. *Trichomonas vaginalis* (overgrowth of protozoan normally present in vaginal tract)—normal pH altered and overgrowth occurs.

✦ F. *Candida albicans*—fungal infection caused by yeast, also called monilia.
   1. 500,000 Americans get this infection—majority are women.
   2. Widespread use of antibiotics increasing epidemic—these destroy protective organisms normally present.
   3. *Candida* thrives in sugar–carbohydrate-rich environment.
   4. Symptoms: itching; swelling; white, cheesy discharge from vagina or thrush in mouth; may have systemic symptoms of fatigue, allergies, depression, flatus.
G. Evaluate for related conditions, psychological factors, endocrine disorders, and reactions to chemical substances that the client may be using.

Implementation

A. Give soothing compresses, colloidal baths.
B. Apply medicated creams.
C. Nystatin and Monistat are drugs of choice systemically; vaginal inserts and ointment.
D. Gyne-Lotrimin and terazol creams (vaginal) are inserted at night.
E. Fluconazole (oral agent) is given one time. Results appear in 3 days.

Endometriosis

✦ *Definition:* The abnormal growth of endometrial tissue outside the uterine cavity. A common cause of infertility.

Characteristics

A. Embryonic tissue that remains dormant until ovarian stimulation after menarche.
B. Endometrial tissue transported from the uterine cavity through the fallopian tubes during menstruation.
C. Endometrial tissue transported by lymphatic tissue during menstruation.
D. Accidental transfer of endometrial tissue to pelvic cavity during surgery.

Assessment

✦ A. Evaluate lower abdominal and pelvic pain during menstruation due to distention of involved tissue and surrounding area by blood; symptoms are acute during menstruation.
B. Assess for dysmenorrhea: usually steady and severe.
C. Assess for abnormal uterine bleeding.
D. Ask about pain during intercourse.
E. Assess for back and rectal pain.

Implementation

A. Explain to client that pregnancy may delay growth of lesions. Symptoms usually recur after pregnancy.

B. Instruct that hormone therapy with oral contraceptives usually eliminates menstrual pain and controls endometrial growth.

C. Discuss use of in vitro fertilization in cases where pregnancy is desired.

D. Prepare client for surgical intervention; total hysterectomy may be indicated.

Pelvic Inflammatory Disease (PID)

✦ *Definition:* An inflammatory condition of the pelvic cavity that may involve ovaries, fallopian tubes, vascular system, or pelvic peritoneum.

Assessment

✦ A. Assess for cause of disease.
1. Gonorrheal and chlamydial organisms most common causes.
2. Caused by sexual transmission.

B. Assess for elevated temperature, general malaise, headache.

C. Evaluate for nausea and vomiting.

D. Assess for lower pelvic pain and tenderness following menses.

E. Pain increases during voiding and defecation.

F. Observe for purulent, foul-smelling vaginal discharge.

G. Evaluate for leukocytosis.

✦ Implementation
A. Instruct client on controlling spread of infection.
B. Place in semi-Fowler's position: dependent drainage.
C. Apply heat to abdomen for comfort.
D. Administer warm douches to improve circulation.
E. Take and record vital signs every 4 hours.
F. Administer antibiotics as ordered.
G. Note nature and amount of vaginal discharge.
H. Instruct to avoid use of tampons and urinary catheterization to prevent spread of infection.
I. Instruct on good nutrition and fluid intake.

Toxic Shock Syndrome (TSS)

✦ *Definition:* An uncommon but serious illness reported by menstruating women, usually under age of 30, who use tampons. TSS may also occur in women using sanitary napkins.

Assessment

✦ A. Assess for two primary symptoms: sudden high fever (may be as high as 103–105°F) and rash that looks like a sunburn.

B. Other symptoms commonly observed: vomiting and diarrhea; dizziness, fainting or near fainting when standing up, headache, and sore throat.

C. Red macular rash occurs in many women first on torso.

Implementation

✦ A. When toxic shock suspected, client is hospitalized—the development of severe circulatory compromise cannot be predicted.

✦ B. Blood, urine, and vaginal cultures determine sites of focal *Staphylococcus aureus* infection; a beta-lactamase–resistant antibiotic with bactericidal activity is administered; when there is no focal infection site, Betadine vaginal douches are given 3 times a day for 2–3 days.

C. Monitor blood pressure and administer IV colloids and vasopressor agents as ordered.

D. Administer sodium bicarbonate for acidosis.

E. Monitor for signs of respiratory distress.

Conditions of the Uterus

Definition: May include displacement of the uterus, prolapse of the uterus, or fibroid tumors of the uterus.

Assessment

A. Assess for displacement.
1. Retroversion and retroflexion: backward displacement of the uterus.
2. May cause difficulty in becoming pregnant.

✦ B. Assess for prolapse.
1. Weakening of uterine supports causes the uterus to slip down into the vaginal canal; the uterus may even appear outside the vaginal orifice.
2. Prolapse may cause urinary incontinence or retention.

Implementation

A. Instruct in good perineal hygiene if pessary is used.
B. Follow nursing care for hysterectomy clients.

Fibroid Tumors

✦ A. Fibroid tumors are benign.
B. Occur in 20–30 percent of all women between the ages of 25 and 40.
✦ C. Symptoms include menorrhagia, back pain, urinary difficulty, and constipation.
D. Fibroid tumors may cause sterility.
E. Treatment.
1. Removal of tumors, if they are small.
2. Hysterectomy, if tumors are large.

SURGICAL INTERVENTIONS

Tumors of the Breast

Definition: Tumors or neoplasms are composed of new and actively growing tissue. They are classified in many ways, the most common according to origin and whether they are malignant or benign. The second highest cause of death in females is malignant tumors of the reproductive system.

✦ **Assessment**

A. Assess for lump in upper outer quadrant of breast, usually nontender, but may be tender.

B. Observe for dimpling of breast tissue surrounding nipple or bleeding from nipple.

C. Check for presence of asymmetry with affected breast being higher.

D. Check for prominent venous pattern—can signal increased blood suply to tumor.

E. Erythema can indicate benign local infection or superficial lymphatic invasion by a neoplasm.

F. Evaluate staging from Stage I to Stage IV.

✦ G. Evaluate types of surgery to be done:
  1. Breast-conserving therapy.
     a. Surgical procedures: lumpectomy, wide excision, partial mastectomy, segmental mastectomy, quadrantectomy.
     b. Removal of involved breast tissue and some surrounding tissue and axillary lymph nodes.
  2. Total mastectomy.
     a. Removal of breast tissue only.
     b. Performed for carcinoma in situ, typically ductal.
  3. Modified radical mastectomy.
     a. Removal of breast tissue and axillary lymph nodes.
     b. Pectoralis major and minor muscles remain intact.
  4. Radical mastectomy.
     a. Removal of breast tissue and pectoralis major and minor.
     b. Axillary lymph node dissection.

✦ **Implementation: Mastectomy**

✦ A. Begin emotional support preoperatively and continue in postoperative period.
  1. Client may have altered body image.
  2. Client may be extremely depressed.

✦ B. Place in semi-Fowler's position with affected arm elevated to prevent edema.

✦ C. Turn, cough and deep-breathe to prevent respiratory complications.

D. Turn only to back and unaffected side.

E. Jackson–Pratt or Hemovac may be placed postoperatively.

✦ F. Prevent complications of contractures and lymphedema by encouraging range-of-motion exercises early in postoperative period.

G. Provide IV fluids. Should not be administered in affected arm.

H. Monitor vital signs for prevention of complications such as infection and hemorrhage. Take blood pressure on unaffected arm only.

I. Reinforce pressure dressings. Observe for signs of restriction from dressing.
  1. Impaired sensation.
  2. Color changes of skin.

J. If skin grafts were applied, provide nursing care as for any other graft.

K. Encourage visit from Reach for Recovery Group.

L. Instruct to perform self-breast exam monthly at a regular time, 7 days after start of menstruation.

M. Discuss need for mammography.

Breast Reconstruction

A. Emotional and psychological implications of loss of a breast are severe.
  ✦ 1. Loss has impact on body image, self-esteem, sense of being sexually attractive, and intimate relationships.
  2. Reconstructive surgery following a mastectomy may positively affect the woman's adjustment to loss of a breast.

✦ B. Reconstruction may be immediate (following surgery) or delayed.

C. Mastectomy without reconstruction—client uses a breast prosthesis.

✦ D. Types of procedures.
  1. Implants are soft sacs or a tissue-expander prosthesis filled with silicone gel.
     a. Expander sac is gradually expanded via a needle until breast matches remaining breast; takes several months to complete process.
     b. Following expansion, prosthesis may be removed and replaced by silicone implant.
  2. Silicone implants may result in complications.
     a. Fibrous capsular contractions around implant.
     b. Infection is usually a rare complication.
     c. Debate about use of silicone led, in 1992, to the FDA's limiting use of silicone to breast reconstruction.
  ✦ 3. Autogenous tissue flaps—second type of breast reconstruction.
     a. Tissue flaps eliminate need for implant—unless there is insufficient skin available (TRAM flap, latissimus dorsi).
     b. Involves use of tissue from upper portions of back or lower abdomen.

E. Performing immediate breast reconstruction eliminates need for second hospitalization and surgery.

Cancer in the Reproductive System

Characteristics

A. Cancer of the cervix.
  ✦ 1. Most common type of cancer in the reproductive system.
  2. Usually appears in females between the ages of 30 and 50.
  3. Signs and symptoms include bleeding between periods—may be noted especially after intercourse or douching; leukorrhea.
  4. May become invasive and include tissue outside the cervix, fundus of the uterus, and the lymph glands.
  ✦ 5. Treatment—depends on extent of the disease.
    a. Hysterectomy.
    b. Radiation.
    c. Radical pelvic surgery in advanced cases.
B. Cancer of the endometrium, fundus, or corpus of uterus.
  1. Usually not diagnosed until symptoms appear—Pap smear inadequate for diagnosis.
  2. Progresses slowly—metastasis occurs late.
  3. Treatment.
    a. Early—hysterectomy.
    b. Late—radium and x-ray therapy.
C. Cancer of the vulva.
  1. Long-standing pruritus (itching) and local discomfort—itching occurs in half of women.
  2. Foul-smelling and slightly bloody discharge.
  3. Early lesions. May appear as chronic vulval dermatitis (cancerous lesions grow slowly).
  4. Surgical interventions.
    a. Vulvectomy is the preferred treatment.
    b. Radiation therapy is used in the inoperable lesions.
✦ D. Cancer of the ovary.
  1. Malignancy may occur at all ages—risk increases after age 40.
  ✦ 2. The most deadly form of reproductive cancer; lack of warning symptoms; etiology not understood.
  ✦ 3. Early diagnosis and surgical removal important (survival rate is 93 percent).
    a. Usually detection is by chance, not screening.
    b. Tumor marker, CA-125, may be useful, but many false negatives occur.
  ✦ 4. Cancer is staged according to the involvement of tissue and may involve one or both ovaries.
    a. Stage I—limited to the ovaries.
    b. Stage II—pelvic extension.
    c. Stage III—metastasis outside pelvis or positive retroperitoneal lymph nodes.
    d. Stage IV—distant metastasis.

5. Laparotomy is used for diagnosis and treatment—surgery is primary treatment.
6. Chemotherapy may be used for Stage I; radioactive instillation for Stage II.
    a. Chemotherapeutic drugs include cyclophosphamide, cisplatin, carboplatin and paclitaxel.
    b. Cisplatin and paclitaxel most commonly used because of clinical benefits and manageable toxicity.
    c. Leukopenia, neurotoxicity, and fever may occur with treatment.
    d. Paclitaxel can cause cardiac effects.
7. Bone marrow transplantation or stem cell transplantation may be used.
8. Nursing care is the same as for any major abdominal surgery with the exception of psychosocial implications of cancer.

Implementation

✦ A. Provide immediate postoperative care.
  1. Observe dressings for signs of hemorrhage.
  2. Check vital signs until stable.
  3. Assist client to turn, cough, and deep-breathe every 2 hours.
  4. Give pain medications as ordered.
  5. Observe drainage and empty Hemovac as necessary.
  6. Record intake and output.
  7. Maintain IV.
  8. Maintain catheter care to reduce incidence of infection.
  9. Position for comfort.
B. Provide convalescent care.
  1. Encourage verbalization regarding change in body image.
  2. Irrigate wound as ordered, using solution as prescribed (usual solution is either sterile saline or hydrogen peroxide), which cleans area and improves circulation.
  3. Prevent wound infection.
C. Instruct client on discharge teaching.
  1. Signs of infection—foul-smelling discharge, elevated temperature, swelling.
  2. Nutritious diet and planned rest periods.
  3. Wound irrigation and dressing change.
  4. Importance of follow-up care by physician.

Hysterectomy

✦ Characteristics

A. Total hysterectomy—removal of the uterus including the cervix; fallopian tubes and ovaries are not removed.

B. Total abdominal hysterectomy and bilateral salpingo-oophorectomy—involves removal of the entire uterus, ovaries, and fallopian tubes.

C. Radical hysterectomy—partial vaginectomy with dissection of lymph nodes in the pelvis.

Assessment

◆ A. Observe for hemorrhage—vaginal and at the incision site.

◆ B. Observe for signs of infection—elevated temperature, foul-smelling vaginal discharge, and pelvic congestion.

C. Assess for changes in body image—feelings of loss.

D. Evaluate for pneumonia.

E. Auscultate for paralytic ileus.

F. Observe for thrombophlebitis.

Implementation

◆ A. Immediate postoperative care.
   1. Observe incision site for bleeding and reinforce dressings as needed.
   2. Monitor vital signs frequently.
   3. Administer pain medications as ordered (assist with PCA use).
   4. Administer IV fluids as ordered.
   5. Observe for signs of thromboembolism—administer heparin if ordered.
   6. Provide for hygienic care.
   7. Give catheter care to prevent infection—observe amount and color of drainage.
   8. Assist client to cough, turn, and deep-breathe.
   9. Promote methods to decrease pelvic congestion.
      a. Apply antiembolic stockings.
      b. Avoid high-Fowler's position.
      c. Promote range of motion.

◆ B. Provide convalescent care.
   1. Increase activity as tolerated.
   2. Ambulate with assistance.
   3. Auscultate chest for breath sounds.
   4. Auscultate abdomen for bowel sounds.
   5. Allow client to verbalize feelings of loss of femininity, childbearing ability, disfigurement, fear of cancer.
   6. Provide for emotional support.
   7. Increase diet as tolerated—fluids to 3000 mL/day provided no cardiac or renal problems.
   8. Administer laxatives and stool softeners as ordered, and rectal tubes or Harris flush for flatus—diet modification to prevent constipation.

C. Prepare client for discharge.
   ◆ 1. Encourage expression of feelings with significant other.
   2. Explain that menstruation will no longer occur.
   3. Explain that estrogen therapy may be ordered by the physician, if the ovaries were removed, to control menopausal symptoms.

   ◆ 4. Instruct the client to observe for signs of complications.
      a. Elevation of temperature.
      b. Foul-smelling vaginal discharge.
      c. Redness, swelling, or drainage from the incision site.
      d. Abdominal cramping.
   5. Explain the importance of follow-up visits with the physician.
   6. Explain the importance of taking medications as ordered.
   7. Douching and coitus are usually avoided for 6 weeks.
   8. Remind client to avoid both lifting heavy objects and prolonged sitting for several weeks as instructed by physician.

Anterior and Posterior Colporrhaphy

Characteristics

◆ A. Repair of cystocele—downward displacement of the bladder toward the vaginal entrance, caused by tissue weakness, injuries in childbirth, and atrophy associated with aging.

◆ B. Repair of rectocele—anterior sagging of rectum and posterior vaginal wall caused by injuries to the muscles and tissue of the pelvic floor during childbirth.

Assessment

A. Observe for foul-smelling discharge from vaginal area or operative site.

B. Observe for urinary retention and catheterize as necessary.

Implementation

A. Provide postoperative care to decrease discomfort.

◆ B. Provide care of perineal sutures—two methods:
   1. Sutures left alone until healing begins; thereafter, daily vaginal irrigations with sterile saline.
   2. Sterile saline douches twice daily, beginning with the first postoperative day.

C. Preparation of client for discharge. Client should be instructed in perineal hygiene (no douching or coitus until advised by physician), and to watch for signs of infection.

Pelvic Exenteration

Definition: A surgical procedure that is performed when cancer is widespread and cannot be controlled by other means—life-saving in certain malignancies.

Characteristics

◆ A. Total pelvic exenteration—removal of the reproductive organs, pelvic floor, pelvic lymph nodes, perineum, bladder, rectum, and distal portion of sigmoid colon.

B. A substitute bladder is made from a segment of the ileum. Client will have a permanent colostomy.

C. When cancer has spread beyond the pelvis, this procedure will not be done.

✦ Implementation

A. Provide general postoperative procedures; in addition, give care for abdominal–perineal resection of the bowel and an ileoconduit.

B. Observe surgical site for drainage and reinforce dressings as necessary; client may have drainage tubes connected to suction from incision area.

C. Observe for complications (occur in 25–50 percent), usually involving urinary and GI systems.

D. Encourage client to express feelings—especially important considering the diagnosis.

E. Refer client to cancer support group, which studies have shown improve life expectancy.

GENITOURINARY SYSTEM REVIEW QUESTIONS

1. A client is scheduled for a voiding cystogram. Which nursing intervention would be essential to carry out several hours before the test?

   1. Maintaining NPO status.
   2. Medicating with urinary antiseptics.
   3. Administering bowel preparation.
   4. Forcing fluids.

2. A retention catheter for a male client is correctly taped if it is

   1. On the lower abdomen.
   2. On the umbilicus.
   3. Under the thigh.
   4. On the inner thigh.

3. A client with a diagnosis of gout will be taking colchicine and allopurinol BID to prevent recurrence. The most common early sign of colchicine toxicity that the nurse will assess for is

   1. Blurred vision.
   2. Anorexia.
   3. Diarrhea.
   4. Fever.

4. A client's laboratory results have been returned and the creatinine level is 7 mg/dL. This finding would lead the nurse to place the highest priority on assessing

   1. Temperature.
   2. Intake and output.
   3. Capillary refill.
   4. Pupillary reflex.

5. After the lungs, the kidneys work to maintain body pH. The best explanation of how the kidneys accomplish regulation of pH is that they

   1. Secrete hydrogen ions and sodium.
   2. Secrete ammonia.
   3. Exchange hydrogen and sodium in the kidney tubules.
   4. Decrease sodium ions, hold on to hydrogen ions, and then secrete sodium bicarbonate.

6. Conditions known to predispose to renal calculi formation include

   1. Polyuria.
   2. Dehydration, immobility.
   3. Glycosuria.
   4. Presence of an indwelling Foley catheter.

7. The most appropriate nursing intervention, based on physician's orders, for treating metabolic acidosis is to

   1. Replace potassium ions immediately to prevent hypokalemia.
   2. Administer oral sodium bicarbonate to act as a buffer.
   3. Administer IV catecholamines (Levophed) to prevent hypotension.
   4. Administer fluids to prevent dehydration.

8. The IV is attached to a controller to maintain the flow rate. If the alarm sounds on the controller, which of the following actions would the nurse *not* perform?

   1. Ensure that the drip chamber is full.
   2. Assess that height of IV container is at least 30 inches above venipuncture site.
   3. Ensure that the drop sensor is properly placed on the drip chamber.
   4. Evaluate the needle and IV tubing to determine if they are patent and positioned appropriately.

9. A 76-year-old woman who has been in good health develops urinary incontinence over a period of several days and is admitted to the hospital for a diagnostic work-up. The nurse would assess the client for other indicators of

   1. Renal failure.
   2. Urinary tract infection.
   3. Fluid volume excess.
   4. Dementia.

10. A 60-year-old male client's physician schedules a prostatectomy and orders a straight urinary drainage system to be inserted preoperatively. For the system to be effective, the nurse would

    1. Coil the tubing above the level of the bladder.
    2. Position the collection bag above the level of the bladder.
    3. Check that the collection bag is vented and distensible.
    4. Determine that the tubing is less than 3 feet in length.

11. During a retention catheter insertion or bladder irrigation, the nurse must use

    1. Sterile equipment and wear sterile gloves.
    2. Clean equipment and maintain surgical asepsis.
    3. Sterile equipment and maintain medical asepsis.
    4. Clean equipment and technique.

12. The physician has ordered a 24-hour urine specimen. After explaining the procedure to the client, the nurse collects the first specimen. This specimen is then

    1. Discarded, then the collection begins.
    2. Saved as part of the 24-hour collection.
    3. Tested, then discarded.
    4. Placed in a separate container and later added to the collection.

13. You are assigned to a client with a retention catheter. You will assess for contamination, which could be caused by

    1. Insertion technique.
    2. Catheter removal.
    3. Urethral/catheter interface.
    4. Migration to the bladder.

14. A client in acute renal failure receives an IV infusion of 10% dextrose in water with 20 units of regular insulin. The goal of this therapy is to

    1. Correct the hyperglycemia that occurs with acute renal failure.
    2. Facilitate the intracellular movement of potassium.
    3. Provide calories to prevent tissue catabolism and azotemia.
    4. Force potassium into the cells to prevent arrhythmias.

15. A client with chronic renal failure is on continuous ambulatory peritoneal dialysis (CAPD). Which nursing diagnosis should have the highest priority?

    1. Powerlessness.
    2. High risk for infection.
    3. Altered nutrition: less than body requirements.
    4. High risk for fluid volume deficit.

16. The nurse is assigned a client undergoing chronic peritoneal dialysis. The priority assessment is

    1. Pulmonary embolism.
    2. Hypotension.
    3. Dyspnea.
    4. Peritonitis.

17. To formulate a care plan for a client receiving dialysis, the nurse understands that the physiological mechanism associated with peritoneal dialysis is that the

    1. Peritoneum allows solutes in the dialysate to pass into the intravascular system.
    2. Peritoneum acts as a semipermeable membrane through which solutes move via diffusion and osmosis.
    3. Presence of excess metabolites causes increased permeability of the peritoneum and allows excess fluid to drain.
    4. Peritoneum permits diffusion of metabolites only from intravascular to interstitial spaces.

18. A client is on dialysis treatments three times per week. The nurse explains that the main advantage of using an internal arteriovenous fistula rather than an external arteriovenous cannula for dialysis is

    1. Accessing the internal fistula is less uncomfortable for the client.
    2. The internal fistula can be utilized immediately after insertion.
    3. There is less risk of hemorrhage from the internal fistula.
    4. It is easier to access the blood flow with the internal fistula than through the external cannula.

19. The main complication following a nephrostomy that the nurse must assess for is

    1. Bleeding from the nephrostomy site.
    2. Cardiopulmonary involvement following the procedure.
    3. Difficulty in restoring fluid and electrolyte balance.
    4. Contamination of the site.

20. Client instructions following a vasectomy will include

    1. No sexual activity for 2 weeks.
    2. Application of ice for pain or swelling.
    3. Bedrest for several days.
    4. Returning for suture removal in 1 week.

21. The nurse explains to the client that decreasing dietary oxalate intake can reduce the formation of calcium–oxalate renal stones. The client is prepared to make correct diet choices when he tells the nurse he knows that foods to avoid on such a diet include

    1. Red meats, butter, cheese.
    2. Carrots, spinach, tomatoes, green beans.
    3. Bananas, apples, apricots.
    4. Rice, potatoes, breads.

22. The nurse is doing discharge teaching to a client who will be discharged on diuretics. Measures to prevent hypokalemia will include

    1. Eating one banana a day.
    2. Taking 1 teaspoon of salt substitute a day.
    3. Eating 10 prunes a day.
    4. Drinking an 8-ounce glass of orange juice every day.

23. A client is scheduled for a kidney transplant. A medication she will probably take on a long-term basis that will require specific client teaching to ensure compliance is

    1. Corticosteroids.
    2. Antibiotics.
    3. Anticoagulants.
    4. Gamma globulin.

24. The client who is receiving Furadantin for a urinary tract infection may also receive ascorbic acid. The rationale for this additional agent is to

    1. Promote tissue repair.
    2. Fortify mucosal resistance.
    3. Acidify the urine.
    4. Alkalinize the urine.

25. A client is to start on finasteride (Proscar) for the treatment of benign prostatic hypertrophy (BPH). Which statement by the client indicates that he needs more teaching?

    1. "This drug will eliminate the need for prostate surgery."
    2. "I will not be surprised if I experience a decreased interest in sex."
    3. "It may take 6 or more months before this drug works."
    4. "I should be able to empty my bladder better while I'm on this drug."

GENITOURINARY SYSTEM

Answers with Rationale

1. (4) Forcing fluids ensures a continuous flow of urine to provide adequate urine output for specimen collection. High fluid intake also prevents multiplication of bacteria that may have been introduced during the procedure.

   NP:I; CN:PH; CL:A

2. (1) The catheter should be taped on the upper thigh or lower abdomen to prevent a penoscrotal angle that can cause fistula development.

   NP:AN; CN:PH; CL:C

3. (3) Diarrhea is by far the most common early sign of colchicine toxicity. When given in the acute phase of gout, the dose of colchicine is usually 0.6 mg (PO) QH (not to exceed 10 tablets) until pain is relieved or gastrointestinal symptoms develop.

   NP:A; CN:PH; CL:A

4. (2) The elevated creatinine level suggests impaired renal function. Assessing intake and output will provide data related to renal function. The other assessments are not indicative of renal function.

   NP:A; CN:PH; CL:A

5. (4) By decreasing NA^- ions, holding on to hydrogen ions, and secreting sodium bicarbonate, the kidneys can regulate pH. Therefore, this is the most complete answer. While this buffer system is the slowest, it can completely compensate for acid–base imbalance.

   NP:AN; CN:H; CL:C

6. (2) Urinary stasis, renal infection, and dehydration predispose the client to the formation of renal calculi, which may or may not require surgery.

   NP:AN; CN:PH; CL:C

7. (4) Causes of metabolic acidosis include dehydration, diarrhea, and diabetes mellitus. Fluid administration is a priority. Hyperkalemia results as cells are dehydrated; therefore, potassium will not be administered until hydration has occurred.

   NP:P; CN:PH; CL:A

8. (1) The drip chamber should be only one-third full so that the sensor can "pick up" the drops. All of the other actions would be appropriate to carry out.

   NP:I; CN:S; CL:C

9. (2) Urinary tract infections in the elderly often present as urinary incontinence that develops suddenly. Renal failure (1) and fluid volume excess (3) typically are characterized by oliguria. High uric acid level would result in symptoms of gout, not urinary incontinence.

   NP:A; CN:PH; CL:A

10. (3) The collection bag must be able to fill easily; therefore, it needs to be distended. The bag must be vented with a filter so that urine can be drained from the chamber. The tube must not be allowed to coil or become kinked above the level of the bladder. The collection bag is positioned below the level of the bladder to allow for continuous urine drainage and prevent urine backflow into the bladder. To prevent reflux of urine, the tubing must be of sufficient length, usually 5 feet.

    NP:E; CN:PH; CL:C

11. (1) To prevent introduction of pathogens into the urinary tract, sterile equipment is used and its sterility maintained.

    NP:P; CN:S; CL:C

12. (1) The first specimen is discarded because it is considered "old urine" or urine that was in the bladder before the test began. After the first discarded specimen, urine is collected for 24 hours.

    NP:I; CN:PH; CL:C

Coding for Questions/Answers Abbreviations: **Nursing Process: NP,** Assessment: A, Analysis: AN, Planning: P, Implementation: I, Evaluation: E; **Client Needs: CN,** Safe, Effective Care Environment: S, Health Promotion and Maintenance: H, Psychosocial Integrity: PS, Physiological Integrity: PH; **Clinical Area: CA,** Medical Nursing: M, Surgical Nursing: S, Maternal/Newborn Nursing: MA, Pediatric Nursing: P, Psychiatric Nursing: PS; **Cognitive Level: CL,** Knowledge: K, Comprehension: C, Application: A, Analysis: AN.

13. (4) Infection due to catheter presence is most commonly associated with migration to the bladder along the internal lumen of the catheter after contamination. Keeping the collection bag dependent of the tubing is important to prevent reflux and contamination. The other answers are potential, but not as common, causes of infection.

    NP:P; CN:PH; CL:C

14. (2) Dextrose with insulin helps move potassium into cells and is immediate management therapy for hyperkalemia due to acute renal failure. An exchange resin may also be employed. This type of infusion is often administered before cardiac surgery to stabilize irritable cells and prevent arrhythmias; in this case KCl is also added to the infusion.

    NP:P; CN:PH; CL:A

15. (2) There is a high risk of infection in clients receiving CAPD because microorganisms can enter the body by migrating around, or through, the peritoneal dialysis catheter. They may also enter through contaminated dialysate solutions. The other diagnoses are not as life-threatening in a client on CAPD.

    NP:AN; CN:PH; CL:A

16. (4) Peritonitis is a grave complication with peritoneal dialysis. Hemodialysis may be necessary until infection clears. Excess fluid and protein effluent into the peritoneum also complicate care. Use of aseptic technique is essential.

    NP:E; CN:PH; CL:AN

17. (2) The peritoneum acts as a semipermeable membrane across which the substances move by osmosis from an area of high concentration (the blood) to an area of lower concentration (the dialysate). The dialysate contains small amounts or none of the substances that are to be removed from the body. This process takes 48 to 72 hours to be effective, and this time frame must be considered in planning for care.

    NP:AN; CN:PH; CL:C

18. (3) There is an increased incidence of hemorrhaging with the external cannula. Hemorrhage results from the cannula becoming disconnected. One advantage of the external cannula is that it is painless to use. Surgery is required to establish the internal fistula, and it should be allowed to heal for several weeks before being utilized.

    NP:I; CN:PH; CL:C

19. (1) While all the other conditions may be complications, bleeding from the site is the main concern. The procedure is done to achieve relief from infection caused by urinary stasis, which may have resulted in kidney congestion.

    NP:A; CN:PH; CL:A

20. (2) If the client has pain or swelling, application of ice will help reduce symptoms. Sexual activity can be resumed, but the client will not be clear of sperm from the ductus for 4 to 6 weeks. Bedrest is not indicated, and sutures are absorbable.

    NP:I; CN:S; CL:C

21. (2) Foods high in oxalate include spinach, green and wax beans, beets, and chocolate.

    NP:E; CN:PH; CL:A

22. (2) To prevent hypokalemia, the client should take supplemental potassium. One teaspoon of salt substitute provides 50 mEq of potassium chloride. Potassium supplement tablets are also acceptable. While many texts advocate food for replacement, many foods have to be eaten in large quantities to provide sufficient potassium (50 mEq/day): four to six bananas, 1000 mL of orange juice, or 30 to 40 prunes. Often these foods are high in calories.

    NP:I; CN:H; CL:A

23. (1) Prednisone, a corticosteroid, is the usual drug of choice. The other medication classifications are not used in the routine care of transplant clients.

    NP:P; CN:PH; CL:C

24. (3) Furadantin antimicrobial activity is more potent in acidic urine. Ascorbic acid or vitamin C tablets acidify the urine.

    NP:AN; CN:PH; CL:C

25. (1) Because this statement is incorrect, the client will need more teaching. Finasteride is an androgen inhibitor that may promote a reduction of prostatic hypertrophy, thereby improving bladder emptying. It may take 6 to 12 months to become effective and it does not work for all clients. Some clients, therefore, will need surgery to relieve the obstructive symptoms of BPH. One of the side effects of the drug is decreased libido.

    NP:E; CN:PH; CL:A

MUSCULOSKELETAL SYSTEM

The musculoskeletal system provides the support and protective mechanism of the body. Bones, joints, and skeletal muscles comprise the system.

ANATOMY AND PHYSIOLOGY

Bone Structure

A. Types of bones.
1. Long: legs, arms.
2. Short: wrists, ankles.
3. Flat: skull, sternum, ribs.
4. Irregular: vertebrae, face, scapulae, pelvic girdle.
B. Bone surfaces.
1. Grooves and holes provide passage for nerves and blood vessels.
2. Protrusions at the ends of the bone form parts of the joints.
3. Shallow depressions and ridges are attachment points for fibrous tissue.
C. Bone function.
1. Support and protect structures of the body skeleton.
2. Provide attachments for muscles that move the skeleton.
3. Central cavity of some bones contain hematopoietic tissue (connective tissue), which forms blood cells.
4. Assist in regulation of calcium and phosphate concentrations.

Long Bones

A. Diaphysis: long, central shaft.
B. Epiphysis: the end of a long bone.
1. Covered by hyaline cartilage.
2. Auricular surface: the part of the epiphysis that contacts other bones.
C. Periosteum: adhering sheath of connective tissue covering bone.
D. Internal structures.
1. Central medullary cavity: contains yellow marrow composed of fat.
2. Surface layer: an ivory-like, dense, compact bone.
3. Cancellous bone: a spongy layer below the surface layer. It contains small cavities that merge with a large central cavity.
4. Red marrow: consists of hematopoietic tissue, macrophages, and fat cells. Fills the spaces between spongy bone.

Joints

Definition: Joints, also called articulations, are regions where two or more bones meet. Joints hold bones together while allowing movement.
A. Classification.
1. Synarthrosis: fibrous or fixed joints (immovable).
2. Amphiarthrosis: cartilaginous or slightly movable joint.
3. Diarthrosis: synovial or freely movable joint.
   a. Ball and socket.
   b. Condyloid.
B. Function.
1. Articulation is the meeting place of two or more joints.
2. Assist in type and range of movement between bones.
C. Synovial fluid.
1. Function.
   a. Lubricate the cartilage.
   b. Cushion shocks.
   c. Provide a nutrient source.
2. Structure.
   a. Fluid formed by the synovial membrane.
   b. Synovial membrane lines the joint capsule, which contains the fluid.

System Assessment

A. Observe for signs of a fracture.
1. Assess for specific type of fracture.
✦ 2. Observe all suspected fracture sites for edema, pain, and obvious deformities.
B. Assess for possible complications associated with a cast.
C. Evaluate client for complications associated with joint disorders.
D. Observe for complications of amputation.
1. Observe for presence of phantom limb pain.
2. Assess stump dressings for bleeding and/or signs of infection.
E. Observe for complications of hip surgery.
1. Observe position in bed of clients with hip fractures to identify potential complications associated with hip flexion.
2. Assess for signs of shock and hemorrhage following surgery.
3. Evaluate need for client instruction on exercises, positioning, and crutch walking.

CMS

- Circulatory assessment: check digits for color, temperature, capillary refill and edema.
  a. Inadequate arterial flow: pallor, slow capillary filling (> 2 seconds) and coolness to touch.
  b. Inadequate venous return: cyanosis, mottling, and increased temperature.
- Neurologic assessment: motion and sensation.

---

    4.   Evaluate client's need for rehabilitation program.

F. Observe circulation, motion, and sensation (CMS) for all orthopedic clients.

G. Assess skin and neurovascular status before, during and after any immobilizing modality—compare contralateral extremity and baseline data.

H. Inspect and palpate the client's bones for any sign of obvious deformity or changes in size or shape. Palpation will elicit pain and tenderness; assess for warmth and crepitation.

I. Measure extremities for length and circumference—compare bilaterally.

J. Assess muscle mass and strength—compare bilaterally.

JOINT AND NERVE DISEASES

Rheumatoid Arthritis

Definition: Chronic, systemic, autoimmune, inflammatory disease affecting the joints. Usual onset is from 30 to 50 years of age, but can occur at any age. Etiology remains a mystery.

Assessment

A. Evaluate for bilateral joint involvement (erythema, warm, tender, painful).

B. Assess for insidious onset of malaise, weight loss, paresthesia, stiffness.

C. Assess pain and stiffness early in morning (subsides with moderate activity).

D. Observe for subcutaneous nodules.

E. Assess low-grade temperature.

F. Observe for anemia with fatigue and weakness.

G. Check for pattern of joint involvement—from small joints to knees, spine, etc.

H. Assess for limitation of function and deformities of hands and feet.

I. Laboratory and diagnostic tests.
    1. Rheumatoid factor (RF)—present in about 80 percent of people with RA. High levels are associated with progressive disease and poorer prognosis.

    2. ANA titer, CRP, and ESR are elevated due to active inflammation.

    3. CBC—usually shows anemia.

    4. Synovial fluid—shows inflammatory changes: increased turbidity, decreased viscosity, increased protein levels, 3000 to 50,000 WBCs/μL with PMNs (circulating neutrophils) predominating.

    5. X-ray—few changes with early disease. As disease progresses there are joint changes.

Implementation

A. Instruct client on medications and side effects. Chemotherapy reduces inflammation and relieves pain.
    1. Salicylates.
      a. ASA most common.
      b. Side effects include tinnitus, GI upset, prolonged bleeding time.
    2. Nonsteroidal anti-inflammatory drugs (NSAIDs).
      a. Phenylbutazone, indomethacin, Motrin, Naprosyn, Nalfon, Ansaid.
      b. Side effects include GI disturbances, CNS manifestations, skin rashes.
    3. Antimalarials.
      a. Remission-inducing agents.
      b. May cause ocular toxicity—ophthalmic exam twice yearly indicated.
    4. Gold salts (chrysotherapy).
      a. Effective after 3–4 months.
      b. Toxicity can be severe.
    5. Alternative to gold is an oral chelating agent, pencillamine (Cuprimine). Drug has an anti-inflammatory action.
    6. Antimetabolics—for clients who don't respond to NSAIDs.
      a. Methotrexate.
      b. Azathioprine (Imuran).
      c. Cyclophosphamide (Cytoxan).
    7. Corticosteroids: adjunct therapy only.
      a. Used during exacerbations or severe involvement.
      b. Low dose to prevent toxicity.
      c. Prednisone, Cortef.

B. Instruct client how to preserve joint function.

C. Provide rest periods throughout day.

D. Instruct client in diet control.

E. Provide psychological support for altered body image and living with chronic disease.

F. Prevent flexion contractures and promote exercise.
    1. Initiate range-of-motion exercises.
    2. Avoid weight bearing for inflamed joints.
    3. Give warm baths and exercises.

G. Prepare for surgery if severe joint involvement.

Table 8-6. COMPARISON OF RHEUMATOID ARTHRITIS AND OSTEOARTHRITIS

Characteristics	Rheumatoid Arthritis	Osteoarthritis
Disease	Systemic with exacerbations and remissions	Localized; course varies and is progressive
Laboratory findings	RF + in 80% of clients Elevated ESR, CRP indicating active inflammation	RF negative Transient elevation of ESR related to synovitis
X-ray	Joint space narrowing and erosion with bony overgrowths, subluxation with advanced disease; osteoporosis related to corticosteroid use	Joint space narrowing, osteophytes, subchondral cysts, sclerosis
Age of onset	Young to middle age	Usually > 40
Gender	Female/male 2:1 or 3:1, less marked differences after age 60	< 50 more men than women, > 50 more women than men
Weight	Lost or maintained	Often overweight
Joints affected	Usually bilateral and symmetric small first joints, wrists, elbows, shoulders, and knees	Often asymmetric response seen in weight-bearing joints of knees and hips, small joints, cervical, lumbar spine
Pain	Stiffness lasts 1 hour to all day and may decrease with use; pain is variable and may disrupt sleep	Stiffness occurs on arising but usually subsides after 30 minutes; pain gradually worsens with joint use and time, lessens with rest
Effusions	Common	Uncommon
Nodules	Present, especially on extensor surfaces	Heberden's and Bouchard's nodes
Synovial fluid	WBC > 20,000 μL with mostly neutrophils	WBC < 2000 μL mild leukocytosis
Drug therapy	Disease-modifying antirheumatic drugs (DMARDs) NSAIDs Intra-articular or systemic corticosteroids Biologic/targeted therapy	Acetaminophen NSAIDs Antibiotics Intra-articular hyaluronic acid Intra-articular corticosteroids Opioid analgesics
Surgery	Reconstructive joint surgery Implants Arthroplasty	Reconstructive joint surgery

1. Synovectomy.
2. Joint replacement.

Osteoarthritis

Definition: Hypertrophic degeneration of joints. Cartilage that covers the ends of bones disintegrates.

Characteristics

A. Disorder strikes joints that receive the most stress (e.g., knees, toes, lower spine). Distal finger joint involvement is usually seen in women.
B. Pain and stiffness in the joints.

Implementation

A. Instruct client on well-balanced diet.
✦ B. Prevent permanent disability.
   1. Plan exercise to prevent joint fixation.
   2. Provide exercise periods to increase muscle tone.
   3. Control exercise periods to prevent fatigue.
C. Maintain proper positioning.
   1. Align and frequently change position to prevent complications.
   2. Encourage and support client as frequent movements cause pain.
✦ D. Apply heat for relief of pain.
   1. Dry heat with a heat lamp to relieve stiffness.
   2. Moist heat with hot tubs, hot towels, or paraffin baths for the hands.
E. Provide adequate rest—10–12 hours per day.
F. Administer medications as ordered and teach client about side effects.
✦   1. Salicylates most common for relief of pain.
   2. Side effects of ASA include tinnitus, nausea and prolonged bleeding time.
   3. Anti-inflammatory drugs (cortisone) reduce the effects of inflammation thus decreasing pain, swelling and stiffness.
   4. NSAIDs.
     a. COX-2 inhibitors: Celebrex.
     b. Ibuprofen.

G. Physicians now prescribing natural Rx—glucosamine—for pain and stiffness.

Gout

✦ *Definition:* A disease caused by a defect in purine metabolism marked by urate deposits, which cause painful arthritic joints. Affects men over 50 years of age.

Assessment

✦ A. Assess joints (especially big toe) for pain, inflammation, tenderness, presence of urate deposits, and warm to touch.

B. Assess for low-grade temperature.

✦ C. Evaluate serum uric acid and elevated urinary uric acid.

Implementation

A. Maintain bedrest during acute attack.

B. Immobilize inflamed, painful joints.

✦ C. Administer ordered medications.
   1. Analgesics for pain.
   ✦ 2. Anti-inflammatory agents.
       a. Colchicine PO or IV every hour × 8 hours until pain subsides or nausea, vomiting, cramping, or diarrhea occurs.
       b. Phenylbutazone or indomethacin may be used.
       c. Corticosteroids.
   ✦ 3. Allopurinol to decrease serum uric acid levels.
   4. Uricosuric agents to promote uric acid excretion and inhibit uric acid accumulation (Probenecid, Sulfinpyrazone).

✦ D. Instruct client on low-purine diet and avoidance of alcohol.
   1. *See* Chapter 4 for foods on a low-purine diet.
   2. If client is obese, place on weight-reduction diet.

✦ E. Force fluids to at least 2000 mL to prevent stone formation.

F. Maintain urine pH above 6 with alkalinizing agent.

Carpal Tunnel Syndrome

✦ *Definition:* A syndrome caused by compression of the median nerve as a result of inflammation and swelling of the synovial lining of the tendon sheaths. Repetitive use causes irritation of the tendon sheaths.

Assessment

A. Pain in the wrist.

✦ B. Numbness and tingling of the fingers, especially the thumb, index finger and lateral ventral surface of the middle finger.

C. Pain often worse at night, awakens client; may be relieved by shaking hand or massage.

D. Diagnosis.
   1. History.
   2. Physical exam.
   3. Electrodiagnostic study—use of probe to measure carpal tunnel.

✦ Implementation

A. Surgery (more painful, slow recovery).

B. Endoscopic carpal tunnel release (ECTR).

C. Activity modification, splinting, injection of steroids, NSAIDs.

D. Alternative therapy: vitamin B_6 supplementation.

ORTHOPEDIC AND VASCULAR CONDITIONS

Osteoporosis

Definition: Decrease in the amount of bone capable of maintaining structural integrity of the skeleton. Etiology is unknown. Loss of bone mass is associated with aging and increases fragility and risk of fractures.

Characteristics

A. Factors that contribute to condition.
   1. Bone remodeling results in increased bone mass until age 35; thereafter, bone mass decreases.
   ✦ 2. Nutritional factors.
       a. Lack of vitamin D.
       b. Deficient calcium (minimum 800 mg; for women with decreased bone mass, 1200 mg).
       c. Low estrogen levels after menopause.
   ✦ 3. Excessive intake of drugs (corticosteroids).
   4. Coexisting medical conditions (malabsorption, lactose intolerance, alcohol abuse, renal failure).
   5. Immobility causes bone to be reabsorbed faster than it is formed.

B. Diagnostic tests.
   1. Routine x-ray when there is 25–45 percent demineralization.
   2. Single-photon absorptiometry identifies degree of bone mass in wrist.
   3. Dual-photon absorptiometry identifies bone loss at hip or spine.
   4. Laboratory studies exclude other diagnoses.
   ✦ 5. Quantitative computed tomography (QCT) of the spine is the most sensitive test to detect osteoporosis.
   6. Dual-energy x-ray absorptiometry (DEXA) of the lumbar spine or hip is the most accurate method for measuring bone density—it is highly accurate and delivers negligible radiation.
   7. Serum bone Gla-protein (osteocalcin) is used as a marker for osteoclastic activity and indicates

rate of bone turnover. It is most useful to evaluate treatment rather than as an indicator of the severity of the disease.

Assessment

A. Assess for backache with pain radiating around trunk.
B. Evaluate for skeletal deformities.
C. Assess for pathologic fractures.
✦ D. Evaluate lab findings.
   1. Serum calcium, phosphorus, and alkaline phosphatase are usually normal.
   2. Parathyroid hormone may be elevated.

Implementation

A. Provide pain control.
   1. Application of heat/cold.
   2. Medications to prevent pain—NSAIDs.
✦ B. Prevent fractures.
   1. Instruct in safety factors—watch steps, avoid use of scatter rugs.
   2. Keep siderails up to prevent falls.
   3. Move gently when turning and positioning.
   4. Assist with ambulation if unsteady on feet.
✦ C. Administer medications.
   1. Estrogen replacement therapy decreases osteoporosis (Estratab, Estroderm, Premarin); currently controversial as study suggests that Premarin and Provera (synthetic progesterone) significantly increase risk of cancer.
   2. Calcium—prevents osteoporosis; found in milk, dairy products, yogurt, oysters, canned sardines, salmon, dark green leafy vegetables.
   3. Calcitonin—prevents further bone loss and increases bone mass.
   4. Fluoride—decreases solubility of bone mineral and rate of bone reabsorption.
   5. Fosamax—a form of bisphosphonate. FDA warning—osteonecrosis of the jaw (jaw death) from taking this drug.
   6. Calcium and vitamin D—support bone metabolism.
D. Instruct in regular exercise program.
  ✦ 1. Range-of-motion and weight-bearing exercises.
   2. Ambulation several times per day.
E. Instruct in good use of body mechanics.
F. Provide diet high in protein, calcium, vitamin D (adequate sunlight); avoid excesses of alcohol and coffee.

Compartment Syndrome

Definition: Following an injury that causes swelling, pressure increases in a muscle fascial compartment. Muscles, nerves and blood vessels are compressed, causing ischemia.

Characteristics

A. Pressure in the muscle compartment can be increased by edema or hematoma.
B. Stricture around the limb or reperfusion following restoration of blood flow can result in this condition.

Assessment

A. Monitor extremity for
   1. Pain: Is it out of proportion to the injury? Does it increase on active and passive motion or elevation of extremity?
   2. Pallor.
   3. Paresthesia or numbness.
   4. Cold extremity compared to the other extremity.
   5. Pulselessness in affected extremity.
   6. Pain unrelieved by medication.
B. Measure compartment pressure using an intracompartmental monitor (normal is less than 10 mm Hg; 20 mm Hg or more may cause ischemia).

Implementation

A. Position limb at level of client's heart (elevation higher may increase ischemia).
B. Initiate IV line and administer pain medication.
C. Do not apply cold or heat without orders—may further compromise circulation.
D. Prepare for surgery—fasciotomy to release pressure and skin grafting to decrease risk of sepsis.

Osteomyelitis

✦ *Definition:* An infection of the bone—it may occur as an acute, subacute or chronic process. Cause is usually bacterial, with *Staphylococcus aureus* the most common organism. May be caused by fungi, parasites, and viruses.

✦ ### Assessment

A. Signs of infection.
   1. Tachycardia.
   2. Nausea, vomiting, anorexia.
   3. Involved extremity is limp.
   4. Localized tenderness, especially in epiphyseal area.
   5. Drainage and ulceration at involved site.
   6. Swelling, erythema, and warmth at involved site.
   7. Lymph node involvement, especially in involved extremity.
   8. High temperature, abrupt onset of pain, malaise.
B. Laboratory and diagnostic tests.
   1. X-rays.
   2. MRI—shows epidural abscess.
   3. CT—detects sequestra, sinus tract, and soft-tissue abscess.

4. Bone scan—determines if infection is active.
5. Ultrasound—detects fluid collection, abscesses, and thickening.
6. ESR—elevated in acute episode, normal in chronic osteomyelitis.
7. WBC—elevated.
8. Blood and tissue culture—determines infecting organism—directs antibiotic therapy.

Implementation

✦ A. Prevent transmission of infection.
   1. Strict hand hygiene.
   2. Administer antimicrobials.
   3. Maintain calorie and protein intake.
✦ B. Prevent hyperthermia.
   1. Monitor temperature every 4 hours.
   2. Maintain cool environment.
   3. Ensure daily fluid intake 2000–3000 mL daily.
C. Improve physical mobility.
   1. Maintain limb in a functional position.
   2. Maintain rest, avoid subjecting affected extremity to weight-bearing activities.
   3. Ensure active or passive range of motion (ROM) every 4 hours.
D. Control of pain.
   1. Splint or immobilize to decrease pain caused by movement.
   2. Provide pain medications 20–30 minutes prior to planned activities.
   3. Warm moist packs.
   4. Assistive devices.
   5. Gentle handling and minimal manipulation.
E. Provide emotional support.
✦ F. Medications.
   1. Parenteral antibiotics begun as soon as cultures are obtained.
   2. Penicillinase-resistant medication (methicillin, oxacillin) may be given until culture and sensitivity results are known.
   3. IV therapy usually given for 4–6 weeks.
   4. Ciprofloxacin PO BID is effective and sometimes used.
G. Surgical treatment.
   1. Needle biopsy or aspiration.
   2. Surgical debridement.

Osteomalacia

✦ *Definition:* A metabolic bone disorder characterized by inadequate mineralization of bone matrix.

Characteristics

A. Rarely occurs in the United States; now increasing in older adults and those on vegetarian diet.
✦ B. Causes.
   1. Vitamin D deficiency.
   2. Phosphate depletion.
   3. Systemic acidosis.

Assessment

A. Evaluate bone pain.
B. Assess for difficulty changing from lying to sitting position.
C. Muscle weakness.
D. Waddling gait.
E. Dorsal kyphosis.
F. Pathological fractures.
G. Lab and diagnostic tests.

Implementation

A. Maintain adequate nutrition.
B. Minimize risk for injury.
C. Promote physical mobility.
✦ D. Administer medications.
   1. Vitamin D to raise serum calcium.
   2. Pain medication.

Fractures

Definition: A break in the continuity of bone caused by trauma, twisting, or as a result of bone decalcification.

Assessment

A. Signs of a fracture.
   ✦ 1. Cardinal signs of a fracture.
      a. Pain or tenderness over involved area.
      b. Loss of function of the extremity.
      c. Deformity.
         (1) Overriding.
         (2) Angulation: limb is in an unnatural position.
   2. Crepitation: sound of grating bone fragments.
   3. Ecchymosis or erythema.
   4. Edema.
   5. Muscle spasm.
B. Evaluate cause of fracture.
   1. Fatigue—muscles are less supportive to bone and, therefore, cannot absorb the force being exerted.
   2. Bone neoplasms—cellular proliferations of malignant cells replace normal tissue causing a weakened bone.
   3. Metabolic disorders—poor mineral absorption and hormonal changes decrease bone calcification which results in a weakened bone.
   4. Bedrest or disuse—atrophic muscles and osteoporosis cause decreased stress resistance.
C. Identify whether break is intracapsular: bone broken inside the joint; or extracapsular: fracture outside the joint.

D. Identify whether fracture is stable or unstable.
   1. Stable (nondisplaced)—a fracture in which the bones maintain their anatomic alignment.
   2. Unstable (displaced)—a fracture in which the bones move out of correct anatomic alignment.

Implementation

A. Evaluate type of treatment used for fracture.
   1. Traction.
   ✦ 2. Reduction (restoring bone to proper alignment).
      a. Closed reduction.
         (1) Manual manipulation.
         (2) Usually done under anesthesia to reduce pain and relax muscles, thereby preventing complications.
         (3) Cast is usually applied following closed reduction.
      b. Open reduction.
         (1) Surgical intervention.
         (2) Usually treated with internal fixation devices (screws, plates, wires, etc.).
         (3) Following surgery, client can be placed in traction; however, client is usually placed in cast.
   3. Cast.
✦ B. Fracture healing.
   1. Occurs over several weeks.
   2. New bone tissue occurs in region of break.
   3. Repair is initiated by migration of blood vessels and connective tissue from periosteum in break area.
   4. Dense fibrous tissue fills in the break and forms a callus (temporary union).
   5. Types of cells.
      a. Osteoblast: near the broken area.
      b. Chondroblast: farther away from broken area.
   6. Cells deposit cartilage between broken surfaces.
   7. Cartilage is slowly replaced by mineralized bone tissue, which completes repair.
   8. Fractures are a common injury in children even though bones can be bent 45 degrees before breaking.
✦ C. Emergency care of fractures.
   1. Immobilize affected extremity to prevent further damage to soft tissue or nerve.
   2. If compound fracture is evident, do not attempt to reduce it.
      a. Apply splint.
      b. Cover open wound with sterile dressing.
   3. Splinting.
      a. External support is applied around a fracture to immobilize the broken ends.

✦ TYPES OF FRACTURE

- Greenstick.
  1. A crack; the bending of a bone with incomplete fracture. Affects only one side of the periosteum.
  2. Common in skull fractures or in young children when bones are pliable.
- Comminuted.
  1. Bone completely broken in a transverse, spiral or oblique direction (indicates the direction of the fracture in relation to the long axis of the fracture bone).
  2. Bone broken into several fragments.
- Open or compound.
  1. Bone is exposed to the air through a break in the skin.
  2. Can be associated with soft-tissue injury as well.
  3. Infection is common complication due to exposure to bacterial invasion.
- Closed or simple.
  1. Skin remains intact.
  2. Chances are greatly decreased for infection.
- Compression.
  1. Frequently seen with vertebral fractures.
  2. Fractured bone has been compressed by other bones.
- Complete: bone is broken with a disruption of both sides of the periosteum.
- Impacted: one part of fractured bone is driven into another.
- Depressed fracture.
  1. Usually seen in skull or facial fractures.
  2. Bone or fragments of bone are driven inward.
- Pathological: break caused by disease process.

---

      b. Materials used: wood, plastic (air splints), magazines.
   4. Function of splinting.
      a. Prevent additional trauma.
      b. Reduce pain.
      c. Decrease muscle spasm.
      d. Limit movement.
      e. Prevent complications, such as fat emboli if long bone fracture.
D. Provide specific care for fracture treatment.
   1. Traction.
   2. Cast.
   3. Surgical intervention.

Traction

Definition: The application of a pulling force to an injured or diseased part of the body or extremity while countertraction pulls in the opposite direction.

Purposes of Traction

A. Prevent or reduce muscle spasm.
B. Immobilize a joint or part of the body.
C. Reduce a fracture or a dislocation.
D. Treatment of a joint condition.

✦ Table 8-7. TYPES OF TRACTION

Type	Position	Purpose
✦ Skin Traction—usually short term; 48–72 degrees, until skeletal traction is applied or surgery is done		
Cervical	Flat in bed or head of bed elevated 15–20 degrees	Relieve muscle spasms and compression in upper extremities and neck
Buck's	Head of bed elevated 10–20 degrees for ADLs, knee flexed	Immobilize hip when fractured; relieve muscle spasms before hip surgery
Bryant's	Flat with 45- to 90-degree hip flexion; buttocks raised 1 inch from mattress, legs extended	Stabilize fractured femur; correct congenital hip in young children weighing less than 30 lb
Russell's	Head of bed can be elevated 30–45 degrees; hip flexion at 20 degrees	Stabilize fractured femur prior to surgery; some knee injuries
Pelvic girdle	Head of bed elevated, knee gatch elevated to same level (William's position)	Relieve low back, hip, or leg pain; reduce muscle spasm; herniated disc
✦ Skeletal Traction—used for longer periods of treatment than skin traction		
Blackburn, Gardner–Wells, Crutchfield, Vinke Tongs	Spine immobilized; bedrest, supine position	Provide for hyperextension; traction allows vertebrae to slip back into position
Halo traction	Flat, low-Fowler's in bed, ambulate, or sit up	Stabilize fractured or dislocated cervical vertebrae
✦ Balanced Suspension		
Steinmann pin, Kirschner wires, used with Thomas splint and Pearson attachment	Low-Fowler's, either side or back; bedrest in supine position	To align bone and approximate fractures of femur, tibia, fibula
External Fixation Devices Hoffman Synthes	Any position possible with device—allows client mobility and active exercise of uninvolved part	Manages complex fractures with soft-tissue damage; offers stability for comminuted fractures

E. Prevent soft-tissue damage by immobilization.

F. Reduce muscle spasm associated with low back pain or cervical whiplash.

G. Expand joint space during arthroscopic procedures.

H. Expand joint space during major joint reconstruction.

Assessment

A. Assess for type of traction ordered. (*See* Table 8-7 for types of traction devices.)

✦ B. Skeletal traction.

   1. Mechanical traction applied to bone, using pins (Steinmann), wires (Kirschner), or cervical tongs (Crutchfield, Gardner–Wells, halo external fixation).

   2. Most often used in fractures of femur, tibia, humerus, cervical spine.

   3. Balanced suspension traction.

      a. Thomas's splint with Pearson attachment is used in conjunction with skin or skeletal traction (used particularly with skeletal traction for fractured femur).

      b. Balanced suspension traction is produced by a counterforce other than the client.

✦ C. Skin traction.

   1. Traction applied by use of elastic bandages, moleskin strips, or adhesive.

   2. Used most often in alignment or lengthening (for congenital hip displacement, etc.) or to relieve muscle spasms in preop hip clients.

   3. Most common types.

      a. Russell traction.

      b. Buck's extension.

      c. Cervical traction (used for whiplashes and cervical spasm).

         (1) Pull is exerted on one plane.

         (2) Used for temporary immobilization.

      d. Pelvic traction (used for low back pain).

D. External fixation devices.

   1. Devices used for stabilizing bone or joint.

   2. Device has metal frame and percutaneous pins.

   3. Provides traction without ropes or weights so client has mobility.

E. Assess for complications of immobility.

F. Assess for signs and symptoms of infection with skeletal traction.

G. Assess condition of skin for possible breakdown.

Implementation

A. Check traction equipment.
1. Check the ropes for fraying.
2. Make sure ropes are in the center of the pulley.
3. Check the weights for correct number of pounds and if weights are hanging free.

✦ B. Maintain body alignment through proper care of traction.
 ✦ 1. Ensure that weights remain hanging freely and do not touch the floor.
 2. Ensure that pulleys are not obstructed.
 ✦ 3. Check that ropes in the pulley move freely.
 4. Secure knot in rope to prevent slipping.
 ✦ 5. Keep client up in bed, in direct line with traction and proper countertraction.
 6. Do not remove or lift weights without specific order. (Exceptions are pelvic and cervical traction that clients can remove at intervals.)
 ✦ 7. Cover sharp edges on traction apparatus with hollowed-out rubber balls to prevent injury to personnel.
 ✦ 8. Maintain counterbalance or correct pull.
  a. Pull is exerted against traction in opposite direction (balanced suspension).
  b. Pull is exerted against a fixed point.
  c. Bed is elevated under area involved to provide the countertraction.

C. Provide firm mattress or bedboards.

D. Monitor for complications.
1. Neurovascular compromise.
2. Inadequate bone alignment.
3. Skin or soft-tissue injury.
4. Pin-site infection.
5. Osteomyelitis.

E. Provide range-of-motion exercises for unaffected extremities.

✦ F. Prevent footdrop.
1. Provide footplate.
2. Encourage dorsiflexion exercises.

G. Provide overhead trapeze to allow client to assist in activities (turning, moving up in bed, using bedpan, etc.).

H. Prevent complications associated with immobility (p. 368).

✦ Balanced Skeletal Traction

A. Maintain proper alignment and check traction mechanism.
1. Weights hanging freely, off floor and bed.
2. Knots secure in all ropes.
3. Rope should move freely through pulleys.
4. Pulleys not constrained by knots.

B. Protect skin from excoriation.
1. Check around top of Thomas splint.
2. Pad with cotton wadding or ABDs.

C. Prevent pressure points around the top of Thomas splint keeping client pulled up in bed.

✦ D. Provide pin-site care.
1. Observe pin or tong insertion site for migration or drainage, odors, erythema, edema (usually indication of inflammatory process of infection).
2. Watch for skin breakdown if bandage is used to apply traction.
3. Cover ends of pins or wires with rubber stoppers or cork to prevent injury to nursing personnel or client.
4. Cleanse area surrounding insertion site of pin or tongs with antimicrobial solution. Some physicians order antibiotic ointments to be applied to area or order "no pin-site care."

E. Maintain at least 20-degree angle from thigh to the bed.

F. Provide footplate to prevent footdrop.

G. Keep heels clear of Pearson attachment to prevent skin breakdown and pressure sores.

H. Position client frequently from side to side (as ordered). Place table on unaffected side.

I. Unless contraindicated, elevate head of bed for comfort and to facilitate adequate respiratory functions.

J. Do not remove traction without a physician's order.

Halo Traction

A. Complete a neurologic assessment.
1. Cranial, peripheral nerves at base of skull—this area is prone to injury.
2. Check motion and sensation.

B. Check alignment—neck should not be flexed or extended.

C. Safety issues.
 ✦ 1. Keep Allen wrench taped to front of vest in case of emergency (need for CPR).
 2. Client is top heavy with limited view—remove obstacles when walking.
 3. Have emergency tracheostomy tray and bag-valve-mask available on unit.
 4. Never use bars of halo brace to move client.

D. Inspect pin site for drainage, crusting or inflammation.

E. Provide skin care under vest.

✦ Skin Traction

✦ A. Buck's extension.
1. Apply foam boot appliance with Velcro fastener.
2. Attach a foot block with a spreader and rope that goes into a pulley.

3. Attach weight to pulley and hang freely over edge of bed (not more than 8–10 pounds of weight can be applied).

4. Observe and readjust bandages for tightness and smoothness (can cause constriction that leads to edema or even nerve damage).

5. Do not apply Buck's traction over or under a calf compression device. Foot pumps are allowed to prevent DVT.

✦ B. Cervical traction.
   1. Use head harness (or halter).
      a. Pad chin.
      b. Protect ears from friction rub.
   2. Elevate head of bed and attach weights to pulley system over head of bed.
   3. Observe for skin breakdown.
      a. Be sure to keep skin dry in areas encased in the halter.
      b. Place back of head on padding.

C. Pelvic traction.
   1. Apply girdle snugly over client's pelvis and iliac crest; attach to weights.
   2. Observe for pressure points over iliac crest.
   3. Keep client in good alignment.
   4. May raise foot of bed slightly (30 cm) to prevent client from slipping down in bed.

External Fixation Devices

A. Check pin site for signs of infection.

B. Provide pin site care (*see* p. 367).

C. Check neurovascular status (circulation, motion, and sensation) every 4 hours; client may have extensive soft-tissue and vessel damage.

D. Instruct client to keep extremity elevated if edema is present.

Cast Care

A. After application of cast, allow 24–48 hours for drying. For synthetic cast, allow 30 minutes; 60 minutes for weight bearing.
   ✦ 1. Cast will change from dull to shiny substance when dry.
   2. Heat can be applied to assist in drying process.

✦ B. Do not handle cast during drying process, because indentation from fingermarks can cause skin breakdown under cast.

✦ C. Keep extremity elevated to prevent edema and promote venous return.

✦ D. Provide for smooth edges surrounding cast.
   1. Smooth edges prevent crumbling and breaking down of edges.
   2. Stockinet can be pulled over edge and fastened down with adhesive tape to outside of cast.

> ### CMS INTERVENTION
>
> • **Circulation**—report if
>   a. Digits are swollen despite elevation and active exercise.
>   b. Digits are pale, blue, or cool to touch.
>   c. There is delayed capillary refill (> 2 seconds).
> • **Motion**—report if
>   a. There is pain on passive movement.
>   b. Strength of action is unequal in both extremities.
> • **Sensation**—report if
>   a. Pain increases; there is pain with passive motion of digits or when extremity is elevated.
>   b. Client complains of numbness or paresthesia (pins and needles sensation).

E. Observe casted extremity for signs of circulatory impairment. Cast may have to be cut if edematous condition continues.

✦ F. Always observe for signs and symptoms of complications: pain, swelling, discoloration, tingling or numbness, diminished or absent pulse, paralysis, pain, cool to touch.

G. If there is an open, draining area on the affected extremity, a window (cut-out portion of cast) can be utilized for observation and/or irrigation of wound.

H. Keep cast dry.
   1. Breaks down when water comes in contact with plaster.
   2. Use plastic bags or plastic-coated bed Chux during the bath or when using bedpan, to protect cast material.
   3. Synthetic cast can be cleaned—does not easily break down.

I. Utilize isometric exercises to prevent muscle atrophy and to strengthen the muscle. Isometrics prevent joint from being immobilized.

J. Position client with pillows to prevent strain on unaffected areas.

K. Turn every 2 hours to prevent complications. Encourage client to lie on abdomen 4 hours a day.

Complications of Immobilization

✦ A. Prevent respiratory complications.
   1. Have client cough and deep-breathe every 2 hours.
   2. Turn every 2 hours if not contraindicated.
   3. Provide suction if needed.

✦ B. Prevent thrombus and emboli formation.
   1. Apply antiembolic stockings.
   2. Initiate isometric and isotonic exercises.
   3. Start anticoagulation therapy, if indicated.
   4. Turn every 2 hours.
   5. Observe for signs and symptoms of pulmonary and/or fat emboli.

COMPLICATIONS OF IMMOBILIZATION

Many nursing interventions will prevent complications of immobilization.

Interventions	Purpose
Turn and position client every 2 hours if not contraindicated	Prevent respiratory complications Prevent thrombus and emboli formation Prevent contractures Prevent skin breakdown
Encourage fluids	Prevent skin breakdown Prevent urinary retention and calculi Prevent constipation
Monitor intake and output	Prevent skin breakdown Prevent urinary retention and calculi

◆ C. Prevent contractures.
 1. Start range-of-motion exercises to affected joints QID, all joints BID.
 2. Provide foot board and/or foot cradle.
 3. Position and turn every 2 hours.
◆ D. Prevent skin breakdown.
 1. Massage with lotion once a day to prevent drying.
 2. Use alcohol for back care to toughen skin.
 3. Massage elbows, coccyx, heels BID.
 4. Turn every 2 hours.
 5. Alternate pressure mattress, sheepskin.
 6. Use Stryker boots or heel protectors.
 7. Use elbow guards.
E. Prevent urinary retention and calculi.
 1. Encourage fluids.
 2. Monitor intake and output.
 3. Administer urinary antiseptic (Mandelamine, etc.).
 4. Offer bedpan every 4 hours.
F. Prevent constipation.
 1. Encourage fluids.
 2. Provide high-fiber diet.
 3. Administer laxative or enema as ordered.
 4. Offer bedpan at same time each day—encourage to establish good bowel habits.
G. Provide psychological support.
 1. Allow client to vent about feelings of dependence.
 2. Encourage independence when possible (bathing, self-feeding, etc.).
 3. Encourage visitors for short time periods.
 4. Provide diversionary activities (television, newspapers, etc.).

Fractured Ribs

◆ Assessment

A. Assess lung sounds for pneumothorax or hemothorax.

B. Examine chest excursion for asymmetry.
◆ C. Assess for shock.
 1. Monitor vital signs every hour until stable.
 2. Check color and warmth every 2 hours.
 3. Check LOC.
 4. Observe for restlessness.
D. Evaluate pain and need for analgesic.
E. Evaluate need for chest tubes.

Implementation

A. Provide nursing intervention for shock.
 1. Administer oxygen as indicated.
 2. Administer IV if signs of shock present.
 3. Keep lightly covered.
 4. Have chest tube insertion tray available.
B. Relieve pain from muscle spasms and fractures.
 ◆ 1. Give pain medication 30 minutes before any movement.
 2. Change position every 2 hours.
 3. Use pillows for support.
 4. Place client in semi-Fowler's position.
◆ C. Prevent complications of immobility.
 1. Cough and deep-breathe every 2 hours to prevent hypostatic pneumonia.
 2. Turn to unaffected side and back every 2 hours.
 3. Maintain skin care to prevent pressure sores and circulatory impairment.
  a. Back care.
  b. Heel, elbow, coccyx massage.
 4. Institute leg exercises to prevent circulatory impairment.
 5. Prevent constipation and flatus.
  a. Insert rectal tube (no more than 20 minutes at a time).
  b. Provide stool softener.
  c. Maintain diet high in bulk and fiber.
  d. Force fluids.
 6. Chest strapping is avoided as much as possible because it limits expansion and may lead to pneumonia and atelectasis.

Hip Conditions

Characteristics

A. High incidence in elderly group—hip fractures most common cause of traumatic death after age 75.
B. Fractures caused by brittle bones (osteoporosis) and frequent falls in the elderly.
C. Elderly clients with hip fractures frequently have associated medical conditions (cardiovascular, renal disorders).

Assessment

◆ A. Evaluate types of fracture.

✦ 1. *Intracapsular* (within the joint capsule); head or neck of the femur.
   a. Treated by internal fixation—replacement of femoral head with Austin Moore prosthesis.
   b. Occasionally, primary total hip replacement.
   c. Usually placed in skin traction first for immobilization and relief of muscle spasm.
   d. Client can be out of bed without weight bearing in 1–2 days postoperatively (depending on other physical problems).

✦ 2. *Extracapsular:* trochanteric fracture outside the joint.
   ✦ a. Fracture of greater trochanter.
      (1) Can be treated by balanced suspension traction if little displacement of bone. Full weight bearing usually in 6–8 weeks, when healing takes place.
      (2) Surgical intervention is necessary if large displacement or extensive soft-tissue damage; usually internal fixation with wire.
   ✦ b. Intertrochanteric fracture.
      (1) Extends from medial region of the junction of the neck and lesser trochanter toward the summit of the greater trochanter.
      (2) Treated initially by balanced suspension traction.
      (3) Surgically treated early due to debilitated physical condition of most of these clients (usually 70 years and older with other system diseases like diabetes, hypertension, etc.).
      (4) Internal fixation used with nailplate, screws, and wire.
   ✦ c. Not allowed to flex hip to the side, on the side of the bed, or in a low chair. When hip is flexed, displacement can occur.

B. Assess for complications of immobility.

Implementation

✦ FOR CLIENTS OTHER THAN HIP PROSTHESIS

A. Hemovac will usually be in place to drain off excessive blood and fluid accumulation.
   1. Compute intake and output.
   2. Keep Hemovac compressed to facilitate drainage.

B. Have client perform bed exercises at least four times per day.
   1. Flex and extend foot, tense muscles, and straighten knee.
   2. Tighten buttocks, straighten knee, and push leg down in bed.
   3. Tighten stomach muscles by raising neck and shoulders.
   4. Stretch arms to head of bed and deep-breathe.

C. Change positions by raising head of bed.
   1. Gatch knees slightly to relieve strain on hips and back.
   2. Turn to unaffected side.
   3. Pivot into chair within 1–2 days postoperatively.

✦ HIP PROSTHESIS

A. Replacement of head of femur by Austin Moore prosthesis.

✦ B. Keep affected leg abducted to prevent dislocation of the prosthesis—use Charnley pillow.

✦ C. Make sure hip flexion angle does not exceed 60–80 degrees.

✦ D. Forbid client to flex hip while getting out of bed; forbid client to sit in low chair.
   1. Use high stools.
   2. Use wheelchairs with adjustable backs.
   3. Use commode extenders.

E. Elevate head of bed 30–40 degrees for meals only.

F. Turn client to unaffected side with pillow support between legs.

G. Ambulate in 2–4 days with partial weight bearing.

✦ TOTAL HIP REPLACEMENT

A. Replacement of both the acetabulum and the head of the femur with metal or plastic implants.

B. Used in degenerative diseases or when fracture of head of femur has occurred with nonunion.

✦ C. To prevent flexion, keep operative leg in abduction by use of pillows or abductor splints.
   1. Positioning is important (every 2 hours).
   2. Turn client about 45 degrees with aid of trapeze and pillows. Do not elevate bed more than 30–45 degrees.
   3. Do not turn to affected side unless specific orders.
   4. Maintain anti-rotation boot (if indicated) while client is supine, but remove when client is turned.
   5. When using fracture bedpan, instruct client to flex unoperated hip and use trapeze.

✦ D. Keep Hemovac in place until drainage has substantially decreased (24–96 hours).
   1. By 48 hours, drainage should be 30 mL in 8 hours.
   2. Check dressing to ensure patency of Hemovac.
   3. Observe drainage for signs of hemorrhage or infection.

E. Prevent edema and thrombus formation from venous stasis.

1. Incidence of deep vein thrombosis is 45–70 percent; of these, 20 percent develop pulmonary emboli.
2. Readjust antiembolic stockings at least every 4–8 hours.
3. Change position frequently by raising and lowering head of bed. When ordered, tilt bed to change positions.
4. Promote leg exercises—flexing feet and ankles.

F. Prevent infections—may be very dangerous.
   1. Monitor prophylactic antibiotics.
   2. Remove wand suction device as soon as possible to prevent infection.

G. Continuous passive motion (CPM) first day postop with increasing degrees of flexion to 90 degrees.

✦ H. Ambulate client carefully at bedside—first or second postoperative day.
   1. Do not allow client to bear weight on affected hip.
   2. Up with walker second postoperative day.
   ✦ 3. Avoid positions with greater than 90 degrees flexion such as sitting straight up in a chair.
   4. Use commode extenders.
   5. Use wheelchair with adjustable back.
   6. Use high stools.

I. Start physical therapy after 3–4 days.

INSTRUCT CLIENT NOT TO

- Cross legs at ankle or knee.
- Stand with toes turned in.
- Flex hips greater than 90 degrees or sit with knees lower than hips.
- Sit in bathtub—use showers.
- Bend over.
- Use low chairs or sit on edge of bed.

J. Observe for neurovascular problems in affected leg.
   1. Capillary refill response in toes; pedal pulses in feet.
   2. Color and temperature in leg and toes.
   3. Edema in leg.
   4. Pain on passive flexion of foot.
   5. Numbness—ability to move leg.

KNEE SURGERY

Arthroscopy

Definition: Small incision in knee joint through which cartilage fragments are removed.

Assessment
A. Assess for pain, tenderness, decreased range of motion, clicking noise—torn cartilage (meniscus).
B. Assess for joint instability and pain—torn ligaments.

Implementation
A. Instruct client in surgical procedure for postoperative care.
   1. Arthroscopic meniscectomy—removal of torn cartilage fragments through small incision in knee joint using arthroscope.
   2. Open meniscectomy—direct surgical technique to knee joint for repair.
✦ B. Elevate leg to minimize swelling.
✦ C. Start client on quad-setting, straight-leg raising exercises. Should be done for 5 minutes every 30 minutes.
   1. Quad-setting: tightening or contracting the muscles of anterior thigh (kneecap is drawn up toward thigh).
   2. Straight-leg raising: lifting leg straight off the bed, keeping knee extended and foot in neutral position.
D. Apply ice bags to knee to reduce edema.
E. Ambulate first postoperative day without weight bearing (use three-point, crutch-walking gait).
F. In addition, give routine postoperative care.
G. Monitor for pulmonary embolism—complication of surgery.

Total Knee Arthroplasty

Definition: Implantation of a metallic upper portion that substitutes for the femoral condyles and a high-polymer plastic lower portion that substitutes for the tibial joint surfaces.

Assessment
A. Assess incisional area for drainage.
B. Observe for infection.
C. Observe for circulation, sensation, movement.

✦ Implementation
A. Control pain; client may have epidural or PCA for first 24 hours, then oral analgesic.
B. Monitor dressing and drainage if closed-wound drainage system is used.
C. Promote mobility.
   1. Continuous passive motion (CPM) may be ordered postop—moderate flexion and extension—increases circulation, movement, and prevents adhesion formation.
   ✦ 2. Have client perform quad-setting and straight-leg raising exercises every hour.
   3. Have client perform passive range-of-motion exercises.
D. Soft foam knee immobilizer, brace or splint is usually applied. (Nursing care is same as for any client in a splint.)
   1. If hinged splint (Bledsoe) is ordered, do not open or adjust without physician's order.

2. Assess skin and CMS every 4 hours.
◆ E. *Do not dangle* to prevent dislocation.
F. Monitor for signs of infection—a serious complication.
　1. Clients should remind physicians and dentists about prosthesis for prescribed antibiotics.
　2. Infection could occur 3 months or even a year after surgery.
G. Instruct client in crutch walking.
H. Client will be out of bed in 2–3 days.
I. Provide general postoperative care—monitor for pulmonary embolism. Anticoagulant therapy may be ordered prophylatically.

Crutch Walking

◆ A. Measure client for crutches.
　1. Distance between axilla and arm pieces on crutches should be two fingerwidths in axilla space—incorrect measurement could damage brachial plexus.
　2. Elbows should be slightly flexed when walking.
◆ B. Teach gait sequence.
　◆ 1. Four-point; crutch-foot sequence.
　　a. Move right crutch; move left foot; move left crutch; move right foot.
　　b. Gait is slow, but stable; client can bear weight on each leg.
　2. Three-point gait.
　　a. Client can bear little or no weight on one leg—two crutches support affected leg.
　　b. Move both crutches and affected leg forward; then move unaffected leg forward.

SPINAL SURGERY

Laminectomy, Discectomy, Etc.

Definition: Disorders of the vertebrae that require excision of vertebral posterior arch, removal of the nucleus of the disc or enlargement of the opening between discs.

◆ **Characteristics**
A. Laminectomy—removal of part of vertebral lamina.
B. Discectomy—removal of the nucleus pulposus of the intervertebral disc (may be performed alone or with laminectomy).
C. Foraminotomy—enlargement of the opening between the disc and the facet joint to remove overgrowth compressing the nerve.
D. Microdiscectomy—microsurgical techniques to remove nucleus pulposus of disc.

Assessment
◆ A. Evaluate for circulatory impairment.
　1. Check blanching.
　2. Observe color.

3. Check warmth of lower or upper extremities (depends on surgical site).
◆ B. Observe for sensation and motion in lower extremities (nerve root damage).
　1. Assess sensation.
　2. Check client's ability to wiggle toes and move feet; record ability to do plantar flexion, dorsiflexion of feet, toes and ankles.
◆ C. Observe dressings for spinal fluid leak, hemorrhage and infection. If present, notify physician.
　1. Use Dextrostix to test leakage. If positive for glucose, it is a very strong indicator that this is cerebrospinal fluid (CSF).
　2. Leaking CSF increases risk of infection to wound and meninges.
D. Note bowel sounds and bladder function.
E. Observe for respiratory problems—especially with cervical laminectomy.
◆ F. Assess for hematoma formation as manifested by severe incisional pain not relieved by medication. If left untreated, it may cause irreversible neurologic deficits.
◆ G. Assess for laryngeal nerve damage—may cause permanent hoarseness. Impaired ability to swallow puts the client at risk for aspiration.

Implementation
◆ A. Change client's position every 2 hours (by log-rolling) for at least 48 hours.
　1. Turn client as one unit by using drawsheet (or pull sheet), placing pillows between legs.
　2. Turn client to either side and back (unless contraindicated). Use support mechanisms when on side.
◆ B. Keep NPO until flatus and bowel sounds present.
C. Promote general range-of-motion exercises.
D. Ambulate client or have client lie in bed; sitting puts strain on surgical site.
E. Ambulate in 1–2 days postoperatively, unless contraindicated.
F. Provide general postoperative care.
G. Administer stronger pain medication postop, if on medication for a long time preoperatively.
H. Encourage fluid intake and diet rich in nutrients.
　1. Suggest increased intake of fruits and vegetables.
　2. Increased fiber to prevent constipation.
I. Encourage use of incentive spirometer.

Spinal Fusion

◆ *Definition:* The fusion of spinous processes—stabilizing the spine by removing bony chips from iliac crest and grafting them to fusion site.

For spinal cord injury, *see* page 183; for scoliosis, *see* page 699.

Assessment

A. Assess for spinal fluid leak or hemorrhage.
B. Measure vital signs; identify symptoms of infection.
C. Evaluate for circulatory, motion, sensation impairment.
D. Evaluate bladder and bowel function.

Implementation

✦ A. Maintain postoperative positioning.
    1. Some physicians keep client supine for first 8 hours to reduce possibility of compression.
    2. Most physicians keep client off back for first 48 hours.
✦ B. Provide ambulation. Starting ambulation varies with physicians, from 3–4 days to 8 weeks, depending on extent of fusion.
    1. Brace is applied when client is ambulated.
    2. Spine should be immobilized for early healing of bone graft and for new callus to form.
✦ C. Instruct client to *not* lift, bend, stoop, or sit for prolonged periods for at least 3 months.
D. Inform client grafts are stable by the end of the first year.
E. Explain there are some limitations to flexion of spine, depending on extent of fusion.
F. Provide additional interventions same as for laminectomy.

Harrington Rod Instrumentation

Used to treat scoliosis—*see* Chapter 13, page 699.

AMPUTATION

Definition: The surgical removal of a limb, a part of a limb, or a portion of a bone elsewhere than at the joint site. Removal of a bone at the joint site is termed disarticulation.

✦ Characteristics

A. Open type—guillotine—performed when infections are present, wound left open to drain; once infection is cleared, wound is closed.
B. Closed type—flap—wound is closed with a flap of skin.

Assessment

A. Evaluate dressings for signs of infection or hemorrhage.
B. Observe for signs of a developing necrosis or neuroma in incision.
C. Evaluate for phantom limb pain.
D. Observe for signs of contractures.

Implementation

✦ A. Provide preoperative nursing management.
    1. Have client practice lifting buttocks off bed while in sitting position.
    2. Provide range of motion to unaffected leg.
    3. Inform client about phantom limb sensation.
       a. Pain and feeling that amputated leg is still there; caused by nerves in the stump.
       b. Exercises lessen sensation.
✦ B. Provide postoperative nursing management.
    1. Observe stump dressing for signs of hemorrhage, infection or wound that will not heal.
       a. Keep tourniquet at bedside to control hemorrhage if necessary.
       b. Mark bleeding by circling drainage with pencil and marking date and time.
       c. Elevate foot of bed to prevent hemorrhage and to reduce edema first 24 hours ONLY. (Elevating the stump itself can cause a flexion contracture of hip joint.)
       d. Avoid dependent positioning of stump—to prevent edema and discomfort.
    2. Observe for symptoms of a developing necrosis or neuroma in area of incision.
✦   3. Provide stump care.
       a. Rewrap Ace bandage 3–4 times daily.
       b. Wash stump with mild soap and water.
       c. While washing stump, tap and massage skin toward incision line to prevent development of adhesions.
✦   4. Teaching related to stump care.
       a. Below-the-knee amputation—prevent edema formation.
         (1) Do not hang stump over edge of bed.
         (2) Do not sit for long periods of time.
       b. Above-the-knee amputation—prevent external or internal rotation of limb.
         (1) Place rolled towel along outside of thigh to prevent rotation.
         (2) Use low-Fowler's position to provide change in position.
✦   c. Position client with either type of amputation in prone position to stretch flexor muscles and to prevent flexion contractures of hip. Done usually after first 24–48 hours postoperative.
         (1) Place pillow under abdomen and stump.
         (2) Keep legs close together to prevent abduction.
       d. Teach use of ambulatory aids—crutch walking (started when client achieves stable balance) and wheelchair transfer.
✦   e. Prepare stump for prosthesis.
         (1) Stump must be conditioned for proper fit.
         (2) Shrinking and shaping stump to conical form by applying bandages or an elastic stump shrinker.

(3) A cast readies stump for the prosthesis.

  f. Provide care for temporary prosthesis, which is applied until stump has shrunk to permanent state.

5. Recognize and respond to client's psychological reactions to amputation.
    a. Feelings of loss, grieving.
    b. Loss of independence.
    c. Lowered self-image.
    d. Depression.

✦ 6. Continue discussing phantom limb pain with client.
    a. Feelings of pain in the part that has been amputated *will* eventually disappear.
    b. Occurs more frequently in above-the-knee amputation.
    c. TENS may provide relief.

FIBROMYALGIA (FMS)

Definition: A syndrome that effects about 2 percent of the population. The triad of symptoms that are the hallmark of the syndrome include long-lasting widespread pain (with tender points), sleep disturbances and fatigue.

Characteristics

A. Cause unknown—may be caused by genetic predisposition, a stressor such as an acute injury, an illness with fever, surgery, immune system depression or long-term psychosocial stress (sometimes childhood trauma).
B. Disease is difficult to diagnose because symptoms are common and laboratory results generally are normal.
C. Affects women between the ages of 30 and 50 years, and about 0.5 percent of men.
D. Central nervous system in people with fibromyalgia is not functioning properly and components of the body's stress response are responsible for symptoms.
   1. Sensory processing: experience great sensitivity not just to pain, but also to loud noises, bright lights, odors, drugs, temperature changes and chemicals.
   2. Substance P: threefold higher concentration in spinal fluid of this chemical that amplifies pain signals.
   3. Serotonin: low or processed poorly.

4. HPA axis: several abnormalities in the hypothalamic–pituitary–adrenal axis.

Assessment

A. General symptoms: pain and tenderness, fatigue, sleep disturbance, frequent headaches, cognitive difficulties, irritable bowel syndrome, urinary urgency and frequency, dry eyes and mouth, temporomandibular joint syndrome (TMJ), sensitivity to loud noises, unusual and uncontrollable eye movements.
B. Constitutional symptoms: weight fluctuations, heat and cold intolerance, night sweats, weakness.
C. "Allergic" symptoms: multiple chemical sensitivity, nasal congestion, rhinitis.
D. Depression and anxiety.
E. Painful menstrual periods; itching, burning sensations around the vaginal opening.

Implementation

A. There is no "one" treatment—treatment is geared toward relieving symptoms.
B. Monitor medications.
   1. Analgesics: Pregabalin (Lyrica) has been shown to reduce pain and improve sleep for up to six months; acetaminophen (Tylenol); tramadol (Ultram)—stronger analgesic than acetaminophen, rarely as addictive as narcotics; NSAIDs—often used for pain relief rather than for their anti-inflammatory effects (ASA, Advil, Aleve).
   2. Tricyclic antidepressants.
       a. Work by raising the levels of norepinephrine in the brain.
       b. Given in doses lower than required for antidepressant effects—drugs can improve the quality of sleep.
   3. SSRIs.
       a. Increase amount of serotonin in brain, reducing fatigue and possibly pain.
       b. Often prescribed in combination with a tricyclic antidepressant.
C. Nutrition, vitamin and mineral supplements: limit caffeine, sugar and alcohol—muscle irritants.
D. Exercise—eases the symptoms of fibromyalgia.
E. Coping skills—techniques to help ease tension, anxiety and pain.
F. Complementary therapies—massage, movement therapies (such as Pilates), chiropractic manipulations and acupuncture, among others.

MUSCULOSKELETAL SYSTEM REVIEW QUESTIONS

1. A client has sustained an intertrochanteric fracture of the hip and has just had a nailplate inserted for internal fixation. The client has been instructed that she should not flex her hip. The best explanation of why this movement would be harmful is

   1. It will be very painful for the client.
   2. The soft tissue around the site will be damaged.
   3. Displacement can occur with flexion.
   4. It will pull the hip out of alignment.

2. When the client is lying supine, the nurse will prevent external rotation of the lower extremity by using a

   1. Trochanter roll by the knee.
   2. Sandbag to the lateral calf.
   3. Trochanter roll to the thigh.
   4. Footboard.

3. A client has just returned from surgery after having his left leg amputated below the knee. Physician's orders include elevation of the foot of the bed for 24 hours. The nurse observes that the nursing assistant has placed a pillow under the client's amputated limb. The nursing action is to

   1. Leave the pillow, as his stump is elevated.
   2. Remove the pillow and elevate the foot of the bed.
   3. Leave the pillow and elevate the foot of the bed.
   4. Check with the physician and clarify the orders.

4. A client has sustained a fracture of the femur and balanced skeletal traction with a Thomas splint has been applied. To prevent pressure points from occurring around the top of the splint, the most important intervention is to

   1. Protect the skin with lotion.
   2. Keep the client pulled up in bed.
   3. Pad the top of the splint with washcloths.
   4. Provide a footplate in the bed.

5. The major rationale for the use of acetylsalicylic acid (aspirin) in the treatment of rheumatoid arthritis is to

   1. Reduce fever.
   2. Reduce inflammation of the joints.
   3. Assist the client in range-of-motion activities without pain.
   4. Prevent extension of the disease process.

6. Following an amputation, the advantage to the client for an immediate prosthesis fitting is

   1. Ability to ambulate sooner.
   2. Less chance of phantom limb sensation.
   3. Dressing changes are not necessary.
   4. Better fit of the prosthesis.

7. One method of assessing for signs of circulatory impairment in a client with a fractured femur is to ask the client to

   1. Cough and deep-breathe.
   2. Turn himself in bed.
   3. Perform biceps exercises.
   4. Wiggle his toes.

8. The morning of the second postoperative day following hip surgery for a fractured right hip, the nurse will ambulate the client. The first intervention is to

   1. Get the client up in a chair after dangling at the bedside.
   2. Use a walker for balance when getting the client out of bed.
   3. Have the client put minimal weight on the affected side when getting up.
   4. Practice getting the client out of bed by having her slightly flex her hips.

9. A client is in the hospital with his left leg in Buck's traction. The team leader asks the nurse to place a footplate on the affected side. The purpose of this action is to

   1. Anchor the traction.
   2. Prevent footdrop.
   3. Keep the client from sliding down in bed.
   4. Prevent pressure areas on the foot.

10. When evaluating all forms of traction, the nurse knows that the direction of pull is controlled by the

    1. Client's position.
    2. Rope/pulley system.
    3. Amount of weight.
    4. Point of friction.

11. Russell's traction incorporates a

    1. Sling under the knee.

2. Cervical halter.
3. Pelvic girdle.
4. Pearson attachment.

12. Which of the following statements is true of skeletal traction?

1. Neurovascular complications are less apt to occur than with skin traction.
2. The client has less mobility than he or she does with skin traction.
3. Fractures can be reduced because more weight can be used than with skin traction.
4. It is preferred for children because fracture fragment alignment is so important.

13. Following a fracture of the right hip, a client has an open reduction with internal fixation using an Austin Moore prosthesis. Postoperatively the affected leg should be maintained in a position of

1. Adduction.
2. External rotation.
3. Internal rotation.
4. Abduction.

14. A cast placed on a client's leg has dried. If the drying process were completed, the nurse would observe the cast to be

1. Dull and gray in appearance.
2. Shiny and white in appearance.
3. Cool to the touch and gray in appearance.
4. Warm to the touch and white in appearance.

15. When a client is being instructed in crutch walking using the swing-through gait, the most appropriate directions are

1. "Look down at your feet before moving the crutches to ensure you won't fall as you move them."
2. "Place one crutch forward with the opposite foot and then place the second crutch forward followed by the second foot."
3. "Move both crutches forward, then lift and swing your body past the crutches."
4. "Use the crutch bar to balance yourself to prevent falls."

16. A client's physician orders a Charnley pillow. The nurse understands that the purpose of using this type of pillow is to

1. Support the ball-and-socket joint.
2. Maintain abduction.

3. Maintain adduction.
4. Encourage internal rotation of the hips.

17. Before the nurse assists the client to crutch walk, a critical assessment is to

1. Evaluate the desire to be independent.
2. Assess the lower extremity muscle tone.
3. Determine the ability to ambulate alone.
4. Evaluate the need for other assistive devices.

18. The nurse is preparing a client for a myelogram using metrizamide (Amipaque), a water-soluble contrast material. The nurse will know the client understands the postmyelogram care regimen when she says

1. "I will need to keep my head elevated for at least 8 hours."
2. "I will need to lie flat for 12 to 24 hours."
3. "I will not be allowed to drink much liquid for 12 hours."
4. "I expect to have some itching and a stiff neck for a few days."

19. To achieve the desired outcome of functional healing of a fracture, which nursing goal should receive the highest priority?

1. Maintain immobilization and alignment.
2. Provide optimal nutrition and hydration.
3. Promote independence in activities of daily living.
4. Provide relief from pain and discomfort.

20. A young male client has had a cast placed on his right leg. While caring for the client, the nurse identifies a "hot spot" or area on the cast that feels warm. The nurse reports the findings to the physician because the data indicates possible

1. Poor circulation.
2. Pressure from the cast.
3. Uneven cast drying.
4. Infection.

21. When a client has cervical halter traction to immobilize the cervical spine, countertraction is provided by

1. Elevating the foot of the bed.
2. Elevating the head of the bed.
3. Application of the pelvic girdle.
4. Lowering the head of the bed.

22. After falling down the basement steps in his house, a client is brought to the emergency room. His physician confirms that his leg is fractured. Following ap-

plication of a leg cast, the nurse will first check the client's toes for

1. Increase in temperature.
2. Change in color.
3. Edema.
4. Movement.

23. A 23-year-old female client was in an automobile accident and is now a paraplegic. She is on an intermittent urinary catheterization program and diet as tolerated. The nurse's priority assessment should be to observe for

1. Urinary retention.
2. Bladder distention.
3. Weight gain.
4. Bowel evacuation.

24. A female client with rheumatoid arthritis has been on aspirin gr. xx TID and prednisone 10 mg BID for the last 2 years. The most important assessment question for the nurse to ask related to the client's drug therapy is whether she has

1. Headaches.
2. Tarry stools.
3. Blurred vision.
4. Decreased appetite.

25. A 7-year-old boy with a fractured leg tells the nurse that he is bored. An appropriate intervention would be to

1. Read a story and act out the part.
2. Watch a puppet show.
3. Watch television.
4. Listen to the radio.

26. Which nursing interventions should the nurse teach the client with fibromyalgia? Choose all that apply.

1. Stress the importance of participating in an ongoing rehabilitation program.
2. Teach that sugar and coffee provide energy and should be included in the diet.
3. Encourage checking with the primary care provider about vitamin and mineral supplements.
4. Increase the amount of sleep the client receives each day.

27. Which of the following is *not* a symptom associated with fibromyalgia?

1. Joint damage caused by inflammation.
2. Noncardiac chest pain.
3. Migraine.
4. Irritable bowel syndrome.

MUSCULOSKELETAL SYSTEM

Answers with Rationale

1. (3) If the hip if flexed to the side, on the side of the bed or in a low chair, hip displacement can occur. Displacement could result in pain, but this is not the primary reason for the instructions. The remaining two answers are not specific or adequate explanations.

   NP:AN; CN:PH; CL:C

2. (3) External rotation of the lower leg is a result of external rotation at the hip. Neutral rotation of the trochanter is promoted by placing a thigh trochanter roll that extends from the upper hip to the knee.

   NP:P; CN:PH; CL:A

3. (2) The orders state bed elevation (this is done to reduce edema and prevent hemorrhage). A pillow under the stump may lead to a flexion contracture of the hip joint, so it is contraindicated. Also, further teaching by the RN is indicated so that the NA understands why the pillow is contraindicated.

   NP:I; CN:PH; CL:A

4. (2) The most important intervention for preventing pressure points is to keep the client pulled up in bed. The nurse may also pad the top of the splint with soft material such as cotton wadding or ABDs to prevent excoriation. The footplate would prevent footdrop.

   NP:I; CN:PH; CL:A

5. (2) Aspirin acts as an anti-inflammatory drug and, thus, reduces the inflammation of the joint. In doing so, it also relieves pain. Aspirin does not prevent extension of the disease. While aspirin reduces fever, this is not the major reason for its use in the treatment of rheumatoid arthritis.

   NP:AN; CN:PH; CL:K

6. (1) When the prosthesis is in place immediately following surgery, the client can stand up several hours postoperatively and walk the next day. The operative site is closed to outside contamination and benefits from improved circulation due to ambulation.

   NP:P; CN:PH; CL:C

7. (4) The only activity that will indicate a complication directly related to circulatory impairment due to a fractured femur is the inability to wiggle his toes.

   NP:A; CN:PH; CL:A

8. (2) Postoperative hip replacement clients may get up the first day, but need to use a walker for balance. They should not bear any weight on the affected side, dangle or sit in a chair, flexing their hips. Positions with 60- to 90-degree flexion should be avoided.

   NP:I; CN:PH; CL:A

9. (2) The purpose of the footplate is to prevent footdrop while the client is immobilized in traction. This will not anchor the traction, keep the client from sliding down in bed, or prevent pressure areas.

   NP:P; CN:PH; CL:C

10. (2) The rope/pulley and weight system is arranged so that fracture fragments are in the desired approximate position for healing. The client's position should always rest in line with the traction pull. The line of pull must never be interfered with by changing the position of a pulley and extension bar.

    NP:E; CN:PH; CL:C

11. (1) Russell's traction is a type of skin traction that incorporates a sling under the knee that is connected by a rope to an overhead bar pulley. It is frequently used to treat femoral shaft fractures in the adolescent.

    NP:AN; CN:PH; CL:K

Coding for Questions/Answers Abbreviations: **Nursing Process: NP,** Assessment: A, Analysis: AN, Planning: P, Implementation: I, Evaluation: E; **Client Needs: CN,** Safe, Effective Care Environment: S, Health Promotion and Maintenance: H, Psychosocial Integrity: PS, Physiological Integrity: PH; **Clinical Area: CA,** Medical Nursing: M, Surgical Nursing: S, Maternal/Newborn Nursing: MA, Pediatric Nursing: P, Psychiatric Nursing: PS; **Cognitive Level: CL,** Knowledge: K, Comprehension: C, Application: A, Analysis: AN.

12. (3) Because more weight can be applied with skeletal traction, it can be used to reduce fractures and maintain alignment. It is not used commonly in the elderly because of prolonged immobilization. It is not preferred for children because some displacement of fracture fragments is desirable to prevent growth disturbance. Frequently, clients have more mobility than they do with skin traction.

    NP:AN; CN:PH; CL:K

13. (4) To prevent dislocation of the prosthesis, the legs are kept abducted with neutral rotation. Adduction (1), flexion, and internal rotation (3) are to be avoided.

    NP:P; CN:PH; CL:C

14. (2) The cast will be shiny and cool to the touch when dry. It will have a dull appearance when wet.

    NP:A; CN:PH; CL:K

15. (3) This is the procedure for using the swing-through gait. Clients are instructed to look straight ahead when walking with crutches. Looking down can lead to falls and uneven gait. Putting pressure from the arm on the crutch bar can cause nerve damage.

    NP:I; CN:S; CL:C

16. (2) A Charnley pillow is applied to maintain abduction (*not* adduction) and external (*not* internal) rotation of the hips. This is most commonly used when the head of the femur is replaced by an Austin Moore prosthesis. Hip flexion angle should not exceed 60 to 90 degrees.

    NP:AN; CN:PH; CL:C

17. (3) The ability to ambulate alone or the requirement of personnel to assist with ambulation is the most critical step in assisting a client in crutch walking. Lower muscle strength needs to be evaluated to determine readiness to ambulate and need for assistance.

    NP:A; CN:PH; CL:A

18. (1) The head must be kept elevated because this drug could provoke a seizure if it reaches the brain in a bolus form. After myelography using an oil-based contrast medium (Pantopaque), clients are kept flat. Forcing fluids helps prevent postmyelogram headache by replacing lost spinal fluid. Itching suggests an allergic reaction, while a stiff neck suggests meningeal irritation; neither is an expected response to a myelogram.

    NP:E; CN:PH; CL:C

19. (1) Maintaining the prescribed immobilization and body alignment will keep the fracture fragments in close anatomical proximity, thereby promoting functional fracture healing. This goal should receive the highest priority. The other goals, although applicable in the care of a client with a fracture, do not have as high a priority in meeting this particular desired outcome.

    NP:P; CN:PH; CL:C

20. (4) Infection can be identified by "hot spots," or areas on the cast that feel warm to the touch. A hot spot is not evidence of poor circulation (1) or too tight a cast (2).

    NP:I; CN:PH; CL:A

21. (2) To keep the client from migrating toward the head of the bed while the cervical halter traction is used, the head of the bed is slightly elevated. Lowering the head of the bed (4) would aggravate such migration, as would elevating the foot of the bed (1).

    NP:P; CN:PH; CL:C

22. (2) A cast is rigid and used to maintain alignment. If it is too tight, it will press on blood vessels. The color of the toes will change first, then temperature, when blood supply is decreased. As the blood flow slows through the walls of the vessels, edema will occur.

    NP:A; CN:PH; CL:A

23. (2) Bladder distention indicates the need for catheterization. Catheterizations are usually performed every 4 to 6 hours. The danger of not intervening when the bladder is distended is that it could lead to overdistention or stretching.

    NP:A; CN:PH; CL:A

24. (2) Aspirin impedes clotting by blocking prostaglandin synthesis, which can lead to bleeding. A side effect of prednisone is gastric irritation, also leading to bleeding. Tarry stools indicate bleeding in the upper GI system.

    NP:A; CN:PH; CL:A

25. (1) This activity involves the child so that he is actively, if not physically, participating in play. It also allows the child to use his creativity, unlike watching a puppet (2) or television show (3) or listening to the radio (4).

    NP:I; CN:H; CL:A

26. (1, 3, 4) Once a client has fibromyalgia, it is a lifelong noncurable disease that requires continued rehabilitation. Caffeine, sugar, and alcohol (which are muscle irritants) should be avoided. Vitamins, minerals, and supplements should not be taken without physician guidance as they may interact with other

prescription drugs. In many clients, the pain of fibromyalgia occurs as a direct response to lack of sleep. Assisting the client to get a better night's sleep can reduce the amount of pain experienced.

NP:AN; CN:S; CL:C

27. (1) There is no inflammation associated with fibromyalgia. Choices (2), (3), and (4) are all common symptoms of fibromyalgia.

NP:A; CN:S; CL:C

INTEGUMENTARY SYSTEM

The integumentary system comprises the enveloping membrane, or skin, of the body and includes the epidermis, the dermis, and all the derivatives of the epidermis, such as hair, nails, and various glands. It is indispensable for the body, as it forms a barrier against the external environment and performs many vital body functions.

ANATOMY AND PHYSIOLOGY

Skin

Definition: The organ that envelops the body. It accounts for approximately 15 percent of the body weight and forms a barrier between the internal organs and the external environment.

Characteristics
A. Consists of three layers: epidermis, dermis, and subcutaneous.
B. It is the largest sensory organ, equipped with nerves and specialized sensory organs sensitive to pain, touch, pressure, heat, and cold.
C. Chief pigment is melanin, produced by basal cells.
D. Functions of skin.
   1. Protection.
   2. Temperature regulation.
   3. Sensation.
   4. Storage.

✦ Bacterial Flora on the Skin
A. Normally present in varying amounts are coagulase-positive *Staphylococcus,* coagulase-negative *Staphylococcus, Mycobacterium, Pseudomonas,* diphtheroids, nonhemolytic *Streptococcus,* hemolytic *Streptococcus* (group A).
B. The organisms are shed with normal exfoliation of skin; bathing and rubbing may also remove bacteria.
C. Normal pH of skin (4.2–5.6) retards growth of bacteria.
D. Damaged areas of skin are potential points of entry for infection.

Hair

Definition: A threadlike structure developed from a papilla in the corium layer.

A. Hair goes through cyclic changes: growth, atrophy, and rest.
B. Melanocytes in the bulb of each hair account for color.
C. All parts of the body except the palms, soles of the feet, distal phalanges of fingers and toes, and penis are covered with some form of hair.

Sweat Glands

Definition: Aggregations of cells that produce a liquid (perspiration) having a salty taste and a pH that varies from 4.5 to 7.5.
A. Eccrine sweat glands.
   1. Located in all areas of the skin except the lips and part of the genitalia.
   2. Open onto the surface of the skin.
   3. Activity controlled by the sympathetic nervous system.
   4. Secrete sweat (perspiration).
      a. The chief components of sweat are water, sodium, potassium, chloride, glucose, urea, and lactate.
      b. Concentrations vary from individual to individual.
B. Apocrine sweat glands.
   1. Located in the axilla, genital, anal, and nipple areas.
   2. Located in ear and produce ear wax.
   3. Develop during puberty.
   4. Respond to adrenergic stimuli.
   5. Produce an alkaline sweat.

Sebaceous Glands

A. Develop at base of hair follicle.
B. Secrete sebum.
C. Hormone controlled. Increased activity with androgens; decreased activity with estrogen.

System Assessment

✦ A. Assess color.
   1. Assess color of skin, including deviations from the normal range within the individual's race.
      a. Use a nonglare daylight or 60-watt bulb.
      b. Note especially the bony prominences.
      c. Observe for pallor (white), flushing (red), jaundice (yellow), ashen (gray), or cyanotic (blue) coloration.
      d. Check mucous membranes to be accurate.
   2. Observe for increased or decreased areas of pigmentation.
   3. Observe for various skin discolorations: ecchymosis, petechiae, purpura, or erythema.

B. Evaluate skin temperature.
   1. Palpate skin (especially areas of concern) for temperature.
   2. Note changes in different extremities.
C. Assess turgor.
   1. Observe skin for its ease of movement and speed of return to original position.
   2. Observe for excessive dryness, moisture, wrinkling, flaking, and general texture.
   3. Observe for a lasting impression or dent after pressing against and removing finger from skin—indicates edema or fluid in the tissue.
D. Assess skin sensation.
   1. Observe the client's ability to detect heat, cold, gentle touch, and pressure.
   2. Note complaints of itching, tingling, cramps, or numbness.
E. Assess signs of poor nutrition.
   1. Rough, dry, scaly skin.
   2. Pigmented or irritated.
   3. Bruises or petechiae.
F. Observe cleanliness.
   1. Observe general state of hygiene. Note amount of oil, moisture, and dirt on the skin surface.
   2. Note presence of strong body odors.
   3. Investigate hair and scalp for presence of body lice.
G. Assess integrity (intactness of skin),
   1. Note intactness of skin. Observe for areas of broken skin (lesions) or ulcers.
   2. Assess any lesion for its location, size, shape, color(s), consistency, discomfort, odor, and sensation associated with it.
H. Assess for presence of skin lesions.

Skin Lesions

A. *Macule:* a flat, circumscribed, discolored lesion less than 1 cm in diameter.
B. *Papule:* a raised, solid lesion less than 1 cm in diameter.
C. *Nodule:* similar to a papule except greater depth.
D. *Vesicle:* an elevated lesion of skin or mucous membrane filled with fluid.
E. *Pustule:* a pus-filled vesicle.
F. *Wheal:* an irregularly shaped and elevated lesion of skin or mucous membrane due to edema; diameter variable.
G. *Plaque:* a collection of papules.
H. *Erosion:* a moist depressed area due to partial or full loss of epidermis.
I. *Ulcer:* the complete loss of dermis leaving irregular depression; scars on healing.

System Implementation

A. Monitor client's most vulnerable body areas for ischemia, hyperemia, or broken areas.

B. Encourage a well-balanced diet, especially protein-rich foods.
C. Promote high fluid intake to maintain hydration status and prevent skin breakdown.
D. Change the client's body position at least every 2 hours to rotate weight-bearing areas and prevent pressure ulcers.
   1. Observe all vulnerable areas at this time.
   2. Include right and left lateral, prone, supine, and swimming-type positioning if possible.
E. Massage skin to increase circulation.
F. Keep skin clean.
G. Protect healthy skin from drainage and environmental pollutants.
H. Encourage active exercise or range of motion to promote circulation.
I. Monitor medications for various skin conditions or lesions.
J. Instruct clients about appropriate skin care.

COMMON SKIN LESIONS

Pressure Ulcers

See Gerontological Nursing chapter.

Paronychia

Definition: Infection and inflammation of the tissue around the nailplate.

Characteristics

A. High incidence in middle-aged women.
B. High incidence in diabetics.

Assessment

A. Evaluate acute infection from a hangnail.
B. Observe for cellulitis.

Implementation

A. Implement warm soaks.
B. Apply antibiotic or fungicidal ointment.
C. Care for incision and drainage of affected area.

Acne Vulgaris

Definition: A disorder of the skin with eruption of papules or pustules primarily due to increased production of sebum from the sebaceous glands. Affects adolescents and young adults.

Characteristics

A. Non-inflammatory type composed of whiteheads and blackheads in the follicular duct.
B. Inflammatory acne pustules with possible scarring.

TYPES OF ACNE	
Types of Acne	**Treatment**
I Comedomal (numerous comedones)	Retin-A
II Papulopustular (red papules with pus)	Retin-A, topical antibiotics
III Cystic acne (nodules and cysts)	Retin-A with oral antibiotics
IV Pustulocystic (nodular cysts severe, resistant to treatment)	Accutane

C. Affected by hormone levels (androgen), which lead to blocking of secretions with subsequent blackheads.

◆ D. Treatment options.
   1. Oral contraceptives are FDA approved.
   2. Desquamation preparations, which allow free flow of sebum.
   3. Accutane—specifically for severe acne.
      a. Active ingredient is risotretinoin, a retinoid and relative of vitamin A.
      ◆ b. Absolutely contraindicated during pregnancy—causes birth defects.
      ◆ c. Blood tests recommended every few weeks to monitor for liver damage or high fat levels in the blood.
      d. May be an association between drug and mental health problems such as suicide.
   4. Retin-A (tretinoin)—a topical cream to reduce scarring from acne.
   5. Mechanical removal by an extractor.
   6. Complete cleansing with regular or Neutrogena soap and clean towels.
   7. Mild facial erythema via sunlight or lamp.
   8. Topical antibiotics.
   9. Systemic oral tetracycline for some cases.
   10. Dermabrasion for selected cases, to reduce scarring.

Implementation

A. Teach good skin and scalp hygiene.
B. Have client avoid squeezing, rubbing, picking.
C. Have client avoid greasy cleansing creams and cosmetics.
◆ D. Support a high-protein, low-fat diet.
   1. Fatty foods, white sugar, nuts, and chocolate are best avoided, but research has not verified this.
   2. Diet not as important a therapy as in the past.
   3. Eliminate seaweed products, which aggravate condition.
E. Encourage client to get adequate rest and sunshine.
F. Provide emotional support for body image and relationship problems.

Cellulitis

Definition: Infection of the dermis or subcutaneous tissue caused by either streptococcal or staphylococcal organisms—may follow surgical wound, impetigo, trauma, or otitis media.

Assessment

◆ A. Swelling, erythema.
B. Leukocytosis.
C. Pain and itching.

Implementation

◆ A. Monitor systemic antibiotics—effective for the condition.
B. Elevate the extremity to reduce dependent edema.
C. Apply heat to extremity to promote blood circulation.
D. Encourage rest to decrease muscular contractions to limit extension of organism into circulatory system.

Impetigo

◆ *Definition:* A bacterial disease caused by *Streptococcus, Staphylococcus* or both.

Characteristics

A. Lesions are intraepidermal vesicles.
B. Lesions progress to pustules, which become crusted.

Implementation

◆ A. Instruct client that the most important intervention is the prevention of the spread of the disease.
   1. Complete cleansing with hexachlorophene soap and other hygienic care materials.
   2. Separate towels.
B. Instruct that lesions dry by exposure to air; use compresses of Burow's solution to remove the crusts to allow faster healing.
C. Apply antibiotic ointments.
   1. Bacitracin or mupirocin (Bactroban).
   2. If no response to topical antibiotic cream, systemic drug (erythromycin) is used.

Furuncle (Boil)

◆ *Definition:* A bacterial disease caused by *Staphylococcus* pyrogen infection of a hair follicle.

Assessment

A. Evaluate furuncle. Onset is sudden; the skin becomes red, tender, and hot around the hair follicle.
B. Observe furuncle. The center forms pus, and the core may be extruded spontaneously or by excision and manipulation.
◆ C. Check for presence of diabetes mellitus. Should be ruled out only after tests prove negative.

D. Instruct client in necessity of scrupulous cleanliness: isolation of towels, soap, and clothing.

E. Administer systemic antibiotics if a series of carbuncles occur.

Herpes Simplex

Definition: A viral disease (cold sore) caused by herpes virus, hominis types I and II.

Characteristics

◆ A. Herpes I.
1. Most common type.
2. Causes burning, tingling, and itching; soon followed by tiny vesicles.
3. Most frequently occurs on lips, but can occur on the face and around the mouth.

◆ B. Herpes II. (*See* Chapter 12, page 553.)
1. Most often the cause of genital infection.
2. Transmitted primarily through sexual contact.
3. Difficult to treat and to prevent recurrence.

Implementation

A. Herpes simplex virus, type I.
1. Keep area dry; apply drying agent (ether).
◆ 2. L-Lysine amino acid: 1 g/day for 6 months.

◆ B. Herpes genitalis, type II.
1. Avoid sexual contact with active lesion.
2. Use acyclovir cream; recurrence give acyclovir 200 mg PO × 5 for 5 days.

Herpes Zoster (Shingles)

Definition: Acute invasion of the peripheral nervous system due to reactivation of *Varicella zoster* virus.

Assessment

A. Evaluate eruption with fever, malaise, and pain.
B. Assess vesicles (exudate contains virus) that appear in 3–4 days.
C. Assess client's status—if immunosuppressed, condition can be life-threatening.

Implementation

A. Isolate client.
B. Apply lotions—calamine, cayenne pepper cream.
C. Administer drugs: analgesics for pain; antiviral agents (acyclovir) and anti-inflammatory drugs such as NSAIDs.
D. Instruct client on preventive measures to enhance immune system.

SYPHILIS

◆ *Definition:* A contagious venereal disease that leads to many structural and cutaneous lesions. Caused by the spirochete *Treponema pallidum*. The disease is transmitted by direct, intimate contact or in utero.

Characteristics

◆ A. Transmitted commonly by sexual intercourse, but infants may become infected during birth process. Early-stage syphilis up 29 percent from 2000, largely among gay men.
B. No age or race is immune to the disease.
C. Diagnosed by serum studies and/or darkfield examination of secretions of the chancre.
◆ 1. Wassermann test.
2. Kahn test.
D. No immunity develops, and reinfection is common.
E. Types of syphilis.
1. Early syphilis—two stages.
a. Primary stage.
(1) Incubation period is 10 days to 3 weeks.
◆ (2) Characteristic lesion is red, eroded, indurated papule; the sore or ulcer at the site of the invasion by the spirochete is called a *chancre*.
(3) Accompanied by enlarged lymph node in drainage area of chancre.
(4) May be painless or painful.
(5) This stage is highly infectious.
◆ b. Secondary stage.
(1) Develops if the individual is not treated in the primary stage. Occurs in 2–6 months and may last 2 years.
(2) May be mild enough to pass unnoticed or may be severe, with a generalized rash on skin and mucous membrane.
(3) Headache, fever, sore throat, and general malaise are common.
(4) Disappears by itself if untreated in 3–12 weeks.
◆ 2. Late syphilis—tertiary stage.
a. Symptoms may develop soon after secondary stage or lie hidden for years.
b. Blood test may be negative.
c. Less contagious but very dangerous to individual.
d. If untreated, cardiovascular problems may ensue.
e. Blindness or deep ulcers may occur.
f. May be treated with antibiotics but cure is more difficult.

Implementation

A. Advise client that strict personal hygiene is an absolute requirement.
B. Educate client in prevention: symptoms, mode of transmission, and treatment.

C. Assist in case finding; encourage use of clinics for diagnosis and treatment.

D. Administer long-acting penicillin G benzathine (still primary treatment in the early stages).

E. Instruct client to avoid sexual contact until clearance is given by physician.

ALLERGIC RESPONSES

Eczema (Atopic Dermatitis)

Definition: A superficial inflammatory process involving primarily the epidermis.

Characteristics

A. Eczema is a chronic condition with remissions and exacerbations.

B. Eczema occurs at all ages and is common in infancy, especially in those with hereditary allergic tendencies.

C. Treatment is dependent on cause (foods, emotional problems, familial tendencies).

D. Child is isolated from recently vaccinated children; child is *not* vaccinated.

Assessment

A. Assess for eruptions that are erythematous, papular, or papulovesicular.
   1. May be edematous, weeping, eroded, crusted, and/or dry.
   2. Chronic form may cause skin to be thickened, scaling, and fissured.

B. Assess if regional lymph nodes are swollen.

C. Assess if irritability is present.

Implementation

A. There is no cure—goal is to reduce pruritus and inflammation, and to hydrate and lubricate the skin.
   1. Have clients keep fingernails short; provide gloves to prevent scratching.
   2. Apply wet dressings soaked in aluminum acetate or therapeutic baths (no soap during acute stages).
   3. Apply mild lotion (calamine) when no oozing or vesiculation is present.
   4. Use cornstarch paste to remove crusts.

B. Apply corticosteroids 1% to 2½% (fluticasone propionate) as anti-inflammatory agent.

C. Oral corticosteroids may be given for acute reaction.

D. Topical treatment of zinc spray shows excellent results.

Contact Dermatitis

Definition: A skin reaction caused by contact with an agent to which the skin is sensitive.

Characteristics

A. Causes.
   1. Clothing (especially woolens).
   2. Cosmetics.
   3. Household products (especially detergents).
   4. Industrial substances (i.e., paints, dyes, cements).

B. Treatment.
   1. Avoidance of irritant or removal of irritating clothing.
   2. Avoidance of contact with detergent (use of rubber gloves for household chores).
   3. Avoidance of contact with industrial agent (use of protective clothing or, for highly sensitive individuals, change of job locations).

Poison Oak or Poison Ivy

Definition: Dermatitis caused by contact with poison oak, poison ivy, or poison sumac, which contain urushiol, a potent skin-sensitizing agent.

Assessment

A. Assess for papulovesicular lesions.

B. Assess for severe itching.

Implementation

A. Cleanse skin of plant oils (alcohol products, such as vodka, work well).

B. Administer steroids for severe reactions; topical cortisone to reduce inflammation and itching.

C. Apply cold, wet dressings of Burow's solution to relieve itching.

SKIN CONDITIONS

Malignant Skin Tumors

Assessment

A. Evaluate lesion that starts as a papule and spreads; central area may become depressed and ulcerated.

B. Assess extent of local invasion or extensive local destruction.

C. Evaluate lesions that enlarge rapidly (may indicate basal cell epithelioma, and can metastasize).

D. Assess for any nodular tumor that appears, usually on the lower lip, tongue, head, or neck.

✦ E. Assess for specific type of skin tumor.
   1. Basal cell epithelioma is a tumor arising from the basal layer of the epidermis formed because of basal cell keratinization. The typical lesion is a small, smooth papule with telangiectasis and atrophic center.
   ✦ 2. Melanoma is the most malignant of all cutaneous lesions. It arises from melanocytes and is often fatal. It occurs most frequently in

light-skinned people when they are exposed to sunlight.

3. Squamous cell carcinoma is a tumor of the epidermis that frequently comes from keratosis and is considered an invasive cancer. The lesion begins as erythematous macules or plaques with indistinct margins, and the surface often becomes crusted.

Implementation

A. Assist with surgical excision, the most effective treatment.
B. Administer cancer drugs if ordered.
C. Assist with irradiation if ordered.
1. Counsel client on side effects of treatment.
2. Offer emotional support throughout treatment.
D. Advise client to prevent occurrence of skin cancer by using sunscreening devices.
E. Advise client to avoid prolonged exposure to sun.
✦ F. Educate client to observe any changes in color or form of moles.
G. Watch for potential malignancy in other locations.

Lupus Erythematosus

Definition: A chronic, multisystem autoimmune disease of the connective tissue that may involve any organ of the body—500,000 people in the United States are afflicted with the disease, mostly women. Etiology unknown.

Characteristics

A. Affects women nine times more than men.
B. May affect every cell in the body.
C. Prognosis poor when cardiac, pulmonary or renal involvement early in disease.

Assessment

A. Onset may be insidious or acute.
✦ B. Assess for discoid eruption—a chronic, localized, scaling erythematous skin eruption over the nose, cheeks and forehead, giving a characteristic "butterfly" appearance.
C. Evaluate for fever, malaise, and weight loss.
D. Observe for exacerbation and remission of symptoms.
E. Assess for sensitivity to sunlight.
✦ F. Systemic (disseminated) lupus erythematosus may have multiple organ involvement that can lead to death.
1. Pericarditis is common manifestation (30 percent); myocarditis also present (25 percent of clients).
2. Lung and pleural involvement common (40 to 50 percent).

3. Vascular system often involved with inflammation, producing lesions on fingertips, elbows, toes, etc.
4. Lymphadenopathy occurs in half of all clients.
5. Neuropsychiatric symptoms are often present and require intervention.

Implementation

A. Goal of treatment is to prevent loss of organ function—involves careful monitoring.
✦ B. Administer corticosteroid treatment to prevent progression of the disease—most important class of drugs used for treatment.
✦ C. Instruct client to avoid sunlight and local antibiotic ointments that spread the lesions.
D. Apply topical sunscreen preparations (i.e., Covermark, Pabanol, etc.)
E. Advise client of possible side effects of prescribed medications; advise client to notify physician promptly if side effects occur so drugs may be discontinued before serious complications.
F. Counsel client to avoid fatigue.
G. Cover up disfigurement from scarring with opaque or tinted cosmetics as recommended by physician.

BURNS

Definition: Destruction of layers of the skin by thermal, chemical, or electrical agents.

Degree of Burn According to Depth

A. Classified by depth of tissue destruction. Categories are similar to, but not the same as, prior categories of first-, second-, and third-degree burns.
✦ B. Superficial, partial-thickness (first degree).
1. Involves epidermis.
2. Area is red or pink.
3. Moderate pain.
4. Spontaneous healing.
✦ C. Deep, partial-thickness (second degree).
1. Involves epidermis and dermis to the basal cells.
2. Blistering.
3. Severe pain.
4. Regeneration in 1 month.
5. Scarring may occur.
✦ D. Full-thickness (third degree).
1. Involves epidermis, dermis, and subcutaneous tissue and may extend to the muscle in severe burns.
2. White, gray, or black in appearance.
3. Absence of pain.
4. Edema of surrounding tissues.
5. Eschar formation.

6. Grafting needed due to total destruction of dermal elements.

Extent of Burn

✦ A. Rule of nines—good for rapid estimation of extent of body surface area (BSA) involved.
   1. Head and neck   9%
   2. Anterior trunk   18%
   3. Posterior trunk   18%
   4. Arms (9% each)   18%
   5. Legs (18% each)   36%
   6. Perineum   1%
B. Lund/Browder method.
   1. More accurate and appropriate to use when calculating fluid replacement.
   2. A chart is necessary to compute percentages assigned to body areas.
   3. Percentages vary for different age groups.
C. Palm method.
   1. Client with scattered burns may have percentage calculated with this method.
   2. Size of client's palm is 1% of BSA—this percentage is used to assess injury.
✦ D. Fluid replacement formulas.
   1. Brooke Army formula—colloids, electrolytes, and glucose first 24 hours.
   2. Parkland/Baxter—lactated Ringer's only first 24 hours; day 2, colloid is added.
   3. Consensus formula—lactated Ringer's solution first 24 hours.
   4. Evans formula—colloids, electrolytes, and glucose first 24 hours.
E. Associated factors that determine seriousness of burn.
   1. Age.
      a. Younger than 18 months.
      b. Older than 65 years.
   2. General health.
   3. Site of burn.
   4. Associated injuries (fractures).
   5. Causative agents.
   6. Other medical problems.

Category of Burn Classification

✦ A. Classification according to the percentage of body area destroyed.
   1. *Major burns:* 25 percent or more of the body has sustained second-degree burn, and 10 percent has sustained third-degree burn; further complicated by fractures, respiratory involvement, and smoke inhalation. Burns of feet, hands, face, and genitalia.
   2. *Moderate burns:* less than 10 percent of the body has sustained third-degree burn, and 15 to 25 percent has sustained second-degree burn.

3. *Minor burns:* less than 15 percent of the body has sustained second-degree burn, and less than 2 percent has sustained third-degree burn.
B. Classification according to cause.
   1. *Thermal burns:* flame burns, scalding with hot liquids, or radiation.
   2. *Chemical burns:* strong acids or strong alkali solutions.
   3. *Electrical burns.*
      a. Most serious type of burn.
      b. Body fluids may conduct an electrical charge through body (look for entrance and exit area).
      c. Cardiac arrhythmias may occur.
      d. Toxins are created postburn that injure kidneys.
      e. Voltage and ampere information important in history taking.

Assessment

A. Assess extent of injury.
   1. Assess for superficial burn: involves only reddening of the skin.
   2. Assess for partial-thickness burn: skin blisters, regeneration of epithelium without grafting.
   3. Assess for full-thickness burn: destruction of most of the epidermal tissue; unable to regenerate without graft.
B. Assess type of treatment appropriate to extent of burn.
   ✦ 1. First aid.
      a. Provide comfort and prevent chilling.
      b. Wash area with cool, sterile solution or water if no sterile solution is available.
      c. Cover with a sterile cloth to prevent liquid contamination.
      d. Do not apply greasy substances until burn is evaluated.
      e. Wash surrounding area thoroughly with mild detergent.
   2. Exposed method: No dressing is used so that hard eschar forms, protecting wound from infection. This method is excellent for areas difficult to bandage effectively. Requires isolation and is difficult for a child.
   3. Closed method: Sterile occlusive dressing is applied frequently, usually with topical medications. Debridement occurs every time the dressing is changed, preventing a large loss of blood at one time, as when eschar is removed.
C. Continued assessment during acute burn phase.
   1. Respiratory status.
   2. Fluid status.
   3. Vital signs.

4. pH from NG tube and residual gastric volume; gives data on need for antacid therapy.
5. Pain level and need for pain relief.
6. Wound assessment—color, odor, exudate, eschar, etc.
7. Body weight; need for adjusted caloric intake.
8. Psychosocial response to injury.

Implementation

✦ A. Maintain patent airway. Monitor for tracheal–laryngeal edema.

B. Provide fluid replacement therapy.
 ✦ 1. Resuscitative phase.
   a. First 24 to 48 hours postburn, fluid shifts from plasma to interstitial space.
   b. Potassium levels rise in plasma.
   c. Blood hemoconcentration and metabolic acidosis occur.
   d. Fluid loss is mostly plasma.
   e. Nursing responsibilities.
    (1) Monitor vital signs frequently.
    (2) Monitor urinary output (50 to 100 mL/hr—minimum output 30 mL/hr).
    (3) Give one-half of total fluids in first 8 hours or as ordered. (The first 8 hours starts at the time the burn occurs, *not* the time the client arrives at the healthcare facility.)
    (4) Notify physician if urine output less than 30 mL/hr, weight gain, jugular vein distention, crackles or increased arterial pressure.
 ✦ 2. Acute or intermediate phase.
   a. Capillary permeability stabilizes and fluid begins to shift from interstitial spaces to plasma.
   b. Hypokalemia, hypernatremia, hemodilution, and pulmonary edema are potential dangers.
   c. Nursing responsibilities.
    (1) Monitor CVP.
    (2) Observe lab values.
    (3) Maintain adequate urine output.

C. Assess pain level frequently and relieve pain with morphine sulfate IV as ordered. Give small doses frequently.

✦ D. Prevent infection.
 1. Provide aseptic technique and environment.
   a. Use meticulous hand hygiene technique or antiseptic gel before and after client care.
   b. Use clean or sterile gloves.
   c. Use isolation protocol. (*See* Table 8-8.)
 2. Observe for signs of infection, increased temperature and pulse, wound drainage.

✦ TREATMENT

A. Immediate care.
 1. Put out the flames—have client drop to floor or ground and roll.
 2. Apply cold water for brief duration in second-degree burn if seen within 10 minutes of injury.
 3. Do not apply any ointment.
 4. Cover burns with sterile or clean cloth.
 5. Irrigate chemical burns thoroughly.

B. Emergency care.
 ✦ 1. Patent airway and IV line are established.
 2. 100% oxygen if burn occurred in enclosed area.
 3. Degree and extent of burn are determined—adequate pain relief given.
 ✦ 4. Fluid balance is maintained.
   a. First day, give formula of choice according to percent of body burn and weight plus 2000 mL D_5W.
   b. Second day, give colloids with solutions.
   c. Urine output is maintained at least 50 mL/hr.
   d. Vital signs—CVP line usually inserted.
 5. Nasogastric tube (inserted to prevent vomiting from paralytic ileus).
 6. Tetanus toxoid.
 7. Escharotomy or fasciotomy if needed.

C. Long-term care.
 1. Wound debridement.
 2. Wound care: ointment and/or dressing.
 3. Skin grafting.

✦ D. Types of skin grafting.
 1. Homograft or allograft: from cadaver or other person.
 2. Xenograft: from an animal (usually pigs).
 3. Autograft: from self.
 4. Biosynthetic covering (Biobrane): mimics skin's most important function—protecting against trauma and infection.
 5. Cultured epithelial autograft (CEA): provides permanent covering (client's cells are harvested and grown in laboratory, then grafted).
 6. Integra—artifical skin approved by FDA in 1996—permanent, immediate covering that reproduces skin's normal function and stimulates regeneration of dermal tissue.
   a. Consists of two layers that completely adhere to wound bed and mimic dermis and epidermis.
   b. As dermis is regenerated, the matrix is absorbed and a "neodermis" forms in 14–21 days—once dermis has healed, silicone layer is removed and replaced by thin, meshed epidermal graft.

✦ Table 8-8. ISOLATION PROTOCOL		
Protocol for Entering Isolation Room	**Protocol for Leaving Isolation Room**	
1. Complete hand hygiene.	1. Untie gown at waist.	5. Take off goggles or face shield.
2. Put on gown and tie.	2. Take off gloves.	6. Take off mask.
3. Put on and tie mask.	3. Untie gown at neck.	7. Leave room and complete hand hygiene.
4. Don goggles or face shield.	4. Pull gown off and place in laundry hamper.	
5. Don gloves.		

3. Provide prophylactic measures: tetanus and antibiotics.
✦ E. Prevent pulmonary complications.
1. Establish and observe for adequate airway.
2. Suction PRN.
3. Provide humidified oxygen PRN.
4. Teach coughing and deep-breathing.
5. Provide frequent position changes.
✦ F. Establish adequate circulatory volume to prevent shock.
1. Observe for signs of hypovolemia (e.g., thirst, vomiting, increased pulse, decreased blood pressure, and decreased urinary output).
2. Observe for signs of circulatory overload, particularly around the second to fifth days, when fluid in extracellular tissues returns to circulation. There is danger of congestive heart failure.
3. Monitor intravenous fluid therapy.
4. Monitor intake and output.
G. Monitor for complications.
1. Congestive heart failure and/or pulmonary edema.
2. Sepsis.
3. Acute respiratory failure.
✦ H. Promote good body alignment—prevent contractures.
1. Keep body parts in alignment.
2. Elevate burned extremities.
3. Provide active and/or passive range of motion to all joints.
✦ I. Provide adequate nutrition (TPN or enteral feedings).
1. Give high-protein, high-caloric diet—goal is to provide positive nitrogen balance.
2. Give nutritional supplements (Ensure) and vitamin/mineral supplements.
3. Provide small, frequent, and attractive meals.
4. Encourage child, who is frequently anorexic, to eat.
J. Provide adequate heat to maintain temperature.
✦ K. Administer antacids, H_2-receptor antagonists, and sucralfate (Carafate) to prevent stress ulcer, as ordered.
✦ L. Maintain wound dressings.
1. Initial excision: mainly for electrical burns.

2. Occlusive dressings.
a. Painful and costly.
b. Decrease water loss.
c. Limit range-of-motion exercises.
d. Help to maintain functional position.
e. Advent of topical antibiotics has led to decreased use.
3. Exposure method.
a. Allows for drainage of burn exudate.
b. Eschar forms protective covering.
c. Use of topical therapy.
d. Skin easily inspected.
e. Range-of-motion exercises easier to perform.
✦ M. Apply topical preparations to wound area.
1. Mafenide (Sulfamylon 5% to 10%).
a. Exerts bacteriostatic action against many organisms.
b. Penetrates tissue wall.
c. Dressings not needed when used.
d. Agent of choice for electrical burns.
e. Breakdown of drug provides heavy acid load. Inhibition of carbonic anhydrase compounds situation.
f. Monitor ABGs for acidosis. Individual compensates by hyperventilating.
g. Alternate use with Silvadene.
✦ 2. Silver sulfadiazine (Silvadene 1%).
a. Broad antimicrobial activity.
b. Effective against yeast.
c. Inhibits bacteria resistant to other antimicrobials.
(1) Not usually used prophylactically.
(2) Given for specific organism.
(3) Not helpful first 48 hours due to vessel thrombosis.
d. Can be washed off with water.
e. Assess for leukopenia after 2–3 days—may resolve automatically.
3. Silver nitrate 0.5%.
a. Used for many years but decreasing in popularity.

    b. Controls bacteria in wound and reduces water evaporation.

    c. Disadvantages are that it acts only on surface organisms, dressings are messy and must be kept wet, and bulk of dressing decreases ROM.

N. Administer systemic antibiotics when there is wound sepsis or positive cultures.

O. Debridement and eschar removal daily.

P. Provide long-term care.
1. Maintain good positioning to prevent contractures.
2. Prevent infection.
3. Maintain adequate protein and caloric intake to promote healing.
4. Monitor hydration status.
5. Protect skin grafts.
6. Provide psychological support (as important as physical care).
    a. Deal with the client's fear of disfigurement and immobility from scarring.
    b. Provide constant support, as plastic repair is lengthy and painful.
    c. Involve the family in long-term planning and day-to-day care.

✦ Q. Design activities for the burned child while child is hospitalized.
1. Actively involve the child (e.g., acting out part of a story verbally).
2. Provide television, books, and games.
3. Allow the child to associate with friends.

R. Counsel parents.
1. Parents and child have difficulty dealing with disfigurement and need assistance.
2. Parents frequently feel guilty, although they are usually not at fault and need assistance working out these feelings.

LYME DISEASE

✦ *Definition:* A multisystem inflammatory disorder caused by an infection acquired through ticks that live in wooded areas and survive by attaching themselves to animal and human hosts.

Assessment

A. Disease is caused by the spirochete *Borrelia burgdorferi*.

B. This disease has many and varied symptoms and is difficult to diagnose because it masquerades as other illnesses.

✦ C. Following a tick bite, the first symptoms occur several days to a month following the bite.
1. Assess for a small red pimple, macule, or papule that spreads into a ringed-shaped rash in 4–20 days. Rash may be large or small, or not occur at all (making diagnosis difficult).
2. Assess for flu-like symptoms: headache, stiff neck, muscle aches, and fatigue.

D. Assess for the second stage occurring several weeks following the bite: central nervous system abnormalities (about 15 percent); heart disease symptoms (8 percent), or joint pain (arthritis).

E. Assess for third-stage symptoms: arthritis progresses and large joints are usually involved (50 percent).
1. Lingering Lyme arthritis may be caused by lingering infection or immune response.
2. A test called the polymerase chain reaction (PCR) identifies persistent Lyme arthritis that may persist even after aggressive antibiotic therapy.

Implementation

✦ A. Blood test may detect the disease but is usually negative during the early phases.
1. Once diagnosis is confirmed, administer antibiotics—dosage depends on severity of symptoms.
2. Penicillin-type drugs given as soon as possible—shortens course of disease.
3. IV Rocephin is prescribed for severe cardiac and neurologicic problems.

B. Prevention is the best treatment.
1. Avoid areas that contain ticks—those that are wooded, grassy, especially in the summer months. There is no vaccine.
2. Wear tight-fitting clothing and spray body with tick repellent.
3. Examine entire body for ticks upon return home; if tick is located, remove with tweezers and wash skin with antiseptic, and preserve tick for examination.

INTEGUMENTARY SYSTEM REVIEW QUESTIONS

1. When administering a tepid bath, a client begins to shiver. The intervention would be to

   1. Continue with the bath, as this helps dissipate the heat.
   2. Stop the bath for a few minutes and place a warm blanket on the client to stop shivering.
   3. Stop the bath, as the body is attempting to produce heat.
   4. Warm the solution, continue the bath, and change the location of cloth placement.

2. A client has interrupted skin integrity. All of the nursing actions below would be appropriate. Which intervention would have the highest priority as a skin protection measure?

   1. Use of appropriate skin care products.
   2. Use of a therapeutic bed (continuous air-flow mattress).
   3. Aseptic technique during skin care.
   4. Pressure ulcer care for the specific stage of the ulcer.

3. The nurse will know a client with lupus erythematosus understands principles of self-care when she can discuss

   1. Drying agents.
   2. Moisturing agents.
   3. Antifungal creams.
   4. Solar protection.

4. The treatment prescribed for the burned area of skin before skin grafting can take place will include

   1. Silver nitrate soaks for 24 hours.
   2. Burn irrigations with Sulfamylon.
   3. Warm soaks with sterile water.
   4. Germicidal soap scrubs to the affected area.

5. While assessing a client with systemic lupus erythematosus, the nurse should keep in mind that the disease affects multiple systems. The nurse should assess for the most common symptoms of

   1. Psychiatric disorders.
   2. Photosensitivity.
   3. Glomerulonephritis.
   4. Joint symptoms.

6. When a client has suffered severe burns all over his body, the most effective method of monitoring the cardiovascular system is

   1. Cuff blood pressure.
   2. Arterial pressure.
   3. Central venous pressure.
   4. Pulmonary artery pressure.

7. The client's skin becomes irritated from the bed linen. A possible nursing intervention that could alleviate the problem is to

   1. Change the linen.
   2. Switch to a pressure-relieving mattress.
   3. Use lotion on the skin.
   4. Keep the client out of bed as much as possible.

8. All of the following are objectives for bathing clients. Which one is the most important?

   1. Maintain muscle tone.
   2. Provide comfort.
   3. Assess the client's overall status.
   4. Improve the client's sense of self-worth.

9. Monitoring the client's skin condition involves several specific nursing actions. Which action would be the *least* important?

   1. Check the skin color.
   2. Assess the skin temperature.
   3. Observe skin turgor.
   4. Examine skin for dryness.

10. When the nurse is completing an assessment of a burned client, second-degree burns would appear as

    1. Full-thickness with extension to underlying muscle and bone.
    2. Partial-thickness with erythema and often edema, but no vesicles.
    3. Partial-thickness with involvement of epidermis and dermis, showing edema and vesicles.
    4. Full-thickness with dry, waxy, or leathery appearance without vesicles.

11. A client has chronic dermatitis involving the neck, face, and antecubital creases. She has a strong family

history of varied allergy disorders. This type of dermatitis is probably best described as

1. Contact dermatitis.
2. Atopic dermatitis.
3. Eczema.
4. Dermatitis medicamentosa.

12. An employee at the local factory comes to the nurse's office with a large furuncle (boil) on his left upper arm. He has come to the office with this same complaint over the past 6 months. In addition to specific care for the boil itself, the nursing intervention should include

1. Advising the client to bathe more regularly.
2. Doing nothing else, as furuncles are not related to any other disease process.
3. Calling in all employees and checking them for furuncles.
4. Encouraging the client to see his family physician as recurrent boils may be a sign of underlying disease.

13. Burn clients require continuous emotional support. Evaluating the nursing care for this male client, the nurse will know that he will receive therapeutic support by which of the following nursing actions?

1. The staff's keeping his room neat and clean.
2. Rotating the staff so he could have varied interactions.
3. Reacting to him as an individual by spending time with him.
4. Keeping family members aware of his condition.

14. A client sustains a 30 percent burn over her lower extremities. When she arrives in the emergency room, the most important intervention is to

1. Clean and dress the wound.
2. Immediately perform endotracheal intubation.
3. Administer a tetanus booster.
4. Start an IV.

15. The following types of clients all require similar diets: a young client with second- and third-degree burns; a middle-aged client following abdominal surgery; and an elderly client prior to elective surgery. The most appropriate diet is one high in

1. Fat and vitamin C.
2. Protein and calories.
3. Carbohydrates and low in fat.
4. Protein and low in carbohydrates.

INTEGUMENTARY SYSTEM

Answers with Rationale

1. (3) Stop or modify the bath to prevent shivering. Shivering is a method of producing body heat.

   NP:I; CN:S; CL:A

2. (4) The most important intervention is to implement pressure ulcer care. The specific ulcer stage treatment is necessary to stop the ulcer from increasing and institute healing therapy. The other interventions are more important for prevention of skin breakdown, even though they should be carried out after skin integrity has been interrupted.

   NP:I; CN:PH; CL:A

3. (4) It is most important that the client with lupus protects herself from sun exposure with large-brimmed hats, long sleeves, and sunscreen cream. Keeping the skin moist and clean are also important, but lesions are best prevented by sun protection.

   NP:E; CN:H; CL:C

4. (4) In addition to the germicidal soap scrubs, systemic antibiotics are administered to prevent infection of the wound. Silver nitrate is not a common treatment today.

   NP:P; CN:PH; CL:C

5. (4) Joint involvement (with or without synovitis) is seen in almost all clients with lupus. Glomerulonephritis (3) develops in about 50 percent of clients and may lead to renal failure. Photosensitivity (2) is less common, and psychiatric disorders (1) due to neurologic involvement are seen in clients with severely active disease.

   NP:A; CN:PH; CL:C

6. (4) Pulmonary artery pressure is the most effective method. Clients with a large percentage of burned body surface often do not have an area where a cuff can be applied. Cuff blood pressures (1) are also affected more by peripheral vascular changes. Pulse monitoring is not accurate enough to detect subtle changes in the system. Central venous pressures (3) are less than optimal because changes in left heart pressure (sign of pulmonary edema) are often not reflected in the right heart pressures.

   NP:A; CN:PH; CL:C

7. (2) A pressure-relieving mattress could help to lessen the irritated skin. Changing the linen (1) would help only if the linen were hypoallergenic. The other two answers are not therapeutic and would not solve the problem. It is important to keep the linen free from wrinkles, which contribute to irritation.

   NP:I; CN:S; CL:A

8. (3) Assessing the client's overall status, including physical and mental, is the broadest and most important because it gives cues to the total condition of the client. The other objectives will be fulfilled as this activity is completed.

   NP:P; CN:S; CL:A

9. (4) Dryness of the skin is the least important because the other parameters give more information about the client's overall condition. Color (1) helps to identify poor circulation or oxygen exchange; skin temperature (2) may indicate increased temperature; and turgor (3) may indicate dehydration.

   NP:A; CN:PH; CL:C

10. (3) A second-degree burn involves the epidermis and dermis. Answer (1) is the definition of a fourth-degree burn, (2) is characteristic of a first-degree burn, and (4) is the definition of a third-degree burn.

    NP:A; CN:PH; CL:C

Coding for Questions/Answers Abbreviations: **Nursing Process: NP,** Assessment: A, Analysis: AN, Planning: P, Implementation: I, Evaluation: E; **Client Needs: CN,** Safe, Effective Care Environment: S, Health Promotion and Maintenance: H, Psychosocial Integrity: PS, Physiological Integrity: PH; **Clinical Area: CA,** Medical Nursing: M, Surgical Nursing: S, Maternal/Newborn Nursing: MA, Pediatric Nursing: P, Psychiatric Nursing: PS; **Cognitive Level: CL,** Knowledge: K, Comprehension: C, Application: A, Analysis: AN.

11. (2) Atopic dermatitis is chronic, pruritic, and allergic in nature. Typically, it has a longer course than contact dermatitis (1) and is aggravated by commercial face or body lotions, emotional stress, and, in some instances, particular foods.

    NP:AN; CN:PH; CL:K

12. (4) Sometimes recurrent boils are symptoms of an underlying disease process such as glycosuria. Bathing (1) will not influence the course of the boils.

    NP:I; CN:PH; CL:A

13. (3) Reacting to each client as an individual and spending time with him shows that the nurse is aware of the client's personal situation and will make an effort to support the client.

    NP:E; CN:PS; CL:C

14. (4) Fluid resuscitation is critical to maintain circulation and prevent hypovolemic shock. Fluid is lost as it shifts from the vessels as a result of increased vascular permeability. If the burn were around the face and neck, intubation (2) may be done to preserve a patent airway. A tetanus booster (3) would be given, but it is not the first intervention.

    NP:I; CN:PH; CL:A

15. (2) Kilocalories and protein are essential for tissue repair and healing. These clients are in a hypermetabolic state and will require increased protein and kilocalories to prevent negative nitrogen balance.

    NP:P; CN:PH; CL:AN

<table>
<tr><td>

BLOOD AND LYMPHATIC SYSTEM

The circulatory system, a continuous circuit, is the mechanical conveyor of the body constituent called blood. Blood, composed of cells and plasma, circulates through the body and is the means by which oxygen and nutritive materials are transported to the tissues and carbon dioxide and metabolic end products are removed for excretion. The lymphatic system collects toxins from the tissues and carries it to the blood.

</td><td>

BLOOD AND BLOOD FACTORS

Blood Components

Plasma

✦ A. Plasma accounts for 55 percent of the total volume of blood.

  B. It is composed of 92 percent water and 7 percent proteins.
   1. Proteins include serum, fibrinogen, albumin and gamma globulin.
   2. Less than 1 percent are organic salts, dissolved gases, hormones, antibodies, and enzymes. (*See* Table 8-9.)

Solid Particles

  A. Solid particles account for 45 percent of the total blood volume.

</td></tr>
</table>

Table 8-9. BLOOD COMPONENT THERAPY

Type	Use	Alerts	Administration Equipment
Fresh plasma	To replace deficient coagulation factors To increase intravascular compartment	Hepatitis is a risk Administer as rapidly as possible Use within 6 hours	Any straight-line administration set
Platelets	To prevent or treat bleeding problems, especially in surgical clients To replace platelets in clients with acquired or inherited deficiencies (thrombocytopenia, aplastic anemia) To replace when platelets drop below 20,000 mm^3 (normal 150,000 to 350,000 mm^3)	Administer at rate of 10 minutes per unit (usually comes in multiple platelet packs)	Platelet transfusion set with special filter to allow platelets to infuse through filter
Granulocytes	To treat oncology clients with severe bone marrow depression and progressive infections To treat granulocytopenic clients with infections that are unresponsive to antibiotics To treat clients with gram-negative bacteremia or infections where marrow recovery does not develop	Administer slowly, over 2–4 hours Give one transfusion daily until granulocytes increase or infection resolves Use within 48 hours after drawn Give when granulocytes are below 500 Observe for shaking, chills and fever (treat with Tylenol before transfusions) Observe for hives and laryngeal edema (treat with antihistamines)	Use Y-type blood filters and prime with physiological saline A microaggregate filter is not used, as it filters out platelets
Serum albumin	To treat shock To treat hypoproteinemia	Available as 5% or 25% solution Infuse 25% solution slowly at 1 mL/min to prevent circulatory overload	Special tubing accompanies albumin solution in individual boxes

✦ B. Blood cells.
   1. Erythrocytes (red blood cells).
      ✦ a. Normal count in an adult is 4–6 million cells/mm³.
         b. They contain hemoglobin, which carries oxygen to cells, and carbon dioxide from cells to lungs.
         c. Red blood cells originate in bone marrow and are stored in the spleen.
         d. Average life span is 10–120 days.
   2. Leukocytes (white blood cells).
      ✦ a. Normal count in an adult is 4500 to 11,000/mm³.
      ✦ b. Primary defense against infections.
         c. Neutrophils play an active role in the acute inflammatory process and have phagocytic action.
         d. Macrophages—both fixed and wandering cells—act as scavengers and phagocytize foreign bodies, cellular debris, and more resistant organisms (i.e., fungi and *Mycobacterium tuberculosis*).
         e. Lymphocytes play an important role in immunologic responses.
         f. Monocytes are the largest of the leukocytes and are less phagocytic than macrophages.
   3. Platelets (thrombocytes).
      ✦ a. 100,000–400,000/mm³ are needed for clot retraction. (*See* Table 8-10.)
         b. Less than 60,000/mm³ may lead to a tendency to bleed.

System Assessment

A. Assess onset of symptoms, whether insidious or abrupt.
B. Assess for petechiae, ecchymosis.
C. Evaluate bleeding time.
D. Assess for fatigue and general weakness.
E. Assess for chills or fever.
F. Assess for dyspnea.
G. Observe for ulceration of oral mucosa and pharynx.
H. Assess for pruritus.
I. Check skin color—pallor, yellow cast, or reddish-purple hue.
J. Assess for visual disturbances.
K. Palpate for hepatomegaly or splenomegaly.
L. Assess for dietary deficiencies—ask questions about daily intake of foods.
M. Assess for neurological symptoms.
   1. Numbness and tingling in the extremities.
   2. Personality changes.
N. Evaluate cardiovascular signs and symptoms.
   1. Hypotension or hypertension.
   2. Character of pulse.

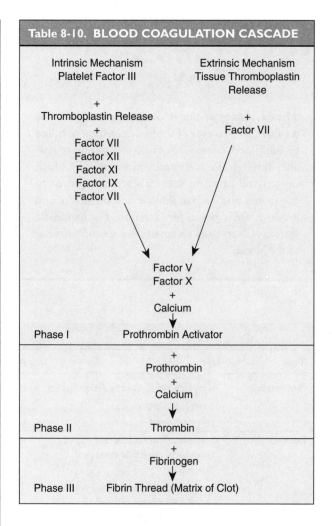

Table 8-10. BLOOD COAGULATION CASCADE

Intrinsic Mechanism Platelet Factor III	Extrinsic Mechanism Tissue Thromboplastin Release
+ Thromboplastin Release + Factor VII Factor XII Factor XI Factor IX Factor VII	+ Factor VII

Factor V
Factor X
+
Calcium
↓

Phase I   Prothrombin Activator
+
Prothrombin
+
Calcium
↓

Phase II   Thrombin
+
Fibrinogen
↓

Phase III   Fibrin Thread (Matrix of Clot)

3. Capillary engorgement.
4. Venous thrombosis.
O. Assess for gastric distress and weight loss.

System Implementation

✦ A. Prevent infections.
   1. Maintain isolation, if indicated, and meticulous medical asepsis.
   2. Suggest bedrest.
   3. Provide high-protein, high-vitamin, and high-calorie diet.
   4. Administer antibiotics as ordered.
✦ B. Promote rest for fatigue and weakness.
   1. Conserve client's strength.
   2. Suggest frequent rest periods.
   3. Ambulate as tolerated.
   4. Decrease disturbing activities and noise.
   5. Provide optimal nutrition.
✦ C. Provide care for hemorrhagic tendencies.
   1. Provide rest during bleeding episodes.
   2. Apply gentle pressure to bleeding sites.
   3. Apply cold compresses to bleeding sites when indicated.

4. Do not disturb clots.
5. Use small-gauge needles to administer medications by injection.
6. Support the client during transfusion therapy.
7. Observe for symptoms of internal bleeding.
8. Have tracheostomy set available for client who is bleeding from mouth or throat.

D. Give care for ulcerative lesions of the tongue, gums, and/or mucous membranes.
   1. Provide nonirritating foods and beverages.
   2. Give frequent oral hygiene with mild, cool mouthwash and solutions.
   3. Use applicators or soft-bristled toothbrush.
   4. Lubricate lips.
   5. Give mouth care both before and after meals.

✦ E. Monitor and treat oxygen deficit.
   1. Elevate head of the bed.
   2. Support client in the orthopneic position.
   3. Administer oxygen when indicated.
   4. Prevent unnecessary exertion.

F. Provide measures to alleviate bone and joint pain.
   1. Use cradle to relieve pressure of bedding.
   2. Apply hot or cold compresses as ordered.
   3. Immobilize joints when ordered.

G. Apply cool sponges if fever present.

H. Administer antipyretic drugs as ordered.

I. Encourage fluid intake unless contraindicated.

J. Provide care for pruritus and/or skin eruptions.
   1. Keep client's fingernails short.
   2. Use soap sparingly, if at all.
   3. Apply emollient lotions for skin care.

K. Attempt to decrease client's anxiety.
   1. Explain nature, discomforts, and limitations of activity associated with diagnostic procedures and treatments.
   2. Listen to client.
   3. Treat client as an individual.
   4. Allow family to participate in client's care.
   5. Encourage family to visit with client; provide privacy for family and client.

TRANSFUSION ADMINISTRATION

Implementation

✦ A. Follow rules for preventing transfusion reaction.
   ✦ 1. Check physician's orders—type and number of units.
   ✦ 2. Identify client and blood bag. Check:
      a. Client's room number; check that ID band number matches transfusion record number; and have client state name. (Client must have blood ID bracelet.)
      b. Name spelled correctly on transfusion record and consent form is signed.
      c. Patency of IV.
      d. Blood type matches on transfusion record and blood bag (A, B, O, and Rh). (*See* Table 8-11.) Note expiration date.

✦ B. Observe blood bag for bubbles, cloudiness, dark color, or black sediment—indicative of bacterial invasion.

✦ C. Check blood with another RN before infusing. Sign transfusion form with another RN according to hospital policy.

✦ D. Ask client about allergy history and report any previous blood reactions.

✦ E. Start infusion with normal saline and appropriate blood tubing. Start blood within 30 minutes from time it is removed from refrigeration. (Blood should not remain at room temperature for long period of time.)

✦ F. Do not allow duration of blood infusion to exceed 4 hours.

✦ G. Use blood filter to prevent fibrin and other materials from entering the bloodstream.

✦ H. Maintain aseptic technique during procedure.

✦ I. Start transfusion slowly at 20–25 drops per minute and observe for transfusion reaction— usually occurs during the first 5–15 minutes.

✦ J. Take baseline vital signs at start of transfusion and again 5 minutes later.

✦ K. Complete the transfusion in no less than 2 hours.
   1. After initial slow rate, infuse at a rate of 60–80 drops/min. (Administration set—10 gtt/mL.)
   2. Hypovolemic client.
      a. Administer blood at the rate of 500 mL in 10 minutes by use of a blood pump or as ordered.
      b. Observe for pulmonary edema and hypervolemia.

TRANSFUSION REACTIONS

Hemolytic or Incompatibility Reaction

Characteristics

A. Most severe complication.
B. Caused by mismatched blood.

✦ C. The reaction is caused by agglutination of the donor's red cells.
   1. The antibodies in the recipient's plasma react with the antigens in the donor's red cells.
   2. The clumping blocks off capillaries and, therefore, obstructs the flow of blood and oxygen to cells. (*See* Table 8-12.)

✦ Table 8-11. SUMMARY OF ABO BLOOD GROUPING

Blood Type	Antigen in RBCs	Antibodies in Plasma	Incompatible Donor Blood	Compatible Blood Donor
A	A	Anti-B	AB and B	A and O
B	B	Anti-A	A and AB	B and O
AB	A and B	None	None	All blood groups
O	None	Anti-A and anti-B	All blood groups	O

✦ Table 8-12. TRANSFUSION REACTIONS

Type	Clinical Manifestations	Nursing Interventions
Bacterial	Sudden increase in temperature Hypotension Dry, flushed skin Abdominal pain Headache Lumbar pain Sudden chill	Stop transfusion immediately Maintain IV site; change tubing as soon as possible Observe for shock Monitor vital signs every 15 minutes until stable Obtain urine specimen Insert Foley if necessary Notify physician and obtain order for broad-spectrum antibiotic Draw blood cultures before antibiotic administration Send blood tubing and bag to lab for culture and sensitivity Control hypothermia
Allergic	Mild: urticaria and hives, pruritus Severe: respiratory wheezing, laryngeal edema Anaphylactic reaction	Stop transfusion immediately Monitor vital signs for possible anaphylactic shock Obtain order for antihistamine Monitor for signs of progressive allergic reaction as transfusion continues
Hemolytic	Severe pain in kidney region and chest Pain at needle insertion site Fever (may reach 105°F), chills Dyspnea and cyanosis Headache Hypotension Hematuria Nausea	Stop transfusion immediately and remove blood tubing Maintain patent IV, start normal saline infusion at "keep open" rate Obtain vital signs Notify blood bank STAT Reconnect tubing to needle and obtain new tubing as soon as possible Administer oxygen Send two blood samples from different sites, urine sample (catheterize if necessary), blood, and transfusion record to lab Obtain orders for IV volume expansion and diuretic (Mannitol) to ensure flushing of kidneys to prevent acute renal tubular necrosis Monitor vital signs every 15 minutes for shock Monitor urine output hourly for possible renal failure Foley catheter may need to be inserted

Assessment

✦ A. Assess for increased temperature.
✦ B. Evaluate for decreased blood pressure.
✦ C. Observe for pain across chest and at site of needle insertion.
✦ D. Assess for chills.
  E. Observe for hematuria.
  F. Evaluate if backache in the kidney region is present.
  G. Assess dyspnea and cyanosis.
  H. Observe for jaundice in severe cases.

Implementation

✦ A. Stop transfusion immediately upon appearance of symptoms.
✦ B. Return remaining blood and client's blood sample to the laboratory for type and cross-match.
✦ C. Keep IV patent after changing blood tubing with either normal saline or D$_5$W, as ordered.
✦ D. Take vital signs every 15 minutes.
  E. Insert Foley catheter for a urine sample for red blood cells and an accurate output record.

F. Check for oliguria.

G. Administer medications such as vasopressors if indicated.

H. Administer oxygen as necessary.

Allergic Reactions

Characteristics

A. Allergic response to any type of allergen in the donor's blood.

✦ B. Common reaction, usually mild in nature.

✦ Assessment

A. Assess for hives.

B. Assess for urticaria.

C. Observe for wheezing.

D. Check for laryngeal edema.

✦ Implementation

A. Administer an antihistamine like Benadryl to control itching and to relieve edema.

B. Slow infusion rate, evaluate and, if reaction is severe, discontinue the transfusion immediately and keep vein open with normal saline.

Bacterial Contamination

Assessment

✦ A. Check blood to see if it is cloudy or discolored or appears to have bubbles present.

B. Assess for sudden increase in temperature.

C. Check for dry, flushed skin.

D. Assess for abdominal or lumbar pain.

E. Assess for hypotension.

F. Assess for headache and sudden chills.

Implementation

✦ A. If transfusion has been started, discontinue immediately.

B. Send remaining blood to laboratory for culture and sensitivity. It is usually advisable to send client's blood sample as well, if transfusion has been started.

C. Change IV tubing and keep line patent.

D. Check vital signs, including temperature, every 15 minutes.

E. Insert Foley catheter for accurate output and urine specimen as ordered.

F. Control hyperthermia, if present, with antipyretics, cooling blankets, or sponge baths.

G. Draw blood cultures before antibiotics.

Transmission of AIDS

A. Blood donations are now screened for the AIDS virus.

✦ B. AIDS antibody test keeps potentially infectious blood and blood products out of the U.S. blood supply.

1. AIDS antibody is a protein naturally produced in body in response to presence of the AIDS virus.

2. Positive test indicates the AIDS antibody is in blood.

3. Blood that tests positive will not be accepted (even if result may be a false positive).

C. Based on the AIDS antibody test for all blood and blood products, transfusion-related AIDS is now extremely rare.

(*See also* Chapter 6, Infection Control.)

Transmission of Viral Hepatitis

Characteristics

✦ A. Donors are screened to prevent transmission.

1. If blood shows positive for hepatitis B surface antigen (formerly Australian antigen), donor is rejected.

2. If donor has had jaundice or hepatitis, donor is rejected permanently.

B. Hepatitis transmitted through blood is usually not fatal.

C. Nursing management is related to the care of clients with hepatitis, based on the seriousness of the condition. (Refer to Gastrointestinal System, page 302, for specific nursing actions.)

Circulatory Overload

Characteristics

✦ A. Transfusion is administered too rapidly.

✦ B. Quantity is in excess of the amount the circulatory system can accommodate.

C. Usually occurs when transfusion is administered to debilitated clients, elderly or young clients, or clients with cardiac or pulmonary disease.

Assessment

✦ A. Observe CVP for increased reading.

✦ B. Assess for tachycardia, sudden increase in blood pressure.

✦ C. Evaluate for respiratory difficulty (i.e., dyspnea, shortness of breath, cough, rales, rhonchi).

D. Assess for hemoptysis and/or pink frothy sputum.

E. Evaluate edema, especially pulmonary edema.

Implementation

✦ A. Discontinue transfusion.

✦ B. Provide for patent airway and adequate ventilation.

1. Administer oxygen at 2 L/min/nasal cannula.

2. Intubate as needed.

✦ C. Place client in semi- to high-Fowler's position to facilitate respiration.

✦ D. Give diuretics (Lasix) as ordered.

1. Drugs will help to decrease blood volume.

2. Reduces effects of hypervolemia on the heart.

E. If client is in congestive heart failure, may need to digitalize.

F. Be prepared for ECG and chest x-ray.

Massive Blood Transfusion Reaction

Definition: Massive transfusion is a transfusion of a volume of blood greater than or equal to one's blood volume in 24 hours (e.g., 10 units in a 70-kg adult). If a client receives stored blood in such large volumes, his or her own blood may be, in effect, "washed out."

Assessment

A. Hypothermia due to rapid transfusion of large amounts of cold blood.

B. Arrhythmias or cardiac arrest.

C. Liver failure clients may have difficulty metabolizing citrate.

D. Hypocalcemia.

Implementation

A. Hypothermia can be avoided by using a heat-exchange device that gently warms blood. All other means of warming blood are contraindicated due to hemolysis.

B. Treatment for hypocalcemia (rarely required) is 10 mL of a 10% solution of calcium gluconate IV diluted in 100 mL D_5W given over 10 minutes.

C. Do not transfuse blood stored for longer than 1 week if client has renal failure because client may have elevated K^+.

Transfusion-Related Acute Lung Injury (TRALI)

Definition: TRALI is a syndrome that includes dyspnea, hypotension, bilateral pulmonary edema, and fever.

Characteristics

A. TRALI has surpassed hemolytic reactions as the leading cause of transfusion-related death. Mortality rate is reported to be 5 to 10 percent.

B. Sudden development of noncardiogenic pulmonary edema (acute lung injury).

C. Usually occurs within 2–6 hours after transfusion of blood product; can occur up to 48 hours later.

D. As many as one-third of all clients who develop acute lung injury have been exposed to blood products.

E. TRALI may be an important and potentially preventable cause of acute lung injury.

Assessment

A. Clients present with findings similar to that of adult respiratory distress syndrome.

B. Symptoms.
   1. Hypotension.
   2. Fever.
   3. Dyspnea and tachycardia.
   4. Noncardiogenic pulmonary edema with diffuse bilateral pulmonary infiltrates on chest radiography is characteristic.

C. Assess for presence of TRALI with transfusions of all types of blood products.

Implementation

A. Generally supportive and similar to that for adult respiratory distress syndrome.

B. Ventilatory and hemodynamic assistance are utilized as required. Most symptoms resolve within 96 hours after ventilatory support.

C. There are no clear indications for the use of corticosteroids, and their use remains controversial in this setting.

D. Additional blood component therapy should not be withheld if clear indications for transfusion exist.

DISORDERS OF THE BLOOD

Purpuras

Definition: The extravasation of blood into the tissues and mucous membranes.

Characteristics

A. Idiopathic thrombocytopenic purpura is characterized by platelet deficiency due to either hypoproliferation, excessive destruction, or excessive pooling of platelets in the spleen.

B. Vascular purpura is characterized by weak, damaged vessels, which rupture easily.

Assessment

✦ A. Observe for petechiae; bruising.

B. Assess postsurgical bleeding.

C. Evaluate increased bleeding time.

D. Evaluate abnormal platelet count (less than 20,000).

E. Assess for ecchymosis.

Implementation

A. Identify underlying cause (medication) if possible.

B. Complete steps to control bleeding.

C. Monitor transfusion of platelets.

D. Monitor administration of corticosteroids.

E. Monitor client with postsurgical splenectomy for idiopathic thrombocytopenia.

Agranulocytosis

✦ *Definition:* An acute, potentially fatal blood disorder characterized by profound neutropenia; most commonly caused by drug toxicity or hypersensitivity.

✦ **Assessment**
   A. Assess for chills and fever.
   B. Assess for sore throat.
   C. Assess for exhaustion and depletion of energy.
   D. Observe for ulceration of oral mucosa and throat.

Implementation
✦ A. Discontinue suspected chemical agents or drugs.
   B. Isolate client to reduce exposure to infections.
   C. Administer corticosteroids only if client appears to be toxic.

Polycythemia Vera

✦ *Definition:* A chronic disease of unknown etiology characterized by overactivity of bone marrow with overproduction of red cells and hemoglobin. Hematocrit is elevated (55% males and 50% females).

Assessment
✦ A. Assess skin.
   1. Reddish-purple hue.
   2. Pruritus.
   B. Diagnosis made by elevated RBC mass, normal O_2 saturation level and enlarged spleen.
✦ C. Assess for complications.
   1. Increased blood volume.
   2. Capillary engorgement.
   3. Hemorrhage, nose bleeds.
   4. Risk for venous thrombosis.
   5. Hypertension.
   D. Assess for signs of hypervolemia: visual disturbances, congestion of conjunctiva, headache, tinnitus, and vertigo.
   E. Assess for gastric distress and weight loss.

Implementation
✦ A. Monitor administration of radiophosphorus (^{32}P) in dosages based on body weight; initially IV, then orally, to suppress marrow function.
✦ B. Monitor alkylating agent—busulfan.
✦ C. Assist with phlebotomy to remove 500 to 2000 mL of blood per week until hematocrit reaches 50 percent; procedure is repeated when hematocrit rises.
   1. Monitor blood pressure, pulse, and respirations for tachycardia during procedure and postprocedure.
   2. Promote client comfort by positioning in prone position to prevent vertigo and syncope.
   3. Instruct clients to avoid iron supplements (especially in multivitamins).
   4. Instruct clients to avoid aspirin and aspirin-containing drugs; alters platelet functioning.
   D. Monitor for complications (impending CVA, thrombocytosis).
   E. Instruct client to monitor symptoms of iron deficiency.

   F. Instruct client to watch common bleeding sites (nose, skin) and report immediately.

Anemia

✦ *Definition:* A condition that occurs when there is a decrease in either quantity or quality of blood. The deficiency may be a decrease in erythrocytes or a lower than normal level of hemoglobin.

Characteristics
✦ A. Common causes of anemia.
   1. Acute or chronic blood loss (hemorrhage, bleeding ulcers, malignancy).
   2. Destruction of red blood cells (hemolysis).
   3. Abnormal bone marrow function—drugs, chemicals, chemotherapy.
   4. Decreased erythropoietin due to renal damage.
   5. Inadequate maturation of red blood cells.
✦ B. Classifications.
   ✦ 1. Hemolytic anemias—premature destruction of RBCs.
      a. Thalassemia.
      b. Sickle cell disease.
      c. Acquired hemolytic anemia.
   ✦ 2. Hypoproliferative (inadequate production) anemias.
      a. Vitamin B_{12} deficiency or folic acid deficiency.
      b. Result of marrow damage caused by medications or chemicals.
   3. Secondary to blood loss.
      a. Chronic blood loss.
      b. Acute blood loss.

Assessment
✦ A. Assess for signs related to tissue hypoxia.
   1. Weakness and fatigue.
   2. Need for sleep and rest.
   3. Lethargy.
   4. Dyspnea.
   5. Tachycardia and tachypnea.
   6. Pallor.
   7. Cold extremities.
✦ B. Assess for signs related to the central nervous system.
   1. Vertigo.
   2. Irritability.
   3. Depression.
   C. Evaluate poor wound healing.
   D. Assess for dietary deficiencies.

Implementation
✦ A. Provide diet high in protein, iron, and vitamins to increase production of erythrocytes; remember that client is sensitive to hot, cold and spicy foods.

B. Maintain adequate fluid intake.

C. Protect from infection.

D. Manage fatigue (most common symptom). Provide complete bedrest if necessary.

E. Promote good skin care to prevent pressure ulcers.

F. Protect from falls and injury (due to vertigo).

G. Avoid extremes of heat and cold (due to disturbance in sensory perception).

H. Provide good mouth care with diluted mouthwash and soft toothbrush.

I. Provide emotional support for long-term therapy.

Iron-Deficiency Anemia

Definition: The most common type of anemia in the world, slowly progressive, related to a deficiency in iron.

Characteristics

A. Occurs most often in infants, adolescents, pregnant females, alcoholics, and the elderly.

B. Results from chronic blood loss, inadequate nutritional intake, defective absorption, improper utilization of iron, prolonged drug therapy, or improper cooking of foods.

Assessment

A. Assess for cheilosis—corners of the mouth are cracked, red, and painful.

B. Assess for exertional dyspnea.

C. Check glossitis.

D. Assess for papillae atrophy of tongue (shiny).

E. Check for pica syndrome (abnormal craving for sand, clay, ice).

F. Observe for concave, brittle nails.

G. Assess for fatigue and lack of energy.

H. Observe for signs of anaphylactic shock, particularly with IV medications.
   1. Headache.
   2. Urticaria.
   3. Hypotension.

Implementation

A. Provide diet high in iron: liver, lean meats, egg yolk, dried fruit, whole-wheat bread, wheat germ, red beans, asparagus, and molasses.

B. Administer iron preparations for 6 to 12 months.
   1. Oral.
      a. Administer ferrous sulfate, 300 mg TID.
      b. Give liquid iron with straw to avoid staining of teeth.
      c. Administer oral iron on empty stomach to increase absorption; or, because it is irritating to the GI tract, suggest client take iron after meals.
      d. Give iron with orange juice or vitamin C, because iron absorption is aided by vitamin C.

      e. Watch for side effects: epigastric distress, abdominal cramps, nausea, and diarrhea or constipation.
      f. Warn client that stools will be black.
   2. Parenteral.
      a. Administer Imferon (IV, IM), Sorbitex (IM).
      b. Use Z-track (deep IM) to prevent pain and discoloration.

C. Monitor fluid and electrolyte balance.

D. Provide frequent rest periods for intense fatigue.

Megaloblastic Anemia

Definition: A group of anemias that have morphologic changes caused by defective DNA synthesis and abnormal RBC maturation.

Characteristics

A. The primary cause is a deficiency of vitamin B_{12} or folic acid.

B. Sources.
   1. Absence of intrinsic factor (pernicious anemia).
   2. Surgical resection of the stomach.
   3. Atrophy of gastric mucosa.
   4. Dietary deficiency—malabsorption disease.
   5. Bacterial or parasitic infections.
   6. Drugs: methotrexate, oral contraceptives, and anticonvulsants.
   7. Alcohol abuse and anorexia.

C. Genetic predisposition (especially in northern Europe).

Assessment

A. Assess for neurological disturbance—tingling of extremities, peripheral neuropathy.
   1. These symptoms do not ocur with folic acid deficiency.
   2. Distinction between deficiency in vitamin B_{12} must be made with deficiency in folic acid.

B. Assess for symptoms of spinal cord degeneration—alterations in gait (loss of balance).

C. Check any loss of finger movement.

D. Evaluate personality and behavioral changes.

E. Assess for glossitis—beefy, red tongue.

F. Assess for anorexia.

G. Assess for fatigue, weakness, pallor.

H. Observe yellow cast to skin.

Implementation

A. Obtain blood work for RBC count and megaloblastic maturation.

B. Prepare client for the following tests.
   1. Bone marrow aspiration (assist physician during test).
   2. Upper GI series (administer bowel prep).

3. Schilling test (maintain NPO for 12 hours; collect 24-hour urine) for pernicious anemia.
4. Gastric analysis—insertion of nasogastric tube, collection of aspirant, injection of histamine.

✦ C. Administer vitamin B$_{12}$ deep IM—usually once a month; usual dose of folic acid is 1 mg/day PO or 5 mg/day for malabsorption.

✦ D. Change in diet and oral folic acid if anemia is caused by folic acid deficiency (chronic alcoholism, malabsorption syndrome, or medications).

E. Provide emotional support during bone marrow aspiration.

F. Provide safety measures if a neurological deficiency is present—assist with ambulation.

G. Provide support and explain behavior changes to client and family.

Aplastic Anemia

✦ *Definition:* Deficiency of marrow stem cells resulting from bone marrow suppression. Pancytopenia frequently accompanies RBC deficiency.

Characteristics

✦ A. Etiology.
1. Toxic action of drugs: Chloromycetin, sulfonamides, Dilantin, alkylating agents, antimetabolites, and anticonvulsants (Mesantoin).
2. Chemicals: DDT, benzene.
3. Exposure to radiation.
4. Diseases that suppress bone marrow activity (leukemia and metastatic cancer).

B. Treatment.
1. Removal of causative agent.
2. Hematopoietic stem cell transplant (HSCT).
3. Bone marrow or stem cell transplant is treatment of choice for clients younger than age 40.
4. Immunosuppressive therapy.
   a. Antithymocyte globulin (ATG).
   b. Cyclosporine.
   c. High-dose cyclophosphamide (Cytoxan).
   d. Steroids.

Assessment

A. Exposure to chemicals and/or drugs.
B. Assess for increased fatigue.
C. Assess for ability to complete activities of daily living.
D. Assess for dyspnea, fatigue.
E. Evaluate blood for low platelet and leukocyte count.
F. Assess for infection.

Implementation

✦ A. Avoid use of toxic chemical agents—DDT, carbon tetrachloride, etc.

B. Administer androgens and/or corticosteroids—now not commonly used due to toxic side effects.

✦ C. Monitor transfusion of fresh platelets (RBC transfusion may be introduced also).

✦ D. Protect from infections—avoid contact with others who have infection; provide meticulous hygiene, clean environment.
1. Administer antibiotics when infection occurs.
2. Place client in private room.

E. Prevent fatigue—provide for adequate rest periods. Avoid activities that are stressful.

F. Observe for complications.

G. Provide physical comfort measures.

H. Provide emotional support for client and family.

I. Educate client how to protect from infection and excessive bleeding.

J. Educate public in use of toxic pesticides and chemicals.

Thrombocytopenia

Definition: Condition that is a lower than normal number of circulating platelets.

Characteristics

✦ A. Normal platelet count is 150,000 to 400,000/mm^3. A count lower than 100,000 leads to this condition; lower than 60,000 may result in tendency to bleed.

B. Condition results from decreased platelet production, destruction of platelets (most common), decreased platelet survival, or sequestration of blood in the spleen.

✦ C. Common causes of platelet destruction.
1. Idiopathic thrombocytopenic purpura—production of an antibody that works against platelet antigen.
2. Heparin induced—may develop with client's receiving heparin for more than 5 days. (Use of low-molecular-weight heparin may prevent this complication.)
3. Certain drugs (alcohol, aspirin, chemotherapeutic agents, gold salts, sulfonamides, thiazides, penicillin, etc.) induce this condition, which usually resolves in 1–2 weeks after drug is withdrawn.

Assessment

✦ A. Assess skin signs: petechiae (occurring only in platelet disorders), ecchymoses, and purpura.
B. Assess for history of menorrhagia, epistaxis.
C. Check low platelet count, bleeding time, and bone marrow examination.

Implementation

A. Monitor corticosteroid therapy—decreases antibody production. Inform client not to stop medication suddenly.

B. Administer care following a splenectomy—removal of the organ responsible for destruction of antibody-coated platelets.

C. Monitor use of immunosuppressive drugs.

✦ D. Monitor platelet transfusion—may be done for certain clients, especially for thrombocytopenic bleeding.

✦ E. Constantly monitor for bleeding tendency—when platelet count is less than 60,000, avoid
   1. Infections.
   2. Rectal temperature.

✦ F. Apply pressure to venipuncture sites for 5 minutes.

✦ G. Educate client on how to recognize signs and measures to prevent injury.
   1. Avoid trauma and contact sports.
   2. Use soft toothbrush—avoid trauma to gums.
   3. Use electric shaver.
   4. Avoid drugs that thin blood (aspirin).

Note: For sickle cell anemia and thalassemia, *see* Pediatric Nursing, Chapter 13.

SPLEEN

✦ *Definition:* A gland-like organ located in the upper left part of the abdominal cavity; it is a storage organ for red corpuscles and, because of a large number of macrophages, acts as a blood filter.

Characteristics

A. Functions as a blood reservoir.

B. Purifies blood by removing waste and infectious organisms.

C. Destroys old red blood cells.

D. Is the primary source of antibodies in infants and children.

E. Produces lymphocytes, plasma cells, and antibodies in adults.

F. Produces erythrocytes in fetus.

G. Destroys erythrocytes when they reach the end of their life span.

Hypersplenism

Definition: The premature destruction of erythrocytes, leukocytes, and platelets.

Characteristics

✦ A. The most common form of hypersplenism is congestive splenomegaly, usually due to portal hypertension secondary to cirrhosis.

✦ B. Other causes are idiopathic thrombocytopenia, thrombosis, stenosis, or atresia.

C. Secondary hypersplenism occurs in association with leukemias, lymphomas, Hodgkin's disease, and tuberculosis.

D. Treatment: correct underlying condition and/or splenectomy.

Rupture of the Spleen

Definition: Traumatic rupture following violent blow or trauma to the spleen.

Assessment

✦ A. Assess weakness due to blood loss.

✦ B. Evaluate abdominal pain and muscle spasm particularly in the left upper quadrant.

C. Assess for rebound tenderness.

D. Assess for referred pain to left shoulder.

E. Palpate for tenderness.

F. Check leukocytes (well over 12,000).

G. Assess for progressive shock with rapid, thready pulse; drop in blood pressure; and pallor.

Implementation

✦ A. Prepare for surgical intervention—splenectomy.

B. Prevent infection.

C. Monitor vital signs closely.

Splenectomy

Definition: Excision of the spleen.

Assessment

✦ A. Evaluate indications for surgical intervention.
   1. Trauma.
   2. Hypersplenism.
   3. Idiopathic thrombocytopenia.
   4. Hodgkin's disease.
   5. Lymphoma.
   6. Preceding renal transplantation (reduces rejection).

B. Observe for signs of infection.

C. Assess vital signs for baseline data.

Implementation

✦ A. Prevent thrombus formation.
   1. Initiate bed exercises.
   2. Ambulate early.
   3. Provide adequate hydration.

✦ B. Prevent respiratory complications due to reduced expansion of left lung and location of spleen near diaphragm.
   1. Turn, cough, and deep-breathe every 2 hours.
   2. Maintain IPPB if prone to URI.

C. Prevent infection if rupture occurs.
   1. Observe for signs of infection.
   2. Administer antibiotics.

NEOPLASTIC BLOOD DISORDERS

Leukemia

✦ *Definition:* A malignant disorder of blood-forming tissue characterized by neoplastic proliferation of hematopoietic cells or their precursors.

CHEMOTHERAPY PRINCIPLES

- Combination of drugs used.
  1. Limits toxicity of individual drugs.
  2. Increases destruction of cells sensitive to various agents.
- Induction therapy used after initial diagnosis.
- Maintenance therapy used during remission.

✦ **Characteristics**

A. The increased proliferation process alters the cell's ability to mature and/or function correctly.

B. In acute processes the predominant cell is poorly differentiated, but in chronic processes the leukemic cell is well defined.

C. Anemia results from an increased number of white blood cells that are immature and do not function normally, and a decreased number of red blood cells, hemoglobin, and platelets.

D. Diagnostic tests.
   1. Bone marrow aspiration/biopsy.
   2. Differential count.

E. Etiology—predisposing factors.
   1. Excess radiation exposure.
   2. Viral factors.
   3. Immune alteration.
   4. Noxious chemicals and drugs.
   5. Bone marrow alterations.

Assessment

✦ A. Assess for sudden high fever with abnormal bleeding.

✦ B. Assess for nosebleeds, purpura, ecchymosis, petechiae, or prolonged menses.

C. Evaluate general nonspecific symptoms such as weakness, lethargy, low-grade fever.

D. Evaluate recurrent infections if any of the above symptoms are present.

Implementation

✦ A. Administer chemotherapeutic agents.
   1. Specific drugs and combinations are ordered according to the specific type of leukemia and whether it is acute or chronic.
   2. *See* chemotherapy drugs and protocol in Chapter 9, Oncology Nursing.

✦ B. Prevent complications related to the side effects of drugs.
   1. Proper mouth care (ulcerations and bleeding).
   2. Anorexia.

C. Maintain fluid and electrolyte balance.

D. Administer allopurinol to combat problems associated with increased serum uric acid (from rapid destruction of body tissue).

E. Provide high-calorie, high-vitamin diet to prevent weight loss, weakness, debilitation.

✦ F. Provide emotional support for
   1. Alopecia.
   2. Altered body image.
   3. Fear of dying.
   4. Depression.
   5. Financial burden.

G. Provide client education.
   1. Drugs—dosage and side effects.
   2. Associated treatments.
   3. Disease process.

H. Prevent infections, ulcerations, hemorrhage.

Acute Myeloid Leukemia (AML)

Characteristics

A. Incidence: occurs more commonly at adolescence and after age 55. Slightly higher incidence in males. Onset can be insidious or rapid.

B. Pathophysiology: uncontrolled proliferation of myeloblasts (precursors of granulocytes), which replace normal cells in the marrow.

Assessment

✦ A. Assess for anemia and symptoms of dyspnea, fatigue, pallor, palpitations.

✦ B. Assess for symptoms of platelet deficiency: epistaxis, gingival bleeds, purpura, petechiae, or bleeding in major systems.

C. Assess for symptoms of local abscesses, elevated temperature, chills.

D. Palpate for splenomegaly.

✦ E. Assess for lymph node enlargement and difficulty with respiration and swallowing.

F. Assess for bone pain.

G. Evaluate CNS involvement with signs of increased ICP.

H. Check for hyperuricemia (excessive uric acid).

Implementation

✦ A. Administer chemotherapy, called induction therapy.
   ✦ 1. Cytarabine, Daunomycin, mitoxantrone, or idarubicin.
   2. 70 percent of clients suffer a relapse and long-term survival is only 5 percent.

B. Bone marrow transplant is another option for treatment.

C. Administer antibiotics for increased temperature.

D. Monitor platelet administration when bleeding occurs.

E. Administer allopurinol when hyperuricemia occurs.

Chronic Myeloid Leukemia (CML)

Characteristics

✦ A. Incidence: primarily a disease of young adults (age 30 to 50). Thought to have a genetic origin. Philadelphia chromosome is involved.

B. Pathophysiology: abnormal stem cell leading to a marked increase of granulocytes and megakaryocytes (platelet cells). The mature neutrophil is the cell that is predominant.

C. Clients may be without symptoms.

✦ **Assessment**

A. Assess for fatigue and malaise.

B. Palpate for large, tender spleen.

C. Observe skin for pallor, purpura, nodules.

D. Assess for abdominal discomfort.

E. Evaluate fever, heat intolerance, or increased perspiration.

F. Assess for retinal hemorrhage.

G. Assess for bone pain.

H. Assess anemia.

I. Evaluate increased uric acid level.

Implementation

✦ A. Administer oral alkylating agent busulfan (Myleran) and hydroxyurea.

B. Prepare for splenectomy or irradiation.

C. Instruct client and family in preventive principles.
1. Good nutrition.
2. Prevention of infection.
3. Complicating signs.
4. Skin care.
5. Adequate rest to minimize weakness.

Chronic Lymphocytic Leukemia (CLL)

Characteristics

✦ A. Incidence—insidious onset, most common in ages 50 to 70.

✦ B. Pathophysiology—the small lymphocyte (B cell) is the predominant cell type and eventually leads to decreased production of other hematopoietic cells.

Assessment

A. Many clients are asymptomatic but diagnosed by increased lymphocyte count.

✦ B. Assess classic signs.
1. Weakness, fatigue, and lymphadenopathy.
2. Anemia.
3. Weight loss.
4. Abdominal discomfort with hepatomegaly/ splenomegaly.
5. Vesicular skin lesions.

C. Assess less common signs.
1. Excessive diaphoresis.
2. Infection.

✦ **Implementation**

A. Administer drugs: chlorambucil (Leukeran), cyclophosphamide (Cytoxan), and glucocorticoids.

1. Clients who don't respond may go into remission with fludarabine.
2. Fludarabine may cause bone marrow depression; clients at risk for infections.

B. Prepare for splenectomy in some cases.

C. Prevent infection, be especially oriented toward maintaining clean skin.

D. Observe for complications: thrombocytopenia.

E. Provide emotional support.

Acute Lymphocytic Leukemia (ALL)

Characteristics

✦ A. Incidence—usually appears before age 15 but is highest in 3- to 4-year-olds. Males slightly more at risk. More than 80 percent of all children survive 5 years or more.

B. Pathophysiology—uncontrolled proliferation of lymphoblasts with eventual reduction of other blood cells.

✦ **Assessment**

A. Assess for malaise, fatigue, and fever.

B. Assess bone involvement, and lymph and spleen alterations.

C. Check for bleeding gums, skin, and nose.

D. Evaluate CNS symptoms, especially stiff neck and headache.

Implementation

A. Prepare for induction therapy.

B. Maintain therapy when in remission.

✦ C. Administer drugs.
1. Mercaptopurine (6-MP) and methotrexate.
2. Vincristine and prednisone intermittently.

D. Complete remission occurs in more than 90 percent of clients treated with drug protocols.

MALIGNANCY OF THE LYMPHATIC SYSTEM

Hodgkin's Disease

✦ *Definition:* A chronic, progressive, neoplastic, invariably fatal reticuloendothelial disease involving the lymphoid tissues of the body. It is most common between the ages of 20 and 40. While the exact etiology is unknown, the suspected sources are viral (20 percent of clients are infected with Epstein-Barr virus), environmental, genetic, and immunologic. Onset is often insidious.

✦ **Assessment**

A. Assess for painless enlargement of cervical lymph nodes.

B. Assess for severe pruritus.

C. Evaluate irregular fever, night sweats.

D. Palpate for splenomegaly and hepatomegaly.

✦ MEDICAL IMPLICATIONS

A. Radiation is used for stages I, II, and IIE in an effort to erad-icate the disease (80–90 percent cure rate).

B. Wide-field megavoltage radiation with doses of 3500 to 4000 roentgens over a 4- to 6-week period.

C. Recent results show improvement with a 2- to 4-month course of chemotherapy followed by radiation.

D. Combination chemotherapy for stages III and IV and all B symptoms: doxorubicin, bleomycin, vinblastine and dacar-bazine (ABVD).

E. Observe for jaundice, weight loss.

F. Assess edema and cyanosis of the face and neck.

G. Evaluate pulmonary symptoms including dyspnea, cough, chest pain, cyanosis, and pleural effusion.

H. Assess for fatigue, malaise, and anorexia, which indi-cate progressive anemia.

I. Evaluate bone pain and vertebral compression.

J. Assess nerve pain and paraplegia.

K. Assess laryngeal paralysis.

L. Evaluate increased susceptibility to infection.

✦ M. Assess degree of staging—crucial to treatment regimen.

1. *Stage I:* disease is restricted to single anatomic site, or is localized in a group of lymph nodes; asymptomatic.
   Treatment: if nodes are above diaphragm, radia-tion alone. Depending on size of nodes, chemotherapy may be added.

2. *Stage II:* two or three adjacent lymph nodes in the area on the same side of the diaphragm are affected.
   Treatment: same as above. If lymph nodes are large, combination radiation and chemotherapy.

3. *Stage II(E):* localized extralymphatic site on same side of diaphragm.

4. *Stage III:* disease is widely disseminated on both sides of diaphragm into the lymph areas and organs.
   Treatment: full-dose chemotherapy and radia-tion to areas of enlarged nodes.

5. *Stage IV:* involvement of bone, bone marrow, pleura, liver, skin, gastrointestinal tract, central nervous system, and gradually the entire body.
   Treatment: Six rounds of chemotherapy with CT and PET scans for monitoring; may also get radiation.

N. B symptoms: fever over 38°C (100.4°F), night sweats, more than 10% weight loss.

Implementation

✦ A. Provide supportive relief from effects of radiation and chemotherapy.

1. Side effects include nausea and vomiting.

2. Controlled by premedication of sedatives and antiemetic agents.

✦ B. Assist client to maintain as normal a life as possible during course and treatment of disease.

1. Counsel client and family to accept process of treatment.

2. Provide supportive assistance in dealing with feelings of anger, depression, fear, and loneliness.

C. Prevent infection as body's resistance is lowered.

D. Continually observe for complications: pressure from enlargement of lymph glands on vital organs.

Non-Hodgkin's Lymphoma (NHL)

✦ *Definition:* A malignant disorder (involving malignant B cells) that originates from lymphoid tissues but is not characterized as Hodgkin's disease.

Assessment

✦ A. Assess for enlarged lymph nodes; painless.

B. Unexplained fever, night sweats, weight loss, fatigue.

✦ C. Assess for gastrointestinal involvement—jaundice, ab-dominal cramping, bloody diarrhea, bowel obstruction.

D. Ureteral obstruction may cause hydronephrosis.

E. Compression of the spinal cord may impair neuro-logic function.

F. Hemolytic anemia may occur late in the disease.

✦ G. Diagnosis.

1. Biopsy of suspicious node.

2. Staged like Hodgkin's disease.

3. Once diagnosis is made, chest x-ray, CT scan, bone marrow, and blood work are done to determine stage.

4. Treatment is based on these features.

H. Prognosis—varies among types.

1. Good survival rate with low-grade localized lymphomas.

2. Aggressive type—one-third survival rate.

Implementation

✦ A. Based on actual classification of disease—same as for Hodgkin's disease.

1. Radiation treatment of choice for non-aggressive form.

2. Chemotherapy combination is used for aggres-sive form.

3. Interferon recently approved for follicular low-grade lymphomas.

B. Remission may occur but typically the disease recurs more aggressively.

C. Bone marrow and blood stem transplants may pro-long survival—considered for clients younger than age 60.

BLOOD AND LYMPHATIC SYSTEM REVIEW QUESTIONS

1. The client has orders to draw blood for serum electrolytes. She is on bedrest and has an IV in the basilic vein of the right forearm. The most appropriate site for blood withdrawal is the

   1. Left upper arm (brachial vein).
   2. Right forearm (radial vein).
   3. Foot (greater saphenous vein).
   4. Left forearm (median cubital vein).

2. For client safety, it is essential to check data on the requisition form against the blood unit. The essential data would *not* include

   1. Client's name.
   2. Blood group and type.
   3. Blood unit number.
   4. Blood bank that issued the blood.

3. LVNs/LPNs are allowed to withdraw blood specimens according to nurse practice guidelines if they

   1. Have received in-service education in this area.
   2. Practiced the skill in their nursing program.
   3. Are IV certified.
   4. Are the team leader in a facility.

4. A client is about to be discharged on the drug bishydroxycoumarin (Dicumarol). Of the principles below, which is the most important to teach the client before discharge?

   1. He should be sure to take the medication before meals.
   2. He should shave with an electric razor.
   3. If he misses a dose, he should double the dose at the next scheduled time.
   4. It is the responsibility of the physician to do the teaching for this medication.

5. A client's laboratory results are returned and the hemoglobin is 10 g/dL and the hematocrit is 30 percent. The highest-priority nursing goal should be to

   1. Promote skin integrity.
   2. Conserve the client's energy.
   3. Prevent constipation.
   4. Encourage mobility.

6. When a client with a high fever and a diagnosis of viral infection is admitted to the hospital, the nurse would expect the lymphocyte (T cell) count to be

   1. Higher than normal.
   2. Lower than normal.
   3. Within normal limits.
   4. Absent.

7. A client receiving a blood transfusion begins to wheeze and her skin becomes flushed with hives. The nurse knows that these symptoms are characteristic of a(n)

   1. Allergic reaction.
   2. Hemolytic reaction.
   3. Thrombic crisis.
   4. Transfusion reaction.

8. A client with acute lymphocytic leukemia is scheduled to receive methotrexate. The most important nursing goal when caring for this client is to

   1. Prevent infection.
   2. Maintain fluid balance prior to and following drug administration.
   3. Observe for signs of gastrointestinal disturbance.
   4. Observe for changes in mental alertness.

9. A client has just had a blood infusion started. The nurse suspects a possible hemolytic reaction to the blood. After stopping the blood transfusion, which nursing intervention would *not* be carried out?

   1. Return the blood bag to the laboratory.
   2. Obtain frequent urine specimens.
   3. Send a blood specimen to the laboratory for detection of intravascular hemolysis.
   4. Start another unit of blood to prevent further hemolysis.

10. A general guideline for starting a blood transfusion is to start it at how many macrodrops per minute, for how long a time?

    1. 10 drops for 10 minutes.
    2. 20 drops for 10 minutes.
    3. 25 to 50 drops for 15 minutes.
    4. 120 drops for 15 minutes.

11. You are caring for a client who has been on Prevacid, trazadone, and Zoloft for the past 8 weeks. This client has an absolute neutrophil count of 300/mm^3 and a white blood cell count of 1500/mm^3. The nurse should consider which of the following implementations as the priority?

1. Rapid administration of packed cells to raise blood count.
2. Frequent vital signs.
3. Maintaining neutropenic precautions.
4. Regularly scheduled administration of Prevacid, trazadone, and Zoloft to maintain blood levels.

12. A client has lost about 30 percent of his total blood volume. Blood has been replaced, but his blood pressure remains low. Which of the following drugs would the nurse anticipate the physician's ordering?

1. A vasopressor.
2. A vasodilator.
3. An adrenergic-blocking drug.
4. A parasympatholytic drug.

13. The nurse has orders to administer blood to a client. The primary IV solution to which the nurse will add the blood is normal saline (NS). The rationale for using this solution rather than D$_5$W is

1. NS prevents cell hemolysis.
2. NS is more compatible with blood.
3. The dextrose in D$_5$W inactivates the blood.
4. NS is more common as a primary IV solution.

14. When assessing a client for Coumadin therapy, the condition that will exclude this client from Coumadin therapy is

1. Diabetes.
2. Arthritis.
3. Pregnancy.
4. Peptic ulcer disease.

15. While monitoring a client's blood transfusion, the nurse determines that a hemolysis reaction is occurring. The first nursing intervention is to

1. Slow down the transfusion.
2. Administer IV Benadryl.
3. Stop the transfusion.
4. Notify the physician.

16. A client has aplastic anemia secondary to radiation exposure. What is the pathologic process involved in aplastic anemia?

1. Decreased intake of iron.
2. Increased rate of red blood cell destruction.
3 Decreased liver function.
4. Decreased bone marrow production of red blood cells.

17. The nursing diagnosis with the highest priority for the client with aplastic anemia who is being treated with both prednisone and cyclophosphamide (Cytoxan) is a risk for

1. Activity intolerance.
2. Infection.
3. Injury.
4. Impaired skin integrity.

BLOOD AND LYMPHATIC SYSTEM

Answers with Rationale

1. (4) The most appropriate site is the other (left) arm given that the IV is running in the right arm. The median cubital vein is the easiest vein from which to draw blood and, because the nurse will need to use a tourniquet, the left arm is appropriate—otherwise, this procedure would interfere with the IV.

   NP:P; CN:PH; CL:A

2. (4) The blood bank source is not part of the essential data that must be checked. Additional items that should be checked are ID number and expiration date of the blood.

   NP:P; CN:S; CL:C

3. (3) If LVNs or LPNs are IV certified, they will be able to withdraw blood according to most nurse practice act guidelines. In-service education (1) or practice (2) is not enough training for this skill.

   NP:P; CN:S; CL:K

4. (2) Dicumarol is an anticoagulant drug and one of the dangers involved is bleeding. Using a safety razor can lead to bleeding through cuts. The drug should be given at the same time daily but not related to meals (1). Due to danger of bleeding, missed doses (3) should not be made up.

   NP:P; CN:H; CL:A

5. (2) These test results indicate anemia. Impaired oxygen-carrying capacity of red blood cells causes cellular hypoxia and results in fatigue. Conserving energy limits oxygen expenditure and minimizes fatigue. Increased mobility (4) increases the demand for oxygen and contributes to fatigue. Although hypoxic tissues are more vulnerable to breakdown, protecting the integumentary system (1) is not as high a priority as is the promotion of the body's overall oxygenation. Constipation (3) is not a problem in anemia.

   NP:P; CN:PH; CL:AN

6. (1) A high T-cell count (above 3400/mm^3, lymphocytosis) would occur with a viral infection or influenza. These are the cells (along with B cells) that fight chronic bacterial and acute viral infections.

   NP:A; CN:PH; CL:C

7. (1) These signs, in addition to laryngeal edema, are characteristic of an allergic reaction that is, less specifically, a transfusion reaction. Chills, increased temperature, and pain in the kidney region are indications of a hemolytic reaction.

   NP:AN; CN:PH; CL:C

8. (1) A serious side effect of methotrexate is leukopenia—fewer white blood cells than normal, which results in neutropenia. This condition could lead to infection, in which case the client would have to be admitted to the hospital and the drug stopped. Antibiotics would be started.

   NP:I; CN:PH; CL:AN

9. (4) The nurse would not start another unit of blood; a normal saline infusion would be started at a "keep open" rate with new IV tubing. The blood, IV tubing, urine specimen, and transfusion record would be sent to the lab. Urine specimens (2) would be checked to monitor for acute renal tubular necrosis caused by the incompatibility of the blood.

   NP:I; CN:PH; CL:A

10. (3) A blood transfusion should be started slowly (from 25 to 50 drops per minute) for the first 15 minutes because slow administration allows time to observe for an adverse reaction. Most reactions occur in the first 15 minutes. The continuing rate is 100 mL/hr.

    NP:P; CN:PH; CL:C

11. (3) Maintaining neutropenic precautions is the most important implementation for this client. The client is

---

Coding for Questions/Answers Abbreviations: **Nursing Process: NP,** Assessment: A, Analysis: AN, Planning: P, Implementation: I, Evaluation: E; **Client Needs: CN,** Safe, Effective Care Environment: S, Health Promotion and Maintenance: H, Psychosocial Integrity: PS, Physiological Integrity: PH; **Clinical Area: CA,** Medical Nursing: M, Surgical Nursing: S, Maternal/Newborn Nursing: MA, Pediatric Nursing: P, Psychiatric Nursing: PS; **Cognitive Level: CL,** Knowledge: K, Comprehension: C, Application: A, Analysis: AN.

at risk for infection. Low neutrophil and white blood cell counts are often found in clients with aplastic anemia or malignancies or in clients who have received cytotoxic therapy. These low blood counts are most likely due to the Prevacid, trazadone, and Zoloft. Administration of blood (1) is not indicated; frequent vital signs (2) are important, but not the highest priority; continuing the medications that are the most likely cause of the low blood count (4) will merely make the situation worse.

NP:I; CN:PH; CL:AN

12. (2) Vasodilator drugs are given when volume replacement has been completed. They decrease vascular resistance, decrease the work of the heart, and improve cardiac output and tissue perfusion. Vasopressor drugs (1) intensify shock by increasing vasoconstriction in the microcirculatory beds.

NP:P; CN:PH; CL:A

13. (1) Normal saline does prevent cell hemolysis, so it is the solution of choice. Answer (2) is also correct, but it is not as specific.

NP:AN; CN:PH; CL:A

14. (3) Coumadin therapy is contraindicated in the pregnant woman because it crosses the placenta. The pregnant client should be taught heparin administration with a heparin lock if anticoagulation therapy must be continued. The arthritic client (2) may take aspirin or NSAIDs, which potentiate the effects of Coumadin, and should be watched for gastrointestinal bleed, as should the client with ulcer disease (4).

NP:A; CN:PH; CL:A

15. (3) The first action would be to stop the transfusion to avoid administering any additional incompatible cells. The incompatible cells can lead to agglutination, oliguric renal failure, pulmonary emboli, and death if administered in large quantities. Some resources state that as little as 50 mL of incompatible blood can lead to severe complications and death.

NP:I; CN:S; CL:A

16. (4) The term *aplastic* indicates arrested development. Aplastic anemia is a rare and serious condition in which the bone marrow stops producing enough red and white blood cells to keep the body healthy, resulting in an increased risk of infection and uncontrollable bleeding.

NP:AN; CN:PS; CL:K

17. (2) Both prednisone and cyclophosphamide increase the risk for infection and decrease the body's immune function.

NP:AN; CN:S; CL:C

ENDOCRINE SYSTEM

The endocrine system consists of a series of glands that function individually or conjointly to integrate and control innumerable metabolic activities of the body. These glands automatically regulate various body processes by releasing chemical signals called hormones.

ANATOMY AND PHYSIOLOGY

Function

A. Maintenance and regulation of vital functions.
   1. Response to stress or injury.
   2. Growth and development.
   3. Reproduction.
   4. Fluid, electrolyte, and acid–base balance.
   5. Energy metabolism.
B. Endocrine glands.
   1. Have specific functions.
   2. Influence one another.
   3. Secrete hormones directly into the bloodstream.
   4. Controlled by autonomic nervous system.
   5. Located in various parts of body.
C. Hormones. (*See* Table 8-13.)
   1. Chemical messengers that stimulate or inhibit life processes.
   2. Transmitted via the bloodstream to target tissues.
   ✦ 3. Regulated through negative feedback control system (hypothalamic–pituitary axis). For example, the TSH-releasing hormone (TRH) is secreted by the hypothalamus, which causes the pituitary to secrete TSH. TSH stimulates the thyroid to secrete thyroxine. Thyroxine feeds back on the pituitary and inhibits production of TSH.
   4. Also regulated by renin–angiotensin–aldosterone, insulin–glucose, and calcium–parathormone.
   5. Endocrine disorders are caused by a deficit or excess in hormone production.

Structure

✦ A. Hypothalamus connects pituitary gland to central nervous system.
✦ B. Pituitary gland divided into three lobes.
   1. Anterior pituitary control (master gland).
      a. Tropic hormones exert effect through regulation of other endocrine glands—ACTH, TSH, FSH, LH.
      b. Target tissues: hormones have direct effect on tissues—growth hormone, prolactin, MSH.
   2. Posterior lobe (neurohypophysis)—ADH (also called vasopressin), oxytocin, melanophore-stimulating hormone.
   3. Intermediate lobe.
C. Adrenal gland—located on the top of each kidney.
   1. Cortex produces glucocorticoids, mineralocorticoids, sex hormones.
   2. Medulla produces epinephrine and norepinephrine.
D. Thyroid gland—located anterior to the trachea. Produces thyroxine, triiodothyronine, and thyrocalcitonin.
E. Parathyroid gland—located near thyroid. Produces parathormone (PTH).
F. Pancreas—located between stomach and small intestine. Produces insulin and glucagon.
G. Ovaries—located in female pelvic cavity. Produce estrogen and progesterone.
H. Testes—located in male scrotum. Produce testosterone.

System Assessment

A. Assess for growth imbalance.
   1. Excessive growth.
      a. Pituitary or hypothalamic disorders.
      b. Excess adrenal, ovarian, or testicular hormone.
   2. Retarded growth.
      a. Endocrine and metabolic disorders; difficult to distinguish from dwarfism.
      b. Hypothyroidism.
B. Evaluate for obesity.
   1. Sudden onset suggests hypothalamic lesion (rare).
   2. Cushing's syndrome (with characteristic buffalo hump).
C. Assess abnormal skin pigmentation.
   1. Hyperpigmentation may coexist with depigmentation in Addison's disease.
   2. Thyrotoxicosis may be associated with spotty brown pigmentation.
   3. Pruritus is a common symptom in diabetes.
D. Check for hirsutism.
   1. Normal variations in body occur on nonendocrine basis.
   2. First sign of neoplastic disease.
   3. Indicates changes in adrenal status.
E. Evaluate appetite changes.
   1. Polyphagia is a common sign of uncontrolled diabetes.
   2. Indicates thyrotoxicosis.

◆ Table 8-13. ENDOCRINE SYSTEM			
Endocrine Gland	**Hormones Produced**	**Function**	**Endocrine Disorder**
Pituitary Location: base of the brain	*Anterior Lobe* Adrenocorticotropic hormone (ACTH) Thyrotropic hormone (TSH) Somatotropic growth-stimulating hormone (STH) Gonadotropic hormones (FSH, LH, LTH) *Posterior Lobe* (neurohypophysis) Vasopressin (ADH) Oxytocin Melanophore-stimulating hormone (MSH) *Intermediate Lobe*	Termed "master gland" as it directly affects the function of other endocrine glands Regulates thyroid gland and metabolism Promotes growth of body tissues Controls sexual development and function Influences water absorption by kidney Influenced by hypothalamus	*Anterior pituitary* Gigantism Acromegaly Dwarfism *Posterior pituitary* Diabetes insipidus
Adrenal Location: on top of each kidney	*Cortex* Glucocorticoids Cortisol Cortisone Corticosterone Mineralocorticoids Aldosterone Deoxycorticosterone Corticosterone Sex hormones Androgens Estrogens *Medulla* Epinephrine (adrenaline) Norepinephrine (nonadrenaline)	Regulates sodium and electrolyte balance Affects carbohydrate, fat, and protein metabolism Influences the development of sexual characteristics Stimulates "fight or flight" response to danger Increases blood glucose levels Stimulates release of ACTH from pituitary, which then stimulates adrenal cortex to release glucocorticoids Increases rate and force of cardiac contractions *Constricts* blood vessels in skin, mucous menbranes, and kidneys *Dilates* blood vessels in the skeletal muscles, coronary arteries, and pulmonary arteries Increases heart rate and force of contraction Vasoconstricts blood vessels throughout the body	Addison's disease Cushing's syndrome Pheochromocytoma Primary aldosteronism
Thyroid Location: anterior part of the trachea just inferior to the larynx	Thyroxine Triiodothyronine Thyrocalcitonin	Controls rate of body metabolism, growth and nutrition Secretes calcitonin, a hormone that decreases excessive levels of calcium in the body by slowing the calcium-releasing activity of bone cells	Goiter Cretinism Myxedema Hyperthyroidism (Graves' disease)
Parathyroid Location: near thyroid	Parathormone (PTH)	Controls calcium and phosphorus metabolism	Hypoparathyroidism Hyperparathyroidism

Continues

✦ Table 8-13. ENDOCRINE SYSTEM *(Continued)*			
Endocrine Gland	**Hormones Produced**	**Function**	**Endocrine Disorder**
Pancreas Islets of Langerhans Location: between the stomach and small intestine	Insulin Glucagon	Influences carbohydrate metabolism Indirectly influences fat and protein metabolism	Diabetes mellitus Hyperinsulinism
Ovaries Location: pelvic cavity **Testes** Location: scrotum	Estrogen and progesterone Testosterone	Controls development of secondary sex characteristics	Lack of acceleration or regression of sexual development

3. Nausea and weight loss may indicate Addisonian crisis or diabetic acidosis.

F. Check for polyuria and polydipsia.
1. Symptoms usually of nonendocrine etiology.
2. If sudden onset, suggest diabetes mellitus or insipidus.
3. May be present with hyperparathyroidism or hyperaldosteronism.

G. Assess mental changes.
1. Though often subtle, may be indicative of underlying endocrine disorder.
   a. Nervousness and excitability may indicate hyperthyroidism.
   b. Mental confusion may indicate hypopituitarism, Addison's disease, or myxedema.
2. Mental deterioration is observed in untreated hypoparathyroidism and hypothyroidism.

H. Assess metabolic status.
1. Changes in energy level.
2. Fatigue.
3. Changes in heat or cold tolerance.
4. Recent weight changes.
5. Changes in sleep pattern.

I. Assess for coma state.
1. Drowsiness.
2. Hyperpnea.
3. Tachycardia.
4. Subnormal temperature.
5. Fruity odor to breath.
6. Acetone in urine.
7. Stupor leading to coma.

J. Assess diagnostic tests (radioactive iodine uptake, T_3 and T_4, thyroid stimulation, and glucose tolerance test), *see* Chapter 11, Laboratory Tests.

System Implementation

A. Administer hormone replacement on time to keep blood level stable.
✦ B. Monitor for side effects of hormone replacement therapy.

✦ CONDITIONS ASSOCIATED WITH HORMONAL IMBALANCES

A. Tumors of the glands.
   1. Benign (common).
   2. Malignant (rare).
   3. Ectopic.
B. Absence of gland.
C. Autoimmune factors.
D. Infections.
E. Side effects of replacement hormones.
F. Dysfunction of the pituitary gland, which affects functioning of the target glands.

C. Identify clinical manifestations indicating hyperfunction or hypofunction of endocrine glands.
✦ D. Monitor for fluid and electrolyte imbalances due to hormone imbalance.
E. Provide appropriate diet specific for endocrine disorder.
F. Promote rest and reduce stress.
G. Prepare client physically and psychologically for surgical removal of endocrine gland.
H. Instruct client on methods to prevent infection.
✦ I. Differentiate diabetic coma from other causes.
   1. Urinalysis for sugar and acetone.
   2. Blood sugar level.
   3. Eyeballs—soft due to loss of intracellular fluid.
   4. Undigested food is found in stomach if Levin tube is inserted.

PITUITARY GLAND DISORDERS

Acromegaly (Anterior Pituitary Hyperfunction)

✦ *Definition:* The hypersecretion of growth hormone by the anterior pituitary. Occurs in adulthood after closure of the epiphyses of the long bones.

Assessment

A. Assess for excessive growth of short, flat bones.
   1. Large hands and feet.
   2. Thickening and protrusion of the jaw and orbital ridges that cause teeth to spread.
   3. Increased growth of soft tissue.
   4. Coarse features.
   5. Pain in joints.
   6. Forehead enlarges.
   7. Tongue enlarges.
   8. Hypertension.
   9. Peripheral nerve damage.
   10. Congestive heart failure.
   11. Seizures.
B. Evaluate voice, which becomes deeper.
C. Assess increased diaphoresis.
D. Assess for oily, rough skin.
E. Assess increased hair growth over the body.
F. Evaluate menstrual disturbances; impotence.
G. Assess for symptoms associated with local compression of brain by tumor.
   1. Headache.
   2. Visual disturbances; blindness.
H. Check any related hormonal imbalances.
   1. Diabetes mellitus (growth hormone is insulin antagonist).
   2. Cushing's syndrome.
I. Evaluate laboratory values—increased growth hormone level.

Implementation

A. Provide emotional support.
   1. Encourage client's expression of feelings.
      a. Loss of self-image and self-esteem.
      b. Fears about brain surgery.
      c. Consequences of surgery (sterility and lifetime hormone replacement).
   2. Have client avoid situations that may be embarrassing.
   3. Encourage support of and communication with family.
B. Provide frequent skin care.
C. Position and support painful joints.
D. Test urine for glucose and acetone.
E. Administer supportive care for irradiation of pituitary.
F. Provide preoperative and postoperative care for hypophysectomy.

Gigantism (Anterior Pituitary Hyperfunction)

✦ *Definition:* The hypersecretion of growth hormone by the anterior pituitary. Occurs in childhood prior to closure of the epiphyses of the long bones.

Assessment

A. Assess for symmetrical overgrowth of the long bones.
✦ B. Evaluate increased height in early adulthood (may be 8–9 feet).
C. Check for deterioration of mental and physical processes, which may occur in early adulthood.
D. Assess for other tissue responses similar to acromegaly.

Implementation

A. Supportive care for irradiation of pituitary.
B. Provide preoperative and postoperative care for hypophysectomy.

Hypophysectomy

✦ *Definition:* The removal of the pituitary gland because of tumor formation. If tumors are small, an adenectomy may be performed.

Treatment

A. Surgical procedures.
   1. Craniotomy—for large, invasive tumors.
   2. Microsurgery.
   3. Cryohypophysectomy.
B. Medical treatment.
   1. Radiation therapy.
   2. Stereotactic radiosurgery.
   3. Drugs.
      a. Somatostatin analogs.
      b. GH receptor antagonists.
      c. Dopamine antagonists.

Implementation

A. Preoperative care.
   1. Provide general preoperative care.
   2. Provide emotional support.
✦ B. Postoperative care.
   1. Administer corticosteroids on time.
   ✦ 2. Monitor fluid and electrolyte balance.
      a. Hypernatremic due to ADH disturbance leading to fluid imbalance and diabetes insipidus.
      b. Avoid water intoxication.
      c. Encourage fluid intake of 2500–3000 mL/day unless otherwise ordered.
   3. Carefully monitor vital signs.
   4. Monitor blood gas determinations.
   5. Provide routine care for craniotomy. Observe for
      a. Vital signs.
      b. Increased intracranial pressure.
      c. Shock.
      d. LOC.
   6. Initiate client education.

    a. Compensate for altered stress response.

    b. Avoid contact with infectious individuals.

    c. Carry emergency adrenal hormone drugs.

    d. Use Medic-Alert band.

✦ C. Monitor for complications.

    1. Craniotomy—bleeding in acromegaly (due to excessive growth of frontal bones).

    2. Microsurgery—rhinorrhea and meningitis (due to interruption of CSF during surgery).

    3. Cryohypophysectomy—probe hits other vital structures.

Dwarfism (Anterior Pituitary Hypofunction)

✦ *Definition:* Dwarfism is the hyposecretion of growth hormone by the anterior pituitary. Growth is symmetrical but decreased.

✦ **Assessment**

A. Assess for retarded physical growth.

B. Evaluate premature body-aging processes.

C. Assess for pale, dry, smooth skin.

D. Check poor development of secondary sex characteristics and external genitalia.

E. Evaluate slow intellectual development.

Implementation

✦ A. Administer human growth hormone (HGH) injections if the imbalance is diagnosed and treated in early stage.

B. Monitor for complications.

Diabetes Insipidus (DI—Posterior Pituitary Hypofunction)

✦ *Definition:* An antidiuretic hormone (ADH) deficiency, usually seen in young adults, resulting from damage or tumors in the posterior lobe of the pituitary gland. May develop following brain surgery, head injury, infection of the central nervous system.

✦ **Characteristics**

A. Neurogenic diabetes—can result from a disruption of the hypothalamus and pituitary gland (i.e., head trauma or cranial surgery) or can be idiopathic.

B. Nephrogenic—disorder that occurs when renal tubules are not sensitive to ADH. May be familial or the result of renal failure.

Assessment

✦ A. Assess for severe polyuria (as much as 20 L/day) and polydipsia.

B. Evaluate fatigue and muscle pain.

C. Assess for dehydration.

D. Assess weight loss, muscle weakness, headache.

✦ E. Check laboratory values—low urinary specific gravity (< 1.006 or less).

F. Evaluate for inability to concentrate urine.

G. Monitor laboratory values.

    1. Urine specific gravity.

    2. Serum sodium.

    3. Serum vasopressin.

✦ **Implementation**

A. Maintain adequate fluids.

B. Measure intake and output and weight.

✦ C. Stress importance of Medic-Alert band.

D. Avoid liquids or foods with diuretic-type action.

E. Provide comfort measures if client is on radiation therapy.

F. Provide preoperative and postoperative care for hypophysectomy.

✦ G. Administer vasopressin tannate (Pitressin Tannate), IM, or nasal spray if ordered (often given for temporary DI after head trauma or surgery).

✦ H. Monitor diet: low sodium, low protein with diuretics.

I. Administer benzthiazide diuretics for mild cases.

J. Administer Diabinese to potentiate vasopressin or act as antidiuretic.

K. Administer Clofibrate for antidiuretic effect.

L. Monitor administration of nonsteroidal anti-inflammatory agents to increase urinary concentration.

M. Give supportive care for irradiation of tumor.

ADRENAL CORTEX DISORDERS

Addison's Disease (Adrenocortical Insufficiency)

✦ *Definition:* The hypofunction of the adrenal cortex of the adrenal gland, resulting in a deficiency of the steroid hormones. It often has a slow and insidious onset, and is eventually fatal if left untreated.

Assessment

A. Assess for normal dietary intake.

✦ B. Assess for lassitude, lethargy, fatigue, and muscular weakness.

C. Check out any gastrointestinal disturbances, nausea, diarrhea, and anorexia.

D. Assess for hypotension.

E. Evaluate increased pigmentation of the skin of nipples, buccal mucosa, and scars. This condition occurs in 15 percent of clients.

F. Evaluate emotional disturbances, depression.

G. Assess for weight loss, emaciation.

H. Assess laboratory values and diagnostic tests.
1. Elevated potassium; decreased sodium; elevated BUN levels due to decreased glomerular filtration rate.
2. Low blood glucose.
3. Lack of normal rise in urinary output of 17-ketosteroids and 17-hydroxycorticosteroids following IV administration of ACTH over 8 hours.
4. Lack of normal rise in blood level of plasma cortisol following IM injection of ACTH.
5. Serum cortisol levels—decreased.
6. ACTH stimulation test—cortisol levels rise with pituitary deficiency but do not rise in primary adrenal insufficiency.
7. CT of head—identify intracranial problems impinging on the pituitary gland.
8. ECG—look for characteristic changes associated with hyperkalemia (peaked T waves, widening QRS complex, and an increased PR interval).

Implementation

A. Monitor daily weight and record accurate intake and output—restoration of fluid and electrolyte balance priority.
B. Take vital signs QID (more often if client unstable).
C. Check for inadequate or overdosage of hormones.
1. Cortisone and hydrocortisone.
a. Sodium and water retention.
b. Potassium depletion or hyperkalemia (may disappear with cortisol therapy).
c. Drug-induced Cushing's syndrome.
d. Gastric irritation (give medication with meal or antacid).
e. Mood swings.
f. Local abscess at injection site when given IM (inject deeply into gluteal muscle).
g. Addisonian crisis, which might be produced by sudden withdrawal of medication.
2. Fludrocortisone acetate (Florinef)—the same side effects as cortisone and hydrocortisone, particularly sodium retention and potassium depletion.
D. Protect from exposure to infection.
E. High-protein, high-carbohydrate diet in small, frequent feedings.
F. Provide emotional support; assist client to avoid stress.
G. Provide client education.
1. Safe self-administration of replacement hormones. Lifelong replacement therapy with synthetic corticosteroid drugs is necessary.
2. Avoidance of over-the-counter drugs.

3. Care to avoid infections; report promptly to physician if infections appear.
4. Medic-Alert band.
5. Regular exercise; avoid strenuous activity, particularly in hot weather.
6. Importance of continuous medical supervision.
7. Avoidance of stress.
8. Avoidance of exposure to cold.

Addisonian Crisis

Definition: A condition caused by adrenal insufficiency that may be precipitated by infection, trauma, stress, surgery, or diaphoresis with excessive salt loss. Death may occur from shock, vascular collapse, or hyperkalemia.

Assessment

A. Assess for severe headache and abdominal, leg, and lower back pain.
B. Assess for extreme, generalized muscular weakness.
C. Assess for manifestations of shock.
1. Hypotension.
2. Rapid, weak pulse.
3. Pallor.
4. Rapid respiratory rate.
5. Extreme weakness.
D. Assess for irritability and confusion.

Implementation

A. Administer parenteral fluids for restoration of electrolyte balance.
B. Administer adrenocorticosteroids; do not vary dosage or time from that ordered.
C. Continually monitor vital signs and intake and output until crisis passes.
D. Protect client from infection.
E. Keep client immobile and as quiet as possible; avoid unnecessary nursing procedures.

Cushing's Syndrome (Adrenocortical Hyperfunction)

Definition: Clinical condition resulting from the combined metabolic effects of persistently elevated blood levels of glucocorticoids.

Characteristics

A. Etiology.
1. Overactivity of adrenal cortex.
2. Benign or malignant tumor of adrenal gland.
B. Cause may be iatrogenic—drug therapy for other conditions.

Assessment

A. Assess for abnormal adipose tissue distribution.
1. Moon face.

2. Buffalo hump.
3. Obese trunk with thin extremities.
B. Assess skin—color and texture.
    1. Florid facies.
    2. Red striae of skin stretched with fat tissue.
    3. Fragile skin, easily bruised.
✦ C. Assess for osteoporosis—susceptible to fractures, renal stones.
✦ D. Assess for hyperglycemia—may eventually develop diabetes mellitus.
E. Evaluate mood swings—euphoria to depression.
F. Assess for high susceptibility to infections; diminished immune response to infections once they occur.
G. Evaluate lassitude and muscular weakness.
H. Assess for masculine characteristics in females.
I. Assess for thin extremities.
J. Assess for hypertension.
✦ K. Evaluate electrolyte imbalance.
    1. Potassium depletion.
    2. Sodium and water retention.
    3. Metabolic alkalosis.
✦ L. Assess laboratory values.
    1. Elevated blood glucose and glycosuria.
    2. Elevated white blood count with depressed eosinophils and lymphocytes.
    3. Elevated plasma cortisone levels.
    4. Elevated 17-hydroxycorticosteroids in urine.

Implementation

✦ A. Protect from infections.
B. Protect from accidents or falls.
C. Provide meticulous skin care, avoiding harsh soaps.
D. Provide low-calorie, high-protein, high-potassium diet.
✦ E. Provide emotional support.
    1. Allow for venting of client's feelings.
    2. Avoid reactions to client's appearance.
    3. Anticipate the needs of the client.
    4. Explain that changes in body appearance and emotional lability should improve with treatment.
✦ F. Measure intake and output and daily weights; test blood glucose.
G. Follow specific nursing measures posthypophysectomy.
H. Provide comfort measures during radiation therapy, cobalt irradiation of the pituitary or implants.
✦ I. Provide postsurgery care for adrenalectomy, unilateral or bilateral.
    1. Bilateral—lifetime replacement of steroids.
    2. Unilateral—temporary steroid replacement (6–12 months).
✦ J. Monitor drug therapy.
    1. Aminoglutethimide—inhibits cholesterol synthesis.
    2. Metyrapone—inhibits adrenal cortex steroid synthesis.

3. Mitotane—usually for inoperable, cancerous tumors.
4. Cyproheptadine—serotonin antagonist that inhibits ACTH.
K. Provide client teaching.
    1. Importance of continuous medical supervision.
    2. Safe self-administration of replacement hormones.
    3. Side effects of medications.
    4. Avoidance of infections and stress.
    5. Need for adequate nutrition and rest.

Primary Aldosteronism

Definition: A disorder due to the hypersecretion of aldosterone from the adrenal cortex of the adrenal gland. It is usually caused by tumors. Females are at greater risk.

Assessment

✦ A. Assess for hypokalemia.
    1. Weakness of muscles.
    2. Excessive urine output (polyuria); excessive thirst (polydipsia).
    3. Metabolic alkalosis.
✦ B. Assess for hypertension, postural hypotension, headache.
✦ C. Assess for positive Chvostek's sign (muscle twitching when area over facial nerves is tapped).
D. Assess laboratory values.
    1. Lowered potassium level.
    2. Elevated serum sodium level.
    3. Increased urinary output of aldosterone.
    4. Metabolic alkalosis.

✦ **Implementation**

A. Provide quiet environment.
B. Measure intake and output and daily weights.
C. Check muscular strength and presence of Chvostek's sign.
D. Measure blood pressure in supine and standing positions.
E. Provide same postoperative care as for adrenalectomy.
F. Monitor administration of potassium salts and spironolactone.

ADRENAL MEDULLA DISORDERS

Pheochromocytoma (Hyperfunction)

Definition: A small tumor in the adrenal medulla of the adrenal gland that secretes large amounts of epinephrine and norepinephrine. Familial autosomal dominant.

Assessment

A. Observe that condition occurs primarily in children and middle-aged women.

✦ B. Assess for hypertension—primary manifestation.

✦ C. Observe for sudden attacks that resemble overstimulation of the sympathetic nervous system.
   1. Hypertension (intermittent or persistent).
   2. Severe headache.
   3. Excessive diaphoresis.
   4. Palpitation, tachycardia.
   5. Nervousness and hyperactivity.
   6. Nausea, vomiting, and anorexia.
   7. Dilated pupils.
   8. Cold extremities.
   9. Tremors.
   10. Flushing.
   11. Anxiety.
   12. Vertigo.
   13. Blurred vision.
   14. Dyspnea.
   15. Cardiac failure or cerebral hemorrhage leading to death if not treated.

D. Assess for increased rate of metabolism and loss of weight.

E. Assess for hyperglycemia.

F. Assess laboratory values.
   1. Findings common to hypertension, cardiac disease, and loss of kidney function.
   2. Elevated vanillylmandelic acid (VMA) and catecholamine levels in urine.
   3. Elevated blood levels of catecholamines.
   4. Elevated blood glucose and glycosuria.

G. Presence of tumor may be found on x-rays or identified during surgical exploration.

Implementation

✦ A. Monitor for evidence of hypertensive attacks; keep Regitine at bedside for hypertensive crisis.

✦ B. Monitor for normal vital signs and absence of glycosuria after alpha-adrenergic-blocking agents (phenoxybenzamine) are given—1–2 weeks before surgery.

✦ C. Assess daily for glucose and acetone in urine.

D. Provide high-calorie, nutritious diet omitting stimulants.

E. Promote rest and reduce stress.

F. Provide preoperative care for surgical excision of tumor.
   1. Give Regitine 1–2 days before surgery to counteract hypertensive effects of epinephrine and norepinephrine.
   2. Closely monitor blood pressure (every 15 minutes) during interval of phentolamine administration.

G. Provide postoperative care—observe for precipitous shock, hemorrhage, persistent hypertension.

H. Administer drugs if ordered: alpha blocker; phentolamine, phenoxybenzamine, sodium nitroprusside.

I. Surgical removal of the tumor is the treatment of choice.

Adrenalectomy

✦ *Definition:* Surgical removal of an adrenal gland when overproduction of adrenal hormone is evident (Cushing's syndrome, pheochromocytoma) or in metastatic breast or prostatic cancer.

Assessment

A. Assess test results that indicate whether radiation, drug therapy, or surgery is appropriate to reverse Cushing's syndrome or restore hormone balance.

✦ B. Surgical intervention requires special management—CVP, BP, P.
   1. Assess hypertension.
   2. Assess degree of edema.
   3. Evaluate for signs of diabetes—blood glucose levels.
   4. Assess for cardiovascular manifestations.

C. Assess client's knowledge of disorder and understanding of management.

D. Assess all laboratory reports before surgery.
   1. Check for signs of hypernatremia and hypokalemia.
   2. Assess for hyperglycemia or glycosuria.

E. Assess dietary intake and fluid intake and output.

F. Assess for complications.
   1. Wound infections.
   2. Hemorrhage.
   3. Peptic ulcers.
   4. Pulmonary disorders.

Implementation

A. Preoperative care.
   1. Provide general preoperative care.
   2. Administer exogenous glucocorticoids.

✦ B. Postoperative care.
   1. Monitor vital signs and intake and output.
   2. Minimize effects of postural hypotension.
   3. Strictly adhere to sterile techniques when changing dressings; assess for infections.
   4. Observe for shock, hypoglycemia, hypotension.
   5. Maintain IV cortisol replacement (24–48 hours); mineralocorticoids.
   6. Monitor for paralytic ileus as this may develop from internal bleeding.
   7. Administer IV fluids to maintain blood volume.
   8. Monitor ECG changes.
   9. Monitor electrolytes.
   10. Monitor blood glucose levels.

THYROID GLAND DISORDERS

Cretinism (Thyroid Hypofunction)

Definition: A condition caused by inadequate secretions from the thyroid gland in the fetus, in utero, or soon after birth caused by congenital hypothyroidism.

✦ **Assessment**

A. Assess for severe retardation of physical development, resulting in grotesque appearance, sexual retardation.
B. Assess for severe mental retardation, apathy.
C. Check for dry skin; coarse, dry, brittle hair.
D. Assess for constipation.
E. Evaluate slow teething.
F. Evaluate poor appetite.
G. Observe for large tongue.
H. Observe for pot belly with umbilical hernia.
I. Evaluate sensitivity to cold.
J. Assess for yellow skin.
K. Assess laboratory values.
 1. T_4 less than 3 µg/100 mL.
 2. Elevated serum cholesterol.
 3. Low radioactive iodine uptake.

Implementation

✦ A. Administer desiccated thyroid or Synthroid.
B. Administer Cytomel; effects more difficult to monitor.

Hypothyroidism (Myxedema)

Definition: The decreased synthesis of thyroid hormone in adulthood, resulting in a hypothyroid state—acquired hypothyroidism. Occurs primarily in older age group, five times more frequent in women than in men.

Assessment

✦ A. Assess for slowed rate of body metabolism.
 1. Lethargy, apathy, and fatigue.
 2. Intolerance to cold, hypothermia.
 3. Hypersensitivity to sedatives and barbiturates.
 4. Weight gain.
 5. Cool, dry, rough skin.
 6. Coarse, dry hair; hair loss; brittle nails.
 7. Numbness and tingling of fingers.
 8. Hoarseness.
B. Assess for personality changes.
 1. Forgetfulness and loss of memory.
 2. Complacency.
 3. Slowed speech.
✦ C. Assess for anorexia, constipation, and fecal impactions.
D. Observe for interstitial edema.
 1. Nonpitting edema in the lower extremity.
 2. Generalized puffiness.

E. Observe for decreased diaphoresis.
✦ F. Check for reproductive disturbances.
 1. Menorrhagia (females).
 2. Infertility (females).
 3. Decreased libido (males).
G. Assess for cardiac complications.
 1. Coronary heart disease.
 2. Angina pectoris.
 3. MI and congestive heart failure.
 4. Bradycardia
 5. Dysrhythmias.
H. Evaluate anemia.
I. Assess laboratory findings.
 1. Low serum thyrotoxin concentration.
 2. Hyponatremia.
 3. Elevated serum cholesterol.

✦ **Implementation**

A. Allow time for client to complete activities.
B. Provide warm environment: extra blankets, etc.
C. Provide meticulous skin care.
D. Orient client as to date, time, and place.
E. Prevent constipation.
✦ F. If sedatives or narcotics are necessary, give one-half to one-third normal dosage, as ordered by physician.
G. Monitor thyroid replacement (initial small dosage, increased gradually).
H. Maintain individualized maintenance dosage.
 1. Desiccated thyroid.
 2. Thyroxine (Synthroid).
 3. Triiodothyronine (Cytomel).
 4. Natural combinations from animal thyroid.
I. Monitor for overdosage symptoms of thyroid preparations.
 1. Myocardial infarction and angina and cardiac failure, particularly in clients with cardiac problems.
 2. Restlessness and insomnia.
 3. Headache and confusion.
J. Monitor arterial blood gases.
K. Monitor pulse oximetry.
L. Monitor oxygen administration.

Myxedema Coma

✦ *Definition:* A serious condition resulting from persistent low thyroid production.

✦ **Assessment**

A. Assess for hypoventilation, compromised respiratory function.
B. Observe for hypotension leading to cardiac abnormalities; bradycardia.
C. Evaluate cold sensitivity leading to severe hypothermia.
D. Evaluate mood swings.

♦ **Implementation**
  A. Monitor administration of thyroid hormone IV.
  B. Provide total supportive care.
  C. Provide psychological support.
     1. Body image change.
     2. Complete dependency.
     3. Mental depression.
  D. Closely observe for problems of immobility.
  E. Provide low-calorie diet.
  F. Provide ventilatory support if needed.
  G. Measure vital signs frequently, especially temperature.
  H. Monitor fluid intake to prevent dilutional hyponatremia.
  I. Avoid use of sedatives and hypnotics.

Hashimoto's Thyroiditis

♦ *Definition:* An autoimmune disorder in which antibodies develop that destroy thyroid tissue.

♦ **Characteristics**
  A. Functional tissue is replaced with fibrous tissue and TH level decreases.
  B. Decrease in TH levels prompt the gland to enlarge in an effort to compensate, causing goiter.

Assessment and Implementation
See Graves' Disease below.

Thyrotoxicosis/Hyperthyroidism/ Graves' Disease

♦ *Definition:* A condition that results from the increased synthesis of thyroid hormone. When associated with ocular signs and a diffuse goiter, it is called Graves' disease. Occurs four times more frequently in women than in men; usually occurs between 20 and 40 years of age.

Assessment
♦ A. Evaluate laboratory tests.
     1. Thyroid antibodies (TAs)—used to determine if thyroid autoimmune disease is causing symptoms. TA is elevated in Graves' disease.
     2. Thyroid suppression test. RAI and T_4 levels are measured. The client then takes TH for 7 to 10 days, after which the tests are repeated. Failure of hormone therapy to suppress RAI and T_4 indicates hyperthyroidism.
     3. Above-normal test results: PBI, ^{131}I, and T_3, T_4.
     4. Relatively low serum cholesterol.
♦ B. Assess increased rate of body metabolism.
     1. Weight loss despite ravenous appetite and ingestion of large quantities of food.
     2. Intolerance to heat.
     3. Nervousness, jitters, and fine tremor of hands.
     4. Smooth, soft skin and hair.

♦ **MEDICAL IMPLICATIONS**

A. Antithyroid drugs.
   1. Propylthiouracil (PTU, Propyl-Thracil).
   2. Methimazole (Tapazole).
   3. Side effect: agranulocytosis.
♦ B. Iodine preparations.
   1. Saturated solution of potassium iodide (SSKI).
   2. Lugol's solution—give in milk or juice.
   3. PIMA (potassium iodide).
C. Alternative to iodines: lithium—blocks hormone release.
D. Propranolol and calcium antagonists.
   1. Rapidly reverse toxic manifestations.
   2. Used preoperatively.
♦ E. Radioiodine therapy.
   1. Safer therapy and useful in clients who are poor surgical risks.
   2. Uptake of ^{131}I by thyroid gland results in destruction of thyroid cells. This is contraindicated in pregnant women because radioactive iodine crosses the placental barrier and can have negative effects on the thyroid of the developing fetus.
   3. Myxedema may occur as a complication.
   4. Because the amount of gland destroyed is not readily controllable, the client may become hypothyroid and require lifelong TH replacement.
F. Thyroidectomy.

     5. Tachycardia, palpitations, atrial fibrillation, angina, and congestive heart failure.
     6. Diarrhea.
     7. Diaphoresis.
     8. Flushed, moist skin.
     9. Muscular weakness.
♦ C. Assess personality changes.
     1. Irritability and agitation.
     2. Exaggerated emotional reactions.
     3. Mood swings—euphoria to depression.
     4. Quick motions, including speech.
♦ D. Assess any enlargement of the thyroid gland (goiter).
     1. Toxic multinodular goiter is characterized by small, discrete independently functioning nodules in thyroid gland that secrete TH.
     2. May be benign or malignant. Slow to develop. Usually found in women in 60s or 70s.
  E. Observe for exophthalmos.
   ♦ 1. Fluid collects around eye sockets, causing eyeballs to protrude (may be unilateral or bilateral).
     2. Not always present.
     3. Usually does not improve with treatment.
  F. Assess for cardiac arrhythmias.
  G. Evaluate difficulty focusing eyes.

✦ Implementation

A. Provide adequate rest.
1. Bedrest.
2. Diversionary activities.
3. Sedatives.
B. Provide cool, quiet, stable environment.
C. Maintain high-calorie, high-protein, high-carbohydrate, high-vitamin diet without stimulants—six small meals/day and snacks.
D. Monitor daily weights.
E. Provide emotional support.
1. Be aware that exaggerated emotional responses are a manifestation of hormone imbalance.
2. Be sensitive to needs.
3. Avoid stress-producing situations.
F. Adhere to regular schedule of activities.
G. Provide client education.
1. Protection from infection.
2. Safe self-administration of medications.
3. Importance of adequate rest and diet.
4. Avoidance of stress.
✦ H. When giving iodine solutions in milk or juice, have client drink through a straw to prevent discoloration of the teeth.

Thyroidectomy

Definition: Removal of thyroid gland for persistent hyperthyroidism.

Assessment

A. Assess type of surgery to be done: total resection or subtotal resection of the gland.
B. Assess vital signs and weight for baseline data.
C. Assess serum electrolytes for hyperglycemia and glycosuria.
D. Assess level of consciousness.
E. Evaluate for signs of thyroid storm.

Implementation

✦ A. Preoperative care—prevent thyrotoxicosis.
1. Administer antithyroid drugs to deplete iodine and hormones (5–7 days).
2. Administer iodine to decrease vascularity and increase size of follicular cells (5–7 days).
3. Provide routine preoperative teaching.
4. Reassure client.
5. Maintain nutritional status.
6. Monitor for evidence of iodine toxicity.
✦ B. Postoperative care.
1. Check frequently for respiratory distress—keep tracheostomy tray at bedside.
2. Maintain semi-Fowler's position to avoid strain on suture line.
3. Observe for bleeding.

a. Vital signs—tachycardia, hypotension.
b. Pressure on larynx.
c. Hematoma around wound.
4. Observe for damage to laryngeal nerve.
a. Respiratory obstruction.
b. Dysphonia.
c. High-pitched voice.
d. Stridor.
e. Dysphagia.
f. Restlessness.
5. Observe for signs of hypoparathyroidism (causes an acute attack of tetany).
a. Chvostek's sign and Trousseau's sign.
b. Convulsions.
c. Irritability and anxiety.
d. Stridor, wheezing, and dyspnea.
e. Photophobia, diplopia.
f. Muscle and abdominal cramps.

Thyroid Storm (Thyrotoxic Crisis)

✦ *Definition:* An acute, potentially fatal hyperthyroid condition that may occur as a result of surgery, inadequate preparation for surgery, severe infection, or stress.

Characteristics

A. Cause not known; symptoms reflect exaggerated thyrotoxicosis.
B. Infrequent due to premedication of iodine and antithyroid drugs.
C. Can be precipitated by stressors.
1. Infection.
2. Abrupt withdrawal of medication.
3. Metabolic causes.
4. Emotional stress.
5. Pulmonary embolism.
6. Trauma.
7. Surgery.
8. Pregnancy.
9. Vigorous palpation of thyroid.

Assessment

✦ A. Assess for increased temperature (> 101°F).
B. Assess diaphoresis.
C. Assess for dehydration.
✦ D. Evaluate cardiopulmonary symptoms.
1. Tachycardia (> 120).
2. Arrhythmias.
3. Congestive heart failure.
4. Pulmonary edema.
✦ E. Assess gastrointestinal symptoms.
1. Abdominal pain.
2. Nausea, vomiting, and diarrhea.
3. Jaundice.
4. Weight loss.

◆ MEDICAL IMPLICATIONS

A. Large doses of IV propranolol to control thyroid storm.

B. Adrenergic- and catecholamine-blocking agents to decrease heart activity.

C. Glucocorticoids to allay stress effects.

D. Sodium iodide to slow IV infusion.

E. SSKI PO.

F. Antithyroid drugs.

F. Assess central nervous system symptoms.
1. Tremors.
2. Severe agitation, restlessness, and irritability.
3. Apathy leading to delirium and coma.
4. Altered mental state.

Implementation

◆ A. Do not palpate thyroid gland (stimulus increases symptoms).

◆ B. Decrease temperature: acetaminophen, external cold (ice packs, cooling blanket). Salicylates contraindicated—increase free thyroid hormone levels.

C. Protect from infection, especially pneumonia.

D. Monitor vital signs.

◆ E. Maintain fluid and electrolyte balance.
1. Electrolyte shifts cause brittle situation of over- and underhydration.
2. Maintain adequate output.
3. Observe for sodium and potassium imbalance due to vomiting and diarrhea.
4. Observe for signs of overhydration if cardiopulmonary complications are evident.

◆ F. Monitor ECG for arrhythmias if
1. Adrenergic blockers are used.
2. Diuretics are given.
3. Electrolyte imbalance is present.
4. Cardiovascular medication is given.

G. Humidify oxygen.

H. Administer IV glucose diet with glucose and large doses of vitamin B complex.

I. Protect for safety if agitated or comatose.

J. Provide calm, quiet environment.

K. Reassure client and family.

PARATHYROID GLAND DISORDERS

Hypoparathyroidism

◆ *Definition:* A condition caused by acute or chronic deficient hormone production by the parathyroid gland. Usually occurs following thyroidectomy.

◆ MEDICAL IMPLICATIONS

A. Acute condition.
1. Slow drip of IV calcium gluconate or calcium chloride.
2. Anticonvulsants and sedatives (phenytoin and phenobarbital).
3. Parathyroid hormone IM or sub q.
4. Aluminum hydroxide (decreases phosphate level).
5. Rebreathing bag to produce mild respiratory acidosis.
6. Tracheostomy if laryngospasm causes obstruction.

B. Chronic condition.
1. Oral calcium carbonate (Os-Cal)—1–3 g/day.
2. Active form of vitamin D preparations (Calciferol).
3. High-calcium, low-phosphorus diet.
4. Warning—many high-calcium foods are also high in phosphorus.

Assessment

◆ A. Assess for acute hypocalcemia.
1. Numbness, tingling, and cramping of extremities.
◆ 2. Acute, potentially fatal tetany.
   a. Painful muscular spasms.
   b. Seizures.
   c. Irritability.
   d. Positive Chvostek's sign.
   e. Positive Trousseau's sign.
   f. Laryngospasm.
   g. Cardiac arrhythmias.

◆ B. Assess for chronic hypocalcemia.
1. Poor development of tooth enamel.
2. Mental retardation.
3. Muscular weakness with numbness and tingling of extremities.
4. Tetany.
5. Loss of hair and coarse, dry skin.
6. Personality changes.
7. Cataracts.
8. Cardiac arrhythmias.
9. Renal stones.

C. Assess laboratory values.
1. Low serum calcium levels.
2. Increased serum phosphorus level.
3. Low urinary calcium and phosphorus output.
4. Increased bone density on x-ray examination.

Implementation

◆ A. Same as for seizures and epilepsy.

B. Administer parenteral parathormone.

◆ C. Frequently check for increasing hoarseness.

D. Observe for irregularities in urine.

E. Force fluids as ordered.

F. Observe for dystonic reactions if on phenothiazines.
G. Maintain environment free of bright lights and noise.
H. Provide psychological support.
   1. Altered body image.
   2. Emotional instability.
   3. Extreme weakness.

Hyperparathyroidism

✦ *Definition:* A condition caused by overproduction of the parathyroid hormone by parathyroid gland.

Characteristics

✦ A. Primary hyperparathyroidism—occurs when there is hyperplasia or adenoma in one of the parathyroid glands.
✦ B. Secondary hyperparathyroidism (caused primarily from malabsorption and renal failure) results in chronic hypocalcemia (which stimulates excessive production of PTH).
C. Tertiary hyperparathyroidism (usually the result of long-term secondary parathyroidism) results in hypercalcemia.
✦ D. Treatment focus—decrease elevated serum calcium levels.
   1. When cause is malabsorption, there is decreased absorption of calcium from the intestine and a deficiency in vitamin D. Treatment is calcium supplements and vitamin D.
   2. When cause is renal failure, phosphate is retained causing serum calcium levels to decrease and PTH levels to rise. Treatment is aimed at lowering phosphorus level, increasing calcium with oral supplements and vitamin D.
   3. If lowering phosphate level (thus, elevating calcium level, which stops chronic stimulation of parathyroid gland) does not work, surgery is performed.

Assessment

A. Assess for bone demineralization with deformities; pain; high susceptibility to fractures.
✦ B. Assess for hypercalcemia.
   1. Mild hypercalcemia may not evidence symptoms.
   2. Calcium deposits in various body organs: eyes, heart, lungs, and kidneys (stones).
   3. Gastric ulcers.
   4. Personality changes, depression, apathy, and paranoia.
   5. Nausea, vomiting, anorexia, and constipation.
   6. Polydipsia and polyuria.
   7. Hypertension.
   8. Cardiac dysrhythmias.
   9. Skeletal pain.
   10. Pathologic fractures.

✦ C. Assess laboratory values.
   1. Elevated serum calcium level; lowered serum calcium.
   2. Normal to elevated serum phosphorus levels.
   3. Elevated urinary calcium and phosphorus levels.
   4. Evidence of bone changes on x-ray examinations.
   5. Normal to increased alkaline phosphatase.

Implementation

✦ A. Force fluids for hypercalcemia. Include juices to make urine more acidic.
B. Provide normal saline IV infusion.
✦ C. Observe for electrolyte imbalance with Lasix administration.
D. Measure intake and output.
E. Closely observe urine for stones and gravel.
✦ F. Observe for digitalis toxicity if client is taking digitalis.
G. Prevent accidents and injury through safety measures.
H. Provide surgical care if subtotal surgical resection of parathyroid glands is done.
I. Oral supplements of calcium and vitamin D will be administered with malabsorption, renal failure, or for bone rebuilding processes (several months).
J. Administer calcitonin and corticosteroids if ordered.

Parathyroidectomy

Definition: Removal of one or more of the parathyroid glands, usually as a result of thyroidectomy.

Assessment

✦ A. Assess for positive Chvostek's and Trousseau's signs.
✦ B. Assess for CNS signs of psychomotor or personality disturbances.
✦ C. Evaluate laboratory results for baseline data.
   1. Serum potassium, calcium, phosphate, and magnesium.
   2. Renal magnesium function tests (renal damage from hyperplasia).
D. Evaluate urine for presence of stones.
E. Assess lung sounds for prevention of pulmonary edema.
F. Assess muscle weakness, ability to walk, and range of movement for minimizing bone stress.

Implementation

✦ A. Observe for tetany and treat accordingly.
✦ B. Maintain patent airway.
   1. Observe for respiratory distress.
   2. Keep a tracheostomy tray at the bedside.
✦ C. Provide diet high in calcium, vitamin D, and magnesium salts.

Table 8-14. COMPARISON OF TYPE 1 AND TYPE 2 DIABETES

	Type 1	Type 2
Etiology	Unknown; autoimmune process involved	Heredity more relevant (100% of children contract Type 2 when both parents have it)
Cause	Absence of circulating insulin (in some cases, disease is mild and benign)	Insulin insufficient, not totally deficient; defective glucose-mediated insulin secretion
Onset	Usually abrupt—under age 35	Insidious, often over age 35
Weight	History of failure to gain despite voracious appetite	Linked to obesity and inactivity
Sex	Found in girls and boys equally	Most common in females
Cardinal signs	Polydipsia, polyphagia, polyuria	Polydipsia, polyphagia, polyuria
Other signs	Weakness, tiredness, urinary tract infections, skin infections, blurred vision	Overweight, fatigue, frequent infections, blurred vision, impotence, absence of menstration
Stability	Unstable; brittle—difficult to control	Stable with compliance; less difficult to control
Distinguishing feature	Honeymoon phase—symptoms decrease with a short remission	No honeymoon phase
Complications	Hyperglycemia, diabetic ketosis, and ketoacidosis	Neuropathy, retinopathy, uropathy
Treatment	Insulin and ADA diet, exercise	ADA diet alone; ADA and insulin, or ADA and oral hypoglycemic agents

D. Increase fluids to prevent formation of urinary stones—monitor intake and output for low levels of calcium, magnesium and phosphate.

✦ E. Monitor IV administration of calcium gluconate if given for postoperative emergency.

F. Monitor for postoperative complications.
1. Renal colic.
2. Laryngeal nerve damage.
3. Acute psychosis (look for listlessness).

✦ G. Position client in semi-Fowler's and support head and neck to decrease edema.

H. Ambulate client as soon as possible to speed up recalcification of bones.

PANCREAS DISORDERS

Diabetes Mellitus (Types 1 and 2)

Definition: A group of disorders that have a variety of genetic causes, but have glucose intolerance as a common thread.

Characteristics

A. Classifications (*see* Table 8-14).

1. Type 1—insulin-dependent diabetes mellitus with beta cell destruction or defect in function affects about 5 percent of all diabetics.
   a. *Immune mediated*—presence of islet cell or insulin antibodies that identify the autoimmune process leading to beta cell destruction.
   b. *Idiopathic*—no evidence of autoimmunity.
2. Type 2—non–insulin-dependent diabetes mellitus is the most common. Results when body produces insufficient insulin or there is insulin resistance with relative insulin deficiency. Affects 90 percent of all diabetics. Twenty-one million Americans have Type 2 and 41 million are prediabetic.
   a. Type 2 accounts for half of all cases in young people.
   b. Incidence in young has risen dramatically last 10 years.
3. Gestational (GDM)—increased blood glucose levels during pregnancy.
4. Other specific types—genetic defects of beta-cell function or insulin action, pancreatic diseases, endocrinopathies or drug- or chemical-induced diabetes.

✦ **MEDICAL IMPLICATIONS**

A. Diet.
  ✦ 1. The cornerstone of management, interdependent with medication and exercise.
  2. Attainment of normal weight may clear symptoms in Type 2 diabetes.
  3. Total calories are individualized.
  ✦ 4. ADA general dietary guidelines.
    a. High complex carbohydrates, high-soluble-fiber foods (oat bran cereals, beans, peas, fruits with pectin) assist in controlling blood glucose; fiber: up to 40 g/day. Focus is now on total carbohydrate— not source of carbohydrate (such as sugar).
    b. Protein—10–20 percent of total calories from both animal and vegetable sources.
    c. Fat—less than 30 percent of daily calories.
    d. Limit saturated fat to 10 percent or less of daily calories. Emphasize low-saturated fats and mono- and polyunsaturated fats.
  5. The goal of the diet is to improve overall health through optimal nutrition using "exchange lists," "Dietary Guidelines for Americans" or the new food pyramid called "My Pyramid."
  6. ADA exchange diet; six exchange lists.
    a. Starch/bread, meat and meat substitutes, vegetables, fruit, milk, and fat.
    b. Foods can be substituted or exchanged for each other.
    c. Diet prescribed as to total calories and number of exchanges from each group.
  7. The Revised Food Pyramid.
    a. Grains, half should be whole grain.
    b. Vegetables, fresh or frozen.
    c. Fruits, fresh or frozen, dried or juices.
    d. Oils, liquid, not solid.
    e. Milk, low fat or nonfat.
    f. Meat and beans: poultry, fish, eggs, nuts and seeds.
  8. Carbohydrate counting—grams consumed are monitored and adjusted daily according to blood glucose levels.
  9. Calorie counting—more appropriate for obese client. Emphasizes food choices based on number of calories.
  10. Glycemic index—diet based on how much a certain food raises the blood glucose level as compared to an equivalent amount of glucose. (See Chapter 4.)
✦ B. Medications.
  1. Insulin type: See Table 8-15.
  2. Oral hypoglycemic drugs—improve sensitivity to insulin.
    a. Effective for those with some functioning beta cells in islets of Langerhans.
    b. Used for older clients, noninsulin dependent with normal weight, and diet will not control hyperglycemia.

  c. First-generation sulfonylureas.
    (1) Thought to stimulate beta cells to increase insulin release.
    (2) Tolbutamide (Orinase), short acting (6–12 hours).
    (3) Chlorpropamide (Diabinese), long acting (36–60 hours).
    (4) Acetohexamide (Dylemor), intermediate acting (10–20 hours).
    (5) Tolazamide (Tolinase), intermediate acting (12–24 hours).
  d. Second-generation (longer-acting drugs) sulfonylureas.
    (1) Glyburide (Diabeta, Micronase, Glynase), intermediate acting (12–24 hours).
    (2) Glipizide (Glucotrol), short acting (12–24 hours).
    (3) Glimepinide (Amaryl).
  e. Nonsulfonylureas to improve insulin resistance: metformin (Glucophage), acarbose (Precose), rosiglitazone, pioglitazone, and Avandia and Actos.
  f. A new class of oral medications, DDP-4 inhibitors, sitagliptin (Januvia), lower blood glucose levels by increasing and prolonging action of GLP-1.
✦ C. Insulin pump—new method of insulin administration.
  1. Continuous delivery of fixed small amounts of diluted insulin—mimics release of insulin by pancreas.
  2. Uses regular insulin: 50% continuous delivery and 50% divided into three premeal bolus doses.
  3. Amount calculated by blood glucose monitoring; done 2–4 times per day.
  4. Usually pump and syringe with needle placed in abdomen and taped in place.
  5. Method useful for conscientious, active person who does not want to adjust life to coincide with insulin peaks.
  6. Client disadvantages.
    a. Requires conscientious client commitment to understand and learn pump use.
    b. Requires extensive client teaching.
    c. Regimen is complicated and may require more time than client can spend.
D. Insulin pens.
  1. Prefilled insulin cartridges loaded into pen-like holder.
  2. Dial dose.
  3. No need to carry insulin or draw up before administration.
E. Jet injectors.
  1. Delivers insulin through skin.
  2. No needles.
F. Exercise.
  1. Decreases body's need for insulin.
  2. Moderate activity recommended.
  3. Administer 10 g CHO before exercise.

B. Etiology.
  1. Genetic factors.
     a. Presence of HLA antigens.
     b. Individual genes located on "short arm" of sixth chromosome.
  2. Viruses.
     a. Type 1 diabetes occurs at time viral diseases are prevalent—autumn and spring.
     b. Type 1 onset often preceded by viral attack.
     c. Coxsackie B$_4$ is found in pancreas.
     d. Twenty viruses associated with diabetes.
✦ C. Pathophysiology.
  ✦ 1. Type 1 (insulin-dependent).
     a. Rapid onset—requires insulin due to absence of circulating insulin.
     b. Autoimmune response or idiopathic.
     c. Presence of anti-islet cell antibodies.
     d. Pancreatic beta cells die.
     e. Ketosis unless treated.
  ✦ 2. Type 2 (non–insulin-dependent), formerly adult-onset type.
     a. Gradual onset—may be controlled by diet.
     b. Ninety percent of diabetes cases are this type.
     c. Impaired beta-cell response to glucose (client usually nonobese).
     d. Tissues insensitive to insulin (client usually obese).
        (1) Extrapancreatic defect.
        (2) Normal or high levels of circulating insulin.
✦ D. *Somogyi phenomenon.* Hypoglycemia usually at night followed by compensatory rebound hyperglycemia in the morning (lasts 12–72 hours).
  1. Usually caused by too much insulin or an increase in insulin sensitivity.
  2. Client may be stabilized by gradual lowering of insulin dose and increase in diet at the time of the hypoglycemia reaction.
✦ E. *Dawn phenomenon.*
  1. Blood glucose normal until 3 AM—begins to rise in early morning hours.
  2. Common problem—glucose released from liver in early AM—needs to be controlled.
  3. Algorithm for hyperglycemia—altering time and dose of insulin (NPH or Ultralente) by one or two units stabilizes client.

Assessment

✦ A. Assess for early symptoms.
  ✦ 1. Common to both Type 1 and Type 2.
     a. Polyuria.
     b. Polydipsia.
     c. Polyphagia.
     d. Blurred vision.
     e. Fatigue.
     f. Abnormal sensations (prickling, burning).
     g. Infections (vaginitis).
     h. Weakness.
     i. Tingling or numbness in hands or feet.
     j. Dry skin.
  2. Type 1.
     a. Postural hypotension.
     b. Decreased muscle mass.
     c. Weight loss in spite of increased appetite.
  3. Type 2.
     a. Often asymptomatic.
     b. Often obese.
     c. Slow wound healing.
     d. Blurred vision.
     e. Fatigue.
     f. Paresthesias.
  4. Type 2 in young people.
     a. Hyperglycemia.
     b. Hypertension.
     c. Dyslipidemia.
     d. Small number have sleep apnea.
B. Assess for distinguishing features of Type 1 and Type 2 diabetes.
C. Assess for risk factors.
  1. Client history—hereditary predisposition.
  2. Weight—presence of obesity.
  3. High stress levels.
✦ D. Diagnosis of diabetes: assess results of laboratory values.
  ✦ 1. Fasting blood sugar > 126 mg/dL on two separate occasions, postprandial blood sugar > 200 mg/dL and at least once between meals at 2 hours PC; abnormal glucose tolerance test or tolbutamide (Orinase) tests.
  2. Impaired glucose tolerance (IGT) is a fasting blood sugar of 100–125 mg/dL. Current ideal normal fasting level of 80–100 mg/dL.
  3. Acetest and Ketostix—may be positive for presence of acetone and ketones in urine.
  4. Elevated cholesterol and triglyceride levels.
  5. Capillary blood glucose (finger-stick) is most common method.
  6. *Glycosylated hemoglobin test* (HgbA$_1$).
     a. Monitors blood sugar and hemoglobin; determines how well diabetes is controlled.
     b. Reflects glycemic state over preceding 8 to 12 weeks.
     c. Abnormally high in diabetics with chronic hyperglycemia.
     d. Values: normal 4 to 6 percent; good control less than 7 percent; fair control 7 to 8 percent; poor control more than 9.0 percent.

✦ **Table 8-15. INSULIN TYPES AND ACTION**

Types	Source	Onset	Peak	Duration
Rapid Acting				
Humalog (Lispro)	Human	5–15 min	60–90 min	3–5 hr
Novolog (Aspart)				
Short Acting				
Novolin R	Human	0.5–1 hr	2–4 hr	5–7 hr
Humulin R	Human			
Intermediate Acting				
Humulin N (NPH)	Human	1–2 hr	6–12 hr	16–24 hr
Novolin N (NPH)	Human	2 hr	6–8 hr	16–22 hr
Mixture				
Humulin 70/30	Human (70% NPH, 30% regular)	30 min	2–12 hr	24 hr
Novolin 70/30	Human (70% NPH, 30% regular)			
Humulin 50/50	Human (50% NPH, 50% regular)			
Humalog 75/25	(75% lispro protamine suspension, 25% lispro)	15 min	1 hr	24 hr
NovolinL	Human	3–4 hr	4–12 hr	16–20 hr
Long Acting				
Humulin Ultralente	Human	6–8 hr	12–16 hr	20–30 hr
Lantus (glargine)		4–6 hr	No peak	24 hr

NPH = neutral protamine Hagedorn. *Note:* The time of insulin onset, peak, and duration may vary in different clients.
Human insulin is biologically engineered through the process of recombinant DNA technology; it is modified human insulin.
Source: Smith, S., Duell, D., & Martin, B. (2008). *Clinical nursing skills,* 7th ed. Upper Saddle River, NJ: Prentice Hall Health.

✦ **Implementation**

A. When diabetic client is hospitalized:
1. Administer IV fluids and medications as ordered.
2. Adhere to procedures for other laboratory tests.
3. Provide meticulous skin care, particularly for lower extremities.
4. Observe for signs of insulin reactions and ketoacidosis.
5. Measure intake and output.

B. Provide emotional support.
1. Allow for verbalization of client's feelings.
   a. Necessary changes in lifestyle, diet and activities.
   b. Changes in self-image and self-esteem.
   c. Fear of future and complications.
2. Provide special counseling for adolescents because of their heightened sensitivity to being different and their frequently unusual dietary habits.
   a. Diet should be adequate for normal growth and development, and regulated according to diabetic needs.
   b. The type of diet prescribed is influenced by the philosophy of the physician.
   c. Diets vary from free diets to strict dietary control.
3. Encourage involvement of family.

✦ C. Provide client education (key to effective self-management).
1. Assessment.
   a. Level of knowledge.
   b. Cultural, socioeconomic, and family influences.
   c. Daily dietary and activity patterns.
   d. Emotional and physical status and effect on client's current ability to learn.
✦ 2. Insulin and insulin injections.
   a. Keep insulin at room temperature; refrigerate extra supply of insulin.
   b. Turn insulin bottle top to bottom several times prior to drawing up insulin.
   c. Use sterile injection techniques.
   d. Choose injection sites to prevent injection in dystrophic areas.
   e. Watch for signs of hypo- and hyperglycemia.
✦ 3. Self-monitoring of blood glucose level (SMBG).
   a. Balancing blood glucose levels results in fewer complications.
   b. Protocol is taking blood glucose levels 2 to 4 times/day.
      (1) Glucose monitors are small and easy to use. Lancets and lasers are used to obtain blood samples.

(2) A monitor that measures glycated protein is now available—indicator of overall glucose control during previous 2 weeks.

(3) FDA approved the smallest diabetes testing system available, Sidekick.

c. Pattern control is goal.

d. Use algorithms as guidelines for amount of insulin.

e. Clients should use a diary or log to record results.

4. Continuous glucose monitoring systems (CGMS) are now available.

a. Sensor implanted under skin in abdomen sends continuous readings to a pager device clipped on belt.

b. Glucose readings occur every few seconds for close monitoring.

c. Appropriate for those with "brittle diabetes," in a health crisis, or who display a wide range of levels.

5. Oral medications.

a. Take medications regularly.

b. Watch for hypoglycemic reactions occurring with sulfonylureas.

c. Remember that alcohol ingestion in conjunction with sulfonylureas causes an Antabuse-like reaction.

6. Avoidance of infection and injury.

a. Report infection or injury promptly to physician.

b. Maintain meticulous skin care.

◆ c. Maintain proper foot care.

(1) Wash with mild soap—dry well.

(2) Use lanolin to prevent cracking.

(3) Cut toenails straight across, or have nails trimmed by podiatrist.

(4) Use clean cotton socks.

(5) Inspect feet daily—report skin breaks.

(6) Avoid "bathroom surgery" for corns and calluses.

d. Be aware that insulin requirements may increase with infections.

e. Be prepared for healing process impairment.

f. Avoid tight-fitting garments and shoes.

◆ 7. Diet.

a. Do not vary meal times.

b. Incorporate diet with individual needs, lifestyle, cultural, and socioeconomic patterns.

c. Most adults require 30 calories/kg of ideal body weight.

◆ 8. Exercise.

a. Regulate time and amount.

◆ CURRENT TRENDS IN INSULIN ADMINISTRATION

- Abdominal injection sites preferred for consistent and rapid rate of absorption.
- Rotating injection areas is recommended, for clients using pork or beef insulin. Rotation *within* sites is recommended for those using human or purified pork insulin.
- Injection site should be 1 inch from the previous injection site.
- Wait 30 seconds after slowly injecting insulin to prevent insulin leakage.
- Aspirating before and massaging after injection are no longer recommended.

---

b. Avoid sporadic, vigorous activities; use aerobic exercise.

c. Give 10 g CHO before exercise and every hour during exercise.

d. Do not exercise during peak action time of insulin.

e. Rigorous exercise while blood sugar is 240–300 percent may precipitate ketoacidosis.

9. Medic-Alert band.

10. Provide constant availability of concentrated sugar.

Syndrome X—Metabolic Syndrome

Definition: A group of risk factors that, in combination, put someone at higher risk of coronary artery disease. These risk factors include central obesity (excessive fat tissue in the abdominal region), glucose intolerance, high triglycerides and low HDL cholesterol, and hypertension.

Characteristics

A. Underlying cause is resistance to insulin.

1. Normally, blood carries the glucose to the body's tissues, where the cells use it as fuel. Glucose enters the cells with the help of insulin.

2. In insulin resistance, cells don't respond to insulin and glucose can't enter the cells. The body reacts by putting out more and more insulin to help glucose get into the cells.

3. This results in higher than normal levels of insulin and glucose in the blood.

4. Increased insulin raises triglycerides level and interferes with how the kidneys work, leading to increased blood pressure.

B. Combined effects of insulin resistance put a client at risk of heart disease, stroke, diabetes and other conditions.

C. Risk factors.

1. Age—increases with age.

2. Race—greater in Hispanics and Asians.
3. Obesity—body mass index (BMI) > 25, abdominal obesity, having an apple shape rather than a pear shape.
4. History of diabetes—family history of Type 2 diabetes or a history of gestational diabetes.
5. Other diseases—high blood pressure, cardiovascular disease, polycystic ovary syndrome.

Treatment

A. Screening and diagnosis.
   1. Elevated waist circumference, greater than 35 inches for women and 40 inches for men.
   2. Elevated level of triglycerides of 150 mg/dL or higher, or client receiving treatment for high triglycerides.
   3. Reduced HDL < 40 mg/dL in men or < 50 mg/dL in women.
   4. Elevated blood pressure ≥ 130 mm Hg systolic, ≥ 85 mm Hg diastolic.
   5. Elevated fasting blood glucose of 100 mg/dL or higher.
B. Intervention.
   1. Exercise.
   2. Weight loss.
   3. Stop smoking.

COMPLICATIONS

✦ Ketoacidosis (DKA)

Definition: One of the most serious results of poorly managed diabetes. The two major metabolic problems that are the source of this condition are hyperglycemia and ketoacidemia, both due to insulin lack associated with hyperglucagonemia.

Characteristics

A. Without insulin, carbohydrate metabolism is affected.
B. Hyperglycemia results from increased liver production of glucose and decreased glucose uptake by peripheral tissues.
C. The liver oxidizes fatty acids into
   1. Acetoacidic acid (increased ketone bodies lead to ketoacidosis).
   2. Beta-hydroxybutyric acid (acetone is volatile and is blown off by lungs).
   3. As glucose levels increase, there is osmotic overload in kidneys, resulting in dehydration and electrolyte losses.
   4. As ketone bodies increase, acidosis and comatose states occur.

Assessment

A. Assess for ketoacidotic coma—usually preceded by a few days of polyuria and polydipsia with associated symptoms (classic symptoms of hyperglycemia).
B. Assess for ill appearance.
C. Assess for anorexia, nausea, and vomiting.
D. Assess for drowsiness, confusion, and mental stupor.
E. Assess for dehydration; deep, rapid breathing; and fruity odor of acetone to breath.
F. Observe for complications of circulatory collapse or respiratory distress.

Implementation

✦ A. Maintain fluid and electrolyte balance.
   1. Normal saline IV until blood sugar reaches 250–300 mg/dL%; then a dextrose solution (5% glucose) is started.
   2. Potassium added to IV after renal function is evaluated and hydration is adequate.
✦ B. Provide insulin management.
   1. Give one-half dose IV during acute phase and one-half dose sub q or low-dose protocol; IV bolus of 5–10 U of regular insulin followed by infusion of 5–10 U/hr until plasma glucose level is 250 mg/100 mL.
   2. Regulating level takes 4–6 hours; regulation of pH takes 8–12 hours.
   3. Monitor for onset of insulin reaction.
✦ C. Maintain patent airway and adequate circulation to brain (cardiac monitoring if status indicates).
D. Monitor vital signs every 1–2 hours; arterial blood gases hourly until pH is 7.2+.
E. Monitor urine frequently for glucose and acetone.
F. Test blood glucose level every 1–2 hours.
G. Perform hourly urine measurements.
H. Maintain personal hygiene.
I. Keep client warm.
J. Protect from injury.

Insulin Reaction/Hypoglycemia

✦ *Definition:* An abnormally low blood glucose, usually below 50 mg, resulting from too much insulin, not enough food, or excessive activity.

Assessment

A. Assess for symptoms, especially before meals.
✦ B. Assess for sweating, tremors, pallor, tachycardia, palpitations, or nervousness.
✦ C. Evaluate for headache, confusion, emotional changes, memory lapses, slurred speech, numbness of lips and tongue, alterations in gait, loss of consciousness.
D. Evaluate lab tests.
   ✦ 1. Blood glucose, usually below 50–60 mg/dL.
   2. Urine for acetone (usually negative).

INSULIN RESISTANCE

- Definitions
    1. People (25% of the U.S. population) who produce insulin but the quality of its action is inadequate.
    2. The body does not respond to insulin the way a normal body would (high insulin level or decreased insulin action).
- The underlying disorder is a prediabetic state, called metabolic syndrome—a precursor to coronary artery disease and diabetes.
- The major symptoms of metabolic syndrome are obesity, high blood pressure, low HDL and high triglycerides, mildly elevated blood sugar (not high enough to be called diabetes), and family history of diabetes.
- Treatment
    1. Reversing primary symptoms (weight loss, exercises, stress reduction, etc.).
    2. Medications: Metformin improves insulin resistance by decreasing glucose production in the liver; rosiglitazone and piolitazone improve insulin resistance by improving glucose uptake by muscles and fat cells.

Implementation

◆ A. Administer oral carbohydrate in form of dextrosol tablet, unsweetened orange juice or 8 oz. of skim milk if client is alert; administer glucagon (sub q or IV) if client is not alert.

B. Administer carbohydrates by mouth when client awakens.

◆ C. Provide client teaching.
   1. Maintain regimen of diet, medications, and exercise.
   2. Treat the symptoms early to prevent complications.
   3. Instruct client to always carry simple carbohydrates for treatment of early symptoms.
   4. Take 200-calorie snack 30 minutes before peak time of insulin to prevent hypoglycemia.
   5. Extra food should be taken before engaging in heavy physical exercise.

D. Prevent compensatory rebound hyperglycemia (Somogyi phenomenon).
   1. Caused by the body's attempt to oppose the excessive action of insulin through liver glycogenolysis.
   2. Insulin dose is reduced and client returned to stabilized rate.

E. Provide instruction in use of portable insulin pump if ordered.

F. Provide instruction in use of blood sugar monitors.
   1. Prick finger and smear drop of blood on reagent strip.
   2. Compare results with monitor or chart and record.

Chronic Complications

Definition: Chronic complications of diabetes are becoming more common as diabetics live longer. Included in this category are blindness, renal disease, and vascular conditions. (*See* Table 8-16.)

◆ A. *Diabetic retinopathy:* progressive impairment of retinal circulation that eventually causes vitreous hemorrhage with vision loss.
   1. Assessment.
      a. Duration and degree of disease (incidence increases with length of time disease is present).
      b. Impaired vision.
      c. Ability to carry out daily tasks: blood glucose testing and insulin injections.
      d. Need for assistance from others.
   2. Implementation.
      a. Assist in ways to maintain independence and self-esteem.
      b. Support client when treatment is implemented: photocoagulation or vitrectomy.
      c. Instruct in actions that prevent or reduce complications: stable blood glucose levels.
      d. Instruct client to have frequent eye examinations.

◆ B. *Diabetic nephropathy:* the specific renal disease, intercapillary glomerulosclerosis, is called Kimmelstiel–Wilson syndrome. It is the result of chronic diabetes.
   1. Assessment.
      a. Urine alterations; proteinuria, azotemia, frequent urinary tract infections, neurogenic bladder.
      b. Serum lab values; BUN, creatinine.
      c. Thirst and fatigue.
      d. Hypertension.
   2. Implementation.
      a. Administer medications to prevent urinary tract infections.
      b. Instruct client to keep blood glucose levels within normal limits.
      c. Maintain adequate fluid intake.
      d. Instruct in 20- to 40-g protein diet.
      e. Restrict sodium and potassium in diet.
      f. Prepare client for dialysis therapy if appropriate.
      g. Administer medications to control hypertension.

◆ C. *Neuropathy:* general deterioration that affects the peripheral and autonomic nervous systems.
   1. Assessment.
      a. Peripheral neuropathy.
         (1) Pain in the legs.

◆ **Table 8-16. COMPLICATIONS ASSOCIATED WITH DIABETES**

Clinical Manifestations	Hypoglycemia	Diabetic Ketoacidosis (DKA)	Hyperglycemic Hyperosmolar Nonketotic Coma (HHNK)
	Type I	**Type I**	**Type II**
Cause	Too much insulin or too little food	Absence or inadequate insulin	Uncontrolled diabetes or oral hypoglycemic drugs
Onset	Rapid (within minutes)	Slow (about 8 hours)	Slow (hours to days)
Appearance	Exhibits symptoms of fainting	Appears ill	Appears ill
Respirations	Normal	Hyperpnea (Kussmaul's breathing) from metabolic acidosis	No hyperpnea unless lactic acidosis is present
Breath odor	Normal	Sweetish due to acetone	Normal
Pulse	Tachycardia	Tachycardia	Tachycardia
Blood pressure		Hypotension	Hypotension
Hunger	Hunger pangs in epigastrium	Loss of appetite	Hunger
Thirst	None	Increased	Increased, dehydration
Vomiting	Nausea; vomiting rare	Common	Common
Eyes	Staring, double vision	Appear sunken	Visual loss
Headache	Common	Occasionally	Occasionally
Skin	Pallor, perspiration, chilling sensation	Hot, dry skin	Hot, dry skin
Muscle action	Twitching common, unsteady gait	Twitching absent	Twitching absent
Pain in abdomen	None	Common	Common
Mental status	Confusion, erratic, change in mood, unable to concentrate	Malaise, drowsy, confusion, coma	Confused, dull, coma
Lab findings			
Sugar in urine	None after residual is discarded	Present	Present
Blood sugar	Below 50–70 mg/dL	High, 350–900 mg/dL	Very high, 800 mg/dL up to 2400 mg/dL
Ketones	Absent	High	Absent
Ketones in blood plasma	Absent	4+ present	Absent

(2) Aching and burning sensations in lower extremities.
  b. Alterations in bowel and bladder function.
    (1) Bowel dysfunction: constipation, diarrhea, nocturnal fecal incontinence.
    (2) Urinary dysfunction: infrequent voiding, weak stream, dribbling, signs of urinary infection.
  c. Autonomic nervous system impairment.
    (1) Sexual dysfunction.
    (2) Orthostatic hypotension.
    (3) Pupillary changes.
  d. Circulatory abnormalities.
    (1) Skin breakdown and signs of infection.
    (2) Thick toenails: suggestive of circulatory impairment.

(3) Low temperature and poor color in feet; athlete's feet.

(4) Thin, shiny, atrophic skin.

(5) Weak peripheral pulses.

2. Implementation.

a. Assist client to deal with pain.

(1) Encourage walking for exercise.

(2) Provide foot cradle when in bed.

b. Assist client to deal with bladder–bowel problems.

(1) Provide privacy for toileting.

(2) Provide psychological support.

(3) Administer Lomotil as ordered for diarrhea.

(4) Administer neomycin as ordered to prevent bacterial growth in an atonic bowel.

(5) Administer Urecholine as ordered.

(6) Establish 2-hour voiding schedule to prevent urinary stasis.

(7) Encourage fluids.

c. Counsel client who has sexual dysfunction.

(1) Allow client to vent feelings about sexual impotence.

(2) Observe for depression (sexual impotence is usually permanent).

d. Provide excellent foot care.

(1) Wash with soap and warm water or antibacterial gel, dry thoroughly.

(2) Massage feet with lanolin or mineral oil to prevent scaling or cracking.

(3) File or cut toenails across nail. Do not injure soft tissue around nail (check hospital policy for nail care).

(4) Prevent moisture from accumulating between toes; use lamb's wool.

(5) Instruct in well-fitting shoes. Do not go barefoot.

(6) Wear loose-fitting socks.

(7) Exercise feet daily.

(8) See podiatrist regularly.

(9) Notify physician if cuts, pain, or blisters appear on feet.

Functional Hyperinsulinism/Hypoglycemia

✦ *Definition:* A condition that occurs as the result of excess secretion of insulin by the beta cells of the pancreas gland.

Characteristics

✦ A. May be associated with "dumping syndrome" following gastrectomy.

B. May occur prior to development of diabetes mellitus.

Assessment

A. Assess for personality changes.

1. Tenseness.

2. Nervousness.

3. Irritability.

4. Anxiousness.

5. Depression.

B. Assess for excessive diaphoresis.

C. Assess for excessive hunger.

D. Evaluate muscle weakness and tachycardia.

E. Assess laboratory values—low blood sugar during hypoglycemic episodes.

Implementation

✦ A. High-protein, low-carbohydrate diet.

B. Counseling may reduce anxiety and tenseness.

ENDOCRINE SYSTEM REVIEW QUESTIONS

1. Following brain surgery, the client suddenly exhibits polyuria and begins voiding 15 to 20 L/day. Specific gravity for the urine is 1.006. The nurse will recognize these symptoms as the possible development of

   1. Diabetes insipidus.
   2. Diabetes, Type 1.
   3. Diabetes, Type 2.
   4. Addison's disease.

2. A person with a diagnosis of Type 2 diabetes should understand the symptoms of a hyperglycemic reaction. The nurse will know this client understands if she says these symptoms are

   1. Thirst, polyuria, and decreased appetite.
   2. Flushed cheeks, acetone breath, and increased thirst.
   3. Nausea, vomiting, and diarrhea.
   4. Weight gain, normal breath, and thirst.

3. The Type 2 diabetic who is obese is best controlled by weight loss because obesity

   1. Reduces the number of insulin receptors.
   2. Causes pancreatic islet cell exhaustion.
   3. Reduces insulin binding at receptor sites.
   4. Reduces pancreatic insulin production.

4. A nursing assessment for initial signs of hypoglycemia will include

   1. Pallor, blurred vision, weakness, behavioral changes.
   2. Frequent urination, flushed face, pleural friction rub.
   3. Abdominal pain, diminished deep tendon reflexes, double vision.
   4. Weakness, lassitude, irregular pulse, dilated pupils.

5. Which of the following nursing diagnoses would be *most* appropriate for the client with decreased thyroid function?

   1. Alteration in growth and development related to increased growth hormone production.
   2. Alteration in thought processes related to decreased neurologic function.
   3. Fluid volume deficit related to polyuria.
   4. Hypothermia related to decreased metabolic rate.

6. The RN should assess for which of the following clinical manifestations in the client with Cushing's syndrome?

   1. Hypertension, diaphoresis, nausea, and vomiting.
   2. Tetany, irritability, dry skin, and seizures.
   3. Unexplained weight gain, energy loss, and cold intolerance.
   4. Water retention, moon face, hirsutism, and purple striae.

7. The client with hyperparathyroidism should have extremities handled gently because

   1. Decreased calcium bone deposits can lead to pathologic fractures.
   2. Edema causes stretched tissue to tear easily.
   3. Hypertension can lead to a stroke with residual paralysis.
   4. Polyuria leads to dry skin and mucous membranes that can break down.

8. Which of the following is the priority nursing implementation for a client with a tumor of the posterior lobe of the pituitary gland who has had a urine output of 3 L in the last hour with a specific gravity of 1.002?

   1. Measure and record vital signs each shift.
   2. Turn client every 2 hours to prevent skin breakdown.
   3. Administer Pitressin Tannate as ordered.
   4. Maintain a dark and quiet room.

9. A client has the diagnosis of diabetes. His physician has ordered short- and long-acting insulin. When administering two types of insulin, the nurse would

   1. Withdraw the long-acting insulin into the syringe before the short-acting insulin.
   2. Withdraw the short-acting insulin into the syringe before the long-acting insulin.
   3. Draw up in two separate syringes, then combine into one syringe.
   4. Withdraw long-acting insulin, inject air into regular insulin, and withdraw insulin.

10. Certain physiological changes will result from the treatment for myxedema. The symptoms that may indicate adverse changes in the body that the nurse should observe for are

1. Increased respiratory excursion.
2. Increased pulse and cardiac output.
3. Hyperglycemia.
4. Weight loss, nervousness, and insomnia.

11. A client with myxedema has been in the hospital for 3 days. The nursing assessment reveals the following clinical manifestations: respiratory rate of 8/min, diminished breath sounds in the right lower lobe, crackles in the left lower lobe. The most appropriate nursing intervention is to

   1. Increase the use of ROM, turning, and deep-breathing exercises.
   2. Increase the frequency of rest periods.
   3. Initiate postural drainage.
   4. Continue with routine nursing care.

12. In an individual with the diagnosis of hypoparathyroidism, the nurse will assess for which primary symptom?

   1. Fatigue, muscular weakness.
   2. Cardiac arrhythmias.
   3. Tetany.
   4. Constipation.

13. The nurse explains to a client who has just received the diagnosis of Type 2 diabetes mellitus that sulfonylureas, one group of oral hypoglycemic agents, act by

   1. Stimulating the pancreas to produce or release insulin.
   2. Making the insulin that is produced more available for use.
   3. Lowering the blood sugar by facilitating the uptake and utilization of glucose.
   4. Altering both fat and protein metabolism.

14. A client has been admitted to the hospital with a tentative diagnosis of adrenocortical hyperfunction. In assessing the client, an observable sign the nurse would chart is

   1. Butterfly rash on the face.
   2. Moon face.
   3. Positive Chvostek's sign.
   4. Bloated extremities.

15. The nurse is teaching a diabetic client to monitor her blood glucose using a glucometer. The nurse will know the client is competent in performing her finger-stick to obtain blood when she

   1. Uses the ball of a finger as the puncture site.
   2. Uses the side of a fingertip as the puncture site.
   3. Avoids using the fingers of her dominant hand as puncture sites.
   4. Avoids using the thumbs as puncture sites.

ENDOCRINE SYSTEM

Answers with Rationale

1. (1) Diabetes insipidus is an antidiuretic deficiency and may occur following brain surgery or head injury. It also occurs in young adults resulting from damage to the posterior lobe of the pituitary gland. Severe polyuria occurs when there is an inability to concentrate urine. These are not symptoms of Types 1 and 2 diabetes (2, 3) or Addison's disease (4) (which is adrenocorticol hypofunction).

   NP:AN; CN:PH; CN:C

2. (2) All the other choices have one wrong answer or symptom: (1) hunger, not decreased appetite; (3) pain in abdomen, not diarrhea; (4) breath odor of acetone, not normal. Answers such as this are tricky, because you have to pick out the wrong answers from among several right answers.

   NP:E; CN:PH; CL:A

3. (3) Obesity causes reduced insulin binding at receptor sites, which leads to pancreatic hypersecretion of insulin and eventual pancreatic cell exhaustion.

   NP:AN; CN:H; CL:C

4. (1) Weakness, fainting, blurred vision, pallor, and perspiration are all common symptoms when there is too much insulin or too little food—hypoglycemia. The signs and symptoms in answers (2) and (3) are indicative of hyperglycemia.

   NP:A; CN:PH; CL:C

5. (4) Because the thyroid gland regulates the metabolic rate, a decrease in thyroid function would result in a decreased metabolic rate.

   NP:AN; CN:PH; CL:C

6. (4) Clinical manifestations of Cushing's syndrome include water retention, moon face, hirsutism, and purple striae.

   NP:A; CN:PH; CL:C

7. (1) The parathyroid glands regulate calcium in the body. Excessive activity results in calcium leaving the bones and teeth to enter the bloodstream. This makes the bones more brittle and susceptible to fracture.

   NP:P; CN:PH; CL:A

8. (3) The client is experiencing antidiuretic hormone deficiency. Pitressin produces concentrated urine by increasing tubular reabsorption of water, thus preserving up to 90 percent of water.

   NP:I; CN:PH; CL:AN

9. (2) Short-acting insulin is withdrawn first to prevent possible contamination of the short-acting insulin bottle by the longer-acting insulin.

   NP:P; CN:PH; CL:A

10. (2) The increased pulse rate and increased cardiac output caused by thyroid compounds can cause angina, arrhythmias, or, in extreme cases, heart failure. The older the client, the more compromised the cardiovascular system may become.

    NP:E; CN:PH; CL:A

11. (1) Clients with myxedema often experience a decreased respiratory rate and chest excursion, so they require extra care to prevent atelectasis. Encouraging moving, turning, and coughing exercises will open the alveoli, thus decreasing the risk of atelectasis. Postural drainage (3) will not prevent atelectasis because the treatment does not expand the alveoli.

    NP:I; CN:PH; CL:A

12. (3) Tetany occurs mainly in the distal extremities, manifested by flexion of the fingers, hands, and toes (carpopedal spasms). Increased mechanical irritability exists especially with attempts at voluntary move-

Coding for Questions/Answers Abbreviations: **Nursing Process: NP,** Assessment: A, Analysis: AN, Planning: P, Implementation: I, Evaluation: E; **Client Needs: CN,** Safe, Effective Care Environment: S, Health Promotion and Maintenance: H, Psychosocial Integrity: PS, Physiological Integrity: PH; **Clinical Area: CA,** Medical Nursing: M, Surgical Nursing: S, Maternal/Newborn Nursing: MA, Pediatric Nursing: P, Psychiatric Nursing: PS; **Cognitive Level: CL,** Knowledge: K, Comprehension: C, Application: A, Analysis: AN.

ments. Laryngeal spasms, convulsions, and death will result if the tetany is not treated promptly.

NP:A; CN:PH; CL:C

13. (1) Sulfonylurea drugs (e.g., Orinase) lower the blood sugar by stimulating the beta cells of the pancreas to synthesize and release insulin.

NP:I; CN:H; CL:C

14. (2) Moon face, thin extremities, and buffalo hump are characteristics of Cushing's syndrome (adrenocor-

tical hyperfunction). A positive Chvostek's sign (3) is seen with primary aldosteronism; butterfly rash (1) is seen with lupus.

NP:A; CN:PH; CL:C

15. (2) The sides of fingertips have fewer nerve endings than do the balls of the finger, so less discomfort will result from selecting the sides as puncture sites. Both hands, including the thumbs, can be used as puncture sites.

NP:E; CN:PH; CL:A

PERIOPERATIVE CARE CONCEPTS

The term *perioperative* refers to all phases of surgical care: preoperative, intraoperative, and postoperative. This section outlines the nursing care measures for surgical clients and covers the principles of care, anesthesia, postoperative complications, and fluid replacement therapy.

PREOPERATIVE AND POSTOPERATIVE CARE

Routine Preoperative Care

Psychological Care

✦ A. Reinforce the physician's teaching regarding the surgical procedure.
  B. Identify client's anxieties; notify physician of extreme anxiety.
  C. Listen to client's verbalization of fears.
  D. Provide support to the client's family (where family can wait during surgery, approximately how long the surgery takes, etc.).

✦ **Preoperative Teaching**
  A. Postoperative exercises: leg, coughing, deep-breathing, etc.
  B. Equipment utilized during postoperative period: intermittent positive-pressure breathing machine (IPPB), NG tube for suctioning, etc.
✦ C. Pain medication and when to request it.
    1. Epidural patient-controlled analgesia (PCA or PCEA) instructions.
    2. Client needs to be taught use of PCA before surgery with instructions reinforced after surgery.
  D. Explanation of NPO.

✦ **Physical Care**
✦ A. Completed before surgery.
    1. Observe and record client's overall condition.
       a. Nutritional status.
       b. Physical defects, such as loss of limb function, skin breakdown.
       c. Hearing or sight difficulties.
    2. Obtain chest x-ray, ECG, and blood and urine samples, as ordered.
    3. Take preoperative history and assess present physical condition.
    4. Determine if any drug allergies.
✦ B. Completed early morning of surgery after client is admitted.

  1. Perform skin prep and clip excess hair (shaving the operative site is no longer recommended); clean operative site with topical antiseptics (povidone-iodine, chlorhexidine) to reduce bacterial count.
  2. Give enema, if ordered.
  3. Insert indwelling catheter, nasogastric tube, IV.
  4. Administer preoperative medications.
  5. Provide quiet rest with siderails up and curtains drawn.
  6. Monitor blood glucose levels, if ordered (nosocomial infections increased when blood glucose level is more than 220 mg/dL).

✦ **Nurse's Responsibility**
  A. Perform or supervise skin prep and cleansing.
  B. Carry out preoperative nursing interventions.
  C. Notify physician of drug allergies, overwhelming anxiety, unusual ECG findings, abnormal lab findings (blood glucose level).
  D. Ensure that consent form is signed.
  E. Administer preoperative medications on time.
  F. Complete preoperative checklist.
  G. Check if history and physical examination findings are on chart.
  H. Chart preoperative medications.
  I. Check Identaband, provide quiet environment.
  J. Remove dentures, nail polish, hairpins, etc.

Postanesthesia Unit

✦ **Assessment**
✦ A. Assess patent airway.
  B. Assess need for oxygen.
    1. Administer humidified oxygen by mask or nasal cannula as ordered.
    2. Monitor oxygen saturation using finger probe monitor.
  C. Check gag reflex.
  D. Observe for adverse signs of general anesthesia or spinal anesthesia.
✦ E. Assess vital signs—initially every 5–15 minutes according to condition.
    1. Pulse rate, quality, and rhythm.
    2. Blood pressure.
    3. Respirations, rate, rhythm, and depth.
  F. Evaluate temperature for heat control.
✦ G. Observe dressings and surgical drains.
    1. Mark any drainage on dressings by drawing a line around the drainage; note date and time.
    2. Note color and amount of drainage on dressings and in drainage tubes.
    3. Ensure that dressing is secure.
    4. Reinforce dressings as needed.
  H. Assess IV fluids—type and amount of solution, flow rate, IV site.

I. Measure urine output hourly.

J. Observe client's overall condition.
   1. Check skin for warmth, color, and moisture.
   2. Check nailbeds and mucous membranes for color and blanching; report if cyanotic.
   3. Observe for return of reflexes.

K. Assess client for return to room.
   1. Be sure vital signs are stable and within normal limits for at least 1 hour.
   2. See if client is awake and reflexes are present (gag and cough reflex). Check for movement and sensation in limbs of clients with spinal anesthesia.
   3. Take oral airway out (if not out already). Observe for cyanosis.
   4. Be sure dressings are intact and there is no excessive drainage.

Implementation

✦ A. Maintain patent airway—leave airway in place until gag reflex returns.

B. Administer humidified SpO_2 by mask or nasal cannula at 6 L/min.

C. Monitor O_2 saturation finger probe.

D. Position client for adequate ventilation—side-lying is best, if not contraindicated.

E. Observe for adverse signs of general anesthesia or spinal anesthesia.
   1. Level of consciousness.
   2. Movement of limbs.

✦ F. Monitor vital signs every 10–15 minutes.
   1. Pulse—check rate, quality, and rhythm.
   2. Blood pressure—check pulse pressure and quality as well as systolic and diastolic pressure.
   3. Respiration—check rate, rhythm, depth, and type of respiration (abdominal breathing, nasal flaring).
   4. Vital signs are sometimes difficult to obtain due to hypothermia.
   5. Movement from operating room table to gurney can alter vital signs significantly, especially with cardiovascular clients.

G. Maintain temperature (operating room is usually cold)—apply warm blankets.

H. Maintain patent IV.
   1. Check type and amount of solution being administered.
   2. Adjust correct flow rate.
   3. Check IV site for signs of infiltration.
   4. Check blood transfusion.
      a. Blood type and blood bank number. Time transfusion started.
      b. Client's name, identification number, expiration date.
      c. Amount in bag upon arrival in recovery room. Color and consistency of blood.

I. Monitor urine output if indwelling catheter in place.

J. Monitor dressings and surgical drains for drainage.
   1. Empty drainage collection device as needed.
   2. Report unusual amount of drainage.

K. Administer medications.
   1. Begin routine drugs and administer all STAT drugs.
   2. Pain medications are usually administered sparingly and in smaller amounts.

L. Discharge client from postanesthesia unit.
   1. Call anesthesiologist to discharge client from recovery room (if appropriate).
   2. Give report on client's condition to floor nurse receiving client.
   3. Ensure IV is patent.
   4. Reinforce or change dressings as needed.
   5. Ensure all drains are functioning.
   6. Record amount of IV fluid remaining and amount absorbed.
   7. Record amount of urine in drainage bag.
   8. Record all medications administered in recovery room.
   9. Clean client as needed (change gown, wash off excess surgical scrub solution).

M. Use Postanesthesia Recovery Scoring System in addition to vital signs.
   1. Ability to move extremities.
   2. Ability to cough and deep-breathe.
   3. Normal blood pressure maintained within 20 mm Hg preanesthesia.
   4. Fully awake.
   5. Normal skin color.

Phase II Surgical Unit

✦ **Assessment**

A. Assess for patent airway; administer oxygen as necessary.

B. Assess vital signs—usual orders are every 15 minutes until stable; then every 30 minutes × 2, every hour × 4; then every 4 hours for 24–48 hours.

C. Check IV site and patency frequently.

D. Observe and record urine output.

E. Assess intake and output.

F. Observe skin color and moisture.

✦ **Implementation**

✦ A. Maintain patent airway. Position client for comfort and maximum airway ventilation.

✦ B. Turn every 2 hours and PRN—avoid sharply bent knees and hips. (*See* Table 8-17.)

C. Apply elastic stockings and compression device if ordered.

D. Encourage coughing and deep-breathing every 2 hours (may use IPPB or blow bottles).

✦ Table 8-17. SURGICAL PROCEDURES: POSTOPERATIVE POSITIONS AND AMBULATION

System	Postop Position* or as Ordered	Ambulation*
Neurosurgical		
Craniotomy		
Surgery involving: posterior fossa	Supine or low-Fowler's (10 degrees) side to side only	Evening or first day
Anterior or middle fossa	Low- or semi-Fowler's side to back to side unless bone flap removed, then nonoperative side and back only	Evening or first day
Ventriculoperitoneal shunt	Supine, back to unoperative side	First to second day
Respiratory		
Laryngectomy	Semi-Fowler's; side–back–side	First or second day
Tracheostomy	Semi-Fowler's; side–back–side	Evening of surgery
Nasal surgery	Semi-Fowler's; back	First day
Tonsillectomy	Semi-Fowler's if local anesthesia used; modified Trendelenburg, side-lying or prone with head turned to side if general anesthesia used	Evening of surgery
Lung surgery (lobectomy)	Semi- to high-Fowler's; unaffected side–back–side	Evening of surgery or first day
Pneumonectomy	Semi- to high-Fowler's; affected side–back–side	First day
Circulatory		
Open-heart surgery for atrial and ventricular septal defects	Low-Fowler's or supine; turn side–back–side	First to third day
Valve replacement surgery	Supine or low-Fowler's until vital signs stable; turn side–back–side	First to second day
Coronary artery bypass	Supine or low-Fowler's until vital signs stable; turn side–back–side	First to second day
Ear		
Stapedectomy	Low-Fowler's; unoperative side only	Evening of surgery or first day
Eye		
Cataract removal	Low-Fowler's; unoperative side only	Day of surgery; usually within 2–4 hours postop
Repair of detached retina	Varies with site of detachment; unoperative side only or as ordered	Evening of surgery or first day
Enucleation	High-Fowler's; unoperative side only or as ordered	First day
Gastrointestinal		
Gastric resection	Minimum low-Fowler's; turn side–back–side	Evening of surgery or first day
Ileostomy; colostomy	Sims', lateral recovery, semi-Fowler's	First day
Appendectomy	Semi-Fowler's	Evening of surgery or first day
Cholecystectomy—open	Semi- to low-Fowler's	First day
Cholecystectomy—laparoscopic	Sims' to relieve gas pockets near diaphragm	Evening of surgery
Small bowel resection	Low-Fowler's; turn side–back–side	First day
Portacaval shunt	Semi-Fowler's	Evening of surgery or first day
Partial pancreatectomy	Semi-Fowler's	First day
Hemorrhoidectomy	Supine; turn side to side	First day
Radical neck	Fowler's, side-lying either side	First to second day

♦ Table 8-17. SURGICAL PROCEDURES: POSTOPERATIVE POSITIONS AND AMBULATION *(Continued)*		
System	**Postop Position* or as Ordered**	**Ambulation***
Genitourinary		
Nephrostomy	Semi- to high-Fowler's; unoperative side only	Evening of surgery
Nephrectomy	Semi- to high-Fowler's; side–back–side	Evening of surgery
Kidney transplant	As ordered	First day
Ureterolithotomy	Low-Fowler's; side–back–side	Evening of surgery
TURP	Low- to semi-Fowler's	Evening of surgery
Orchiectomy	As ordered	First day
Cystectomy and ileal conduit	Low-Fowler's; side–back–side	First day
Gynecologic		
Hysterectomy	Low-Fowler's; side–back–side	Evening of surgery
Radical hysterectomy	Supine or low-Fowler's; side–back–side	First day
Pelvic exenteration	As ordered	First day
Vulvectomy	As ordered	First day
Mastectomy	Fowler's; unoperative side or back	Evening of surgery
Musculoskeletal		
Amputation	Low-Fowler's; unoperative side and back; prone once per shift	Evening of surgery use adaptive devices (i.e., crutches)
Open reduction and internal fixation	Fowler's; side–back–side	Evening of surgery or first day
Hip prosthesis	Low-Fowler's; back or unoperative side only. DO NOT FLEX hips, keep in abduction and external rotation	First or second day, non–weight-bearing
Hip nailing	Low-Fowler's; unoperative side and back only	First day, non–weight-bearing
Total knee replacement	As ordered	First day with client
Total hip replacement	Supine or side to side with orders; DO NOT FLEX hips, keep in abduction and external rotation	First to third day, non–weight-bearing
Laminectomy	Low-Fowler's; turn side to side, may position on back, logroll	Evening of surgery or first day
Spinal fusion	Flat, side to side only, logroll	Second or third day with brace

* Postop positioning and ambulation are dependent on client condition and type of anesthesia used.

E. Keep client comfortable with medications (monitor PCA if ordered).

F. Check dressings and drainage tubes every 2–4 hours; if abnormal amount of drainage, check more frequently.

G. Give oral hygiene at least every 4 hours; if nasogastric tube, nasal oxygen, or endotracheal tube is inserted, give oral hygiene every 2 hours.

H. Bathe client when temperature can be maintained—bathing removes the antiseptic solution and stimulates circulation.

I. Keep client warm and avoid chilling, but do not increase temperature above normal.
   1. Increased temperature increases metabolic rate and need for oxygen.
   2. Excessive perspiration causes fluid and electrolyte loss.

J. Irrigate nasogastric tube every 2 hours and PRN with normal saline to keep patent and to prevent electrolyte imbalance.

K. Maintain dietary intake—type of diet depends on type and extent of surgical procedure.

1. Minor surgical conditions—client may drink or eat as soon as he or she is awake and desires food or drink.
2. Major surgical conditions.
   ✦ a. Maintain NPO until bowel sounds return or start enteral feedings for non-GI surgery.
   b. Clear liquid advanced to full liquid as tolerated.
   c. Soft diet advanced to full diet within 3 to 5 days (depending on type of surgery and physician's preference).
L. Place on bedpan 2–4 hours postoperatively if catheter not inserted.
M. Start activity as tolerated and dictated by surgical procedure. Most clients are ambulatory first 24 hours. (*See* Table 8-17.)

ANESTHESIA

Preoperative Medications

General Action

A. Decreases secretions of mouth and respiratory tract.
B. Depresses vagal reflexes—slows heart and prevents complications with excitation during intubation.
C. Produces drowsiness and relieves anxiety.
D. Allows anesthesia to be induced more smoothly and in smaller amounts.

✦ Types of Drugs

A. Barbiturates.
   1. Short-acting barbiturate at bedtime (Seconal or Nembutal).
   2. Short-acting tranquilizer 1 hour preoperatively (decreases blood pressure and pulse and relieves anxiety).
B. Belladonna alkaloids.
   1. General action.
      a. Decreases salivary and bronchial secretions.
      b. Allows inhalation anesthetics to be administered more easily.
      c. Prevents postoperative complications such as aspiration pneumonia.
   2. Scopolamine is used in conjunction with morphine or Demerol to produce amnesic block.
   3. Atropine blocks the vagus nerve response of decreased heart rate, which can occur as a reaction to some inhalation anesthetics.
C. Nonnarcotic analgesic.
   1. Actions.
      a. Stadol used as component of balanced anesthesia.
      b. Given IM.
      c. Does not cause dependence or respiratory depression with increased dose.

> ### ✦ PREOPERATIVE MEDICATION TYPE AND ACTION
>
> - Hypnotic or opiate—given night before surgery
>   Decreases anxiety
>   Promotes good night's sleep
> - Tranquilizers and sedative-hypnotics—preoperative medication
>   Decreases anxiety
>   Allows smooth anesthetic induction
>   Provides amnesia for immediate perioperative period
> - Anticholinergic—preoperative medication
>   Decreases secretions
>   Counteracts vagal effects during anesthesia

      d. Contraindicated in narcotic addiction.
   2. Side effects.
      a. Sedation, lethargy.
      b. Headache, vertigo.
      c. Nervousness, palpitations, diplopia.
      d. Nausea, dry mouth.

Anesthetic Agents

A. Anesthesia produces insensitivity to pain or sensation.
B. Dangers associated with anesthesia depend on overall condition of client.
   1. High risk if associated cardiovascular, renal, or respiratory conditions.
   2. High risk for unborn fetus and mother.
   3. High risk if stomach is full (chance of vomiting and aspiration).
C. Types of anesthesia.
   1. General—administered IV or by inhalation. Produces loss of consciousness and decreases reflex movement.
   2. Local—applied topically or injected regionally. Client is alert, but pain and sensation are decreased in surgical area.

✦ General Anesthesia

✦ A. Balanced anesthesia (combination of two or more drugs) is used to decrease side effects and complications of anesthetic agents.
B. Goals of general anesthesia.
   1. Analgesia.
   2. Unconsciousness.
   3. Skeletal muscle relaxation.
C. Stages of general anesthesia.
   1. Stage one: early induction—from beginning of inhalation to loss of consciousness.
   2. Stage two: delirium or excitement.
      a. No surgery is performed at this point—dangerous stage.
      b. Breathing is irregular.

3. Stage three: surgical anesthesia.
   a. Begins when client stops fighting and is breathing regularly.
   b. Four planes, based on respiration, pupillary and eyeball movement, and reflex muscular responses.
4. Stage four: medullary paralysis—respiratory arrest.

◆ D. Anesthetic agents.
1. Tranquilizers and sedative-hypnotics (benzodiazepines).
   a. Given IV (Midazolan, Versed, diazepam, lorazepam).
   b. Generally short acting—used preoperatively.
2. Opioids (narcotics) morphine, Fentanyl.
   a. Given IV (Demerol IM)—fast onset.
   b. Does not provide amnesia.
3. Neuroleptanalgesics (sufentanil).
   a. Combination of short-acting opioid (Fentanyl) and droperidol—called a narcotic agonist analgesic.
   b. Analgesia is profound with this combination.
4. Dissociative agents (ketamine).
   a. Given IV or IM—rapid induction.
   b. Client is not asleep, but dissociated.
5. Barbiturates (Pentothal, Brevital).
   a. Given IV—rapid induction.
   b. High doses required for prolonged induction; may lead to respiratory depression.
6. Nonbarbiturate hypnotics (Amidate, Diprivan).
   a. Given IV—rapid induction.
   b. Few respiratory or cardiovascular side effects—used for fragile clients.
7. Inhalation agents.
   a. Volatile liquids (halothane, Penthrane, Ethrane). Rapid induction—used for every type of surgery. Possible respiratory depression.
   b. Gases—nitrous oxide—used for short-term procedures.

◆ E. Adjuncts for general anesthesia.
1. Preoperative medications.
2. Neuromuscular blocking agents (tubarine, Pavulon, Flaxedil)—used to facilitate intubation.
3. Depolarizing neuromuscular blocking agents (Anectine, Syncurine)—mimic action of acetylcholine at neuromuscular junction.

◆ **Local Anesthesia**

A. Topical anesthetics (Lidocaine).
1. Poorly absorbed through skin but usually rapid through mucous membranes (mouth, gastrointestinal tract, etc.).

2. Systemic toxicity is rare but local reactions common, especially if used for long periods of time on clients allergic to chemicals.
3. Used for hemorrhoids, episiotomy, nipple erosion, and minor cuts and burns.
4. Used on eye procedures extensively—removing foreign bodies and tonometry.

B. Infiltrated local anesthesia or field block (Marcaine, Xylocaine, Duranest).
1. Anesthesia directly applied to surgical area.
2. Drug is injected into tissue.
3. Can have systemic effects if injected into highly vascular area.

C. Regional anesthetics, central nerve blocks (Pontocaine, Novocaine).
1. Types: spinal, caudal, saddle, epidural.
2. Precautions.
   a. Spinal and epidural anesthesia: position client with head and shoulders elevated (prevents diffusion of anesthesia to the intercostal muscles, which could produce respiratory distress).
   b. Epidural (continuous anesthesia used in obstetrics): make sure catheter is securely fastened to prevent it from slipping out.

Conscious Sedation

◆ A. Form of IV anesthesia—depressed level of consciousness with the ability to respond to stimuli and verbal commands.
1. Combined sedation and analgesic effect so client is pain free during procedure.
2. Client can maintain patent airway.

B. Specific drugs used vary with credentials of person administering agents.
1. Versed or Valium IV frequently used.
2. Other drugs used are analgesics (morphine, Fentanyl) and reverse agonists (Narcan, naloxane).
3. Client must never be left alone and must be closely monitored for respiratory, cardiovascular, or CNS depression.
4. Client is monitored by ability to maintain airway and respond to verbal demands.

C. Agents may be used alone or in combination with local, regional, or spinal anesthesia.

D. Levels of sedation.
1. Minimal: client relaxed and may be awake—understands direction.
2. Moderate: client drowsy—may sleep, but easily awakened.
3. Deep: client sleeps through procedure; has little or no memory; oxygen given because breathing is slowed.

POSTANESTHESIA

Implementation

✦ A. General anesthesia.
1. Maintain patent airway.
2. Promote adequate respiratory function (position client for lung expansion).
3. Have client deep-breathe and cough frequently, especially if inhalation anesthesia used, to promote faster elimination of gases.
4. Turn frequently to promote lung expansion and to prevent hypostatic pneumonia and venous stasis.

✦ B. Spinal and epidural anesthesia.
1. Take precautions to prevent injury to lower extremities (watch heating pad, position limb correctly, etc.).
2. Provide gentle passive range of motion to prevent venous stasis.
3. Keep head flat or slightly elevated to prevent spinal headache (client may turn head from side to side).
4. Increase fluid intake, if tolerated, to increase cerebral spinal fluid.

Postoperative Medications

A. Evaluate need for pain relief.
B. Provide nonmedication measures for relief of pain such as relaxation techniques, back care, positioning.
C. Identify the pharmacological action of the medication.
D. Review the general side effects of the medication.
1. Drowsiness.
2. Euphoria.
3. Sleep.
4. Respiratory depression.
5. Nausea and vomiting.
E. Administer medications as ordered, usually at 3- to 4-hour intervals for first 24–48 hours for better action and pain relief. Assess for pain relief.
F. Know the action of the following drugs.
1. Opioids.
2. Synthetic opiate-like drugs.
3. Nonnarcotic pain relievers.
4. Narcotic antagonists.
5. Antiemetics.

Narcotic Analgesics

A. Pharmacological action—reduces pain and restlessness.
B. General side effects.
1. Drowsiness.
2. Euphoria.
3. Sleep.
4. Respiratory depression.
5. Nausea and vomiting.

C. Given at 3- to 4-hour intervals for first 24–48 hours for better action and pain relief.
D. Types of analgesics.
✦ 1. Opioids (narcotics).
✦ a. Morphine sulfate—potent analgesic.
(1) Specific side effects: miosis (pinpoint pupils) and bradycardia.
(2) Usual dosage: ¼–⅛ gr IM every 3–4 hours PRN.
✦ b. Hydromorphone (Dilaudid)—potent analgesic.
(1) Specific side effects: hypotension, constipation, euphoria.
(2) Usual dosage: 2–4 mg PO, IM, or IV every 4–6 hours.
c. Oxymorphine (Numorphan)—potent analgesic.
(1) Specific side effects: urinary retention, ileus, euphoria.
(2) Usual dosage: 1–1.5 mg sub q or IM every 4–6 hours; 0.5 mg IV every 4–6 hours.
d. Hydrocodone (Vicodin)—potent analgesic.
(1) Specific side effects: dizziness, drowsiness, sedation, nausea, and vomiting.
(2) Usual dosage: 10 mg orally every 3–4 hours.
e. Codeine sulfate—mild analgesic.
(1) Specific side effect: constipation.
(2) Usual dosage: 30–60 mg every 3–4 hours IM.
f. Oxycodone HCl (OxyContin); also Percocet (with acetaminophen) and Percodan (with aspirin).
(1) Potent opioid analgesic that is very addictive, especially with high dosage and long-term use.
(2) Usual dosage is 20–80 mg PO daily.
(3) This drug is very popular "on the street" and is dangerous because of its addictive quality.
✦ 2. Synthetic opiate-like drugs.
a. Demerol (meperidine)—potent analgesic (rarely used as of 2000).
(1) Specific side effects: miosis or mydriasis (dilatation of pupils), hypotension, and tachycardia.
(2) Usual dosage: 25–100 mg every 3–4 hours IM.
(3) Used less frequently today.
b. Talwin (pentazocine)—potent analgesic.
(1) Specific side effects: gastrointestinal disturbances, vertigo, headache, and euphoria.

(2) Usual dosage: 50 mg oral tablets every 3–4 hours; 30 mg IM every 3–4 hours PRN.

✦ 3. Nonnarcotic pain relievers.
 a. Salicylates (aspirin).
  (1) Decrease pain perception without causing drowsiness and euphoria. Act at point of origin or pain impulses.
  (2) Side effects.
   (a) Gastrointestinal irritation (give client milk and crackers).
   (b) Gastrointestinal bleeding.
   (c) Increased bleeding time. Use special precaution if client is on anticoagulants.
   (d) Hypersensitivity reactions to aspirin.
   (e) Tinnitus indicates toxic level reached.
   (f) Thrombocytopenia can occur with overdose (especially in children).
  (3) Usual dosage: 300–600 mg every 3–4 hours, orally or rectally.
 b. Nonsalicylate analgesics (acetaminophen).
  (1) Action similar to aspirin.
  (2) Side effects: hemolytic anemia and kidney damage.
  (3) Usual dosage: 325–650 mg every 3–4 hours orally.
 c. Nonsteriodal anti-inflammatory.
  (1) Action: analgesic and antipyretic for moderate to severe pain.
  (2) Side effects: nausea, gastrointestinal disturbances, vertigo, drowsiness, rash.

Antiemetics
A. Pharmacological action.
 1. Reduces the hyperactive reflex of the stomach.
 2. Makes the chemoreceptor trigger zone of medulla less sensitive to nerve impulses passing through this center to the vomiting center.
B. General side effects.
 1. Drowsiness.
 2. Dry mouth.
 3. Nervous system effects.
✦ C. Common drugs.
 1. Phenothiazines.
  a. Compazine (prochlorperazine).
   (1) Specific side effects: amenorrhea, hypotension, and vertigo.
   (2) Normal dosage: 5–10 mg every 3–4 hours IM.
  b. Phenergan (promethazine).
   (1) Specific side effects: dryness of mouth and blurred vision.

  (2) Normal dosage: 12.5–50 mg every 4 hours PRN.
 2. Nonphenothiazines.
  a. Dramamine (dimenhydrinate).
   (1) Specific side effect: drowsiness.
   (2) Normal dosage: 50 mg IM every 3–4 hours.
  b. Tigan (trimethobenzamide).
   (1) Specific side effects (rare); hypotension and skin rashes.
   (2) Normal dosage: 200 mg (2 mL) TID or QID IM.

COMMON POSTOPERATIVE COMPLICATIONS

See Table 8-18.

Respiratory Complications

✦ Assessment

A. Evaluate complaint of tightness or fullness in chest.
B. Assess for cough, dyspnea, or shortness of breath.
C. Evaluate increased vital signs, particularly temperature and respiratory rate.
D. Observe for restlessness.
E. Assess for decreased breath sounds, crackles.

Implementation

✦ A. Turn, cough, hyperventilate at least every 2 hours.
✦ B. Have client use incentive spirometer to provide motivation and evaluation of sustained inspiration.
 1. Inhale deeply and hold 3 seconds.
 2. Repeat hourly.
 3. Yawning also accomplishes same goal of stimulating surfactant and opening collapsed alveoli.
✦ C. Provide pharmacological therapy (through nebulization or oral route).
 1. Antibiotics—to fight infection by causative organism.
 2. Bronchodilators—act on smooth muscle to reduce bronchial spasm.
  a. Sympathomimetics (beta$_2$ agonists preferred).
  b. Anticholinergics (atropine sulfate inhalant).
  c. Theophyllines.
 3. Adrenocorticosteroids—to reduce inflammation (prednisone).
 4. Enzymes—to liquefy thick, purulent secretions through digestion.
  a. Dornavac.
  b. Varidase.

5. Expectorants—to aid in expectoration of secretions.
   a. Mucolytic agents reduce viscosity of secretion (Mucomyst).
   b. Detergents liquefy tenacious mucus (Tergemist, Alevaire).

D. Medicate for pain to facilitate TCH and use of mechanical devices.

Pneumonia

See page 256.

✦ Table 8-18. POSTOPERATIVE COMPLICATIONS

Potential Complication	Clients at Risk	Indicative Findings

Atelectasis: collapse of alveoli; may be diffuse and involve a segment, lobe, or entire lung
 	
Potential onset:
First 48 hours
	All with general anesthesia
	Special-risk clients:
	Smokers
	Chronic bronchitis
	Emphysema
	Obesity
	Elderly
	Upper abdominal surgery
	Chest surgery
	Abdominal distention
		Fever to 102°F
		Tachycardia
		Restlessness
		Tachypnea 24–30 minutes
		Altered breath sounds
		    Dullness to percussion
		    Diminished or absent breath sounds
		Crackles
		ABGs: decreased PaO_2

Pneumonia: inflammatory process in which alveoli are filled with exudate
 	
Potential onset:
First 36–48 hours
	Clients with unresolved atelectasis
	Following aspiration
	Smokers
	Elderly
	Chronic bronchitis
	Emphysema
	Heart failure
	Debilitated
	Alcoholic
	Immobile
	Cough suppressant medications
	Respiratory depressant medications
		Client complains of dyspnea; tachycardia; increasing temperature; productive cough, and increasing amount of sputum becoming tenacious, rusty or purulent
		Tactile fremitus
		Dullness to percussion
		Bronchial breath sounds
		Increased crackles or rhonchi
		Voice sounds present
		    Bronchophony
		        Egophony
		            Whispered pectoriloquy
		ABGs: decreased PaO_2

Pulmonary embolism: foreign object has migrated to branch of pulmonary artery *Potential onset:* Seventh to tenth day *Massive embolism:* Pulmonary hypertension, dyspnea, right heart failure, shock, ABGs: decreased PaO_2, increased $PaCO_2$	Superficial vein thrombosis: rare Deep vein thrombosis: 40–60% Air emboli: intraperitoneal surgery Fat emboli: long bone fracture, split sternum	Only 10% recognized clinically Pain sharp and stabbing, occurs with breathing, localized (right lower lobe most frequent) Marked shortness of breath Increased heart rate—tachycardia Restlessness and other symptoms of hypoxia (severe anxiety)
Pulmonary infarction: necrosis of lung tissue due to occlusion of blood supply (less than 10% develop) *Potential onset:* * 2–72 hours after arterial obstruction	Pulmonary embolism	Hemoptysis Cough Fever 101–102°F Pleural friction rub Pleuritic pain

Atelectasis

Definition: Collapse of pulmonary alveoli caused by mucus plug or inadequate ventilation.

Assessment

✦ A. Assess for clinical manifestations that usually develop 24–48 hours postoperatively. (Most common cause of early postoperative temperature increase.)

B. Assess respiratory symptoms.
   1. Observe for asymmetrical chest movement.
   2. Auscultate lung sounds. Decreased or absent breath sounds over affected area; crackles; bronchial breathing over affected area.

Prevention	Intervention	Drug Therapy

Preoperative: Have client practice turning, coughing, and deep-breathing
Discuss importance of exercises
Postoperative clients at risk:
  Turn every 30 minutes
  Deep-breathe and cough
Other clients:
  Initiate turning and deep-breathing exercises every 1–2 hours
Ambulate as soon as possible
Medicate to reduce pain, splinting and resistance to treatment
	Deep-breathing and incentive spirometry
	Administer supplemental oxygen as ordered
	Monitor response to treatment
	Monitor for onset of pneumonia
	If entire lobe of lung is involved, prepare for bronchoscopy to remove plug
	Change position q2h
		Analgesics: pain control
		Bronchodilators (nebulized through IPPB); liquefy secretions
		Water or saline (nebulized through IPPB): liquefy secretions

Provide vigorous treatment for atelectasis Prevent aspiration Ambulate as soon as possible	Turn, cough and deep-breathe every 1 hour May need to stimulate cough with nasotracheal suctioning Send sputum for culture and sensitivity Frequent mouth care for comfort Administer oxygen as ordered Increase fluid intake Monitor for response to treatment	Antibiotics: Cephalosporin or ampicillin prophylactically for 48 hours for high-risk clients Cephalosporin IV or parenteral for infections Antipyretics: decrease temperature
Provide range of motion Encourage early ambulation Prevent thrombophlebitis Do not massage an area with potential for or suspected thrombus Elastic stockings or leg compression devices	Administer oxygen to relieve hypoxia Reduce anxiety Position client on left side with head dependent to prevent air embolus Prevent recurrent embolization; prepare for fibrinolysis; prepare for anticoagulation Prepare for x-ray, angiography, and/or ventilation/perfusion scan Encourage adequate hydration	Anticoagulation therapy: IV heparin to maintain therapeutic APTT Sodium prophylactically for high-risk clients Urokinase, t-PA, streptokinase: thrombolytic effect (24 hours) Analgesics: pleuritic pain control
Prevent thromboembolic pulmonary artery occlusion *See* prevention of thrombophlebitis	Describe indicative findings to physician Institute relaxation techniques to decrease client's anxiety Administer oxygen Support and comfort client	Antibiotics: prevention of infection

Continues

◆ **Table 8-18. POSTOPERATIVE COMPLICATIONS** *(Continued)*

Potential Complication	Clients at Risk	Indicative Findings

Thrombophlebitis: inflammation of vein with clot formation
 	
Potential onset:
Seventh to fourteenth day
	Abnormal vein walls:
	Varicose veins
	Previous thrombophlebitis
	Trauma to vein wall
	Tight strap on operating room table
	Surgery on hips or in pelvis
	Age over 60 years (arteriosclerosis)
	
	Venous stasis:
	Immobility, long-duration surgery
	Casts, restrictive dressings
	Constant Fowler's position
	Prolonged dependent lower
	  extremities
	Knee gatch elevated
	Pillows under knees, calves
	Obesity
	Abdominal distention
	Shock
	Heart failure
	
	Hypercoagulability:
	Surgical stress response
	Anesthesia
	Decreased circulation
	Hypovolemia, dehydration
	Malignant neoplasms
	Postpartum
	Oral contraceptives
	Insert rectal tube
		Superficial vein thrombophlebitis:
		Pain, redness, tenderness, and
		  induration along course of vein
		Palpable "cord" corresponding to course
		  of vein
		History of trauma including IV site
		
		Deep small-vein thrombophlebitis:
		Increased muscle turgor and
		  tenderness over affected vein
		Deep muscle tenderness
		Most frequent site: vessels at calf
		Affected limb warm to touch with
		  occasional swelling
		Client complains of tightness or
		  stiffness in affected leg
		Positive Homan's sign (dorsiflexion
		  of foot leads to calf pain)
		Fever rarely more than 101°F
		
		Major deep vein thrombophlebitis:
		No superficial signs of inflammation
		Homan's sign unreliable
		
		Femoral vein thrombosis:
		Pain and tenderness in distal thigh
		  and popliteal region
		Swelling extends to level of knee

Ileus: failure of peristalsis
 	
Potential onset:
First 24–36 hours
	All surgical clients
	Stress response to surgical trauma
		No bowel sounds or fewer than
		  5/min (normal: 5–35 clicks or
		  gurgles/min)
		Vomiting
		Abdominal distention

Paralytic ileus: paralysis of intestinal peristalsis *Potential onset:* First 3–4 days	Intraperitoneal surgery Peritonitis Kidney surgery Decreased cardiac output Pneumonia Electrolyte imbalance Wound infection	No bowel sounds Abdominal distention No passage of flatus or feces Nasogastric drainage green to yellow, 1–2 L in 24 hours Anorexia, nausea Complaints of fullness and diffuse pain

Intestinal obstruction: adhesions, trap or kink in segment of intestine
Potential onset:
Third to fifth day
The lower the obstruction, the
  more gradual the onset
	Abdominal surgery	No postoperative bowel movement
		Abdominal distention
		Client complains of periodic sharp,
		  colicky pains
		Hyperactive, high-pitched, tinkling
		  bowel sounds
		Abdominal tenderness
		Nasogastric drainage: dark brown or black

Prevention	Intervention	Drug Therapy
Avoid injury to vein wall: Use care when strapping to operating room table Avoid IVs in lower extremities Pad siderails for restless, convulsive, and/or combative client Avoid restraints *Avoid venous stasis:* Encourage early ambulation Provide feet and leg exercises Elastic stockings; sequential-compression devices Increase frequency of exercise for client at risk Prevent client's sitting with legs in dependent position Place pillow between legs while client is lying on side to prevent pressure from upper leg on lower Provide deep-breathing exercises Provide active and passive range of motion Increase velocity of blood flow: No standing Steady IV flow Antiembolic stockings (controversial) Decrease hypercoagulability: Provide adequate hydration Prevent infections Maintain circulation Decrease stress/anxiety	*Superficial vein thrombophlebitis:* Treat symptoms Continue ambulation unless accompanied by deep venous involvement Monitor for progression toward saphenafemoral junction (may need ligation) *Deep vein thrombophlebitis:* Provide adequate bedrest Elastic stockings Sequential-compression devices Elevate foot of bed with 6- to 8-inch blocks Administer warm moist compresses to relieve venospasm and help resolve inflammation Monitor for pulmonary embolism	Streptokinase: thrombolytic effect (24 hours) Heparin IV or sub q: decrease clotting time (short-term) Nonorthopedic surgery—low-dose sub q heparin (or low-molecular-weight heparin) Coumadin PO: decrease clotting time (long-term) Analgesics: pain control Low-molecular-weight dextran IV on operative day and 2 days postoperative Aspirin 1.2 g/day in divided doses
Do not feed until bowel sounds return Offer only sips of water until return of bowel sounds Maintain normal serum potassium level	Monitor for return of normal bowel sounds (enteral feeding following non-GI surgeries will resolve ileus faster) Monitor for distention Monitor for passage of flatus signaling return of peristalsis Monitor signs of hypokalemia	Switch to nonopioid analgesic (opioids slow GI motility), NSAIDs and acetaminophen
Maintain electrolyte balance, especially potassium Maintain cardiac output Prevent pneumonia Provide early ambulation	Treat cause Maintain nasogastric suction until peristalsis returns Monitor for intestinal obstruction	Potassium chloride if serum level is low Dexpanthenol (Ilopan) to stimulate return of peristalsis, total parenteral nutrition (TPN) if indicated
None	Identify condition early Report to physician immediately Reduce client anxiety Maintain patent nasogastric tube Prepare for insertion of intestinal tube Prepare for surgery if necessary	Antibiotic therapy: for prevention of infection (optional) Analgesics: pain control Never give laxative or purgative if obstruction is suspected

Continues

✦ Table 8-18. POSTOPERATIVE COMPLICATIONS (Continued)

Potential Complication	Clients at Risk	Indicative Findings
Urinary tract infection *Potential onset:* Third to fifth day or 48 hours after removal of catheter	*Decreased resistance:* History of bladder distention History of urinary retention Previous urinary tract infection History of prostatic hypertrophy History of catheterization Diabetic Debilitated Immobile	Dysuria Frequency Urgency High fever: up to 104°F with fewer systemic toxic symptoms than would be expected Change in urine odor Pus in urine Sediment May be asymptomatic
Wound infection *Potential onset:* Streptococcal: 24–48 hours after contamination *Staphylococcus* gram-negative rods, etc.: 5–7 days postoperatively	*Slow to heal:* Obese Diabetic *Poor nutrition:* Debilitated Elderly Ulcerative colitis *Poor circulation:* Elderly Hypovolemic Heart failure *Lack of oxygen to wound:* Vasoconstriction Severe anemia Depressed immunity Cancer Renal failure Preoperative steroid therapy Prolonged complex surgery (stress response leading to increased ACTH) Malnutrition Elderly At risk for transmission Proximity of another client with infection Transmission by hands of personnel	Initial inflammation: 36–48 hours Wound tender, swollen, warm, increased redness Increasing heart rate Increasing temperature (100.4°F or more) Increasing or recurring serous drainage; drainage becomes purulent, foul odor There may be no local signs if infection is deep Elevated WBC Malaise

3. Evaluate shortness of breath.
4. Assess for painful respirations; splinting of diaphragm.

✦ C. Assess for increased vital signs: temperature (fever to 102°F), respiration, pulse (tachycardia).

D. Observe for anxiety and restlessness.

E. ABGs: decreased PaO_2.

✦ Implementation

A. Administer O_2 as ordered.

B. Encourage sustained inspiration exercises.

C. Instruct in proper cough technique (splint incision).

D. Turn frequently (every 2 hours) and position to facilitate expectoration.

E. Do clapping, percussion, vibration, if ordered.

F. Do postural drainage every 4 hours.

G. Administer expectorants and other medications, as ordered.

H. Suction as necessary.

I. Encourage oral fluid intake to reduce tenacious sputum and to facilitate expectoration.

J. Place client in cool room with mist mask or vaporized steam.

K. Mobilize client as soon as possible.

L. Medicate for pain to allow for respiratory ventilation.

Prevention	Intervention	Drug Therapy
Maintain sterile technique with catheterization and catheter removal Provide competent indwelling catheter care Encourage early ambulation to decrease retention and stasis	Encourage fluid intake; cranberry juice to decrease urine pH Increase activity to enhance bladder emptying Encourage voiding every 2 hours while awake Send specimen for culture and sensitivity Monitor for residual urine of more than 100 mL	Urinary antiseptics (sulfonamides); bacterial suppression Antibiotics (ampicillin, tetracycline); bacterial suppression Anticholinergics: antispasmodic Topical urinary analgesic: pain relief
Practice meticulous hand hygiene and gloving Practice aseptic technique in wound care Separate from infected clients Use special caution for a new wound, easily contaminated Maintain nutrition Provide frequent turning Ambulate as soon as possible Maintain PaO$_2$ Increase attention to prevention for clients with depressed immunity Operative site: clip excess hair and cleanse with povidone-iodine (reduces bacterial counts)	Maintain nutrition Maintain oxygenation Maintain circulation and blood volume Maintain pulmonary toilet Cleanse wound or irrigate as ordered Apply wet-to-moist dressings Monitor for systemic response to infection, fever, malaise, headache, anorexia, nausea Treat symptoms	Administer antibiotics as ordered New cyanoacrylate adhesives (Dermabond, Indermil) close wounds and promote healing Send wound drainage specimen for culture and sensitivity

Deep Vein Thrombophlebitis

See page 233.

Pulmonary Embolism

Definition: The movement of a thrombus from site of origin to lung.

Assessment

✦ A. Assess for mild condition (involves smaller arteries).
   1. Signs mimic pleurisy or bronchial pneumonia.
   2. Transient dyspnea.
   3. Mild pleuritic pain.
   4. Tachycardia.
   5. Increased temperature.
   6. Cough with hemoptysis.
✦ B. Assess for severe condition (involves pulmonary artery).
   1. Chest pain.
   2. Severe dyspnea leading to air hunger.
   3. Shallow, rapid breathing.
   4. Sharp substernal chest pain.
   5. Vertigo leading to syncope.
   6. Hypovolemia.
   7. Cardiac arrhythmias.
   8. Generalized weakness.

9. Feelings of doom—severe anxiety.
10. Hypotension.

Implementation

✦ A. Prevention.
1. Ambulatory as soon as possible after surgery.
2. Range-of-motion exercises.
3. Pneumonic compression boots.
✦ B. Maintain patent airway.
1. Place in semi- to high-Fowler's position if vital signs allow.
2. Administer oxygen as needed (nasal cannula).
3. Assist with intubation as needed.
4. Auscultate breath sounds every 1–2 hours.
5. Obtain arterial blood gases to ascertain acid–base imbalance and/or pulse oximetry to monitor SaO_2 level.
6. Turn as directed by physician; do not do percussion or clapping or administer back rubs.
7. Encourage client to cough and deep-breathe every 1–2 hours.
✦ C. Administer medications as ordered.
1. Administer anticoagulants (check lab values each day before administering medication, following initial anticoagulation).
   a. Heparin: 5000–15,000 units IV bolus, then continuous infusion of 1000 units every hour to maintain therapeutic APTT.
   b. Long-term: warfarin 5–10 mg daily.
2. Give narcotics for pain (watch for respiratory depression).
3. Administer diuretics or cardiotonics, as necessary.
4. Thrombolytic therapy for acute right ventricular failure or refractory hypoxemia.
   a. Immediate dissolution of embolus, but danger of bleeding.
   b. Usual medications: urokinase, t-PA, streptokinase.
✦ D. Take vital signs every 2–4 hours.
✦ E. Maintain bedrest; have client avoid sudden movements.
✦ F. Observe for signs of shock.
✦ G. Observe for possible extension of emboli or for occurrence of other emboli.
1. Check urine for hematuria or oliguria.
2. Check legs, especially calf.
3. Check sputum for blood.
H. Prepare for surgical intervention when client is not responsive to heparin therapy.
1. Surgical intervention carries high risk.
2. Types of surgery.
   a. Femoral vein ligation.
   b. Ligation of inferior vena cava.
   c. Pulmonary embolectomy.

Fat Embolism Syndrome (FES)

Definition: Release of medullary fat droplets into bloodstream following trauma.

Characteristics

✦ A. Embolism occurs after long bone or sternum fractures (particularly from mishandling of client or incorrect splinting of fracture).
1. Fat droplets that are released from the marrow enter the venous circulation and usually become lodged in the lungs.
2. If the fat droplets become lodged in the brain, the embolism is severe and usually fatal.
3. Usually occurs within first 24 hours following injury.
B. Major cause of death from fractures.
C. Prevent by adequate splinting at accident scene and careful handling of fractured extremity.

Assessment

✦ A. Assess for classical sign (occurs 50–60 percent): petechiae from fat globule deposits across chest, shoulders and axilla. Petechiae do not blanch, but fade out within hours. Can involve conjunctiva.
✦ B. Evaluate related pulmonary signs: shortness of breath, leading to pallor, cyanosis and hypoxemia.
C. Evaluate related brain involvement.
1. Restlessness (may be first symptom—occurs within 24 to 72 hours), memory loss, confusion.
2. Headache, hemiparesis.
D. Observe for related cardiac involvement.
1. Tachycardia.
2. Right ventricular failure.
3. Decreased cardiac output.
E. Assess for other signs and symptoms.
1. Diaphoresis.
2. Change in level of consciousness.
3. Shock.
4. Increased temperature (if involvement of hypothalamus).
F. Presence of unexplained fever, petechiae, and change in mental status; be alert for possibility of FES.

Implementation

✦ A. Preventive measures important: immobilization of fracture with minimal manipulation.
✦ B. Maintain oxygenation.
1. Position client in high-Fowler's position to allow for respiratory exchange. Maintain bedrest.
2. Administer oxygen to decrease anoxia and to reduce surface tension of fat globules (IPPB may be needed).

C. Obtain arterial blood gases to maintain sufficient PO$_2$ levels.

D. Physician may intubate and place on respirator if respirations are severely compromised.

E. Institute preventive treatment to avoid further complications, such as shock and heart failure.

F. Monitor administration of medications.
1. Cortisone therapy to reduce inflammation.
2. Restoration of blood volume.

Adult Respiratory Distress Syndrome (ARDS)

Characteristics

✦ A. A medical emergency that may have many causes.
1. Can be secondary to bacterial or viral pneumonia.
2. Massive trauma and hemorrhagic shock.
3. Fat emboli.
4. Sepsis.

✦ B. Pathophysiology—damage to pulmonary capillary membrane that produces a leak, diffuse interstitial edema, and intra-alveolar hemorrhage.
1. Decrease in surfactant.
2. Intrapulmonary shunting with decreased oxygen saturation—hypoxia.
3. Decreased lung compliance.

C. Multiple organ system failure.

Assessment

✦ A. Assess for clinical manifestations. Usually seen within first 24 hours following shock or injury.

✦ B. Observe for extreme dyspnea, tachypnea, and cyanosis.

✦ C. Assess for pulmonary edema.

D. Auscultate lungs for atelectasis (many small emboli throughout lungs).

E. Evaluate blood gas alterations.
1. PO$_2$ decreased.
2. PCO$_2$ normal or decreased due to tachypnea.
3. pH normal to slightly alkalotic.

Implementation

✦ A. Prevent overhydration in severe trauma cases.

✦ B. Provide early treatment of severe hypoxemia (can be life-threatening).

C. Keep clients "dry," as they have excess fluids in their lungs. (Restrict fluid intake.)

✦ D. Administer medications.
1. Corticosteroids to reduce inflammation and to prevent further capillary membrane deterioration.
2. Diuretics to decrease fluid overload.
3. Sedatives to prevent client from resisting respirator.

4. Heparin to reduce platelet aggregation.
5. Antibiotics guided by Gram stains of sputum.

✦ E. Maintain adequate ventilation and oxygenation.
1. Provide intubation and mechanical ventilation with volume respirator.
2. Obtain frequent arterial blood gases.
3. Suction frequently with "bagging." Ambu bag increases alveolar expansion.
4. Prone position improves oxygenation.

F. Provide tracheostomy care, if appropriate, every 4 hours.

G. Provide oral hygiene every 4 hours.

H. Prevent further complications, such as shock and septicemia.

I. Provide adequate nutrition.

Wound Infections

See also Chapter 6, Infection Control.

Characteristics

A. Usual causative agents.
1. *Staphylococcus.*
2. *Pseudomonas aeruginosa.*
3. *Proteus vulgaris.*
4. *Escherichia coli.*

B. Usually occur within 5–7 days of surgery.

✦ Assessment

A. Observe for slowly increasing temperature (greater than 100.4°F), tachycardia, chills, and malaise.

B. Evaluate pain and tenderness surrounding surgical site.

C. Observe for edema and erythema surrounding suture site.

D. Feel for increased warmth around suture site.

E. Observe for purulent drainage.
1. Yellow if *Staphylococcus.*
2. Green if *Pseudomonas.*

F. Elevated white blood count.

Implementation

✦ A. Use meticulous hand hygiene and gloving techniques.

✦ B. Take cultures before starting medication; administer specific antibiotics for causative agent.

C. Irrigate wound with solution as ordered (usually normal saline).

D. Keep dressing and skin area dry to prevent skin excoriation and spread of bacteria.

E. Observe standard precautions. CDC is still recommending sterile technique in changing dressings (wet-to-moist).

F. If excoriation occurs, use karaya powder and drainage bags around area of wound.

CLIENTS AT RISK FOR POSTOPERATIVE INFECTION

Uncontrolled diabetes
Renal failure
Obesity
Receiving corticosteroids
Receiving immunosuppressive agents
Prolonged antibiotic therapy
Poor nutrition—protein and/or ascorbic acid deficiencies
Marked dehydration and hypovolemia
Decreased cardiac output
Edema and fluid and electrolyte imbalances
Anemia
Preoperative infection

Note: See also Chapter 6, Infection Control.

Wound Dehiscence and Evisceration

✦ *Definition: Dehiscence* is the splitting open of wound edges. *Evisceration* is the extensive loss of pinkish fluid (purulent if infection is present) through a wound and the protrusion of a loop of bowel through an open wound. Client feels like "everything is pulling apart."

Assessment

A. Observe for usual causes.
  1. General debilitation.
    a. Poor nutrition.
    b. Chronic illness.
    c. Obesity.
  2. Inadequate wound closure.
  3. Wound infection.
  4. Severe abdominal stretching (by coughing or vomiting).
  5. Immunosuppression.
B. Evaluate wound daily. Condition occurs about seventh postoperative day.
C. Assess for sensation of "giving" at the incision, pain, and saturated dressing with clear, pink drainage.
✦ D. Protrusion of viscera through wound edges (evisceration).

Implementation

A. Wound dehiscence.
  1. Apply butterfly tapes to incision area.
  2. Increase protein in diet.
  3. Observe for signs of infection and treat accordingly.
  4. Apply abdominal binder when ambulating.
  5. Keep client on bedrest.
✦ B. Evisceration.
  1. Lay client in supine or low-Fowler's position.

2. Cover protruding intestine with moist, sterile, normal saline packs; change packs frequently to keep moist.
3. Notify physician.
4. Take vital signs for baseline data and detection of shock.
5. Notify operating room for wound closure.
6. Provide patent IV.
7. Keep client NPO; place NG tube if ordered.

Disseminated Intravascular Coagulation (DIC)

✦ *Definition:* Simultaneous activation of the thrombin (clotting) and fibrinolytic system.

Characteristics

✦ A. Excessive intravascular thrombin is produced, which converts fibrinogen to fibrin clot.
  1. After fibrinogen is depleted, circulating thrombin continues to be present and will continue to convert any form of fibrinogen to fibrin.
  2. Fibrinogen enters system by transfusion or by body production of fibrinogen. This process intensifies the hemorrhagic state.
B. DIC is associated with extracorporeal circulation seen in obstetric complications and disseminated cancer.
C. Major defect is widespread microvascular thrombosis.

Assessment

✦ A. Observe for excessive bleeding (caused by depletion of clotting factors) through genitourinary tract, following injections, etc.
B. Evaluate lab results for low hemoglobin, low platelets.
C. Evaluate arterial blood gases for acidosis.
D. Observe for skin lesions, such as petechiae, purpura, subcutaneous hematomas.

Implementation

✦ A. Treat cause of DIC symptomatically.
  1. Antibiotics for infections.
  2. Fluids and colloids for shock.
  3. Steroids for endotoxins.
  4. Dialysis for renal failure.
B. Administer heparin IV to stop cycle of thrombosis—hemorrhage. Usage is controversial because it often promotes bleeding; used in combination with fluid replacement therapy.
  1. Neutralizes free circulating thrombin.
  2. Inhibits blood clotting in vivo, due to effect on factor IX.
  3. Prevents extension of thrombi.
  4. Keep clotting time two to three times normal.
  5. Give 10,000–20,000 units every 2–4 hours.

✦ C. Give transfusion of platelets, cryoprecipitate, and fresh frozen plasma to replace clotting factors.
  1. Monitor blood transfusion carefully.
  2. Be alert for fluid overload—increasing CVP; slow, bounding pulse.
D. Administer oxygen as needed.
E. Take precautions to prevent additional hemorrhage.
  1. Avoid chest tube "milking."
  2. Take temperature orally or axillary, not rectally.
  3. Avoid administration of parenteral medications if possible.
  4. Avoid trauma to mucous membranes.
  5. If nasogastric tube inserted, prevent bleeding by administering antacids and keeping NG tube connected to low suction. Do not irrigate unless absolutely necessary.

FLUID REPLACEMENT THERAPY

Fluid Replacement Solutions

✦ A. Types of IV solutions.
  ✦ 1. Hypertonic solution—a solution with higher osmotic pressure than blood serum.
    a. Cell placed in solution will crenate.
    b. Used in severe salt depletion, very rare.
    c. Used in intracranial pressure therapy—reduces edema by rapid movement of fluid out of ventricles into bloodstream.
    d. Used as a nutrient source (10% D).
    e. Common types of solution: normal saline, dextrose 10% in saline, dextrose 10% in water, and dextrose 5% in saline.
    f. Should not be administered faster than 200 mL/hr.
  ✦ 2. Hypotonic solution—a solution with less osmotic pressure than blood serum.
    a. Causes cells to expand or increase in size.
    b. Used to correct diarrhea and dehydration.
    c. Common types of solution: dextrose 5% in half-strength (0.45%) NS; dextrose 5%; one-third strength (0.33%) NS; and dextrose 5% in water.
    d. Should not be administered faster than 400 mL/hr.
  ✦ 3. Isotonic solution—a solution with the same osmotic pressure as blood serum.
    a. Cells remain unchanged.
    b. Used for replacement or maintenance (expands extracellular volume); especially used to expand circulating intravascular volume.
    c. Common type of solution: lactated Ringer's solution; 5% dextrose in NS, 5% D in water.

✦ B. Choice of fluid replacement solution—depends on client's needs.
  1. Fluid and electrolyte replacement only.
    a. Saline solution.
    b. Lactated Ringer's solution.
  2. Calorie replacement—dextrose solutions.
  3. Restriction of dietary intake, such as low sodium.
  4. IV medications that are insoluble in certain IV fluids.
  5. Rate of administration of IV solution to correct fluid imbalance.
  6. Dextrose plays no part in tonicity. It is metabolized off.
C. Purpose of fluid and electrolyte therapy.
  1. To replace previous losses.
  2. To provide maintenance requirements.
  3. To meet current losses.

Implementation

A. Check circulation of immobilized extremity.
B. Check label of solution against physician's order.
C. Check rate of infusion.
D. Observe vein site for signs of swelling.
E. Take vital signs at least every 15 minutes for replacement fluid administration.

✦ **Intravenous Calorie Calculation**

A. 1000 mL D_5W provides 50 g of dextrose.
B. 50 g of dextrose provides 4 calories per gram (actually 3.4 calories).
C. 1000 mL D_5W provides 200 calories.
D. Usual IV total/day is 2000–3000 mL (400–600 calories/day).

✦ **Intravenous Regulation**

✦ A. Calculation of drip factor.
  1. Microdrip—60 gtt/mL fluid.
  2. Adult drop factor usually depends on administration set—10 to 20 gtt/mL fluid.
✦ B. General formula.

$$\text{Drops/min} = \frac{\text{Total volume infused} \times \text{drops/mL}}{\text{Total time for infusing in minutes}}$$

Example: Ordered 1000 mL D_5W administered over 8-hour period of time.
  1. With microdrip, it is easy to remember that the number of drops per minute equals the number of milliliters to be administered per hour.

Example: $\dfrac{1000}{8} = 125$ mL/hr

Using formula: (8×60) $\dfrac{1000 \times 60}{480} = \dfrac{60,000}{480} = \dfrac{125}{\text{gtt/min}}$

2. With administration set that delivers 10 gtt/min.

$$\frac{1000 \times 10}{480} = \frac{10,000}{480} = 20.8 \text{ or } 21 \text{ gtt/min}$$

3. With administration set that delivers 15 gtt/min.

$$\frac{1000 \times 15}{480} = \frac{15,000}{480} = 31 \text{ gtt/min}$$

✦ C. Calculation of medication as dose per hour.

Example: Add 20,000 units heparin to 500 mL D$_5$W. Give 1000 units/hr, using a 20 gtt/mL set.

$$\frac{1000 \text{ units}}{60} \times \frac{500 \text{ mL}}{20,000 \text{ units}} \times \frac{20 \text{ gtt/mL}}{1}$$

$$\frac{\overset{25}{\underset{3}{\cancel{\underset{\cancel{60}}{\cancel{1000}}}}}}{} \times \frac{\overset{1}{\cancel{500}}}{\underset{40}{\underset{2}{\cancel{20,000}}}} \times \frac{\overset{1}{\cancel{20}}}{1} = \frac{25}{3} = 8 \text{ gtt/min}$$

✦ D. Calculation of medication as dose per minute.

Example: Add 2 g lidocaine to 500 mL D$_5$W. Give 2 mg/min, using a 60 gtt/mL set.

$$\frac{2 \text{ mg}}{1} \times \frac{500 \text{ mL}}{2 \text{ g}} \times \frac{60 \text{ gtt/mL}}{1}$$

$$\frac{\overset{1}{\cancel{2}}}{1} \times \frac{\overset{1}{\cancel{500}}}{\underset{4}{\underset{2}{\cancel{2000}}}} \times \frac{\overset{30}{\cancel{60}}}{1} = 30 \text{ gtt/min}$$

PERIOPERATIVE CARE REVIEW QUESTIONS

1. Evaluating the effectiveness of preoperative teaching before colostomy surgery, the nurse expects that the client will be able to

   1. Describe how the procedure will be done.
   2. Exhibit acceptance of the surgery.
   3. Explain the function of the colostomy.
   4. Apply the colostomy bag correctly.

2. The nurse understands that it is important to obtain baseline vital signs for her client preoperatively to

   1. Establish a baseline postoperatively.
   2. Inform the anesthetist so he can administer appropriate preanesthesia medication.
   3. Judge the client's recovery from the effects of surgery and anesthesia when taking postoperative vital signs.
   4. Prevent operative hypotension.

3. The physician tells a client that he will need exploratory surgery the next day. As the nurse determines the preoperative teaching plan, which one of the following interventions is most important?

   1. Answer questions the client has about his condition or the forthcoming surgery.
   2. Explain the routine preoperative procedures: NPO, shower, medication, shave, etc.
   3. Describe the surgery and what the client will experience following surgery.
   4. Assure the client there is nothing to worry about because the physician is very experienced.

4. Before a client goes to surgery, it is necessary to sign an operative permit. The most appropriate sequence for signing the permit is to

   1. Have the client sign the permit as soon as he is admitted, so he will know what surgery he will be having.
   2. Prepare the client for surgery, give the preoperative narcotics, and have him sign the permit before he goes to sleep.
   3. Ensure that the surgeon has explained the surgery to the client, answer his questions, have him sign the permit, and then complete the final preparations for surgery.

   4. Have the client sign the operative permit and then notify the physician that the permit has been signed.

5. While the nurse is orienting a client scheduled for surgery in the morning, the client states that she is afraid of what will happen the next day. The most appropriate response is to

   1. Assure her that the surgery is very safe and problems are rare.
   2. Let her talk about her fears as much as she wishes.
   3. Explain that she has an excellent doctor and she has nothing to worry about.
   4. Explain that worrying or anxiety has been proven to prolong hospitalization.

6. A client scheduled for surgery is given a spinal anesthetic. Immediately following the injection, the nurse will position the client

   1. On his abdomen.
   2. In semi-Fowler's position.
   3. In slight Trendelenburg position.
   4. On his back or side, with head raised.

7. Following spinal anesthesia, a client is brought into the postanesthesia unit. The assessment data that indicate a complication of anesthesia has developed include

   1. Hiccoughs.
   2. Numbness in legs.
   3. Headache.
   4. No urge to void.

8. A client has just arrived at the postanesthesia unit from surgery. The priority assessment is to

   1. Assess the client's need for oxygen.
   2. Check the gag reflex.
   3. Assess vital signs.
   4. Assess airway for patency.

9. Assessing a postoperative client who has developed unresolved atelectasis, the priority assessment will be

   1. Hemorrhage.
   2. Infection.
   3. Pneumonia.
   4. Pulmonary embolism.

10. Following surgery, the client's surgeon orders a Foley catheter to be inserted. Which one of the following interventions would the nurse carry out first?

    1. Clean the perineum from front to back.
    2. Check the catheter for patency.
    3. Explain to the client that she will feel slight, temporary discomfort.
    4. Arrange the sterile items on the sterile field.

11. Following surgery for repair of an inguinal hernia, the nurse establishes a postoperative fluid intake goal for the client. The most appropriate amount would be _____ mL/day.

12. Following abdominal surgery, which clinical manifestation is indicative of negative nitrogen balance?

    1. Poor skin turgor from dehydration.
    2. Edema or ascites of the abdomen and flank.
    3. Pale color to skin.
    4. Diarrhea.

13. Hemorrhage is a major complication following oral surgery and radical neck dissection. If this condition occurs, the most immediate nursing intervention would be to

    1. Notify the surgeon immediately.
    2. Treat the client for shock.
    3. Put pressure over the common carotid and jugular vessels in the neck.
    4. Immediately put the client in high-Fowler's position.

14. A client has sustained multiple injuries and fractures in a motor vehicle accident (MVA). During which period would the nurse be most vigilant in assessing for the development of a fat embolism?

    1. During the first 24 to 48 hours after the MVA.
    2. 72 to 96 hours after the MVA.
    3. During the first week after the MVA.
    4. During the second week after the MVA.

15. Assessing the client following abdominal surgery, the nurse observes pinkish fluid and a loop of bowel through an opening in the incision. The first nursing action is to

    1. Notify the physician.
    2. Notify the operating room for wound closure.
    3. Cover the protruding bowel with a moist, sterile, normal saline dressing.
    4. Apply butterfly tapes to the incision area.

16. Following laminectomy surgery, the client returns from the recovery room to the surgical unit. The nurse would anticipate that the most common complication following anesthesia would be

    1. Atelectasis.
    2. Pneumonia.
    3. Paralytic ileus.
    4. Edema.

17. Following a missed abortion, a client has developed disseminated intravascular coagulation (DIC). The most critical nursing intervention for this client is to

    1. Administer ordered medications.
    2. Allay anxiety—provide emotional support.
    3. Administer oxygen at 6 L/min.
    4. Encourage fluid intake.

18. Following surgery for an abdominal hysterectomy, a 50-year-old client is unable to void. She was catheterized 8 hours ago in the recovery room and she is now complaining that she has the urge to void frequently but voids only a few mL of urine each time. The nurse will plan the next intervention based on the understanding that this symptom is most commonly associated with

    1. Bladder damage.
    2. Kidney infection.
    3. An inadequate intake of fluids.
    4. Retention of urine with overflow.

19. A client recently had outpatient surgery on his knee and has just been admitted to the ED with the following symptoms: marked shortness of breath, tachycardia, chest pain, and severe anxiety. The nurse will recognize that these symptoms must be reported immediately to the physician. The next intervention will be to prepare to administer

    1. Oxygen.
    2. Heparin.
    3. Urokinase.
    4. Coumadin.

20. Which of the following statements regarding postoperative nutrition is correct?

    1. Clients may have water on awakening from major surgical procedures.
    2. Clear liquid diets are provided for 2–3 days following minor surgical procedures.
    3. Soft diets are initiated the first postoperative day for major surgical conditions.
    4. Clear liquids are started after bowel sounds are assessed following major surgical procedures.

PERIOPERATIVE CARE

Answers with Rationale

1. (3) Successful teaching can be validated when the client is able to repeat the information. A description of the surgery is irrelevant and application of the bag will be done later. Acceptance of the surgery is an emotional issue.

   NP:E; CN:H; CL:C

2. (3) It is important to have presurgery vital signs so that the client's progress can be monitored to assure that his postoperative condition is stable. A baseline is completed presurgery for evaluation postsurgery.

   NP:A; CN:PH; CL:C

3. (1) It is most important to begin at the client's level of understanding, so answering questions is more essential than giving explanations until the client is ready to listen. Describing the surgery (3) is not the nurse's responsibility, and giving false reassurance by assuring the client there is nothing to worry about (4) is nontherapeutic.

   NP:P; CN:S; CL:A

4. (3) Informed consent by a client who is mentally competent is required to have an operative permit signed. This means the physician must talk to the client and the client must not be under the influence of narcotics. The operative permit does not have to be witnessed.

   NP:P; CN:S; CL:C

5. (2) Allowing the client to express her fears results in a decrease in anxiety and a more realistic and knowledgeable reaction to the situation. Answers (1) and (3) close off communication because they are false reassurance. Answer (4) may increase her anxiety.

   NP:I; CN:PS; CL:A

6. (3) Usually, the client is positioned on the back following the injection. If a high level of anesthesia is desired, the head and shoulders can be lowered to slight Trendelenburg position. After 20 minutes the anesthetic is set, and the client can be positioned in any manner.

   NP:I; CN:PH; CL:A

7. (3) When spinal fluid is lost through a leak or the client is dehydrated, a severe headache can occur, which may last several days. Numbness (2) and no urge to void (4) would be expected with spinal anesthesia unless it continues for several hours postop. The complication of hiccoughs (1) can be associated with abdominal surgery, but is not attributable to spinal anesthesia.

   NP:A; CN:PH; CL:A

8. (4) The priority assessment is to determine if the airway is patent. All of the other nursing actions will follow this assessment: need for oxygen (1), gag reflex (2), and vital signs (3).

   NP:A; CN:PH; CL:A

9. (3) Pneumonia is a major complication of unresolved atelectasis and must be treated along with vigorous treatment for atelectasis. Hemorrhage (1) and infection (2) are not related to this condition. Pulmonary embolism (4) could result from deep vein thrombosis.

   NP:A; CN:PH; CL:AN

10. (3) It is necessary to give the client an adequate explanation for any procedure. This will result in less anxiety and more cooperation from the client.

    NP:I; CN:PH; CL:A

11. The answer is 2000–3000 mL/day, maintenance level postsurgery. The client's body will require additional fluids over the minimum due to fluid loss and the recovery process after surgery. Minimum fluid intake is considered 1500 mL per day.

    NP:P; CN:PH; CL:C

Coding for Questions/Answers Abbreviations: **Nursing Process: NP,** Assessment: A, Analysis: AN, Planning: P, Implementation: I, Evaluation: E; **Client Needs: CN,** Safe, Effective Care Environment: S, Health Promotion and Maintenance: H, Psychosocial Integrity: PS, Physiological Integrity: PH; **Clinical Area: CA,** Medical Nursing: M, Surgical Nursing: S, Maternal/Newborn Nursing: MA, Pediatric Nursing: P, Psychiatric Nursing: PS; **Cognitive Level: CL,** Knowledge: K, Comprehension: C, Application: A, Analysis: AN.

12. (2) Edema is due to insufficient nitrogen for synthesis. When this occurs, it leads to a change in the body's osmotic pressure, resulting in oozing of fluids out of the vascular space. This phenomenon results in the formation of edema in the abdomen and flanks.

    NP:AN; CN:PH; CL:AN

13. (3) Putting pressure over the vessels in the neck may be life-saving because a severe blood loss can occur rapidly, leading to shock and death. The surgeon would be notified as soon as possible.

    NP:I; CN:PH; CL:A

14. (1) Approximately 85 percent of cases of fat embolism occur within 48 hours of injury, making this the most critical time for monitoring the client for manifestations of this complication.

    NP:P; CN:PH; CL:A

15. (3) The first nursing action, before notifying the physician (1), is to cover the open wound. Evisceration will eventually have to be closed in the operating room, but this is a later step. Butterfly tapes (4) would be applied to the wound area to prevent further dehiscence.

    NP:I; CN:PH; CL:A

16. (1) Even before pneumonia (2), atelectasis may occur as a result of the alveoli not being expanded. This leads to an alteration in gas exchange. Paralytic ileus (3) could result from any surgery, especially if the client ingests food before the bowel is functioning properly.

    NP:AN; CN:PH; CL:C

17. (1) In DIC, the client begins to hemorrhage after the initial hypercoagulability uses up the clotting factors in the blood. Administering heparin, therefore, is a critical nursing intervention. Heparin prevents clot formation and increases available fibrinogen, coagulation factors, and platelets. The other actions have lesser priority. Oxygen would be administered at 2 to 3 L/min.

    NP:P; CN:PH; CL:A

18. (4) Ten to 15 percent of postoperative clients who have undergone general anesthesia require urinary catheterization. Urinary retention must be treated immediately to prevent a urinary tract infection.

    NP:P; CN:PH; CL:AN

19. (3) The client's condition suggests pulmonary embolism (PE), which is not uncommon following orthopedic surgery on the knee. The physician will order urokinase delivered through a PICC to dissolve the clot (the primary goal in treating PE). Heparin (2) and Coumadin (4) (the oral form of warfarin) are anticoagulants and will only prevent further clots from forming. Oxygen (1) may well be ordered, but the critical intervention is the thrombolytic agent, which must be given within a few hours of the onset of the symptoms.

    NP:I; CN:PH; CL:AN

20. (4) Liquids are not started until bowel sounds have returned; if there is no motility in the bowel, blockage could result. Clear liquid diets are started as soon as bowel sounds return. Diet protocol following major surgery begins with clear liquid to full liquid to soft to regular diet as tolerated.

    NP:P; CN:PH; CL:C

Oncology Nursing

✦ The icon denotes content of special importance for NCLEX.

DETECTION AND PREVENTION OF CANCER

Cancer Incidence and Trends

A. Cancer—a definition.
   1. Term represents a group of more than 200 neoplastic diseases that involve all body organs.
   2. One or more cells lose their normal growth-controlling mechanism and continue to grow uncontrolled. They tend to invade surrounding tissue and to metastasize to distant body sites.

✦ B. Second leading cause of death in United States after heart disease.
   1. Ranks fourth for males and first for females as cause of death; second after accidents as cause of death for children.
   2. Greatest increase seen in lung cancer—consistent with smoking patterns.

C. Incidence rate.
   1. 1.2 million in United States are diagnosed with cancer every year. It is predicted that the incidence of cancer in the United States could double by the middle of the century, due to growth and aging of population.
   2. Number of cancer deaths increased by 11 percent during past 40 years.
   ✦ 3. Leading causes of cancer death are lungs, prostate, and colorectal for males; lungs, breast, and colorectal for females.

Identified Causes and Risk Factors

A. Multiplicity theory: multiple factors lead to the development of cancer; 60–90 percent thought to be related to environmental factors.

B. Carcinogens: agents known to increase susceptibility to cancer.
   1. Chemical carcinogens: asbestos, benzene, vinyl chloride, by-products of tobacco, arsenic, cadmium, nickel, radiation and mustard gas.
   2. Iatrogenic chemical agents: DES; chemotherapy; hormone treatment; immunosuppressive agents, radioisotopes, cytoxic drugs.
   3. Radiation carcinogens: x-rays; sunlight (ultraviolet light); nuclear radiation.
   4. Viral factors: herpes simplex; Epstein–Barr; hepatitis B and retroviruses.
   5. Genetic factors: hereditary or familial tendencies.
   6. Demographic and geographic factors.
   7. Dietary factors: obesity; high-fat diet; diets low in fiber; diets high in smoked or salted foods; preservatives and food additives; alcohol.
   8. Psychological factors: stress.
   9. Age.

Primary Prevention Measures

✦ A. Optimal dietary patterns and lifestyle changes.*
   1. Dietary factors are related to 50 percent of all environmental cancers.
   2. Avoid obesity (at 40 percent overweight, there is a 55 percent increased risk of cancer in females and 33 percent increased risk in males).
   3. Decrease fat intake of both saturated and unsaturated fats—maximum 30 percent of total calories.
   4. Increase total fiber in diet—decreases risk of colon cancer.
   5. Increase cruciferous vegetables (cabbage, broccoli, carrots, Brussels sprouts).
   6. Increase vitamin A—reduced incidence of larynx, esophagus, and lung cancers.
   7. Increase vitamin C—aids tumor encapsulation and promotes longer survival time.
   8. Increase vitamin E—inhibits growth of brain tumors, melanomas, and leukemias.
   9. Decrease alcohol consumption.
   10. Avoid salt—cured, smoked, or nitrate-cured foods.

   Core curriculum for Oncology Nursing.

✦ B. Minimize exposure to carcinogens.
   1. Avoid smoking—thought to be a cause of 75 percent of lung cancers in United States.
   2. Avoid oral tobacco—increases incidence of oral cancers.
   3. Avoid exposure to asbestos fibers and constant environmental dust.
   4. Avoid exposure to chemicals.
   5. Avoid radiation exposure and excessive exposure to sunlight.

C. Obtain adequate rest and exercise to decrease stress.
   1. Chronic stress associated with decreased immune system functioning.
   2. Strong immune system responsible for destruction of developing malignant cells.
   3. Participate in a regular exercise program.
   4. Get adequate rest (6–8 hours per night).
   5. Have a physical exam on a regular basis, including recommended diagnostic tests.

Secondary Prevention—Early Detection

A. Risk assessment (*see* Risk Factors).
B. Health history and physical assessment.
✦ C. Screening methods.
   1. Mammography, Pap test, prostate exam, prostate-specific antigen (PSA) blood test, etc.
   2. Self-care practices: breast self-examination (BSE) done every month; testicular self-examination (TSE) done every month; skin inspection.

THE SEVEN EARLY WARNING SIGNS OF CANCER

C **C**hange in bowel or bladder habits.
A **A**ny sore that does not heal.
U **U**nusual bleeding or discharge from any body orifice.
T **T**hickening or lump in breast or elsewhere.
I **I**ndigestion or difficulty swallowing.
O **O**bvious change in wart or mole.
N **N**agging cough or hoarseness.

---

3. Sigmoidoscopy for males and females 50 years and older.
4. Fecal occult blood test for males and females 40 years and older.

Characteristics

A. *Benign neoplasms:* usually encapsulated, remain localized, and are slow growing.
B. *Malignant neoplasms:* not encapsulated, will metastasize and grow, and exert negative effects on host. (*See* Table 9-1.)
C. Categories of malignant neoplasms.
   1. Carcinomas—grown from epithelial cells; usually solid tumors (skin, stomach, colon, breast, rectal).
   2. Sarcomas—arise from muscle, bone, fat, or connective tissue—may be solid.
   3. Lymphomas—arise from lymphoid tissue (infection-fighting organs).
   4. Leukemias and myelomas—grow from blood-forming organs.
D. Mechanisms of metastases.
   1. Transport of cancer cells occurs through the lymph system and either the cells reside in lymph nodes or pass between venous and lymphatic circulation.
      a. Tumors that begin in areas of the body that have extensive lymph circulation are at high risk for metastasis (breast tissue).
      b. The speed of metastasis is directly related to the vascularity of the tumor.
      c. Angiogenesis: cancer cells induce growth of new capillaries; thus cells can spread through this network.
      d. Hematogenous: cancer cells are disseminated through the bloodstream. The bloodstream may carry cells from one site to another (liver to bone).
   2. Direct spread of cancer cells (seeding) where there are no boundaries to stop the growth (e.g., ovary and stomach).
   3. Transplantation is the transfer of cells from one site to another.

Table 9-1. COMPARISON OF CHARACTERISTICS OF BENIGN AND MALIGNANT TUMORS

	Malignant	Benign
Cell type	Abnormal, more unlike parent cells	Close to those of original tissues
Growth	Variable and usually rapid; infiltrates surrounding tissues in all directions	Slow and noninfiltrating, expansive
Encapsulated	Rare	Usually
Metastasis	Frequent, through blood, lymph, or new tumor sites	Absent
Effect	Terminal without treatment	Can become malignant or obstruct vital organs
Differentiation	Poorly	Partially
Recurrence	Frequent	Rare
Vascularity	Moderate to marked	Slight

Diagnosis

A. Diagnostic studies will depend on suspected primary site.
B. Laboratory and radiologic tests often identify a problem first.
   1. Radiographic procedures (e.g., tomography, computed tomography [CT], contrast studies).
   2. Ultrasonography.
   3. Radioisotopic scanning studies (e.g., brain scan, gallium imaging).
   4. Magnetic resonance imaging (MRI).
   5. Biologic response markers (useful for diagnosing primary tumors).
   6. Positron emission tomography (PET).
      a. PET scans reveal cellular-level metabolic changes occurring in an organ or tissue. This is important and unique because disease processes often begin with functional changes at cellular level.
      b. PET scan can measure such vital functions as blood flow, oxygen use, and glucose metabolism, which helps doctors identify abnormal- from normal-functioning organs and tissues.
      c. Scan can also be used to evaluate the effectiveness of a treatment plan, allowing client's course of care to be adjusted if necessary.
C. Other laboratory tests.
   1. Enzyme tests, such as acid phosphatase.

2. Tumor marker: ID analysis of substances found in blood or body fluids.

Cancer Classification

Grading

A. Grading refers to classifying tumor cells—done by biopsy, cytology, or surgical excision. (*See* Table 9-2.)
   1. Tumor grade is one of many factors that doctors consider when they develop a treatment plan for a cancer client.
   2. Tumor grade refers to the degree of abnormality of cancer cells compared with normal cells.
B. Biopsy: definitive diagnosis of cancer.
   1. Excisional biopsy—removes all suspicious tissue. Used for small tumors < 2 cm.
   2. Incisional biopsy—removes a sample of tissue from a mass.
   3. Needle aspiration—aspiration of small amount of core tissue from a suspicious area.
   4. Exfoliative cytology—cells in tissue or secretions are evaluated by Pap method.
C. Tissue specimens are evaluated by frozen or permanent sections by a pathologist.
D. Results from biopsy and other diagnostic procedures (blood tests, x-ray studies, endoscopic procedures) will determine extent of disease staging.

Staging

✦ A. Staging describes the size of the tumor and extent or metastasis of a malignant tumor; also quantifies severity of disease.
✦ B. A useful system of staging for carcinomas is the TNM system.
   1. T: Primary tumor.
   2. N: Regional nodes.
   3. M: Metastasis.
C. The extent to which malignancy has increased in size
   1. Primary tumor (T).
      a. T_X: tumor cannot be assessed.
      b. T_0: no evidence of primary tumor.
      c. T_{IS}: carcinoma in situ.
      d. T_1, T_2, T_3, T_4: progressive increase in tumor size and involvement.
   2. Involvement of regional nodes (N).
      a. N_X: regional lymph nodes cannot be assessed clinically.
      b. N_0: regional lymph nodes not abnormal.

GRADING AND STAGING

It is important for physicians and clients to know cancer's grade and stage because both the extent to which the disease has progressed (stage) and its microscopic features (grade) are important factors in planning treatment and estimating a client's prognosis.

Table 9-2. GRADING TUMORS

The American Joint Commission on Cancer has recommended the following guidelines for grading tumors:

Grade	Differentiation	Dysplasia
GX	Cannot be assessed	
G1-Low	Well differentiated	Mild dysplasia, cells differ slightly from normal cells
G2-Intermediate	Moderately well differentiated	Moderate dysplasia, more abnormal
G3-High	Poorly differentiated	Severe dysplasia
G4-High	Undifferentiated	Anaplasia, cell of origin unable to be determined

Some cancers also have special grading systems. For example, the Gleason system to describe the degree of differentiation of prostate cancer cells uses scores ranging from Grade 2 to Grade 10. Lower Gleason scores describe well-differentiated, less aggressive tumors. Higher scores describe poorly differentiated, more aggressive tumors.

---

   c. N_1, N_2, N_3, N_4: increasing degree of abnormal regional lymph nodes.
   3. Metastatic development (M).
      a. M_X: not assessed.
      b. M_0: no evidence of distant metastasis.
      c. M_1 to M_4: increasing degree of distant metastasis.
D. Another method of staging is clinical staging of tumors.

TREATMENT METHODS

✦ A. Broad goals.
   1. Goal of therapy is to cure the client—eradicate the tumor.
   2. When cure is not possible, controlling or arresting the tumor growth becomes the goal—to prolong survival.
   3. Palliation or alleviation of symptoms.
✦ B. The gold standard for cancer treatment remains surgery, radiation therapy, chemotherapy, and combined approaches.
C. The newest weapon against cancer is adaptive immunotherapy (AIT).
   1. AIT uses principles of vaccine therapy.
      a. Cells from tumor tissue are cloned, treated in a lab, and injected back into the client for increased immune response.

Table 9-3. CLINICAL STAGING OF TUMORS	
Stage	**Treatment**
Stage 0 Cancer in situ—abnormal cells confined to lobule (LCIS) or duct (DCIS) lining. Considered a marker for increased risk of invasive cancer.	No treatment for LCIS but close monitoring of both breasts. Lumpectomy for DCIS and radiation.
Stage I Earlier stage of invasive breast cancer: tumor no larger than 2 cm and cancer cells have not spread. More than 70% with Stage I have no evidence of axillary node involvement.	Treated with lumpectomy followed by radiation or mastectomy with dissection of nodes. Alternative treatment is sentinel lymph node biopsy.
Stage II One of the following conditions is present: tumor no larger than 2 cm and has spread to axillary nodes; tumor is 2–5 cm with or without regional spread; tumor larger than 5 cm with negative axillary nodes.	Treatment similar to procedures above with one or more adjuvant therapies recommended.
Stage III This stage involves extensive local and regional spread to axillary nodes, chest wall, breast skin or substernal nodes.	Treated with chemotherapy before surgery to shrink tumor. After mastectomy, additional chemotherapy and radiation is given.
Stage IV Cancer has metastasized to distant organs, most often lungs, bones, liver or brain.	Therapy is systemic chemotherapy, hormonal or biological therapy; other treatments may be used to alleviate symptoms.

  b. Days after the vaccine is administered, lymph nodes are harvested so the T cells can replicate; these are then infused into the client.

  c. Method is currently in clinical trials; side effects minimal (as opposed to radiation and chemotherapy).

 2. With AIT, the biologic response modifier is the reactive T-cell solution; activated T cells in the body fight the tumor.

Surgery

✦ A. Useful as primary treatment for localized cancer (breast, colon, melanoma of skin, etc.).

 1. Highest rate of cure for localized disease.

 2. Disadvantage—deforming or debilitating to client.

✦ B. Types of treatment.

 1. Local excision: simple surgery with small margin of normal tissue surrounding tumor—used when tumor is small.

 2. En bloc dissection or wide excision; removal of tumor, nodes, tissues, and any contiguous structures.

 3. Video-assisted endoscopic surgery is replacing surgery with long incisions; surgery is done through 2 or 3 short incisions via a camera to remove tumor.

 4. Surgery on cancer in situ.

  a. Electrosurgery—application of electrical current to destroy cancerous cells.

  b. Cryosurgery—deep freezing with liquid nitrogen to cause cell destruction.

  c. Chemosurgery—applied chemotherapeutic agents layer by layer with surgical excision.

  d. CO_2 laser—use of laser for local excision.

C. Other forms of surgery.

 1. Prophylactic: removal of tissue or organs that may develop cancer.

 2. Cosmetic surgery: follows radical surgery.

  a. May be performed immediately following surgery, postsurgery, or in stages.

  b. Method is appropriate for breast, head, neck, and skin cancers.

D. Palliative surgery—promotes comfort and quality of life without cure.

Implementation

A. Preoperative care.

 1. Promote health status prior to surgery.

  a. Malnourished client is at risk for infection, delayed wound healing, and dehiscence.

  b. Mental status may impact surgery results.

 2. Provide emotional support prior to surgery.

  a. Encourage talking about fears and anxieties.

  b. Provide accurate information—clarify levels of knowledge.

    c. Assess family needs and provide information and support.

B. Postoperative care.
  1. Provide traditional postop care.
  2. Provide for physical comfort.
     a. Enteral feeding.
     b. Pain relief.
     c. Positioning and activity.
     d. Wound care and healing.
  3. Provide emotional support.
     a. Allow for grief process—encourage expression of fears.
     b. Discuss change in body image—support increase in self-esteem.
     c. Provide accurate information.
  4. Support rehabilitation process.
     a. Encourage family involvement.
     b. Make referrals to appropriate resources.
     c. Complete discharge planning.

Radiation Therapy

✦ *Definition:* Use of high energy moving through space or medium to interrupt cellular growth at a local level.
A. Indications.
  1. Used to treat solid tumors—ionizing radiation transfers energy to molecules present in cancer cell.
  2. Different tissues have different radiosensitivities—rapidly dividing tissues (testes, ovaries, lymphoid tissues, and bone marrow) are more sensitive.
✦ B. Types of ionizing radiation.
  1. Electromagnetic—radiation in wave form.
     a. X-rays—linear accelerators deposit maximum dose 5 cm or more below the skin.
     b. Electrons—delivered by machines.
     c. Gamma rays—delivered by machines that contain radioactive sources (cobalt-60, cesium-137) or radioactive substances (seeds, threads, or liquids).
  2. Particulate—radiation in the form of heavy particles.
     a. Beta particles—high speed electrons (phosphorus-32; strontium-90).
     b. Protons, neutrons, and alpha particles accelerate subatomic particles through the body tissue.
C. Newest option in radiation is intensity-modulated radiation therapy (IMRT).
  1. Delivers a high dose of radiation to the tumor, but spares vital, healthy tissue around it.
  2. Method targets large or small tumors; type of beam can mold to tumor shape.
  3. Therapy is administered by Peacock system.

    a. Conventional radiation delivers single, large beams of uniform intensity.
    b. IMRT bombards tumor with small beams of different intensity from all sides.
  4. Heralded as greatest breakthrough in cancer management in 25 years.

External Radiation

✦ A. Teletherapy—external source of radiation. (Machine is a distance from client.) Most common type of treatment.
B. Types.
  1. Natural radioactive source—gamma rays delivered via machine to lesion.
  2. Machine is the linear accelerator—high-voltage electric current delivers electrons to client.
✦ C. Side effects: fatigue—major systemic effect; headache; nausea and vomiting; skin irritation or injury; scaling, erythema; dryness.

Implementation

A. Offer psychological support and teaching.
  1. What to expect from treatment.
  2. Explanation of radiotherapy room.
  3. Possible side effects and ways to minimize them.
✦ B. Promote diet: high protein, high carbohydrate, fat free, and low residue.
  1. Foods to avoid: tough, fibrous meat; poultry; shrimp; all cheeses (except soft); coarse bread; raw vegetables; irritating spices.
  2. Foods allowed: soft-cooked eggs, ground meat, pureed vegetables, milk, cooked cereal.
  3. Increase fluids.
  4. Diet supplement to increase calorie and fluid intake.
  5. Do not eat several hours before treatment.
C. Administer medications.
  1. Compazine—nausea.
  2. Lomotil—diarrhea.
✦ D. Provide skin care—radiodermatitis occurs 3–6 weeks after start of treatment.
  1. Avoid creams, lotions, perfumes to irradiated areas unless directed to apply by physician. Aloe vera cream or gel may be recommended.
  2. Wash with lukewarm water, pat dry (some physicians allow mild soap).
  3. Avoid exposure to sunlight or artificial heat such as heating pad.
✦ E. Observe for "wet" reaction.
  1. Weeping of skin due to loss of upper layer.
  2. Promote rest after therapy.
  3. Cleanse area with warm water and pat dry BID.
  4. Apply antibiotic lotion or steroid cream if ordered.
  5. Expose site to air.

Internal Radiation/Brachytherapy

A. Implantation of radioactive substance within the tumor or close to it.

✦ B. Types.
   1. Unsealed sources: isotopes (^{131}I and ^{32}P).
      a. Liquid and administered orally.
      b. Half-life generally short but varies with isotope.
      c. Precautions important during high-risk period (usually first four days).
   2. Sealed sources: radium needles, radon seeds, and ^{137}Cs.
      a. Radioactive substance encased in metal capsule placed in body cavity.
      b. Delivers radiation directly to tumor.
      c. Even though implant is sealed, special precautions are instituted.

C. Side effects.
   1. Occur when normal cells are damaged.
   2. Acute side effects occur during or shortly after radiation therapy; chronic effects occur months or years following therapy.
   ✦ 3. Common side effects from radiation therapy: alopecia, mouth dryness, mucositis, esophagitis, nausea and vomiting, diarrhea, cystitis, erythema, and dry and wet desquamation.
   4. Factors influencing degree of side effects.
      a. Body site irradiated.
      b. Radiation dose—the higher the dose given, the more potential side effects.
      c. Extent of body area treated (larger area, more potential for side effects).
      d. Method of radiation therapy.

Implementation

✦ A. Maintain bedrest when radiation source in place.
   1. Restrict movement to prevent dislodging radiation source.
   2. Do not turn or position client except on back (when cesium needle in tongue or cervix).

B. Administer range-of-motion exercises QID.

C. Take vital signs every four hours (report temperature over 100°F).

D. Observe for untoward effects: dehydration or paralytic ileus (if cervical implant).

✦ E. Observe and report skin eruption, discharge, abnormal bleeding; teach client to avoid using lotions, ointments, and powder.

F. Provide clear liquid diet (low residue is sometimes ordered) and force fluids.

G. Insert Teflon Foley catheter (radiation decomposes rubber) to avoid necessity of bedpan.

✦ H. Observe frequently for dislodging of radiation source (especially linen and dressings).
   1. Avoid direct contact around implant site.

✦ 2. When radiation source falls out, do not touch with hands. Pick up source with foot-long applicator.
✦ 3. Put source in lead container and call physician.
4. If unable to locate source, call physician immediately and bar visitors from room.

I. After source is removed, give the following care.
   1. Administer Betadine douche if cervical implant.
   2. Give Fleets enema.
   3. Client may be out of bed.
   4. Avoid direct sunlight to radiation areas.
   5. Administer cream to relieve dryness or itching.

J. Instruct that client may resume sexual intercourse within seven to ten days.

✦ K. Notify physician if nausea, vomiting, diarrhea, frequent urination or bowel movements, or temperature above 100°F is present.

Safety Measures

✦ A. Implement radiation safety measures. (*See* above.)

✦ B. Follow special principles of time, distance, and shielding.
   1. Minimize time.
      a. Radiation exposure proportional to amount of time spent with client.
      b. Plan care to be delivered in shortest amount of time to meet goals—be efficient with time.
      c. Review procedures before beginning them.
   2. Maximize distance.
      a. Intensity of radiation is related to distance from client.
      b. Duration of safe exposure increases as distance is increased; work as far away from source as possible.

3. Utilize shielding.
    a. Use lead shields or other equipment to reduce transmission of radiation.
    b. Store radioactive material in lead-shielded container when not in use.
✦ C. Follow radiation precautions for isotope implant.
    1. All body secretions considered contaminated—use special techniques for disposal.
    2. If client vomits within first four hours—everything vomitus touches is considered contaminated.
    3. Use disposable gown, dishes, etc.
    4. Limit contact with hospital personnel and visitors.

Chemotherapy

Characteristics

A. The medical management of cancer includes the use of chemotherapy. First used in the early 1950s, there are now more than 80 effective drugs available.
    1. Chemotherapy is method of choice when there is suspected or confirmed spread of malignant cells.
    2. Method used when the risk of recurrence is high.
    3. May be used as palliative measure to relieve pain or increase comfort.
B. Mechanism of action.
    ✦ 1. Functions at cellular level by interrupting cell life—modifies or interferes with DNA synthesis.
    2. Chemotherapeutic agents eradicate cells, both normal and malignant, that are in the process of cell reproduction.

Drug Classification

A. Drugs classified by group into those that act on a certain phase of cell reproduction (cell cycle specific) or those that do not reproduce (cell cycle nonspecific).
✦ B. Cell cycle–specific agents: antimetabolics and mitotic inhibitors.
    1. Act on the cell during a particular phase of reproduction.
    2. Most effective in tumors where a large number of cells are dividing.
    3. Divided doses produce greater cytotoxic effects (not all cells will be in the same phase at the same time).
    4. Antimetabolites.
        a. Specific for the S phase—replaces building blocks of DNA so cell can't divide.
        b. Examples of antimetabolites: methotrexate, 6-mercaptopurine, 5-fluorouracil, azacytidine, cytarabine, Hydrea.

5. Plant alkaloids.
    a. Specific for the M phase—prevent cell division by destroying the mitotic spindle.
    b. Examples of mitotic inhibitors: plant alkaloids—vincristine, vindesine, vinblastine, teniposide.
✦ C. Cell cycle–nonspecific drugs: alkylating agents, antitumor antibiotics, and nitrosoureas.
    1. Act on cells during any phase of reproduction—some drugs will attack cells in the resting phase (not actively dividing).
    ✦ 2. Agents are dose dependent—the more drug given, the more cells destroyed.
    3. These drugs are more toxic to normal tissue because they are less selective.
    4. Alkylating agents.
        a. These drugs prevent cell division by damaging the DNA "ladder" structure and are effective in all phases of the cell cycle.
        b. Usually included in almost all chemotherapy regimens.
        c. Examples of alkylating agents: Cytoxan, Myleran, melphalan (L-PAM), Thiotepa, Platinol.
    5. Antitumor antibiotics.
        a. These drugs attack DNA (they act like alkylating drugs) by slipping between the DNA strands and preventing replication.
        b. Examples of antitumor antibiotics: adriamycin, Cosmegen, dactinomycin.
    6. Nitrosoureas.
        a. Alkylating agents that are stronger and have a greater ability to attack cells in the resting phase of cell growth.
        b. These drugs can cross the blood–brain barrier.
        c. Examples of nitrosoureas: streptozocin, methyl CCNU, BCNU, DCNU.
D. Other miscellaneous agents (such as procarbazine) are used in the chemotherapy group, but their exact mechanism of action is unknown.
✦ E. Hormonal agents (estrogens, androgen, progestins) work in all cycles and are used in therapy to affect the hormonal environment (Decadron, DES, Halotestin, tamoxifen, prednisone).
    1. Affect the growth of hormone-dependent tumors.
    2. Steroids interfere with the synthesis of protein and alter cell metabolism (lymphomas and leukemias).
    3. Antihormones (Tamoxifen and Evista) block tumor growth by depriving the tumor of the necessary hormones.
✦ F. Combination chemotherapy.

1. Most often administered in combination, which enhances the response rate: for example, doxarubicin, bleomycin, vinblastine and dacarbazine (ABVD) used for Hodgkin's lymphoma.
2. Studies at Stanford University now suggest ABVD and a fifth or sixth chemotherapy drug be combined with prednisone (for its anti-inflammatory effect) for 3 months for Hodgkin's disease.
3. Cancer cells divide erratically on different schedules; thus drugs that are effective alone and have different mechanisms of action can combine to destroy even more cells.
4. Drugs used in combination for synergistic activity.
5. Guidelines for drug administration are carefully planned and referred to as protocols or regimens.
   a. Package inserts are based on single-agent therapy, so it is important to adhere to the ordered protocol.
   b. Dosages of drugs are based on height and weight calculated as body surface area.

G. Other chemotherapeutic agents that do not fall into specific categories.
   1. Elspar—an enzyme used to treat lymphocytic leukemia; ulexin—antiandrogen used to treat prostate cancer; and Taxol—used to treat ovarian, breast, and cell lung cancers.
   ✦ 2. Chemotherapeutic drugs cause myelosuppression; nursing interventions include blood counts and instituting precautions if blood count falls below normal, and assess for infection.

Goals of Treatment

A. The major goal is to cure the malignancy.
   1. Chemotherapy, as primary mode of treatment, may include curing certain malignancies such as acute lymphocytic leukemia, Hodgkin's disease, lymphosarcomas, Wilms' tumor.
   2. Cure may also occur in combination with other modes of treatment, radiation, or surgery.
B. Control may be the goal when cure is not realistic; the aim is to extend survival and improve the quality of life.
C. Palliation may be the goal when neither cure nor control may be achieved; this goal is directed toward client comfort.

Chemotherapeutic Administration

A. Chemotherapeutic agents are administered through a variety of routes.
   1. Oral route—used frequently. Safety precautions must be observed.
   2. Intramuscular and subcutaneous used infrequently, as drugs are not vesicants.
   ✦ 3. Intravenous is the most common route—provides for better absorption.
      a. Potential complications: infection, phlebitis.
      b. Prevention of complications: use smallest-gauge needle possible; maintain aseptic technique; monitor IV site frequently; change IV fluid every 4 hours.
   ✦ 4. Central venous catheter infusion—used for continuous or intermittent infusions.
      a. Potential complications: infection, catheter clotting, sepsis, malposition of needle.
      b. Prevention of complications: maintain aseptic technique and monitor site daily; flush catheter daily and between each use with heparin solution; assess client for signs of sepsis.
   ✦ 5. Venous access devices (VADs)—used for prolonged infusions.
      a. Potential complications: infection and infiltration from malposition.
      b. Assess site frequently and assess for systemic infection.
   6. Intra-arterial route—delivers agents directly to tumor in high concentrations while decreasing drug's systemic toxic effect.
      a. Potential complications: infection or bleeding at catheter site, catheter clotting, or pump malfunction.
      b. Change dressing site daily and assess for signs of infection; irrigate catheter with heparin solution and avoid kinks in tubing.
   7. Intraperitoneal—used for ovarian and colon cancer. High concentration of agents delivered to peritoneal cavity via catheter, then drained.
   8. Other less frequently used routes are intrapleural, intrathecal, and ventricular reservoir.

B. Factors for deciding dosage and timing of drugs.
   1. Dosage calculated on body surface area and kilograms of body weight.
   2. Time lapse between doses to allow recovery of normal cells.
   3. Side effects of each drug and when they are likely to occur.
   4. Liver and kidney function, as most antineoplastics are metabolized in one of these organs.

Chemotherapy Safety Guidelines

✦ A. Antineoplastic drugs are potentially hazardous to personnel and may have teratogenic and/or carcinogenic effects.
✦ B. Safety guidelines have been issued by the Occupational Safety and Health Administration (OSHA).

1. Obtain special training for drug administration.
2. Use two pairs of powder-free, dispensable chemotherapy gloves, and a disposable, closed, long-sleeved gown with outer pair of gloves covering gown cuff whenever there is risk of exposure to hazardous drugs.
3. Provide syringes and IV sets with Luer-Lok fittings for preparing and administering hazardous drugs. Also provide containers for their disposal.
4. Use a closed-system drug-transfer device and needleless system to protect nursing personnel during drug administration.
5. Label all prepared drugs appropriately.
6. Double-bag chemotherapy drugs once prepared, before transport.
7. Have equipment ready to clean up any accidental spill (spill kit).
8. Dispose of all materials in marked containers labeled hazardous waste.
9. Dispose of all needles and syringes intact.
10. Follow facility's policies and procedures when preparing to administer chemotherapy.
11. Double-check chemotherapy orders with another oncology nurse.
12. Read material safety data sheets (MSDS) prior to administration.
13. Use personal protective equipment (PPE).
14. Wash your hands both before you put on and after you take off gloves.
15. After infusion is complete, promptly dispose of any equipment that contained the drug in a puncture-proof container that is clearly marked.
16. Chemotherapy agents may be excreted in body fluids; these may be contaminated for 48 hours after the last drug dose. Wear PPE when handling such excreta, and wash your hands after removing gloves.
17. Check facility's policies about handling linen that's been contaminated with chemotherapy.
18. If a chemotherapy drug comes into contact with your skin or a client's skin, thoroughly wash the affected area with soap and water, but don't abrade the skin with a scrub brush.
19. If the drug gets in your eyes, flush with copious amounts of water for at least 15 minutes while holding back your eyelids. Then get evaluated by employee health or the ED.

✦ C. When infusing vesicant drugs, monitor IV carefully—at first sign of extravasation, remove IV and implement Rx protocol.

Side Effects and Nursing Management

✦ A. Side effects occur primarily due to the mechanism of action of potent drugs on normal cells.

1. Normal cells most affected are bone marrow cells, epithelial cells of the GI tract and hair follicles, and cells of the gonads.
2. Since other normal cells are not actively reproducing (except with tissue injury and repair), they are not severely affected.
3. Time of most severe depression of cells (termed *nadir*) is different for each type of cell.

B. Skin and mucosa, protective linings of the body, are damaged.

✦ 1. Mucositis (cells of the mucosa are affected)—may extend from oral cavity and stomach through GI tract.
   a. Symptoms may be nausea, vomiting, anorexia, fluid and eletrolyte imbalance, dietary insufficiency, and stomatitis.
   b. Assess for erythema, tenderness, and ulceration.
2. Clients at high risk are those with dental caries, those with gum disease, smokers, and those who drink alcohol.
3. Nursing interventions include good oral hygiene, mouthwashes, avoiding foods that are sharp, spicy, or acidic—diet should be soft, bland, tepid.

✦ C. Alopecia, or hair loss, caused by damage to rapidly dividing cells of the hair follicles.

1. Hair loss begins 2–3 weeks after chemotherapy and continues through the cycles of chemotherapy; regrowth occurs following the course of therapy.
2. Nursing interventions include scalp hypothermia (ice cap) and scalp tourniquet; both reduce the amount of drug reaching the hair follicle and may prevent hair loss.

✦ D. Nausea, vomiting, and anorexia are common in clients receiving chemotherapy.

1. Antiemetic regimens (Reglan) may counteract these symptoms.
2. Nursing interventions include supporting changes in food preferences, additional or less seasoning, small and more frequent meals.
3. Offer high-calorie and protein supplements.

✦ E. Elimination disturbance occurs when the client does not eat well, is not exercising, or has mucositis.

1. Diarrhea is related to toxicity of the drugs on the mucosal lining; diet bland and low residue.
2. Constipation may be related to the drugs (especially vinblastine and vincristine) that affect nerve endings in the GI tract.
   a. Add more fiber and liquid to diet (3000 mL/day).
   b. Avoid milk and dairy products.

c. Include low-residue foods and foods high in potassium.

d. Stool softeners are ordered to minimize constipation; may add vegetable laxative.

F. Elevated uric acid and crystal urate stone formation may occur.

✦ G. Hematological disruptions: damage to normal cells in the bone marrow can be life-threatening and is, therefore, the most dangerous side effect.

1. White blood cells and platelets have a shorter life span than red blood cells so they are more susceptible to damage.

2. White blood cell suppression—leukopenia (less than 5000/mm³ when normal white blood cell count is 5000–10,000/mm³).

   a. Granulocytes are the most suppressed, which places client at risk for bacterial infection.

   b. Common sites of infection are the lung, urinary tract, skin, and blood.

   c. Implementation includes meticulous aseptic technique for IV therapy as well as hand hygiene; avoid exposure to infected persons.

   d. Assess for fever, chills, and sore throat.

   e. Teach signs and symptoms of infection to the cancer client with instructions to report symptoms to the doctor or nurse.

✦ 3. Platelet suppression to below normal (less than 150,000–300,000/mm³) is called thrombocytopenia.

   a. A number less than 50,000/mm³ makes the client susceptible to bleeding gums and/or nose, easy bruising, heavier menstrual flow, etc.

   b. Teach client precautions: soft toothbrush, avoidance of douches and enemas, care with trimming nails, avoiding venipunctures when possible, and avoidance of any activity that might increase intracranial pressure (ICP).

4. Red blood cell suppression—anemia is not usually a severe toxicity.

H. All hormonal agents cause fluid retention: monitor weight gain, I&O, edema, and administer diuretics as ordered.

Nutrition in Oncology

A. Maintaining a healthy diet with supplements can affect cancer diagnosis.

1. Nutrition is a factor in the cause of some cancers.

2. Poor diet increases cancer risk.

3. High-fat meat and low fiber is linked to breast, prostate and colon cancer. Alcohol and tobacco connected to head and neck cancers.

4. Low calcium is linked to colon cancer, and low vitamin D is linked to prostate cancer.

B. Recommended diets.

1. Low fat and high fiber—high intake of fruits and vegetables with limited alcohol intake.

2. Avoid high weight gain and add physical activity.

C. Cancer cachexia—weight loss associated with certain types of cancer.

1. With this type of weight loss, weight is lost equally from muscle and fat.

2. Most often seen with lung and pancreatic cancer, but is present with other cancers.

D. Certain nutrients may be deficient in cancer clients—nutrient supplement (vitamins and minerals) recommended.

Psychosocial Impact of Chemotherapy

A. Assessment.

1. Client's reaction to illness and chemotherapy.

2. Prior experience with those receiving chemotherapy.

3. Coping style under stress.

4. Support network.

5. Psychosocial changes resulting from cancer.

   a. Threats to the roles client has in life: career, marriage, parent, etc.

   b. Threat to life goals.

   c. Altered independence.

B. Implementation.

1. Support client's coping style without attempting to change style.

2. Provide accurate information, encourage questions, and expression of concerns.

3. Allow time for client to communicate, express fears, concerns, and adjustment to both disease and treatment.

4. Refer client to appropriate healthcare providers and to help groups.

Targeted Medicine: Pharmacogenomics

A. Medicine targeted to illness and genetic makeup.

1. Advances in genetics are transforming medicine.

2. Genetic markers can predict how drugs are absorbed and metabolized and how clients will respond.

3. Increase in serious adverse drug reactions, costs, morbidity and mortality provide impetus for advancing targeted drugs.

B. Oncology is one area targeted drugs now being used.

1. Breast cancer: Herceptin targets a protein found in certain type of cancer; blocks growth of tumor cells.

2. Has far fewer side effects than traditional chemotherapy.

Pain in Cancer

Characteristics

✦ A. Incidence.
   1. Various studies suggest that 50 percent of persons with cancer will not experience significant pain.
   2. Severe pain is experienced by about 60–80 percent of hospitalized clients.
   3. In early stages of cancer there is little pain—pain that is felt is associated with treatment (surgery).
B. Causes of pain in cancer.
   1. Physiological causes.
      a. Bone destruction with infraction results from metastatic lesions secondary to primary carcinomas.
      b. Obstruction of an organ by tumor growth (intestinal obstruction).
      c. Compression of peripheral nerves produces sharp, continuous pain—pain follows nerve distribution.
      d. Infiltration or distention of tissue produces a localized, dull pain that increases in intensity as tumor grows.
      e. Inflammation, infection, and necrosis cause pain from pressure or dilatation and distention of tissue distal to an obstruction.
   2. Psychological causes.
      a. This form of pain depends on client's perceived threat from the condition or stress reaction to it.
         (1) Fear or anxiety generated from the effects the disease may have on the person's lifestyle or relationships.
         (2) Loss or threat of loss may produce a reactive depression with feelings of despair.
         (3) Frustration of drives or lack of need satisfaction may also contribute to psychological pain.
      b. Perception of threat or stress is influenced by client's personality characteristics: self-concept, independence–dependence, emotional stability, education, age, etc.
C. The nature of cancer pain falls into two general categories: chronic and intractable pain.

Assessment of Pain

✦ A. Physical dimension of cancer pain is variable.
   1. The severity of pain is assessed using a 0- to 10-point scale—0 being pain free and 10 being the worst pain.
   2. Teach "pain tasks" to client.
      a. Encourage client to identify and state what, where, and when pain occurs.
      b. This method will help determine which symptoms are most troublesome.
   3. Evaluate the meaning of the pain experienced by the client—understand pain as the client views it.
B. Scope of pain assessment must encompass several factors (Rowlingson).
   1. Severity and duration of pain.
   2. Nature of the disease process.
   3. Probable life expectancy.
   4. Temperament and psychological state.
   5. Occupational, domestic, and economic background of the client.
C. Assess vital signs as indicators of pain.
   1. Low to moderate pain and superficial in origin—the sympathetic nervous system is stimulated.
      a. Increased blood pressure and pulse.
      b. Increased respiratory rate and muscle tension.
   2. Severe pain or visceral in origin—the parasympathetic nervous system is affected.
      a. Decreased blood pressure and pulse.
      b. Nausea, vomiting, and weakness.
   3. Pain present for a month or longer (late-stage pain); there will probably be no change in vital signs.
D. Assess client's behavior as an indicator of pain.
   1. Alterations in body posture/gestures.
   2. Alterations in activities of daily living.
✦ E. Assess verbalizations, both verbal and nonverbal, as indicators of pain.
   1. Ask systematic questions to determine degree of pain: location, radiation, onset, frequency, duration, quality.
   2. Determine situational factors that influence pain level: level of consciousness, meaning of pain, attitudes and feelings of others, presence of secondary gains, fatigue level, and stressful life events.
   3. Assess and document client's pain often and regularly.

Treatment Methods

Medication Management

✦ A. Drug therapy is considered the cornerstone of cancer pain management—begins with least invasive and progresses to opioids as pain intensifies.
   1. Acetaminophen, aspirin, NSAIDs relieve mild pain.
   2. Opioids (codeine or hydrocodone) added to regimen as pain progresses.
      a. Given in fixed-dose combinations with aspirin.

Table 9-4. WORLD HEATH ORGANIZATION THREE-STEP ANALGESIC LADDER

Drug therapy is the cornerstone of cancer pain management. The three-step analgesic ladder proposed by the World Health Organization (WHO) is often followed in managing pain.

Step	Pain Intensity on a 0- to 10-Point Pain Scale	Drugs of Choice	Pain Management
1	Pain is mild and is described by client at 1–3	Non-opioids for mild pain (e.g., aspirin, acetaminophen, NSAIDs)	Provide appropriate and concurrent treatment for cause of pain; use adjuvant drugs as needed
2	Pain is moderate and is described by client at 4–6	Opioids for mild to moderate pain (e.g. codeine, oxycodone)	**Pain persists or increases** Add Step 2 opioid; continue Step 1 drugs and add adjuvant drugs as needed.
3	Pain is moderate to severe and is described by client at 7–10	Opioids for moderate to severe pain (e.g., morphine, hydromorphone, methadone)	**Pain persists or increases** Replace Step 2 opioid with Step 3 opioids; continue Step 1 drugs and add adjuvant drugs as needed.

Examples of adjuvant drugs: Tricyclic antidepressants, antiseizure drugs, anxiolytics, antihistamines, benzodiazepines, caffeine, dextroamphetamine, corticosteroids.

   b. Progresses to higher dose or more potent opioid (morphine, hydromorphone).
   c. Drugs can be given 24/7 with additional "rescue" doses as needed.
  3. Intraspinal morphine administration.
   a. An implantable infusion pump delivers a continual supply of opiate to the epidural or subarachnoid space.
   b. Useful for eliminating intractable pain below the mid- to low-thoracic level where spinal cord opiate receptors respond to morphine.
 B. Evaluate client continually for opioid side effects (constipation, nausea, vomiting, sedation, respiratory depression, and urinary retention) that interfere with the goal of the therapy.

Surgical Management

A. Various neurological and neurosurgical interventions effectively manage pain experienced by cancer clients.
  1. Nerve blocks, either peripheral or intrathecal, can relieve pain.
  2. Procedures involve interruption of pain pathways someplace along the path of transmission from the periphery to the brain.
B. Electrical stimulation of the periventricular gray matter in the brain is used for pain relief.
  1. An electrode is implanted through a burr hole on the side opposite the most intense pain.
  2. Electrical pulses are then sent periodically into the brain.

Noninvasive Modalities

A. Electrical stimulation may be used for pain relief.
  1. Transcutaneous methods (TENS): stimulation to the skin surface over the painful area.
  2. A peripheral nerve implant applies stimulation to peripheral nerves.
  3. Electrodes implanted in the dorsal column stimulate spinal column fibers.
B. Hypnosis is currently viewed as one component of pain management.
  1. A hypnotic state can achieve significant analgesia.
  2. Self-control over pain and its associated anxieties can be assisted with hypnosis.

Psychosocial Implications

A. Key stress periods for client with cancer are time of diagnosis, period of hospitalization, and release from the hospital.
  1. Shock and fear are the major reactions.
  2. Severe depression is experienced by some clients.
  3. The emotional pain of the diagnosis initially outweighs the physical component of the cancer.
B. Adjustment to cancer depends on past life experiences.
  1. A client's previous attitude toward medical practices, hospitalization, and treatment methods influence adjustment.
  2. The manner in which a client has coped with previous stress or crises will determine, in part, how this stress is handled.

C. Phases of psychological adaptation to terminal illness include denial, anger, bargaining, depression, and acceptance.
   1. These phases may be experienced differently, clients may experience them in a different order, or they may not experience all of the phases.
   2. It is important for the nurse to understand the characteristics of these phases and to recognize which phase the client is in.
D. The client will experience a range of feelings and defense mechanisms.
   ✦ 1. Denial may occur initially with the diagnosis; this is a protective mechanism necessary until the diagnosis can be confronted.
      a. Allow the client to be in denial until he or she is ready to face reality.
      b. Provide opportunities for the client to confront her illness—be open to questions and clarification.
   2. Fear and anxiety may manifest in physical symptoms: insomnia, nausea, vomiting, diarrhea, headaches, etc.
   3. Anger and resentment, especially in the initial phases of the disease, may be a healthy way of expressing feelings.
      a. Encourage expression of anger—let the client know that you are able to listen to anger, resentment, and frustration.
      b. Encourage client to focus anger on external problem solving and more adaptive coping patterns.
   4. Depression may be considered normal for a period of time following surgery.
      a. Observe for the signs of depression.
      b. Because suicide is always a risk with depression, interventions should be aimed at safety for the client.

Psychosocial Care for the Cancer Client

✦ A. Develop a collaborative relationship with the client.
   1. Identify and attempt to solve problems together.
   2. Engage with clients so that they do not feel they have to cope alone.
   3. Provide emotional support to help allay fears and anxieties.
✦ B. Always be honest with the client.
   1. Truth is easier to cope with than uncertainty and the unknown.
   2. Honesty provides the foundation for a nurse–client relationship.
   3. Accurate information can be followed by an open discussion of the disease, the prognosis, the client's feelings, etc.

   4. Knowing the truth enables the client to begin to accept and work out the future without being immobilized by fears.
C. Assist the client to cope with pain.
   1. Stay with the client, especially when the pain is severe.
   2. Explore the nature of pain with the client.
   3. Respect the client's response to pain and believe what the client tells you.
D. Provide general comfort measures.
   1. Position for proper alignment.
   2. Use touch and massage for painful areas.
   3. Exercise extremities gently to maintain range of motion.
   4. Maintain patency of tubes and keep free of infection using meticulous hand hygiene and aseptic techniques.
   5. Preserve the client's energy by prioritizing activities.
   6. Assist the client to obtain adequate rest at night and during the day to reduce fatigue.
✦ E. DO NOT undermedicate for cancer pain.
   1. Undertreatment with analgesics has been identified as a major problem (70 to 80 percent) for cancer clients—and nursing has a crucial responsibility to correct this problem.
   2. Two forms of undertreatment: physicians underprescribe and nurses routinely administer less than half the amount clients could receive.
   3. The danger of overuse of narcotics is a potential problem.
      a. This concern *should not* result in undertreatment.
      b. Only a very small percentage of clients are overmedicated.
F. Support family of the client as they move through the grieving process.
   1. Be honest with family members to establish a firm relationship.
   2. Encourage expression of feelings.
✦ G. Introduce the hospice concept—provides care for the terminally ill client and family.
   1. Primary goal is to provide emotional support for the client and family.
   2. An accompanying goal is to provide for physical care.
   3. Relief of pain is just as important to a dying person as emotional support.

Hospice Care

A. Hospice care provides treatment, comfort, and support for the terminally ill client, as well as relief and solace for the family. Approximately 1 in 3 elderly Americans uses hospice service.

B. Hospice neither speeds up nor slows down the dying process—it provides a specialized environment where a dying client may receive medical care in addition to emotional and spiritual support during the dying process.

   1. One of the real advantages of hospice is that the personnel are trained to treat pain aggressively.
   2. The client should be as pain free as possible, while at the same time remaining as alert as possible.

C. Hospice care includes an interdisciplinary team that includes a registered nurse, a social worker, a home health aide, a chaplain, and trained volunteers.

D. Hospice is reimbursed by Medicare in all states and by Medicaid in some states; for most other insurers, the percentage of care paid for varies by insurance carrier.

E. There are several barriers to hospice care.

   1. The client's physician must certify that the life expectancy of the client is six months or less.
   2. Some insurance carriers require clients to waive their rights to medical benefits if they are receiving hospice care.
   3. The largest obstacle is that there is a problem with communication—between physician and client, client and family, and family and client.
   4. When the finality of dying cannot be discussed, hospice care may not present itself as an option.

ONCOLOGY NURSING REVIEW QUESTIONS

1. When the nurse is counseling a client about preventive measures for cancer, one of the most important behaviors to emphasize is to

   1. Decrease fat intake.
   2. Avoid exposure to the sun.
   3. Avoid smoking.
   4. Obtain adequate rest and avoid stress.

2. Of the following screening methods for prevention of cancer, the most important one for the client to be aware of is

   1. Magnetic resonance imaging (MRI).
   2. Breast self-examination.
   3. Risk assessment.
   4. Sigmoidoscopy.

3. A client has just received a report from her physician that describes a tumor that was recently biopsied. If the result she receives is listed as "T_0, N_0, M_0," the client will know that she has

   1. No evidence of a primary tumor, lymph node involvement, and metastasis.
   2. No primary tumor, but evidence of a degree of distant metastasis.
   3. A primary tumor and regional nodes involved.
   4. Carcinoma in situ.

4. A client has just completed a course in radiation therapy and is experiencing radiodermatitis. The most effective method of treating the skin is to

   1. Wash the area with soap and warm water.
   2. Apply a cream or lotion to the area.
   3. Leave the skin alone until it is clear.
   4. Avoid applying creams or lotions to the area.

5. You are assigned a client who is to be treated with a cobalt implant for intracavity irradiation for cervical cancer. Her treatment will be completed in 72 hours. Which protective measures are indicated for personnel and visitors? List all of the numbers that apply _____.

   1. Place a "Radiation Treatment" sign on the door to the client's room and on the front of the client's chart.
   2. All nurses and visitors must wear a protective shield. (Keep a lead shield at the client's doorway.)

   3. Complete care of the client as fast as possible and leave the room quickly.
   4. Do not allow pregnant women to visit or to be assigned as staff for this client, but children under age 18 may visit.
   5. Visitors must limit exposure to 1 hour/day and keep a distance from the client.

6. The nurse is assessing a client with a radiation implant and observes that the implant has been dislodged. The nurse cannot immediately locate the implant. The first nursing action is to

   1. Search for the implant in the bed covers and place it in a lead container.
   2. Call the physician and bar all visitors from the room.
   3. Pick up the source with a foot-long applicator.
   4. Notify the radiation safety team.

7. A client with cancer that has metastasized to the liver is started on chemotherapy. His physician has specified divided doses of the antimetabolite. In discharge planning, the nurse instructs the client to take the drug in divided doses. What is the rationale for this instruction?

   1. "There really is no reason; your doctor just wrote the orders that way."
   2. "This schedule will reduce the side effects of the drug."
   3. "Divided doses produce greater cytotoxic effects on the diseased cells."
   4. "Because these drugs prevent cell division, they are more effective in divided doses."

8. Intravenous is the most common route for the administration of chemotherapy drugs because it provides for better absorption. When a client is receiving drugs via this route, one of the most important assessments the nurse will perform is for the complication(s) of

   1. Catheter clotting.
   2. Infection and phlebitis.
   3. Malposition of the needle.
   4. Sepsis.

9. A client experiencing severe, intractable pain from cancer complains that the pain medication is not handling the pain at all. The nurse has given the client all

the medicine she can receive. The next nursing action is to

1. Emotionally support the client and tell her she will receive the next dose of medication as soon as possible.
2. Contact the physician immediately and intervene on the client's behalf to increase the pain dose or change the medication.
3. Suggest the client try breathing or other alternative techniques to cope with the pain.
4. Explore the nature of the pain and help the client perceive it in a different way.

10. A client has been receiving chemotherapy for the treatment of breast cancer. She is now to start receiving daily injections of filgrastim (Neupogen). The nurse would assess for a therapeutic response to this drug by monitoring which laboratory test result?

1. Blood urea nitrogen (BUN).
2. Potassium.
3. Platelets.
4. White blood cell count (WBC).

11. For a client who has received a diagnosis of skin cancer, the type that has the poorest prognosis because it metastasizes so rapidly and extensively via the lymph system is

1. Basal cell epithelioma.
2. Squamous cell epithelioma.
3. Malignant melanoma.
4. Sebaceous cyst.

12. Cancer is the second major cause of death in the United States. What is the first step toward effective cancer control?

1. Increasing government control of potential carcinogens.
2. Changing habits and customs that predispose the individual to cancer.
3. Conducting more mass-screening programs.
4. Educating public and professional people about cancer.

13. Alkylating drugs are used as chemotherapeutic agents in cancer therapy. The nurse understands that these drugs stop cancer growth by

1. Damaging DNA in the cell nucleus.
2. Interrupting the production of necessary cellular metabolites.
3. Creating a hormonal imbalance.
4. Destroying messenger RNA.

14. Antineoplastic drugs are dangerous because they affect normal tissue as well as cancer tissue. Normal cells that divide and proliferate rapidly are more at risk. Which of the following areas of the body would be least at risk?

1. Bone marrow.
2. Nervous tissue.
3. Hair follicles.
4. Lining of the GI tract.

15. To educate clients, the nurse should understand that the most common site of cancer for a female is the

1. Uterine cervix.
2. Uterine body.
3. Vagina.
4. Fallopian tubes.

16. A 45-year-old client has just been admitted to the hospital for an abdominal hysterectomy following a diagnosis of uterine cancer. Results of lab tests indicate that the client's WBC is 9800/mm^3. The nursing intervention is to

1. Call the operating room and cancel the surgery.
2. Notify the surgeon immediately.
3. Take no action as this is a normal value.
4. Call the lab and have the test repeated.

17. While the nurse is orienting a client scheduled for surgery, the client states she is afraid of what will happen the next day. What is the most appropriate response?

1. Assure her that the surgery is very safe and problems are rare.
2. Encourage her to talk about her fears as much as she wishes.
3. Explain that her physician is one of the best and she has nothing to worry about.
4. Explain that worrying will only prolong her hospitalization.

18. A 52-year-old client has had a lobectomy for cancer of the left lower lobe of the lung. He is 18 hours postoperative. The nurse understands that for this client the most appropriate position immediately postoperatively is

1. Flat bedrest.
2. Turned to the unoperative side only.
3. Turned to the operative side only.
4. Semi-Fowler's position, turned to either side.

19. A client has had a partial colectomy and is 2 days postop. During a 6:00 PM assessment, the nurse

observed all of the following. A priority concern that would require the earliest intervention is a

1. Dressing that is moderately saturated with serosanguineous drainage.
2. Warm and reddened area on the client's left calf.
3. Distended bladder that is firm to palpation.
4. Decrease in breath sounds on the right side.

20. A client has possible malignancy of the colon, and surgery is scheduled. The rationale for administering Neomycin preoperatively is to

1. Prevent infection postoperatively.
2. Eliminate the need for preoperative enemas.
3. Decrease and retard the growth of normal bacteria in the intestines.
4. Treat cancer of the colon.

21. A client has just learned that he has a diagnosis of cancer of the lung. His physician has recommended that the lung be removed. The client says to the nurse that he is sure the doctor made a mistake because he can breathe just fine. The nurse interprets this response as

1. Depression.
2. Denial.
3. Avoidance.
4. Reaction formation.

22. A female client is to be discharged following a simple mastectomy of the right breast for cancer. Discharge instructions should include

1. Follow-up visits with a physical therapist.
2. Referral to a Reach for Recovery group.
3. Returning to her physician for monthly breast exams.
4. How to perform a breast self-exam monthly.

23. Which nursing diagnosis should receive highest priority in a client who is receiving the chemotherapeutic agent cisplatin (Platinol)?

1. Risk of infection.
2. Activity intolerance.
3. Altered oral mucous membranes.
4. Altered nutrition: less than body requirements.

24. A client is experiencing diarrhea as a side effect of chemotherapy. Which nursing diagnosis should receive the highest priority?

1. Fluid volume deficit.
2. Impaired skin integrity.
3. Body image disturbance.
4. Activity intolerance.

25. A female client with a diagnosis of cancer of the cervix has a radon seed implanted. Which data would it be important for the nurse to assess every few hours?

1. Presence of nausea and vomiting.
2. Hydration status.
3. Ability of the client to change position.
4. Dislodging of radiation source.

ONCOLOGY NURSING

Answers with Rationale

1. (3) Avoiding smoking is a primary cancer preventive behavior. Smoking is believed to be the cause of 75 percent of lung cancers in the United States. All of the other behaviors are also important preventive measures, but tobacco is a known carcinogen.

   NP:I; CN:H; CA:M; CL:C

2. (2) Breast self-examination (BSE) is the most important method to instruct the client about because it is a primary prevention method. It is performed every month (whereas a mammogram is done every year after age 50), and many breast lumps are first found by the woman when she is examining her breasts. An MRI (1) would be done for diagnosis. Risk assessment (3) and sigmoidoscopy (4) are also important preventive measures, but in priority fall below a BSE.

   NP:P; CN:H; CA:MA; CL:A

3. (1) The staging of the cancer according to cancer classification means that there is no evidence of a primary tumor (T_0), regional lymph nodes are not abnormal (N_0), and there is no evidence of distant metastasis (M_0).

   NP:AN; CN:PH; CA:S; CL:C

4. (4) Irradiated areas are very sensitive; all creams and lotions, which would serve to irritate the skin, should be avoided. The area should be washed with lukewarm water; a mild soap may be used, but most physicians prefer clear water.

   NP:I; CN:PH; CA:M; CL:A

5. Answers are (1), (2), and (5). (3) and (4) are incorrect. Completing care as soon as possible is not the point—limiting exposure to 15 minutes/day is the advised protocol. It is true that pregnant women cannot be exposed; anyone under 18 also cannot be admitted.

   NP:P; CN:S; CA:M; CL:A

6. (2) The first nursing action is to bar all visitors from the room and notify the physician. It is important not to contaminate yourself by searching for the implant (1). The physician will notify the radiation team and make decisions about reimplanting the radiation source in the client.

   NP:I; CN:S; CA:S; CL:AN

7. (3) Because not all cells will be in the same phase at the same time, divided doses will produce greater cytotoxic effects. This schedule will not reduce the side effects of the drug. Even though the drugs may prevent cell division (4), divided doses will not affect this characteristic.

   NP:I; CN:PH; CA:M; CL:C

8. (2) Infection and phlebitis are two of the most common complications of receiving chemotherapy drugs via IV. The other complications are seen with central venous catheter insertion, used for continuous infusions.

   NP:A; CN:PH; CA:M; CL:A

9. (2) It is the nurse's responsibility to intervene with the physician and report that the pain medication is not providing adequate pain relief. Undertreatment with analgesics has been identified as a major problem for cancer clients, and studies have shown that physicians frequently underprescribe. The other responses will help support the client, but they will not be effective enough to relieve severe pain.

   NP:I; CN:PH; CA:M; CL:AN

10. (4) Filgrastin stimulates the production of WBCs. It is given to clients experiencing bone marrow depression with leukopenia secondary to cancer chemotherapy.

    NP:E; CN:PH; CA:M; CL:AN

11. (3) Malignant melanoma has the poorest prognosis. Basal cell epithelioma (1) and squamous cell epithelioma (2) are both superficial, easily excised, slow-

Coding for Questions/Answers Abbreviations: **Nursing Process: NP,** Assessment: A, Analysis: AN, Planning: P, Implementation: I, Evaluation: E; **Client Needs: CN,** Safe, Effective Care Environment: S, Health Promotion and Maintenance: H, Psychosocial Integrity: PS, Physiological Integrity: PH; **Clinical Area: CA,** Medical Nursing: M, Surgical Nursing: S, Maternal/Newborn Nursing: MA, Pediatric Nursing: P, Psychiatric Nursing: PS; **Cognitive Level: CL,** Knowledge: K, Comprehension: C, Application: A, Analysis: AN.

growing tumors. A sebaceous cyst (4) is a benign (nonmalignant) growth.

NP:AN; CN:PH; CA:M; CL:K

12. (4) The most important step in controlling cancer is educating the public about cancer and its warning signs. Education will have an effect on early diagnosis and treatment.

NP:AN; CN:PH; CA:M; CL:C

13. (1) Alkylating agents affect production of DNA, which, in turn, disrupts cell growth and division.

NP:AN; CN:PH; CA:M; CL:C

14. (2) Nervous tissue is least at risk. Bone marrow (1), hair follicles (3), and the lining of the GI tract (4) are the cells that are most vulnerable because they have rapid cell division and proliferation similar to cancer cells. The nervous tissue cells do not have rapid cell division.

NP:AN; CN:PH; CA:M; CL:K

15. (1) Cervical cancer is the most common site and squamous cell cancer is the most common cell type.

NP:AN; CN:H; CA:M; CL:C

16. (3) The normal WBC count is 5000 to 10,000/mm^3. If the results were abnormally high or low, the surgeon would have to be notified (2) and the surgery may be canceled (1). Tests with abnormal results are not routinely repeated (4) unless the results are grossly abnormal.

NP:I; CN:H; CA:S; CL:A

17. (2) Allowing the client to express her fears results in a decrease in anxiety and a more realistic and knowledgeable reaction to the situation. Studies have shown that the less anxiety the client has about the surgery, the more positive the postoperative results. (1) and (3) are false reassurances and nontherapeutic.

NP:I; CN:PS; CA:S; CL:A

18. (4) Postoperatively, the client can be turned to both sides to increase full expansion of lung tissue. It is best to place him in semi-Fowler's position when his vital signs are stable to ensure full lung expansion.

NP:P; CN:PH; CA:S; CL:A

19. (3) Inability to void after the Foley catheter has been removed is a common problem resulting from anesthesia or pain medication and requires an early intervention. It is important to be aware of the client's output for several reasons: to ensure adequate intake, to detect renal problems, and to assess for blood pressure problems. The solution to this problem is catheterization, based on a physician's order. The dressing should be closely observed but is not presently a problem (1). The area on the calf may be developing thrombophlebitis (2) and should be reported to the physician immediately. The breath sounds (4) can be improved by turning, coughing, and deep-breathing.

NP:I; CN:PH; CA:S; CL:AN

20. (3) Neomycin suppresses normal bacterial flora, thereby "sterilizing" the bowel preoperatively to decrease the possibility of postoperative infection. It cannot prevent infection (1). Neomycin does not influence the need for preoperative enemas (2) or treat cancer of the colon (4).

NP:P; CN:PH; CA:S; CL:C

21. (2) The first phase of psychological adaptation to terminal illness is denial. It is important for the nurse to recognize this as a natural reaction and support the client until he can deal with the reality of the diagnosis.

NP:AN; CN:PS; CA:S; CL:A

22. (4) It is most important for the client to perform a breast self-exam monthly at a regular time because she would not make monthly visits to her physician. Telling her how to contact a support group (2) would also be helpful.

NP:P; CN:H; CA:S; CL:A

23. (1) Cisplatin may depress the bone marrow, thereby interfering with the production of WBCs. The resultant leukopenia can be life-threatening; therefore, risk of infection is the highest priority. The other nursing diagnoses, although appropriate for this client, would be of lower priority.

NP:AN; CN:PH; CA:M; CL:A

24. (1) Although all of these nursing diagnoses could apply to a client with diarrhea, fluid volume deficit is the priority diagnosis because it is potentially life-threatening.

NP:AN; CN:PH; CA:M; CL:C

25. (4) Frequently checking that the radiation source has not become dislodged is the most important assessment. The seed may get lost in the linen or dressing. If the radiation source is dislodged, it must be placed in a lead container for safety. The other assessment parameters are important, but do not have to be done every few hours.

NP:A; CN:S; CA:M; CL:AN

Emergency Nursing 10

✦ The icon denotes content of special importance for NCLEX.

ASSESSING LIFE-THREATENING CONDITIONS

Initial Status Assessment

A. Airway.
   1. Open airway—if airway is obstructed, victim cannot get oxygen.
     a. Move fast—time is critical because brain damage could occur after 4 minutes.
     b. Check if tongue is obstructing airway—this is the most common obstruction.
   2. Check if spine stabilization or immobilization is needed.
   3. Check for respiratory distress.
B. Breathing.
   1. Assess breathing by watching rise and fall of chest.
   2. Listen for air being expelled.
   3. Use head-tilt/chin-lift method if victim is not breathing and airway is not obstructed.
     a. Feel or hear for air movement, which is a reliable indicator of an open airway.
     b. If no response, repeat procedure (if AED is available, apply to victim).
C. Circulation.
   1. Check carotid or femoral pulse.
   2. Assess bleeding—if not controlled within a short period of time, victim will go into shock. (*See* Loss of Blood box.)
   3. Assess color, temperature, and moisture of skin.
   4. Assess capillary refill.
   5. Identify type of bleeding.
     a. Arterial bleeding (spurting blood).
     b. Venous bleeding (flowing blood).
     c. Capillary bleeding (oozing blood).
   6. Choose appropriate method to control bleeding.
     a. Direct local pressure—place direct pressure over wound and press firmly (95 percent of bleeding can be controlled by direct pressure with elevation).
     b. Maintain compression by wrapping wound firmly with pressure bandage.
     c. Elevate wound above level of heart.
     d. Use pressure point to slow blood flow to wound—brachial point for arm, femoral point for leg.
     e. Use tourniquet if bleeding cannot be controlled by other methods—this is a last resort because it can present a serious risk to the affected limb if no circulation is present.

Secondary Status Assessment

A. Remove clothes or helmet for total examination of victim.

   1. Move client to private room or area.
   2. Cover client to keep warm.
B. Obtain vital signs, T,P,R, and BP, including pain level.
C. Check initial intervention into an emergency situation (e.g., open wound, bleeding).
D. Follow up major assessment interventions.
   1. Heart or ECG assessment.
   2. Oxygen saturation.
   3. Urinary catheter if necessary.
   4. GI tube insertion if necessary.
   5. Blood and laboratory studies.
   6. Pain/anxiety level.
   7. General appearance and demeanor, including mental status.
E. Pay attention to family accompanying client.
F. Obtain full history from client or family.
   1. Current problem or complaint.
   2. Allergies.
   3. Medications/herbs client is taking.
   4. Past health history, including surgeries.
   5. Physical assessment of client.

COMMON EMERGENCIES

Wounds

Definition: Break in the continuity of the tissue of the body, either internal or external.
A. Classification.
   1. Open—break in the skin or mucous membrane.
   2. Closed—injury to underlying tissues without a break in the skin or mucous membrane.
B. Types of open wounds.
   1. Incised.
   2. Contused.
   3. Lacerated.
   4. Punctured.
C. The RYB wound classification classifies open wounds that are healing—not usually an emergency.
   1. Red wounds (R) are in the inflammatory, proliferative, or maturation phase of healing.
   2. Yellow wounds (Y) are infected or contain fibrinous slough and aren't ready to heal.
   3. Black wounds (B) contain necrotic tissue and aren't ready to heal.
   4. Treatment options are based on wound color.
✦ D. First aid for open wounds.
   1. Stop bleeding immediately.
   2. Protect wound from contamination and infection.
   3. Provide shock care.
   4. Obtain medical attention.
✦ E. Techniques to stop severe bleeding.

1. Direct pressure.
2. Elevation.
3. Pressure on supplying artery.
4. Tourniquet.

F. Characteristics of closed wounds.
   1. No break in skin.
   2. Blood loss may be from outer openings of body cavities.
   3. Usually caused by an external force.
   4. Victim demonstrates signs of internal bleeding.

✦ G. First aid for closed wounds.
   1. Check for fractures and other internal injuries.
   2. Treat for shock.
   3. Do not give fluids by mouth if internal injuries are suspected.
   4. Apply ice to small areas of closed wounds.

✦ H. Measures to prevent contamination or infection of wounds.
   1. Do not remove cloth pad initially placed on wound.
   2. Do not cleanse deep wounds that require medical attention.
   3. Use sterile dressing or cleanest dressing available.
   4. Do not remove deeply embedded objects.

Choking

Definition: Temporary or permanent asphyxia due to obstruction of the airway.

✦ A. Signs and symptoms.
   1. Violent choking.
   2. Alarming attempts at inhalation.
   3. Cyanosis of face, neck, and hands.
   4. Cessation of breathing.
   5. Inability to speak.
   6. Unconsciousness.

✦ B. First aid measures.
   1. Remove object if possible.
   2. Allow victim to assume position of comfort.
   3. Encourage coughing.
   4. Use Heimlich maneuver (*see* p. 492).
   5. Artificial respirations if breathing ceases.
   6. Obtain medical assistance.

Poisoning

Definition: Introduction into the body or onto the skin surface of any solid, liquid, or gas that tends to impair health or to cause death.

✦ A. First aid treatment.
   1. Call doctor or poison control center (800-222-1222). Give the following information.
      a. Age of victim.
      b. Name and amount of poison taken.
      c. Whether victim vomited.

2. If victim is conscious, give antidote, if known.
3. Induce vomiting if material ingested is not strong acid or petroleum product. With these substances, use activated charcoal.
   a. 50–100 g activated charcoal or prepackaged charcoal/sorbitol product mixed with water.
   b. The earlier charcoal is given, the more effective it is.
4. If inhaled gases, remove victim to fresh air.
5. If contact poison, wash exposed areas.

B. Follow-up treatment as prescribed.

Frostbite and Cold Exposure

Definition: Tissues are frozen, which results in the formation of ice crystals in tissue and cells.

✦ A. Signs and symptoms.
   1. White or grayish-yellow skin.
   2. Pain or burning sensation.
   3. Blisters.
   4. Area cold and numb.
   5. Mental confusion.
   6. Tingling or numbness.

✦ B. First aid treatment.
   1. Cover area.
   2. Rewarm area quickly in water bath (102 to 108°F.
   3. Do not rub.
   4. Elevate affected area.

Dehydration

See Chapter 13, Pediatric Nursing.

Heat Exhaustion

Definition: Response to heat characterized by fatigue and weakness; occurs when intake of water cannot compensate for loss of fluids through sweating.

✦ A. Signs and symptoms.
   1. Pale, clammy skin.
   2. Profuse perspiration.
   3. Headache.
   4. Nausea.
   5. Dizziness.
   6. Fainting.

✦ B. First aid treatment.
   1. Offer victim sips of fluid and electrolyte replacement—one-half glass every 15 minutes for 1 hour.
   2. Remove restrictive clothing and have victim lie down and elevate feet.
   3. Place in cool environment.
   4. Apply cool, wet cloths.
   5. Monitor for airway, breathing, and circulation (ABCs).

Heatstroke

Definition: Response to heat characterized by extremely high body temperature due to disturbance in sweating mechanism—a medical emergency.

◆ A. Signs and symptoms.
1. High body temperature—104°F or higher.
2. Hot, red, dry skin.
3. Rapid, strong pulse.
4. Neurological symptoms—hallucinations, confusion.
   B. First aid treatment—stabilizing ABCs.
   C. Cool body quickly using whatever methods are available (remove clothing, ice water bath, pan, wet sheets, cool fluids, etc.).

Burns

Definition: Injury of the skin, subcutaneous tissue, muscle, and/or bones caused by heat, chemical agent, or radiation.

◆ A. Classification of burns.
1. Superficial (first-degree)—red skin, mild swelling and pain, rapid healing.
2. Deep, partial thickness (second-degree)—red or mottled skin, blisters, considerable swelling, wet appearance due to loss of plasma, and severe pain.
3. Full thickness (third-degree)—deep tissue destruction, white or charred appearance, complete loss of all layers of skin. Skin graft needed for healing.

◆ B. First aid treatment for superficial burn.
1. Apply cold water or submerge in cold water.
2. Prevent contamination.
3. Avoid greasy substances.
4. Apply aloe vera gel if available.
   C. First aid treatment for deep, partial-thickness burn.
1. Immerse burn, if fairly small area, in cold water for 1–2 hours.
2. Apply clean cloths.
3. Blot area dry.
4. Do not break blisters.
5. Do not apply antiseptic preparations or home remedies.
6. Elevate affected extremities.
7. Seek medical attention.

◆ D. First aid treatment for full-thickness burns.
1. Do not attempt to remove clothing from burned area.
2. Cover burn with sterile dressing.
3. Elevate involved extremities.
4. Do not immerse burn in water or apply ice water.
5. If medical help is not quickly available, and victim is conscious and not vomiting, give victim,

---

EMERGENCY BURN TREATMENT

A. Immediate care.
1. Put out flames—have client drop to floor or ground and roll.
2. Apply cold water for brief duration in second-degree burn if seen within 10 minutes of injury.
3. Apply no ointment.
4. Cover burns with sterile or clean cloth.
5. Irrigate chemical burns thoroughly.

B. Emergency care.
◆ 1. Patent airway and IV line are established.
2. 100% oxygen given if burn occurred in enclosed area.
3. Degree and extent of burn is determined—adequate pain relief given.
◆ 4. Fluid balance is maintained.
a. First day, give formula of choice according to percentage of body burned and weight plus 2000 mL D_5W.
b. Second day, give colloids with solutions.
c. Urine output is maintained at least 50 mL/hr.
d. Vital signs—CVP line usually inserted.
5. Nasogastric tube (inserted to prevent paralytic ileus).
6. Tetanus toxoid given.

---

at 15-minute intervals, a solution of fluid and electrolytes if available or ½ teaspoon of salt and ½ teaspoon of soda in a quart of water.

Fractures

Definition: A break or crack in a bone.
   A. Types of fractures.
1. Open—bone ends protrude through skin.
2. Closed—bone cracked or broken but does not protrude through skin.
◆ B. Signs and symptoms.
1. Victim heard or felt bone snap.
2. Abnormal or false motion in body area.
3. Differences in shape and length of corresponding bones.
4. Obvious deformities.
5. Swelling.
6. Discoloration.
7. Pain or tenderness to touch.
◆ C. First aid measures.
1. Prevent motion of injured parts and adjacent joints.
2. Elevate involved extremities.
3. Apply splints.
   D. Splinting—device used to immobilize extremity or trunk when a fracture is suspected.

1. Purpose.
   a. Immobilize part.
   b. Decrease pain.
   c. Reduce chance of shock.
   d. Protect against further injury during transportation.
2. Principles.
   a. Ensure splint is long enough to extend past joint on either side of suspected fracture.
   b. Place pad between splint and skin.
   c. Immobilize joints above and below location of suspected fracture.
   d. Apply splint to extremity; do circulation checks to fingers/toes.

See Fractures in Chapter 8.

Sprains

Definition: Injury to a joint ligament or a muscle tendon in region of a joint.
◆ A. Signs and symptoms.
   1. Swelling.
   2. Tenderness.
   3. Pain on motion.
   4. Discoloration.
◆ B. First aid measures.
   1. Do not allow walking if ankle or knee sprained.
   2. Elevate limb above heart level for 24 hours.
   3. Apply ice first 24 hours.
   4. If swelling and pain persist, seek medical attention.
C. Common athletic injuries (even those that require clinical attention) use the formula RICE.
   1. Rest—immobilize injured part.
   2. Ice—apply ice to dull pain and reduce blood flow.
   3. Compression—apply pressure with towel or elastic bandage.
   4. Elevation—for first day or two keep injured area elevated.

Strains

Definition: Injury to a muscle and its facial sheath as a result of overstretching.
◆ A. Signs and symptoms.
   1. Pain on motion.
   2. Discoloration.
   3. Edema.
   4. Decrease in function.
B. First aid measures.
   1. Bedrest.
   2. Ice, then after the acute phase (24+ hours), heat may be applied.
   3. Bed board (with back sprain).
   4. Elastic wrap.

Dislocations

Definition: Injury to capsule and ligaments of a joint that results in displacement of a bone end at a joint.
◆ A. Signs and symptoms.
   1. Swelling.
   2. Obvious deformity.
   3. Pain upon motion.
   4. Tenderness to touch.
   5. Discoloration.
B. First aid measures.
   1. Splint and immobilize affected joint in position as found.
   2. Do not reduce dislocation or correct deformity near a joint.
   3. Apply sling if appropriate.
   4. Elevate affected part if possible.

SHOCK STATES

Definition: A syndrome in which there is insufficient circulating blood volume for the size of the vascular bed, thereby resulting in inadequate tissue perfusion and impaired cellular metabolism.

Classifications of Shock States

A. Low blood flow states.
   ◆ 1. Hypovolemic shock.
      a. Absolute hypovolemia—lowered intravascular volume.
         (1) Blood loss—from trauma, surgery, etc., is most common cause.
         (2) Plasma loss from burns; fluid loss from diarrhea, vomiting, etc.
      b. Relative hypovolemia—shift of fluid volume out of vascular space into extravascular space.
         (1) Etiology: pooling of fluids.
         (2) Internal bleeding or massive vasodilation.
   ◆ 2. Cardiogenic shock.
      a. Myocardial dysfunction that results in compromised cardiac output.
      b. Causes.
         (1) Systolic dysfunction: inability to pump blood forward.
         (2) Diastolic dysfunction: ventricles unable to adequately fill (cardiac tamponade).
         (3) Arrhythmias.
         (4) Structural abnormalities (valvular stenosis or regurgitation).
◆ B. Maldistribution of blood flow.

CLINICAL SIGNS OF BLOOD LOSS

Less than 1000 mL loss
- Blood pressure normal
- Heart rate normal
- Respiratory rate normal
- Capillary refill time normal
- No mental status changes

1000 to 2000 mL loss
- Blood pressure 70–90 mm Hg systolic
- Heart rate—more than 120 beats/min
- Cool, pale skin
- Respiratory rate increased
- Mental status changes

More than 2000 mL loss
- Blood pressure—less than 90 mm Hg systolic
- Heart rate—more than 140 beats/min
- Cold, clammy skin
- Respiratory rate increased—hyperventilation
- Mental staus confused

---

1. Distribution shock is caused by massive vasodilation and pooling of blood.
2. Types of distributive shock include septic, neurogenic, and anaphylactic shock.
3. Results in decreased cardiac output.

Hypovolemic Shock

✦ **Characteristics—Stages of Shock**

A. Initial—15 percent volume loss: no signs/symptoms; body begins to respond to imbalance of O_2 supply and demand.

B. Compensatory or second stage—volume loss increases from 15 percent to 30 percent: body activates mechanisms to maintain homeostasis. Clinical symptoms manifest.

C. Progressive or third stage—30 percent to 40 percent blood loss: as the compensatory mechanisms fail, requires immediate interventions. Decreased perfusion and altered cellular permeability.

D. Refractory—more than 40 percent volume loss: profound hypotension and hypoxemia; life-threatening.

E. If victim remains in shock, it will lead to death of cells, tissue, and organs.
   1. Body initially compensates for blood loss—check signs carefully.
   2. Continually evaluate client's condition.

Assessment

✦ A. Assess for early signs due to
   1. Anxiety, thirst, postural changes in vital signs.
   2. Tachycardia, tachypnea, narrow pulse pressure.
   3. Increased sympathetic nervous system activity.

B. Observe for signs/symptoms of shock.
   1. Rapid, shallow breathing.
   2. Cold, pale skin (capillary refill > 2/second).
   3. Failure to respond to simple commands.

✦ C. Observe for oliguria.
   1. Kidneys normally receive 20 percent of cardiac output, so if urine volume drops acutely, assume cardiac output has dropped.
   2. If urine output falls below 30 mL/hr, notify physician immediately.

✦ D. Note Kussmaul breathing—as blood pH is lowered, the respiratory rate increases in an effort to blow off excess carbon dioxide and return body to acid–base balance.

E. Assess if cool, dry, or moist skin is present.
   1. Caused by peripheral vasoconstriction.
   2. Blood is diverted to vital organs rather than to skin.

F. Observe sensorium changes—due to brain hypoperfusion.
   1. Restlessness/anxiety.
   2. Lethargy.
   3. Confusion.

G. Note fatigue and muscle weakness—result of shift from aerobic to anaerobic metabolism leading to lactic acid buildup.

✦ H. Assess for severe shock
   1. Blood pressure—systolic below 80 mm Hg and narrowing of pulse pressure to 20 mm Hg or below (body loses ability to compensate and blood pressure drops rapidly).
   2. Shallow, irregular respirations.
   3. Sustained tachycardia.
   4. Level of unconsciousness; progresses to coma as blood supply to brain decreases.
   5. Dilated, fixed pupils due to brain hypoxia.
   6. Anuria as perfusion to kidneys decreases sharply.
   7. Cyanotic skin, mucous membranes, and nailbeds—indicates poor prognosis.

Implementation

A. Treat the cause of shock (stop bleeding).

✦ B. Maintain open airway—provide oxygen via mask or cannula—monitor pulse oximetry.

✦ C. Administer fluids to treat shock state.
   1. First-line treatment is crystalloids (isotonic fluids).
   2. Prepare client for IV fluid, colloids–plasma expanders, blood replacement.

✦ D. Place client in supine position with legs elevated (6–10 inches), head on pillow.

✦ E. Insert Foley catheter for hourly urine monitoring.
   1. Record intake and output.

2. Notify physician if urine output is less than 30 mL/hr.

✦ F. Record vital signs every 15 minutes.
1. Blood pressure.
   a. Orthostatic hypotension develops before systemic hypotension.
   b. Decreased BP is usually late sign of shock.
   c. Progressive drop in BP (SBP < 90 mm Hg) with a thready, increasing pulse indicates hypovolemia.
2. Respirations.
   a. Rapid early in shock (compensation for tissue hypoxia).
   b. Emergency equipment for intubation/ventilator should be available.
3. Central venous pressure.
   a. CVP reflects volume status (preload).
   b. If below 5 cm H_2O, indicates hypovolemia.
G. Monitor client responses.
1. Change in skin temperature and color reflect changes in tissue oxygenation and perfusion.
   a. Cold, clammy, pale skin indicates peripheral vascular constriction.
   b. Pallor and cyanosis indicate tissue hypoxia.
2. Restlessness indicates cerebral hypoxia.
3. Assess for improvement in vital signs.
H. Maintain body temperature.
I. Avoid rough or excessive handling.
J. Do not allow client to eat or drink.

Cardiogenic Shock

Characteristics

A. *Definition:* Myocardial dysfunction that results in reduced cardiac output and compromised tissue perfusion.
1. Systolic dysfunction: inability to pump blood forward (MI).
2. Diastolic dysfunction: ventricles are unable to adequately fill (cardiac tamponade).
B. Causes.
1. Decrease in cardiac output—loss of myocardial contractility.
2. Most common cause is myocardial infarction with greater than 40 percent muscle necrosis.
✦ C. Pathophysiology.
1. Decreased cardiac output causes sympathetic nervous system stimulation, which produces vasoconstriction and inadequate tissue perfusion, resulting in anaerobic metabolism.
   a. Result is increased lactate.
   b. Increased lactate causes metabolic acidosis.
2. Decreased cerebral perfusion.
3. Decreased renal perfusion, resulting in decreased urine production.

Assessment

✦ A. Differentiate from hypovolemic shock.
1. Pulmonary capillary wedge pressure and CVP are increased in cardiogenic shock.
2. Pulmonary capillary wedge pressure and CVP are low in hypovolemic shock.
B. Hypotension (less than 90 mm Hg, or 300 mm Hg less than client's normal BP) and a low cardiac index (< 2.2 L/min/m^2) are classic signs of shock.
✦ C. Measure urinary output. May be less than 30 mL/hr due to poor renal perfusion (oliguria).
✦ D. Assess for signs and symptoms of decreased cardiac output.
1. Pallor or cyanosis.
2. Hypoxia (decreased PO_2).
3. Orthopnea.
4. Dyspnea.
5. Dependent pitting edema.
6. Distended neck veins.
7. Pulmonary congestion.
8. Cool, pale, moist skin.
9. Decreased orientation, fatigue.
10. Tachycardia; arrhythmias.
E. Assess for acidemia—decreased pH of the blood.

Implementation

✦ A. Oxygen therapy or mechanical ventilation to increase PO_2, decrease work of breathing.
B. Monitor medications.
1. Diuretics for pulmonary congestion.
2. Morphine sulfate for pain; vasopressors for hypotension unresponsive to fluid therapy.
3. Vasodilators (nitroglycerin) or nipride to decrease ventricular afterload.
4. Dobutamine—causes less vasoconstriction and tachycardia and may be ordered following stabilization of blood pressure.
C. Intra-aortic balloon pump (IABP) is used for internal counterpulsation.
1. Regular inflation and deflation of the balloon augments pumping action of the heart.
2. Hemodynamic monitoring is important to monitor status of client.
D. Establish fluid and electrolyte acid–base balance.
1. Replace fluid if hypovolemic.
2. Correct acidosis (improve cardiac output).
3. Maintain urinary output—greater than 30 mL/hr.
E. Control pain and restlessness by IV analgesia.
F. Treat arrhythmias—result of hypoxia, acidosis, electrolyte imbalance, underlying disease, and drug therapy.
G. Decrease cardiac workload.
1. Physical and emotional rest.
2. Psychological support.

3. Comfortable position—flat with pillow, or semi-Fowler's position if client has difficulty breathing.

DISTRIBUTIVE (VASOGENIC) SHOCK

Definition: Three types—septic, neurogenic, and anaphylactic. In all three, shock occurs as a result of vasodilation and abnormal distribution of fluids within the circulatory system.

Septic Shock

Characteristics

✦ A. Most common type of distributive shock—caused by infection (gram-negative or gram-positive bacteria).

✦ B. Progresses to bacteremia—bacteria enter bloodstream directly from site of infection or from toxic substances released by bacteria into the bloodstream.

C. Nonspecific inflammatory response and specific immune responses initiated with release of biochemical mediators.
   1. Secondary mediators cause release of proinflammatory cytokines.
   2. Cytokines cause endothelial cell damage and multiple organ dysfunction.

✦ D. Usually occurs in two phases.
   1. *Phase 1:* high cardiac output with vasodilation. Client is overheated and demonstrates warm, flushed skin.
   2. *Phase 2:* low cardiac output with vasoconstriction. Blood pressure drops; skin is cool and pale.

E. Multiple-organ dysfunction syndrome (MODS)—mortality rate high—40% (sepsis is 11th highest cause of death in United States).

Assessment

✦ A. Phase 1—may appear to be mild infection.
   1. Vital signs and mental confusion may be first sign with increased heart rate or increased respiratory rate.
   2. Assess for flushed, pink face warm to the touch; dry skin.
   3. Observe for low blood pressure and pulse.
   4. Check results of complete blood count—blood culture to determine organism.

✦ B. Phase 2.
   1. Assess for tachycardia; blood pressure decreases; PO_2 is dropping.
   2. Does not appear pink and warm—cool skin.
   3. Observe for tachypnea.
   4. Assess urine output—may drop to 30 mL per hour.
   5. Assess for thirst.

Implementation

A. Goal of treatment for septic, neurogenic, and anaphylactic shock includes hemodynamic support.
   1. Fluid replacement (and blood products).
   2. Vasopressors and inotropes.
      a. Inotropic drugs (dopamine)—if tissue perfusion is inadequate.
      b. Norepinephrine (Levophed)—potent vasoconstrictor if dopamine does not raise mean arterial blood pressure.
      c. Naloxone (Narcan)—may be ordered to treat gram-negative septic shock; attacks bacterial endotoxin that causes cellular destruction.

✦ B. Administer broad-spectrum antibiotics as ordered—begin STAT (do not wait for regular medication times).
   1. Continue to check IV site frequently—if evidence of infection, restart IV in a new site.
   2. Check BUN level regularly.

C. Administer activated drotrecogin alfa (Xigris), a recombinant form of activated protein c.
   1. Drug will combat inflammation to altered coagulation; interrupts body's response to severe sepsis, including bleeding and clotting.
   2. Should be used early in beginning of organ system dysfunction.

✦ D. Administer oxygen as ordered (mechanical ventilation)—concentration should be moderate; pulse oximeter reading useful for SaO_2.

✦ E. Take vital signs hourly. Stages can progress rapidly.

F. Observe continually for change in pattern: blood pressure down, pulse and respirations up. Notify physician immediately.

✦ G. Check PO_2 and pH—client may go into metabolic acidosis. Notify physician if pH falls below 7.35.

H. Give frequent skin care and perfusion to prevent breakdown.

✦ I. Check I&O frequently; pay attention to amount of urine from catheter.
   1. If urine output falls below 30 mL/hr, notify physician immediately.
   2. Prevent fluid overload by calculating previous hourly urine output plus 30 mL/hr.

J. Provide appropriate psychological support.
   1. Client is frightened, so remain in the room.
   2. Explain all procedures and attempt to alleviate anxiety.

K. Observe for complications or reversal in improvement of shock state.
   1. Respiratory: dyspnea, cyanosis, intercostal retractions (shock lung).
   2. Cardiac: heart failure—may require digitalis.
   3. Renal: oliguria—may require mannitol.

Neurogenic (Spinal) Shock

Definition: Massive vasodilation and pooling of blood due to failure of peripheral vessels; imbalance of parasympathetic/sympathetic vascular tone (*also see* Spinal Cord Injury, page 183).

Characteristics

A. Interference with sympathetic nervous system (head injury).
B. Injury to spinal cord or as a result of spinal anesthesia.
C. Severe pain, drugs, or hypoglycemia causing vaso-motor center depression.

Assessment

A. Assess for hypoglycemia, bradycardia or hypothermia.
B. Assess vital signs; hypotension.
C. Loss of reflex activity in spinal cord below injury level (areflexia).
D. Paralytic ileus.

Implementation

A. Monitor airway, breathing, circulation (ABC) mea-sures (hypotension, bradycardia).
B. Fluid resuscitation to increase blood pressure.
C. Monitor vasoconstrictors to increase blood pressure.
D. Monitor atropine-like drugs to block vagal effects causing bradycardia.
E. If hypothermia present, requires warming measures.

Anaphylactic Shock

Characteristics

✦ A. A whole-body allergic reaction caused by hypersen-sitivity to allergen (allergic reaction to medication, bee sting, etc.).
B. Antigen–antibody reaction.
C. Increased cell membrane permeability—histamine is released, causing marked vasodilatation.
D. Bronchiolar constriction and hypoxia.
E. Pooling of blood, causing decreased venous return.
F. Decreased cardiac output and hypoxia.

Assessment

✦ A. Assess for dyspnea, respiratory difficulty, cyanosis, wheezing (can be life-threatening).
✦ B. Observe for vertigo, decreased blood pressure, increased pulse.
C. Evaluate local edema, skin rash, flushing, urticaria (occasional), and restlessness.
D. Evaluate if apprehension is present.

Implementation

✦ A. Goal is ABC—maintain patent airway, breathing, circulation.
B. Identify causative agent.

✦ C. Position client for optimal cerebral perfusion (flat or 30-degree elevation if dyspneic).
✦ D. Administer epinephrine subcutaneously.
   1. Dilates bronchioles and constricts arterioles.
   2. Side effects: tachycardia, CNS stimulation.
   3. Rapid acting.
E. Administer oxygen.
F. Administer antihistamine (Benadryl).
   1. Relieves itching, wheals, congestion of nasal mucosa.
   2. Side effect: dries mucous membranes.
G. Maintain IV of NS or lactated Ringer's to support perfusion.
H. Administer corticosteroids—reduce formation of cellular proteins and decrease edema.
I. Administer aminophylline—bronchodilator; con-trols bronchospasms.

Snake Bite

Assessment

A. Assess extent of envenomation.
   1. Rattlesnakes, copperheads, cottonmouths (pit vipers) are responsible for 98 percent of venomous bites.
      a. Pit vipor venom is hemolytic.
      b. Coral snake venom is neurotoxic.
   2. Reactions to poisonous snakes occur within 5–15 minutes.
   ✦ 3. Signs.
      a. One or two distinct puncture wounds, fang marks.
      b. Burning pain.
      c. Edema and erythema.
      d. Serosanguineous fluid oozing from wound.
      e. Numbness around bite within 5–15 min-utes.
B. Assess systemic signs.
   1. Diaphoresis, chills.
   2. Anxiety.
   3. Tachycardia, hypotension.
   4. Temperature elevation.
   5. Tingling of tongue, rubber or metal taste.
   6. Visual disturbance; seizure.
   7. Nausea/vomiting.
   8. Dizziness.
   9. Muscle fasciculations.
   10. GI bleeding.
   11. Respiratory problems.

Implementation

✦ A. Emergency treatment: seek medical help immediately.
   1. Immobilize area with support or sling and posi-tion below heart.
   2. Remove constrictive clothing or jewelry.

3. Do not apply a tourniquet or ice.
4. Do not allow client to physically exert self, as this hastens spread of venom. Keep client still.
5. Do not incise area or apply suction.

B. In-hospital treatment.
   1. Skin test for sensitivity to horse serum.
   2. Administer prescribed antivenin intravenously.
      a. Dilute antivenin dose in saline (250–500 mL).
      b. Dose based on severity of envenomation.
      c. Have epinephrine available in case of allergic reaction.
   3. Monitor vital signs.
   4. Monitor for decreased swelling.
   5. Monitor blood coagulation studies.
   6. Type and cross-match blood.
   7. Administer analgesics for pain.
      a. ASA for mild pain.
      b. Codeine or Demerol for severe pain.
   8. Administer antibiotics.
      a. Initial dose: ampicillin, erythromycin, or tetracycline 500 mg.
      b. Maintain 250 mg every 4 hours for 24 hours.

C. Monitor for complications.
   1. Respiratory arrest due to neurotoxin.
   2. Acute renal failure due to hemolysis.
   3. Disseminated intravascular coagulation (DIC).
   4. Compartment syndrome; gangrene.
   5. Infection.
   6. Delayed serum sickness.

Bee Sting

Assessment

A. Tightness in chest, difficulty swallowing or breathing.
B. Generalized swelling and itching.
C. Erythema and hives.
D. Feeling of heat throughout body.
E. Weakness, vertigo.
F. Nausea, vomiting, abdominal cramps.

Implementation

✦ A. Remove stinger with tweezers or by scraping motion with fingernail. Do not squeeze venom sac.
B. Cleanse sting area and apply ice to relieve pain and edema.
✦ C. Observe for signs of laryngospasm or bronchospasm. Be prepared to assist with a tracheostomy.
D. Keep client warm and positioned supine with head and feet slightly elevated.
✦ E. For client going into full-blown anaphylactic shock, implement following orders.
   ✦ 1. Immediately administer epinephrine 1:1000 solution sub q.

a. Adult: 0.25–0.3 mL at sting site and same amount in unaffected arm.
b. Child: 0.01 mL/kg (maximum 0.25 mL at each site).

2. Repeat injections one to three times at 20-minute intervals until blood pressure and pulse rise toward normal.
   a. Adult: 0.3–0.4 mL.
   b. Child: less than 20 kg, 0.10–0.15 mL; over 20 kg, 0.15–0.3 mL.
3. Administer pressor agents if blood pressure does not stabilize following 2–3 sub q injections of epinephrine.
   a. Aramine and Levophed are drugs of choice.
   b. Administer IV drip at 30–40 drops/min.
4. Begin IV solution of D_5W with 250 mg aminophylline and 30–40 mg Solu-Cortef to support circulation and prevent shock.
5. Administer rapid-acting antihistamine: Benadryl 50 mg IM.

CARDIOPULMONARY RESUSCITATION (CPR)

Indications

A. Respiratory arrest with pulse present—establish airway, breathing.
B. Cardiac arrest with ineffective breathing.
C. No movement or response.

Assessment and Actions

✦ A. Determine unresponsiveness—"Are you okay?"
✦ B. Call for help (911 or emergency number); get AED.
C. Position supine on firm surface.
✦ D. Establish airway; check breathing.
   1. Kneel beside victim's shoulders.
   2. Open airway—head-tilt/chin-lift maneuver.
   3. Look, listen, and feel.
   4. If not breathing, give two rescue breaths, each over 1 second with enough volume to produce a visible rise of the chest.
   5. Observe for chest rising. If not, reposition head.
   6. Perform rescue breathing.

E. **American Heart Association current CPR guidelines.**
   1. If no pulse, use 30 compressions for every 2 rescue breaths until AED arrives.
   ✦ 2. Use harder and faster chest compressions (100 times/minute), allowing chest to recoil after each compression.
   3. Check for pulse—if no pulse present, immediately attach AED if available.

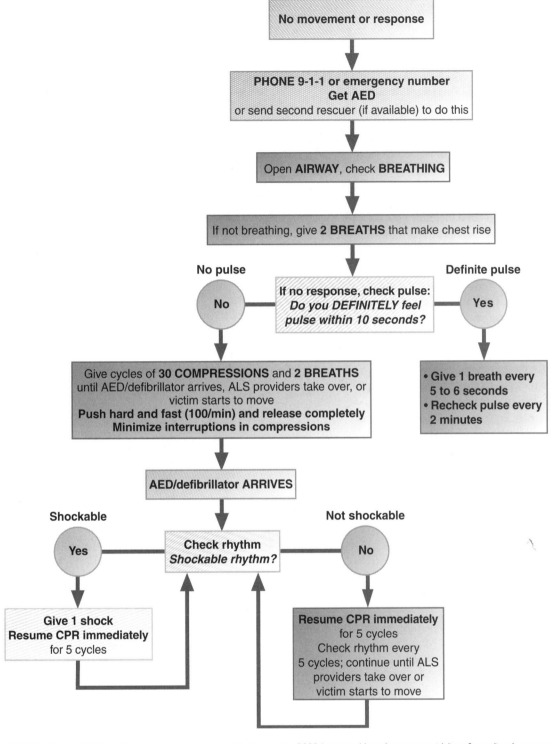

F. Steps of compression (if AED not available) for CPR.

1. Heel of hand on lower half of sternum.
2. Other hand on top—hands parallel—may interlace fingers, but keep fingers off chest.
3. Straighten arms and lock elbows—shoulders directly over hands so thrust is straight down on sternum.
4. Depress sternum 1.5–2 inches (compressions and release of equal duration).

PERFORMING RESCUE BREATHING

- Pinch nose with thumb of hand on forehead.
- Take deep breath and seal your lips around victim's mouth—airtight seal.
- Give two slow breaths (1.5–2 seconds each).
- Observe that each ventilation causes chest to rise and fall, and hear and feel exhalation.
- Check carotid pulse for 5–10 seconds.
- Continue rescue breaths if pulse is present.
- If no pulse, begin CPR.

UNIVERSAL STEPS OF AED OPERATION

1. Open AED, which automatically turns on power. If not, press power button on. Once power is on, AED will direct you through the steps.
2. Remove clothing from chest. Dry chest.
3. Attach AED to victim's chest with electrode pads.
4. "Snap" on connecting cables to adhesive electrode pads.
5. Stop CPR. Do not touch victim.
6. Analyze rhythm.
7. Loudly state, "Stand clear of victim."
8. Give one shock (if shock is indicated).
9. Begin CPR for 5 cycles or 2 minutes.
10. Analyze and repeat shock and CPR.
11. Check for presence of pulse.
12. Follow protocol for rescue breathing.

---

5. Release pressure between compressions, but do not lift hands from chest or change position.
6. Provide chest compressions at 100/minute. Recommend a one-syllable mnemonic: e.g., first 15 letters of the alphabet, "a, b, c, d, ... m, n, OFF."
7. Check for carotid pulse after one minute of compressions—if absent, continue CPR.
8. Stop and check for return of pulse and spontaneous breathing every few minutes.

G. Termination of CPR.
  1. Successful resuscitation.
     a. Spontaneous return of adequate life support.
     b. Assisted life support.
  2. Transfer to emergency vehicle (other trained rescuers assume care).
  3. Pronounced dead by physician.
  4. Exhaustion of rescuer(s).

Using an AED

A. Initial steps.
  1. Place AED near victim's left ear.
  2. Open AED, turn on power switch and lift monitor screen up.
  3. Open defibrillatory pads and connect to cables and to victim's chest.
  4. Stop CPR (if second rescuer performing).
  5. Shout, "Stand clear."
B. Check rhythm.
  1. Shockable rhythm—give 1 shock, resume CPR immediately for 5 cycles.

2. Not shockable rhythm—resume CPR immediately for 5 cycles.
3. Check rhythm every 5 cycles and continue until ALS provider takes over or victim moves.

Heimlich Maneuver

A. Airway obstruction management.
  1. Victim standing or sitting.
     a. Make fist with one hand.
     b. Place thumb side of fist against victim's abdomen, between umbilicus and xiphoid process.
     c. Grasp fist with other hand and press fist into victim's abdomen with quick upward thrust.
     d. Repeat thrusts until object expelled from victim's airway.
  2. Victim lying down.
     a. Place victim supine.
     b. Kneel astride victim's thighs and place heel of one hand against victim's abdomen (between xiphoid process and umbilicus).
     c. Place other hand on top of first.
     d. Press into abdomen with quick upward thrust.

Table 10-1. AMERICAN HEART ASSOCIATION SUMMARY OF BLS ABCD MANEUVERS FOR INFANTS, CHILDREN AND ADULTS (NEWBORN INFORMATION NOT INCLUDED)			
Maneuver	**Adult** (Adolescent and Older)	**Child** (1 Year to Adolescent)	**Infant** (Younger Than 1 Year of Age)
Airway	Head-tilt/chin-lift (suspected trauma, use jaw thrust)		
Breathing Initial	2 breaths at 1 second/breath	2 effective breaths at 1 second/breath	
HCP: Rescue breathing without chest compressions	10 to 12 breaths/min (approximate)	12 to 20 breaths/min (approximate)	
HCP: Rescue breaths for CPR with advanced airway	8 to 10 breaths/min (approximately)		
Foreign-body airway obstruction	Abdominal thrusts		Back slaps and chest thrusts
Circulation **HCP:** Pulse check ($\leq$ 10 seconds)	Carotid		Brachial or femoral
Compression landmarks	Lower half of sternum, between nipples		Just below nipple line (lower half of sternum)
Compression method: Push hard and fast, allow complete recoil	Heel of one hand, other hand on top	Heel of one hand or as for adults	2 or 3 fingers (2 rescuers): 2 thumb-encircling hands
Compression depth	1½ to 2 inches	Approximately one-third to one-half the depth of the chest	
Compression rate	Approximately 100/min		
Compression–ventilation ratio	30:2 (one or two rescuers)	30:2 (single rescuer), 15:2 (2 rescuers)	
Debfibrillation AED	Use adult pads	Use AED after 5 cycles of CPR (out of hospital) Use child pads for child 1 to 8 years if available **HCP: For sudden collapse (out of hospital) or in-hospital arrest, use AED as soon as available.**	No recommendation for infants < 1 year of age

Note: Maneuvers used by only healthcare providers are indicated by "HCP."

Source: Handbook of emergency cardiovascular care, Guidelines CPR/ECC 2005, p. 1. American Heart Association.

EMERGENCY NURSING REVIEW QUESTIONS

1. On duty in the emergency room, the nurse is concerned when a client continues to bleed from severe lacerations even after applying direct pressure. The next action is to

   1. Apply ice to lower the body temperature.
   2. Monitor closely for signs of shock.
   3. Elevate the upper extremities and apply blankets to raise body temperature.
   4. Maintain a patent airway and prevent vomiting.

2. A client enters the emergency department complaining of severe chest pain. A myocardial infarction is suspected. A 12-lead ECG appears normal, but the doctor admits the client for further testing until cardiac enzyme studies are returned. All of the following will be included in the nursing care plan. Which activity has highest priority?

   1. Monitoring vital signs.
   2. Completing a physical assessment.
   3. Maintaining cardiac monitoring.
   4. Maintaining at least one IV access site.

3. A client enters the emergency department complaining of chest pressure and severe epigastric distress. His vital signs are BP 158/90, P 94, R 24, and T 99°F. The doctor orders cardiac enzyme studies. If this client were diagnosed with a myocardial infarction, the nurse would expect which cardiac enzyme to rise within the next 2 to 3 hours?

   1. Creatine kinase (CK)—3 to 8 hours.
   2. Lactic dehydrogenase (LDH)—24–48 hours.
   3. Troponins—3–6 hours.
   4. Myoglobins—2–3 hours.

4. The nurse knows that the most informative measurement for determining cardiogenic shock is

   1. Arterial blood pressure.
   2. Central venous pressure.
   3. Pulmonary artery pressure.
   4. Cardiac output index.

5. A 35-year-old male was knifed in a street fight, was admitted through the emergency room, and is now in the ICU. An assessment of his condition reveals the following symptoms: respirations shallow and rapid, paradoxical pulse, CVP 15 cm H_2O, BP 90 mm Hg

systolic, skin cold and pale, urinary output 60–100 mL/hr for the last 2 hours. Analyzing these symptoms, the nurse will base a nursing diagnosis on the conclusion that the client has which one of the following conditions?

   1. Hypovolemic shock.
   2. Cardiac tamponade.
   3. Wound dehiscence.
   4. Atelectasis.

6. CPR cannot prevent possible brain damage unless initiated within _____ minutes of an arrest.

7. You enter a client's room and find him unresponsive. What is your first action?

   1. Call for an AED.
   2. Assess the client's respiratory and pulse status.
   3. Deliver four back blows to the client.
   4. Finger probe for a possible obstruction.

8. What is the second nursing action when the client remains unresponsive, as described in question 7?

   1. Call for help and retrieve an AED.
   2. Start CPR.
   3. Administer rescue breathing.
   4. Check carotid pulse.

9. For a client who has just been stung by a bee and has gone into anaphylactic shock, what is the priority assessment?

   1. Observe for vertigo.
   2. Evaluate for local edema.
   3. Assess for dyspnea or respiratory difficulty.
   4. Check for skin rash.

10. When circumstances require first aid care to several people at once, what is a priority action?

   1. Make rapid initial evaluation of the victims.
   2. Enlist other persons in the area to help.
   3. Call 911 or an emergency number.
   4. Improvise—decide on what material is available.

11. An earthquake has just occurred and the hospital has sustained a great deal of damage. The first action is to

1. Call for help for the clients who are the most critical.
2. Find the disaster instructions posted on every unit in the hospital and follow instructions.
3. Return to the central staff room for instructions.
4. Wait until you receive instructions.

12. If medical care is not available and someone is injured, the first nursing intervention should be to

1. Determine the priority action.
2. Call 911 or an emergency number.
3. Don't get involved because of legal ramifications.
4. Improvise—make do according to the circumstances.

13. A 6-year-old child is brought into the emergency department with a jellyfish sting on his leg. He is screaming with pain. The first emergency intervention is to

1. Bathe the lesion in vinegar and apply shaving cream.
2. Bathe the area with fresh water.
3. Administer an antihistamine as ordered.
4. Administer a tetanus shot, as ordered.

14. A female client comes to the emergency room. The nurse's immediate assessment reveals that the client is bleeding profusely from a deep laceration on her left lower forearm. The first action is to

1. Apply a tourniquet just below the elbow.
2. Apply pressure directly over the wound.
3. Call for the physician to check the wound.
4. Place the client in shock position.

15. The first maneuver for the nurse to use when checking for airway obstruction is to

1. Tilt the head and lift the chin.
2. Attempt to ventilate.
3. Turn the client to the side.
4. Do a jaw thrust.

16. The intervention that can best establish whether a client is unconscious is by observing the client's response to

1. Verbal stimuli.
2. Light in the eyes.
3. Pinching the earlobe.
4. Opening the airway.

17. Administering care to a client in hypovolemic shock, the sign that the nurse would expect to observe is

1. Hypertension.

2. Cyanosis.
3. Oliguria.
4. Tachypnea.

18. When a client experiences a severe anaphylactic reaction to a medication, the nurse's initial action is to

1. Start an IV (standard orders)
2. Assess vital signs.
3. Place the client in a supine position.
4. Prepare equipment for intubation.

19. A client has burns on the front and back of both his legs and arms. The approximate percentage of his body that has been involved is

1. 27 percent.
2. 36 percent.
3. 45 percent.
4. 54 percent.

20. While assessing a client who is being treated with a heating pad or hot compress, the first sign of possible thermal injury is

1. Tingling sensation in the extremities.
2. Redness in the area.
3. Edema.
4. Pain.

21. Proper depth of compressions for an infant (under 12 months) who is receiving CPR would be

1. ⅓ to ½ depth of chest.
2. ¼ to ¾ inch.
3. 1 to 1½ inches.
4. 1½ to 2 inches.

22. A systolic blood pressure of 60 mm Hg or less would indicate shock in which of the following client age groups?

1. 5 years old or younger.
2. 5 to 12 years old.
3. 12 to 16 years old.
4. 16 to 20 years old.

23. The nurse assessing a client for shock observes that the earliest symptom of shock is

1. Hypertension.
2. Increased urine output.
3. Narrowing pulse pressure.
4. Warm, moist skin.

24. A 20-year-old female client is admitted in a comatose state to the emergency room. Her vital signs are BP

140/80, P 110, R 30 and labored. A Medic-Alert bracelet indicates that she is a diabetic. If the nurse were assessing her for ketoacidosis, one significant symptom would be

1. Oliguria.
2. Acetone odor to breath.
3. Kussmaul breathing.
4. Sensorium change.

25. When caring for an unconscious client, the nurse's primary concern must always be

1. Airway protection and adequate respiratory status.
2. Decreasing intracranial pressure.
3. Fluid balance and cardiac stability.
4. Maintaining range of motion and muscle tone.

EMERGENCY NURSING

Answers with Rationale

1. (2) Blood loss results in shock; therefore, close monitoring of vital signs and shock symptoms is essential. Applying ice (1) would not be appropriate. With hemorrhage, the temperature will be below normal, but should be monitored.

    NP:I; CN:PH; CA:M; CL:A

2. (3) Even though initial tests seem to be within normal range, it takes at least 3 hours for the cardiac enzyme studies to register. In the meantime, the client needs to be watched for bradycardia, tachycardia, heart block, ventricular irritability, and other arrhythmias. The other activities can be accomplished around the MI monitoring.

    NP:AN; CN:PH; CA:M; CL:AN

3. (1) Creatine kinase (CK, formerly called CPK) rises in 3–8 hours if an MI is present. When the myocardium is damaged, CK leaks out of the cell membranes and into the bloodstream. Lactic dehydrogenase rises in 24–48 hours, and LDH-1 and LDH-2 rise in 8–24 hours.

    NP:P; CN:PH; CA:M; CL:A

4. (4) The cardiac output is that amount of blood pumped by the left ventricle each minute. It is a good indicator of left ventricular function. As the left ventricle fails, the pressure in the chamber rises. Then the arterial blood pressure falls. The CVP would increase later when peripheral flow is impeded into the right atrium due to pulmonary congestion.

    NP:P; CN:PH; CA:M; CL:C

5. (2) All of the client's symptoms are found in both cardiac tamponade and hypovolemic shock except the increase in urinary output. In shock, urinary output decreases to less than 30 mL/hr; thus this is the symptom that would distinguish hypovolemic shock

    from cardiac tamponade and form the basis for a nursing diagnosis.

    NP:AN; CN:PH; CA:M; CL:C

6. CPR should be initiated within 3 minutes, because after 4 minutes, there may be brain damage because of lack of O_2 getting to the brain.

    NP:AN; CN:S; CA:M; CL:K

7. (2) An immediate assessment is needed, so the first action is to see if the client is breathing by observing for rise and fall of the chest. The remaining answers are incorrect.

    NP:I; CN:S; CA:M, CL:A

8. (1) After finding a client unresponsive, the first action is to call for help and retrieve the AED, because AEDs should be used as soon as possible. CPR should then be started with rescue breathing.

    NP:I; CN:S; CA:M; CL:AN

9. (3) The priority assessment is respiratory difficulty because this condition can be life-threatening and requires an immediate intervention. The other assessments are important and are present with this condition, but may not be life-threatening, unless the throat is swelling.

    NP:A; CN:S; CA:M; CL:A

10. (1) A priority is to quickly evaluate victims to determine which victim is most seriously injured so that first aid can be administered. The other actions would follow answer 1.

    NP:I; CN:S; CA:M; CL:AN

11. (2) The first action is to follow instructions posted in the Disaster Planning poster. If everyone follows these guidelines, there will be less confusion and clients will

Coding for Questions/Answers Abbreviations: **Nursing Process: NP,** Assessment: A, Analysis: AN, Planning: P, Implementation: I, Evaluation: E; **Client Needs: CN,** Safe, Effective Care Environment: S, Health Promotion and Maintenance: H, Psychosocial Integrity: PS, Physiological Integrity: PH; **Clinical Area: CA,** Medical Nursing: M, Surgical Nursing: S, Maternal/Newborn Nursing: MA, Pediatric Nursing: P, Psychiatric Nursing: PS; **Cognitive Level: CL,** Knowledge: K, Comprehension: C, Application: A, Analysis: AN.

receive the care they require. The other options would all follow the first action.

NP:I; CN:S; CA:M; CL:AN

12. (1) Setting the priority is the first action; if a person is bleeding, then stopping the bleeding is a critical action that could save a life. Calling for help or calling 911 (2) would come after assessing the priorities. It is a professional responsibility to get involved (3) if circumstances are critical. Improvising (4) would also come after setting priorities.

NP:I; CN:S; CA:M; CL:A

13. (1) A standard jellyfish kit contains vinegar and shaving cream. The vinegar is to bathe the lesion to reduce pain, and the cream is applied so that cysts will adhere to the cream and be scraped off. Seawater, not fresh water (2), is used to bathe the lesion because fresh water will cause the cysts to fire. Later, the child may be given an antihistamine (3) if the sting was severe; he would require a tetanus shot (4) only if he were not up-to-date with tetanus.

NP:I; CN:S; CA:M; CL:A

14. (2) The first action is to apply direct pressure to the wound. If the bleeding continues, additional actions must be taken. They include placing the client in a shock position (4) and perhaps applying a tourniquet (1).

NP:I; CN:S; CA:M; CL:A

15. (1) If airway obstruction is suspected, the first action is to tilt the head by pressing backward and lifting the chin. Then, the nurse would attempt to ventilate (2). To open the airway, a jaw thrust (4) is done.

NP:I; CN:S; CA:M; CL:A

16. (1) A client's response (or lack thereof) to verbal stimuli is the best indicator of unconsciousness. An unconscious client's pupils may continue to react to light. Pinching the lobe of the ear (3) offers little in the way of pain stimuli. Opening the airway (4) is not an appropriate stimulus.

NP:A; CN:PH; CA:M; CL:C

17. (3) In shock, there is decreased blood volume through the kidneys. This is evidenced by a decrease in the amount of urine excreted. The body has numerous compensatory mechanisms that assist in keeping the blood pressure normal for a short time.

NP:AN; CN:PH; CA:M; CL:A

18. (3) The shock position is necessary to maintain vital signs. The other interventions would be implemented in order (2), then (1) start an IV and prepare for intubation.

NP:I; CN:S; CA:M; CL:A

19. (4) The client's burns cover approximately 54 percent of his body surface. Each arm is 9 percent (18 percent) and each leg is 18 percent (36 percent).

NP:AN; CN:PH; CA:M; CL:C

20. (2) Redness, or erythema, is the first sign of possible injury. This is an important observation to prevent a burn injury.

NP:A; CN:S; CA:M; CL:A

21. (1) The proper depth of compression for infant and child CPR is $\frac{1}{3}$ to $\frac{1}{2}$ inch. This is done midsternum, using only two fingers or the thumbs, if the chest is encircled by the rescuer's hands. Compression depth for an adult (answer 4) is $1\frac{1}{2}$ to 2 inches.

NP:P; CN:S; CA:M; CL:K

22. (2) A systolic blood pressure of 60 mm Hg or less found in children 5 to 12 years old would indicate shock.

NP:P; CN:S; CA:M; CL:C

23. (3) Narrowing pulse pressure and hypotension are two early signs of shock. Decreased, not increased, urine output is present as well as cool, moist skin caused by vasoconstriction.

NP:AN; CN:S; CA:M; CL:A

24. (2) As acetone is liberated through the breakdown of fat, it is volatile and, therefore, is blown off by the lungs, creating the characteristic fruity odor of the breath. Polyuria (not oliguria), polydipsia, and polyphagia are early symptoms. Kussmaul breathing is a sign of early shock as the body attempts to return to acid–base balance. Sensorium change would occur later.

NP:A; CN:PH; CA:M; CL:A

25. (1) As neurological status deteriorates, the airway must be assured to avoid compromising oxygenation or aspiration. Hypoxia will exacerbate brain injury. The other answers are appropriate goals after airway patency is assured.

NP:I; CN:PH; CA:M; CL:AN

Laboratory Tests 11

✦ The icon denotes content of special importance for NCLEX.

◆ Table 11-1. ROUTINE BLOOD CHEMISTRY TESTS*

Test	Purpose	Normal Values
Erythrocytes		
Red blood cell count (RBC or erythrocytes)	Determines actual number of formed blood elements in relation to volume Identifies abnormalities; monitors RBC count	Males: 4.5–6.2 million/mm^3 Females: 4.0–5.5 million/mm^3 Children: 3.2–5.2 million/mm^3
Hematocrit (HCT)	Measures percentage of red blood cells per fluid volume of whole blood	Males: 40–54/100 mL Females: 37–47/100 mL Children: 29–54/100 mL
Hemoglobin (Hgb)	Measures amount of hemoglobin/100 mL blood to determine oxygen-carrying capacity; assists in diagnosing anemia	Males: above 13–18 g/100 mL Females: above 12–16 g/100 mL
Platelet count	Determines number of platelets	Adults: 150,000–450,000/mm^3
Prothrombin time (PT) (see pages 506 and 507 for INR)	Evaluates thrombin generation or how long it takes for a fibrin clot to form Detects deficiencies in extrinsic clotting mechanism; monitors anticoagulant therapy	10–13 seconds Prolonged values seen in liver disease, vitamin K deficiency, specific drugs, etc.
Activated partial thromboplastin time (APTT)	Evaluates adequacy of plasma-clotting factors—intrinsic clotting mechanism	20–38 seconds Prolonged values indicate coagulation factor deficiency, cirrhosis, vitamin K deficiency
Thrombin time	Screening test to detect abnormalities in thrombin fibrinogen reaction (Conversion to fibrin in stage 3 of clotting sequence)	10–15 seconds
Leukocytes		
White blood cell count (WBC or leukocytes)	Establishes quantity and maturity of white blood cell elements If WBC is abnormal, it is important to learn which of five types is increased or decreased Tests of five WBC types is called a differential	Adults: 4500–11,000/mm^3 Children: 5000–13,000/mm^3 Neutrophils: 3000–7500/mm^3 Band neutrophils: 150–700/mm^3 Basophils: 25–150/mm^3 Eosinophils: 50–450/mm^3 Lymphocytes: 1500–4500/mm^3 Monocytes: 100–800/mm^3
Erythrocyte sedimentation rate (ESR)	Measures rate of red blood cells settling from plasma—reflects inflammatory conditions	*Wintrobe Method* Males: 0–9 mm/hr Females: 0–15 mm/hr Children: 0–13 mm/hr *Westergren Method* Males: 0–15 mm/hr Females: (under 50 years) 0–20 mm/hr; (over 50 years) 0–30 mm/hr Children: 0–20 mm/hr

*Blood chemistry–renal tests change with age—see Gerontological Nursing, Chapter 15.

SERUM ELECTROLYTE LEVELS

Potassium (K⁺)

A. Normal adult range 3.5–5.0 mEq/L. Child range 3.5–5.0 mEq/L.
B. Purpose—test for electrolyte imbalance.
C. Indications.
    1. Increased K⁺—acute renal disease, burns, crushing injuries, adrenal insufficiency, dehydration, anorexia nervosa, excessive intake caused by specific drugs (potassium penicillin), salt substitute, or, the most common, too-rapid infusion of IV solution containing potassium.
    2. Decreased K+—renal loss (due to diuretics), loss from the GI tract via NG tube, vomiting or diarrhea, reduced potassium intake, hypomagnesemia, endocrine causes.
D. Treatment implications.
    1. Critical values may lead to fatal cardiac arrhythmias.
    2. Assess for signs and symptoms of potassium excess or loss (*see* below).
◆ E. *Hyperkalemia.*
    1. Removal of excess potassium per physician's orders.
        a. Administer diuretics if kidney function is adequate.
        b. Administer exchange resins through NG tube or via sodium polystyrene sulfonate (Kayexalate) enema.
        c. Administer hypertonic IV glucose with insulin as ordered—moves potassium back into cells.
        d. Administer sodium bicarbonate—shifts potassium back into cells.
        e. Hemodialysis or peritoneal dialysis.
    2. Nursing considerations.
        a. Restrict potassium intake.
        b. Calcium will counteract negative effects of potassium on the heart.
        c. Frequently check cardiac monitor placed on client with hyperkalemia.
        d. Penicillin in form of potassium should not be administered to clients with hyperkalemia.
◆ F. *Hypokalemia.*
    1. Replacement of lost potassium.
        a. Administer oral potassium, monitor IV infusion of potassium.
        b. Replace no more than 20 mEq of KCl in 1 hour.
    2. Nursing considerations.
        a. Observe ECG monitor if possible to observe for cardiac effect of KCl.
        b. Give foods rich in potassium—bananas, molasses, oranges, raisins, seafood.
        c. Assess for hypokalemia in clients who require frequent NG suctioning.

Sodium (Na⁺)

A. Normal adult range 135–145 mEq/L. Child range 135–145 mEq/L.
B. Purpose—test for deficiency or excess of electrolyte seen in some endocrine disorders and monitor fluid balance in IV electrolyte therapy.
C. Indications.
    1. Increased level is a very high concentration of sodium in the extracellular fluid—dehydration, severe vomiting or diarrhea, decreased water intake, fever, renal failure, and ingestion of sodium chloride.
    2. Decreased level is a very low concentration of sodium in the extracellular fluid—diuretics, excessive perspiration, GI loss (vomiting, diarrhea), lack of sodium in diet, Addison's disease or adrenal insufficiency, burns, and excessive IV solutions without NaCl replacement.
D. Treatment implications.
    1. Assess for signs and symptoms of sodium excess or loss.
    2. Assess for critical levels (< 120 mEq/L or > 155 mEq/L).
◆ E. *Hypernatremia.*
    1. Removal of excess sodium.
        a. Administer salt-free IV solutions (dextrose), monitor for hyponatremia, and administer 0.45% NaCl to prevent hyponatremia.
        b. Restrict sodium in diet.
        c. Discontinue drugs that cause sodium retention.
    2. Nursing considerations.
        a. Weigh daily and record intake and output.
        b. Assess blood pressure level in terms of fluid retention.
◆ F. *Hyponatremia.*
    1. Replacement of lost sodium.
        a. Administer IV fluids with sodium (3% or 5% saline)—monitor venous pressure to prevent circulatory overload.
        b. Restrict water intake—monitor intake and output.
    2. Nursing considerations.
        a. Clients who excrete excess sodium must be advised how to increase sodium intake.
        b. Assist client to identify symptoms of sodium depletion.

Calcium (Ca⁺⁺)

A.   Normal serum level is 4.5–5.8 mEq/L.

B.   Purpose—test for deficit or excess of calcium electrolyte.

C.   Indications.

1.   Increased level—excess of calcium in the extracellular fluid. Excess of vitamin D (from milk), hyperparathyroidism, cancer (neoplasm of parathyroid, multiple myeloma), immobilization, Paget's disease, thyrotoxicosis, acromegaly, specific drugs (thiazide diuretics), and calcium supplements with inadequate assimilation.

2.   Decreased level—deficit of calcium in the extracellular fluid. Vitamin D deficiency, magnesium deficiency, excessive laxatives, malabsorption syndrome, hypothyroidism, chronic renal insufficiency, burns, acute pancreatitis, removal of the parathyroid glands, blood transfusions (over 2000 mL) without calcium supplements, and specific drugs (anticonvulsant therapy).

D.   Treatment implications.

1.   Assess for signs and symptoms of excess or loss of calcium.

2.   Assess for critical levels of calcium (< 7.0 or > 13.5 mg/100 mL). Notify physician immediately.

   a.   Assess for tetany and convulsions indicating hypocalcemia.

   b.   Excess calcium may lead to coma.

✦ E.   *Hypercalcemia.*

1.   Removal of excess calcium.

   a.   Increase fluid intake, which decreases tubular reabsorption of calcium and prevents stone formation.

   b.   Promote calcium excretion (sodium salts IV and diuretics).

2.   Nursing considerations.

   a.   Limit dietary intake of calcium.

   b.   Avoid milk and milk products, which contain high levels of calcium.

✦ F.   *Hypocalcemia.*

1.   Replacement of low levels of calcium.

   a.   Administer calcium gluconate IV or serum albumin if low levels are due to low serum albumin concentration.

   ✦ b.   Monitor for tetany—major symptom of hypocalcemia.

2.   Nursing considerations.

   a.   Monitor by checking for positive Trousseau's test or Chvostek's sign.

   b.   Administer oral calcium supplements and a diet high in calcium (dairy products, bone meal, molasses, yogurt) with vitamin D. Instruct client to take supplements before bed with vitamin C for greater absorption.

Magnesium (Mg⁺⁺)

A.   Normal serum level is 1.5–2.5 mEq/L.

B.   Purpose—test for excess or deficit serum levels of magnesium to evaluate kidney function and metabolic disorders.

C.   Indications.

1.   Increased magnesium—renal insufficiency, severe dehydration, adrenal insufficiency, hypothyroidism, leukemia, overuse of antacids with magnesium (Gelusil), specific drugs.

2.   Decreased magnesium—acute pancreatitis, chronic nephritis, diuretic phase of renal failure, gastric drainage, abnormal loss due to diarrhea, impaired absorption, specific drugs (diuretics), hypercalcemia, acute alcoholism and cirrhosis, prolonged IV (3 weeks) without magnesium.

D.   Treatment implications.

1.   Assess for signs and symptoms of magnesium excess or loss.

2.   Assess for critical values indicating immediate interventions.

   a.   Increased level—above 2.5 mEq/L. The higher the level of magnesium, the more sedative the effect.

   b.   Assess for loss of deep tendon reflexes, respiratory decrease, and cardiac arrest.

✦ E.   *Hypermagnesemia.*

1.   Removal of excess magnesium.

   a.   Increase fluid intake—for magnesium intoxication, give IV calcium gluconate slowly in peripheral veins (do not use a CVP line) to promote excretion of excess magnesium.

   b.   Administer diuretics with possible renal dialysis if renal function is impaired.

2.   Nursing considerations.

   a.   Monitor for increased levels, which potentiate cardiac effect of increased potassium.

   b.   Monitor for renal failure, often associated with high levels of magnesium.

✦ F.   *Hypomagnesemia.*

1.   Replacement of magnesium.

   a.   Assess for severe deficiency—muscle twitching indicates neurological signs; nausea and vomiting indicate GI signs.

   b.   Administer magnesium sulfate IV (10–40 mEq/L in IV fluid) or IM slowly. Observe for urine output and keep antidote (calcium gluconate) available.

2.   Nursing considerations.

   a.   Monitor daily ingestion of magnesium PO and promote diet high in magnesium—nuts, green vegetables, seafood.

b. Check for hidden conditions affecting magnesium levels such as alcoholism, GI malabsorption.

Chloride (Cl⁻)

A. Normal serum value is 100–106 mEq/L.
B. Purpose—test for excess or deficit levels.
C. Indications.
1. Increased chloride—prolonged diarrhea leading to metabolic acidosis, acute renal failure, respiratory alkalosis (hyperventilation, CNS damage), diabetes insipidus, dehydration, specific drugs (salicylate intoxication, steroids).
2. Decreased chloride—prolonged vomiting or NG suction, loss of HCl, diarrhea, metabolic acidosis, adrenocortical insufficiency, renal disease that loses salt, specific drugs.
D. Treatment implications.
1. Assess for signs and symptoms of chloride excess and loss.
2. Assess for critical values, below 70 mEq/L or above 120 mEq/L.
3. Assess for conditions that cause increased sodium levels—may also cause increased chloride.
E. Nursing considerations.
1. Record intake and output and daily weights to monitor electrolyte imbalances.
2. Prolonged vomiting or uncontrollable diabetes may lead to abnormally low levels of chloride.

Phosphorus (P)

A. Normal serum value is 2.3–4.7 mg/dL.
B. Purpose—test for excess or deficit levels.
C. Indications.
1. Increased phosphorus—hypocalcemia, tetany, hypoparathyroidism, headaches, GI irritation, kidney disease, specific drugs, and vitamin D excess.
2. Decreased phosphorus—hypocalcemia, hypomagnesemia, hyperparathyroidism, vitamin D deficiency, alcohol intoxication, malabsorption.
D. Treatment implications.
1. Assess for signs and symptoms of phosphorus excess and loss.
2. Assess for critical values—hyperphosphatemia may occur with hypocalcemia and cardiac complications (arrhythmias).
E. Nursing considerations.
1. Hyperphosphatemia.
   a. May require dialysis to lower serum phosphorus.
   b. Gastric lavage with potassium may lower level of phosphorus.

c. Blood transfusions may be necessary.
2. Hypophosphatemia.
   a. Administer phosphate salt tablets or foods high in phosphorus (eggs, fish, meat, poultry, grains, peas, peanuts, walnuts, whole wheat, rye, and chocolate).
   b. Administer IV potassium phosphate.

Chem 7 (SMA 7)

A. Measure serum levels of seven substances: electrolytes (potassium, sodium, and chloride), carbon dioxide, glucose, BUN, and creatinine.
1. Tests fluid balance and renal function, as well as acid–base status.
2. When combined with CBC, these tests give a view of how entire body is functioning.
3. Chem 7 is also part of preoperative workup.
✦ 4. Standard values of Chem 7 (may vary from lab to lab; check own facility values).
   a. Potassium: 3.5–5.3 mEq/L.
   b. Sodium: 135–145 mEq/L.
   c. Chloride: 98–106 mEq/L.
   d. CO_2: 23–30 mmol/L.
   e. Glucose (fasting): 65–110 mg/dL.
   f. BUN: 7–18 mg/dL.
   g. Creatinine: 0.5–1.5 mg/dL.
B. How these values may be interpreted.
1. Postassium: an electrolyte that helps maintain acid–base balance.
2. Sodium: an electrolyte that helps maintain acid–base balance and osmotic pressure.
3. Chloride: an electrolyte that helps maintain extra electrical neutrality; combines with sodium to form a salt.
4. CO_2: reflects value of bicarbonate in arterial blood.
5. Glucose: fasting blood glucose levels may identify diabetes.
6. BUN: reflects liver's ability to make urea and the kidney's ability to excrete it. With renal disease, the BUN goes up.
7. Serum creatinine: more specific test of renal function; elevated levels indicate renal disease.

CARDIAC FUNCTION TESTS

Serum Cardiac Markers

A. Enzyme activity evaluation denotes heart muscle damage.
1. When the heart muscle is without oxygen for 30–60 minutes, the cells are damaged, which results in necrosis. Intracellular enzymes leak

out of cell membranes and are released into the bloodstream as the cells die.

2. Specific enzymes are released into the bloodstream at varying intervals; as myocardial cells die, they release chemicals that can be measured. The times of detection in the bloodstream, peak levels, and return to normal time vary greatly.

  ✦ a. Creatine kinase (CK), formerly called creatine phosphokinase or CPK-isoenzymes (CPK-MB)—most valuable measurement; level rises within 4–6 hours of initial heart muscle damage, peaking at 18–24 hours. More than 6 times normal value with damage—returns to normal within 3–4 days.

  b. Compare CK-MB with following two tests (SGOT and LDH) to determine myocardial damage.

  ✦ c. Lactate dehydrogenase LDH_1, LDH_2-isoenzymes—level rises in 12–24–48 hours; persists longer, can be as long as 2 weeks. When the physician analyzes these two levels (LDH_1 and LDH_2), he or she will look for a *flipped ratio*—when LDH is the highest, it indicates an MI.

  ✦ d. Serum glutamic oxaloacetic transaminase SGOT+ or aspartate aminotransferase (AST). High levels peak following an acute MI or liver damage.

3. CK-MB: one of three isoenzymes that make up the total creatine kinase (CK).

  a. Diagnostically cardiac specific.

  b. Present in bloodstream within 3–8 hours.

  c. Peaks within 24 hours.

  d. Returns to normal within 48–72 hours.

4. Normal cardiac enzyme ranges.

  a. Total creatine kinase—15–99 units/L; CKMB, 0–6% heart value.

  b. Total lactate dehydrogenase—either 100–190 units/L or 48–95 units/L; isoenzymes LDH_1, 14–26 percent and LDH_2, 27–37 percent.

  ✦ c. The greater the peak in enzymes and the longer the level remains, the more serious the heart damage.

B. Troponin test.

1. Tested for myocardial injury; when infarction occurs, this substance is released in the bloodstream.

2. Made up of three proteins found in striated muscle. Cardiac troponin T rises in 3–6 hours and remains up for 14–21 days; troponin 1 rises in 7–14 hours and remains up 5–7 days. Both are accurate assessments for myocardial damage.

3. Normally values are low (troponin T 0.0–0.2 ng/mL and troponin 1 less than 0.6 ng/mL); any rise may indicate myocardial cell damage. Serial tests are important.

C. Myoglobin test.

1. Oxygen-binding protein found in cardiac muscle (and skeletal muscle).

2. Level rises shortly after cell dies; peaks in 4–6 hours and returns to normal in 24–36 hours.

Blood Lipid Tests

✦ A. Normal values.

1. Cholesterol—below 200 mg/100 mL is desirable (teenager's level should be below 180 mg/100 mL). Levels over 239 mg/100 mL classified as high.

2. Triglycerides—cluster of fatty acids formed from breakdown of dietary fat and simple sugar (40–150 mg/100 mL).

3. Low-density lipoproteins (LDLs, the "bad" cholesterol)—60–180 mg/100 mL.

  a. LDLs burrow into the arterial walls to form plaque.

  b. Factors that lead to elevated LDL: diet (saturated fat and cholesterol); obesity; poorly controlled diabetes; genetic predisposition.

4. Very-low-density lipoproteins (VLDLs)—25–50 percent of total cholesterol.

5. High-density lipoproteins (HDLs, the "good" cholesterol)—male level, 30–70 mg/100 mL; female level, 30–80 mg/100 mL.

6. The "ideal" lipoprotein profile: high on high-density lipoprotein (HDL); low on low-density lipoprotein (LDL).

7. The greater amount of HDL cholesterol in proportion to total cholesterol value, the lower the risk for developing coronary artery disease.

B. Purpose—total cholesterol, lipoproteins, and triglycerides are screening tests to determine risk of atherosclerosis and heart disease.

1. High cholesterol—increased risk of heart disease.

2. High-density lipoprotein—lower risk of heart disease.

3. Low-density lipoprotein—higher risk of heart disease.

4. Hyperecholesterolemia combined with low levels of high-density lipoprotein—increases risk of arteriosclerosis.

5. High triglycerides—higher risk of acute myocardial infarction.

C. Variations.

1. Serum cholesterol increased in biliary obstruction (cirrhosis), hypothyroidism, pancreatic disease, uncontrolled diabetes, and pregnancy.
2. Serum cholesterol decreased in liver disease, hyperthyroidism, malnutrition, anemias, malabsorption of cholesterol.
3. Triglycerides increased in hepatitis, pancreatitis, cirrhosis due to alcoholism, renal failure, acute myocardial infarction.
4. Triglycerides decreased in hyperparathyroidism, pulmonary disease, malnutrition.

Arterial Blood Studies

+ A. Arterial blood gases.
  1. Assesses respiratory function.
     + a. Oxygen (pO_2).
        (1) Increased may indicate polycythemia.
        (2) Decreased may indicate COPD, cancer of lung, sickle cell anemia, anemias, cystic fibrosis.
     + b. Carbon dioxide (pCO_2).
        (1) Increased may indicate COPD, emphysema, bronchitis, asthma attack, pneumonia, cerebral trauma, neuro disorder.
        (2) Decreased may indicate anxiety, hysteria, tetany, increased temperature, DTs, hyperthyroidism, salicylate poisoning.
     + c. pH—high is alkalotic, low is acidotic.
     + d. Oxygen saturation and bicarbonate (HCO_3).
        (1) Oxygen saturation should be viewed with hemoglobin value.
        (2) Bicarbonate—if low (< 23) or high (> 27), indicates malfunction of metabolic process.
  2. Determines state of acid–base balance.
  3. Reveals adequacy of the lungs to provide oxygen and to remove carbon dioxide.
  4. Assesses degree to which kidneys can maintain a normal pH.
+ B. Normal arterial values.
  1. Oxygen saturation—93–98 percent.
  2. PaO_2—95 mm Hg.
  3. Arterial pH—7.35–7.45 (7.4).
  4. pCO_2—35–45 mm Hg (40).
  5. HCO_3 content—22–26 mEq/L.
  6. Base excess— −3 to +3 (0).
+ C. Acid–base imbalances.
  1. Respiratory acidosis.
     a. pH—< 7.35.
     b. pCO_2—< 45 mm Hg.
     c. pO_2—90 mm Hg.
     d. HCO_3—24 mEq/L.

2. Respiratory alkalosis.
   a. pH—> 7.45.
   b. pCO_2—35 mm Hg.
   c. pO_2—95 mm Hg.
   d. HCO_3—< 22 mEq/L.
3. Metabolic acidosis.
   a. pH—< 7.35.
   b. HCO_3—< 22 mEq/L.
   c. pCO_2—38 mm Hg.
   d. pO_2—95 mm Hg.
   e. Cl—120 mEq/L.
   f. K—5.5 mEq/L.
4. Metabolic alkalosis.
   a. pH—> 7.45.
   b. HCO_3—> 26 mEq/L.
   c. pCO_2—38 mm Hg.
   d. pO_2—95 mm Hg.
   e. K—3.0 mEq/L.
   f. Cl—88 mEq/L.

HEMATOLOGICAL TESTS

+ ## Blood Grouping

A. Normal values summary of ABO blood grouping.
B. Purpose—to correctly match donated blood with recipients.
+ C. Rh blood group.
  1. Positive (85 percent of the population).
  2. Negative (15 percent of the population).

Antigens and Antibodies

A. Based on type of antigens present in red blood cells as well as type of antibodies in the serum.
+ B. A and B antigens.
  1. Clients with type A blood have antigen A present; clients with type B blood have antigen B present.
  2. Clients with type AB blood have both A and B antigens present.
  3. Clients with type O blood have no antigens present.
+ C. Anti-A and anti-B antibodies present.
  1. Clients with type A blood do not have anti-A antibodies because the blood cells would be destroyed by agglutination; they have anti-B antibodies.
  2. Type B blood has anti-A antibodies.

Blood Coagulation

A. Clotting takes place in three phases.

1. Phase I—prothrombin activator formed in response to ruptured vessel or damage to blood.
2. Phase II—prothrombin activator catalyzes conversion of prothrombin into thrombin.
3. Phase III—thrombin acts as an enzyme to convert fibrinogen into fibrin thread.

B. Types of clotting factors.
   1. Calcium ions.
      a. Cofactor in coagulation.
      b. Does not enter into reaction.
      c. If absent, neither extrinsic nor intrinsic system will operate.
   2. Phospholipids.
      a. Necessary for formation of final prothrombin activator.
      b. Thromboplastin is phospholipid in extrinsic system.
      c. Platelet factor III is phospholipid for intrinsic system.
   3. Plasma protein—all clotting factors from V to XIII.

✦ C. Coagulation mechanisms.
   1. Extrinsic mechanisms.
      a. Extract from damaged tissue is mixed with blood.
      b. Trauma occurs to tissue or endothelial surface of vascular wall, releasing thromboplastin.
   2. Intrinsic mechanisms.
      a. Blood itself comes into contact with roughened blood vessel wall.
      b. Platelets adhere to vessel and disintegrate, which releases blood factor III containing thromboplastin.

D. Fibrinolytic system.
   1. Adequate function is necessary to maintain hemostasis.
   2. Dissolves clots through formation of plasmin.

Prostate-Specific Antigen (PSA) Test

A. Values.
   1. Normal: 0 to 4–6 ng/mL.
   2. Benign prostatic hypertrophy: 4 to 9 ng/mL.
   3. Prostate cancer: 10 to 120 ng/mL.
B. Purpose—shows concentration of glycoprotein from prostate tissue.
   1. Increases with benign prostatic hypertrophy (BPH).
   2. Markedly increases with cancer of the prostate.
   3. Used to diagnose or to monitor effect of treatment with chemotherapy or radiation.
   4. Collect 5 mL of venous blood before rectal or prostate exam (exam irritates tissue).

Prothrombin Time (PT)

✦ A. Normal values—10–13 seconds (some labs use 11–16 seconds).
B. Purpose—prothrombin time provides data on thrombin generation or how long it takes for a fibrin clot to form after reagent tissue and calcium are added to citrated plasma.
   1. It is a screening test to detect deficiencies in the extrinsic clotting mechanism.
   2. Useful for control of long-term anticoagulant therapy.
C. Critical values.
   1. If value is greater than 30 seconds, hemorrhage may occur—observe for bleeding.
   2. Administer vitamin K as ordered.
D. Possible causes of prolonged clotting time.
   1. Inadequate vitamin K in premature and newborn infants or in diet.
   2. Poor fat absorption (obstructive jaundice).
   3. Liver disease (cirrhosis, hepatitis).
   4. Specific drugs (heparin, Coumadin, salicylates).

Activated Partial Thromboplastin Time (APTT)

✦ A. Normal values—20–38 seconds with standard technique; different activators will yield different values.
B. Purpose—best single screening test for coagulation disorders.
   1. Test evaluates adequacy of plasma clotting factors—intrinsic clotting mechanism.
   2. Test of choice for monitoring heparin therapy.
   3. Used for clients with hemophilia.
C. Arterial values—if APTT is very prolonged (100 seconds), assess for spontaneous bleeding coagulant disorder.
D. Possible causes of prolonged clotting time.
   1. Vitamin K deficiency.
   2. Liver disease.
   3. Hemophilia.
   4. Specific drugs (heparin, warfarin, Coumadin, salicylates).
✦ E. When APTT is prolonged, M.D. may order protamine sulfate (or in severe cases, whole blood or plasma transfusion).

✦ International Normalized Ratio (INR)

A. Designed to standardize values and improve monitoring process. Test provides a more accurate assessment of client's anticoagulant; a uniform value in which client's PT is expressed as a ratio.
B. Standardizes PT ratio by allowing all thromboplastin reagents to be compared to an international

standard thromboplastin (sensitivity index) provided by the World Health Organization (WHO).

1. INR is a mathematical correction to prothrombin time ratio (PTR).
2. Value is calculated using client's PT divided by the mean normal PT. Target range is 2.5 to 3.5.
3. INR is calculated by raising the observed PT ratio to the power of the sensitivity index, depending on the reagent used.

C. The INR is the best lab value for monitoring anticoagulation therapy; improves the effectiveness of the medication.
D. Should be used only after client has been stabilized on warfarin (which takes at least a week).
E. Often, both PT and INR values are reported for monitoring Coumadin therapy.

Serum Protein Electrophoresis Test

A. Normal values:
Total serum protein: 6.3 to 7.9 g/dL.
Albumin: 3.5 to 5.0 g/dL.
Alpha$_1$ globulin: 0.1 to 0.4 g/dL.
Alpha$_2$ globulin: 0.4 to 1.0 g/dL.
Beta globulin: 0.5 to 1.1 g/dL.
Gamma globulin: 0.5 to 1.7 g/dL.
B. Purpose: To differentiate between protein fractions—serum proteins are made up of albumin and globulins. Test indicates the size, shape, and electrical charge of the major blood proteins (fractions) to diagnose certain diseases.
C. Abnormal results.
   1. Elevated levels.
      a. Albumin: dehydration, exercise.
      b. Alpha$_1$ and alpha$_2$, globulins: myocardial infarction, hepatic disease, myeloma, collagen diseases and acute and chronic infections.
   2. Decreased levels: liver disease, malnutrition, leukemia, renal failure, emphysema, anemia.

RENAL FUNCTION TESTS

◆ A. Phenolsulfonphthalein (PSP) test indicates the functional ability of the kidney to
   1. Excrete waste products.
   2. Concentrate and dilute urine.
   3. Carry on absorption and excretion activities.
   4. Maintain body fluids and electrolytes.
◆ B. Renal concentration tests.
   1. Evaluate the ability of the kidney to concentrate urine.
   2. As kidney disease progresses, renal function decreases. Concentration tests evaluate this process.
   3. Renal concentration is measured by specific gravity readings.
◆ C. Specific gravity.
   1. Normal value—range is 1.003–1.030, usually 1.010–1.025.
   2. If specific gravity is 1.018 or greater, it may be assumed that the kidney is functioning within normal limits.
   3. Specific gravity that stabilizes at 1.010 indicates kidney has lost ability to concentrate or dilute urine.
◆ D. Blood urea nitrogen (BUN).
   1. Normal value—10–20 mg/100 dL.
   2. Purpose—tests for impaired kidney function by testing the body's urea production and urine flow.
   3. BUN level affected by protein intake and tissue breakdown.
◆ E. Serum creatinine.
   1. Normal value—male: 0.8–1.2 mg/dL; female: 0.6–0.9 mg/dL. If normal value doubles, overall renal function and glomerular filtration rate (GFR) have decreased by half.
      a. When elevated, suggests hypertension or drugs such as steroids.
      b. Decreased indicates mild to severe renal impairment, muscular dystrophy, or use of certain drugs.
   2. Purpose—tests renal function by evaluating the balance between production and filtration of glomeruli.
   3. This is the most sensitive of renal function tests.
◆ F. Concentration and dilution tests.
   1. Fishberg concentration test—high-protein dinner with 200 mL fluid is ordered. Next AM on arising, client voids q 1/hr. One specimen should have specific gravity more than 1.025.
   2. Dilution test—NPO after dinner. Morning voiding discarded. Client drinks 1000 mL in 30 to 45 minutes. Four specimens at 1-hour intervals are collected. Specific gravity of one specimen will fall below 1.003.
   3. Specific gravity—urine range 1.003 to 1.030. Increased solutes cause increased specific gravity (*see* above).
◆ G. Glomerular filtration rate (GFR) or endogenous creatinine clearance.
   1. Normal values—125 mL/min (male) and 110 mL/min (female).
   2. Purpose—kidney function is assessed by clearing a substance from the blood such as inulin, a polysaccharide found in plants (filtration in the glomerulus).

3. Common test is the amount of blood cleared of urea per minute.
4. Test done on 12- or 24-hour urine specimen.

H. Electrolyte tests.
1. Kidney function is essential to maintain fluid and electrolyte balance.
2. Tests for electrolytes (sodium, potassium, chloride, and bicarbonate) measure the ability of the kidney to filter, reabsorb, or excrete these substances.
3. Impaired filtration leads to retention, and impaired reabsorption leads to loss of electrolytes.
4. Tests are performed on blood serum, so venous blood is required.

Urine Analysis

✦ A. Normal values.
1. Specific gravity—1.010–1.025.
2. Urine pH—4.5–8.0.
3. Color—straw.
4. Odor—aromatic.
5. Appearance—clear.
6. Protein—negative or zero.
7. Glucose—negative or zero.
8. Ketones—negative or zero.
9. Red blood cells—0–3.
10. White blood cells—0–4.
11. Casts—none; occasional.
12. Crystals—negative.
13. Yeast cells—none.
14. Parasites—none.

B. Urinalysis is a critical test for total evaluation of the renal system and for indication of renal disease.

✦ C. Specific gravity shows the degree of concentration in urine.
1. Normal value—1.010–1.025.
2. Indicates the ability of the kidney to concentrate or dilute urine.
3. Change from normal range.
   a. Elevated (greater than 1.030) indicates fluid depletion—diabetes mellitus, dehydration, vomiting/diarrhea, contrast media (1–2 days).
   b. Low (less than 1.010) indicates fluid excess—diabetes insipidus, overhydration, renal disease.
4. Renal failure—specific gravity constant at 1.010.

D. Analysis of urine pH.
1. pH is the symbol for the logarithm of the reciprocal of the hydrogen ion concentration.

2. A measurement of hydrogen ion concentration is taken—the lower the number, the higher the acidity of urine.
   ✦ a. Normal value range—4.5 to 8.0 (normal pH is 6 to 7).
   b. Lower than 6 is acidic urine, and higher than 7 is alkaline urine.
3. Regulation of urine pH is important for treatment of certain conditions.
   a. When the pH is alkaline, it suggests urinary tract infection, metabolic or respiratory alkalosis, drug influence, a vegetarian or highly alkaline diet.
   b. When the pH is acidic, it may reflect renal TB, PKU, pyrexia, acidosis.
   c. Acid urine may be desired when treating blood infections or phosphate stones.

✦ E. Chemical analysis of urine.
1. Protein or albumin—zero is normal for a 24-hour specimen.
   a. Presence may indicate kidney dysfunction or renal disease, such as nephritis or nephrosis.
   b. Inflammatory processes any place in the body may result in proteinuria.
   c. Toxemia of pregnancy yields a finding of proteinuria.
   d. Renal calculi indicate positive test results.
   e. Appearance in urine may be due to dehydration, strenuous exercise, high-protein diet.
2. Glucose—normal range is zero.
   a. Presence of glucose may indicate head injury, diabetes, Cushing's, hyperthyroidism.
   b. Test is usually done by test strips or tablets; change in color indicates presence of glucose. (Urine testing for glucose has been primarily replaced by testing blood for glucose.)
3. Ketone bodies—normal range is zero. Positive is +1 to +3.
   a. Ketonuria primarily indicates diabetic acidosis but is also present with starvation and pernicious vomiting.
   b. Test is usually done by strip or powder mixed with urine; purple color indicates positive test.
4. Bilirubin—normal range is zero.
   a. Presence in urine may indicate liver disease and may appear before the clinical symptom of jaundice.
   b. Detected in the urine by qualitative methods, such as inspection of color.
5. Blood—normal range is zero.

    a. If red blood cells are present, may indicate disease of kidney or urinary tract, and the source of hemorrhage must be determined.

    b. Specific diagnosis is made by complete urine analysis for casts and epithelial cells.

F. Microscopic examination of urine.
1. Evaluation of urinary sediment is important for diagnostic purposes.
2. Test for cellular elements (epithelial cells, white and red blood cells).
3. Test for casts, fat bodies, and crystals.

G. Levels of albuminuria.
1. 30 mg/100 mL = 1+.
2. 100 mg/100 mL = 2+.
3. 300 mg/100 mL = 3+.
4. 1000 mg/100 mL = 4+.

Schilling Urine Test

A. Determines absorption of vitamin B_{12} necessary for erythropoiesis—definitive test for pernicious anemia and intestinal malabsorption syndrome.

B. 7% excretion of radioactive B_{12} in urine within 24 hours. (When less than 3 g is excreted, diagnosis is confirmed.)

ANALYSIS OF GI SECRETIONS

A. Contents of the GI tract may be examined for the presence or absence of digestive juices, bacteria, parasites, and malignant cells.

B. Stomach contents may be aspirated and analyzed for volume and free and total acid.

✦ Gastric Analysis

A. Performed by means of a nasogastric tube.
1. Maintain NPO 6–8 hours prior to the test.
2. Pass NG tube; verify its presence in the stomach; tape to client's nose.

B. Collect fasting specimens.
1. Administer agents, such as alcohol, caffeine, histamine (0.2 mg subcutaneous), as ordered, to stimulate the flow of gastric acid.
    a. Watch for side effects of histamine, including flushing, headache, and hypotension.
    b. Do not give drug to clients with a history of asthma or other allergic conditions.
2. Collect specimens as ordered, usually at 10- to 20-minute intervals.
3. Label specimens and send to laboratory.
4. Withdraw NG tube; offer oral hygiene; make client comfortable.

5. Gastric acid is high in the presence of duodenal ulcers and is low in pernicious anemia.

✦ C. Tubeless gastric analysis.
1. Enables the determination of acidity or its absence.
2. Have client fast for 6–8 hours prior to the examination.
3. Administer gastric stimulant followed by Azuresin or Diagnex Blue, as ordered.
4. Acid in the stomach displaces the dye, which is then released, absorbed by the bowel mucosa, and excreted in the urine.
5. The bladder is emptied; the specimen saved. One hour after taking dye resin, client is instructed to void again. Urine is analyzed, and an estimation is made of the amount of free acid in the stomach.

✦ D. Gastric washings for acid-fast bacilli.
1. Instruct client to fast 6–8 hours prior to the procedure.
2. Insert nasogastric tube and secure gastric washings.
3. Send specimens to the laboratory to determine the presence of acid-fast bacilli.
4. Wash your hands carefully and protect yourself from direct contact with specimens.
5. This procedure is performed on suspected cases of active pulmonary tuberculosis when it is difficult to secure sputum for analysis.

Stool Analysis

✦ A. Stool specimens are examined for amount, consistency, color, shape, blood, fecal urobilinogen, fat, nitrogen, parasites, food residue, and other substances.
1. Stool cultures are also done for bacteria and viruses.
2. Some foods and medicines can affect stool color—spinach, green; cocoa, dark red; senna, yellow; iron, black; upper GI bleeding, tarry black; lower GI bleeding, bright red.

B. Stool abnormalities.
1. Steatorrhea—bulky, greasy and foamy, foul odor.
2. Biliary obstruction—light gray or clay-colored.
3. Ulcerative colitis—loose stools, with copious amounts of mucus or pus.
4. Constipation or obstruction—small, hard masses.

C. Specimen collection.
1. Specimens for detection of ova and parasites should be sent to the laboratory while the stool is still warm and fresh.

2. Examinations for blood are performed on small samples. A tongue blade may be used to place a small amount of stool in a disposable waxed container, or place a drop on a commercial card, which will turn color if blood is present in the stool.

3. Stools for chemical analysis are usually examined for the total quantity expelled, so the complete stool is sent to the laboratory.

LIVER FUNCTION TESTS

A. Pigment studies.
1. Serum bilirubin—abnormal in biliary and liver disease causing jaundice.
   a. Direct (conjugated)—normal: 0–0.3 mg/100 mL, soluble in H_2O.
   b. Indirect (unconjugated)—normal: 0.8–1.0 mg/100 mL, insoluble in H_2O.
   c. Total serum bilirubin—normal: 0–0.9 mg/100 mL.
2. Urine bilirubin—normally none is found.
3. Urine urobilinogen—0–4 mg/24 hours.
4. Fecal urobilinogen—40–280 mg/24 hours.
5. Serum cholesterol—150–250 mg/100 mL.

B. Protein studies.
1. Total protein—6–8 g/100 mL.
2. Serum albumin—3.5–5.0 mg/100 mL.
3. Serum globulin—1.5–3.0 mg/100 mL.
4. Prothrombin time—11–15 seconds.
5. Cephalin—0–1+.
6. In liver damage, fewer plasma proteins are synthesized; thus albumin synthesis is reduced.
   a. Serum globulins produced by the plasma cells are increased.
   b. PT is reduced in liver cell damage.

C. Cholesterol (see page 504).

D. Detoxification.
1. Bromsulphalein excretion (BSP).
2. Less than 5 percent dye retention after 1 hour.
   a. Dye is injected intravenously and removed by the liver cells, conjugated, and excreted.
   b. Blood specimen is obtained at 30-minute and 1-hour intervals after injection.
   c. Increased retention occurs in hepatic disorders.

E. Enzyme (transaminase) indicators.
1. Elevations reflect organ damage.
2. Levels.
   a. AST (formerly SGOT)—10–40 units/mL.
   b. ALT (formerly SGPT)—5–35 units/mL.
   c. LDH—100–200 units/mL.
   d. GGT—10–48 units/mL.

F. Alkaline phosphatase.
1. 2–5 units (varies with method used).
2. Elevated in obstructive jaundice, liver disease, Paget's disease, and cancer with bone metastasis.

G. Blood ammonia.
1. 20–120 µg/dL.
2. Ammonia level rises in liver failure because liver converts ammonia to urea.
3. Metabolic alkalosis increases the toxicity of NH_3.

THYROID FUNCTION TESTS

Radioactive Iodine (RAI) Uptake (Radioiodine ^{131}I)

A. Normal values—5–35 percent in 24 hours (recently lowered values in United States due to increased ingestion of iodine).
1. Elevated values indicate hyperthyroidism, thyrotoxicosis, hypofunctioning goiter, iodine lack, excessive hormonal losses.
2. Depressed values indicate low T_4, antithyroid drugs, thyroiditis, myxedema, or hypothyroidism.

B. Purpose—measures the absorption of the iodine isotope to determine how the thyroid gland is functioning.

C. Principles.
1. The use of ^{123}I rather than ^{131}I is now preferred because of its lower radiation hazard. (^{123}I can be used on pregnant women; ^{131}I is contraindicated.)
2. The amount of radioactivity is measured at 2, 6, and 24 hours after ingestion of the capsule.
3. ^{131}I (as does ^{123}I) evaluates the storage of iodine and gives a distribution pattern.

Thyroid-Stimulating Hormone (TSH) Ultrasensitive Assay

A. Normal values were 0.5–5.0 µU/mL—new, narrower TSH normal range of 0.3–3.0 µU/mL is a more accurate level and is recommended to become the standard of practice for therapeutic management.
1. Increased values, more than 20 µU/mL indicates hyperthyroidism, Addison's disease, goiter, and toxicity from certain drugs.
2. Decreased values: first-degree (secondary) hypothyroidism is less than 0.3 µU/mL, and second- to third-degree hypothyroidism is less than 0.1 µU/mL.

B. Test is an ultrasensitive indicator that has mostly replaced all other thyroid tests.
 1. If assay is normal, no other test is indicated.
 2. If test is abnormal, it should be validated by a T_4 assay.

✦ T_3 and T_4 Resin Uptake Tests

A. Normal values.
 1. T_4—3.8–11.4 percent.
 2. T_3—25–35 percent.
 3. T_4.
  a. Elevated—hyperthyroidism, early hepatitis, exogenous T_4.
  b. Decreased—hypothyroidism, abnormal binding, exogenous T_4.
 4. T_3.
  a. Elevated—hyperthyroidism, T_3 toxicosis.
  b. Decreased—advancing age.
B. Purpose—both of these in vitro tests are used as screening tests for diagnosis in thyroid disorders. T_4 is 90 percent accurate in diagnosing hyperthyroidism and hypothyroidism.
C. Decreased T_4 and normal or elevated TSH level can indicate thyroid disorder; decreased T_4 and decreased TSH level can indicate pituitary disorder.
D. Principles.
 1. Levels of T_3 and T_4 in the blood regulate TSH.
 2. These levels change according to a balancing system of negative feedback.
 3. Venous blood sample is obtained to directly measure concentration of unsaturated thyroxine-binding globulin in the serum.
 4. Thyroid function tests should be interpreted according to the clinical situation.

✦ TSH

A. Normal values 0–6 μU/mL or < 10 μU/mL (may vary with laboratory).
 1. Increased values indicate primary hypothyroidism.
 2. Decreased values indicate Hashimoto's thyroiditis, hyperthyroidism, large doses of glucocorticoids, secondary hypothyroidism.
B. Purpose—differentiates primary from secondary hypothyroidism and assesses level of thyroid gland activity.
C. Principles.
 1. Administration of IM TSH (thyrotropin) measures the responsiveness of the thyroid gland.
 2. Blood samples are obtained at intervals.

BLOOD GLUCOSE STUDIES

✦ Fasting Plasma Glucose (FPG)

A. Normal fasting glucose is 70 to 100 mg/100 mL; indicates good metabolic control.
B. > 125 mg/dL can signify diabetes.
 1. This is a new number based on recent guidelines that lowered the threshold for diabetes.
 2. Fasting is defined as no calorie intake for 8 hours.
C. FPG is used to diagnose hypoglycemia, confirm a diagnosis of prediabetic state, confirm diabetic mellitus, or monitor blood glucose levels.

✦ Random (Casual) Plasma Glucose Levels

A. Levels of more than 200 mg/dL on more than one occasion are diagnostic of diabetes.
B. Casual is any time of day without regard to when the last meal was eaten.

✦ Glucose Tolerance Test

A. Normal values are between 70–105 mg fasting blood glucose and no sugar in the urine.
 1. Greater than 140 mg/dL fasting and 200 mg/dL 2 hours postprandial are diagnostic of diabetes.
 2. The oral glucose tolerance test and IV glucose are no longer recommended for routine clinical use.
B. Purpose—primary aim is to diagnose or rule out diabetes, but also important for unexplained hypoglycemia and malabsorption syndrome.
C. Principles.
 1. This test determines rate of removal of a concentrated dose of glucose from the bloodstream.
 2. Test is indicated when there is sugar in the urine or when fasting blood sugar is elevated.
 3. This is a timed test done in the morning after fasting for at least 12 hours. Blood and urine samples are taken at intervals up to 3 hours.
 4. This test is contraindicated for recent surgical clients or clients with history of myocardial infarctions.

IMMUNODIAGNOSTIC TESTS

HIV-1 Antibody Test (ELISA)

✦ A. The ELISA (enzyme-linked immunosorbent assay) test was developed to screen donor blood on a national scale.
 1. This test does not test for AIDS, but rather antibodies to the HIV virus.

2. Once exposed to a virus, it takes the body time to produce antibodies. A person may already be infected and if the body has not yet produced antibodies, the ELISA test will be negative.

3. The test is not perfect because it may produce a false positive or false negative.

4. When performed at least 12 weeks after infection, the test has a 99.5 percent sensitivity and will show a positive result.

B. All positive results must be retested.

C. The Western blot test is given for final confirmation; used to confirm seropositive blood as identified by ELISA.

D. The indirect immunofluorescence assay (IFA) is being used by some physicians rather than the Western blot to confirm positive HIV. This test is rapid and easy to complete.

✦ Coombs' Test

A. Normal values—negative.

B. Purpose—test to discover presence of antibodies present in Rh-negative mother's blood.
1. Test also will confirm diagnosis of hemolytic disease in the newborn.
2. Titration determines extent to which antibodies are present.

C. Types of test for Rh incompatibility.
1. Indirect Coombs'—mother's blood reveals antibodies as result of previous transfusion or pregnancy.
2. Direct Coombs'—tests newborn's cord blood—determines presence of maternal antibodies attached to baby's cells.

✦ Venereal Disease Research Laboratory (VDRL) Test

A. Normal values—serum is nonreactive.

B. Purpose—to screen for primary or secondary syphilis and for diagnosis.

C. Differential diagnosis.
1. Biological false-positive tests may occur with hepatitis, mononucleosis, leprosy, malaria, rheumatoid arthritis, lupus erythematosus.
2. A nonreactive result does not rule out syphilis, as it takes up to 4 weeks after infection to cause an immunologic response.

D. The rapid plasma reagin circle card test (RPR-CT) is also used to screen for diabetes.

E. The treponemal test (FTA-ABS) is used to verify the screening test and determine that it was not a false positive.

Epstein-Barr Virus (EBV) Antibodies

A. Normal values—negative (antibodies appear within first 3 weeks, then decline rapidly).

B. Purpose—to diagnose infectious mononucleosis or to determine the antibody status of EBV-infected people.

C. Test—serum is tested for heterophile antibodies (Monospot test).

D. Differential diagnosis.
1. Positive results may occur with infectious mononucleosis, hepatitis A and B, cancer of the pancreas.
2. A negative Monospot does not always rule out acute or past EBV.

✦ Serologic Tests for Hepatitis A and B

A. Normal values—negative for hepatitis A, B, non-A, non-B, and D.

B. Purpose—serologic tests diagnose and differentiate different forms of hepatitis and detect presence in client's or donor's blood.

C. Test variations.
1. Hepatitis A (HAV).
   a. Anti-HAV IgM presence confirms recent infection of hepatitis A—detectable for 3 to 12 weeks.
   b. Anti-HAV IgG indicates previous exposure to HAV, recovery, and immunity. Appears after acute infection and is detectable for life.
2. Hepatitis B (HBV).
   a. Hepatitis B surface antigen—appears in 27 to 41 days and is the earliest indicator of HBV.
   b. Antibody to hepatitis B surface antigen indicates clinical recovery with subsequent immunity.
3. Hepatitis C (non-A, non-B) has no serologic or laboratory test to establish diagnosis—usually made by excluding other causes of hepatitis.
4. Hepatitis D or delta is associated with hepatitis B and depends on HBV for replication. It is found in the serum 7 to 14 days during acute infection.
5. Hepatitis E virus—fecal–oral route; similar to HAV.
6. Hepatitis G—also known as GB virus C.

✦ Rubella (German Measles) Viral Serologic Test

A. Normal values.

1. Negative titer of less than 1.8 or 1.10 (depending on test)—no antibody detected, therefore not immune.
2. Positive titer of more than 1.10—antibody detected, therefore immune.

B. Purpose—exposure to rubella is important to detect because exposure to this virus—if a woman is in the first trimester of pregnancy—may result in congenital abnormalities, abortion, or stillbirth.

✦ Papanicolaou (Pap) Smear

A. Diagnosis to identify preinvasive and invasive cervical cancer.
B. Vaginal secretions and secretions from posterior fornix are swabbed and smeared on a glass slide.

C. Pathological classifications (early cellular changes may be detected before disease becomes clinically observable).
1. Class I—no abnormal or atypical cells present.
2. Class II—atypical or abnormal cells present but no malignancy found; repeat Pap smear and follow up if necessary.
3. Class III—cytology, suggestive of malignancy; additional procedures indicated (biopsy, dilation and curettage [D&C]).
4. Class IV—cytology, strongly suggestive of malignancy; additional procedures indicated (biopsy, dilation and curettage [D&C]).
5. Class V—cytology results conclusive of malignancy.

LABORATORY TESTS REVIEW QUESTIONS

1. A client has just had his anticoagulant therapy monitored via the International Normalized Ratio (INR). The rationale for using this laboratory value is

   1. It is less expensive than doing a PT or PH test.
   2. It is the only test available for anticoagulant therapy monitoring.
   3. The client chooses the test and this test is easier for him to do.
   4. It is the most efficient lab value for monitoring anticoagulant therapy.

2. A client with suspected HIV will receive which test(s) to verify the diagnosis?

   1. Home Access HIV-1 Test System.
   2. Enzyme-linked immunosorbent assay (ELISA) and Western blot assay.
   3. Indirect immunofluorescence assay (IFA).
   4. ELISA and DNA.

3. A 57-year-old, postmenopausal female client complaining of chest pain is admitted. She is suspected of having a myocardial infarction. Which of the following isoenzyme values would be indicative of specific myocardial damage?

   1. CK (formerly CPK).
   2. CK–MB band.
   3. CK–MM band.
   4. CK–BB band.

4. A client has been advised to take a bile acid sequestrant (Colestid) to lower his LDL. It comes in powder form or tablets. The nurse should inform the client that if he chooses tablet form, he should

   1. Take milk with the medication.
   2. Take up to 30 tablets per day for the medication to be effective.
   3. Take the tablet every 6 hours.
   4. Not take the medication with citric acid (orange juice).

5. A client with symptoms of nausea and vomiting is admitted to the emergency department. He states that before he came to the hospital, when he tried to lie down, his abdominal pain got worse and was not relieved by antacids. When questioned, he states that he had consumed a large meal and two glasses of wine.

The tentative diagnosis is acute pancreatitis. The physician orders lab work. With this complaint picture and diagnosis, the nurse would expect lab results to include

   1. Decreased WBC.
   2. Elevated serum amylase and lipase.
   3. No change in serum bilirubin level.
   4. Elevated alkaline phosphatase.

6. When a physician orders ABGs on a client, which results will tell the nurse if an acid–base problem is present and whether it is respiratory or metabolic?

   1. pH and CO_2.
   2. CO_2 and HCO_3.
   3. pH, CO_2, and HCO_3.
   4. pH and $PaCO_2$.

7. Which group of cells is the first line of defense against bacterial infection working primarily through phagocytosis?

   1. Monocytes.
   2. Platelets.
   3. Neutrophils.
   4. Basophils.

8. Kayexalate is ordered for a client with a serum potassium of 5.5 mEq/L. If this substance is effective, the nurse should expect to see an ECG with

   1. Return of T-wave width and amplitude to normalcy.
   2. Broad, flat P waves.
   3. Absence of P waves.
   4. Return of QRS to upright configuration.

9. A client is scheduled to take a serum creatinine test, and she asks the nurse what this test shows. The most appropriate response would be

   1. "This test will tell your doctor how your kidneys are functioning."
   2. "You'll have to ask your doctor."
   3. "It will tell if you have severe renal impairment or a disease."
   4. "Results will indicate if certain drugs, such as steroids, are interfering with kidney functioning."

10. The nurse is assigned to a male client who was admitted with flu symptoms of nausea and vomiting. He is receiving IV therapy. The lab has sent his early-morning blood results, which are: BUN 32, creatinine 1.1, hematocrit 50. The initial nursing intervention is to

    1. Notify the physician STAT.
    2. Do nothing because the results are within normal limits.
    3. Decrease the IV rate and notify the physician, as lab results indicate overhydration.
    4. Evaluate urine output for amount and specific gravity.

11. The nurse would expect to find an improvement in which of the blood values as a result of dialysis treatment?

    1. High serum creatinine levels.
    2. Low hemoglobin.
    3. Hypocalcemia.
    4. Hypokalemia.

12. Which of the following blood chemistry results would the nurse expect to find elevated in a client with right-sided congestive heart failure?

    1. Ammonia.
    2. Albumin.
    3. LDH.
    4. CK.

13. A client with a long-standing history of alcoholic cirrhosis with ascites is admitted to the hospital. His diagnosis is acute bleeding from esophageal varices secondary to cirrhosis with portal hypertension. Which of the following laboratory findings indicates that blood is being digested and absorbed by the GI tract?

    1. Elevated BUN.
    2. Elevated serum ammonia.
    3. Decreased hemoglobin.
    4. Elevated bilirubin.

14. An 80-year-old client has been admitted to the hospital with influenza and dehydration. Which of the following blood urea nitrogen (BUN) levels would indicate to the nurse that the client has received adequate fluid volume replacement?

    1. 40 mg/dL.
    2. 29 mg/dL.
    3. 17 mg/dL.
    4. 3 mg/dL.

15. A client who sustained head trauma in a motor vehicle accident has been diagnosed and treated for having syndrome of inappropriate antidiuretic hormone (SIADH) secretion. Which of the following urine specific gravity values would indicate that the situation had not resolved?

    1. 1.005.
    2. 1.018.
    3. 1.025.
    4. 1.035.

16. As part of an annual physical exam, a 60-year-old adult male has had lab work done. Which of the following serum creatinine levels would indicate that the client has a mild degree of renal insufficiency?

    1. 4.0 mg/dL.
    2. 3.3 mg/dL.
    3. 1.7 mg/dL.
    4. 0.8 mg/dL.

17. The nurse should explain to a client who takes Lasix and has a potassium of 3.2 mEq/L that he should

    1. Avoid apple juice, orange juice, and instant coffee.
    2. Eat three servings daily of fruits and meat or fish.
    3. Maintain a fluid intake of 2 L/day.
    4. Avoid driving or operating electrical equipment.

18. Of the following blood gas values, the one the nurse would expect to see in the client with acute renal failure is

    1. pH 7.49, HCO_3 24, pCO_2 46.
    2. pH 7.49, HCO_3 14, pCO_2 30.
    3. pH 7.26, HCO_3 24, pCO_2 46.
    4. pH 7.26, HCO_3 14, pCO_2 30.

19. The premenstrual hemoglobin of a 24-year-old client with no history of trauma, recent surgery, or hemorrhage is 9.8 g/dL. The nurse interprets that this value is due to

    1. Iron-deficiency anemia.
    2. Hypovolemia.
    3. Dehydration.
    4. Cardiogenic shock.

20. A client is scheduled for a carotid endarterectomy in 3 days. Which of the following preadmission lab test results must be immediately reported to the physician?

    1. Sodium of 151 mEq/L.
    2. Chloride of 105 mEq/L.
    3. Potassium of 3.8 mEq/L.
    4. Bicarbonate of 23 mEq/L.

21. A client is admitted to the hospital for evaluation. His physician writes in the chart "rule out liver cancer" and schedules a liver biopsy. Before the procedure, the nurse reviews the PT results just back from the lab: 24—INR, 4.0. The nurse also notes that this client is not on an anticoagulant. The nursing intervention is to

    1. Do nothing—the results of the PT are normal.
    2. Notify the physician before the biopsy procedure.
    3. Ask the lab to repeat the test tomorrow and notify the physician.
    4. Ask the client if he has been eating foods high in vitamin K.

22. A 60-year-old client is admitted to the surgery unit for removal of fibroid tumors. When the nurse checks the lab results for routine blood chemistry, she notes that the sedimentation rate is 29 mm/dL. The appropriate intervention is to

    1. Ask the client if she has been sick with a fever.
    2. Do nothing—the value is normal.
    3. Notify the physician.
    4. Ask the lab to repeat the test.

23. A TSH ultrasensitive assay has been ordered for a client, and she asks the nurse the purpose of this test. The most appropriate reply is

    1. "This test is a screening test to diagnose thyroid disorders."

    2. "The doctor is testing whether you have Hashimoto's disease."
    3. "This test measures the absorption of iodine and how it relates to the thyroid gland."
    4. "The test indicates whether your thyroid gland is over- or under-active."

24. At the physician's office, the client has a random plasma glucose test. The results were 250 mg/dL. The client asked the office nurse why the doctor told him to come back the next day to repeat the test. The best answer is

    1. "The doctor always repeats this test."
    2. "You may have diabetes and the doctor wants to be sure."
    3. "This test must be done at least twice for accurate results."
    4. "It was a little high, so the doctor wants to check the results."

25. A client has a gastric analysis done and results showed that gastric acid was high. This test result would indicate to the nurse that the client may receive the diagnosis of

    1. Pernicious anemia.
    2. Peptic ulcer.
    3. Tuberculosis.
    4. Duodenal ulcer.

LABORATORY TESTS

Answers with Rationale

1. (4) INR is the most efficient lab value test to use because it provides a more accurate and standardized value and, therefore, improves the effectiveness of the medication. It is not less expensive (1); the client does not choose the test (3) and it is not the only test available (2).

   NP:P; CN:PH; CA:M; CL:C

2. (2) ELISA is the first test used to confirm the presence of antibody to HIV and indicates the person has been exposed to or infected by HIV. The Western blot assay is used to confirm seropositivity as identified by ELISA. The Home Access kit (1) has been approved by the FDA, but false-positive test results are possible and must be verified. The IFA (3) is an indirect test and must be confirmed by the Western blot. DNA (4) may be used to track HIV.

   NP:AN; CN:H; CA:M; CL:K

3. (2) CK is a cellular enzyme that is fractionated out into MB, MM, and BB bands. The MB bands are specific to cardiac muscle, the MM bands (3) relate to skeletal muscle, and the BB bands (4) relate to CK in the brain. Although an elevated CK (1) may indicate cardiac muscle damage, it is only the MB portion that is specific to cardiac muscle.

   NP:A; CN:PH; CA:M; CL:A

4. (2) If the client chooses to take the tablets rather than the powder, he will have to take up to 30 tablets per day. The powder can be taken with a beverage or cereal.

   NP:I; CN:PH; CA:M; CL:A

5. (2) These elevated serum levels (amylase and lipase) are the hallmark of acute pancreatitis. Increased WBC (1) and serum bilirubin level (3) are also seen with acute pancreatitis. Elevated alkaline phosphatase (4) is found in chronic pancreatitis.

   NP:AN; CN:PH; CA:M; CL:AN

6. (3) If an acid–base problem is present, the nurse will note it from the pH result (if blood pH is below 7.4, it is acid; if above 7.4, it is base). The matching component, CO_2, indicates whether the problem is respiratory; HCO_3, the other matching value, reflects a metabolic problem. $PaCO_2$ represents only the respiratory part of acid–base balance, but the CO_2 and HCO_3 values must be present. For example, if an acid–base problem is present, the nurse will note pH and either $PaCO_2$ (respiratory) or HCO_3 (metabolic).

   NP:AN; CN:PH; CA:M; CL:AN

7. (3) Neutrophils are the first line of defense against infection. They live in the circulation for about 6 hours after bacteria are ingested. The cells die and become the main component of pus. Monocytes (1) are the second group to defend the body. Platelets (2) are blood components that go to the site of injury and stem blood loss. Basophils (4) release heparin and histamine in areas that are invaded by antigens.

   NP:AN; CN:S; CA:M; CL:K

8. (1) The Kayexalate should bring the potassium level down. When this occurs, the effects on the T wave reverse and the ECG will return to normal.

   NP:E; CN:S; CA:M; CL:AN

9. (1) This response is preferred because it answers the question rather than avoiding it, as in answer (2). It does not give information that may frighten the client (3), nor does it suggest an outcome that will be negative (4).

   NP:I; CN:PH; CA:M; CL:A

10. (4) These lab results indicate that the client is dehydrated. Specific gravity and urine output are indicators used to support the laboratory findings. The higher the specific gravity, the more dehydrated the client.

    NP:I; CN:PH; CA:M; CL:AN

Coding for Questions/Answers Abbreviations: **Nursing Process: NP,** Assessment: A, Analysis: AN, Planning: P, Implementation: I, Evaluation: E; **Client Needs: CN,** Safe, Effective Care Environment: S, Health Promotion and Maintenance: H, Psychosocial Integrity: PS, Physiological Integrity: PH; **Clinical Area: CA,** Medical Nursing: M, Surgical Nursing: S, Maternal/Newborn Nursing: MA, Pediatric Nursing: P, Psychiatric Nursing: PS; **Cognitive Level: CL,** Knowledge: K, Comprehension: C, Application: A, Analysis: AN.

11. (1) High creatinine levels will be decreased as a result of dialysis. Anemia is a result of decreased production of erythropoietin by the kidney and is not affected by hemodialysis (2). Hyperkalemia and high base bicarbonate levels are present in renal failure clients.

NP:E; CN:PH; CA:M; CL:A

12. (3) The liver becomes engorged with blood in right-sided congestive heart failure. Liver function studies, such as the LDH, an enzyme production test for the liver, will be abnormally elevated in 40 percent of these clients. Serum bilirubin is also frequently increased. Ammonia (1) and albumin (2), also liver tests, will not be elevated. CK isoenzymes (4) (CK–MB) are a valuable indicator of myocardial infarction.

NP:AN; CN:PH; CA:M; CL:AN

13. (1) As blood is digested, the BUN rises rapidly. A result of bleeding may also be a lowered hemoglobin (3), but this does not indicate digestion and absorption of blood nitrogen. An elevation of serum ammonia (2) may ensue if the liver is unable to handle the protein load of digested blood.

NP:AN; CN:PH; CA:M; CL:A

14. (3) The normal BUN is 10–20 mg/dL. Values of 40 mg/dL (1) and 29 mg/dL (2) indicate unresolved dehydration. A value of 3 mg/dL (4) is significantly lower than normal and may indicate fluid overload.

NP:A; CN:PH; CA:M; CL:AN

15. (4) This value is above normal limits (the normal range of a urine specific gravity is 1.010–1.025). A value of 1.005 (1) may be seen when the client was in the diuretic phase of a head injury or insult. Values of 1.018 (2) and 1.025 (3) are within normal limits, but 1.025 is indicative of concentrated urine.

NP:A; CN:PH; CA:M; CL:AN

16. (3) The normal serum creatinine level for a male is 0.6–0.9 mg/dL. A client with a mild degree of renal insufficiency would have a slightly elevated level, which in this case would be 1.7. Levels of 3.3 (2) and 4.0 (1) may be associated with acute or chronic renal failure.

NP:A; CN:PH; CA:M; CL:A

17. (2) The normal potassium level is 3.5–5.0 mEq/L. The client's potassium level is low, and he needs to replenish what has been lost as a result of taking the Lasix. In addition to taking potassium supplements, the client should be given a list of the appropriate foods that have an average of 7 mEq potassium per serving. Fruit, meat, fish, instant coffee, and milk are high in potassium.

NP:P; CN:PH; CA:M; CL:AN

18. (4) The client with acute renal failure would be expected to have metabolic acidosis (low HCO_3) resulting in acid blood pH (acidemia) and respiratory alkalosis (lowered PCO_2) as a compensating mechanism. Normal values are pH 7.35–7.45; HCO_3 23–27 mEq; and PCO_2 35–45 mm Hg.

NP:A; CN:PH; CA:M; CL:AN

19. (1) The normal Hgb for a female is above 12–16 g/dL. With the data given, the nurse would suspect anemia. Hypovolemia (2) will alter Hgb if the loss of blood volume was due to hemorrhage. Dehydration (3) may increase the level by hemoconcentration. Cardiogenic shock (4) may increase the Hgb because of the need for increased oxygen-carrying capacity.

NP:A; CN:PH; CA:M; CL:A

20. (1) The normal electrolyte values for an adult are as follows: sodium 135–145 mEq/L, chloride 100–106 mEq/L (2), potassium 3.5–5.0 mEq/L (3), and bicarbonate 22–29 mEq/L (4). The serum sodium is the only abnormal value.

NP:A; CN:PH; CA:M; CL:AN

21. (2) Because the client is not on anticoagulant therapy, the results are abnormal (normal PT is 11–15 seconds). It is important to notify the physician before the biopsy; bleeding could be life-threatening. The client will probably be given vitamin K therapy; when the PT results return to the normal range, the procedure can be done. Liver disease likely caused the prolonged PT.

NP:I; CN:PH; CA:M; CL:AN

22. (2) This is a normal sed rate for a female over age 60. Under age 50, normal is 20 mm/hr. If it were increased, it would indicate the presence of infection or inflammation and surgery might have to be postponed.

NP:I; CN:PH; CA:M; CL:A

23. (4) The clearest and best reply is a general description of the test, but one that is not specific enough to frighten the client, as in (1) and (2). Answer (3) is inaccurate because this answer refers to the radioactive iodine uptake test.

NP:I; CN:PS; CA:S; CL:C

24. (3) The best answer is to be truthful, but not to frighten the client by telling him that he may have diabetes (this is the domain of the physician). Levels of more than 200 mg/dL on more than one occasion would, however, be diagnostic of diabetes, so the doctor would order at least two tests.

NP:I; CN:PH; CA:M; CL:C

25. (4) High gastric acid levels may indicate duodenal ulcer. Pernicious anemia (1) would yield low results. TB (3) may be diagnosed by gastric washings for acid-fast bacilli, especially if sputum analysis is difficult to procure.

NP:AN; CN:PH; CA:M; CL:A

Maternal–Newborn Nursing 12

✦ The icon denotes content of special importance for NCLEX.

ANATOMY AND PHYSIOLOGY OF FEMALE REPRODUCTIVE ORGANS

✦ Anatomy

✦ Female Reproductive Organs

A. Usually divided into two groups: the external and internal genitalia.

B. External genitalia are collectively called the vulva, which consist of:
1. Mons veneris or mons pubis.
2. Labia majora.
3. Labia minora.
4. Clitoris.
5. Vestibule.
6. Urinary meatus.
7. Skene's ducts and Bartholin's glands.
8. Hymen.
9. Perineum.

C. Internal organs of reproduction are located in the pelvic cavity.
1. Uterus—muscular organ.
   a. Two major functions.
      (1) Organ in which fetus develops.
      (2) Organ from which menstruation occurs.
   b. Consists of two major parts.
      (1) Corpus (body), which has three layers.
         (a) Perimetrium—external layer.
         (b) Myometrium—middle layer.
         (c) Endometrium—internal layer.
      (2) Cervix, composed of three parts.
         (a) Internal os—opens into body of uterine cavity.
         (b) Cervical canal located between internal and external os.
         (c) External os—opens into vagina.
2. Fallopian tubes—two slender muscular tubes that extend laterally from the cornu of the uterine cavity to the ovaries; they are the passageways through which the ova reach the uterus.
3. Ovaries—two flat, oval-shaped organs located on each side of the uterus. (Correspond to the testes in the male.) Two major functions are:
   a. Development and expulsion of ova.
   b. Primary source for secretion of estrogen and progesterone.
4. Vagina—a canal that extends from lower part of the vulva to the cervix; serves three functions for the body:
   a. Passageway for menstrual blood.
   b. Passageway for fetus.
   c. Organ of copulation.

Skeletal Features of the Pelvis

A. The pelvis is important in obstetrics because it is the passage through which the baby passes during birth. Disproportions between fetus and size of pelvis may make vaginal delivery difficult or impossible.

B. Four bones form the pelvis—two innominate bones, the sacrum, and the coccyx.

✦ C. Divisions of pelvis.
1. False pelvis—shallow extended portion above brim that supports abdominal viscera.
2. True pelvis—portion that lies below pelvic brim and is divided into three sections—the pelvic inlet, the midpelvis, and the pelvic outlet.
   ✦ 3. Four main types of pelvic inlets.
      a. Gynecoid—inlet nearly round or blunt, heart-shaped (45 percent of women).
      b. Android—inlet wedge-shaped (15 percent of women).
      c. Anthropoid—inlet oval-shaped (35 percent of women).
      d. Platypelloid—inlet oval-shaped, transversely (5 percent or less of women).

D. Measurements of the pelvis.
1. Diagonal conjugate (CD)—distance between sacral promontory and lower margin of symphysis pubis. Measurement greater than 12.5 cm adequate.
2. True conjugate, or conjugate vera (CV)—distance from upper margin of symphysis to sacral promontory. Measurement greater than 11 cm adequate.
3. Tuberischial diameter (TI)—transverse diameter of outlet. Measurement greater than 8 cm adequate.
4. Size determination.
   a. X-ray pelvimetry is most accurate means of determining size of pelvis.
   b. X-ray pelvimetry is contraindicated to avoid undue exposure of mother and infant unless pelvic contraction is suspected.

Physiology

Menstruation and the Menstrual Cycle

Definition: The periodic discharge of blood, mucus, and epithelial cells from the uterus.

A. Menstrual cycle—usually lasts 28 days, but may vary from 21–35 days with ovulation occurring about 14 days before menstruation begins. Usually occurs between the ages of 12 and 45.

B. Hormonal control—depends on adequate functioning of pituitary, ovaries, and uterus.

C. Hypothalamus exerts control through releasing and inhibiting factors.
  ✦ 1. Proliferative phase—estrogen.
    a. Follicle-stimulating hormone (FSH) (secreted during the first half of the menstrual cycle) stimulates the development of the graafian follicle.
    b. As graafian follicle develops, it produces increasing amounts of follicular fluid containing a hormone called estrogen.
    c. Estrogen stimulates buildup or thickening of the endometrium.
    d. As estrogen increases in the bloodstream, it suppresses secretion of FSH and favors the secretion of the luteinizing hormone (LH).
    e. LH stimulates ovulation and initiates development of the corpus luteum.
  2. Secretory phase—progesterone.
    a. Follows ovulation, which is the release of mature ovum from the graafian follicle.
    b. Rapid changes take place in the ruptured follicle under the influence of LH.
    c. Cavity of the graafian follicle is replaced by the corpus luteum (mass of yellow-colored tissue).
    d. Main function of the corpus luteum is to secrete progesterone and some estrogen.
    e. Progesterone acts upon the endometrium to bring about secretory changes that thicken and maintain the endometrium during the early phase of pregnancy, should a fertilized ovum be implanted.
  3. Menstrual phase.
    ✦ a. Corpus luteum degenerates in about 8 days unless the ovum is fertilized.
    b. There is a cessation of progesterone and estrogen produced by corpus luteum and blood levels drop.
    c. Endometrium degenerates and menstruation occurs.
    d. The drop in blood levels of estrogen and progesterone stimulate production of FSH and a new cycle begins.
    e. Basal body temperature dips then rises about a day after ovulation has occurred (0.5–1°F increase).

Development of the Fetus

Fertilization

Definition: A gamete is a sex cell—ovum or spermatozoon—that has undergone maturation and is ready for fertilization.

A. Fertilization takes place when two essential cells—sperm and ovum—unite.

B. Each reproductive cell (one gamete) carries 23 chromosomes.

C. Sperm carries two types of sex chromosomes, X and Y, which when united with female X chromosome determine the sex of the child (XY—male; XX—female).

D. The site of fertilization is usually in the outer third of the fallopian tubes, and the fertilized egg then descends to the uterus.

Fetal Development

Definition: Embryo is the fertilized ovum during the first 2 months of development. Fetus is the product of conception from 2 months to time of birth. (*See* Table 12-1.)

A. Implantation occurs about the 7th day after fertilization—nidation.

✦ B. First 8 weeks, when all major organs are developing, is the period of greatest vulnerability.

C. Embryonic development—cells arrange themselves into three layers.
  1. Ectoderm—outer layer—gives rise to skin, salivary and mammary glands, nervous system, and other external parts of the body.
  2. Endoderm—inner layer—gives rise to thymus, thyroid, bladder, and other small organs and tubes.
  3. Mesoderm—layer between the other two—gives rise to urinary and reproductive organs, circulatory system, connective tissue, muscle, and bones.

D. Fetal membranes and amniotic fluid.
  1. Fetal membranes—membranes that surround the fetus—are composed of two layers.
    a. Amnion—glistening inner membrane—forms early, about the second week of embryonic development; encloses the amniotic cavity.
    b. Chorion—outer membrane.
  ✦ 2. Amniotic fluid—forms within the amniotic cavity and surrounds the embryo. Usually consists of 500–1000 mL of fluid at the end of pregnancy.
    a. Amniotic fluid is slightly alkaline and contains fetal urine, lanugo from fetal skin, epithelial cells, and sebaceous materials.
    b. Function of the fluid is to provide an optimum temperature and environment for fetus and provide a cushion against injury; fetus also drinks the fluid, probably as much as 600 mL a day near term.
    c. Probably bidirectional maternal-fetal fluid exchange, fetal urine, fetal swallowing, fetal breathing and/or transfer across chorionic plate. By the end of pregnancy,

Table 12-1. FETAL GROWTH DURING PREGNANCY

Age	Development
End of 1 month or 4 weeks	Form of embryonic disc No clearly defined features Body systems rudimentary form Cardiovascular system functioning
End of 2 months or 8 weeks	Head greatly enlarged, about the size of rest of body Some fetal movement due to beginning neuromuscular development Facial features becoming distinct Body covered with thin skin
End of 3 months or 12 weeks	Teeth forming under gums Center ossification appearing in most bones Fingers and toes are differentiated and bear nails Kidneys able to secrete Eyes have lids that are fused shut until 6 months Fetus swallows Sex distinguishable
End of 4 months or 16 weeks	Lanugo appears over body Meconium in intestines Face has human appearance Size: about 15 cm long; weight: about 100 g
End of 5 months or 20 weeks	Skeleton begins to harden Buds of permanent teeth develop Vernix caseosa makes appearance Fetal movements stronger and felt by mother Fetal heartbeat heard Size: about 25 cm long; weight: about 310 g
End of 6 months or 24 weeks	Fat beginning to deposit beneath skin Body and head better proportioned Eyebrows and eyelashes appear Size: about 30 cm long; weight: about 680 g
End of 7 months or 28 weeks	Skin reddish and covered with vernix Size: about 36 cm long; weight: about 1130 g May be viable if born at this time, though still immature
End of 8 months or 32 weeks	Nails are firm and extend to end of digits Lanugo begins to disappear Size: about 41 cm long; weight: about 1810 g Increased chance for survival if born at this time
End of 9 months or 36 weeks	Increased fat deposits under skin Increased development Size: about 46 cm long; weight: about 2270 g Good chance of survival
End of 10 months or 40 weeks	Full term Little lanugo Smooth skin Size: about 50 cm long; weight: 3175–3400 g Optimum time for survival

about 500 mL/hr is replaced (about ½ total fluid volume).

E. Placental function.

1. Placenta—organ that provides for the exchange of nutrients and waste products between mother and fetus and acts as an endocrine organ.
   a. Provides oxygen and removes carbon dioxide from the fetal system.
   b. Maintains fetal fluid and electrolyte, acid–base balance.
   c. Produces hormones necessary to maintain pregnancy.
2. Placenta develops by the third month.
   a. Formed by union of chorionic villi and decidua basalis.
   b. Fetal surface smooth and glistening.
   c. Maternal surface red and fleshlike.
3. Exchange takes place between mother and fetus through diffusion.
4. Placental function is dependent on maternal circulation.
5. In addition to nutrients, materials passed through placenta are drugs, antibodies to some diseases, and certain viruses. Large particles such as bacteria cannot pass through barrier.
6. Placental transfer of maternal immunoglobulin G gives the fetus passive immunity to certain diseases for the first few months after birth.
7. Hormones produced by the placenta.
   a. Human chorionic gonadotropin (HCG)—detected in urine 15 days after implantation. Hormone stimulates the corpus luteum to maintain endometrium and is the basis of immunological test of pregnancy.
   b. Human placental lactogen (HPL)—effect similar to growth hormone; insulin antagonist; mobilizes maternal free fatty acids.
   c. Estrogen and progesterone.
8. The umbilical cord extends from the fetus to center of the fetal surface of the placenta.
   a. Contains two arteries and one vein.
   b. Protected by mucoid connective tissue termed *Wharton's jelly.*
   c. Average cord is 2 cm (0.8 in) diameter and 55 cm (22 in) long.

F. Fetal circulation.

1. Arteries carry venous blood.
2. Vein carries oxygenated blood.
3. Fetal circulation bypass.
   a. Bypass due to nonfunctioning lungs: ductus arteriosus (between pulmonary artery and aorta) and foramen ovale (between right and left atrium).
   b. Ductus venosus bypass—due to fetal liver not being used for exchange of waste; connects umbilical artery to inferior vena cava; allows most of fetal blood to bypass liver.
   c. Bypasses must close following birth to allow blood to flow through the lungs for respiration and through the liver for waste exchange.

G. Calculation of expected date of delivery or confinement (EDC).

1. Nägele's rule: Count back 3 months from first day of last menstrual period and add 7 days.
   Example: LMP July 18
                EDC April 25
2. Pregnancy usually does not terminate on the exact EDC. If using Nägele's rule, it may vary from 1 week before to 2 weeks after the expected date. If ultrasound is used (BPD) between 17–24 weeks' gestation, the expected date is usually ±5–7 days.

H. Multiple pregnancies (uterus contains two or more embryos). May be the result of fertilization of a single ovum or two separate ova. If division takes place very early in monozygotic twins, two placentas and two chorions are formed. (*See* Table 12-2.)

Table 12-2. MULTIPLE PREGNANCIES

Double Ovum	Single Ovum
Dizygotic or fraternal twins	Monozygotic or identical twins
Ova from same or different ovaries	Union of a single ovum and a single sperm
Same or different sex	Same sex
Brother or sister resemblance	Identical genetic pattern
Two placentas but may be fused	One placenta
Two chorions and two amnions	One chorion and two amnions

ANTEPARTUM PERIOD

ANTEPARTAL MATERNAL CHANGES

Physiological Changes

Reproductive Organs

A. Uterus—increases in weight from 57 g to about 907 g at the end of gestation and in size from five to six times larger.
  1. Changes in tissue.
     a. Hypertrophy of muscle cells with limited development of new muscle cells.
     b. Development of connective and elastic tissue, which increases contractility.
     c. Increase in the size and number of blood vessels.
     d. Hypertrophy of the lymphatic system.
     e. Growth of the uterus is brought about by the influences of estrogen during the early months and the pressure of the fetus.
  2. Other changes.
     a. Contractions occur throughout pregnancy, starting from very mild to increased strength.
     b. As the uterus grows, it rises out of the pelvis, displacing intestines, and may be palpated above the symphysis pubis.
◆ B. Ligaments—broad ligaments in the pelvis become elongated and hypertrophied to help support and stabilize uterus during pregnancy.
C. Cervix.
  1. Becomes shorter, more elastic, and larger in diameter.
  2. Marked thickening of mucous lining and increased blood supply.
  3. Edema and hyperplasia of the cervical glands and increased glandular secretions.
  4. Mucous plug expelled from cervix as cervix begins to dilate at onset of labor.
  ◆ 5. Increased vascularity, deepening of color to dark red or purple—*Chadwick's sign*—found in both vagina and cervix.
D. Vagina.
  1. Hypertrophy and thickening of muscle and mucosa.
  2. Loosening of connective tissue.
  3. Increased vaginal discharge.
  4. High pH secretions, less acidic (4.0–6.0 pH).

E. Perineum.
  1. Increased vascularity.
  2. Hypertrophy of muscles.
  3. Loosening of connective tissue.
F. Ovaries and tubes.
  1. Usually one large corpus luteum present in one ovary. Produces hormones (estrogen and progesterone) until week 10–12.
  2. Ovulation does not take place.

Breast

A. Changes in tissue.
  1. Extensive growth of alveolar tissue, necessary for lactation.
  2. Montgomery's glands—enlargement of sebaceous glands of primary areola.
B. Other changes.
  1. Breast increases in size and firmness and becomes nodular.
  2. Nipples become more prominent and areola deepens in color.
  3. Superficial veins grow more prominent.
  4. At the end of third month, colostrum appears.
  5. After delivery, anterior pituitary stimulates production and secretion of milk.

Abdomen

A. Contour changes as the enlarging uterus extends into the abdominal cavity.
B. *Striae gravidarum* usually appear on the abdomen as pregnancy progresses.

Skin

A. Pigmentation increases in certain areas of the body.
  1. Breast—primary areola deepens in color.
  ◆ 2. Abdomen—*linea nigra*, dark streak down the midline of abdomen, especially prominent in brunettes.
  ◆ 3. Face—*chloasma*, the "mask of pregnancy" pigmentation distributed over the face. Usually disappears after pregnancy.
  4. Face and upper trunk—occasionally spider nevi or palmar erythema develops with the increase in estrogen.
B. Increased sebaceous and sweat gland activity.
C. Pigmented areas on abdomen and breast usually do not completely disappear after delivery.

Circulatory System

◆ A. Considerable increase (up to 50 percent) in volume as a result of
  1. Increased metabolic demands of new tissue.
  2. Expansion of vascular system, especially in the reproductive organs.
  3. Retention of sodium and water.

B. Increase in plasma volume is greater than increase in red blood cells and hemoglobin.
   1. Decline in hemoglobin due to hemodilution referred to as "pseudoanemia."
   2. Low hemoglobin in pregnancy, below 11.5 percent, usually caused by iron-deficiency anemia.

✦ C. Folic acid (folate) and iron requirements are increased to meet demands of increased blood supply and growing fetus (need cannot be met by diet alone; supplement usually given).

D. Heart increases in size. Cardiac output is increased (25–50 percent); after 28 weeks reaches maximum volume.

✦ E. Blood pressure *should not* rise during pregnancy. Slight decline is normal in second trimester.

F. Fibrinogen concentration increases to term.

G. Palpitations may be experienced during pregnancy due to sympathetic nervous disturbance and intra-abdominal pressure caused by enlarging uterus.

Respiratory System

A. Thoracic cage is pushed upward and diaphragm is elevated as uterus enlarges.

B. Thoracic cage widens to compensate, so vital capacity remains the same or is increased.

C. Oxygen consumption is increased 15 percent to support fetus and tissue.

✦ D. Shortness of breath may be experienced in latter part of pregnancy due to pressure on diaphragm caused by enlarging uterus and decreased CO_2 levels.

Digestive System

A. Nausea, vomiting, and poor appetite are present in early pregnancy because of decreased gastric motility and acidity; due to effects of progesterone.

B. Constipation is due to a decrease in gastrointestinal motility, reduced peristaltic activity, increased water absorption, the pressure of the uterus, and displacement of intra-abdominal organs; it may be present in latter half of pregnancy.

C. Flatulence and heartburn may be present due to decreased gastric secretion of HCl and pepsin and decreased motility of the gastrointestinal tract; results in delayed gastric emptying time.

D. Cardiac sphincter relaxes.

Urinary System

A. Kidneys.
   1. Kidney and renal function increase.
   2. Renal blood flow and glomerular filtration increase 50 percent.
   3. Renal threshold for sugar is reduced in some women. Glycosuria is an indication of the need to further test for gestational diabetes.

B. Bladder and ureters.
   1. Blood supply to the bladder and pelvic organs is increased.
   2. Pressure of the uterus on the bladder causes frequent urination in early and late pregnancy.
   3. Relaxation of smooth muscles during pregnancy leads to dilatation of ureters and renal pelvis, and may cause urine stasis.
   4. A decrease in bladder tone is caused by hormonal influences, and a decrease in bladder capacity occurs because of crowding; may lead to complications during pregnancy and in the postpartum period (UTI, urinary retention).

Joints, Bones, Teeth, and Gums

A. Softening of pelvic cartilages occurs, probably due to the hormone relaxin, progesterone, and estrogen.

B. Posture changes as upper spine is thrown forward to compensate for increased abdominal size (Lordosis).

C. Demineralization of teeth does not occur as a result of normal pregnancy but may be related to poor dental hygiene.

D. Increased vascularity of gums due to hormonal changes with tendency to bleed easily.

Endocrine System

✦ A. Placenta produces the hormones HCG and HPL.
   1. Production of estrogen and progesterone is taken over from the ovaries by the placenta/fetal unit after the second month.
   2. Normal cycle of production of estrogen and progesterone by ovaries is suspended until after delivery.

B. Anterior lobe of pituitary gland enlarges slightly during pregnancy.

C. Adrenal cortex enlarges slightly.

D. Thyroid enlarges slightly and thyroid activity increases.

E. Aldosterone levels gradually increase beginning about the fifteenth week.

Metabolism

✦ A. Weight gain
   1. Progressive gain to ensure fetal growth and development and stores for successful lactation.
      a. Pattern of weight gain important.
      b. 2nd and 3rd trimester: 0.4 kg/week (normal weight); 0.5 kg/week (underweight); 0.3 kg/week (overweight).
   2. Recommendation determined by prepregnancy weight for height (normal: 11.5–16 kg or 25.3–35.2 pounds).
   3. Weight gain should be from balance of foods from revised (2005) food pyramid.

B. Some of the weight gain is caused by retention of fluid and by deposits of fatty tissue.

C. Water metabolism.

1. Tendency to retain fluid in body tissues, especially in the last trimester.

2. Reversal of fluid retention usually takes place in the form of diuresis in the first 24 hours postpartum.

D. Metabolic rate increases 20 percent.

E. Carbohydrate metabolism.

1. Increased need to spare protein stores.

2. First Half: Glucose readily passes across placenta to meet rapid growth needs of fetus; may experience hypoglycemia and faintness.

3. Second Half: Increased production HPL (insulin antagonist properties) produces a normal maternal hyperglycemia; implications for gestational diabetes or preexisting diabetes.

Psychosocial Changes

Altered Emotional Characteristics

A. Pregnancy may be viewed as a developmental process involving endocrine, somatic, and psychological changes, as a period of increased susceptibility to a maturational crisis.

B. Emotional reactions to pregnancy may vary from early rejection to elation.

C. Mother may be puzzled by changes in her feelings.

D. Mother may have fears and worries about the baby and herself.

E. Quick mood changes are common; some emotional instability usually occurs.

F. Mother may experience dependency-independency conflict.

Socialization for Parental Role

A. Pregnant woman may fantasize or daydream to experience the role of mother before the actual birth.

B. Takes on adaptive behaviors that are best suited to her own personality and situation.

✦ C. Experiences a "letting go" of her former role (e.g., as a career woman).

1. May experience ambivalence about letting go of her old role to take on the new one.

2. Desire to have a baby influences adjustment.

✦ D. Concerns.

1. First and second trimester—concerns about body changes, fear of labor and delivery; beginning conceptualization of fetus as separate individual.

2. Third trimester—emotionally labile, becomes more concerned about labor and delivery; shows readiness to assume care of infant; incorporation of concept of fetus as a separate individual should be complete.

E. Father may also experience ambivalence at taking on new role, assuming increased financial responsibility, and sharing wife's attention with child.

F. Father may experience physiologic changes, such as weight gain, nausea, and vomiting (couvades).

Signs of Pregnancy

Definition: The signs of pregnancy are divided into three groups: presumptive, probable, and positive. Positive signs cannot be detected until after the fourth month.

Assessment (See Table 12-3)

✦ Presumptive Signs (Subjective Changes)

A. Amenorrhea (cessation of menstruation).

B. Breast changes: increased size and feeling of fullness, nipples more pronounced, areola darker.

C. Nausea and vomiting (morning sickness): appears in about 50 percent of pregnant women and usually disappears at the end of the third month.

D. Frequent urination—frequent desire to void: usually occurs in the first 3 to 4 months. Pressure on the bladder from an enlarged uterus gives the sensation of a distended bladder.

✦ E. *Quickening*—first perception of fetal movement: occurs between 16th and 18th week.

F. Fatigue: period of drowsiness and lassitude during first 3 months.

✦ G. *Chadwick's sign:* vaginal changes, discoloration and thickening of vaginal mucosa.

✦ Probable Signs (Objective Changes)

A. Enlargement of the abdomen: usually occurs after the third month when the fetus rises out of the pelvis into the abdominal cavity.

B. Increased pigmentation of skin, *chloasma, linea nigra,* and *striae gravidarum.*

C. Changes in internal organs.

1. Change in shape, size, and consistency of the uterus.

✦ 2. *Hegar's sign*—softening of the isthmus of the uterus: occurs about sixth week.

✦ 3. *Goodell's sign*—softening of the cervix: occurs beginning of the second month.

4. *Chadwick's sign*—vaginal changes, discoloration and thickening of vaginal mucosa.

✦ D. *Braxton Hicks* contractions: usually not felt by the mother until seven months, but contractions begin in the early weeks of pregnancy and continue.

✦ E. *Ballottement*—giving a sudden push to the fetus and feeling it rebound in a few seconds to the original position: usually possible in the fourth to fifth month.

Table 12-3. OBSTETRICAL ASSESSMENT		
Assessment	**Normal**	**Abnormal**
BASELINE DATA		
Assess **breasts** and **nipples**		
Contour and size		
Presence of lumps	No lumps	Lumps
Secretions	Colostrum secretions in late first trimester or early second trimester	Secretions, other than colostrum
Assess **abdomen**		
Contour and size		
Changes in skin color	*Linea nigra* (black line of pregnancy along midline of abdomen) Primiparas: coincidentally with growth of fundus Multiparas: after 13–15 weeks' gestation	
Striae (reddish-purple lines)	On breasts, hips, and thighs during pregnancy After pregnancy, faint silvery-gray	
Scar, rashes, or other skin disturbances	Usually none present	
Fundal height in centimeters (fingerbreadths less accurate): measure from symphysis pubis to top of fundus	Fundus palpable just above symphysis at 8–10 weeks Halfway between symphysis and umbilicus at 16 weeks Umbilicus at 20–22 weeks	Large measurements: EDC is incorrect; tumor; ascites; multiple pregnancy; and polyhydramnios, hydatidiform mole Less than normal enlargement: fetal abnormality, oligohydramnios, placental dysmaturity, missed abortion, fetal death
Perineum: assess for scars, moles, lesions or discharge	None present	Rash, warts, discharge
Evaluate **weight**		
Take **vital signs, blood pressure** (BP), **temperature, pulse,** and **respiration** (TPR)		
Evaluate **lab findings**		
Urine: sugar, protein, albumin	Negative for sugar, protein, and albumin throughout pregnancy	Positive for sugar, protein, and/or albumin
Hematocrit (HCT)	38%–47%	
Hemoglobin (Hgb)	12–16 gm/dL	
Blood type and Rh factor		If Rh negative, father's blood should be typed If Rh positive, titers should be followed; possible RhoGAM at termination of pregnancy
Pap smear STD smears and screening (gonorrhea, chlamydia, bacterial vaginosis) Other: HIV, Hepatitis, TB, Maternal alpha-fetoprotein Serum glucose		

Table 12-3. OBSTETRICAL ASSESSMENT *(Continued)*		
Assessment	**Normal**	**Abnormal**
ANTEPARTUM ASSESSMENT		
Evaluate **weight** to assess maternal health and nutritional status and growth of fetus Weight at conception	First trimester: 3–4 lbs Second trimester: 12–14 lbs Third trimester: 8–10 lbs Minimum weight gain during pregnancy: 24 lbs Underweight: should gain 28–42 lbs. Obese: should gain 15 lb or more	Inadequate weight gain: possible maternal malnutrition Excessive weight gain: if sudden at onset, may indicate preeclampsia; if gradual and continual may indicate overeating
Evaluate **blood pressure** Take in same position, on same arm (right arm, sitting)	Fairly constant with baseline data throughout pregnancy	Increased: possible anxiety (client should rest 20 to 30 minutes before you take BP again) Rise of 30/15 above baseline data: sign of preeclampsia Decreased: sign of supine hypotensive syndrome. If lying on back, turn client on left side and take BP again
Evaluate **fundal height**	Drop around 38th week: sign of fetus engaging in birth canal Primipara: sudden drop Multipara: slower, sometimes not until onset of labor	Large fundal growth: may indicate wrong dates, multiple pregnancy, hydatidiform mole, polyhydramnios, tumors Small fundal growth: may indicate fetal demise, fetal anomaly, retarded fetal growth, abnormal presentation or lie, decreased amniotic fluid
Determine **fetal position** after 32 weeks gestation, using **Leopold's maneuvers.** Complete external palpations of the pregnant abdomen to determine fetal position, lie, presentation, and engagement (see Figure 12-1)		
First maneuver: to determine part of fetus presenting into pelvis	Vertex presentation	Breech presentation or transverse lie
Second maneuver: to locate the back, arms, and legs; fetal heart heard best over fetal back		
Third maneuver: to determine part of fetus in fundus		
Fourth maneuver: to determine degree of cephalic flexion and engagement		

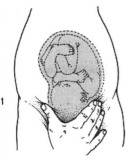 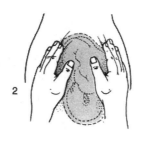 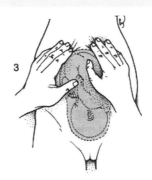 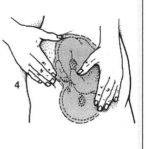

FIGURE 12-1. Steps of Leopold's maneuvers.

Continues

Table 12-3. OBSTETRICAL ASSESSMENT *(Continued)*

Assessment	Normal	Abnormal
Evaluate **fetal heart rate** by quadrant, location, and rate	110–160 beats/min	✦ > 160 or < 110: may indicate fetal distress *Notify physician*
Check for presence of **edema**	In lower extremities toward end of pregnancy	In upper extremities and face: may indicate preeclampsia
Evaluate **urine** (clean catch midstream)	Negative for sugar, protein, and albumin	Positive for sugar: may indicate subclinical or gestational diabetes Positive for protein and/or albumin: may indicate preeclampsia
Evaluate **levels of discomfort** Assess for minor discomforts, danger signs of pregnancy, psychological adaptation, abusive situations		
INTRAPARTUM ASSESSMENT		
Assess for **lightening** and **dropping** (the descent of the presenting part into the pelvis)	Several days to 2 weeks before onset of labor Multipara: may not occur until onset of labor Relief of shortness of breath and increase in urinary frequency	No lightening or dropping: may indicate disproportion between fetal presenting part and maternal pelvis
Check if **mucous plug** has been expelled from cervix	Usually expelled from cervix prior to onset of labor	
Assess for **"bloody show"**	Clear, pinkish, or blood-tinged vaginal discharge that occurs as cervix begins to dilate and efface	
Assess for **ruptured membranes** Time water breaks	Nitrazine paper turns blue Before, during, or after onset of labor	Breech presentation: frank meconium or meconium staining
Color of **amniotic fluid**	Clear, straw color	Greenish-brown: indicates meconium has passed from fetus, possible fetal distress Yellow-stained: fetal hypoxic episode 36 hours or more prior to rupture of membrane or hemolytic disease
Quantity of amniotic fluid	Normal is 500 to 1000 mL of amniotic fluid, rarely expelled at one time	**Polyhydramnios**—excessive amniotic fluid over 2000 mL Observe newborn for congenital anomalies: craniospinal malformation, orogastrointestinal anomalies, Down syndrome, and congenital heart defects **Oligohydramnios**—minimal amniotic fluid, less than 500 mL Observe newborn for malformation of ear, genitourinary tract anomalies, and renal agenesis
Odor of fluid Assess for unusual **vaginal discharge**	No odor	Odor may indicate infection; deliver within 24 hours
Fetal heart rate	110–160 beats/min Regular rhythm	Decreased: indicates fetal distress with possible cord prolapse or cord compression Accelerated: initial sign of fetal hypoxia Absent: may indicate fetal demise

Table 12-3. OBSTETRICAL ASSESSMENT (Continued)

Assessment	Normal	Abnormal
LABOR AND DELIVERY ASSESSMENT		
Evaluate Contractions		
Frequency: from start of one contraction to start of next	3–5 minutes between contractions	Irregular contractions with long intervals between: indicates false labor
Duration: from beginning of contraction to time uterus begins to relax	50–90 seconds	> 90 seconds: uterine tetany; stop oxytocin if running
Intensity (strength of contraction): measured with monitoring device	Peak 25 mm Hg End of labor may reach 50–75 mm Hg	> 75 mm Hg: uterine tetany or uterine rupture
First stage		
Latent phase (0–4 cm dilation)	0–3 to 4 cm average 6.4 hrs (~8.6 hrs nulliparas, 5.3 hrs multiparas)	Prolonged time in any phase: may indicate poor fetal position, incomplete fetal flexion, cephalopelvic disproportion, or poor uterine contractions
Active phase (4–8 cm)	4–6 hours average (~6 hrs nulliparas, 4.5 hrs multiparas)	
Transitional phase (8–10 cm)	Length of time varies (Maximum 3 hr nulliparas, 1 hr multipara)	If total labor < 3 hours: indicates precipitous labor, increasing risk of fetal complications, or maternal lacerations and tears
Assess for **bloody show**		
Observe for presence of **nausea or vomiting**		
Assess **perineum**	Beginning to bulge	
Evaluate **urge to bear down**		Often uncontrolled Multipara: can cause precipitous delivery "Panting" (can be controlled until safe delivery area established)
Second stage (10 cm to delivery)	Primipara: up to 2 hours Multipara: several minutes to 2 hours	> 2 hours: increased risk of fetal brain damage and maternal exhaustion
Assess for **presenting part**	Vertex with ROA or LOA presentation	Occiput posterior, breech, face, or transverse lie
Assess **caput** (infant head) *Multipara:* caput size of dime *Nullipara:* caput size of half-dollar Birth attendant should be present	Visible when bearing down during contraction	"Crowns" in room other than delivery room: delivery imminent (do not move client)
Assess **fetal heart rate**	✦ 110–160/min	Decreased: may indicate supine hypotensive syndrome (turn client on side and take again) Hemorrhage (check for other signs of bleeding; notify physician)
Bradycardia—drop of 20 beats/min below baseline of 110 *Tachycardia*—increase in FHR over 160 beats/min for 10 minutes		Increased or decreased: may indicate fetal distress secondary to cord progression or compression (place client in Trendelenburg's or knee–chest position; give oxygen if necessary; inform physician)
Evaluate **fetal heart rate tracing**	✦ Short-term variability is present Long-term variability ranges from 3–5 cycles/min	Absence of variability (no short term or long term present) Severe variable decelerations (fetal heart rate < 70 for longer than 30–45 seconds with decreasing variability)

Continues

Table 12-3. OBSTETRICAL ASSESSMENT *(Continued)*

Assessment	Normal	Abnormal
Deceleration	Early deceleration (10- to 20-beat drop) Recovery when acme contraction passes—often not serious	Monitor closely—distinguish from late deceleration (10- to 20-beat decrease with hypertonic contraction) leads to fetal distress
Variable deceleration; decrease in FHR, below 120/min	Mild may be within normal parameters—continue to monitor	Cord compression—may result in fetal difficulty
Loss of beat-to-beat variation	If continues less than 15 min, no problem apparent	Late deceleration pattern occurs—monitor for hypertonic contraction; leads to fetal distress
Evaluate **breathing**	Controlled with contractions	Heavy or excessive: may lead to hyperventilation and/or dehydration
Evaluate **pain** and **anxiety**	Medication often required after dilated 4–5 cm unless using natural childbirth methods	Severe pain early in first stage of labor: inadequate prenatal teaching, backache due to position of fetus or position in bed, uterine irritability or uterine tetany
Third stage (from delivery of baby to delivery of placenta)	Placental separation occurs within 30 minutes (usually 3–5 min)	Failure of placental separation Abnormality of uterus or cervix, weak, ineffectual uterine contraction, tetanic contractions causing closure of cervix > 3 hours: indicates retained placenta
Fourth stage (first hour postpartum)		Mother in unstable condition (hemorrhage usual cause) Highest risk of hemorrhage in first postpartum hour
Temperature	36.5–37.5°C	> 37.5°C: may indicate infection Slight elevation: due to dehydration from mouth breathing and NPO
Pulse	Pulse: 60–100	Increased: may indicate pain or hemorrhage
Respiration	Respirations: 12–22	
Blood pressure	Blood pressure: 120–140/80	Increased: may indicate anxiety, pain, or preeclamptic condition Decreased: hemorrhage

POSTPARTUM ASSESSMENT

Assessment	Normal	Abnormal
Assess **vital signs** every 15 minutes for 1 hour, every 30 minutes for 1 hour, every hour for 4 hours, every 8 hours, and as needed	Pulse may be 45–60/min in stage 4 Pulse to normal range about third day	Decreased BP and increased pulse: probably postpartum hemorrhage Elevated temperature > 38°C indicates possible infection Temperature elevates when lactation occurs
Assess **fundus** every 15 minutes for 1 hour, every 8 hours for 48 hours, then daily	Firm (like a grapefruit) in midline and at or slightly above umbilicus Return to prepregnant size in 6 weeks: descending at rate of 1 fingerbreadth/day	Boggy fundus: immediately massage gently until firm; report to physician and observe closely; empty bladder; medicate with oxytocin if ordered Fundus misplaced 1–2 fingerbreadths from midline: indicates full bladder (client must void or be catheterized)

Table 12-3. **OBSTETRICAL ASSESSMENT** *(Continued)*		
Assessment	**Normal**	**Abnormal**
Assess **lochia** every 15 minutes for 1 hour, every 8 hours for 48 hours, then daily		
Color	3 days postpartum: dark red (rubra) 4–10 days postpartum: clear pink (serosa) 10–21 days postpartum: white, yellow brown (alba)	Heavy, bright-red: indicates hemorrhage (massage fundus, give medication on order, notify physician) Spurts: may indicate cervical tear No lochia: may indicate clot occluding cervical opening (support fundus; express clot)
Quantity	Moderate amount, steadily decreases	
Odor	Minimal	Foul: may indicate infection
Assess **breasts** and **nipples** daily	Days 1–2: soft, intact, secreting colostrum Days 2–3: engorged, tender, full, tight, painful Day 3+: secreting milk Increased pains as baby sucks—oxytocin is released causing uterus to contract; common in multiparas	Sore or cracked (clean and dry nipples; decrease breastfeeding time; apply breast shield between feeding) Milk does not "let down": help client relax and decrease anxiety; give glass of wine or beer
Assess **perineum** daily	Episiotomy intact, no swelling, no discoloration	Swelling or bruising: may indicate hematoma
Assess **bladder** every 4 hours	Voiding regularly with no pain and adequate amounts	Not voiding: bladder may be full and displaced to one side, leading to increased lochia (catheterization may be necessary)
Assess **bowels**	Spontaneous bowel movement 2–3 days after delivery	Fear associated with pain from hemorrhoids
Assess mother–infant **bonding**	Touching infant, talking to infant, talking about infant	Refuses to touch or hold infant
Evaluate **Rh-negative status**	Client does not require RhoGAM	RhoGAM administered

✦ MATERNAL HISTORY: DEFINITION OF TERMS

Abortion: pregnancy loss before fetus is viable (usually < 20 weeks or 500 gm) *Gravida:* any pregnancy, including present one *Primigravida:* refers to first-time pregnancy	*Multigravida:* refers to second or any subsequent pregnancy *Para:* past pregnancies that continued past viable age (20 weeks); infants may be alive or dead at birth *Primipara:* refers to female who has delivered first viable infant; born either alive or dead	*Nullipara:* refers to female who has never carried past pregnancy to viable age for fetus *Multipara:* refers to female who has given birth to two or more viable infants; either alive or dead

F. Outline of the fetus by abdominal palpation (a probable sign, because a tumor may simulate fetal parts).

G. Pregnancy tests.

✦ 1. Positive test is based upon the secretion of chorionic gonadotropin in the urine; it is usually detectable 10 days after the first missed period. Test is 95 percent effective.

2. Radioimmunoassay (RIA) test.

a. Test for Beta (B), the subunit of HCG: most sensitive but not readily available.

Pregnancy can be detected before the first period. Test requires 24 hours to complete.

b. 2-hour tube tests: first void specimen; quite reliable.

c. 2-minute rapid-slide test: less sensitive and less reliable.

d. False-positive readings: may be due to protein or blood in urine, neoplasms, ingestion of certain drugs (aspirin, methadone).

H. Amenorrhea by week 4.

✦ **Positive Signs**

A. Apparent after 18th to 20th week.
B. Auscultation of fetal heart rates with stethoscope or ultrasonic equipment (rates: 120 to 160). With ultrasonic equipment, fetal heart rate may be heard at 10 to 12 weeks.
C. Active fetal movements are perceptible by the examiner.
D. Ultrasound examination, showing fetal outline. Transvaginal ultrasound allows identification of gestational sac by 5 weeks' gestation.

Implementation

Physical Examination

A. Initial examination.
    1. Record complete history: past obstetrical history, medical history, family history.
    2. Assist with physical examination: pelvic, breast, chest, abdomen, complete blood count (CBC), Pap smear, rubella titer, slide for gonorrhea and chlamydia, serology for syphilis (VDRL), HIV, hepatitis.
    3. Assess for risk factors: age, socioeconomic, ethnicity, previous pregnancy history, multiple pregnancy, late prenatal care, preexisting or coexisting medical problems, substance abuse.
    4. Establish baseline blood pressure and weight.
    5. Provide client with diet and health instructions.
B. Subsequent examinations: usually once a month until the last trimester, then more frequently. More frequent in high-risk pregnancy.
✦   1. Assess weight, blood pressure, and urine for protein and sugar.
    2. Assist with physical examination.
      a. Measure fundal height.
      b. Palpate abdomen.
      c. Auscultate fetal heart rate.
      d. Observe for signs of complications.
      e. Pap smear and smear for gonorrhea before delivery.
✦   f. Screening and treatment of beta-hemolytic streptococci (GBS) culture-positive women before delivery.

Client Instruction

A. Provide client with diet and health instructions.
    1. It is important that mother maintain adequate nutrition and fluids.
✦   2. Vitamin, folic acid, and iron supplements are usually prescribed.
    3. All drugs can be expected to cross the placenta and affect the fetus.
✦   4. Greatest danger is first trimester, especially when organs are developing.
    5. Many other effects of drugs on the fetus are unknown and may not be evident for years.

    6. Pregnant women should refrain from taking drugs during pregnancy, even commonly used drugs such as aspirin.
✦   7. There is no "safe" level of alcohol consumption during pregnancy.
      a. It is recommended that women abstain from any alcohol during the 1st trimester.
      b. Alcohol passes the placental barrier within minutes of consumption.
      c. Effects of alcohol on the fetus varies according to the stage of fetal development.
✦   8. Nicotine: current research indicates that smoking retards growth of the fetus.
      a. Vasoconstriction of mother's vessels, resulting in decreased placental flow.
      b. Increase in carbon dioxide levels in mother's blood and reduction of oxygen-carrying capacity.
    9. Caffeine: may cause malformations. Suggest limited intake or avoidance of sources of caffeine (i.e., coffee, cola, and chocolate).
B. Inform client regarding activities of daily living.
    1. Exercise in moderation is beneficial but should never be carried on past the point of fatigue.
    2. Sports may be participated in if they are part of the mother's usual activity and there are no complications present.
    3. Fatigue is common in early pregnancy.
    4. Frequent rest periods, at 10–15-minute intervals, are helpful in avoiding needless fatigue.
    5. Dental hygiene should be maintained daily and infections treated promptly.
    6. Tub baths may be taken. Water enters vagina under pressure only. Baths are contraindicated after membranes have ruptured.
    7. Travel.
      a. May travel with physician's permission.
      b. Airlines discourage travel after the eighth month.
      c. When traveling, tell client to elevate feet and walk around periodically to decrease pedal edema.
C. Assess if client is employed and provide instructions as applicable.
    1. May be continued as long as it does not cause overfatigue.
    2. Have client avoid areas where chemicals or gases are used as these may cause congenital malformations in infant.
    3. Have client avoid heavy lifting and individuals with contagious diseases.
D. Provide information to client regarding sexual intercourse.
    1. May be carried on without fear unless bleeding or premature contractions develop.

Table 12-4. MAJOR DISCOMFORTS AND RELIEF MEASURES

Discomfort	Trimester Most Prominent	Relief Measures
Nausea and vomiting	1st	Eat five or six small, frequent meals. Between meals, have crackers without fluid. Avoid foods high in carbohydrates, fried and greasy, or with a strong odor.
Fatigue	1st	Take frequent rest periods during the day.
Frequency voiding	1st, 3rd	Wear perineal pads if there is leakage.
Heartburn	2nd, 3rd	Avoid fatty, fried, and highly spiced foods. Small frequent feedings. *Avoid* sodium bicarbonate.
Abdominal distress	1st, 2nd, 3rd	Eat slowly, chew food thoroughly, take smaller helpings of food.
Flatulence	2nd, 3rd	Maintain daily bowel movement. Avoid gas-forming foods.
Constipation	2nd, 3rd	Drink sufficient fluids. Eat fruit and foods high in fiber and roughage. Exercise moderately. *Do not* use mineral oil.
Hemorrhoids	3rd	Apply ointments, suppositories, warm compresses. Avoid constipation.
Insomnia	3rd	Exercise moderately to promote relaxation and fatigue.
Backaches	3rd	Rest and improve posture; use a firm mattress. Use a good abdominal support; wear comfortable shoes. Do exercises such as squatting, sitting, and pelvic rock.
Varicosities, legs, and vulva	3rd	Avoid long periods of standing or sitting with legs crossed. Sit or lie with feet and hips elevated. Move about while standing to improve circulation. Wear support hose; *avoid* tight garters. Wear peripads with vulva varicosities.
Edema of legs and feet	3rd	Elevate feet while sitting or lying down. Avoid standing or sitting in one position for long periods.
Cramps in legs	3rd	Extend cramped leg and flex ankles, pushing foot upward with toes pointed toward knee. Increase calcium intake.
Pain in thighs or aching of perineum	3rd	Alternate periods of sitting and standing. Rest.
Shortness of breath	3rd	Sit up. Lie on back with arms extended above bed.
Breast soreness	1st, 2nd, 3rd	Wear brassiere with wide adjustable straps that fits well.
Supine hypotensive syndrome	3rd	Change position to left side to relieve pressure of uterus on inferior vena cava.
Vaginal discharge	3rd	Practice proper cleansing and hygiene. Avoid douche unless recommended by physician. Observe for signs of vaginal infection common in pregnancy.

2. May need to vary usual positions as pregnancy advances.

E. Provide information of danger signs during pregnancy and process to follow when labor begins.

Psychosocial Support

A. Reassure client that emotional changes and feelings are normal reactions and that the client need not feel guilty.

B. Provide supportive atmosphere allowing the client to express fears and concerns regarding self, baby, changes in family relationship, etc.

C. Inform client's mate that changes in attitudes, feelings, sexuality, and emotions are temporary and are related to pregnancy. (*See* Table 12-4.)

D. Screen for abusive relationship.

Childbirth Education and Preparation

A. Theories of childbirth.
1. Each method varies somewhat, but basic underlying concepts are similar. Birth is viewed as a natural occurrence. Knowledge about the birth experience dispels fear, tension, and distraction. Concentration during labor and delivery modifies the pain experience.
2. Purpose: to promote relaxation enabling the mother to work with the labor process. Allows parents to take an active part in the birth process, thereby increasing self-esteem and satisfaction.

B. Factors that influence pain in labor.
1. Preconditioning: by "old wives' tales," fantasies, and fears. Accurate information about the childbirth process can often alleviate effects of preconditioning.
2. Pain produces stress, which in turn affects the body's functioning. Interpretations of and reactions to pain can be altered by a refocusing of attention and by conditioning.
3. Feelings of isolation. Social expectations and tension may also include feelings of pain.
4. Expectations for mastery and control.

C. Goals accomplished by means of
1. Education: anatomy and physiology of reproductive system, and the labor and delivery process; replacement of misinformation and superstition with facts. May include classes on nutrition, discomforts of pregnancy, breast-feeding, infant care, etc.
2. Training: controlled breathing and neuromuscular exercises.
3. Presence of father or significant other in labor and delivery rooms to serve as coach and lend support.

D. Common methods presently available.
✦ 1. Read method (natural childbirth): introduced by Grantly Dick-Read in England. Believed pain in childbirth was psychological rather than physiological. Pain brought about by fear and tension. (This theory not subscribed to today.)
2. Lamaze method.
3. Bradley method.
4. Scientific relaxation for childbirth.

E. Other: water birth, LeBoyer Birth Method (introduced in the 1970s to reduce the stress to the infant from birth by providing a quiet, warm environment, soft lights, and a warm bath immediately after birth).

F. Instruction for parents on delivery by C-section.

FETAL ASSESSMENT

Biochemical Measurements

✦ A. Estriol excretion: estrogen metabolism in pregnancy is dependent on a healthy mother, a healthy fetus, and an intact placenta.
1. Estriol level increases as the fetus grows and decreases when growth ceases.
2. Measured by 24-hour urine specimen or serum estriol levels.
3. Provides guide to normalcy of fetoplacental unit.
    a. Placental functioning.
    b. Fetal well-being.
4. Excretion of high estriol levels indicates good function; low levels may indicate fetal jeopardy.
5. Serial assays are usually done, starting at about 32 weeks, to assess the fetal condition.

B. Human placental lactogen (HPL).
1. Product of the placenta.
2. Increased levels during pregnancy correspond with increase in fetal weight.

Amniotic Fluid Studies

A. Amniocentesis is the introduction of a needle through the abdominal and uterine walls and into the amniotic cavity to withdraw fluid for examination.
✦ 1. Amniocentesis indicates
    a. Sex of baby.
    b. Certain congenital defects such as Down syndrome.
    c. State of fetus affected by Rh isoimmunization.
2. Advanced maternal age—over 35, or suspected abnormality.
3. Test provides clearest chromosome profile, but is usually done after 14 weeks—may be done as early as 12 weeks.
4. Procedure.
    a. Amniotic fluid obtained via transabdominal or suprapubic amniocentesis.
        (1) Complications rare (less than 1 percent).
        (2) Rh-negative women would receive Rh-immune globulin after amniocentesis, if not already sensitized.
    b. Performed at about 16 weeks; takes 2 to 4 weeks for results.
    c. Positive test indicates fetus has genetic disorder.
    d. Preceded by ultrasound.

B. Amniotic fluid may be analyzed to determine maturity of fetal lungs.

Evaluation of Fetal Maturity

◆ A. Lecithin/sphingomyelin ratio (L/S ratio).
1. Test for fetal maturity by examining the ratio of two components of surfactant—lecithin and sphingomyelin.
2. Lecithin major constituent of surfactant in the lungs.
3. At 13th week, the concentration of sphingomyelin is higher than lecithin.
4. Thereafter, lecithin increases slowly until the 35th week, when it is two or more times greater than sphingomyelin. At this time, fetal lungs are said to be mature and can maintain stability with the first breath, and the infant is unlikely to develop respiratory distress syndrome (RDS).

◆ B. Phosphatidylglycerol (PG).
1. Second most abundant phospholipid in surfactant.
   a. Appears at 35 to 36 weeks and increases until term.
   b. Presence of this lipid indicates low risk for RDS.
2. Recently, lung maturity is determined by combination of L/S ratio and PG.

Chorionic Villus Sampling (CVS)

Indications

A. Diagnostic capability similar to amniocentesis; results reflect fetal chromosome, enzyme, and DNA content.
B. Advantage is that diagnostic information is available before end of first trimester of pregnancy.
C. Disadvantage—increased risk of pregnancy loss.

Procedure

A. A transcervical approach used to aspirate chorionic villi from the placenta through endocervix.
B. Syringe contents (villi) inspected microscopically and prepared for culture.
C. Results are available in 1–2 weeks.

Alpha-Fetoprotein (AFP)

A. Principal screening procedure for detection of neural tube defect (spina bifida, hydrocephalus; incidence is 1 per 1000–2000 births in United States).
◆ B. Incidence of neural tube defect can be reduced with use of folic acid (0.4 mg/day) prior to and during first trimester of pregnancy.
1. Low levels detect Down syndrome and maternal hypertensive states.
2. High levels detect open neural tube defects, risk of premature delivery, toxemia, fetal distress, Rh isoimmunization.

C. Levels of maternal serum AFP detect possible abnormalities in fetus.
D. Multipurpose test done at 16–18 weeks.
E. Mother's blood is analyzed for amount of AFP that liver normally re-releases at a known and increasing amount as pregnancy proceeds—follow up with amniocentesis or CVS.
F. Procedure allows families to choose whether to have a child with an identified birth defect.

Ultrasound

◆ A. A diagnostic test of intermittent high-frequency sound waves that reflect off tissues according to varying densities.
1. Most common diagnostic procedure—70 percent pregnant women in United States.
2. Evaluates both functional and structural characteristics.
B. Advantages—technique is noninvasive, nondamaging, and painless.
C. Purpose—to differentiate tissue mass and do serial studies. Determines fetal movements, breathing, heart valve capability.
D. Results—detects placental location (for amniocentesis, placenta previa) gestational age, presence of twins, fetal growth, major malformations, amniotic fluid volume, and presence of pelvic masses.
E. Procedure—client instructed to have a full bladder; test takes 20–30 minutes to complete. Near term, anticipate supine hypotension, nausea, and vertigo.

Nonstress Test (NST)

Indications

A. Test designed to measure fetal baseline heart rate and variability. May also include record of fetal movement as reported by the client.
B. Indicated in conditions of known maternal problems such as diabetes, chronic hypertension, and preeclampsia.
C. Usually given after the 32nd week on a weekly or semiweekly schedule and on an outpatient basis.

Procedure

A. Place client in semi-Fowler's position—may use a recliner chair.
B. Take baseline vital signs.
C. Place external monitor over fundus of uterus.
D. Instruct client to press recording button each time she feels fetal movement.
E. Normal test time is 20–40 minutes.
◆ F. Record fetal heart rate and contractile activity.
1. A reactive NST (two or more accelerations of 15 beats/min or more within 20 minutes) shows

a healthy fetus with good reserves—a monitor strip with a normal fetal heart rate, pattern, and good variability.

2. A nonreactive test does not meet the above criteria.

Contraction Stress Test (CST)

Indications

✦ A. Test results determine status of fetoplacental unit—evaluates fetus's ability to tolerate stress of uterine contraction.
   1. If placental flow is normal, fetus remains oxygenated during uterine contractions.
   2. Placental insufficiency produces characteristic late deceleration pattern during contraction. (Fetal bradycardia is less than 110 beats/min or persistent drop of 20 beats below baseline.)
B. Three consecutive contractions of at least 40 seconds in a 10-minute period—may take 1–2 hours.
   1. A positive CST reaction would be persistent late decelerations or bradycardia.
   2. If fetus cannot withstand mild contractions, cesarean delivery is indicated.
C. Following test, observe for complications.
   1. Fetal heart rate below 110.
   2. Sustained uterine contractions.
   3. Supine hypotensive syndrome (check maternal blood pressure).

Procedure

A. Client usually not admitted.
B. Place client in semi-Fowler's or lateral recumbent position to prevent supine hypotensive syndrome.
C. Give liquid nourishment if ordered.
D. Explain procedure to client.
E. Apply external fetal monitor.
F. Observe for uterine activity and fetal heart rate usually for 10–20 minutes to obtain baseline.
G. IV solution with oxytocic drug is started; infusion pump used to administer more accurate dosage.
H. Dosage is increased every 15–20 minutes until client has three good contractions in a 10-minute period. (Oxytocin is discontinued once pattern is established.)
I. Observe client for signs of sensitivity to drug.
J. Record vital signs and oxytocic infusion every 15 minutes on strip.
K. Monitor contractions and fetal heart rate until client returns to preoxytocic state.
L. Discontinue IV and prepare client for discharge.
M. Record all information on chart; monitor strip is considered legal document and becomes part of chart.
✦ N. Discontinue drug immediately if fetal heart rate decreases to below 110 or sustained uterine contraction develops.

Mammary Stimulation Test (MST)

✦ A. Also called Breast Self-Stimulation Test (BSST). Purpose—start contractions without the use of oxytocin.
B. Preferred method—noninvasive.
C. Procedure—manual stimulation of mother's nipples triggers release of oxytocin to induce contractions (follow CST except roll nipples for 5 minutes, then other side if no contractions).
   1. Contractions similar to those with spontaneous labor.
   2. Nerve impulses cause release of endogenous oxytocin.
   3. When three contractions occur in 10 minutes, breast stimulation is stopped.
   4. Assess fetal heart rate for prolonged decelerations.
   5. Perform test in or near delivery room.

Biophysical Profile Score (BPS)

A. Profile identifies fetus in danger and confirms a healthy fetus.
B. A score of 2 for each normal finding and 0 for each abnormal finding for a maximum of 10.
C. Assessment of five parameters by ultrasound for 30 min.
   1. Fetal muscle tone.
   2. Fetal movements—body or limbs (3 per hour).
   3. Breathing movements.
   4. Amniotic fluid volume.
   5. FHR reactivity (assessed with nonstress test).
D. Results of nonstress test—acceleration with fetal movement.
   1. Scores of 8–10 reassuring, but repeat testing is indicated.
   2. Scores of 5–6 equivocal and repeat testing should be done within 24 hours.
   3. Scores of 4 or less worrisome and indicate immediate delivery is necessary.

COMPLICATIONS OF PREGNANCY

Definition: High-risk pregnancy occurs when there is an increased chance of morbidity and/or mortality to the mother and/or fetus due to the presence of a complicating factor.

Characteristics

A. The development of obstetrically related conditions during the pregnancy such as vaginal bleeding, toxic states, and premature labor.
B. Medical conditions such as cardiac disease, diabetes, or infection.
C. Unfavorable obstetrical history as high parity—five or more pregnancies, previous infant death, prema-

ture birth, or infant with congenital malformations, difficulty in conceiving, less than a year since last pregnancy, and Rh incompatibility.

D. Psychosocial conditions such as under 17 years of age, narcotic or alcohol addiction, and poverty.

Assessment

A. Obtain a general assessment of pregnant client for signs indicative of the development of complications. Include an accurate health history.

✦ B. Observe for presence of danger signals.
1. Bleeding from the vagina.
2. Escape of amniotic fluid denoting premature rupture of the membranes.
3. Contractions increasing in strength, duration, and proximity before term.
4. Dizziness or blurred vision or epigastric pain.
5. Edema of the face and fingers.
6. Persistent and severe vomiting.
7. Chills, malaise and/or elevated temperature.
8. Absence of or significant and consistent decrease in fetal movement.
9. Decrease or absence of fetal heart tones.

Implementation

A. Assess, monitor, and control the specific conditions leading to identification of the client as high risk.

B. Refer to following conditions for specific management.

Spontaneous Abortion

✦ Types

A. Spontaneous abortion is defined as the involuntary expulsion of the fetus before viability.

B. Threatened: some loss of blood and pain without loss of products of conception.

C. Imminent: profuse bleeding, severe contractions, bearing-down sensation; without intervention, products of conception will be lost.

D. Inevitable: bleeding, contractions, ruptured membranes, and cervical dilation.

E. Incomplete: portion of products of conception remain in uterine cavity.

F. Complete: all products of conception expelled.

G. Habitual: abortion in three or more succeeding pregnancies.

Characteristics

A. Abnormalities of fetus; blighted embryo.
B. Abnormalities of reproductive tract.
C. Injuries: physical and emotional shocks.
D. Endocrine disturbances.
E. Acute infectious diseases.
F. Maternal diseases.
G. Psychogenic problems.

MEDICAL IMPLICATIONS

- Endocrine disturbances: hormone therapy (estrogen and progesterone), thyroid therapy.
- Incompetent cervical os: McDonald operation, or Shirodkar procedure: internal os constricted by encircling suture, which is removed when labor begins.
- Abnormalities and fibromas: surgical correction of abnormalities, if possible, and removal of fibromas.
- Oxytocic drug may be given to hasten process of abortion, if it is inevitable, and to promote contraction of uterus after abortion.
- Medication for pain if necessary.
- Blood transfusion if necessary.
- Dilatation and curettage in incomplete abortion.
- Administration of RhoGAM to Rh-negative mothers.
- Antibiotic therapy if infection seems possible.

Assessment

A. Observe amount of vaginal bleeding: slight, moderate, or heavy.

B. Evaluate intermittent contractions, pain (usually beginning in the small of the back), and abdominal cramping.

C. Observe for passage of tissue.

D. Evaluate condition of internal cervical os.

E. Evaluate size of uterus and compare estimated length of pregnancy.

F. Assess psychological state of client.

Implementation

✦ A. Save all perineal pads and expelled tissue for examination.

B. Offer emotional support but do not give false reassurance.

C. Observe for signs of shock and institute emergency measures if necessary (type and crossmatch).

D. Maintain client on bedrest.

E. Provide instructions regarding activity restriction.

F. Provide diversional activities while on bedrest.

G. If incompetent cervix is treated with cerclage, provide the following nursing care:
1. Place woman in Trendelenburg's position to keep pressure off cervix.
2. Continuously monitor fetal heart tone and contractions.
3. Observe for premature rupture of the membranes.
4. When woman goes into labor, verify that all sutures are removed and carefully observe labor pattern.

H. Ensure that client receives counseling psychotherapy if needed.

I. Have client restrict activities such as climbing stairs and coitus for at least 2 weeks after bleeding stops.

For Therapeutic Abortions, see page 603.

Extrauterine or Ectopic Pregnancy

Definition: Implantation of the fertilized ovum outside the uterus; usually cannot develop longer than 10 to 12 weeks.

Characteristics

A. Although the fertilized ovum usually attaches to the uterine lining, it may become implanted at any point between the graafian follicle and the uterus.

B. Tubal pregnancy is the most common form (95 percent), but the ovum may attach to an ovary, the abdomen, or interligaments.

C. Implantation.
1. Ovum attaches to tube and erodes into mucosa wall, as it would to the endometrial lining of the uterus.
2. Tube increases in size and stretches.
3. Pregnancy usually terminates during the first 3 months by:
   a. Spontaneous tubal abortion.
   b. Tubal rupture.
   c. Death and disintegration of products of conception within the tube.

D. Abdominal pregnancies have been known to progress to term.

E. Etiology.
1. Progress of ovum through tube is delayed for some reason.
2. Tubal deformities: congenital or due to disease such as gonorrhea.
3. Tumors pressing against the tube.
4. Adhesions from previous surgery.
5. Tubal spasms.
6. Migration of ovum to opposite tube.

Assessment

A. History of missed periods and "spotting."
B. Early signs of pregnancy. (Woman may or may not know she is pregnant.)
C. Anemia—fatigue and pale mucous membranes.
D. Enlarged uterus due to hormonal influence.
E. Slight abdominal pain or sudden excruciating one-sided lower abdominal pain.
1. Often first indication of ruptured tube.
2. 50 percent experience referred right shoulder pain.
F. Fainting and lightheadedness (occurs in 35 to 50 percent).
G. Laboratory tests and ultrasound.

Implementation

A. Institute same care as for postsurgical client.
B. Observe for signs of shock and institute treatment for shock as necessary.

C. Protect client against undue fatigue and infection (energy level and resistance will be low because of severe blood loss).
D. Provide emotional support: client may be frightened and feel the loss of the pregnancy.

Hydatidiform Mole

Definition: A benign neoplasm of the chorion, in which chorionic villi degenerate, become filled with a clear viscous fluid, and assume the appearance of grapelike clusters involving all or parts of the decidual lining of the uterus. Also called trophoblastic disease.

Characteristics

A. Classified in two ways: complete mole (contains no genetic maternal material) and partial mole (contains 69 chromosomes—normal is 46).
B. Incidence is rare—occurs once in every 1000–1500 pregnancies, except in Asia where it is more common.
C. Usually there is no fetus found—may be pathological ova.
D. High incidence (1 in 250) in Asia may be due to dietary protein deficiency.

Assessment

A. Evaluate for vaginal bleeding: may vary from spotting to profuse; anemia as result of blood loss.
B. Assess for intermittent brownish discharge after the 12th week.
C. Check for enlargement of the uterus; may be out of proportion to duration of pregnancy.
D. Check for nausea and vomiting: appears earlier, is more severe, and lasts longer than normal.
E. Evaluate for severe preeclampsia, which develops in the early part of the second trimester.
F. Evaluate for pregnancy-induced hypertension (PIH), which occurs with the rapid expansion of the uterus.
G. Assess for passage of characteristic vesicles.
H. Check fetal heart tones: none may be heard; no fetal parts may be discerned.

MEDICAL IMPLICATIONS

- Test for increased titer of chorionic gonadotropin. A 24-hour specimen is collected for the total daily output.
- Ultrasound: gives positive diagnosis in the first trimester.
- Amniography: x-ray following injection with contrast dye.
- Evacuation of uterus as soon as positive diagnosis is made by dilatation and curettage or vacuum curettage suction.
- Follow-up supervision for one year.
- Continued high hCG titers indicate a pathological condition.
- Pregnancy not advised until one year after tests are negative.

Implementation

A. Observe for uterine hemorrhage following evacuation because the uterus is very fragile and has little tone.

B. Provide emotional support: client may fear a malignancy or may feel the loss of the baby or repulsion at products of conception.

C. Encourage client to have follow-up treatment because of possibility of development of neoplasm.

D. Have client avoid pregnancy for one year from negative test because pregnancy may mask increasing levels of hCG due to development of choriocarcinoma.

Amniotic Fluid Abnormalities

Definition: A minimal or excessive amount of amniotic fluid. Normal amount is 500–1000 mL. The volume in the uterus is an indicator of fetal well-being and placental function.

A. Amount of amniotic fluid can be evaluated by amniotic fluid volume (AFV) or index (AFI).
   1. Ultrasound (AFV) measures pockets of fluid in uterus and calculates normal amount in centimeters.
      a. Pocket measure at least 2 cm across is normal.
      b. Less than 2 cm is associated with oligohydramnios.
   2. AFI measures pockets of amniotic fluid in four quadrants of uterus.
      a. AFI greater than 20 cm (combining amount in all 4 quadrants) indicates hydramnios.
      b. AFI less than 5 cm indicates oligohydramnios.
B. Hydramnios (polyhydramnios).
   1. Actual cause is unknown. Occurs when there is over 2000 mL of amniotic fluid.
   2. Occurs with major fetal malformations.
   3. Diagnosis is usually made through clinical observation of the greatly enlarged uterus.
   4. Assessment.
      a. Observe for greatly enlarged abdomen.
      b. Evaluate edema of the lower extremities.
      c. Question if general abdominal discomfort is present.
      d. Observe for occasional shortness of breath.
      e. Assess for presence of diabetes and Rh sensitization as this condition frequently accompanies it.
   5. Implementation.
      a. Instruct client to empty bladder so it will not distend.
      b. Monitor vital signs.
      c. Place client in semi-Fowler's position to assist in breathing if not contraindicated.
C. Oligohydramnios.
   1. Minimal amniotic fluid—less than 500 mL.
   2. Indicates possible fetal compromise—congenital anomalies of renal aplasia and kidney defects, postmaturity, pulmonary hypoplasia, and placental insufficiency.
   3. Assessment.
      a. Uterus does not increase in size corresponding to age of fetus.
      b. Fetus is easily palpated.
   4. Implementation.
      a. Acute oligohydramnios, rapid infusion of 100 mL lactated Ringer's solution may be given to client to increase blood volume.
      b. Plan for cesarean delivery because with low fluid, fetus may not be able to tolerate pressure of labor.
      c. Continual fetal monitoring (EFM):
         (1) Assess for nonreassuring signs (baseline changes, decreased variability, periodic decelerations from cord compression or placental insufficiency).
         (2) Change positions and/or start amnioinfusion to relieve deceleration pattern.
      d. Fetus is examined immediately for any congenital problem.

Placenta Previa

Definition: A condition in which the ovum implants low in the uterus, toward the cervix, and the placenta develops so that it partially or completely covers the internal os. Occurs once in every 200 pregnancies.

Characteristics

A. Types.
   1. *Complete:* os entirely covered.
   2. *Partial:* only part of os covered.
   3. *Marginal:* margin overlaps os.
B. Occurs more often in multiparas.
C. Occurs more often with increased age of mother.
D. Scarring or tumor of uterus.

Assessment

A. Observe for painless, bright red vaginal bleeding, intermittent or in gushes, after the seventh month without precipitating cause. (As internal os begins to dilate, the part of the uterus that overlies the os separates and leaves gaping vessels, so bleeding occurs.)
B. Evaluate uterine tone and contractibility.
C. Check for signs of hemorrhage.
D. Assess pain if any (generally painless).
E. Assess vital signs.

- History of painless bleeding late in pregnancy.
- Placenta is localized by ultrasound or radioisotope.
- Sterile vagina examination is conducted only when ultrasound is not available, pregnancy is near term, or there is already heavy bleeding.
- Have blood available for transfusion.
- Set up for possible emergency cesarean delivery.
- Determine whether fetal age is adequate for survival.
- Client is hospitalized immediately and placed on bedrest.
- Blood type is determined and crossmatched for possible transfusion.
- Treatment depends on type of placenta previa, condition of mother, and viability of baby.
- ✦ Mechanical pressure is applied to placental site by bringing down baby's head and occluding blood vessels—usually accomplished by the rupture of membranes; vaginal delivery is possible if bleeding is checked.
- Delivery by cesarean method if bleeding is excessive.
- If baby is small and bleeding stops, delivery is usually postponed.

Implementation

✦ A. Maintain client in bed and provide quiet, restful atmosphere and diversion.

✦ B. Count perineal pads and measure blood amounts on bedding, Chux, etc.

C. Give emotional support, explain procedures, and allay fears.

D. *Do not* perform vaginal examination.

E. Have emergency setup for cesarean delivery available.

F. Carefully monitor fetal heart tones with external monitor.

G. Monitor carefully postpartum for bleeding and infection.

Abruptio Placentae

Definition: A condition that occurs when the placenta separates from the normal implantation site in upper segment of uterus before birth of baby; occurs once in 90 pregnancies and accounts for 15 percent of perinatal mortality.

Characteristics

✦ A. Types of separation.
  1. *Complete:* placenta becomes completely detached from uterine wall.
  2. *Partial:* portion of placenta becomes detached from uterine wall.
  3. *Central:* placenta separates centrally and blood is trapped between placenta and uterine wall; concealed bleeding.

B. Hemorrhage.
  1. *External:* blood escapes from the vagina.
  2. *Concealed:* blood is retained in uterine cavity.

- Treatment depends on severity and extent of labor.
- Moderate bleeding: membranes are ruptured to hasten delivery and help control bleeding.
- Severe: immediate cesarean delivery. Treatment for blood loss and shock.
- Blood drawn for coagulation studies (because of risk of DIC).
- Narcotics may be given for severe pain.
- Oxygen may be given.

C. Etiology.
  1. Trauma.
  2. Chronic vascular renal disease.
  3. High parity.
  4. Cocaine use.
  5. Hypertensive disease.

Assessment

✦ A. External assessment: chief symptom is dark vaginal bleeding accompanied by abdominal pain.

✦ B. Evaluate concealed condition.
  1. Intense, cramplike uterine pain.
  2. Uterine tenderness and rigidity.
  3. Lack of alternate contraction–relaxation of uterus.
  4. Fetal heart tones—bradycardia or absent.

C. Assess for early and late signs of shock: restlessness, narrowing pulse pressure, hypotension, increased pulse rate, pallor, changes in levels of consciousness.

D. Continuous evaluation for disseminated intravascular coagulation (DIC).

Implementation

✦ A. Keep client on bedrest.

B. Observe for signs of shock.

✦ C. Carefully monitor contractions (electronic monitor), fetal heart rate, and vital signs.

D. If bleeding is severe, begin administration of intravenous solution: Ringer's lactate @ 150 mL/hr.

E. Order type and crossmatch blood for possible transfusion, and blood tests for platelets, fibrinogen level, prothrombin time (PT), partial thromboplastin time (PTT).

F. Monitor central venous pressure (CVP).

G. Record intake and output (I&O) and observe for anuria or oliguria. (Anuria may develop as a result of decreased kidney perfusion.)

H. Provide emotional support as fetal prognosis is guarded.

✦ I. Observe for hemorrhage after delivery.

J. Observe for DIC (client at risk for uterine atony after birth).

Hyperemesis Gravidarum

✦ *Definition:* Pernicious vomiting during pregnancy. Usually develops during first 3 months of pregnancy.

Characteristics

A. Cause unclear but may be caused by the addition of new substances to the body system—a toxicity or maladjustment of the maternal metabolism.

B. HCG increases and is believed to play a role.

C. Increased incidence of Helicobacteri pylori (stomach ulcers).

Assessment

✦ A. Check for persistent nausea and amount of vomiting.

B. Assess for abdominal pain and hiccups.

C. Measure weight loss (5 percent of pregnancy weight).

D. Evaluate dehydration status caused by excessive vomiting.

E. Assess electrolyte imbalance: depletion of essential electrolytes because of unreplaced loss of sodium chloride and potassium.

F. Assess for metabolic acidosis: acetone odor to breath.

G. Evaluate increase in blood urea nitrogen (BUN).

H. Assess for hypoproteinemia and hypovitaminosis.

Implementation

A. Use tact and understanding of the client's problem.

B. Carefully record I&O; maintain IVs.

C. Provide attractive, small low fat meals, and remove dishes as soon as the client finishes eating.

D. Offer frequent, small feedings: small amounts every 2 hours, dry foods preferred. Offer liquids (herbal teas) between or after meals, rather than with meals.

E. Administer antiemetic, plus a tranquilizer or a sedative as ordered.

F. If vomiting is persistent:
   1. Client is usually hospitalized.
   2. Dehydration and starvation are treated by administration of parenteral fluids, TPN, and vitamin supplements.
   3. Rest and sedatives are prescribed.
   4. Psychotherapy if necessary.

G. Provide rest, reduce stimuli, and restrict visitors.

H. Monitor fetal heart rate.

PREGNANCY-INDUCED HYPERTENSION (PIH)

Preeclampsia

Definition: An acute, hypertensive disease that is peculiar to pregnancy, but most likely to develop in women who already have hypertension or diabetes. PIH occurs in 7 to 10 percent of all pregnancies.

Assessment

A. Assess period in pregnancy that condition appears: usually after the sixth month.

✦ B. Evaluate for major symptoms: hypertension, proteinuria, and edema (may appear separately or together). Two of these three symptoms are usually needed for diagnosis.

✦ C. Assess for mild preeclampsia.
   1. Elevation of blood pressure 30/15 mm Hg on two occasions, 6 hours apart; or > 140/90.
   2. Generalized edema—colloid osmotic pressure lowered.
   3. Proteinuria: 0.3 g/L, 24-hour specimen.
   4. Weight gain: more than 1360 g/wk in second trimester and 450 g/wk in third trimester.
   5. Cardiac output lower than normal.
   6. Hematocrit values elevated; platelet count lowered.

✦ D. Assess for severe preeclampsia.
   1. Blood pressure 160/110 or above, or systolic 50 mm Hg above normal.
   2. Massive edema: excessive weight gain.
   3. Proteinuria: 5 g or more in 24 hours.
   4. Oliguria: 400 mL or less in 24 hours.
   5. Visual disturbances.
   6. Headache.
   7. Vasospasms.
   8. Hemoconcentration.
   9. Epigastric pain (usually a late sign).
   10. CNS irritability (hyperreflexia).

Implementation

✦ A. Maintain client on bedrest (left lateral recumbent usually best) and plan care to promote rest.

✦ B. Monitor magnesium sulfate (given to prevent eclamptic convulsions).
   1. Monitor for toxic dose: hypotonia, loss of deep tendon reflexes, respiratory failure.
   2. Check serum levels of $MgSO_4$: 4–7 mEq/dL.

C. Monitor fetal heart rate and observe for signs of labor.

D. Carefully monitor vital signs and lab values (CBC, biochemical profile).

E. Record intake and output; examine urine for proteinuria, 24-hour urine for total protein and creatinine clearance, and adequate volume.

F. Immediately report increases in signs and symptoms.

G. Check weight at the same time each day.

H. Examine retina daily for arteriole changes or edema.

I. Limit visitors in severe cases.

J. Maintain seizure precautions.

✦ MEDICAL IMPLICATIONS

Mild Preeclampsia

- Treatment aimed at preventing further increase in disease.
- Client usually remains at home.
- Extra rest is prescribed.
- Adequate fluid intake; often hypovolemic.
- Diet: increased protein and carbohydrate, reduced fat, moderate salt.
- Daily weight.
- Increased calcium supplement may reduce vascular and uterine muscle tone.
- Prophylactic use of low-dose aspirin may show small to moderate benefit in reducing risk of preeclampsia (may result in lowered levels of the vasoconstrictor thromboxane). Still needs more research.

Severe Preeclampsia

- Antihypertensives, sedatives, corticosteroids (may be given).
- Diet: high protein; moderate salt, calcium and zinc.
- Bedrest. Admit to high-risk unit.
- Fluid and electrolyte replacement.
- Observe for signs of central nervous system (CNS) irritability and hyperactivity.
- Magnesium sulfate is treatment of choice to help prevent and/or treat convulsions.
- The most reliable treatment is delivery of infant.

K. Final resolution is delivery of the fetus.
L. Prepare client for surgery if indicated.

Gestational Hypertension Home Management

A. Allowed home management when following criteria present.
  1. Blood pressure < 150/100 mm Hg. Able to monitor own BP.
  2. Proteinuria less than 1 g/24 hrs. Able to monitor protein and weight daily.
  3. Normal fetal growth.
  4. No signs of complicating factors (vaginal bleeding).
  5. Mother understands her condition and is able to recognize and report signs and symptoms if condition deteriorates.
  6. Mother is able to count fetal movements and knows when to call doctor.
B. Mother may or may not be on complete bedrest, but is encouraged to rest frequently.
C. Antihypertensive therapy.
  1. Medications—therapeutic goal is to maintain diastolic blood pressure between 90 to 100 mm Hg (maximum).
    a. Methyldopa used for long-term control.

    b. Hydralazine used for acute hypertension.
    c. Labetalol HCl PO should be avoided in women with asthma or chronic hypertensive disease (CHD).
  2. Herbs and supplements.
    a. Herbs: burdock, dandelion, hawthorne.
    b. Nutrients: CoQ10, $MgSO_4$.

Eclampsia

Definition: A more severe form of hypertensive disease, characterized by convulsions and even coma.

Assessment

✦ A. Observe for severe edema.
B. Check urine output and for urine that contains red blood cells, varied casts, and protein (3+ or greater with two random samples).
✦ C. Assess for blood pressure elevation to 160/110 mm Hg or above on two occasions, 6 hours apart.
✦ D. Check for visual disturbances, blurring, or even blindness caused by edema of the retina.
E. Determine if severe epigastric pain is present.
F. Observe convulsions, both tonic and clonic.
G. Assess for signs of labor. (Labor may begin and fetus may be born prematurely or die.)
H. Assess vital signs: temperature and respiratory status.
I. Observe reflex irritability (DTR, clonus).
J. Assess level of consciousness.
K. Determine fetal heart rate and uterine contractibility.
L. Assess for necessity of doing emergency cesarean section.
M. Have emergency medications at bedside—magnesium sulfate and calcium gluconate (antidote for magnesium sulfate toxicity).

Implementation

✦ A. Provide a quiet, darkened room with a constant attendant and bedrest.
B. Check client frequently for edema.
✦ C. Maintain seizure precautions.
D. Suction if necessary.
E. Provide oxygen as necessary.
F. Keep record of vital signs and lab values.
G. Check blood pressure frequently.
H. Keep client NPO.
I. Maintain IV and give medications.
J. Monitor fetal heart tones and contractions.
K. Observe carefully for 24 hours postpartum for anuria, convulsions, headache, and blurred vision.
L. *See* Appendix 12-1 at the end of this chapter for drugs normally used for PIH. Administer magnesium sulfate to prevent seizures—obtain blood levels every 4 hours.

HELLP Syndrome

✦ *Definition:* **H**emolysis, **E**levated **L**iver enzymes, and **L**ow **P**latelet count; syndrome that is an unusual variation of PIH.

Characteristics

A. This syndrome, identified first in 1982, occurs with little warning and may be associated with severe preeclampsia.
B. Epigastric pain may be primary symptom.
C. Ninety percent develop symptoms before the 36th week.

Assessment

✦ A. Check for proteinuria, 1+ to 4+.
B. Question any unusual epigastric pain.
C. Check platelet count (low—less than 100,000/mm^3).
D. Check liver enzymes (elevated).
E. Nausea, vomiting, and malaise may be present.

Implementation

A. Variation of PIH—check implementation under this topic.
B. Women with HELLP should give birth as soon as possible (induced labor or cesarean).
C. With PIH treatment, clients recover in 4 to 5 days.

MEDICAL DISEASES COMPLICATING HIGH-RISK PREGNANCY

Cardiovascular Disease

Characteristics

✦ A. Classification.
   1. *Class I:* no alteration of activity.
   2. *Class II:* slight limitation of activity.
   3. *Class III:* marked limitation of activity.
   4. *Class IV:* symptoms present at rest.
B. Pregnancy expands plasma volume, increasing cardiac output and load on heart.
C. Most deaths are caused by cardiac failure, when blood volume is at a maximum in the last weeks of the second trimester.
D. Heart failure occurs infrequently in labor.
E. Over age 35, there is an increase in the incidence of heart failure and death.

Assessment

✦ A. Observe for signs of cardiac decompensation, especially 28–30 weeks, during labor, and immediate post partum.

✦ MEDICAL IMPLICATIONS

* With proper management, mortality is minimal.
* Client should avoid people with acute infections, especially respiratory infections; antibiotics may be prescribed prophylactically.
* Client should rest frequently; 8–10 hours sleep.
* Strenuous activities, such as stair climbing, heavy cleaning, and straining, should be avoided.
* Clients in classes III and IV may be hospitalized before labor for controlled rest and diet.
* If client decompensates or has distress symptoms with exertion, she should remain on bedrest or in a chair.
* Digitalis treatment when indicated.
* Emotional stress should be avoided and pain and anxiety controlled.

Diet

* Salt intake may or may not be restricted.
* Diuretics (Lasix) may be prescribed if signs of heart failure occur.
* The use of highly salted foods is discouraged.
* Iron, folic acid, and vitamin supplements are important; fluids and high fiber to promote soft stools.

   1. Cardiac function, such as pulse rate over 110 or respiratory rate over 24; heart murmurs.
   2. Decreased vital capacity.
   3. Dyspnea; rales; frequent cough.
   4. Edema.
B. Evaluate for signs of infection, especially respiratory infection.
   1. Elevated temperature.
   2. Sore throat.
   3. Productive cough.
   4. Nasal congestion or discharge.
C. Assess for signs of anxiety or stress.
D. Check vital signs and fetal heart rate.
E. Evaluate activity level.

Implementation

A. Educate client about classifications and effects of pregnancy before conception.
B. Educate client about special needs and danger signals during pregnancy and postpartum.
✦ C. Care for client during labor.
   1. Check vital signs every 15 minutes or more often as needed.
   2. Keep client in bed, preferably lying on one side or in semirecumbent position.
   3. Administer oxygen as necessary.
   4. Provide calm atmosphere and emotional support to alleviate fears.
   5. Administer pain medications as ordered to reduce discomfort during labor.

6. Be alert for signs of impending heart failure.
7. Monitor fetal heart tones.

D. Provide careful observation during postpartum period.

E. Counsel client during postpartum to have help at home and planned rest periods.

Diabetes Mellitus

Definition: A chronic metabolic disease caused by the inability to metabolize glucose properly.

Characteristics

A. Estimated 2 percent of pregnancies seen in large metropolitan areas will have some degree of diabetes.

✦ B. In 3–6 percent of pregnant women, there is a tendency to develop **gestational diabetes** as a result of placental hormones, variations in insulin level, and an increase in free cortisol.
   1. Abnormalities disappear after pregnancy.
   2. Symptoms of hyperglycemia are mild, but may be risky for fetus.
   ✦ 3. Diet is cornerstone of intervention, but insulin therapy is instituted when diet doesn't control condition.

C. Maternal glucose crosses placenta, but insulin does not. Maternal hyperglycemia leads to fetal hyperglycemia, which leads to fetal hyperinsulinemia.

D. Pregnant women should be screened for glucose levels: normal fluctuation is between 60 mg/dL and 120 mg/dL (24–28 weeks).

E. A 3-hour glucose tolerance test will confirm diabetes when two or more values are above normal.

F. Sepsis, eclampsia, and hemorrhage, the most common causes of maternal death, are more common in the pregnant diabetic.

Implications of Diabetes in Pregnancy

A. Diabetes is more difficult to control.

B. There is a tendency for client to develop acidosis.

C. Client is prone to infection.

D. PIH, hemorrhage, and polyhydramnios are more likely to develop.

E. Gestational diabetes may develop into full-blown diabetes.

F. Insulin requirements are increased.

G. Premature delivery is more frequent.

H. Infant may be overweight but have functions related to gestational age rather than size.

✦ I. Infant is subject to hypoglycemia, hyperbilirubinemia, respiratory distress syndrome, and congenital anomalies (incidence 5–10 percent).

J. Stillborn and neonatal mortality rates are high, but may be reduced by proper management and strict control of diabetes.

Assessment

✦ A. All pregnant women should be screened for glucose intolerance between 24 and 28 weeks of pregnancy.
   1. Observe for signs of hypoglycemia.
   2. Observe for signs of hyperglycemia.

✦ B. Major signs and symptoms.
   1. Weight loss.
   2. Excessive hunger or thirst with excess fluid intake.
   3. Polyuria—excess urination.
   4. Recurrent monilial infections.
   5. Maternal hypertension.
   6. Weakness, fatigue, drowsiness.

✦ C. Assess for signs of preeclampsia.
   1. Hypertension.
   2. Proteinuria.
   3. Edema.

D. Check for signs of infection—recurrent and difficult to resolve.
   1. Increased temperature.
   2. Erythematous areas.
   3. Respiratory problems.

E. Check for signs of premature labor.

F. Assess for signs of polyhydramnios.
   1. Respiratory distress.
   2. Fluid stasis in legs.

G. Assess insulin needs.

H. Assess fetal status.

Implementation

A. Educate client on the effects of diabetes on her and the fetus during pregnancy and the reasons for adhering to therapy protocol.
   1. Bimonthly visits for 6 months; weekly visits thereafter.
   2. Maintenance of blood glucose levels according to gestational week.
   ✦ 3. Frequent home monitoring of blood glucose.
   4. Weight control.

- Strict control of diabetes through insulin, dietary, and exercise regulation.
- Frequent (every 1 to 2 weeks) prenatal supervision throughout gestation.
- Control of infection: vaginitis, urinary infections.
- Client may be hospitalized at 36 to 37 weeks' gestation for evaluation and possible early termination of pregnancy.
- Placental function may be evaluated: placental insufficiency (pathological process in placenta resulting in inefficient exchange of waste and gases between mother and fetus) is common in diabetics due to vascular changes.
- Assessment of fetal status: growth, lung maturity, fetal activity, NST, US; if early delivery is indicated.
- Strict control of diabetes is important; HbA$_{1c}$ of 4–7% indicates long-term glucose control over past 4–8 weeks.
- Oral diabetic agents are contraindicated because they may cause congenital malformation.

Mild
- Rest and limitation of activity.
- Curtailment of excessive weight gain.
- Prevention of edema.

Severe
- Hospitalization.
- Bedrest.
- Increased protein diet.
- Adequate fluids.
- Close observation of general condition.
- Daily weight.
- Accurate record of intake and output.
- Check urine for protein.
- Frequent check of vital signs.
- Antihypertensives.
- Serial test is NST after the 32nd week; if nonreactive, OCTs to determine well-being of fetus are completed.

5. Dietary control to increase calorie intake with adequate insulin therapy so glucose will go into the cells. Usually provided with 3 meals and 3 snacks.
   a. Daily calories of 2000–2500 Kcal. (Severe calorie restriction may lead to ketosis.)
   b. Protein: 12–20 percent, 0.8 g/kg unless renal disease is present.
   c. Carbohydrate: 55–60 percent, primarily complex carbohydrates.
   d. Fat: less than 20–30 percent total calories.
   e. Fiber: 300 g/day to control glycemia and constipation—also satisfies appetite.
6. Exogenous insulin if diet cannot control blood sugar levels. Oral hypoglycemics contraindicated; may cause fetal hypoglycemia and abnormalities.
7. Insulin administration.
   a. Human insulin used for more rapid onset and shorter duration of action. Triggers fewer antibodies.
   b. Multiple injections are preferred; mixture of intermediate and regular insulin twice daily.
   c. Pregnant women already using insulin should not change insulin brands.
   d. Methods of administration—*see* insulin administration in Endocrine section of Medical–Surgical chapter.
B. Provide care if client is hospitalized.
   1. Maintain insulin on regular schedule. Insulin may change daily.
   2. Test blood for glucose level as ordered.
   3. Provide adequate diabetic diet as prescribed by physician.

4. Monitor fetal heart rate.
5. Check vital signs, especially blood pressure QID and PRN.
6. Weigh daily at the same time.
7. Keep accurate records of I&O.
8. Provide diversion for client.
9. Provide support and explanations to help allay fears and reduce anxiety.
C. In addition, provide following care to client in labor.
   ✦ 1. Monitor fetal status continuously for signs of distress. If noted, prepare client for immediate cesarean section.
   2. Carefully regulate insulin and provide IV glucose as labor depletes glycogen.
D. Provide postpartum care.
   ✦ 1. Observe client closely for insulin reaction: precipitous drop in insulin requirements usual; hypoglycemic shock may occur.
      a. May require no insulin for first 24 hours.
      b. Reregulate insulin needs following first day according to blood sugar testing.
      c. Diet and exercise must also be reexamined.
   2. Observe for early signs of infection.
   3. Observe for postpartum hemorrhage.

Chronic Hypertension in Pregnancy

Definition: Hypertensive vascular disease is characteristic of hypertension that is already present. It may be aggravated by the pregnancy, or clinical symptoms may first manifest with pregnancy.

Assessment

✦ A. Observe for hypertension: evident before the 20th week; blood pressure is 140/90 at rest.

B. Check for presence of headache; client may otherwise feel weak.

C. Evaluate edema (however, proteinuria usually *not* present).

D. Assess for signs of superimposed preeclampsia.

E. Check for fetal heart rate.

Implementation

A. Maintain bedrest and create an environment conducive to rest.

B. Accurately record vital signs, check urine for protein, and check weight daily.

C. Monitor fetal heart tones.

D. Keep careful record of I&O.

E. Provide adequate diet and fluids.

F. Report any unusual symptoms.

G. Observe for signs of heart failure.

H. Maintain on antihypertensive drugs.

I. Provide supportive atmosphere.

Anemia

Definition: A deficiency in the blood, usually referring to a decrease in the numbers of erythrocytes to a reduction in hemoglobin. Hemoglobin less than 12 g/dL in non-pregnant women and less than 10 g/dL in pregnant women (lower values in pregnancy due to hemodilution).

Assessment

A. Evaluate iron deficiency status. This is cause of anemia in 90 percent of the cases.

B. Observe for client who looks pale, tires easily, and is lethargic.

C. Assess for headache or dizziness.

D. Assess for shortness of breath.

E. Hemoglobin levels 10 g/dL or below, or hematocrit below 37 percent.

Implementation

A. Medical treatment of supplemental iron (ferrous sulfate) 0.3 g TID is given, or in severe cases, Imferon as a parenteral medication is given.
   1. Educate client as to the need to take supplements.
   2. Iron absorption is reduced (40 to 50 percent) when taken with meals; however, when taken after meals, it minimizes gastric upset.
   3. The client may enhance absorption of iron by taking with a food rich in vitamin C.
   4. Client may choose to take oral liquid iron supplement through a straw to protect teeth.

B. Let client know that stools will become dark from iron absorption.

C. Instruct client to use frequent oral hygiene measures to guard against iron deposit on teeth and gums.

D. Administer Imferon, IM as directed.

E. Encourage client to eat foods high in iron (organ meats, blackstrap molasses, egg yolk, seeds, nuts, green leafy vegetables, dried fruits, fish).

Urinary Tract Infection

Definition: Bacteria enter the urinary tract by way of the urethra, causing infection.

Characteristics

A. Usually occurs after the fourth month or in early postpartum; affects 10 percent of maternity clients.

B. Causes.
   1. Pressure on ureters and bladder.
   2. Hormonal effects on tone of ureters and bladder.
   3. Displacement of bladder.
   4. History of urinary infections, vaginitis.

C. Kidneys as well as ureters may be involved.

Assessment

A. Observe for frequent micturition.

B. Check for paroxysms—pain in kidney or "flank pain."

C. Assess for fever and chills.

D. Evaluate catheterized urine specimen to determine if it contains bacteria and pus.

E. Check for burning on urination.

F. Check for signs of premature labor.

Implementation

A. Maintain client on bedrest.

B. Encourage fluid intake by providing client with a variety of fluids.

C. Obtain specimens as ordered.

D. Monitor antibiotic treatment.

E. Monitor urinary antispasmodics and analgesics.

Infectious Diseases

Characteristics

A. Diseases such as influenza, scarlet fever, toxoplasmosis, and cytomegalovirus (type of herpes virus causes cytomegalic inclusion disease) may be transmitted to fetus.

B. Diseases may cause abortions or malformations in early pregnancy, premature labor or fetal death.

✦ C. Rubella in first trimester—a teratogen—may cause congenital anomalies.

Assessment

A. Check for elevation in temperature.

B. Observe for productive cough and nasal secretions.

C. Evaluate for sore throat.

D. Assess for skin rash.

E. Check for contact or exposure of client to persons with infectious disease.

Implementation

A. Educate women before pregnancy to have rubella titer and a vaccination.

B. Educate women to avoid contact with people having known or suspected infectious diseases.

C. Educate women to notify their physician immediately should exposure occur.

Group B *Streptococcus* (GBS)

Characteristics

A. Bacterial infection in GI or urogenital tract.
1. Women may be carriers of GBS yet may be asymptomatic.
2. Women who are symptomatic may experience morbidity from infections.
3. At-risk mothers should receive antimicrobial prophylaxis for GBS disease.

B. Women may transmit GBS to fetus in utero or during childbirth.

C. GBS causes severe invasive disease.
1. Severe respiratory distress.
2. Pneumonia, apnea.
3. Shock.
4. Late onset—infants may develop meningitis.

Assessment

A. Screening procedure: rectal and vaginal swabs for culture obtained at 35–37 weeks for all pregnant women (CDC 2002)—takes 18–48 hours for results.
1. FDA clears new test: 101—Strep B test can provide results in one hour.
2. 10–30 percent of pregnant women have Group B *Streptococcus*; 1–2 percent are colonized, with 1 in 10 developing disease.
3. If test results are positive (colonized), newborn may develop disease.
   a. Early onset—within hours or first week (majority of infants).
   b. Late onset—1 week to 3 months.

B. Fetus becomes infected when traveling through birth canal or from transmission from colonized staff member or other infants.

Implementation

A. Following positive GBS screening results, the mother should receive 4 hours of antibiotic prophylaxis at onset of labor or rupture of membranes.
1. First-line agent—IV penicillin G 5 million units followed by 2.5 million units IV q 4 hr until childbirth.
2. Alternately, ampicillin 2 g IV followed by 1 g IV q 4 hr.

B. Prophylaxis is indicated for
1. Women who have given birth to newborn with GBS.
2. Previous infant born with GBS.
3. Unknown GBS status.

C. Newborn treatment for GBS (*see* Newborn, page 598).

SEXUALLY TRANSMITTED DISEASES (STDS)

Chlamydia

Definition: Caused by *Chlamydia trachomatis*, produces infections in both men and women (fallopian tubes, cervix, urethra) and can develop into pelvic inflammatory disease (PID).

Characteristics

✦ A. Most common STD in the United States.

B. 5 million people contract disease each year, up nearly 6 percent since 2003.

C. High-risk women: young, nonwhites with multiple sex partners and women not using barrier contraceptives.

D. Chlamydia is not a reportable disease in 50 percent of states.

E. Statistics:
1. Twenty percent of men and 40–50 percent of women with gonorrhea also are infected with chlamydia.
2. Twenty-five to fifty percent of PID is caused by chlamydia.
   ✦ 3. Each year 155,000 infants born to mothers with chlamydia are at risk for pneumonia and ophthalmia neonatorum (conjunctivitis).
4. Each year $1 billion spent on infection.

F. *Chlamydiae* are bacteria microorganisms, but have characteristics of both viruses and bacteria.

G. Sensitive to antibiotics (azithromycin or doxycycline).

✦ H. Spread through sexual contact. Incubation period 5–10 days or longer (28 days—gonorrhea is only 2–10 days).

I. Tests for chlamydia include Chlamydiazyme—enzyme immunoassay test; Microtak—direct fluorescent antibody test; and BD Probe Tec—amplified DNP assay.

Assessment

A. Observe for a discharge—vaginal or urethral.
B. Assess for burning.
C. Check for lower abdominal pain or testicular pain.
D. Assess for bleeding or pain with coitus.
E. Assess for rectal pain or discharge.
F. Thirty-three percent of women report no symptoms.

Implementation

✦ A. Administer antibiotics as ordered.
  1. Doxycycline 100 mg 2×/day for 7 days for non-pregnant woman.
  2. Erythromycin 500 mg 4×/day for 7 days for pregnant woman.
  3. Penicillin does not cure chlamydia.
B. Educate men and women about transmission, symptoms, and prevention.
  1. Frequent examinations if people are not monogamous.
  2. If symptoms/signs occur, seek help immediately—teach importance of taking medication as prescribed.
  3. Suggest that sexually active people use barrier methods of contraception.
  4. Avoidance of sex until completion of treatment.
C. Provide accurate information about disease, health care, and prevention.

Syphilis

✦ *Definition:* A chronic infectious disease caused by *Treponema pallidum.*

Characteristics

A. Transmission is by intimate physical contact with syphilitic lesions, which are usually found on the skin or the mucous membranes of the mouth and the genitals.
  1. Since 2000, incidence of early-stage syphilis has increased 29 percent.
  2. Increase is largely among gay men (CDC, 2007).
✦ B. Incubation period is 10 to 90 days following exposure.
C. Primary stage (nonreactive VDRL).
  1. Most infectious stage.
  2. Appearance of chancres, ulcerative lesions.
  3. Usually painless, produced by spirochetes at the point of entry into the body.
D. Secondary stage (reactive VDRL).
  1. Lesions appear about 3 weeks after the primary stage and may occur anywhere on the skin and the mucous membranes.

  2. Highly infectious.
  3. Generalized lymphadenopathy.
E. Tertiary stage.
  1. The spirochetes enter the internal organs and cause permanent damage.
  2. Symptoms may occur 10 to 30 years following the occurrence of an untreated primary lesion.
  3. Invasion of the central nervous system.
    a. Meningitis.
    b. Locomotor ataxia: foot slapping and broad-based gait.
    c. General paresis.
    d. Progressive mental deterioration leading to psychosis.
  4. Cardiovascular: most common site of damage is at the aortic valve and the aorta itself.
F. Characteristics relating to pregnancy.
  1. May cause abortion or premature labor.
  2. Infection is passed to the fetus after the fourth month of pregnancy as congenital syphilis.

Assessment

✦ A. Evaluate serum test (STS) for syphilis on first prenatal visit.
B. May repeat just before fourth month, as disease may be acquired after initial visit.

Implementation

A. Educate women to recognize signs of syphilis.
B. Educate women to seek immediate treatment if known exposure occurs.
C. Educate women as to the need for simultaneous treatment of partner because reinfection may occur.
✦ D. Monitor treatment: during pregnancy, 2.4 million units of procaine penicillin G with 2 percent aluminum monostearate, IM, normally in divided doses.
E. Report all cases of syphilis to health authorities for treatment of contacts.

Gonorrhea

Definition: An infection caused by *Neisseria gonorrhoeae*, which causes inflammation of the mucous membrane of the genitourinary tract.

Characteristics

✦ A. Transmission is almost completely by sexual intercourse.
B. Incidence is of epidemic proportions in the United States.
C. Signs and symptoms.
  1. Male.
    a. Painful urination.
    b. Pelvic pain and fever.

  c. Epididymitis with pain, tenderness, and swelling.
  d. Mucoid or mucopurulent discharge.
  ✦ 2. Female (usually asymptomatic).
    a. Vaginal discharge—greenish-yellow.
    b. Urinary frequency and pain.
D. Complications.
  1. Female: pelvic inflammatory disease (PID) with abdominal pain, fever, nausea, and vomiting.
  2. Male: postgonococcal urethritis and spread of infection to posterior urethra, prostate, and seminal vesicles.
  3. PID can lead to sterility.
  4. A secondary infection can develop in any organ.
✦ E. Infection may be transmitted to baby's eyes during delivery, causing blindness.

Assessment

A. Obtain culture for gonorrhea (usually done on first prenatal visit).
B. Repeat later as infection may occur during pregnancy.

Implementation

A. Educate women to recognize signs of gonorrhea and to seek immediate treatment.
B. Administer prophylactic broad-spectrum antibiotic (erythromycin).
C. Monitor treatment: same as for syphilis.
D. Important to treat sexual partner, as client may become reinfected.

Herpes Simplex Virus (HSV)

Definition: Herpes infection caused by the herpes simplex virus (HSV). Forty-five million people in the United States have been diagnosed.

Characteristics

✦ A. HSV types 1 and 2 both present risk to infant.
B. Type 2 most common as genital herpes.
  1. Involves external genitalia, vagina, and cervix.
  2. Development and draining of painful vesicles.
✦ C. Virus may be lethal to fetus if inoculated during vaginal delivery (50 percent of HSV-infected infants die). Delivery usually by cesarean section.
D. Safe use of acyclovir has not been established for pregnant women.

Assessment

A. Evaluate for presence of painful, draining vesicles on external genitals, vagina, and cervix.
B. Check for increased temperature and vital signs.

Implementation

A. Educate client as to dangers to fetus.

B. Encourage client to report symptoms.
✦ C. Explain to client the possibility of a cesarean section should an outbreak occur around the time of delivery.
  1. Policy regarding time limit of outbreak in relation to time of delivery varies, but usual policy is an outbreak within 2 weeks.
  2. Conservative physicians now advocate cesarean section if condition is present regardless of outbreak.
D. Maintain precautions during vaginal examinations of client.
✦ E. Maintain isolation precautions during hospitalization if disease is active.
F. Postpartum.
  1. Encourage careful handwashing by client.
  2. Avoid direct contact with lesions.
  3. Breastfeeding is not contraindicated unless lesions are on breast.

Human Papillomavirus (HPV)—Genital Warts

Definition: A sexually transmitted infection caused by the human papillomavirus (HPV).

Characteristics

A. The virus affects cervix, urethra, penis, scrotum, and anus.
B. Warts appear 1 or 2 months after exposure, transmitted through intimate sexual contact.

Assessment

A. Assess for small to large wartlike growths on genitals (no symptoms other than lesions).
✦ B. Assess for cervical cell changes—HPV associated with up to 90 percent of cervical malignancies.

Implementation

A. There is no cure for HPV—treatment is cryotherapy, liquid nitrogen, or electrocautery to remove lesions.
B. Key is prevention—similar to any other STD: limit sexual contacts and use condoms.
C. Suggest Pap test every year (cancer risk).
D. A vaccine (Gardasil) was introduced in 2007 that is effective against several strains of this virus that cause 70 percent of all cervical cancers.

Human Immunodeficiency Virus (HIV)

Definition: A retrovirus that may develop into acquired immune deficiency syndrome (AIDS). Contracted through exchange of body fluids, it has a long latency period before progressing to AIDS.

Characteristics

A. History of belonging to high-risk group (drug user, prostitution).

B. Pregnancy associated with slight reduction of helper T cells—may increase possibility of opportunistic infections.

✦ C. HIV transmitted to 30 percent of exposed infants—risk increases with low T-cell count.

Assessment

A. Assess for symptoms of seropositivity (mononucleosis-like symptoms) or AIDS-related complex (ARC) (pre-AIDS condition).

✦ B. Check for severely compromised immune system (indicates presence of AIDS).

C. Take careful history of risk behaviors.

D. Assess for signs of STDs, and CMV.

Implementation

✦ A. Complete post-test counseling if client tests HIV positive.

B. Counsel importance of continued medical care during pregnancy.

C. Maintain body fluid precautions for cell contact with client and teach client precautions.

D. Assess signs and symptoms of illness and serum tests.

✦ E. *See* Newborn with AIDS, page 589.

ASSOCIATED COMPLICATIONS OF PREGNANCY

Pregnancy in Adolescents

Characteristics

A. Crisis of pregnancy compounds the crises of adolescence—physical, social, emotional, social development.

B. More than 1 million teenagers become pregnant every year and 85 percent of these pregnancies are unintended.
1. Trend of teenage pregnancy is going down with more birth control options available.
2. Education about protection from pregnancy as well as STDs is important.

C. Client may be unwed and have no financial resources.

D. Problems associated with teen pregnancy.
1. Physical development may not be complete.
2. High incidence of PIH, preterm labor, SGA infants, anemia, infections, CPD.
3. Diet may be inadequate.

Assessment

A. Assess nutritional status of client.

B. Evaluate any signs of emotional problems, conflicts, or crisis.

C. Evaluate financial status.

D. Assess for signs of premature labor and toxemia.

E. Assess knowledge of pregnancy and infant care.

Implementation

A. Encourage early antepartum care.

B. Provide health instruction on pregnancy, nutrition, hygiene, infant care, and childbirth preparation.

C. Observe frequently for complications.

D. Provide emotional support and counseling.

Disseminated Intravascular Coagulation (DIC)

Definition: A condition in the mother's body that results in an exaggerated clotting process.

Characteristics

✦ A. Possible complication of abruptio placenta, missed abortion, fetal death, amniotic fluid embolism.

B. May result in uncontrolled bleeding.
✦ 1. Thromboplastin from placental tissue and clots enters the bloodstream through open vessels at the placental site and initiates an exaggeration of the normal clotting process.
2. As more thromboplastin is introduced into circulation, more fibrinogen and clotting factors are used up.
3. In addition, the fibrinolytic process that disintegrates fibrin is initiated, resulting in fibrin degradation products, which in turn further interfere with the clotting process.

Assessment

✦ A. Observe for uncontrolled bleeding.

B. Assess for signs of shock: tachycardia, restlessness, anxiety.

C. Be alert for symptoms in women with predisposing factors such as fetal death, abruptio placenta, PIH.

D. Observe for prolonged and uncontrolled bleeding (i.e., skin and mucous membranes, IV sites).

Implementation

A. Provide emotional support to client and family.

B. Assist with medical management and administration of medications.
✦ 1. Heparin solution may prevent clot formation and increases available fibrinogen, coagulation factors, and platelets.
2. Fresh-frozen plasma and/or platelets may be ordered.

C. Monitor IV therapy as ordered.

D. Administer oxygen at 2–3 L/min.

Intrauterine Fetal Death

Assessment

A. Cessation of fetal movement.
B. Absence of fetal heart rate.
C. Failure of uterine growth.
D. Low urinary estriol.
E. Check for negative pregnancy test—may remain positive for a few weeks due to elevated human chorionic gonadotropin.
F. Assess client's external support system (family, friends, priest, etc.).
G. Assess for complications such as disseminated intravascular disease from prolonged retention of the dead fetus.

Implementation

A. Provide emotional support to parents—may feel unfulfilled, incomplete, and depressed.
B. Guide parents in planning future pregnancies.
C. Do not listen for fetal heart rate or do Leopold's maneuvers.
D. Observe for hemorrhage.
E. Observe for psychological disturbances.
F. Prepare emotionally for delivery process and birth of baby.
G. Parents may go through mourning process—encourage them to express feelings; may be angry at staff.
H. Parents may want to see fetus; allow them to do so should they desire.

Pseudocyesis/Pseudopregnancies

✦ *Definition:* A condition that occurs when all the signs of pregnancy develop without the presence of an embryo.

Assessment

A. Observe for amenorrhea, breast changes, and secretion of colostrum.
B. Check for enlargement of abdomen.
C. Ask for reports of quickening.
D. Assess presence of fetal heart rate or visible fetus on sonogram.

Implementation

A. Offer client continued emotional support.
B. Allow client to express her feelings regarding pseudopregnancy.
C. Refer client for continued psychological assistance.

INTRAPARTUM PERIOD

LABOR AND DELIVERY

Definition: Labor is the process by which the products of conception are expelled from the body. Delivery refers to the actual birth.

Adaptive Processes

✦ *Definition:* During latter months of pregnancy, the fetus adapts to the maternal uterus enabling it to occupy the smallest space possible. The term *attitude* refers to the posture the fetus assumes in utero; *fetal lie* is the relationship of the long axis of the body to the long axis of the mother.

Presentation

✦ *Definition:* The part of the fetus that enters the true pelvis first.
✦ A. *Cephalic:* head is presenting part—95–96 percent.
   1. May be vertex, face, or brow.
   2. Vertex is most common and most favorable for delivery. Head is sharply flexed in the pelvis with chin near chest.
✦ B. *Breech:* buttocks or lower extremities are the presenting part.
   1. Types.
      a. Complete or full: buttocks and feet present (baby in squatting position).
      b. Frank: buttocks only presenting, or legs are extended against anterior trunk with feet touching face.
      c. Incomplete: one or both feet or knees presenting, footing single or double, or knee presentation.
   2. May rotate to cephalic during pregnancy but possibility lessens as gestation nears term.
   3. May be rotated by physician but usually returns to breech position.
✦ C. *Transverse lie:* long axis of infant lies at right angles to longitudinal axis of mother (necessitates delivery by C-section).

Position

Definition: Relationship of the fetal presenting part to the maternal bony pelvis.
✦ A. Position is determined by locating the fetal presenting part in relation to the maternal pelvis.

B. Client's pelvis is divided into four imaginary quadrants: right anterior, right posterior, left anterior, and left posterior.
✦ C. Most common positions (abbreviations usually used).
   1. LOA (left occipitoanterior): occiput on left side of maternal pelvis and toward front, face down, favorable for delivery.
   2. LOP (left occipitoposterior): occiput on left side of maternal pelvis and toward rear or face up.
      a. Usually causes back pain during labor.
      b. May slow the progress of labor.
      c. Usually rotates before delivery to anterior position.
      d. May be rotated in delivery room by physician.
   3. ROA (right occipitoanterior): occiput on right of maternal pelvis, toward front, face down, favorable for delivery.
   4. ROP (right occipitoposterior): occiput on right side of maternal pelvis, face up. Same problems as LOP.
D. Means of assessing fetal position during labor.
   ✦ 1. *Leopold's maneuver:* method of palpating the maternal abdomen to determine information about the fetus such as presentation, engagement position, and rough estimate of fetal size.
   2. Vaginal examination.
   3. Rectal examination.

Engagement—Lightening

✦ A. Largest diameter of presenting part has passed the inlet of the maternal pelvis. Usually takes place two weeks before labor in primiparas, but often not until labor begins in multiparas.
B. May be assessed by Leopold's maneuver or vaginal or rectal examination.

Station

✦ A. Degree to which presenting part has descended into pelvis is determined by the station—the relationship between the presenting part and the ischial spines.
B. Assessed by vaginal or rectal examination.
✦ C. Measured in numerical terms.
   1. At level of spines, 0 station.
   2. Cm above level of spines, −1, −2, −3.
   3. Cm below level of spines, +1, +2, +3.
D. Other terms used to denote station.
   1. *High:* presenting part not engaged.
   2. *Floating:* presenting part freely movable in inlet of pelvis or may be movable in inlets of pelvis.
   3. *Dipping:* entering pelvis.

4. *Fixed:* no longer movable in inlet but not engaged.
5. *Engaged:* biparietal plane passed through pelvic inlet.

Fetal Skull

A. Largest anatomical part of the fetus to pass through the birth canal; usually if the head can pass, the rest of the body can be delivered.
B. Made up of seven bones: two frontal, two parietal, two temporal, and one occipital.
◆ C. Sutures: membranous interspaces between bones.
   1. Sagittal: between two parietal bones.
   2. Frontal: between two front bones.
   3. Coronal: between frontal and parietal.
   4. Lambdoidals: between posterior margin of parietal and occipital.
◆ D. Fontanels: points where sutures intersect.
   1. Anterior—diamond shaped. Found at the junction of the sagittal and coronal sutures. Becomes ossified around 12–18 months.
   2. Posterior—smaller triangular shaped. Found at the junction of the sagittal and lambdoid sutures. Becomes ossified by 2–4 months after birth.
   3. Other, smaller fontanels are also present.
   4. Fontanels and sutures allow for fetal skull bones to override, as they adapt to the pelvis.
   5. Important points in vaginal or rectal examination to determine position of fetus— posterior or anterior.

The Labor Process

Cause of Labor

A. Alterations in hormonal balance of estrogen (increases contractility) and progesterone (decreases contractility).
B. Degeneration of the placenta, which no longer provides necessary elements to fetus.
C. Overdistention of uterus creates stimulus— triggering release of oxytocin, which initiates contractions.
D. High levels of prostaglandins near term may stimulate uterine contractions.
E. Hormones secreted by fetus (fetal cortisol).
F. The type of contraction necessary for true labor may be produced by a combination of several of these physiological occurrences although the actual cause is unknown.

Forces of Labor

A. Muscular contractions primarily of muscles of uterus and secondarily of abdominal muscles.

◆ B. Uterine muscles contract during first stages and bring about effacement and dilatation of the cervix.
C. Abdominal muscles come into play after complete cervical dilatation and help expel the baby—voluntary bearing-down effort, urge to push.
D. Contraction of levator ani muscles.

Duration of Labor

A. Varies depending on individual.
B. Average.
   ◆ 1. *Primipara:* up to 18 hours; some may be shorter, others longer.
   ◆ 2. *Multipara:* up to 8 hours; some may be shorter, others longer.
C. Length of labor depends on:
   1. Effectiveness of consistent contractions: contractions must overcome resistance of cervix.
   2. Amount of resistance baby must overcome to adapt to the pelvis.
   3. Stretching ability of soft tissue.
   4. Preparation and relaxation of client. Fear and anxiety can retard progress.
◆ D. Important to judge rate of progress: should be regular progression of uterine contraction, progressive effacement and dilatation of the cervix and progressive descent of the presenting part.

Uterine Contractions

A. Characteristics.
   1. Involuntary: cannot be controlled by will of client.
   2. Intermittent: periods of relaxation between contractions. Intervals allow client to rest and also allow adequate circulation of uterine blood vessels and oxygenation of fetus.
   ◆ 3. Distinguish between true labor (contractions are regular, painful, and continue with walking) and false labor–*Braxton Hicks* (regular, painful, but go away with walking).
   4. Discomfort starts in low back, radiates to abdomen.
   5. As labor progresses, intensity increases.
◆ B. Contractions divided into three periods of intensity.
   1. Increment: increasing intensity.
   2. Acme: peak, or full intensity.
   3. Decrement: decreasing intensity.
C. Contractions are monitored by the following:
   ◆ 1. Place your fingers lightly on the fundus of the uterus (the most contractile portion) and relate what you feel in your fingers to seconds and minutes on a clock. Uterus becomes firm, then hardens, and then decreases in hardness.

✦ 2. Electronic monitoring device.
   a. External: less accurate—done with a pressure-sensitive button placed over the uterine fundus.
   b. Internal: catheter inserted into uterine cavity to measure internal pressures and relay information to a graph.
✦ D. Contractions are monitored for frequency, duration, and intensity.
   1. Frequency: measured by timing contractions from the beginning of one contraction to the beginning of next.
   2. Duration: beginning of contraction to the completion of the contraction. Cannot be measured exactly by feeling with the hand.
   3. Intensity: cannot be measured by feeling; must be measured by internal fetal monitoring device. Usually refers to contraction at the beginning of labor. Peaks at about 25 mm Hg. At the end of labor, it may reach 50 to 75 mm Hg.
   4. Contractions may be described as mild, moderate, or intense.
E. Purpose of contractions.
   1. To propel presenting part forward.
   2. To bring about effacement and dilatation of the cervix.

Effacement and Dilatation

✦ A. Effacement: thinning process by which cervical canal is progressively shortened to complete obliteration. Progresses from a structure of 1 to 2 cm long to almost complete obliteration.
✦ B. Dilatation: process by which external os enlarges from a few millimeters to approximately 10 cm.
C. All that remains of the cervix after effacement and dilatation is a paper-thin circular opening about 10 cm in diameter.
D. Primiparas efface, then dilate; multiparas efface and dilate at the same time.

Changes in the Uterus

A. Uterus usually becomes differentiated in two distinct portions as labor progresses.
   1. Upper portion: contractile, becomes thicker.
   2. Lower portion: passive, becomes thinner and more expanded.
B. Boundary between the two segments is termed the "physiologic retraction ring."

Signs of Labor

Assessment

A. Assess for premonitory signs: physiologic changes that take place the last several weeks of pregnancy, indicating that labor is near.

✦ B. Observe for *lightening*: descent of the uterus downward and forward, which takes place as the presenting part descends into the pelvis.
   1. Time in which it takes place varies from a few weeks to a few days before labor. In multigravida, it may occur during labor.
   2. Sensations.
      a. Relief of pressure on diaphragm. Breathing is easier.
      b. Increased pelvic pressure leading to leg cramps, frequent micturition, and pressure on rectum.
✦ C. Check presence of Braxton Hicks contractions.
   1. May become quite regular but do not effectively dilate cervix.
   2. Usually are more pronounced at night.
   3. May play a part in ripening the cervix.
D. Evaluate for decrease in weight: there is usually a decrease in water retention due to hormonal influences.
E. Assess for cervical changes: cervix usually becomes softer, shorter, and somewhat dilated. May be dilated 1 to 2 cm by the time labor begins.
✦ F. Check presence of bloody show.
   1. Vaginal discharge of tenacious mucus, usually pinkish or streaked with blood, is expelled from the cervix as it shortens and begins to dilate.
   2. Labor usually begins within 24 to 48 hours.
G. Evaluate rupture of membranes.
   ✦ 1. May break any time before labor or during labor. Occasionally, membranes remain intact and are ruptured by the physician during labor (amniotomy).
   2. May gush or trickle.
   3. Client usually advised to come to the hospital as labor may begin within 24 hours.
   4. If labor does not begin spontaneously, it is induced to avoid intrauterine infections.
   5. Confirm rupture by nitrazine paper (turns blue) or ferning.
   6. Note color, amount and odor of amniotic fluid; fetal heart rate.
   7. Assess for signs of prolapsed cord.
H. Assess for beginning of true labor.
   ✦ 1. Contractions increase in frequency, intensity, and duration.
   2. Progressive cervical effacement and dilatation.
   3. Progressive descent of presenting part.
   4. Presence of bloody show.
   ✦ 5. Contractions increase in intensity with walking.
✦ I. Differentiate true from false labor.
   1. Irregular contractions.
   2. Contractions may cause discomfort.
   3. Usually discomfort is located in abdomen.

4. Labor usually does not intensify.
5. Discomfort may be relieved by walking.
6. Contractions do not bring about appreciable changes in cervix.
7. Sometimes difficult to differentiate false labor from true labor, and client is observed for several hours in the hospital.

Implementation

A. Careful monitoring of the client and fetus during the labor and delivery process.
B. Prompt recognition and treatment of complications.
C. Provision of comfort and safety measures during labor and delivery.
D. Supportive assistance to the laboring client or couple to enable them to maintain control during the labor and delivery process.

FETAL ASSESSMENT DURING LABOR

Fetal Monitoring

Characteristics

✦ A. Two types of electronic fetal monitoring: Doppler ultrasound—external; and fetal electrocardiography—internal. Provide for a continuous data readout of fetal heart rate and uterine contraction pattern.
B. Most common method of obtaining an external recording of the fetal heart rate is with an ultrasound transducer that picks up the motion of the fetal heart valves.
C. External monitoring of uterine contraction is done with a pressure sensitive button placed over the uterine fundus.
D. Heart rate sounds and uterine contractions are translated into electrical impulses reproduced on a printout strip on the fetal monitor.
✦ E. External fetal heart rate tracing does not assess fetal heart rate beat-to-beat variability. External uterine contraction monitoring does not quantify the strength of the contractions.
F. Types of external fetal monitors.
  1. Abdominal electrodes: elicits fetal and maternal heart rates.
  2. Phonotransducer: picks up fetal heart tones.
  3. Ultrasonic transducer: picks up fetal heart tones.
  4. Tocotransducer: monitors uterine activity.
G. Types of internal fetal monitors.
  1. Fetal scalp electrode (FSE): attached to presenting part—gives a direct tracing of fetal cardiac activity, which is recorded without interference and indicates beat-to-beat variability.

2. Intrauterine uterine pressure catheter (IUPC): pressure sensitive catheter introduced into the uterus, past the fetal head, and accurately measures frequency, duration, and intensity of uterine contractions.

Assessment

A. Evaluate client's and family's knowledge of rationale for fetal monitoring.
B. Identify client's concerns before procedure is initiated.
C. Assess client's knowledge of procedure.
✦ D. Evaluate position of fetus using Leopold's maneuver. (Fetal heart tone heard best over the fetal back area.)
✦ E. Assess fetal heart rate: normal is 120–160 beats/min.
F. Assess fetal monitor strip for early and late deceleration.

Implementation

A. Preparation: Explain procedure to client.
✦ B. Initiate external fetal monitoring using tocodynamometer (place over the fundus) and ultrasound transducer (usually placed in area of fetal back), or
C. Initiate internal fetal monitoring as indicated (fetal scalp electrode or internal uterine pressure catheter).

✦ **Fetal Monitoring (See Table 12-5)**

A. *Normal fetal heart rate (Baseline):* 110–160 beats/min baseline rate between contractions for a duration of at least 2 minutes (during a 10-minute segment).
B. *Variability (Baseline):* irregular fluctuations in the baseline FHR; usually at least 2 cycles/min (humps) and ranges between 6–25 beats/min (jagged line).
  1. Important indication of fetal oxygenation.
  2. Decrease variability may occur with fetal sleep, fetal hypoxia, medications, or neurologic immaturity.
C. *Periodic accelerations or decelerations:* increase or decrease in FHR lasting at least 30 seconds, usually associated with a contraction. Three types of decelerations: early, late, variable.
D. *Early deceleration:* gradual decrease in FHR in which lowest point (nadir) coincides with peak of contractions.
  1. Onset of deceleration to nadir at least 30 seconds.
  2. Uniform shape.
  3. Usually indicates head compression as result of vagal stimulation.
  4. Not considered ominous.
E. *Late deceleration:* gradual decrease in FHR in which lowest point of deceleration occurs after the peak of the contraction.

Table 12-5. VARIATIONS IN FETAL HEART RATE

Fetal Heart Rate	Possible Etiology	Implementation
Early deceleration Gradual decrease of fetal heart rate (FHR), 10- to 20-beat drop. Rate usually within 110–160. Recovery when acme of contraction passes	Head compression (vagal stimulation) Distinguish from late deceleration	Often not serious—observed late in labor; monitor closely
Late deceleration (in which nadir of deceleration occurs after peak of contraction) 10- to 20-beat decrease in FHR Nadir—occurs after peak contraction	Hypertonic contractions Fetal maternal exchange reduced → hypoxia → fetal distress	Turn client on side to reduce maternal hypotension Administer oxygen Discontinue oxytocin (as ordered) Increase hydration Prepare for immediate delivery (If pattern continues, may result in bradycardia and fetal death)
Variable deceleration Abrupt decrease in FHR of at least 15 beats/min, lasts longer than 15 seconds and less than 2 minutes Usually below 120 beats/min	Cord compression May or may not result in fetal difficulty Hypertonic contractions	Mild variable deceleration may not be dangerous—continue to monitor Change maternal position (knee–chest or Trendelenburg) Discontinue oxytocin, as ordered Administer oxygen Prepare for immediate delivery if continues Increase hydration; prepare for amnioinfusion
Loss of beat-to-beat variation Smooth baseline Less than 6 beats/min	Fetal anoxia (serious sign) Fetal hypoxia and acidosis Maternal medication Immature fetus Fetal malformation	Monitor that variation does not continue more than 15 minutes Monitor maternal hypnotics Decrease stimuli (maternal activity) and recheck rate Observe for late deceleration pattern
Bradycardia Drop of 20 beats/min below baseline (under 120 beats/min)	Fetal hypoxia Fetal distress Congenital heart abnormalities (arrhythmias) Hypothermia (from slow maternal cardiac metabolism)	When preceded by late deceleration or tachycardia—fetus is compromised—prepare for immediate delivery Change maternal position Administer oxygen
Tachycardia Increase in FHR over 160 beats/min for 10-min period	Fetal hypoxia Prematurity—immature autonomic nervous system (ANS) Maternal medication Maternal fever and/or tachycardia Maternal anxiety	Change maternal position Implement maternal relaxation methods to decrease anxiety Administer oxygen Monitor closely to track progress

1. Onset to nadir at least 30 seconds.
2. May indicate fetal hypoxia.
3. Caused by insufficient oxygenation of the uterus and placenta—O_2 reserve for infant to tolerate contractions.

F. *Variable deceleration:* abrupt decrease of at least 15 beats/min, lasting more than 15 seconds and less than 2 minutes.

1. Shape and onset will vary.
2. Indicates cord compression (i.e., cord around neck, baby lying on cord).

G. *Bradycardia:* baseline drop below 110 beats/min for at least 2 minutes (during 10-minute segment) between contractions.

1. May indicate fetal hypoxia.

2. May occur with congenital heart abnormalities, prolapse cord.
3. Maternal causes: medication, maternal bradycardia.

H. *Tachycardia:* baseline increases greater than 160 for at least 2 minutes (during 10-minute segment) between contractions.
   1. Increased maternal BMR (i.e., temperature, pulse) most common.
   2. Increased fetal BMR.
   3. Medications.
   4. Initial response to stress or early hypoxia.

STAGES AND PHASES OF LABOR

◆ *Definition:* Labor is divided into four stages: stage 1—beginning of true labor to complete cervical dilatation; stage 2—complete dilatation to birth of baby; stage 3—birth to delivery of placenta; and stage 4—first 1 to 4 hours after delivery of placenta.

Admission Procedures

◆ A. Check vital signs: temperature, pulse, respirations, and blood pressure.
◆ B. Check fetal heart rate.
C. Determine status of membranes: intact vs. ruptured.
D. Give prep and enema (if ordered by physician).
E. See that appropriate forms are completed.
F. Determine client's psychological state and readiness for coping with labor: some clients may complain of intense pain in very early labor.
G. Encourage client to void, and check urine for sugar, acetone, and protein.
H. Apply external fetal monitor if ordered.
I. Determine frequency, intensity (mild, moderate, severe), and duration of contractions.
J. Determine amount and character of show.
K. Assess cervical dilatation, effacement, station, presentation, position, and vaginal discharge.
L. Keep call bell within easy reach.

Stage 1

◆ *Definition:* Begins with onset of true labor and ends when cervix is completely dilated at 10 cm.

Assessment

A. Following admission procedures, observe for degree of dilatation.
B. Assess contractions: vary from mild and 5–15 minutes apart to intense and close together.
C. Evaluate cervical effacement.
D. Observe presence or increase in bloody show.
E. Assess station.

F. Assess mood of client: comfortable and talkative or tired and irritable.
G. Assess membrane status: intact or ruptured.

Implementation

PHASE ONE: LATENT PHASE

◆ A. Evaluate labor progress.
   1. Begins with onset of regular contractions and ends with dilatation of 3 to 4 cm.
   2. Contractions mild, 5–15 minutes apart, lasting 10–30 seconds. Averages 6.4 hours.
   3. Station varies −2 to −1.
   4. Show varies from brown to pink—scant amount.
◆ B. Observe for ruptured membranes and take fetal heart rate immediately if membranes rupture.
C. Maintain bedrest if membranes have ruptured. (In some hospitals, the client may be allowed out of bed with ruptured membranes if the baby's head is well engaged.)
◆ D. Allow client to walk about if membranes have not ruptured or provide reading material for client.
E. Auscultate fetal heart rate every 30 min–1 hour.
F. Check blood pressure every 30 minutes or PRN.
G. Check vital signs q 4 hrs. or more often if needed.
H. Start IV if ordered. Client usually NPO or clear liquids.
I. Check for bladder distention.
J. Give periodic vaginal examination to determine progress.
K. Provide support based on mother's knowledge of the labor process.
L. Reinforce breathing techniques or teach breathing techniques if client has had no classes.
M. Keep family informed of progress.
N. Encourage the presence of client's husband or a significant other person.
O. Reduce stimuli if client wants to rest.

PHASE TWO: ACTIVE PHASE

◆ A. Begins with acceleration phase.
   1. Cervix dilates from 3–4–8 cm.
   2. Fetal descent is progressive.
   3. Contractions 3–5 minutes apart and lasting 30–45 seconds, moderate intensity.
   4. Increase in bloody show.
   5. Station varies from 0 to +1.
B. Support client as she becomes tired, less talkative, and shows lack of energy.
C. Instruct/support client on breathing/relaxation techniques.
D. Monitor fetal heart rate every 15 minutes (high risk) to 30 min.

E. Apply pressure to sacrum during contraction or encourage baby's father to do so.

✦ F. Encourage client comfort in side-lying position; avoid lying on back to prevent supine hypotension, unless use a wedge to displace pressure from uterus on the vena cava.

G. Administer medications as ordered.
   1. Tranquilizers may be given in early labor.
   2. Analgesics are usually not given until labor is well established—4–6 cm dilatation.

H. Assist with anesthesia, if given, and monitor blood pressure and fetal heart rate.

I. Continue support and keep client informed.

J. Once membranes have ruptured (2–3 cm dilatation), internal fetal monitor may be applied.

PHASE THREE: TRANSITION PHASE

✦ A. Deceleration phase is part of transition.
   1. Dilatation slows as it progresses from 8–10 cm.
   2. Rate of fetal descent increases.
   3. Deceleration should last 3 hours for nulliparas, and 1 hour for multiparas.
   4. Contractions every 1½–2 min, 60–90 seconds duration, strong intensity.
   5. Station +1 to +2—increased amount of bloody show.
   6. Desire to bear down or defecate.

B. Support client as her attention and feelings become inner-directed; she may feel exhausted and no longer able to cope.

C. Care for symptoms of nausea, vomiting, trembling, burping, and crying.

D. Explain progress to client and encourage her to continue with breathing and relaxing techniques.

✦ E. Discourage bearing-down efforts until dilatation is complete.

F. Encourage deep ventilation prior to and after each contraction to avoid hyperventilation.

NURSING ACTIONS FOR DECELERATION

Early—no changes required

Variable—relieve pressure on umbilical cord
- Change position until corrected
- Increase IV fluids
- Give oxygen (3–4 L/min)
- Perform vaginal exam to determine cause

Late—increase uterine and placental blood flow
- Turn mother to left side
- Notify physician immediately
- Increase IV fluids
- Give oxygen (8–10 L/min)
- Maintain maternal blood pressure
- Discontinue oxytocin if used

G. Monitor contractions lightly with fingers as abdomen is sensitive.

H. Accept irritable behavior and aggression and continue supportive care.

I. Help client to push when ready.

J. Observe for signs of imminent delivery and prepare room for delivery or transfer client to delivery room when ready, if utilized.

Stage 2

✦ *Definition:* Begins with complete dilatation of cervix (10 cm) and ends with delivery of infant.

Mechanism of Labor and Delivery

✦ A. Sequence of movements of presenting part through birth canal. Head usually enters transverse and must rotate LOA or ROA for birth.

B. *Engagement:* head enters pelvis.

C. *Descent:* movement that occurs simultaneously with passage of head through pelvis.

D. *Flexion:* occurs as head descends and meets with resistance. In extreme flexion, the smallest diameter of the head presents.

E. *Internal rotation:* head usually enters with long diameter conforming to long diameter of inlet (usually transverse position) and must rotate before it can emerge from outlet; head rotates so that smallest diameter presents to conform to pelvis.

F. *Extension:* follows internal rotation; the head, which is flexed as it passes through birth canal, must extend for birth.

G. *External rotation:* soon after birth, the head rotates to either mother's right or left side, the fetal position before birth.

H. *Expulsion:* with delivery of shoulders, rest of body is expelled spontaneously.

Assessment

A. Observe for signs of imminent delivery.

✦ B. Check contractions every 2–3 minutes; contractions last 60–90 seconds.

C. Auscultate fetal heart rate every 5 minutes (high risk) or 15 minutes.

D. Evaluate vagina and perineum stretching and thinning to allow for passage of baby.

E. Check increase in bloody show.

F. Evaluate urge to push: involuntary bearing down.

G. Observe bulging of perineum.

H. Observe vaginal opening, which distends from a small, narrow opening to a wide, round opening.

I. Observe presenting part as it becomes more visible.

J. Check crowning: widest diameter of baby's head is visible and encircled by vaginal opening.

K. Observe birth of presenting part.

L. Observe rest of body as it is delivered, usually with a gush of fluid.

Implementation

A. If separate delivery room utilized, transfer client carefully from bed to delivery table and place in lithotomy position.

B. On birthing bed or delivery table, pad stirrups to avoid pressure to popliteal veins and pressure areas. Gently raise both legs simultaneously into stirrups to avoid ligament strain. Adjust stirrups and drape client.

C. Provide client with handles to pull on as she pushes.

◆ D. Cleanse vulva and perineum using medical aseptic principles of surgical scrub/prep.

◆ E. Auscultate fetal heart tone every 5 minutes or after each push; transient fetal bradycardia not unusual due to head compression.

F. Check blood pressure and pulse every 15 minutes PRN.

G. Administer oxygen if fetal heart tones decrease.

H. Include baby's father/significant other in birth experience as much as possible; explain what is happening, where to stand, etc.

I. Catheterize if bladder is distended and prevents descent.

J. Encourage mother and keep her informed of advancement of baby.

K. Encourage mother to take a deep breath before beginning to push with each contraction and to sustain push as long as possible; long pushes are preferable to frequent short pushes.

L. Encourage open glottal pushing unless there is a medical indication for rapid delivery.

Stage 3

Definition: From birth to expulsion of the placenta, usually 5–20 minutes after delivery.

Assessment

◆ A. Observe for signs of placental separation.
1. The uterus contracts.
2. The uterus changes from discoid to globular in shape.
3. A slight gush of blood issues from vagina.
4. Lengthening of the umbilical cord occurs.
5. Upward displacement of the uterus occurs.

◆ B. Evaluate placenta after separation.
1. *Schultze* (most common): placenta is inverted on itself, and the shiny fetal surface appears; 80 percent separate in center.
2. *Duncan*: descends sideways, and the maternal surface appears. Separates at edges rather than center.

C. Check to ensure that placental fragments do not remain in uterus.

◆ D. Continually assess both mother and infant for first critical hour after birth.
1. Most common cause of death in first hour is hemorrhage—assess vital signs every 15 minutes.
2. Assess condition of fundus.
3. Check lochia for color and amount.

Implementation

◆ A. Monitor newborn's status and begin bonding with parents.
1. Position baby so that mother and baby may have eye-to-eye contact.
2. Dim lights of birthing room so baby can open eyes fully.

◆ B. Monitor for signs of placental separation.
1. Uterus rises upward in abdomen; as placenta proceeds downward, umbilical cord lengthens.
2. Sudden trickle of blood appears.
3. Uterus changes from discoid to globular shape.

C. Palpate uterus to check for ballooning of uterus caused by uterine relaxation with bleeding into uterine cavity.

D. Splint or support abdominal muscles as mother bears down to assist in delivering placenta.

E. Inspect placental membranes to be sure they are intact after delivery.

◆ F. Palpate fundus of uterus—normal position is at midline and below umbilicus.

Stage 4

Definition: From expulsion of placenta to a period of 1 to 4 hours after delivery or until vital signs are stable.

Assessment

A. Continually assess both mother and infant for first critical hour or two after birth.
◆ 1. Assess firmness and position of fundus and that it remains well contracted to ensure that mother has minimal bleeding.
2. Assess vital signs including blood pressure every 15 minutes.
3. Assess amount and character of vaginal blood flow.

B. Check that blood pressure returns to prelabor levels and pulse is slightly lower than during labor.
1. Return of blood pressure is due to increased volume of blood returning to maternal circulation.
2. Lowered blood pressure and rising pulse may reflect increased blood loss.

COMPLICATIONS OF LABOR AND DELIVERY

Fetal Distress

Assessment

✦ A. Assess fetal heart rate: above 160 or below 120 beats/min indicates distress; signs of oxygen lack or infection. (*See* Table 12-6.)

✦ B. Check for meconium-stained fluid. During hypoxia, bowel peristalsis increases, anal sphincter may relax, and meconium is likely to be passed.

C. Assess for fetal hyperactivity.

D. If labor is monitored, check:
1. Variable deceleration pattern.
2. Late deceleration pattern.
3. Fetal pH below 7.2.

Implementation

✦ A. Discontinue oxytocin if being infused.

✦ B. Turn client to left side; if no improvement, turn to right side. This procedure relieves pressure on umbilical cord during contractions and pressure of uterus on the inferior vena cava.

C. Administer oxygen via mask at 10–12 L/min.

D. Correction of hypotension: increase perfusion of IV fluids.

E. Notify physician.

F. Prepare for emergency cesarean delivery if no improvement.

Vena Cava Syndrome (Supine Hypotensive Syndrome)

✦ *Definition:* Shock-like symptoms that occur when venous return to the heart is impaired by weight of gravid uterus causing partial occlusion of the vena cava.

Assessment

A. Assess for risk factors—multiple pregnancies, obesity, polyhydramnios.

B. Assess shock-like symptoms caused by reduced cardiac output.
1. Hypotension.
2. Tachycardia.
3. Sweating, dizziness, pallor.
4. Nausea and vomiting.
5. Air hunger.

C. Assess for fetal distress; caused by reduced flow of blood to placenta from reduced cardiac output.

Implementation

✦ A. Assist mother to turn to left side (use a wedge pillow) to shift weight of fetus off inferior vena cava.

B. Provide oxygen with tight mask if recovery is not immediate after positioning.

✦ C. Monitor fetal heart rate to determine fetal status.

Premature Rupture of the Membranes (PROM)

Definition: The spontaneous rupture of membranes (before 37 weeks' gestation) prior to the onset of labor.

Assessment

A. Assess latent period: time from rupture of membranes to onset of labor; interval period is time from rupture of membranes to delivery of fetus.

✦ B. Major maternal risks associated with PROM are ascending uterine infection and precipitation of preterm labor.
1. Assess time between membrane rupturing and when labor began—risk of infection may be directly related to time involved.
2. Observe for signs of infection: elevated temperature, chills, malaise, WBC.

✦ C. Assess for signs of labor or prolapsed cord.

D. Observe amniotic fluid for foul odor or signs of fetal distress (meconium staining).

Implementation

A. Monitor for signs of contractions.

Table 12-6. COMPLICATIONS AND SIGNS OF FETAL DISTRESS		
Complication	**Signs of Distress**	**Possible Nursing Implementation**
Hypoxia	Irregular heart rate Heart rate > 160 or < 120 Passage of meconium in the vertex position Absent or minimal variability	Administer oxygen to the mother—turn on left side Constantly observe and monitor fetal heart tone Check for prolapse of the cord Prepare delivery room equipment for possible resuscitation of the baby at birth Increase IV fluids
Generalized infection	Irregular heart rate Heart rate > 160 or < 120	Administer antibiotics to the mother Keep vaginal exams to a minimum Follow same interventions as 1, 2, 4 in hypoxia

✦ B. Monitor for fetal heart tones at least every 4 hours until labor begins.

C. Alleviate client's fears of "dry birth."

D. Record time, amount, color, and odor of ruptured membranes.

E. Record vital signs, especially temperature, every 4 hours.

✦ F. Monitor for most common neonatal risk—respiratory distress syndrome.

Preterm Labor and Delivery

Definition: Labor that occurs prior to the end of the 37th week of gestation.

Characteristics

A. Predisposing factors.
   1. Conditions such as chronic pyelonephritis, cervical incompetence, multiple pregnancies, past history of premature births, sepsis in the fetus, and placental disorders.
   2. Sometimes no specific cause can be identified.

B. Attempts to arrest preterm labor are contraindicated when:
   1. Pregnancy is 37 weeks or over.
   2. Ruptured membranes exist; delivery may be delayed if there are no indications of infection to allow fetus to mature.
   3. Maternal disease exists: abruptio placenta, etc.
   4. Fetal problems such as Rh isoimmunization become threatening.

✦ C. A drug such as betamethasone (Celestone) may be given to the mother to hasten fetal maturity by stimulating development of lecithin when membranes are ruptured and premature labor cannot be arrested—decreases incidence of respiratory distress syndrome.

Assessment

✦ A. Observe for abrupt change in fetal heart tones or signs of distress.

B. Assess vital signs—blood pressure, pulse, temperature, and respirations.

C. Evaluate for signs of infection, respiratory distress, cardiac status.

D. Check intake and urinary output.

E. Examine urine for glucose and protein.

F. Check for presence of edema.

G. Assess maternal emotional state.

Implementation

A. Teach pregnant client early warning signs of preterm labor and to notify healthcare providers early.

B. Encourage adequate hydration, especially if weather is hot, to prevent irritable uterine contractions, which may lead to preterm labor.

MEDICAL IMPLICATIONS

• Tocolysis (use of medications to stop labor) includes beta-mimetics, magnesium sulfate, prostaglandin synthetase inhibitors (indomethacin or sulindac), and calcium channel blockers (nifedipine) are also utilized for premature labor.

• Use of sympathomimetic drugs (ritodrine, terbutaline) are also used—cause an inhibitory effect on uterine smooth muscle and may also cause hypotension, tachycardia, and arrhythmias.

• Cardiac monitor and CVP may be used to monitor maternal cardiac function.

• Trendelenburg's or side-lying position minimizes hypotension.

• Narcotics are usually withheld because of their depressive effect on the infant.

• Drug regimen may be continued on outpatient basis after uterine contractions cease.

✦ C. Maintain bedrest; place client on left side.

✦ D. Continuous monitoring of contractions, vital signs, and fetal heart tones.

E. Administer medications (tocolytics) according to protocol.

F. Keep client informed and provide support: may be fearful, feel guilty, or be anxious; decreasing anxiety is primary goal.

G. Careful observation for signs of complications such as tachycardia.

H. Provide for hygiene and general comfort care.

Prolonged Pregnancy

Definition: Pregnancy over 42 weeks' gestation—degeneration of placenta, thus decreased blood to fetus.

Characteristics

✦ A. Amniotic fluid decreases and vernix caseosa disappears; infant's skin appears dry and cracked.

B. Infant may lose weight.

C. Chronic hypoxia may occur due to placental dysfunction.

D. Determination of gestational age usually made to ascertain actual duration of pregnancy—estriol studies, sonography.

E. Contraction Stress Test (CST) may be done to determine fetus's ability to tolerate labor.

F. Labor stimulated with oxytocin and prostaglandin for cervical ripening.

G. Cesarean delivery if induction contraindicated.

Assessment

A. Determine actual gestational age.

✦ B. Assess results of CST to determine fetus's viability.

C. Assess vital signs of client for baseline data before labor is induced.

D. Assess psychological state of client and need for support.
E. Assess external resources of client.

Implementation

✦ A. Monitor fetal heart rate continuously—report any late or variable deceleration immediately.
B. Support mother during labor process.
C. Prepare for possibility of emergency cesarean section.
D. Monitor induction of labor if natural labor process occurs.
E. Support family during labor and delivery.

Prolapsed Umbilical Cord

Definition: Displacement of the umbilical cord below the presenting part. The cord may protrude through the cervix and into the vaginal canal.

Characteristics

A. Rupture of the membranes before engagement.
B. Abnormal presentation.
C. Premature infant: presenting part does not fill the birth canal, allowing the cord to slip through.
D. Polyhydramnios.

Assessment

✦ A. Observe for presence of cord palpated or seen on vaginal examination.
✦ B. Assess abnormal fetal heart pattern: cord may become compressed and cause fetal hypoxia.

Implementation

✦ A. Place client in knee–chest or modified Sims' position with hips elevated on pillows.
✦ B. Insert fingers of sterile, gloved hand into vagina to lift presenting part off umbilical cord until fetus delivered.
C. Administer oxygen (5 L) to mother by mask.
D. Call for assistance.
E. Notify physician.
✦ F. Continuously monitor fetal heart rate (baseline above 120 beats/min and variable decelerations relieved if cord compression lessened).
G. Do not attempt to push in cord.
H. Stay with client and offer support.
I. Prepare for immediate delivery, by cesarean section if necessary.

Amniotic Fluid Embolism

✦ *Definition:* The escape of amniotic fluid into the maternal circulation. It is usually fatal to the mother.

Characteristics

A. Amniotic fluid contains debris such as lanugo, vernix, and meconium, which may become deposited in pul-

---

> ### MEDICAL IMPLICATIONS
>
> • Oxygen under pressure.
> • Vasopressor to maintain blood pressure.
> • Digitalis for failing cardiac function.
> • Fibrinogen to replace depleted reserves.
> • Heparin to combat fibrinogenemia.
> • Client may be given whole blood or crystalloid.
> • Forceps delivery if cervix is dilated enough to allow for delivery or prepare for cesarean birth.

monary arterioles and result in cardiopulmonary collapse.
B. Usually enters maternal circulation through open venous sinus at placental site.
C. Predisposing factors.
  1. Premature rupture of membranes.
  2. Tumultuous labor.
D. High maternal mortality rate—85 percent.

Assessment

✦ A. Observe for acute dyspnea with hypotension.
✦ B. Assess for sudden chest pain.
C. Check for cyanosis.
D. Assess for CNS hypoxia: changes in LOC, seizures, etc.
E. Observe for pulmonary edema.
F. Check vital signs for indications of shock.
G. Assess for uncontrolled hemorrhage.
H. Assess for uncontrolled hemorrhage (massive DIC).

Implementation

✦ A. Institute efficiency measures to maintain life.
B. If client survives, provide intensive care treatment.
C. Keep family informed and provide emotional support.

Inverted Uterus

Definition: A condition in which the uterus turns inside out, usually during delivery of the placenta.

Assessment

✦ A. Observe for shock, hemorrhage, or severe pain.
B. Check for mild symptoms with incomplete uterine inversion.

Implementation

✦ A. Assist with treatment for shock.
B. Monitor for hemorrhage.
C. Monitor vital signs.
D. Assist client while replacement of uterus (if done vaginally) is done.

Rupture of the Uterus

Definition: The splitting of the uterine wall accompanied by extrusion of all or part of uterine contents into the abdominal cavity. Baby usually dies, and mortality rate in mothers is high due to blood loss.

Assessment

A. Observe for acute abdominal pain and tenderness.

B. Establish that presenting part is no longer felt through cervix.

C. Assess for a feeling in client that something has happened inside her.

D. Evaluate for cessation of labor pains (no contractions).

E. Evaluate for any external bleeding (usually bleeding is internal).

F. Assess for signs of shock: pale appearance, pulse weak and rapid, air hunger, and exhaustion.

G. Evaluate fetal status.

Implementation

A. Be alert for symptoms since immediate diagnosis is necessary if fetus and mother are to survive.

B. Call for assistance, stay with client, and notify physician.

C. Prepare for emergency surgery.

Dysfunctional Labor (Dystocia)

Definition: Dystocia occurs with prolonged and difficult labor and delivery. Labor is considered prolonged when it extends for 24 hours or more after the onset of regular contractions.

Characteristics

A. Dysfunctional uterine contractions.
   1. Uterine contractions inefficient; hence, cervical dilatation, effacement, and descent fail to occur.
   2. Contributing factors.
      a. False labor.
      b. Oversedation or excessive anesthesia.
      c. "Unripe" cervix.
      d. Uterine contractions that are hypertonic or hypotonic.
      e. Uterine abnormalities such as fibroids.
      f. Cephalopelvic disproportion (CPD).
      g. Malpositions.
      h. Uterine or other abnormalities.

B. Abnormal presentations and positions.

1. *Occiput posterior position.*
   a. Usually prolongs labor because baby must rotate a longer distance (135 degrees or more) to reach symphysis pubis.
   b. May lead to persistent occiput posterior (head does not rotate) or deep transverse arrest (head arrested in transverse position).
   c. Treatment.
      (1) Head usually rotates itself with contraction.
      (2) Rotation may be done by physician manually or with forceps.

2. *Breech position* prolongs labor because soft tissue of fetus' bottom does not aid cervical dilatation as does the fetal skull.

3. *Face presentation:* rare; results in increased prenatal mortality.
   a. Chin must rotate so it lies under symphysis pubis for delivery.
   b. If baby is delivered vaginally, the face is usually edematous and bruised, with marked molding.
   c. Cesarean delivery is indicated if face does not rotate.

4. *Transverse lie.*
   a. Long axis of fetus at right angles to long axis of mother.
   b. Spontaneous conversion may occur. Cesarean delivery is the usual treatment.

C. Cephalopelvic disproportion (CPD).
   1. Disproportion between the size of the fetus and size of the pelvis.
   2. Head is large.
   3. Size of shoulders may also complicate delivery.
   4. Causes.
      a. Multiparity: birth weight may progress with each pregnancy.
      b. Maternal diabetes.
      c. Large baby.
      d. Fetal abnormalities.
         (1) Hydrocephalus.
         (2) Tumors.
         (3) Abnormal development.
   5. Size may be determined by sonography and x-ray.
   6. Treatment.
      a. Vaginal delivery if disproportion is not too great. May be fetal injuries: brachial plexus, dislocated shoulder.
      b. Cesarean delivery indicated if disproportion too great.

Assessment

A. Observe rate of progress as well as overall length of labor.

✦DYSTOCIA

A. Dystocia may be classified in several ways, and although the divisions are artificial, they are useful in looking at the processes involved.
   1. Dysfunction of powers or forces with respect to the uterus and abdominal muscles.
   2. Abnormalities of the passengers—fetus and placenta.
   3. Abnormalities of the passages—bony and soft tissue.
   4. May be a combination of two or more dysfunctions and abnormalities.
B. True labor begins but fails to progress. Dystocia may occur during latent or active phase of labor.
C. It is important to look at the rate of progress as well as the overall length of labor; that is, is the client slowly progressing, or is she arrested at one point?

✦ 1. Latent phase may be considered prolonged.
   a. Parous: labor extends 14 hours or longer.
   b. Nulliparous: labor extends 20 hours or longer.
✦ 2. Active phase may be considered prolonged.
   a. Parous: dilatation is lower than 1.5 cm/hr and descent is less than 5 cm/hr.
   b. Nulliparous: dilatation is slower than 1.2 cm/hr and descent is less than 1 cm/hr.
   3. Arrested labor—labor fails to progress beyond a certain point.
✦ B. Signs of distress in the mother.
   1. Infection.
      a. Elevated temperature.
      b. Elevated pulse.
   2. Exhaustion.
      a. Loss of emotional stability.
      b. Lack of cooperation.
      c. Ketonuria.
   3. Dehydration.
      a. Dry tongue and skin.
      b. Concentrated urine.
      c. Acetonuria (ketonuria).
✦ C. Signs of distress in the fetus.
   1. Hypoxia.
      a. Irregular heart rate.
      b. Heart rate above 160 or below 110 or decrease of 20 points below baseline.
      c. Passage of meconium in the vertex position.
   2. Generalized infection.
      a. Irregular heart rate.
      b. Heart rate above 160 or below 110.

Implementation

A. The course of dysfunctional labor varies with cause. If labor is induced:
✦ 1. Promote rest: darken room, reduce noise level.

- Varies with cause.
- Vaginal examination to determine position and station of fetus.
- X-ray pelvimetry or sonography to determine CPD.
- Rest for exhausted client.
- Cautious oxytocic stimulation of labor if malposition, CPD, and other abnormalities are ruled out.
- Cesarean delivery if appropriate.

   2. Position client for comfort.
   3. Give client a back rub.
   4. Provide clean linen and gown, and allow client to bathe or shower if permissible.
   5. Promote oral hygiene.
   6. Give client reassurance and support.
   7. Explain procedures to client.
   8. Let client express feelings and emotions freely.
B. Monitor client's progress.
✦ 1. Watch for signs of exhaustion, dehydration, and acidosis.
✦ 2. Monitor vital signs.
✦ 3. Monitor fetal heart rate.
   4. Monitor progress of labor.
   5. Watch for signs of excessive bleeding and fetal distress.
   6. Encourage client to void q 2 hr and check bladder for distention.
C. Administer medications as ordered.
D. Prepare for cesarean section if necessary.

Precipitate Delivery

Definition: Rapid or sudden labor of less than 3 hours' duration, from onset of cervical changes to delivery of infant.

Assessment

✦ A. Obtain quick admission history by asking focused questions.
   1. "Do you want to push?"
   2. "Have your membranes ruptured?"
   3. "Are you bleeding?"
   4. "Have you had a baby born quickly before?"
B. Assess client's ability to understand your directions.
C. Evaluate resources (proximity of physician and/or other assistance).
D. Assess client's psychological state and need for support at this time. Establish rapport quickly.
✦ E. Assess signs and symptoms of impending delivery.
   1. Desire to push.
   2. Frequency of strong contractions.
   3. Heavy bloody show.
   4. Membranes ruptured.

5. Bulging rectum.
6. Presenting part visible.
7. Severe anxiety.
F. Observe for above signs continually as labor may progress with unexpected rapidity.

Implementation

✦ ASSISTING WITH DELIVERY

✦ A. Never leave the client unattended during this time.
   1. Never hold baby back; allow it to progress naturally.
   2. Ask another employee to notify the physician.
   3. Bring the emergency delivery pack to room.
   4. Have client pant rather than push to avoid rapid delivery of the head.
B. Reassure client that you will remain with her and provide care until the physician arrives.
C. Put on sterile gloves if they are available and if there is time.
D. Break membranes immediately if they have not done so spontaneously.
✦ E. With a clean or sterile towel (if available), support baby's head with one hand, applying gentle pressure to the head to prevent sudden expulsion and undue stretching of the perineum or brain damage to the infant.
✦ F. If cord is draped around baby's neck, with free hand gently slip it over the head.
✦ G. If you have a bulb syringe, gently suction baby's mouth and wipe blood and mucus from mouth and nose with towel, if available. Shoulders are usually born spontaneously after external rotation. If shoulders do not deliver spontaneously, ask client to bear down to deliver them.
H. Support the baby's body as it is delivered.
I. Hold infant level with placenta until cord clamping is done.
   1. If infant is held high, blood may flow back into placenta and cause anemia.
   2. If infant is held below level of placenta, extra blood could cause polycythemia.
J. All manipulation should be gentle to avoid injury to mother and baby.

CARE AFTER DELIVERY

✦ A. After delivery, hold baby securely over hand and arm with the head in a dependent position to allow fluid and mucus to drain.
✦ B. If baby does not cry spontaneously, gently rub baby's back or the soles of baby's feet.
C. Dry baby to prevent heat loss.
D. Place the baby on the mother's abdomen to provide warmth. The weight on the uterus will help it to contract.

E. Palpate mother's abdomen to make sure uterus is contracting.
F. Watch for signs of placental separation.
G. Support placenta in your hand after it is expelled.
✦ H. Clamp the cord after it stops pulsating if clamp or ties are available. Cord need not be cut; there will be no bleeding from the placental surface.
I. Wrap the baby in a blanket.
✦ J. Put the baby to the mother's breast. This reassures the mother that the baby is all right and helps contract the uterus.
K. Check the uterus after delivery of the placenta. Make sure the uterus is contracting.
L. Keep an accurate record of the time of birth and other pertinent data.
✦ M. If baby is delivered unassisted, in bed, before the nurse arrives (precipitate delivery), the nurse should immediately:
   1. Check the baby to make sure breathing is established.
   2. Monitor closely for signs of hemorrhage (increased risk of lacerations, abruptio placenta).
N. Comfort mother and family.
O. Monitor newborn closely for signs of aspiration, asphyxia, or intracranial trauma.

OBSTETRIC MEDICATIONS

Induction of Labor

Definition: To bring about labor through the use of stimulants, such as oxytocin (Pitocin).

Oxytocin Infusion

A. Indications for use.
   1. Post-term gestation (2 weeks or more); placental functions reduced.
   2. Severe preeclampsia.
   3. Diabetes.
   4. Premature rupture of membranes (should deliver within 24 hours).
   5. Uncontrolled bleeding.
   6. Rh sensitization: rising titer.
   7. IUGR.
B. Prerequisites for successful induction.
   1. Fetal maturity.
   2. Cervix amenable for induction (may utilize prostaglandin E_2 gel or misoprostol to assist in ripening cervix); client may be induced for several days with rest at night to ripen cervix, if it is desirable to deliver fetus due to complications.
   3. Normal cephalopelvic proportions.
   4. Fetal head engaged.

Assessment

◆ A. Observe continuous monitoring of contractions and fetal heart rate—danger of ruptured uterus.

◆ B. Evaluate prolonged uterine contractions: over 90 seconds with less than 30-second rest period between. (Safety intervention is to turn off Pitocin.)

C. Assess for uterine relaxation between contractions.

◆ D. Assess for change in fetal heart rate pattern indicating fetal distress.

E. Assess for hemorrhage or shock, which may indicate uterine rupture.

F. Check for rigid abdomen, which may indicate abruptio placenta.

G. Assess vital signs: blood pressure for elevations.

H. Evaluate progress of labor.

Implementation

A. Maintain client on bedrest and explain procedure.

B. Provide supportive care to client in labor.

◆ C. Obtain baseline fetal heart rate and blood pressure; note presence or absence of any contractions.

D. Start IV fluids: usually 50 mL of D_5W in lactated Ringer's solution.

◆ E. Piggyback oxytocin solution into main line: usually 10 units of Pitocin in 1000 mL solution. Controller or Harvard infusion pump may be used to more accurately control drip rate. (Harvard pump may infuse 2.5 units in 50 mL IV fluid.)

◆ F. Begin infusion slowly to test uterine sensitivity to drug: usually begin at rate of 1 to 2 mU/min with dose increased by 1 mU increments every 15 to 30 minutes until regular contraction pattern is established.

G. Monitor labor with external monitor.

H. Discontinue oxytocin solution immediately if hypertonic contractions or signs of fetal distress occur and administer LR solution. Report to physician.

Analgesia During Labor

Assessment

A. Assess client pain status—individual thresholds vary.

B. Check vital signs and fetal heart rate before and after administration.

C. Evaluate allergies to medication.

D. Check time last pain medication was given if any.

E. Assess progress of labor before and after.

Implementation

◆ A. Narcotics are not given until labor is well established in order to avoid retarding progress of labor.

1. Drugs are usually administered between 4 and 6 cm dilatation.

2. Narcotics given to the mother in labor cross placental barrier and affect infant.

◆ B. Do not administer narcotics within 2 hours of delivery because the infant may be born depressed; drugs are at maximum effect 2 hours after ingestion.

1. In the uterus, gas exchange takes place through the placenta; therefore, analgesia given in labor does not pose a threat to infant.

2. After birth, the infants breathe on their own. Analgesics depress the CNS and affect the respiratory and other centers.

3. Some infants do not become fully alert for two to three days after delivery.

C. Continually observe client and keep siderails up.

D. Be familiar with normal dosages and the physiologic effect of preparations used.

E. Record time, type, dosage, route, and client's response.

F. Use precautions for sedatives that are given early in labor to reduce anxiety.

G. For specific drugs, *see* Appendix 12-1.

Anesthesia During Labor

Characteristics

A. No optimum anesthesia exists.

◆ B. One of the major causes of maternal death; other three causes are hemorrhage, infection, and eclampsia.

C. History and physical should be obtained before administering anesthesia.

D. Client should be NPO before use.

E. Anesthesia should be administered by skilled personnel.

F. Choice of anesthesia in obstetrics is determined by the specific client situation and condition.

GENERAL INHALATION ANESTHETICS

A. Advantages.

1. May anesthetize client rapidly.

2. Primary use is for rapid induction for emergency cesarean section.

3. These anesthetics cause uterine relaxation—may be used for manipulation.

4. Inhalation anesthetics may be preferred in hypovolemic client or if the client's condition prohibits the use of regional anesthetics.

B. Disadvantages.

1. Client is not awake for delivery.

2. Brings about respiratory depression of the infant.

3. May cause emesis and aspiration in the client.

4. May be flammable.

C. Common types.

1. Nitrous oxide: danger of aspiration and respiratory depression.

2. Halothane: potent, used in selected cases only.

3. Sodium thiopental (Pentothal): IV anesthesia used as an adjunct; most frequently used for induction; may depress neonate.
4. Trichloroethylene—Trilene: often used in self-administration by mask during labor and delivery. Never leave client alone when she is using self-administered anesthesia.

REGIONAL ANALGESIA AND ANESTHESIA

A. Regional analgesia and anesthesia refer to the drugs given to block the nerves carrying sensation from the uterus to the pelvic region.
1. Some common agents used are: Novocaine, Xylocaine, Pontocaine, and Carbocaine.
2. Vasoconstrictor agents such as epinephrine are only used in conjunction with regional anesthetics to:
   a. Slow absorption and prolong the effect of the anesthetic.
   b. Prevent secondary hypotension.
3. Opioids often used with anesthetic agent to produce analgesia (i.e., morphine, fentanyl).

✦ B. Nerve root block is a principal type of regional anesthesia.
1. General considerations.
   a. Usually relieves pain completely, if administered properly.
   b. Vasodilation below the anesthetic level: may be responsible for a decrease in blood pressure; blood pools in legs.
   c. Does not depress the respiratory center and, therefore, does not harm the client unless hypotension in the client is severe enough to interfere with uterine flow.
   d. May cause postspinal headache.
   e. Contraindicated in a hypovolemic client or in the case of central nervous system disease.
   f. Drug may impede labor if given too early (before 5–6 cm dilatation).
   g. Special skill of anesthesiologist required to administer drug.
   h. Infant may need forceps delivery because the client usually cannot push effectively due to anesthesia.
2. Types.
   a. Epidural–spinal combined.
   b. Lumbar epidural (may be single dose or continuous).
   c. Spinal block.

✦ C. Peripheral nerve block is a second principal type of regional anesthesia.
1. General considerations.
   a. May be done by attending physician—does not require an anesthesiologist.
   b. Local injection of anesthetic to block peripheral nerve endings.
   c. Less effective in relieving pain than nerve root block.
   d. May cause transient bradycardia in fetus, possibly due to rapid absorption of the drug into fetal circulation.
   e. Usually there are no maternal side effects.
   f. Needle guide such as Iowa trumpet usually used.
2. Types.
   a. Local infiltration anesthesia.
   b. Pudendal block.

Assessment

A. Observe progress of labor.
B. Check vital signs and fetal heart rate before and after administration of drug (may cause transient fetal bradycardia).
C. Check drug allergies or hypersensitivity.
D. Observe for signs of dizziness, nausea, faintness, and palpitations.
E. Assess level of anesthesia: relief of pain sensation.
F. Observe for signs of systemic toxic reactions: muscle twitching, convulsions, loss of consciousness, respiratory depression, cardiac arrest.
G. After delivery, check client for return of sensation to lower body.

Implementation

A. Have client void.
B. Bolus IV fluids (500–1000 mL) to help prevent hypotension.
C. Assist client to a knee–chest, side-lying, or sitting position over a bolster or onto left side with head flexed and knees drawn up.
D. Monitor blood pressure every 3–5 minutes until stabilized; then every 30 minutes or PRN.
E. Monitor fetal heart rate.
✦ F. If hypotension occurs:
1. Turn client to left side.
2. Administer oxygen by mask.
3. Increase IV fluids.
4. Notify physician.

OPERATIVE OBSTETRICS

Obstetrical Procedures

Episiotomy

✦ *Definition:* An incision made into the perineum during delivery to facilitate the birth process.
A. Types of episiotomy.

1. *Midline:* incision from the posterior margin of the vaginal opening directly backward to the anal sphincter.
   a. Healing is less painful.
   b. Incision is easy to repair.
   c. May extend to rectal sphincter.
2. *Mediolateral:* incision made at 45-degree angle to either side of the vaginal opening.
   a. Healing process is quite painful.
   b. Incision is harder to repair.
   c. Blood loss greater.
B. Purposes.
   1. Spare the muscles of perineal floor from undue stretching and tearing (lacerations).
   2. Prevent the prolonged pressure of the baby's head on perineum.
   3. Reduce duration of second stage of labor.
   4. Enlarge vagina for manipulation.
C. Method.
   1. Generally done during contraction, as the baby's head pushes against perineum and stretches it.
   2. Blunt scissors are used.
   3. Client is usually given an anesthetic: regional, local, or inhalation.

Lacerations

Definition: Perineal or vaginal lacerations are classified as first-, second-, third-, or fourth-degree tears.
A. Lacerations may involve the perineum, folds of the vagina, urethra tissues, cervical tears, or uterine tears.
   1. May occur with or without an episiotomy.
   2. Repaired with sutures which dissolve.
B. Prevention of lacerations.
   1. Maintain mother in positions with relaxed perineum.
   2. Slow, controlled exit of fetus will promote an intact perineum.

Assisted Delivery: Forceps or Vacuum

Definition: The extraction of a baby from the birth canal by a physician with the use of a specially designed instrument.
A. Types.
   1. Low forceps: presenting part at or below pelvic floor.
   2. Midforceps: presenting part below or at the level of the ischial spine.
   3. Vacuum Extraction: soft silicone cup applied to fetal head; used during prolonged second stage; preferred if borderline CPD.
B. Indications.
   1. Fetal distress.
   2. Poor progress of fetus through the birth canal.
   3. Failure of the head to rotate.

4. Maternal disease (heart disease, acute pulmonary edema, infection) or exhaustion.
5. Client unable to push (as with regional anesthesia).
C. Prerequisite conditions for application of forceps or vacuum cup.
   1. Fully dilated cervix.
   2. Fetal head engaged in maternal pelvis.
   3. Membranes ruptured.
   4. Absence of cephalopelvic disproportion.
   5. Empty bladder.
   6. Fetal heart tones present before and after forceps or vacuum application.
   7. Adequate anesthesia must be given for type of forceps or vacuum applied.
   8. Vacuum: fetus weight < 2500, > 35 week, occiput presentation, no previous fetal scalp blood sampling.
D. Complications.
   1. Lacerations of the vagina or the cervix; there may be oozing or hemorrhage.
   2. Rupture of the uterus.
   3. Intracranial hemorrhage and brain damage to the fetus.
   4. Facial paralysis of the fetus.

Cesarean Delivery

Definition: A surgical delivery of an infant through an incision cut into the abdominal wall and the uterus.
A. Types.
   1. Classical: vertical incision through the abdominal wall and into the anterior wall of the uterus.
   2. Low segment transverse: transverse incision made into lower uterine segment after abdomen has been opened.
      a. Incision made into the part of the uterus where there is less uterine activity and blood loss is minimal.
      b. Less incidence of adhesions and intestinal obstruction.
   3. Cesarean hysterectomy: abdomen and uterus are opened, baby and placenta are removed, and then the hysterectomy is performed. The hysterectomy is performed if:
      a. Diseased tissue or fibroids are present.
      b. There is an abnormal Pap smear.
      c. The uterus ruptures.
      d. There is uncontrolled hemorrhage or placenta abruptio or uterine atony, etc.
B. Indications.
   1. Fetal distress unrelieved by other measures.
   2. Uterine dysfunction.
   3. Certain cases of placental previa and premature separation of placenta.

4. Prolapsed cord.
5. Diabetes or certain cases of toxemia.
6. Cephalopelvic disproportion.
7. Malpresentations such as transverse lie.

Assessment

✦ A. Check vital signs every 5 minutes until stable, then every 15 minutes: blood pressure, temperature, pulse, respirations.
B. Observe site of incision for bleeding.
C. Assess I&O (note appearance as well as amount of urine).
D. Assess level of consciousness or return of sensation with regional anesthesia.
E. Check fundus for tone and location.
F. Evaluate lochia for amount and color every 15 minutes for 2–3 hours.

Implementation

PREOPERATIVE CARE

A. Discuss and reassure to decrease anxiety.
B. Preop teaching if possible.
C. Preop preparation: IV, insert Foley, abdominal prep, operative permit signed, administer antacid (Bicitra).
D. Inform and involve significant other and family as much as possible.

POSTOPERATIVE CARE

A. Institute same care as for the postsurgical client.
B. Institute same care as for the postpartum client.
C. Reinforce abdominal dressing as necessary.
D. Assist client to deep-breathe, cough, and turn.
E. Change perineal pads as needed.
F. Reassure client that the delivery is over and give information regarding the baby. (If something is wrong with the baby, the physician usually discusses this first with the parents.)
G. If mother is able and desires, show her and let her hold the baby. (Client may be too tired or uncomfortable at this time to do so. Be sensitive to her needs.)

LATER CARE

A. Help ambulate client (usually the first postpartum day).
B. Give stool softener as ordered and needed.
C. Encourage client to talk about delivery and baby; incorporate and accept experience.
D. Reinforce physician's teaching about care at home.
   1. Planned rest periods.
   2. No heavy lifting for 4 to 6 weeks.
   3. Signs of infection.
   4. Care of the breast.
   5. Avoidance of constipation.
   6. Nutritious diet.
E. Provide regular postpartum care.

POSTPARTUM PERIOD

PHYSIOLOGY OF THE PUERPERIUM

Definition: The puerperium is the period of 4 to 6 weeks following delivery in which the reproductive organs revert from a pregnant to a nonpregnant state.

UTERUS

A. *Involution:* rapid diminution in the size of the uterus as it returns to a nonpregnant state due primarily to a decrease in size of myometrial cells.
B. *Lochia:* discharge from the uterus that consists of blood from vessels of the placental site and debris from the decidua.
C. *Placental site:* blood vessels of the placenta become thrombosed or compressed.

CERVIX AND VAGINA

A. *Cervix:* remains soft and flabby the first few days, and the internal os closes.
B. *Vagina:* usually smooth walled after delivery. Rugae begin to appear when ovarian function returns and estrogen is produced.

OVARIAN FUNCTION AND MENSTRUATION

A. Ovarian function depends on the rapidity in which the pituitary function is restored.
B. Menstruation usually returns in 4 to 6 weeks in a nonlactating mother.

URINARY TRACT

A. May be edematous and contain areas of submucosal hemorrhage due to trauma.
B. May have urine retention due to loss of elasticity and tone and loss of sensation from trauma, drugs, anesthesia, loss of privacy.
C. Diuresis: mechanism by which excess body fluid is excreted after delivery. Usually begins within the first 12 hours after delivery.
D. Kidney function returns to normal.

BREASTS

A. Proliferation of glandular tissue during pregnancy caused by hormonal stimulation.
✦ B. Usually continue to secrete colostrum the first 2 to 3 days postpartum; enhances immunity and nutrition of infant. Breastmilk (bluish-white, thin) usually produced by 3rd day.

C. Anterior pituitary: stimulates secretion of prolactin after the placental hormones that inhibited the pituitary are no longer present → stimulate alveolar (acini) cells → milk.
D. In 3 to 4 days, breasts become firm, distended, tender, and warm (engorged), indicating production of milk.
E. Breastfeeding woman: apply warm compress, suckle. Nonbreastfeeding woman: apply cold compress, don't express milk.
F. Milk usually produced with stimulus of sucking infant.
G. Posterior pituitary: discharges oxytocin, alveoli contract and milk flows in response to sucking—"let down reflex."

BLOOD

A. White blood cells increase (25,000–30,000/mm^3) during labor and early postpartum period and then return to normal in a few days.
B. Decrease in hemoglobin and red blood cells, and hematocrit usually returns to normal in 1 week.
C. Elevated fibrinogen levels usually return to normal within 1 week.

GASTROINTESTINAL TRACT

A. Constipation due to stretching, soreness, lack of food, and loss of privacy.
B. Postpartum clients are usually ravenously hungry.

Assessment

✦ A. Check vital signs every 8 hours and PRN: decreased blood pressure, increased pulse, or temperature over 100.4°F indicates abnormality; use pain scale to evaluate comfort.
✦ B. Observe fundus for consistency and level: massage fundus lightly with fingers if it is relaxed. Immediately after delivery, fundus is 2 cm below umbilicus, 12 hours later it is 1 cm above umbilicus. Fundus gradually descends into pelvic cavity, and by ninth postpartum day should no longer be palpable (1 cm or 1 finger-breadth QD).
C. Evaluate lochia for amount, color, consistency, and odor. Watch for hemorrhage. Assess color rubra (red, 1–3 days PP), serosa (pink to brownish; 3–7 days PP), alba (creamy white, 10 days).
D. Check perineum for redness, discoloration, or swelling.
E. Check episiotomy for healing and drainage.
F. Check breasts for engorgement or redness; cracking or inverted nipples.
G. Assess emotional status of new mother for depression or withdrawal.
H. Assess for problems with flatus, elimination, hemorrhoids, and bladder or bowel retention.

I. Observe status of mother–infant relationship.

J. Assess mother–infant feeding quality (*see* Breastfeeding).

K. Assess for thrombophlebitis.

L. Assess blood values (i.e., Rh, hemoglobin, hematocrit, WBCs).

Implementation

A. Nursing interventions for first critical hour after birth.

B. Routine postpartum continues after first hour.

C. May administer drug to inhibit lactation if it has not been given immediately postpartum (rarely, if ever, used today).

D. Administer RhoGAM as ordered within 72 hours postpartum to Rh-negative client who has delivered an Rh-positive fetus (direct Coombs' negative) and who is not sensitized.

E. Maintain I&O until client is voiding a sufficient quantity without difficulty.
1. Usually the first three voids are measured.
2. If client fails to void sufficient quantity within 12–24 hours, she is usually catheterized.

F. Teach client perineal care and give perineal care until client is able to do so.

G. Encourage ambulation as soon as ordered and as client is able to tolerate it; give assistance the first time.

H. Encourage verbalization of client's feelings about labor, delivery, and baby.

I. Give warm sitz baths as ordered.

J. Remind client to return for postpartum checkup.

K. Instruct that sexual relations may be resumed as soon as healing takes place and bleeding stops and client feels comfortable with it.

L. Discuss contraception if client so desires.

M. Provide opportunities to enhance mother–infant relationship, rooming-in, early contact, successful feedings, etc.

EMOTIONAL ASPECTS OF POSTPARTUM CARE

Parenting

Postpartum Phases as Outlined by Rubin

A. Taking-in phase: first 2–3 days.
1. Mother's primary needs are her own: sleep, food.
2. Mother is usually quite talkative: focus on labor and delivery experience.
3. Important for nurse to listen and help mother interpret events to make them more meaningful.

B. Taking-hold phase: third postpartum day to 2 weeks—varies with each individual.
1. Emphasis on present—mother is impatient and wants to reorganize self.
2. More in control. Begins to take hold of task of "mothering."
3. Important time for teaching without making mother feel inadequate—success at this time is important in future mother–child relationship.

C. Letting-go phase.
1. Mother may feel a deep loss over the separation of the baby from part of her body and may grieve over this loss.
2. Mother may be caught in a dependent–independent role—wanting to feel safe and secure yet wanting to make decisions. Teenage mother needs special consideration because of the conflicts taking place within her as part of adolescence.
3. Mother may in turn feel resentful and guilty about the baby causing so much work.
4. May have difficulty adjusting to mothering role.
5. May feel conflict between the roles of mother and wife.
6. May feel upset and depressed at times—postpartum blues. If depression continues, client requires referral for therapy—depression may lead to suicide. (*See* Postpartum Depression, page 580.)
7. May be concerned about other children.
8. Important for nurse to encourage vocalization of these feelings and give positive reassurance for task well done.

Assessment

A. Assess maternal and paternal physical and emotional status.

B. Determine what parents know about infant care.

C. Assess parents' own birth—parenting and nurturing.

D. Evaluate impact of parents' cultural back-ground.

E. Assess readiness for parenthood: emotional maturity, pregnancy planned or unplanned, financial status, job status.

F. Assess physical conditions of mother prior to pregnancy, during labor and delivery, and during puerperium.

G. Assess physical conditions of infant at birth, prematurity, congenital defects, etc. (parents may feel guilty, angry, cheated, and so forth).

H. Check for parental career plans.

I. Assess opportunities for early parental–infant interaction.

J. Evaluate parental knowledge of normal growth and development.

Implementation

✦ A. Promote optimum parent–infant interactions during the early postpartum period (crucial time in parent–infant bonding).
  1. Allow periods of time for both mother and father to be alone with infant.
  2. Allow parents to hold infant in delivery and recovery rooms, and provide rooming-in and privacy.
B. Based upon assessment of parents, plan nursing care. Be sure to begin at same level as parents.
C. Be alert to parental cues but be careful not to label.
D. Support mother in infant care activities and use these opportunities to promote her self-esteem.
E. Provide a role model for parents.
F. Plan nursing care to reduce maternal fatigue and anxiety so that time with her infant is pleasurable.
G. Explain to parents that it is normal at this time to feel fatigued, tense, insecure, and sometimes depressed.
H. Anticipatory guidance regarding "Baby Blues," maternal depression, and maternal psychosis.
I. Counsel mother on home care plan.
  1. Rest periods to avoid overfatigue.
  2. Time spent away from baby: to be alone, to be with significant other or husband, to be with other children, and to resume contact with people.
  3. Time for father and baby together.
  4. Enlist support from husband or significant other to listen and validate emotional distress new mothers may experience.
  5. Encourage to seek professional help if symptoms of depression are prolonged or severe.

Breastfeeding

Assessment

✦ A. Review intrapartum medications and possible effects on initial breastfeeding.
B. Assess degree of physical comfort prior to nursing.
C. Assess breasts and nipples for factors that may decrease successful breastfeeding experience (flat or inverted nipples, scarring from breast surgery, significantly asymmetrical breasts, lack of normal pregnancy breast changes, discomfort, engorgement).
D. Observe entire infant feeding and assess infant's position at breast, latch, suck and transfer of milk; confirm correct infant position (nose, cheeks and chin are touching mother's breast).
E. Assess parent's knowledge base: infant feeding cues, maternal response to cues, infant cues of satiety, importance of feeding, proper techniques, breast care, infant weight gain, maternal nutrition, personal

plans, resources for support, coping with return to work while breastfeeding.
F. Assess nutritional and hydration status: increased maternal needs for protein, vitamins, iron and fluids during lactation.
G. Evaluate emotional responses toward nursing: satisfaction, relaxation, mastery.
H. Evaluate LATCH (Latch on, Audible swallow, Type of nipple, Comfort, Help).

✦ Implementation

A. Complete hand hygiene.
B. Provide skin-to-skin contact between mother and child immediately after birth, unless contraindicated.
C. Assist mother with breastfeeding as soon as possible after birth, once mother is comfortable and infant demonstrates feeding cues, usually within the first hour.
D. Assist mother to a comfortable position (sitting or side-lying), using pillows for support to enhance relaxation and proper positioning.
E. Guide baby to breast; stimulate rooting reflex, if necessary; place as much of areola in baby's mouth as possible.
F. Release suction by inserting a finger into side of baby's mouth. The breast will become sore if baby is pulled from it.
G. Burp baby after each breast.
H. Encourage mothers to feed infants at least q 3 hrs or at least 8 times in 24 hrs.
I. When possible, avoid use of pacifier and supplemental water or formula until infant is able to latch on and is successfully breastfed.
J. Teach mother and significant other importance of obtaining adequate rest, breast massage, correct latching, engorgement/nipple soreness, breastfeeding patterns, breastfeeding positions, determining adequate intake.
K. Promote comfort by carefully managing/preventing sore nipples (proper positioning; express colostrum or breastmilk on nipple and areola at end of q feeding—hind milk; moist compresses) and breast engorgement (feed on demand, use warm compresses; breast massage and manual expression prior to nursing; warm shower between feedings; observe for signs of mastitis; wear well-fitting, supportive bra).
L. Nutrition counseling: additional 500 calories in well-balanced diet. Drink 3000 mL fluid qd.
M. Uterine cramping may occur the first few days after delivery while nursing, due to oxytocin stimulation which also causes uterus to contract.
N. Counsel mothers to avoid:

1. Medications or drugs contraindicated unless necessary to client's life—drugs pass to infant through breastmilk.
2. Some foods, such as cabbage or onions, may alter the taste of the milk or cause gas in infant.
3. Birth control pills are often avoided as milk production may be decreased and the medication is passed to infant in the milk.

O. Explain contraindications to breastfeeding:
   1. Active tuberculosis.
   2. Severe chronic maternal disease.
   3. Narcotic addiction—drug abusers must be drug-free for 3 months.
   4. Severe cleft lip or palate in newborn.
   5. HIV-positive status; AIDS.

COMPLICATIONS OF THE PUERPERIUM

Assessment

✦ A. Observe for postdelivery hemorrhage (leading cause of maternal death in the world).
✦ B. Check for uterine atony.
C. Assess for lacerations of birth canal.
D. Assess for postdelivery infection (puerperal sepsis).
E. Evaluate for postpartum alterations in mental state (i.e., depression, psychosis).
F. Assess for mastitis.
G. Check for presence of embolism.

Implementation

✦ A. *Postpartum hemorrhage:* Identify degree of hemorrhage and implement measures to contain it.
B. *Endometritis:* Treat inflammation and prevent further complications.
C. *Urinary tract infection:* Identify presence of infection and initiate treatment.
D. *Mastitis:* Administer antibiotics, support mother during exacerbation, and perform palliative measures.
E. *Subinvolution:* Identify condition and initiate treatment.

Postpartum Hemorrhage

Definition: A condition that occurs when 500 mL or more of blood is lost during or 24 hours after vaginal birth; 1000 mL in cesarean birth.

Characteristics

✦ A. Uterine atony (lack of muscle tone in uterus) is the *primary cause* of early postpartum hemorrhage. Causes for uterine atony include:
   1. Prolonged or precipitous labor.

2. Overdistention: multiple pregnancies, polyhydramnios.
3. Sluggish muscle.
4. PIH.
5. Presence of fibroid tumors.
6. Deep inhalation anesthesia—may inhibit uterine activity.
7. Oxytocin induction of labor.
8. Distended bladder.

✦ B. Lacerations of the reproductive tract is a *second cause* of early postpartum hemorrhage.
   1. Lacerations of the cervix or of the high vaginal walls.
   2. Oozing from blood vessels.

✦ C. Retained placental tissue or incomplete separation of the placenta is a *third cause*. (This is the most frequent cause of late postpartum hemorrhage.)
D. Hematomas.
✦ E. Early postpartum hemorrhage occurs in the first 24 hours after birth. Late postpartum hemorrhage occurs 24 hours to 6 weeks after delivery.
F. Placenta accreta is the abnormal adherence of placenta due to penetration of placental trophoblast into myometrium.
   1. May be partial or complete.
   2. Removal of placenta by hand or hysterectomy if bleeding persists.

Assessment

✦ A. Observe for uterine atony.
   1. Boggy, relaxed uterus.
   2. Dark bleeding.
   3. Passage of clots.
B. Check any lacerations.
   1. Firm fundus.
   2. Oozing of bright red blood.
C. Check for retained placental tissue.
   1. Boggy, relaxed uterus.
   2. Dark bleeding.
✦ D. Evaluate for signs and symptoms of shock.
   1. Air hunger: difficulty in breathing.
   2. Restlessness.
   3. Weak, rapid pulse.
   4. Rapid respirations.
   5. Decrease in blood pressure.
E. Evaluate lab values (compare admission and postpartal)—hemoglobin, hematocrit, clotting time, platelets.

Implementation

A. Remain with client.
✦ B. Monitor vital signs every 15 minutes or PRN until stable.
C. Administer intravenous fluids, blood, volume expanders, or oxytocin as ordered.

LOCHIA ASSESSMENT		
	Normal	**Abnormal**
Color	Lochia rubra—dark red	Lasts longer than 3–4 days
	Lochia serosa—Pinkish-brownish	Lasts longer than 4–10 days
	Lochia alla—yellowish-cream color	Lasts longer than 24 days
Blood composition	Small clots, few in number	Large clots—*requires intervention*
Odor	Musty, stale	Foul smell—*requires intervention*
Volume	240–270 mL/day—decreases gradually	Larger amount—saturated peripad within 1 hour (30–80 mL/hr) *requires intervention*

✦ D. Palpate fundus every 15 minutes or PRN while bleeding continues; then every 2 to 4 hours.

✦ E. Gently massage fundus until firm. Be careful not to overmassage.

✦ F. Administer oxytocin or other uterine stimulants (Methergine, Ergotrate, Hemabate, or Prostin) as ordered for boggy uterus.

G. Have physician notified.

H. Weigh pads and linen.

I. Provide warmth for client.

J. Measure I&O.

K. Explain carefully to client and family to help allay anxiety.

L. Observe for blood reactions and check for clotting defect, monitor lab values (clotting time, platelets, fibrinogen, Hbg, Hct, CBC), and observe for signs of clotting defect.

M. Return client to delivery room or to surgery for removal of placental tissue or repair of laceration.

Postdelivery Infection

Definition: An infection in the uterus within 28 days as a consequence of abortion or labor and delivery.

Characteristics

A. Cause.
   1. Organisms that were introduced during labor and delivery.
   2. Bacteria normally present in vaginal tract.
B. Predisposing factors.
   1. Cesarean birth is major risk.
   2. Weakened resistance due to prolonged labor and dehydration.
   3. Traumatic delivery.
   4. Excessive vaginal examinations during labor.
   5. Premature rupture of membranes.
   6. Excessive blood loss.
   7. Poor health status; anemia.
   8. Intrauterine manipulation.
   9. Retained placental fragments.

Assessment

✦ A. Assess for elevated temperature of 100.4°F or 38.0°C for two or more consecutive days, not counting first 24 hours.

B. Assess any discomfort in the abdomen and perineum.

C. Evaluate burning on urination and character of urine.

✦ D. Check for foul-smelling lochia or discharge.

E. Assess for pelvic pain.

F. Assess for chills.

G. Check for rapid pulse and assess other vital signs.

H. Evaluate malaise, anorexia.

I. Assess boggy, relaxed, and/or tender uterus.

✦ Implementation

A. Administer IV fluids or blood as ordered.

B. Encourage fluid intake: 3000 to 4000 mL if not contraindicated.

C. Administer medications: broad-spectrum IV antibiotics and analgesics as ordered.

D. Offer warm sitz bath for relief of symptoms.

E. Monitor laboratory studies: blood and urine.

F. Provide high-calorie nutritious diet.

G. Place client in Fowler's or semi-Fowler's position as ordered. Position of client promotes drainage.

H. Provide emotional support to mother, who is usually in isolation and unable to see baby.

Deep Vein Thrombosis (Thrombophlebitis)

Definition: A vascular occlusion of vessels of the pelvis or lower extremities. Results from infection, circulatory stasis, and increased postdelivery coagulability of blood.

Assessment

✦ A. Assess for discomfort in abdomen and pelvis.

B. Assess for femoral symptoms—usually do not appear until the second week or later.
   1. Edema and pain in affected leg.
   2. Chills and low-grade fever.
   3. Changes in color and temperature.
   4. Area may feel firm and hard.

C. Assess Homan's sign (now not considered reliable).
D. Use Doppler flow studies.

Implementation

✦ A. Provide specific care for extremity.
1. Maintain bedrest; keep bed clothes off leg.
2. Apply warm compresses, as ordered, for 15 to 20 minutes.
3. Elevate affected leg.
4. Apply bed cradle.
✦ 5. Never massage leg and teach client not to do so.
✦ 6. Apply antiembolic stocking, and teach client its proper use.
B. Encourage fluids.
C. Provide diversion.
D. Administer medications as ordered.
E. Teach client to administer heparin.
F. Teach client to watch for signs of excessive bleeding.
G. Allow client to express fears and concerns.
H. Watch for signs of pulmonary embolism.

Urinary Tract Infection

Definition: Postdelivery urinary tract infections are usually caused by the coliform bacteria and generally occur soon after vaginal delivery.

Characteristics

A. Edema and hyperemia of bladder due to stretching and trauma in labor and delivery.
B. Temporary loss of bladder tone; pressure and injury may result in bladder being less sensitive to fullness.
C. Overdistention and residual urine or inability to void may occur.
D. Trauma to urethra may cause difficulty in voiding.

Assessment

✦ A. Monitor bladder frequently during recovery period to institute preventive measures.
1. Assess for suprapubic or perineal discomfort.
2. Check for frequent urination, burning, dysuria.
B. Check for hematuria.
✦ C. Assess for elevated temperature.
D. Assess for pyelitis—pain in flank.
E. Perform urine cultures and chemical tests to determine presence and number of bacteria.
1. Evaluate microscopic examination for detailed identification of the organism (especially important in chronic infections).
2. Note that a colony count of over 100,000/mL is the most important lab finding and designates infection.

Implementation

✦ A. Observe postpartum client closely for full bladder or residual urine.

1. Palpate bladder for distention.
2. Palpate fundus: full bladder displaces fundus upward and to the sides.
B. Institute measures to help client void.
C. Insert catheter, as ordered, using sterile technique.
✦ D. Encourage fluids to 3000 mL per day.
E. Administer drugs as ordered. (Most common are NegGram, Mandelamine and Furadantin.) May give systemic antibiotics.
F. Obtain urine specimens for microscopic examination.
G. Provide emotional support to client: allow her to express feelings about her illness and the baby.

Mastitis

✦ *Definition:* An infection in breast tissue usually caused by the *Staphylococcus* organism. It occurs in about 1 percent of women who have recently delivered.

Characteristics

A. Infected hands of client or attendants.
B. Bacteria normally present in lactiferous glands.
C. Fissure in nipples.
D. Bruising of breast tissue.
E. Stasis of milk or overdistention may injure tissue, but does not cause infection in itself.
F. Infected baby.

Assessment

A. Assess for chills.
✦ B. Assess for elevated temperature: 103°F or 39.5°C or above.
C. Check for elevated pulse rate.
D. Evaluate breast lobe which may appear hard, red, painful, and evidence localized tenderness.

✦ Implementation

A. Provide support for breast. Make sure client wears snug-fitting, supportive brassiere.
B. Administer antibiotics as ordered (may be based on culture of breastmilk).
C. Bedrest for first few days.
D. Increased fluid intake (2000 to 3000 mL).
E. Apply ice or heat to breast.
F. Teach client to empty breast every 4 hours if nursing is to be discontinued.
G. Wash hands before touching client's breast.
H. Teach client careful handwashing and care of the breast.

✦ Subinvolution

Definition: Failure of the uterus to revert to normal postpartum state, caused by retained placental tissue or fetal membranes, endometritis, or uterine tumors.

✦ Assessment

A. Assess for enlarged, boggy, and tender uterus.
B. Assess for profuse red lochia or hemorrhage.
C. Check for pelvic discomfort and backache.

Implementation

✦ A. Monitor ergonovine (0.2 mg every 4 hours for 3 days) to cause contractions.
B. Administer antibiotics to prevent infection as ordered.
C. Assist physician in manual replacement of mal-position.
D. Explain condition and treatment to client.

Postpartum Depression (PPD)

Definition: Intense and prolonged feelings of sadness, crying, fear, irritability, severe anxiety, panic attacks or spontaneous crying.

Characteristics

A. Lasts longer than postpartum blues, which usually lasts several weeks.
B. Occurs in about 8–26 percent; greatest risk around 4th week postpartum or just prior to initiation of menses, and upon weaning.
C. Not associated with depression during pregnancy.
D. Woman often cannot continue normal parenting tasks, which can increase guilt feelings.
E. Usually requires medical intervention and medication.
F. Symptoms of psychosis (paranoia, hallucinations) require psychiatric interventions.

Assessment

A. Assess for risk factors: primiparity, ambivalence toward pregnancy, history of PPD or psychiatric ill-ness, stressful life events, lack of supportive relation-ships, personal expectations and perceptions of self.
B. Observe for signs of depression.
  1. Note severity and duration.
  2. Ask appropriate questions, which show sensitiv-ity to the negative feelings and thoughts that may occur.
C. May utilize PPD checklists or screening scales.

Implementation

A. Anticipatory guidance: realistic information regard-ing possible negative feelings and reactions that often occur, detrimental effect of the perfect mother or perfect newborn expectations.
B. Encourage family to seek early and/or continue interventions.
  1. Call if notice symptoms.
  2. Take medication (depending on symptoms—tranquilizers, mood elevators, phenothiazines).
  3. Obtain emotional support (encourage verbaliza-tion, support positive self-image, participate in support groups).
C. Implement follow-up interventions to ensure safety (self or newborn).
D. Discuss possible strategies for mother and family to prevent PPD.
  1. Don't be ashamed of having emotional prob-lems after the baby is born—about 15 percent have this problem. Be open and share knowl-edge about PPD with close friends and family.
  2. Adhere to good health habits: well-balanced diet/hydration, exercise regularly, 7–8 hours of sleep.
  3. Have realistic expectations—don't try to be a "supermom."

NEWBORN

NORMAL NEWBORN

✦ Standard Precautions: All newborns must be handled with gloves until after first bath.

Initial Care: Admission/Assessment (0–4 hours after birth)

A. Assess if resuscitation is needed: clear of meconium; breathing or crying; good muscle tone; color pink; term gestation.

✦ B. Assess respirations, heart rate, and color.
   1. Heart < 100 requires positive-pressure ventilation.
   2. Heart < 60 requires additional resuscitation efforts (endotracheal intubation, chest compression, medications).

✦ C. Assign Apgar score at 1 minute and 5 minutes.
   1. If 5-minute score < 7, additional scores should be assigned q 5 minutes up to 10 minutes.
   2. Apgar scoring based on scoring method developed by Virginia Apgar (*see* Table 12-7).

D. Assess height and weight.

E. Assess temperature (axillary or rectal), heart rate (murmurs), respirations and breath sounds, bowel sounds, and capillary refill.

F. Assess for obvious congenital malformations.

G. Check umbilical cord: two arteries and one vein.

H. Obtain head, chest, and abdominal circumference.

I. Observe skin: color, meconium staining, capillary refill; acrocyanosis common for 1–2 hours after birth and when cold.

J. Assess cry: lusty, high pitch, weak.

K. Assess for signs of respiratory distress: tachypnea, nasal flaring, retractions, expiratory grunt, breath sounds decreased.

L. Assess neurological status: reflexes, tremors, twitching.

M. Assess for injuries caused by birth trauma; fractured clavicle, edema of scalp, lacerations, scalp electrode site, dislocated shoulders.

N. Assess for nasal and anal patency.

O. Assess blood glucose when indicated.

P. Complete initial newborn assessment (*see* Table 12-8).

Q. Assess gestational age (*see* Table 12-9).

✦ R. Take vital signs q 30 min, or 1 hr as needed.
   1. Assess temperature: > 100 may indicate infection or dehydration; < 97.6 possibly cold stress, hypoglycemia, temperature instability.
   2. Assess pulse, if > 180 or < 100.
   3. Assess respirations for indications of respiratory distress.

Initial Care: Interventions (0–4 hours after birth)

A. Every delivery should have at least one person present who is primarily responsible for the baby and who has the skills to initiate resuscitation.

B. There should also be one person immediately available who has the skills to perform complete resuscitation (i.e., endotracheal intubation).

C. If resuscitation is not needed: provide warmth; clear airway with bulb syringe; dry infant; and give baby to mother and/or father to hold.
   1. Use warm blankets, hat, or have skin-to-skin contact as infant's body heat is easily lost.
   2. Important to have parents hold infant as soon as possible to promote early bonding.

D. If resuscitation is needed, following steps should be done within 1–2 minutes:
   1. Provide warmth, usually under radiant warmer in open crib/surface.

Table 12-7. **APGAR SCORING**			
Sign	**0**	**1**	**2**
Heart tone	Absent	Slow (less than 100)	Over 100
Respiratory effort	Absent	Slow, irregular	Good crying
Muscle tone	Flaccid	Some flexion of extremities	Active motion
Reflex irritability	No response	Cry, grimace	Vigorous cry
Skin color	Blue, pale	Body pink, extremities blue	Completely pink

Apgar scoring system is a method of evaluating a newborn's condition at 1 and 5 minutes after birth.
- Newborns who score 7–10 are considered free of immediate danger; 8–10 indicates good condition.
- Newborns who score 4–6 are moderately depressed; may require O_2, suctioning, and resuscitation.
- Newborns who score 0–3 are severely depressed; require immediate intervention.

Scores less than 7 at 5 minutes, repeat every 5 minutes for 20 minutes. Infant may be intubated unless 2 successive scores of 7 or more occur.

2. Position—clear airway as necessary.
3. Dry, stimulate, reposition.
4. Give oxygen as necessary.
5. If heart rate < 100, provide positive-pressure ventilation (PPV).

E. If baby does not begin breathing after being stimulated, he or she is probably in secondary apnea and will require PPV.

1. If heart rate < 60 after initial PPV, consider endotracheal intubation and administer chest compressions.
2. If still < 60, administer epinephrine.
3. Overall goal of initial resuscitation is to ensure the baby's lungs are ventilated with oxygen.

F. Administer medications within first 4 hours after birth.

1. Apply broad-spectrum antibiotic erythromycin, or 1% silver nitrate (which is rarely used), within 1 hour after birth to prevent opthalmia neonatorum (blindness from STD).
2. Give Vitamin K IM (usually 1 mg), anterior or lateral thigh, for production of blood clotting factors.
3. Hepatitis B injection if ordered and consent signed by parents (controversial).

G. Check cord clamp is secure and apply if has not been done.

H. Identify baby, mother, and significant other with bands that have the same number.

I. Give initial bath and dress infant when condition and temperature are stable.

J. Care for cord—may use betadine, antibiotic ointment, or alcohol initially.

K. Keep bulb syringe readily available as may accumulate mucus and need suctioning during period of reactivity after deep sleep.

L. Administer feeding as ordered: in some hospitals first feeding is given with supervision (i.e., sterile water) assess for effective swallow, esophageal atresia, etc.

✦ Implementation: Normal Newborn

A. Monitor vital signs, skin color, newborn assessments, stools, and voids during every shift or per hospital policy.

B. Provide circumcision care following procedure as ordered.

1. Observe for bleeding.
2. Change petroleum gauze as necessary.
3. Keep area clean to prevent infection.
4. Teach parents proper care and signs of infection.

C. Teach parents infant care as needed.

1. Feeding.
2. Holding and burping baby.
3. Cord care.
4. Bath.
5. Diapering.
6. Normal vs. abnormal characteristics, when to call doctor, sleeping, weight loss, stools, interactive behaviors, safety, immunizations, car seats.

D. Teach to prevent infections: proper handwashing, avoiding crowded areas or people with colds.

E. Ensure mother plans follow-up visits to the physician: well baby check, immunizations, PKU testing.

✦ F. If infant has feeding (protein source) in hospital, PKU test can be done while in hospital. If not, arrange appointment for phenylketonuria (PKU) test to be done within 2 weeks of birth.

1. Timing is important to prevent buildup of the amino acid phenylalanine.
2. PKU can result in mental retardation.

Schedules of Newborn Feeding

A. First feeding.

1. May be breast-fed immediately following delivery (colostrum is not irritating if aspirated and is absorbed by the respiratory system).
2. Feed in first hour of life.
3. Latest to start feeding is 2–3 hours (when normal low blood sugar occurs).
✦ 4. First feeding—many facilities give sterile water, a few swallows to half ounce to evaluate feeding capability. (Glucose water no longer recommended for first feeding due to danger of aspiration pneumonia.)
5. Give full strength formula or breastmilk as soon as newborn shows an interest.

B. Subsequent feeding.

1. Routine schedule: 2- to 4-hour feedings.
2. Self-demand: baby is fed according to needs, when hungry, usually every 3–4 hours. (Breast-feeding may be 1½–3 hours.)

✦ Calories and Fluid Needs

✦ A. Fluid: 140–160 mL/kg of body weight in 24 hours.

1. Fluid needs are high because the newborn is unable to concentrate urine.
2. More fluids should be given in hot weather or when the baby has an elevated temperature.

✦ B. Caloric needs: approximately 20 kcal/oz formula for term infant or 105–108 kcal/kg/day for newborn.

C. Calorie requirements from the sum of needs for basal metabolic rate (BMR) plus activity, cold stress, loss from feces, digestive and metabolic processes, and growth.

General Infant Assessment

(See Table 12-8)

A. Assess vital signs, including pain.

Table 12-8. SUMMARY CHART OF NEWBORN ASSESSMENT

Assessment	Normal	Abnormal
SKIN ASSESSMENT		
Note skin **color, pigmentation,** and **lesions**	Pink	Cyanosis, pallor, beefy red
	Mongolian spots	Petechiae, ecchymoses, or purpuric spots: signs of possible hematologic disorder
	Capillary hemangiomas on face or neck	Café au lait spots (patches of brown discoloration): possible sign of congenital neurological disorder
		Raised capillary hemangiomas on areas other than face or neck
	Localized edema in presenting part	Edema of peritoneal wall
	Cheesy white vernix	Poor skin turgor: indicates dehydration
	Desquamation (peeling off)	Yellow discolored vernix (meconium stained)
	Milia (small white pustules over nose and chin)	Impetigo neonatorum (small pustules with surrounding red areas)
	Jaundice after 24 hours; gone by second week	Jaundice at birth or within 12 hours
	Skin intact along spine	Dermal sinuses (opening to brain)
		Holes along spinal column
		Low hairline posteriorly: possible chromosomal abnormality
		Sparse or spotty hair: congenital goiter or chromosomal abnormality
Note color of **nails**	Pink	Yellowing of nail beds (meconium stained)
Note **muscle strength** and **tone**	Strong, tremulous	Flaccid, convulsions
		Muscular twitching, hypertonicity
Note **capillary refill**	Brisk 2–3 seconds	> 3 seconds: decreased perfusion; often related to hypovolemia
HEAD AND NECK ASSESSMENT		
Note **shape of head**	Fontanels: anterior open until 18 months; posterior closed shortly after birth	Depressed fontanels indicate dehydration; closed or bulging indicate congenital anomalies; full or bulging indicate edema or increased ICP
	Circumference (32–36.8 cm)	
	Molding—sagittal suture may overlap	Cephalohematoma that crosses the midline
		Microcephaly and macrocephaly
Assess **eyes**	Slight edema of lids	Purulent discharge
		Lateral upward slope of eye with an inner epicanthal fold in infants not of Asian descent
		Exophthalmos (bulging of eyeball): may be congenital anomaly, sign of congenital glaucoma or thyroid abnormality
		Enophthalmos (recession of eyeball): may indicate damage to brain or cervical spine
	Pupils equal and reactive to light by 3 weeks of age	Constricted pupil, unilateral dilated fixed pupil, nystagmus (rhythmic nonpurposeful movement of eyeball): continuous strabismus
	Intermittent strabismus (occasional crossing of eyes)	
	Conjunctival or scleral hemorrhages	Haziness of cornea
	Symmetrical light reflex (light reflects off each eye in the same quadrant): sign of conjugate gaze	Absence of red reflex; asymmetrical light reflex
	Sclera white	

Continues

Table 12-8. SUMMARY CHART OF NEWBORN ASSESSMENT (Continued)

Assessment	Normal	Abnormal
Note **placement of ears,** shape and position	Eyes in line with top of ear Pinna recoils	Low-set ears: may indicate chromosomal or renal system abnormality
Assess **nose**	Discharge, sneezing	Thick, bloody nasal discharge
Assess **mouth**	Sucking, rooting reflexes Retention cysts (pears) Occasional vomiting Intact palate	Cleft lip, palate Flat, white nonremovable spots (thrush) Frequent vomiting: may indicate pyloric stenosis Vomitus with bile: fecal vomiting Profuse salivation: may indicate tracheoesophageal fistula Cleft palate—may be visible or only palpable on hard or soft palate
Assess **neck**	Tonic neck reflex (Fencer's position)	Distended neck veins Fractured clavicle Unusually short neck Excess posterior cervical skin Resistance to neck flexion
Assess **cry**	Lusty cry	Weak, groaning cry: possible neurological abnormality High-pitched cry: newborn drug withdrawal (may occur even 6–12 months after birth); hoarse or crowing inspirations; catlike cry: possible neurological or chromosomal abnormality

CHEST AND LUNG ASSESSMENT

Assess the **clavicles**	Clavicles intact	Fractured clavicle: raised or crepitus
Assess the **chest**	Circular Enlargement of breasts Milky discharge from breasts	1–2 cm less than head circumference Depressed sternum Retractions, asymmetry of chest movements: indicates respiratory distress and possible pneumothorax
Assess the **lungs**	Breath sounds clear bilaterally; fluid clears with crying Abdominal respirations Respiration rate: 30 to 50 Respiration movement irregular in rate and depth Resonant chest (hollow sound on percussion)	Thoracic breathing, unequal motion of chest, rapid grasping or grunting respirations, flaring nares Deep sighing respirations Grunt on expiration: possible respiratory distress Hyperresonance of chest or decreased resonance

HEART ASSESSMENT

Assess the **rate, rhythm,** and **murmurs** of the heart	Rate: 100–160 at birth; stabilizes at 120–140 Regular rhythm Murmurs: significance cannot usually be determined in newborn	Heart rate > 200 or < 100 Irregular rhythm Dextrocardia, enlarged heart

ABDOMEN AND GASTROINTESTINAL TRACT ASSESSMENT

Assess the **abdomen**	Protrudes, soft, no distention	Distention of abdominal veins: possible portal vein obstruction

Table 12-8. SUMMARY CHART OF NEWBORN ASSESSMENT (*Continued*)

Assessment	Normal	Abnormal
Assess the **gastrointestinal tract**	Bowel sounds present	Visible peristaltic waves Increased pitch or frequency: intestinal obstruction Decreased sounds: paralytic ileus Distention of abdomen
	Liver 2 to 3 cm below right costal margin Spleen tip palpable Umbilical cord with one vein and two arteries Soft granulation tissue at umbilicus	Enlarged liver or spleen Midline suprapubic mass: may indicate Hirschsprung's disease One artery present in umbilical cord: may indicate other anomalies Wet umbilical stump or fetid odor from stump
GENITOURINARY TRACT ASSESSMENT		
Assess **kidneys and bladder**	May be able to palpate kidneys Bladder percussed 1 to 4 cm above symphysis pubis	Enlarged kidney Distended bladder; presence of any masses
Assess the **genitalia**	Edema and bruising after delivery Unusually large clitoris in females a short time after birth Vaginal mucoid or bloody discharge may be present in the first week	Inguinal hernia
Urethral orifice	Urethra opens on ventral surface of penile shaft	Hypospadias (urethra opens on the inferior surface of the penis) Epispadias (urethra opens on the dorsal surface of the penis) Ulceration of urethral orifice
Testes	Testes in scrotal sac or inguinal canal	Hydroceles in males
SPINE AND EXTREMITIES ASSESSMENT		
Assess the **spine**	Straight spine	Spina bifida, pilonidal sinus; scoliosis
Assess **extremities**	Freely moveable, full ROM Legs equal length and gluteal folds symmetrical	Asymmetry of movement Sharp click with thigh rotation: indicates possible congenital hip Uneven major gluteal folds: indicates possible congenital hip Polydactyly (extra digits on a hand or foot); syndactyly (webbing or fusion of fingers or toes)
Assess **anus and rectum**	Patent anus Passage of meconium; followed by transitional and then soft, yellow stools	Closed anus: no meconium; intestinal atresia

1. Temperature (36.6°–37.2°C/97.8–99°F); pulse: 120–160; respirations (30–60/minute); blood pressure somewhat unreliable (80–60/45/40 mmHg).
2. Pain assessment should include behavioral, physiologic/autonomic, and metabolic responses (crying, increases oxygen requirement, increased vital signs, expression, and sleeplessness).
3. Facial features: eye squeeze; brow contraction; taut, quivering tongue and open mouth.
4. Pain in children can be life threatening—has more intense, yet shorter response.

✦ B. Assess respiratory status.
　1. Infant's respiratory system must function immediately after loss of placental function; adequate maturation at birth is necessary.
　2. From 20–30 mL of fluid are present in the lungs at birth.
　　a. Approximately one-third is removed as a result of compression of the chest during delivery.
　　b. The remainder is carried off through pulmonary circulation and by the lymph system.

3. Surfactant is a phospholipid found in the lungs.
   a. It reduces surface tension in alveoli and keeps them from collapsing.
   b. Surfactant is necessary to maintain lung expansion and to prevent respiratory distress syndrome.
4. Normal respiration is about 30–50.
   a. Over 60 or below 30 indicates a problem.
   b. Tachypnea is earliest symptom of many neonatal problems (respirations above 60).
   c. Respiration may be slightly elevated during crying episodes or shortly afterward. (Always count for one full minute.)

✦ C. Assess circulatory status.
   ✦ 1. Ductus arteriosus, ductus venosus, and foramen ovale should close (may not be complete for 1 or 2 days).
   2. Peripheral circulation may be sluggish; there may be mottling, acrocyanosis.
   ✦ 3. Heart rate may be variable (normal 120–160).
      a. It may be as high as 180 with crying or below 120 when resting.
      b. Always take apical pulse for one full minute.
   4. Skin color/perfusion.
      a. Brisk capillary refill (2–3 seconds).
      b. > 3 seconds indication of hypovolemia.
      c. Color pink (no pallor, dusky, or central cyanosis); note mucus membranes and skin color when blanched; dark-skinned infants may have grayish hue rather than pallor or cyanosis.
   ✦ 5. Anemia is common in early months because of the decrease in erythropoiesis and breakdown of red blood cells.
      a. Baby may need an iron-supplemented formula.
      b. Recommended daily allowance (RDA) for iron is 6 mg/day from birth to 6 months.
      c. Fetal hemoglobin has a shorter life span (80 days).
   6. Plethora (red coloring to skin) especially visible when baby cries; may be present due to increase in red blood cells.
   7. Physiologic jaundice: normal level less than 1 mg/100 mL blood.
      a. Jaundice visible in skin, sclera.
      b. Begins after first 24 hours of life, usually visible the second or third day after birth.
      c. Caused by impairment in the removal of bilirubin—deficiency in the production of glucuronide transferase, which is needed to convert indirect insoluble bilirubin to direct water soluble bilirubin which is excreted;

transition from fetal to neonatal circulation; and the shorter lifespan of the fetal RBCs.
      d. Jaundice begins to decrease by the sixth or seventh day.
      e. Should be watched carefully although usually does not require treatment.
   ✦ 8. Clinical jaundice that persists beyond 7 days (term infants) or 14 days (premature infants).
      a. Usual treatment is phototherapy (13 mg/100 mL blood; 15 mg/100 mL in premature infants). If the indirect bilirubin continues to go up, a cause other than physiologic jaundice is searched for.
      b. Infant may be on force fluids between feeding to aid in excretion of bilirubin as it is broken down.
   9. Transitory deficiency in the ability of the blood to clot.
      ✦ a. Bacteria in the intestines are necessary for the production of vitamin K.
      b. Bacteria are not present in the intestines during the first few days after birth—newborn infant's bowel is sterile at birth.
      c. Adequate food and bacteria are necessary to produce vitamin K in the bowel.
      ✦ d. Vitamin K IM usually given after birth to aid in blood coagulation.

✦ D. Assess ability of newborn to maintain body heat.
   ✦ 1. Baby suffers loss of heat primarily from head because of being wet and coolness of delivery room.
      a. Place knit cap on head, dry off, and place immediately in a warmer.
      b. Wrap in warm blanket and give infant to mother.
   2. Means of heat production in the newborn.
      a. Increasing metabolism.
      b. Shivering is poor in the newborn.
      c. Metabolism of brown fat (less mature infants have less brown fat).
   ✦ 3. Effects of chilling—cold stress.
      a. Increased consumption of oxygen.
      b. Use of glucose stored as glycogen.
      c. May become hypoglycemic.
      d. May develop metabolic acidosis—products of incomplete metabolism, accumulate with fatty acids from breakdown of brown fat.
      e. Excess fatty acid displaces bilirubin from the albumin binding sites, which can impact jaundice and increase risk of kernicterus.
   4. The baby may have a decrease in the production of surfactant.

a. Glucose, pO$_2$, and proper pulmonary circulation are necessary for the production of surfactant.

b. Decrease in surfactant may lead to respiratory distress.

5. Temperature may be taken by rectum or axilla (latter method is usual).

E. Assess newborn's weight.

✦1. Infants usually lose between 5–10 percent of their body weight the first few days, because of low fluid intake and loss of excess fluid from tissue.

2. Usually regain weight lost within 7–14 days.

F. Assess head size and shape.

1. Head or face may be asymmetrical due to birth trauma.

2. Molding of head may be present (elongation of head as it passes through birth canal to accommodate pelvis); usually disappears in about a week.

✦3. *Caput succedaneum:* diffuse swelling of soft tissues of scalp, caused by an arrest in circulation in those tissues present over the cervix as it dilates; may cross suture lines.

4. *Cephalohematoma:* extravasation of blood beneath periosteum of one of the cranial bones because of a ruptured blood vessel during the trauma of labor and delivery; does not cross suture lines.

✦5. Anterior and posterior fontanel.

a. Should be open.

b. Should neither bulge (may indicate intracranial pressure) nor be depressed (may indicate dehydration).

6. Ears well formed and cartilage present.

G. Assess gastrointestinal system.

1. Salivary glands immature.

2. May have Epstein's pearls; white raised areas on palate caused by an accumulation of epithelial cells.

3. May have transient circumoral cyanosis.

4. Sucking pads; fatty tissue deposits in each cheek that aid in sucking. They usually disappear when no longer needed.

5. Infant stools.

a. *Meconium plug:* thick, gray-white mucus passed before meconium.

✦b. *Meconium:* sticky, black, tarry-looking stools, consisting of mucus, digestive secretions, vernix caseosa, and lanugo; usually passed during the first 24 hours after birth.

✦c. *Transitional stool:* second to fifth day; greenish-yellow color and loose (partly meconium and partly milk).

d. *Breast-fed baby's stools:* formed, non–foul-smelling, and more frequent (yellow, golden, pasty).

e. *Bottle-fed baby's stools:* formed, foul-smelling (pale, yellow-light brown).

f. Observe for color, frequency, and consistency.

6. Regurgitation following feeding is common. It may be reduced by frequent burping during feedings.

H. Assess genitourinary system.

✦1. Urinary functions.

a. Observe ability to concentrate urine and check to see if specific gravity elevated.

b. Uric acid crystals (pink or reddish spot or "brick dust") may appear on diaper due to high uric acid secretion.

2. Female genitalia.

a. May have heavy coating of vernix between labia.

b. Usually has mucus discharge. Mucus may be blood-tinged due to elevated hormonal levels in mother.

3. Male genitalia.

a. Size of penis and scrotum vary.

b. Testicles should be descended or in inguinal canal.

c. Circumcision: surgical removal of foreskin of penis by physician.

(1) Usually performed by the second or third day.

(2) Observe for bleeding from postoperative site.

I. Assess skin.

1. Should be pinkish color or consistent with ethnic background, pink-tinged; may appear dry.

✦2. Acrocyanosis (cyanosis of extremities) may be present for the first hour or two after birth. Persistent blueness may indicate complications such as heart disease.

3. Lanugo and vernix caseosa may be present.

4. Petechiae may be present because of the trauma of birth.

✦5. Milia (secretions of sebaceous materials in obstructed sebaceous glands) may be present and will disappear.

6. Erythema toxicum neonatorum (small harmless eruptions on the skin); transient in nature.

7. Hemangiomas may be present on nape of neck or upper eyelids.

✦8. Mongolian spots (bluish pigmented areas present on the buttocks of babies of Asian, African-American, or Mediterranean heritage, and other dark-skinned races).

9. Mottling may occur if the infant is chilled.

J. Assess for possible effects of maternal hormones.
  ✦1. Maternal hormones may cause enlargement of breast in both male and female infants, and "witches' milk," a milk-like substance, may be excreted from the breasts.
  2. Vaginal bleeding in female infant.
  3. Hypertrophy of labia or scrotum.
K. Assess neurological system.
  ✦1. Reflexes present at birth (sucking, rooting, Moro, grasp, blinking, yawning, tonic neck, Babinski).
  2. Muscle tone.
    a. Fist usually kept clenched.
    b. Baby should offer resistance when change in position is attempted.
    ✦c. Head should be supported when baby is lifted.
    ✦d. Muscles should not be limp.
  3. Cry.
    ✦a. Cry should be loud and vigorous.
    b. Baby should cry when hungry or uncomfortable.
  4. Hunger.
    a. Usually becomes fretful and restless at 3- to 4-hour intervals.
    b. May suck fingers or anything placed near mouth.
  5. Sleep.
    ✦a. Sleeps about 20 out of 24 hours.
    b. Often stirs and stretches while sleeping.
L. Assess functioning of senses.
  1. Eyes.
    a. Eyelids may be edematous or have purulent discharge from the chemical irritation of the antibiotic or silver nitrate.
    b. Light perception is present.
    c. Eye movement is uncoordinated.
    d. Usual color of eyes is blue-gray.
    e. May have subconjunctival hemorrhages, which disappear in a week or two.
    f. May gaze at or follow bright objects.
  2. Nose.
    a. Newborn breathes through nose.
    b. Sense of smell is present.
  3. Ears: hearing is present at birth.
  4. Taste is present at birth.
  5. Touch is present at birth. Responds to stimuli and discomfort.
M. Gestational Age Assessment (using Ballard Tool). (*See* Table 12-9.)
  1. Assess six neuromuscular and six physical characteristics during the first few hours of life. Total score is correlated with weeks of gestation (total of 35 points correlated with 38+ weeks gestation).

  2. Rating is then plotted on graph against weight, length, and head circumference to classify infant's gestational age characteristics and physical growth, which then confirms infant's status as appropriate (10–90th percentile), small (< 10th percentile) or large (> 90th percentile) for gestational age.
  3. Maturity.
    a. Neuromuscular maturity may be unstable during first 24 hours and may need to be repeated. Characteristics include: posture, square window, arm recoil, popliteal angle, scarf sign, and heel-to-ear extension.
    b. Physical maturity is not influenced by labor and birth and does not change significantly. Characteristics observed include: skin, lanugo, plantar surface creases, breast tissue, eye/ear recoil, genitalia (males testes descended, scrotum; females labia tissue).
N. Immunity factors.
  ✦1. May receive from the mother some passive immunity to infectious diseases, such as measles, mumps, and diphtheria.
  2. Capacity to develop own antibodies is slow during first few months.
  3. Has little resistance to infection.
  4. Immunizations: if mother is a carrier both Hepatitis B vaccine and Hepatitis B Immune Globulin (HBIG) should be given within 12 hours of birth.

General Implementation

A. Maintain body temperature.
  ✦1. Place infant in heated incubator or crib with radiant heat.
  2. Wipe off fluid, mucus, and excessive vernix.
  3. Avoid excessive exposure.
  4. Wrap infant in warm blankets.
  5. Transfer to the nursery after parents have seen and held infant.
B. Maintain respiration.
  ✦1. Place infant on side, in modified Trendelenburg's position, to prevent cerebral edema and to facilitate drainage of mucus and blood.
  2. Suction mucus as needed with bulb or suction catheter attached to mucus trap.
  3. Provide oxygen as needed.
C. Prevent infection and injury.
  1. Eye care.
    a. To prevent eye infections (opthalmia neonatorum) from gonorrhea or chlamydia.
    ✦b. Most common treatment: broad-spectrum antibiotic ointment applied to eyes (i.e., erythromycin ointment or tetracycline).

Table 12-9. ASSESSMENT: GESTATIONAL AGE

	Preterm	Term
PHYSICAL CHARACTERISTICS (1st 24 hours)		
Skin	Friable, translucent, visible veins	Few veins, thick, cracking, dry
Lanugo	Abundant	Minimal or none
Soles of feet (creases)	Few creases	Entire sole
Breast	Flat, no bud	Full areola, 10 mm+
Ear	Soft pinna, slow recoil	Thick pinna, instant recoil
Genitals (male)	Small scrotum, few rugae, testes undescended or descending	Scrotum pendulous, rugae, testes usually descended
Genitals (female)	Prominent clitoris, labia open	Large majora, cover clitoris
NEUROMUSCULAR (after 24 hours)		
Posture	Extended, froglike	Flexed
Square Window	90°	0°
Flexion Development		
Arm (flex 5 sec, release)	Slower recoil; angle > 90°	Back to flexed; < 90°
Popliteal Angle (knee flexion)	140°	90° angle
Scarf Sign (arm across chest)	Elbow at midline or past	Elbow will not meet midline
Heel to Ear	Foot goes to ear	Increasing resistance
Ankle dorsiflexion	45° angle	0–20° angle
Head lag	Hypotonia	Good tone
Reflexes		
Moro	Present @ 28 wk; no/weak adduction	Complete; disappears @ 4 mo
Grasp	Begins use arms	Support weight for few seconds; uses hand, arm and shoulder.

c. May use 1 percent silver nitrate (rarely used): two drops in conjunctival sacs; flush eyes with water after about 2 minutes; not effective against chlamydia and can cause chemical conjunctivitis.

2. Cord care—use sterile scissors and clamp. Apply a triple dye or antimicrobial agent such as bacitracin as ordered.

✦ 3. Never handle newborn baby without wearing gloves until after first bath with antibacterial soap—observe Standard Precautions.

Newborn—HIV Positive or AIDS

Characteristics

A. Transmission can occur during utero via the placenta, through breastmilk or contaminated blood.

B. Maternal to newborn transmission rate (20–30 percent of mothers with HIV) decreases by ⅔ when treated with antiviral (zidovudine—antepartal, intrapartal, and to newborn).

C. Tests for newborn antibodies may not show until up to 15 months after birth.

Assessment

A. Assess for physical signs: enlarged spleen and liver, swollen glands.

B. Assess for recurrent respiratory infections, rhinorrhea, interstitial pneumonia, recurrent gastrointestinal problems, failure to thrive, opportunistic infections, developmental delays.

Implementation

✦ A. Don gloves and gown to protect self from contamination. Use Standard Precautions.

B. Wait until newborn's temperature is stable in the nursery to provide care.

✦ C. Wash infant carefully with antibacterial soap wearing gloves and gown.

D. Administer cord care with alcohol, iodine solution, or antibacterial ointment.

E. Wrap infant in clean blanket.

F. Dispose of gloves and gown in plastic bag.

**NEWBORNS REQUIRING INTERVENTION/
STABILIZATION IMMEDIATELY AFTER BIRTH**

- Apgar score less than 8 at 1 minute and less than 9 at 5 minutes or requires resuscitation
- Respirations less than 30 or more than 60
- Cyanosis or circumoral pallor
- Pulse less than 110 or more than 160
- Temperature less than 97.8°F (36.5°C)
- Apparent congenital anomalies
- Late preterm, premature or baby large for gestational age

✦ G. Teach principles of care to mother of HIV baby.
  1. Breastfeeding is discouraged when mother tests positive for HIV.
  2. Circumcisions are not done on infants with HIV-positive mothers until infant's status is determined.
  3. Immunizations with live vaccine (oral polio, measles–mumps–rubella [MMR]) should not be done until infant's status is confirmed. If infant is infected, live vaccine will not be given. Inactivated polio vaccine (IPV) will be administered.
  4. Excellent hygiene procedures should be carried out in the home.
  5. Inform the caregiver exposed to infant's body fluids of the potential for infection transmission.
  6. Teach the importance of good hand hygiene techniques.
  7. Facilitate referral to community agencies and support groups as needed. Mother often unable to assume care because of own illness.

HIGH-RISK INFANTS

Preterm (Premature) Newborn

Definition: An infant born before the end of the 37th week regardless of birth weight.

Characteristics

A. Maternal factors: diabetes, PIH, chronic disease, chronic poor nutrition, premature rupture of membranes, placenta previa, abruptio placenta, incompetent cervix, other premature births, age, multiple gestation, smoking, drugs, infection, etc.
B. Fetal factors: congenital anomalies, infection, other diseases.
C. Socioeconomic factors: low socioeconomic status, poor nutrition, unmarried, under 27 years of age.
D. Other: cause unknown; accounts for large percentage of premature births.
E. Incidence: 8 percent of all live births and 15 percent in socioeconomically deprived populations.

  1. Factors associated with prematurity make it the leading cause of death in neonates.
  2. Primarily due to respiratory distress syndrome, infection, and intracranial hemorrhage.

Assessment

✦ A. Assess digestive system.
  1. Weak swallow/suck reflexes until about 33–34 weeks; poor gag/cough reflex increase risk of aspiration.
  2. Suck and swallow reflexes uncoordinated.
  3. Small stomach capacity.
  4. Poor ability to tolerate fats.
  5. Immature enzyme system.
✦ B. Assess CNS and muscle tone.
  1. Poor muscle tone: muscles appear limp; baby assumes froglike position when placed on abdomen.
  2. Weak, feeble cry.
  3. Weak or absent reflexes.
  4. Heat regulation unstable.
    a. Body temperature below normal, small muscle mass, absent sweat or shiver responses.
    b. Large body surface in proportion to body weight.
    c. Lack of subcutaneous fat.
    d. Poor capillary response to environmental changes.
  5. Susceptibility to brain damage from high levels of bilirubin (kernicterus).
✦ C. Assess respiratory system.
  1. Insufficient production of surfactant allows alveoli to collapse.
  2. Immaturity of alveoli and/or decreased number of functioning alveoli.
  3. Immaturity of musculature and rib cage contributes to increase work to expand alveoli.
  4. Prone to respiratory disease.
  5. Periodic breathing pattern—pauses < 15–20 seconds.
✦ D. Assess integumentary system.
  1. Skin thin and capillaries easily seen.
  2. Little subcutaneous fat.
  3. Lanugo prominent: hair on head is fine and fuzzy.
  4. Vernix may cover body if born between 31 and 33 weeks.
✦ E. Assess immune system: resistance to infection decreased.
  1. Lack of passive immunity from mother (occurs late pregnancy).
  2. Inability to produce own antibodies—immature system.

3. Difficulty localizing infection due to decreased inflammatory response.
4. Skin is thin and offers little protection from disease-causing organisms.

F. Assess hepatic system: liver immature.
1. Poor glycogen stores—increased susceptibility to hypoglycemia.
2. Inability to conjugate bilirubin—susceptible to hyperbilirubinemia.
3. Decreased ability to produce clotting factors.
4. Decreased ability to produce immune factors.

G. Assess circulatory system.
1. Capillary fragility increases susceptibility to hemorrhage, especially intraventricular (ruptures easily leading to signs of increased intracranial pressure—hypotonia, lethargy, bulging fontanels, increasing OFC, bradycardia, apnea, tremors, seizures).
2. Prone to anemia—poor iron stores.

H. Assess renal system.
1. Renal function immature—poor ability to concentrate urine.
2. Fluid and electrolyte balance precarious.
3. Easily dehydrated.
4. Increased time to eliminate drugs.

Implementation

◆ A. Provide immediate care to infant.
1. Give immediate attention in delivery room and transport to nursery to maintain heat.
   a. Maintain skin temperature at 36°C to 37°C or 96.8°F to 97.7°F in isolette or heated crib.
   b. Warming infant too quickly may cause apneic spells.
   c. Gradually wean infant from heated environment and monitor temperature until stable, q 1–3 hours as indicated.
2. Administer humidity (distilled water) usually between 40 and 70 percent as ordered.

◆ B. Evaluate respiratory status.
1. Check respiratory rate—every hour and PRN.
2. Observe for the following signs of respiratory distress:
   a. Color of skin: circumoral pallor, pallor entire body, cyanosis (late).
   b. Flaring of nares.
   c. Expiratory grunting, retractions.
   d. Tachypnea
   e. See-saw movements.
   f. Diminished breath sounds.
3. Auscultate breath sounds with stethoscope.
4. Analyze oxygen concentration (transcutaneous oxygen monitor) every 1–2 hours or as necessary to prevent retrolental fibroplasia and to ensure adequate oxygenation.
5. Observe for periods of apnea and stimulate by gently rubbing chest or tapping foot.
6. Percuss, vibrate, and suction as ordered to remove mucus.

◆ C. Reposition every 2 hours to promote aeration of all lobes of the lung and facilitate drainage.

◆ D. Monitor blood gases and electrolytes frequently; IV regulated by infusion pump to prevent circulatory overload.

◆ E. Initiate feedings—based upon ability to feed.
1. Reflexes
2. Use premie nipple.
3. Monitor for abdominal distention, emesis, tolerating feedings.

F. Monitor closely for early signs of necrotizing enterocolitis (NEC).
1. Often occurs as a result of intestinal ischemia, which may occur with asphyxia when the blood is shunted to the brain or heart.
2. Common symptoms include: abdominal distention, poor feeding, vomiting, blood in stools, temperature, redness.
3. Treatment includes NPO, IV, fluids, antibiotics and surgery.

◆ G. Provide for family's needs.
1. Allow parents to visit baby frequently; as soon as possible, involve parents in infant care to promote parent-to-infant attachment.
2. Answer questions openly, provide up-to-date information on baby's progress.
3. Allow parents to talk freely about infant, give support as needed, and help parents to accept reality of situation.
4. Explain specialized care to parents. Have them report to pediatrician any of the following symptoms: diarrhea, vomiting, lack of appetite, or elevated temperature.
5. Allow mother to feel confident in caring for infant before discharge. Explain to mother infant's special needs.

H. Give gavage feeding if respirations are about 60 breaths per minute.
1. Use premie nipple if bottle feeding.
2. Infants often require alternate feedings of gavage and bottle feeding.

I. Maintain I&O, including stool, and weigh daily.

J. Organize care to conserve energy with rest periods after each feeding.

K. Monitor growth and development: measure head circumference and length at least once a week; check weight daily and note changes and trends.

L. Maintain aseptic technique and strict isolation techniques with infected babies.

M. Prevent skin breakdown: change position frequently; careful cleansing and handling techniques.

N. Observe for signs of infection: vomiting, jaundice, lack of appetite, and lethargy.

O. Check heart rate by apical pulse for a full minute every 1–2 hours.

P. Frequently check for bleeding from umbilical catheter.
1. Apply pressure to puncture site as necessary to prevent bleeding.
2. Administer vitamin K as ordered after birth to prevent hemorrhage.
3. Frequently check monitors if monitored electronically.

Q. Gently stroke and talk to baby when giving care.

✦ R. Hang colorful mobiles or other nonharmful objects in crib for sensory stimulation.

✦ S. Hold baby during feeding as soon as condition permits.

T. Encourage parents to hold, cuddle, feed, and diaper baby as soon as baby's condition permits.

Late Preterm Baby (Born 34 to 37 Weeks)

Characteristics

A. Needs are similar to premature infants.
1. Infants formerly evaluated solely on weight.
2. Gestational age is a better tool to predict problems.

B. Appear as ordinary newborns, but at risk for
1. Respiratory problems.
2. Temperature instability.
3. Hyperbilirubinemia.
4. Hypoglycemia.
5. Infection.
6. Breastfeeding failure.

Assessment

A. Respiratory distress syndrome.
1. Disorder of immature lungs and deficiency of surfactant.
2. Symptoms may appear at birth or after a few hours.
   a. Respirations up to 120 without retractions.
   b. Tachypnea—thought to be related to delayed absorption of lung fluid.
   c. Cyanosis.
   d. Grunting.
   e. Retractions.

B. Hyperbilirubinemia (jaundice)—frequent in late preterm babies.
1. Immature liver mechanisms aggravated by dehydration and poor feeding.

2. Delays clearing of bilirubin in bowel.
3. Phototherapy is treatment in hospital or home.

C. Infections.
1. May be acquired before birth, during delivery or in neonatal period (Group B *Streptococcus*).
2. Signs and symptoms often nonspecific (e.g., respiratory problems, hypothermia, lethargic).
3. Diagnosis may be by blood cultures, CBC, and screening.

D. Hypoglycemia—blood glucose level may fall after birth.

E. Hypothermia—prone to this condition because of large surface area in relation to body weight.

F. Dehydration resulting from poor feeding ability, compounded by phototherapy.

Implementation

A. Constant observation for preterm babies.
1. May require O_2, vital signs, and pulse oximetry.
2. Nutrition via NG tube.
3. IV therapy to prevent dehydration.

B. Preterm infants may have feeding problems—dehydration.
1. Preterm babies being breastfed may have problems latching, sucking and swallowing.
2. May require supplemental bottle formula or expressed breastmilk via NG tube.

C. Late development of cerebral cortex (increases 50 percent between 34 to 40 weeks gestation).
1. Avoid stimulation, light, sound.
2. Avoid painful actions.

D. Hypothermia.
1. Defer bathing and use radiant warmer.
2. Skin-to-skin contact with mother.

Respiratory Distress Syndrome (RDS)

Definition: A group of clinical symptoms signifying that the infant is experiencing problems with the respiratory system—also called hyaline membrane disease.

Characteristics

✦ A. Symptoms are the result of a decrease in the amount of surfactant in the infant's lungs caused by one of the following conditions.
1. Prematurity: immaturity of lungs, decreased number of mature alveoli, and inability to produce surfactant.
2. Hypoxia and acidosis.
3. Hypothermia.
4. High concentration of oxygen.

✦ B. Respiratory distress syndrome is the most common cause of death in infants.

C. Prevention of RDS.

1. Evaluation of amniotic fluids to assess fetal lung capacity.
2. Administration of glucocorticoids (betamethasone) to induce pulmonary maturation.
   a. Prenatal IM injections of 12 mg 1×/day for 2 days.
   b. Birth may be delayed 24 hours after first round of treatment.

Assessment

✦ A. Assess for increased respirations: greater than 60/min.
✦ B. Assess for retractions: sternal and intercostal.
C. Check for presence of cyanosis and expiratory grunting; assess for increased number and length of apnea episodes.
D. Assess for increased apical pulse.
E. Evaluate nasal flaring and chin lag.
F. Evaluate for lack of activity or movement.
G. Assess for inability to take in sufficient oxygen leading to low oxygen and hypoxemia.
H. Assess for hypercarbia due to elevated levels of carbon dioxide.
I. Check for respiratory acidosis due to retention of carbon dioxide as a result of inadequate pulmonary ventilation.
J. Evaluate for decreased body temperature.
K. Check for metabolic acidosis due to increased production of lactic acid and decreased pH.
L. Evaluate x-ray examination, which may reveal
   1. Atelectasis: collapsed portions of lung.
   2. Reticulogranular pattern bilaterally.
   3. Air bronchograms.

Implementation

✦ A. Prevent cold stress: infant is usually placed in isolette or open crib with overhead radiant warmer. Skin temperature is maintained with probe at minimum 97.7°F (36°C)—thermoneutral environment.
B. Provide for nutrition and hydration: usually give IV glucose fluids during acute periods, then gradually increase feedings as tolerated.
C. Do careful monitoring of blood gases and electrolytes, color, and activity.
✦ D. Administer oxygen for hypoxemia.
   1. Maintain paO$_2$ at 50–70 mm Hg warmed and humidified; monitor and record.
   2. Adjust O$_2$ concentration based on ABGs (usually 30–50 percent under an oxyhood).
   3. Administer via hood, nasal prongs, endotracheal tubes, or bag and mask.
   4. Oxygen may be given at atmosphere or increased airway pressure.
   5. Apply continuous positive pressure to lungs during spontaneous breathing. Continuous pos-

---

INFANT WITH ENDOTRACHEAL TUBE

1. Check frequently for correct placement and connection at adapter site.
2. Suction infant with endotracheal tube.
   • Disconnect from respirator at site of adapter.
   • Instill a few minims to 0.5 mL of sterile normal saline into tube to loosen secretions.
   • Suction no longer than 5 seconds using sterile catheter.
   • Ventilate infant as needed during procedure.
   • Reconnect tube to respirator, being sure it is in place and adapter is secure.
   • Auscultate chest for breath sounds.

---

itive airway pressure (CPAP) may be used for moderate cases.
   6. Apply mechanical ventilatory assistance for severe cases.
✦ E. Surfactant replacement therapy is now available to decrease severity of RDS—given via endotracheal tube.
F. Supportive ventilation therapy to prevent hypoventilation and hypoxia.
   1. Mild cases may require only increased O$_2$.
   2. Use of CPAP delivered via endotracheal tube may be required.
   3. Increased urination (weigh diapers) signifies fluid moving out of lungs into bloodstream; kidney perfusion indicates baby's condition is improving.
   4. Monitor chest expansion and ventilator setting (if too high, pneumothorax may occur).
G. Gently handle infant with as little disturbance as possible.
H. Position in side-lying or supine position with neck slightly extended (sniffing position).
I. Keep parents informed of infant's progress.
J. Allow parents to visit infant as much as possible and express their feelings about infant's illness.
K. Gently stroke and talk with infant while giving care.

Small for Gestational Age

Definition: Refers to infants who are significantly undersize for gestational age (below 10th percentile). Also called intrauterine growth retardation (IUGR).

Characteristics

A. Postmature infants.
B. Defective embryonic development.
C. Placental insufficiency.
D. Associated factors: diabetes, toxemia, maternal infection, maternal malnutrition, cigarette smoking, multiple gestation.
✦ E. Infant appearance.

1. Little subcutaneous tissue.
2. Loose, dry, scaling skin.
3. Appears thin and wasted; old for size.
4. May be meconium staining of skin, nails.
5. Sparse hair on head.
6. Active, alert, seems hungry.
7. Cord dries more rapidly than normal infants.

Assessment

◆ A. Assess for hypoglycemia or poor glucose control: nervousness, pallor, apnea, temperature instability, high-pitched, weak cry.

◆ B. Assess for cold stress: lethargy, poor feeding pattern, cold to touch, respirations increased.

C. Assess for asphyxia: may have been deprived while in utero or aspirated amniotic fluid. Infant may require resuscitation at birth.

D. Assess for polycythemia: usually asymptomatic but may have tachycardia, tachypnea, respiratory distress.

Implementation

A. Provide care similar to premature infant until the infant is stabilized.

B. Protect from cold stress: keep warm, usually in isolette.

C. Perform tests for glucose levels.

D. Weigh daily and maintain I&O.

Postmature Infant

Definition: Refers to an infant of over 42 weeks' gestation.

Characteristics

A. Placental function decreased.

B. Nutritional and oxygen needs are not met.

C. Infants exposed to chronic hypoxia.

D. Easily stressed during labor.

E. Increased morbidity and mortality due to above factors.

F. Increased incidence of labor dystocia due to large size of infant.

Assessment

◆ A. Assess that vernix and lanugo are no longer present.

◆ B. Assess skin: appears dry and wrinkled.

C. Check fingernails and toenails: usually long and may be meconium stained.

D. Assess size: may be small for gestational age (SGA) due to nutritional deficiency and chronic hypoxia.

◆ E. Observe for hypoglycemia.

F. Observe for signs of birth injury: dislocated shoulder, fractured pelvis, facial paralysis, and CNS injury.

Implementation

◆ A. Similar to care given to preterm infants if premature characteristics are observed.

1. Requires immediate attention in the delivery room.
2. Suctioning before infant's first breath will prevent meconium aspiration.
3. Heated crib or isolette to prevent cold stress.
4. Evaluate respiratory rate consistently and observe for signs of respiratory distress—administer oxygen and humidification if necessary.
5. Monitor blood gases, electrolytes, and blood sugar.
6. Give oral feedings or check need for IV feedings.
7. Maintain I&O records.
8. Observe for signs of infection; monitor administration of antibiotics.
9. Prevent skin breakdown.

B. Symptoms depend on condition at birth. Care for as SGA in those infants who are underweight for gestational age.

C. Monitor for possible complications (asphyxia neonatorum, polycythemia, birth injuries).

Hyperbilirubinemia

◆ *Definition:* An abnormal elevation of bilirubin in the newborn (above 12.9 mg/100 mL for formula-fed infants and above 15 mg/100 mL for breast-fed infants or prematures).

Characteristics

◆ A. Functional immaturity of the liver: usually appears after 24 hours and disappears after 10 days; physiologic jaundice.

B. Bacterial infections.

C. ABO and Rh incompatibilities: usually show up in the first 24 hours and may be severe.

D. Enclosed bleeding, such as hematoma, from trauma of delivery.

E. Pregnanediol hormone, present in mother's breastmilk, may contribute to jaundice. (Hormone inhibits conjugation of bilirubin by glucuronyl transferase—occurs in fewer than one percent of breastfeeding mothers.)

F. May lead to kernicterus—a deposit of yellow pigmentation in basal ganglia of brain results in irreversible brain damage, caused by high levels of unconjugated, unbound bilirubin.

Assessment

◆ A. Observe for jaundice, which progresses from head to extremities (color of sclera, mucosa, and blanched skin).

1. Physiologic jaundice occurs 3–5 days after birth.
2. When levels reach above 12.9 mg/100 mL in full-term infants and 15 mg/100 mL in premature infants, or persists beyond 7 days, jaundice may be termed pathological.

B. Observe for pallor.

C. Evaluate activity level: infant may be lethargic and feed poorly.

D. Assess if urine is concentrated, or stools are light in color.

✦ E. Assess progress of condition: if untreated, infant may progress from muscular rigidity or flaccidity to increased lethargy, high-pitched cry, respiratory distress, decreased Moro's reflex, and spasms.

F. Evaluate blood tests.

   1. Hemoglobin.

   ✦ 2. Bilirubin: important to measure amount of indirect or unconjugated bilirubin in blood, since unbound bilirubin is free to deposit in body tissues, such as skin, cardiac muscle, brain, and kidney.

   3. Unconjugated bilirubin crosses blood–brain barrier, and when deposited in the brain, can lead to kernicterus and brain damage.

G. Assess fluid balance.

Implementation

A. Observe infant for signs of increased jaundice.

B. Observe for and prevent acidosis/hypoxia and hypoglycemia, which decrease binding of bilirubin to albumin and contribute to jaundice.

✦ C. Maintain adequate hydration and offer fluids between feedings as ordered.

   1. Infant may be on increased fluids to aid in excretion of bilirubin.

   ✦ 2. Phototherapy can cause loose stools so there is a danger of dehydration.

   3. When infant is NPO, the infusion rate may need to be increased.

D. Using skin temperature probe, maintain skin temperature at 97.6°F; avoid cold stress.

E. Prevent infection.

✦ F. Provide phototherapy: phototherapy lamp breaks down bilirubin into water-soluble products.

   1. Do not clothe infant.

   ✦ 2. Cover infant's eyes to prevent retinal damage.

   3. Change baby's position every 2 hours to ensure adequate exposure.

   4. Remove infant from light and remove eye patches during feedings; dress to keep infant warm.

   5. Carefully examine eyes for signs of irritation from eye patches.

   6. Keep an accurate record of hours spent under bili-lights.

G. Meet infant's emotional needs: cuddle, talk to infant, etc.

H. Reinforce physician's teaching to parents and allow parents to express concerns and feelings.

✦ I. Monitor exchange transfusion: considered when bilirubin reaches high levels (20 mg/mL in full-term infant; lower levels in premature infants). No "safe level" of bilirubin to prevent kernicterus—influenced by combination of bilirubin level, neurological age, and condition.

   1. Exchange transfusion is usually performed in operating or delivery room.

   2. Infant is usually placed in radiant warmer and restrained.

   3. Resuscitative equipment and oxygen should be available.

   4. Blood should be no more than 24 hours old and warmed.

   5. Stomach contents are aspirated to prevent vomiting.

   6. Baseline vital signs are obtained and checked every 15 to 30 minutes.

   7. Transfusion is usually given via umbilical catheter.

   8. Exchange usually done by alternately withdrawing and adding blood until about 80 percent of infant's total blood volume has been exchanged—maximum 500 mL Rh-negative blood is given.

   9. Exchange usually takes 45 to 60 minutes.

J. Administer care after transfusion.

   1. Observe for bleeding from the umbilical cord.

   2. Observe vital signs frequently.

   3. Maintain warmth.

   4. Administer oxygen if needed.

   5. Observe for signs of hypoglycemia, sepsis, cardiac arrest, thrombocytopenia, or other irregularities.

   6. Handle infant.

   7. Resume feedings after 4 to 6 hours.

   8. Keep umbilical cord moist in case other transfusions are indicated.

Hemolytic Disease (Erythroblastosis Fetalis)

Definition: The destruction of red blood cells that results from an antigen–antibody reaction and is characterized by hemolytic anemia or hyperbilirubinemia.

Characteristics

✦ A. Rh incompatibility: Rh antigens from the baby's blood enter the maternal bloodstream. The mother's blood does not contain Rh factor, so she produces anti-Rh antibodies. These antibodies are harmless to the mother but attach to the erythrocytes in the fetus and cause hemolysis. Exchange of fetal and maternal blood takes place primarily when the placenta separates at birth.

✦1. Passive immunization or RhoGAM, Rho(D) immune globulin, should be given to the mother within 48 to 72 hours after delivery.
   a. Given if Rh-negative mother (approximately 15 percent of white population have Rh-negative factor) delivers Rh-positive fetus but remains unsensitized.
   b. Currently, the woman receives Rho(D) immune globulin at 28 weeks; it may also be given at 34 weeks' gestation.
   c. Immunization protects mother and fetus.
2. Sensitization rare with first pregnancy.
3. Diagnosis of Rh incompatibility.
   ✦a. Begins in pregnancy, with the discovery of antibodies in an Rh-negative mother's blood by means of *indirect Coombs' test.*
   b. Titration is used to determine the extent to which antibodies are present.
   c. Spectrophotometric analysis of amniotic fluid for bilirubin determines the severity of the disease—the higher the bilirubin content, the more severe the disease.
   ✦d. Testing of cord blood—*direct Coombs' test*—determines the presence of maternal antibodies attached to baby's cells.
B. ABO incompatibility—usually less severe.

Assessment

A. Assess for anemia that is caused by destruction of red blood cells. Severe anemia usually accompanied by cardiac decompensation, edema, ascites, hypoxia, and may result in death.
B. Assess for jaundice, which develops rapidly after birth—before 24 hours.
C. Evaluate for edema—usually seen in stillborn infants or those who die shortly after birth; most likely due to cardiac failure.

Implementation

✦A. Administer immunization to the mother against hemolytic disease with RhoGAM as ordered. (Now given at 28 weeks and postpartum.)
B. Monitor exchange transfusion after birth or intrauterine transfusion. Use Rh negative blood.
C. Follow interventions listed under hyperbilirubinemia.

Sepsis in the Neonate

Definition: Generalized infection resulting from the presence of pathogenic bacteria in the bloodstream—mortality may reach 50 percent when condition appears shortly after birth. May be caused by immature immune system—decreased ability to localize and fight infection.

Predisposing Factors

A. Prolonged rupture of membranes, over 24 hours.
B. Long, difficult labor or prolonged resuscitation after birth.
C. Maternal infection.
D. Aspiration of amniotic fluids or vaginal secretions during birth.
E. Aspiration of formula after birth.
F. Infection within nursery or among nursery personnel (nosocomial).
G. Usually appears within the first 48 hours after birth but may begin prenatally or postdelivery.
H. May quickly lead to septicemia or meningitis if not treated promptly.
I. Beta-hemolytic strep vaginosis most common cause; need to culture antepartally.

✦ Assessment

A. General assessment is important as symptoms may be vague and subtle.
B. Assess feeding, which may be poor, and sucking reflex.
C. Check for presence of diarrhea.
D. Assess for periods of apnea or irregular respirations.
E. Check for jaundice.
F. Assess for low-grade or subnormal temperature—fever rare (temperature instability).
G. Evaluate activity level for lethargy.
H. Assess for irritability, seizure activity.
I. Diagnosis is made from aspiration of gastric contents, which are examined for polymorphonuclear cells, or cultures taken of blood, urine, spinal fluids, throat, skin lesions, and the umbilical area.
J. Assess for results of cervical culture when admitted into labor.

Implementation

✦A. Administer antibiotics if appropriate and observe carefully for toxicity because of liver and kidney immaturity—viral cause is treated symptomatically except herpes simplex and respiratory syncytial virus (RSV).
B. Maintain warmth—usually in an isolette.
C. Administer oxygen as necessary.
D. Administer IV fluids if ordered; otherwise, give fluids as ordered to maintain hydration, electrolytes, and calories.
✦E. Maintain Standard Precautions and proper hand hygiene techniques.
F. Check respiratory rate and apical pulse frequently.
G. Stimulate if apnea is present by gently rubbing chest or foot.
H. Maintain intake and output.
I. Check temperature.
J. Weigh daily.

K. Observe for signs of jaundice.
L. Keep parents informed of infant's progress.
M. Allow parents to visit infant as much as possible.
N. Talk and gently stroke infant while giving care.

Infants of Diabetic Mothers (IDM)

Definition: Infants with blood glucose level of less than 40 mg/dL. Most have been exposed to elevated maternal glucose levels in utero.

Characteristics

A. May be delivered early to prevent intrauterine death; usually delivered after 36 weeks.
B. Often delivered by cesarean section.
C. Children with diabetic mothers have a higher incidence of congenital abnormalities than the general population.
D. High incidence of hypoglycemia, respiratory distress, hypocalcemia, and hyperbilirubinemia.

Assessment

✦ A. Assess for excessive size and weight due to excess fat and glycogen in tissues.
  1. High blood sugar levels in mother cross the placenta and enter the baby's bloodstream, elevating blood sugar levels.
  2. High blood sugar stimulates infant's metabolic system to store glycogen and fat and increase the production of insulin (even though maternal blood sugar supply is lost).
  ✦ 3. High levels of insulin deplete glucose levels, which leads to hypoglycemia (occurs 1–3 hours after birth).
B. Assess infant: birth trauma, LGA, may have puffy face and cheeks, increased risk for congenital defects (cardiac, spine).
✦ C. Observe for signs of hypoglycemia—difficulty feeding, lethargy, apnea, subnormal temperature, tremors, jitteriness, seizures, cyanosis, high-pitched cry.
✦ D. Observe for hypocalcemia (may be caused by prematurity or stress); tremors.
E. Observe for signs of respiratory distress—tachypnea, cyanosis, retractions, grunting, nasal flaring.
F. Hyperbilirubinemia.

Implementation

A. Administer care similar to premature infant.
✦ B. Caloric intake important—early feeding major preventive approach.
  1. Breast or formula feeding started.
  2. Oral glucose given after plasma glucose reading < 40.

3. Infant may need IV therapy depending on condition—5 to 10 percent glucose, the highest safe concentration.
4. 25 to 50 percent dextrose contraindicated because rebound hypoglycemia could occur.
C. Be aware that any infant of a diabetic mother will be started on hypoglycemia protocol regardless of weight.
D. Monitor blood glucose frequently according to orders (usually by 30 min, q 1, 2, 4, 6, 9, 12 & 24 hours after birth).

Hypoglycemia

Definition: Abnormally low level of sugar in the blood (blood glucose value of 40 mg/dL).

Characteristics

A. Placental dysfunction.
B. Diabetes in mother.
C. Cold stress.
D. Renal disease, cardiac disease, preeclampsia, or chronic infection in the mother.
E. Small for gestational age (SGA) infants.
F. Post-term infant.
G. Asphyxia at birth.
H. Infection in infant or any condition that stresses the metabolic rate and increases the need for glucose.

Assessment

A. Assess for presence of cyanosis.
B. Assess for increased respiratory rate.
✦ C. Check any jitteriness, twitching, nervousness, or tremors.
D. Evaluate for lethargy and poor muscle tone.
E. Assess unstable temperature.
✦ F. Assess for shrill or intermittent cry.
G. Check for any feeding problems.
H. Evaluate apneic periods closely.
I. Evaluate blood sugar values: normal is 45 to 100/100 mL of blood; usually around 60 to 75/100 mL.
  1. Term infant: 30/40 mg/100 mL blood.
  2. Preterm: 20 mg/100 mL blood.
✦ J. Monitor screening that is done with heel stick testing, with laboratory studies as a follow-up.

Implementation

✦ A. Prevent low blood glucose through early feedings (immediate breastfeeding, D_5W, or $D_{10}W$).
B. Administer glucose orally or IV, depending on baby's condition—IV started with 10 percent glucose, highest safe concentration.
C. Perform close monitoring of blood sugar values every 1–2 hours.
D. Give care as for other high-risk infants.

Newborn Infected with Group B Streptococcus (GBS)

Characteristics

A. Newborn infected with GBS manifests severe, invasive disease.

B. Risk factors.
1. Prematurity (< 37 weeks).
2. Membranes ruptured more than 12 hours.
3. Intrapartum temperature > 100.4°F.
4. Previously infected infant.
5. GBS bacteriuria identified during pregnancy.

Assessment

A. Assessment critical to survival—infant may deteriorate rapidly in first 12–24 hours if infection present.

B. Early onset—symptoms appear within hours or 1 week.
1. Signs of respiratory distress or aspiration pneumonia.
   a. Grunting, cyanosis.
   b. Apnea.
   c. Temperature instability.
   d. "Shocky" appearance (cyanosis, pallor, clamminess).
2. X-ray to identify pneumonia.

Implementation

A. Clinical therapy is based on detection of carriers and preventive treatment with prophylactic antibiotics for the mother.

B. Newborns with GBS infection are treated as sepsis neonatorum.

C. Two blood cultures are obtained from two peripheral sites.

D. Antibiotics instituted STAT, then altered according to culture sensitivity.
1. Two broad-spectrum antibiotics for 7 to 14 days (penicillin, ampicillin and Kenamycin).
2. Gentamicin may be used if resistance to other antibiotics.

Drug-Dependent Newborn

Characteristics

✦ A. There is a direct relationship between the duration of addiction, dosage, and the severity of symptoms.

B. Cocaine has largely replaced heroin and methadone as addictive substances.

✦ C. Heroin-addicted mother: infant may appear normal at birth with a low birth weight.
1. Onset of withdrawal begins within 72 hours, but may not begin until up to 2 weeks after birth.
2. Infant appears less ill than when mother is taking methadone.

3. Heroin causes early maturity of the liver.

✦ D. Mother on methadone.
1. Onset of withdrawal may be delayed; most evident 48–72 hours and may last 6 days to 8 weeks.
2. Infant may appear to be very ill.
3. May develop jaundice due to prematurity.

✦ E. Mother addicted to cocaine.
1. A stimulant; maternal-to-fetal transfer of cocaine is swift, with the metabolites even more potent than the drug.
2. Infant evidences decreased interactive behavior, feeding problems, irregular sleep patterns, diarrhea.
3. Seven out of 1000 mothers will have infants with major deformities—especially of the kidneys.

Assessment

A. Assess for irritability, jitteriness, tremors, hyperactivity, and hypertonicity.

B. Assess for respiratory distress and ventilatory capacity.

✦ C. Observe for the following signs:
1. Persistent, high-pitched, shrill cry.
2. Sneezing, yawning, nasal stuffiness.
3. Fever.
4. Disruption of normal sleep patterns.
5. Gastrointestinal effects.
   a. Vomiting.
   b. Diarrhea.
   c. Poor feeding.
   d. Hunger, sucking fists.
6. Excessive sweating.
7. Extreme sucking of fists.

D. Assess for convulsions, which are rare.

Implementation

✦ A. Monitor respiratory and cardiac rates every 30 minutes and PRN.

B. Take temperature every 4 to 8 hours and PRN.

C. Reduce external stimuli and handle infant infrequently.
1. Hold infant firmly and close to body during feedings and when giving care.
2. Maintain warmth and swaddle infant in blanket.

D. Pad sides of crib to protect infant from injury.

E. Administer small, frequent feedings by gavage if necessary.

F. Suction if necessary.

G. Provide careful skin care: cleanse buttocks and anal area carefully.

H. Measure I&O.

I. Keep mother informed of infant's progress.

J. Promote mother's interest in infant.

K. Administer medications as ordered, usually paregoric (narcotic opiate), phenobarbital, Valium, tincture of opium.
1. Controls behavioral/neurological and GI symptoms.
2. Drug alleviates substance withdrawal and is slowly withdrawn.

Fetal Alcohol Syndrome (FAS)

Characteristics

A. Maternal alcohol abuse throughout pregnancy results in fetal alcohol syndrome.
1. Most serious cause of teratogenesis.
2. Affected infants.
   a. Prenatal and postnatal growth deficiency (SGA).
   b. CNS dysfunction—mental retardation.
   c. Craniofacial feature: microencephaly, short palpebral (eyelid) fissures, thin upper lip, flat midface.

✦ B. Lesser amount of alcohol ingested throughout pregnancy results in less severe symptoms—identified as fetal alcohol effect (FAE).
1. Studies suggest that 1 ounce/day presents a significant risk to the fetus and 2 ounces almost always affects the fetus.
2. Children suffer long-term neurological effects.
3. Developmental delay and later learning disabilities.
4. May not be diagnosed until early childhood.

Assessment

✦ A. Monitor for respiratory distress and apnea.

B. Observe for cyanosis.

C. Observe for seizures.

D. Check for major brain dysfunction symptoms.

✦ #### Implementation

A. Position on side to facilitate drainage of secretions.
1. Keep resuscitation equipment at bedside.
2. Have suction available, especially following feeding.

B. Administer small feedings and burp well.

C. Avoid heat loss.

D. Reduce environmental stimuli.

FAMILY PLANNING

Infertility

Definition: The inability to conceive after one year of regular intercourse with no contraceptive measures, or the inability to deliver a live fetus after three consecutive conceptions.

Characteristics

✦ A. General statistics indicate that two-thirds of couples achieve pregnancy within 6 months and 90 percent within one year—approximately 8–10 percent of couples in United States are infertile.

B. Approximately 40–50 percent of all infertility is attributed to the female.
1. Following investigation and treatment, 50–70 percent achieve pregnancy.
2. Of the 30–50 percent who do not achieve pregnancy, 10–20 percent have no pathologic basis for infertility.

Assessment

A. Causes of infertility.
1. Female.
   a. Functional: hormonal dysfunction causing insufficient gonadotropin secretions.
   b. Anatomic: ovarian factors, uterine abnormalities, tubal, peritoneal, and cervical factors.
   c. Inflammation or adhesions, chronic infections.
   d. Psychological problems.
   e. Immunologic reaction to partner's sperm.
2. Male.
   a. Semen disorders—volume, motility, or density; abnormal or immature sperm.
   b. Systemic disease such as diabetes.
   c. Genital infection.
   d. Disorders of the testes.
   e. Structural abnormalities.
   f. Genetic defects.
   g. Immunologic disorders.
   h. Chemicals, drugs, and environmental factors.
   i. Psychological problems.
   j. Sexual problems.

B. Tests for infertility.
1. Female.
   a. Complete physical exam and health history.
   b. Basal body temperature graph.
   c. Endometrial biopsy—luteal phase, 2–3 days before menstruation.
   d. Hormone analysis: progesterone, prolactin, FSH, LH, estradiol, blood levels.
   e. Tests to determine structural integrity of the tubes, ovaries, and uterus (ultrasound: abdominal or transvaginal, hysterosalpingogram, laparoscopy).
2. Male.
   a. Detailed history and physical examination.

b. Semen analysis (most conclusive) (> 2.0 mL, pH 7.0–8.0; sperm count > 20 million/mL, > 50 percent motility; > 50 percent normal forms).

c. Other laboratory tests: gonadotropin assay, serum testosterone levels, and urine 17-ketosteroid levels.

d. Testicular biopsy.

e. Ultrasound—structural integrity of spermatic cord, ejaculating ducts, seminal vesicles and vas deferens.

C. Treatment.

1. Female.

a. Identification and correction of underlying abnormality or dysfunction.

b. Hormone therapy (Clomid).

c. Surgical restoration.

d. Drug therapy.

2. Male.

a. Correction of anatomic dysfunctions or infections.

b. Proper nutrition with vitamin supplements.

c. Hormone supplements: testosterone or chorionic gonadotropin.

3. Couples.

a. Male-female interaction studies.

b. Counseling for sexual dysfunctions (education, counseling, or therapy).

c. Intrauterine insemination (using artificial insemination).

(1) Sperm (collected within 3 hours of coitus) inserted via a catheter into uterus.

(2) Option of donor sperm—sperm count &/or motility low or if single woman, etc.

d. In vitro fertilization (IVF)—multiple ova harvested from woman (using large bore needle).

Implementation

A. Education of couple.

1. Information about diagnostic and treatment techniques.

2. Information about reproductive and sexual function and factors that may interfere with fertility.

B. Provide emotional support.

1. Encourage couple to discuss frustration, anger, etc., and express feelings.

2. Suggest couple join groups to share concerns with other couples.

C. Explore alternatives such as adoption.

D. Provide information and preparation for surgery, if necessary or reproductive alternatives (artificial insemination, in vitro fertilization, etc.).

Influences on Parenthood

A. Tendency toward smaller families.

B. Career-oriented women who limit family size or who do not want children.

C. Early sexual experimentation, necessitating sexual education, contraceptive information.

D. Tendency toward postponement of children.

1. Until education is completed.

2. For economic factors.

E. High divorce rates.

F. Alternate family designs.

1. Single parenthood.

2. Communal family.

ISSUES OF CONTRACEPTION

General Concepts

✦ A. General concepts.

1. Dealing with individuals with personal ideas/beliefs regarding contraception.

2. No perfect method of birth control.

3. Method must be suited to individual.

4. Individuals involved must be thoroughly counseled on all available methods and how they work, including advantages and disadvantages.

5. Once a method is chosen both parties should be thoroughly instructed in its use.

6. Individuals involved must be motivated to succeed.

B. Effectiveness depends on:

1. Method chosen.

2. Degree to which couple follows prescribed regimen.

3. Thorough understanding of method.

4. Motivation on part of individuals concerned.

Role of Nurse

A. Education of client in various methods available, their effectiveness, and their side effects.

B. Help clients explore their feelings regarding birth control and what they find acceptable and not acceptable.

C. Create open, relaxed atmosphere, allowing clients to express concerns and feelings about birth control.

D. Thorough explanation of how method works.

E. Instruction of client in possible complications and side effects.

Natural Contraceptive Methods

A. Periodic abstinence: 75 percent effective.

✦ 1. Based on three principles.

a. Ovulation usually occurs 14 days before period begins.

b. An ovum may be fertilized 12–24 hours after release from ovary.

c. Sperm usually survive only 24–48 hours in the uterine environment.

2. If coitus is avoided during the fertile period, pregnancy should not occur.

3. Cervical mucus (Billings): couple avoids intercourse during peak 72-hour period of cycle, when mucus becomes clear, stringy, stretchable, and slippery.

4. Basal body temperature (BBT): avoid intercourse just prior to or day temperature drops and for 72 hours.

a. After temperature drops, during ovulation, and rises and fluctuates until 2–4 days prior to menstruation.

b. BBT thermometer measures in tenths (.1); can use tympanic or digital.

5. Calendar Method—also known as "rhythm."

a. Assumes that ovulation occurs 14 days before menstruation, sperm are viable for 5 days, and ovum can be fertilized for 24 hours.

b. Determine fertile period after recording menstrual cycle for 6 months: subtract 18 days from length of shortest cycle and 11 days from longest cycle; couple abstains during fertile period.

c. Least reliable; should be used together with BBT or Billings.

B. Coitus interruptus: 60 percent effective.

1. Requires withdrawal of penis before ejaculation.

2. Preejaculatory fluid may contain sperm.

C. Lactation—unreliable.

1. Breastfeeding has contraceptive effect.

2. Prolactin's inhibition of luteinizing hormone which maintains menstruation.

3. Provides protection for 3–6 months.

✦ Mechanical Methods

A. Condom (male or female): 95–98 percent effective with proper application.

1. Acts as mechanical barrier by collecting sperm and not allowing contact with vaginal area.

2. Prevents spread of disease.

B. Diaphragm: 80 percent effective; with proper use, 94 percent.

1. Functions by blocking external os and closing access to cervical canal by sperm. It is a mechanical barrier.

2. Must be used in conjunction with vaginal cream or jelly to be effective.

3. Toxic Shock Syndrome may occur; decrease risk by prompt removal 6–8 hours after intercourse and not using during menstruation.

4. Teach client signs of toxic shock: sudden onset of fever > 38.4°C (101.1°F), hypotension (orthostatic dizziness, systolic BP < 90), risk, fatigue, malaise.

C. Contraceptive sponge: 80–90 percent effective.

1. Inserted deep into vagina, sponge releases spermicide.

2. Leave in place for at least 6 hours after intercourse.

3. Decreases risk of STDs.

4. May be risk of developing toxic shock syndrome.

D. Cervical cap: 90 percent effective.

1. Rubber cap with spermicide placed over cervical opening.

2. May decrease risk of STD.

E. Intrauterine devices (IUDs): 95 percent effective.

1. Medicated with copper or progesterone.

a. Copper in place up to 10 years; damages sperm in transit to tubes, prevents fertilization.

b. Progesterone changes cervical mucus and endometrium to prevent fertilization.

c. More rapid transport of ovum through tube reaching endometrium before it is "ready" for implantation.

d. IUD may cause substances to accumulate in uterus and interfere with implantation.

e. IUD may stimulate production of cellular exudate, which interferes with the ability of sperm to migrate to fallopian tubes.

2. Usually made of soft plastic or nickel–chromium alloy.

3. Complications: perforation of uterus; infection: increased incidence of PID; spotting between periods; heavy menstrual flow or prolonged flow; and cramping during menstruation (less with progesterone IUD); allergic rash.

4. Disadvantages: increased risk of PID, need to check for presence of IUD (thread) after menstruation.

✦ Chemical Methods

A. Combined or Single Hormone contraceptive: 99 percent effective.

1. Contraceptive effect occurs by:

a. Artificially raising the blood levels of estrogen and/or progesterone, thereby causing inappropriate release or preventing the release of FSH and LH. Without FSH, the follicle does not mature and ovulation fails to take place.

    b. Endometrial changes.

    c. Alteration in cervical mucus, making it hostile to sperm.

    d. Altered tubal function.

2. Types of birth control pills.

    a. Combined: contains both estrogen and progesterone.

    b. Sequential (mimics normal hormonal cycle): estrogen given alone for 15–16 days, followed by combination of estrogen and progestin for the next 5 days.

    c. Progestin only (99+ percent effective; called mini-pill): inhibits ovulation, thickens and decreases amount of cervical mucus, thins endometrium and alters cilia action in fallopian tubes; contains less progestin and no estrogen so slightly less effective. Good option for women who can't take estrogen or who are over age 35 and smoke.

3. Other types of Combined Hormones.

    a. Injection: Lunelle given q 1 mo.

    b. Transdermal patch: q 1 week × 3.

    c. Vaginal ring: delivers hormones, worn for 3 weeks; self insertion.

4. Minor side effects, which usually diminish within a few months: breast fullness and tenderness; edema, weight gain; nausea and vomiting; chloasma; breakthrough bleeding; and mood changes.

✦ 5. More serious side effects: thrombophlebitis; pulmonary embolism; hypertension. Teach signs and symptoms: pain (chest/abdominal, leg), SOB, headache, dizziness, numbness, visual/speech problems.

6. Contraindications: pregnant, smokes > 20 cigarettes/day; > 35 years, has headaches or neurological symptoms; immobile or surgery on legs; BP > 160/100; diabetes of 20+ years with vascular disease.

B. Chemical agent: Nonoxynol-9 or octoxynol-9.

1. Agent acts by killing or paralyzing sperm; may kill STD agents.

2. Agent acts as a vehicle for spermicide as well as a mechanical barrier through which sperm cannot swim.

3. Available forms are foams, creams, jellies, or suppositories.

4. Should not use nonoxyl-9 if at risk for HIV.

✦ C. Implants: more than 99 percent effective.

1. *Norplant:* six capsules inserted under skin, which release progestin for up to 5 years, suppressing ovulation. Good option for women who are over age 35 and smoke.

2. *Depo-Provera:* IM injection of a progestin administered every 12 weeks. Suppresses ovulation.

D. Emergency Postcoital Contraception.

1. Within 72 hours of sex, a specific number of pills are taken to inhibit ovulation.

2. Copper T-380A IUD is inserted within 5–7 days after sex. Prevents implantation by creating a sterile inflammatory response.

Operative Sterilization Procedures

A. Vasectomy.

1. Surgical procedure with local anesthesia on outpatient basis.

    a. Incision made over ductus deferens on each side of scrotum; sperm ducts isolated and severed.

    b. Ends ligated, lumen coagulated, clipped or polyethylene tubing used with a stopcock for potential reversal.

✦ 2. Client instruction for care.

    a. Apply ice with pain or swelling.

    b. Use scrotal support for 1 week.

    c. Inform client that it takes 4–6 weeks and 3–36 ejaculations to clear sperm from ductus.

    d. Sperm samples (two or three) should be checked for sperm count.

    e. Client rechecked at 6 and 12 months to ensure fertility has not been restored by recanalization.

3. Possible side effects of procedure.

    a. Hematoma, sperm granulomas, and spontaneous reanastomosis.

    b. For those who wish to reverse process, 30–85 percent are successful.

B. Tubal ligation most common method (removal of uterus and ovaries is permanent method of sterilization).

1. Accomplished by abdominal or vaginal procedures; most common method is transection of fallopian tubes.

    a. Tubes are isolated, then crushed, ligated or plugged (newer reversible procedure).

    b. The postpartum and mini-laparotomy procedures require hospitalization.

    c. A newer procedure, laparoscopic sterilization, requires an incision at the umbilicus; the tube is coagulated and may be transected.

2. Complications of procedure include bowel perforation, infection, hemorrhage, and adverse anesthesia effects.

    a. Reversal of tubal ligations results in overall pregnancy rate of 15 percent.

b. Three-quarters of these pregnancies result in live births and 10 percent are tubal pregnancies.

THERAPEUTIC ABORTION

General Considerations

✦ A. Legality.
1. Abortion is now legal in all states as the result of a Supreme Court decision in January 1973.
2. It is regulated in the following manner.
   a. First trimester—decision between client and physician.
   b. Second trimester—decision between client and physician (state may regulate who performs the abortion and where it can be done).
   c. Third trimester—states may regulate and prohibit abortion except to preserve the health or life of the mother.
B. Indications.
1. *Medical:* psychiatric conditions or diseases such as chronic hypertension, nephritis, severe diabetes, cancer, or acute infection such as rubella; possible genetic defects in the infant or severe erythroblastosis fetalis.
2. *Nonmedical:* socioeconomic reasons, unmarried, financial burden, too young to care for infant, rape or incest.
C. Preparation of the individual.
1. Advise client of available sources of abortion.
2. Inform client as to what to expect from the abortion procedure.
3. Provide emotional support during decision-making period.
4. Maintain an open, nonjudgmental atmosphere in which the individual may express concerns or guilt.
5. Encourage and support the individual once the decision is made and after surgery.
6. Give information about contraceptives.
D. Complications and effects.
1. Abortion should be performed before the 12th week, if possible, because complications and risks are lower during this time.
2. Complications.
   a. Infection.
   b. Bleeding.
   c. Sterility.
   d. Uterine perforation.

Techniques

✦ A. First trimester.
1. Dilatation and curettage (D&C).
   a. Cervical canal is dilated with instruments of increasingly large diameter.
   b. Fetus and accessory structure is removed with forceps.
   c. Endometrium is scraped with curette to ensure that all products of conception are removed.
   d. Process usually takes 15–20 minutes.
2. Vacuum aspirator.
   a. Hose-linked curette is inserted into dilated cervix.
   b. Hose is attached to suction.
   c. The vacuum aspirator lessens the chance of uterine perforation, reduces blood loss, and reduces the time of the procedure.
   d. Laminaria tent (cone of dried seaweed): used after 8 weeks gestation helps to dilate cervix; reduces cervical laceration and bleeding during vacuum aspiration.
   e. Prostaglandin gel may also be used to soften the cervix.
3. Mifepristone (RU486)—antiprogestin hormone; can be used up to 9 weeks, more effective earlier; may be combined with a prostaglandin agent (misoprostol).
B. Second trimester.
1. Hysterotomy.
   a. Incision is made through abdominal wall into uterus.
   b. Procedure is usually performed between weeks 14 and 16 of pregnancy.
   c. Products of conception are removed with forceps.
   d. Uterine cavity is curetted.
   e. Tubal ligation may be done at same time.
   f. Client usually requires several days of hospitalization.
   g. Operation requires general or spinal anesthesia.
2. Intra-amniotic injection or amniocentesis abortion (used in less than 1% of all abortions).
   a. Performed after 14–16 weeks of pregnancy.
   b. From 50–200 mL of amniotic fluid are removed from the amniotic cavity and replaced with hypertonic solution of 20–50 percent saline instilled through gravity drip over a period of 45–60 minutes.
   c. Increased osmotic pressure of the amniotic fluid causes the death of the fetus.
   d. Uterine contractions usually begin in about 12 hours and the products of conception are expelled in 24–30 hours.
   e. Oxytocic drugs may be given if contractions do not begin.
   f. Complications.

(1) Infusion of hypertonic saline solution into uterus.

(2) Infection.

(3) Disseminated intravascular coagulation (DIC) disease may develop during procedure.

(4) Hemorrhage.

3. Prostaglandins (most common for 2nd trimester).

    a. These hormonelike acids cause abortion by stimulating the uterus to contract.

    b. May be administered in suppository form, as a gel, or by intrauterine injection.

Abortion Procedure

Assessment

A. Observe for excessive bleeding.

B. Assess for symptoms of infection.

C. Assess for hypernatremia in saline abortions.

D. Check for nausea and vomiting.

Implementation

A. Administer preoperative medications.

B. Ensure that client understands the procedure.

C. Offer emotional support and provide opportunity for client to express feelings.

D. Monitor IV.

E. Check vital signs pre- and postoperatively.

F. Administer pain medications as ordered.

G. Instruct client to watch for signs of excessive bleeding (more than a normal menstrual period) and infection (elevated temperature, foul-smelling discharge, persistent abdominal pain).

H. Administer oxytocic drug as ordered.

I. Administer RhoGAM as ordered for an Rh-negative client.

J. Offer fluids as tolerated, after vital signs are stable and client is alert and responsive.

K. Counsel regarding birth control methods.

L. Stress importance of followup visit to decrease risk of complications; often have a pregnancy test.

Appendix 12-1. COMMON DRUGS IN OBSTETRICS

Name of Drug and Action	Uses and Side Effects	Nursing Implications
Oxytocin, Syntocinon, Pitocin Classification: oxytocic; hormone Produces rhythmic contractions of uterine musculature Dosage: varies with method and purpose of administration. IV: 10–40 USP units in 1000 mL 5% dextrose in saline solution infused at rate 0.5–0.75 mL/min. Calibrated pump 2.5 USP units in 50 mL D$_5$W. Start at 1 mic/min and increase as necessary	Used to induce or augment labor, constrict uterus, and decrease hemorrhage after delivery and postabortion Stimulates contractile tissue in lactating breast to eject milk Side effects: water intoxication, allergic reactions, death due to uterine rupture, pelvic hematomas, bradycardia Excessive contractions more frequent than every 2–3 minutes, duration > 40–60 seconds, or intensity, > 90 mmHg (IUPC)	Observe for signs of sensitivity and overdose Monitor strength and duration of uterine contractions Check FHT every 15 minutes and PRN Take pulse and blood pressure every hour Contractions of 90 seconds with no resting period—stop infusion immediately and notify physician
Methergine Classification: oxytocic; ergot alkaloid Produces constrictive effects on smooth muscle of uterus (more prolonged constrictive effects as compared to rhythmic effects of oxytocin); has vasoconstrictive effect, especially on large arteries Usual IM dose: 0.2 mg; may be repeated in 2–4 hrs; usual oral dose 0.2 mg 3–4 × a day for 2 days	Used primarily after delivery to produce firm uterine contractions and decrease uterine bleeding May be used to prevent postabortal hemorrhage Side effects include nausea, vomiting, dizziness, increased blood pressure, dyspnea, and chest pain	Check blood pressure and pulse before administration of medication, and check vital signs frequently after administration; do not give if BP > 140/90 Injectable form deteriorates rapidly when exposed to light and heat; do not use if discoloration occurs Do not administer with Percodan—hallucinations
Hemabate Classification: oxytocic, prostaglandin Stimulates uterine contractions Used as a method of controlling hemorrhage Usual IM dose: 0.25 mg repeated up to maximum 5 doses, may be repeated q 15–90 min	Contol of refractory causes of postpartum hemorrhage caused by uterine atony; generally used after failed attempts at contol of hemorrhage with oxytoxic agents Side effects include nausea, vomiting, diarrhea, headache, flushing, bradycardia, bronchospasm, wheezing, cough, chills, and fever	Monitor BP, pulse, and respiratory status Administer in deep muscle mass, rotate sites Contraindicated in women with active cardiovascular, renal, liver disease, or asthma

Appendix 12-1. COMMON DRUGS IN OBSTETRICS (Continued)

Name of Drug and Action	Uses and Side Effects	Nursing Implications
Apresoline (hydralazine hydrochloride) Classification: antihypertensive Relaxes vascular smooth muscle, decreases peripheral vascular resistance and increases peripheral vasodilation Dosage: PO 12.5 mg BID, increased incrementally to maximum 100 mg BID	Use to lower blood pressure in severe preeclamsia Side effects: flushing, headache, nausea, vomiting, tachycardia, palpitations, lupus syndrome, and leukopenia	Monitor blood pressure and pulse rate Observe for orthostatic hypotension, tachycardia, palpitations, headache, dizziness, nausea, vomiting Give drug with meals to increase absorption
Magnesium Sulfate Depressive effects on central nervous system; decreases acetylcholine release—neuromuscular transmission of impulses in smooth, skeletal and cardiac muscle Produces peripheral vasodilation Given IV in preeclampsia and eclampsia; dosage varies Loading dose: 4 g in 250 mL D_5W at 5 mL/30 sec (approximately 20 min) or in continuous infusion; then 1–3 g/hr until contractions stop or therapeutic levels are maintained	Used to prevent convulsions in preeclampsia and eclampsia. Also tocolytic to treat preterm labor and uterine tetany Side effects: *Maternal:* warmth, flushing, hypotension, flaccidity, circulatory collapse, depression of CNS and cardiac system. *Fetal:* crosses placenta, lethargy, hypotonia Antidote: Calcium gluconate 10%. Keep 10-mL vial available at bedside	Observe carefully for signs of magnesium toxicity: extreme thirst, feeling hot all over; loss of patellar reflex, muscle weakness Monitor respirations (greater than 12/min), BP (hypotension), and P closely in order to assess effect of drug. Never leave client alone Patellar reflex should be checked frequently Check urine output continuously (greater than 30 mL/hr)
Ritodrine (Yutopar) Analog of beta-adrenergic agonist; alters calcium balance in cells and decreases contractility of smooth muscle, suppresses uterine contractions Usual initial dose is 0.1 mg/min using microdrip chamber at the recommended dilution Effective dose usually between 0.15 and 0.35 mg/min continued for 12 hours after uterine contractions cease Phase in PO dose	Treatment of premature labor or during labor when contractions are unusually frequent and not coordinated; most effective when given in early latent phase of labor; rarely stops active labor Side effects: nausea, vomiting, dizziness, transient hypotension, and tachycardia Hydrate woman prior to infusion with IV solution of 1000 mL normal saline Continuous monitoring (Swan–Ganz) of mother and infant important as mother–infant deaths have occurred	Take blood pressure and pulse every 5 minutes until stable Cardiac monitoring for IV route; notify physician if pulse over 120 Discontinue drug 6 hours before birth Arrhythmias: maintain bedrest—quiet environment Fowler's or side-lying position Monitor uterine activity and FHT Check for toxicity; CNS symptoms, dyspnea, cardiac irregularities; pulmonary edema Screen with ECG prior to beginning therapy Monitor hydration status carefully; limit fluids to 2400–3000 mL/day.
Terbutaline (Brethine) B_2 adrenergic agonist; stimulates B_2 receptors, relaxes smooth muscle of uterus and bronchus 0.25–0.5 mg sub q q1–4h until contractions stop; 5 mg PO maintenance dose	Relaxes uterus in preterm labor Also used for fetal distress to increase placental flow Side effects: tachycardia, palpitations, sweating, tremors, restlessness, lethargy, drowsiness, headache, nausea, vomiting	In addition to above, screen baseline glucose status and follow levels; follow urinary ketones; check for hypertension, muscle cramps, CNS symptoms indicating toxicity
Nifedipine Classification: calcium-channel blocker Reduces the flow of extracellular calcium ions into the intracellular space of the myometrial smooth muscle cells, thereby inhibiting contractile activity Usual dose: PO immediate release 10 mg TID; increase in 10-mg increments q4–6h, not to exceed 180 mg/24 hr Well absorbed either orally or sublingually	Used as a tocolytic Side effects include: hypotension, tachycardia, facial flushing, headache, and pulmonary edema	Monitor BP, pulse, and respiratory status. Encourage client to change position slowly. Instruct to notify nurse of dyspnea, edema of extremities, or nausea/vomiting

Appendix 12-2. RECOMMENDED DAILY DIETARY ALLOWANCES FOR PREGNANCY AND LACTATION

	Pregnancy		Lactation		Function	Sources
	14 to 18	Adult	14 to 18	Adult		
Calories	2400	2300	2600	2500	Meet increased nutritional needs as well as body maintenance	All foods. Important to emphasize values of food groups and avoid empty calories
Protein g	60	60	65	65	Augment maternal tissues—breasts, uterus, blood Growth and development of placenta and fetal tissue Constant repair and maintenance of maternal tissue	All essential amino acids may be found in milk, meat, eggs, and cheeses Other sources, though not complete protein by themselves: tofu, whole grains, legumes, nuts, peanut butter
Iron mg	30+	30+	*	*	Essential constituent of hemoglobin Part of various enzymes Fetal development and storage, especially later part of pregnancy	Good sources: liver, kidney, heart, cooked dry beans, lean pork and beef, dried fruits such as apricots, peaches, prunes, and raisins Fair sources: spinach, mustard greens, eggs
Calcium mg	1200	1200	1200	1200	Skeletal tissue Bones; teeth Blood coagulation Neuromuscular irritability Myocardial function Fetal stores, especially last months	Good sources: milk, cheese, ice cream, yogurt Fair sources: broccoli, canned salmon with bones, dried beans, dark leafy vegetables
Magnesium mg	320	320	355	355	Cellular metabolism Structural growth	Whole grains, milk, nuts, dark green vegetables, legumes
Phosphorus mg	1200	1200	1200	1200	90 percent compounded with calcium. Rest distributed throughout cells—involved in energy production, building and repairing tissue, buffering	Whole-grain items: cereals, whole-wheat bread, brown rice; milk
Sodium g	0.5	0.5	0.5	0.5	Metabolic activities Fluid balance and acid–base balance Cell permeability Muscle irritability	Table salt, meat, eggs, carrots, celery, beets, spinach, salted nuts, carbonated beverages
Iodine μg	175	175	200	200	Necessary for health: mother and fetus; prevents goiter in mother; decreases chance of cretinism in infants	Iodized table salt, cod liver oil
Vitamin A IU	5000	5000	6000	6000	Tooth formation and skeletal growth Cell growth and development Integrity of epithelial tissue Vision—light/dark adaptation Fat metabolism	Good sources: butter, egg yolk, fortified margarine, whole milk, cream, kidney, and liver Fair sources: dark green and yellow vegetables such as sweet potatoes, pumpkins, mustard greens, collards, kale, bok choy, carrots, cantaloupe, apricots

Appendix 12-2. RECOMMENDED DAILY DIETARY ALLOWANCES (*Continued*)

| | Pregnancy | | Lactation | | Function | Sources |
	14 to 18	Adult	14 to 18	Adult		
Riboflavin mg	1.4	1.4	1.6	1.6	Enzyme systems Tissue functioning Tissue oxygenation and respiration Energy metabolism Excreted in breastmilk	Good sources: kidney, liver, heart, milk Fair sources: cheese, ice cream, dark leafy vegetables, lean meat, poultry
Thiamine mg	1.4	1.4	1.4	1.4	Carbohydrate metabolism Normal appetite and digestion Health of nervous system	Good sources: enriched and whole-grain products—bread and cereals, dried peas, beans, liver, heart, kidney, nuts, potatoes, lean pork Fair sources: eggs, milk, poultry, fish, vegetables
Niacin mg	18	18	17	17	Cell metabolism	Good sources: fish, lean meat, poultry, liver, heart, peanuts, peanut butter Fair sources: enriched and whole-grain cereals and bread, milk, potatoes
Folic acid (folate) mg	600	600	500	500	Cell growth Important to prevent neural tube defect Enzyme activities in production of protein Deficiency results in megaloblastic anemia	Dark green and leafy vegetables, liver, peanuts, whole-grain cereals
Vitamin B_{12} mg	2.6	2.6	2.8	2.8	Deficiency may be found in vegans and pernicious anemia	Found only in animal sources
Pyridoxine B_6 mg	1.9	1.9	2.0	2.0	Essential coenzyme with amino acids Deficiency may lead to hypochromic microcytic anemia	Animal and vegetable protein such as meat, fish, beans, nuts and seeds, milk and milk products
Vitamin D IU	500	500	500	500	Influences absorption, retention, and utilization of calcium and phosphorus Formation of bones, teeth, and other tissue	Good sources: fortified milk, butter, egg yolk, liver, fish oils
Vitamin C Ascorbic acid mg	80	85	115	120	Production of intracellular substances necessary for development and maintenance of normal connective tissue in bones, cartilage, and muscles Role in metabolic processes involving protein and tissues Increases absorption of iron	Good sources: citrus fruits and juice, broccoli, cantaloupe, collards, mustard and turnip greens, peppers Fair sources: asparagus, raw cabbage, other melons, spinach, prunes, tomatoes, canned or fresh chilies

* Iron needs during lactation are not different from those of a nonpregnant female (18 mg/day taken with vitamin C to increase assimilation), but continued supplementation following birth is important to replenish iron stores depleted by pregnancy.

Appendix 12-3. NUTRITIONAL GUIDELINES FOR PREGNANCY

A. Influences on dietary habits and nutrition.
1. Food—many emotional connotations originating in infancy.
2. Eating habits influenced by:
   a. Emotional factors.
   b. Cultural factors.
   c. Religious beliefs.
   d. Nutritional information.
   e. Age—especially adolescent and aged.
   f. Physical health.
   g. Personal preferences.
B. Nutritional needs in pregnancy.
1. Influenced by above factors.
2. Must supply caloric and nutritional needs of mother as well as promote optimum fetal growth.
3. May be complicated by:
   a. Poor maternal nutrition before pregnancy.
   b. Medical complications prior to pregnancy (diabetes, anemia).
   c. Complications resulting from pregnancy (toxemia, anemia).
   d. Pica (cravings).
C. Weight gain in pregnancy.
1. Recommendations based on pre-pregnancy weight for height:
   Normal: 11.5–16 kg (25.3–32.2#).
   Underweight: 12.5–18 kg (27.5–39.6#).
   Overweight: 7–11.5 kg (15.4–25.3#).
2. Weight gain during 2nd and 3rd trimesters.
   Normal: 0.4 kg/week (0.88#).
   Underweight: 0.5 kg/week (1.1#).
   Overweight: 0.3 kg/week (0.66#).
✦ 3. Weight gain accounted by

Product of conception	**Pounds**
Fetus—average size	7–8
Placenta	2–2.5
Amniotic fluid	2
Uterus	2
Breasts	1–4
Extracellular fluid	3–5
Blood volume	4–5
	21–30.5 pounds

   b. Rest of weight gain deposited as fat stores or fluid representing energy stored for lactation.
D. Revised daily food guide.
1. This revised daily guide meets RDA standards for daily nutrients except for:
   a. Iron and folacin—cannot be ingested in sufficient quantities by dietary means. Must be supplemented during pregnancy.
✦ b. 300 additional calories needed to meet recommended allowances.
2. Protein intake includes both animal and vegetable protein.
   a. Vegetable protein may be omitted in those whose income will allow by increasing animal servings to three 3-oz. servings.
   b. One serving at least should be red meats.
3. Whole grain items are better choices than leavened breads and cereals. They contain more magnesium, zinc, folacin, and vitamin B_6.
4. At least 2 tablespoons of fat or oils should be consumed daily for vitamin E and essential fatty acids.
E. Special diets.
1. Adolescents.
   a. Have high proportion of low-birth-weight infants.
   b. Dietary habits often poor. Plan menu to include necessary items around foods they like.
   c. Stress balanced diet—avoid empty calories.
2. Low sodium.
   a. Presently sodium restriction is *deemphasized*.
   b. Sodium essential in maintaining increased body fluids needed for adequate placental flow, increased tissue requirements, and renal blood flow.
   c. If moderate salt intake is necessitated, avoid highly salted foods such as canned soups, potato chips, soda pop.
3. Weight control.
   a. Presently, weight loss in pregnancy is discouraged.
   b. Even obese client should gain 15–25 pounds to ensure adequate nutrition for fetal growth.
   c. Strict dieting may lead to ketosis which has proven harmful to fetal brain development.
   d. Stress careful dietary planning to include essential nutrients and avoid empty calories.
   e. Weight reduction program should begin *after* lactation only.
✦ 4. Vegetarians.
   a. Sound nutritional planning to include those combinations of foods, which, when combined, include all essential amino acids. May require iron and zinc.
   b. May require B-complex supplement, especially vitamin B_{12}, which comes only from animal sources.

MATERNAL-NEWBORN NURSING REVIEW QUESTIONS

1. When late decelerations are noted by the nurse, the first action is to

   1. Notify the physician STAT.
   2. Position the client on her left side.
   3. Administer oxygen via face mask.
   4. Increase the drip rate of the intravenous fluid.

2. In assessing a client with potential eclampsia, which cardinal symptom will the nurse assess for?

   1. Weight gain of one pound a week.
   2. Concentrated urine.
   3. Hypertension.
   4. Feeling of lassitude and fatigue.

3. The nurse would anticipate a possible complication in infants delivered by cesarean section. This condition would be

   1. Respiratory distress.
   2. Renal impairment.
   3. ABO incompatibility.
   4. Kernicterus.

4. If a client experiences a ruptured ectopic pregnancy, an expected sign or symptom would be

   1. Elevated blood glucose levels.
   2. Sudden excruciating pain in lower abdomen.
   3. Sudden hypertension.
   4. Extensive external bleeding.

5. A client who is 34 weeks pregnant has just been admitted to the labor room in the first stage of labor. Which of the following clinical manifestations would be considered abnormal and would be reported to the physician immediately?

   1. Expulsion of a blood-tinged mucous plug.
   2. Continuous contraction of 2 minutes duration.
   3. Feeling of pressure on perineum causing her to bear down.
   4. Expulsion of clear fluid from the vagina.

6. An eclamptic client has been receiving magnesium sulfate IV 2g/hour. What symptom would indicate that the current dose can be continued?

   1. Absence of deep tendon reflexes.
   2. A respiratory rate of 16 per minute.

3. Urine output of 50 mL over the last 4 hours.
   4. Heart skipping a beat.

7. An 11 lb. 6 oz. baby girl was delivered by cesarean section to a diabetic mother. The priority assessment of the infant of a diabetic mother would be for

   1. Hypoglycemia.
   2. Sepsis.
   3. Hyperglycemia.
   4. Hypercalcemia.

8. Which of the following conditions is not a result of metabolic error in the fetus?

   1. Phenylketonuria.
   2. Maple syrup urine disease.
   3. Glutamic-acidemia.
   4. Pyloric stenosis.

9. Identify which fetal heart rate pattern shows premature rupture of the membranes on the fetal monitoring rhythm strip.

   1. Early deceleration.
   2. Normal fetal heart rate pattern.
   3. Late deceleration.
   4. Variable deceleration.

10. If you observe the fetal heart rate pattern above, the priority intervention would be to

    1. Do nothing because it is a normal heart rate pattern.
    2. Change the position of the mother until pattern is corrected.
    3. Increase the IV fluids.
    4. Notify healthcare provider immediately.

11. The nurse's understanding of fetal position is that when the baby's head is at station 0 it means that the

    1. Sagittal sutures can be felt in the left posterior position.
    2. Biparietal diameter of the head has passed the outlet.
    3. Posterior fontanels are first palpable.
    4. Level of the head is felt at the ischial spines.

12. A client is gravida 3 para 2 and is in a labor room. After a vaginal exam, it is determined that the presenting head is at station +3. The appropriate nursing action is to

1. Continue to observe the client's contractions.
2. Check the fetal heart rate for a prolapsed cord.
3. Prepare for delivery of the baby.
4. Check with the physician to see if an oxytocin drip is warranted.

13. Pelvic inflammatory disease (PID) is an inflammatory condition of the pelvic cavity and may involve the ovaries, tubes, vascular system, or pelvic peritoneum. The nurse explains to the client that the most common cause of PID is

    1. *M. tuberculosis.*
    2. *Streptococcus.*
    3. *Staphylococcus.*
    4. Gonorrhea.

14. The nurse has just come on duty and is assigned to care for a newborn, born 2 hours ago, who is in an isolette. The nurse checks the temperature of the isolette. In making an assessment, the nurse will know the temperature is too high if the infant's

    1. Pulse is decreased.
    2. Temperature is 101°F rectally.
    3. Temperature is 99.4°F rectally.
    4. Respirations are decreased.

15. As the nurse walks into the newborn nursery, she sees a baby in respiratory distress from apparent mucus. The first nursing action is to

    1. Carefully slap the infant's back.
    2. Thump the chest and start cardiopulmonary resuscitation.
    3. Pick the baby up by the feet and lower the head.
    4. Call the code team.

16. A client, 18 weeks pregnant, is concerned because she had a fever and rash about 2½ weeks ago. The nurse's best response is

    1. "It's best to talk with the physician about that."
    2. "It's unlikely the fetus would have been affected as the first trimester is the most important time."
    3. "What do you think the problems are with that?"
    4. "Are you thinking you may have to terminate the pregnancy?"

17. A 14-year-old came to the clinic for a birth control method. She sat through the class that describes the methods available to her. After class, she asked the nurse, "Which method is best for me to use?" The best response is

    1. "You are so young, are you sure you are ready for the responsibilities of a sexual relationship?"
    2. "Because of your age, we need your parents' consent before you can be examined and then we'll talk."
    3. "Before I can help you with that question, I need to know more about your sexual activity."
    4. "The physician can best help you with that after your physical examination."

18. In assessing a newborn infant, the nurse knows that postmature infants may exhibit

    1. Heavy vernix, little lanugo.
    2. Large size for gestational age.
    3. Increased subcutaneous fat, absent creases on feet.
    4. Small size for gestational age.

19. A primigravida, age 36, delivered an 8 lb. 6 oz. baby girl by cesarean section. Which one of the following nursing actions would *not* be included in the client's immediate postoperative care?

    1. Taking vital signs q 15 min for 2 to 3 hours.
    2. Checking lochia for amount and color q 15 min for 2–3 hours.
    3. Assisting the client to turn, cough, and deep-breathe.
    4. Offering oral fluids q 15 min for 2–3 hours.

20. A client is brought to the maternity unit by her husband. She went into labor at home and, when the contractions were 4 minutes apart and regular, her physician told her to come to the hospital. Her membranes ruptured spontaneously. All of the following actions are appropriate; the *first* nursing action is to

    1. Check the fetal heart rate.
    2. Check the color of fluid.
    3. Assess the quantity of fluid.
    4. Notify the physician.

21. A new mother of a 3-week-old infant comes to the clinic complaining of feeling down, sad, having no energy and wanting to cry. The priority intervention is to

    1. Notify the family that the mother needs more support.
    2. Spend extra time talking to the mother to help her express her feelings.
    3. Notify the physician for medication.
    4. Identify postpartum depression so that appropriate interventions may be made.

22. An appropriate nursing intervention to help a nursing mother care for cracked nipples would be

    1. Applying benzoin to toughen the nipples.
    2. Keeping the nipples covered with warm, moist packs.
    3. Offering to give the baby a bottle.
    4. Rub hind milk on nipples.

23. A client is very concerned because her 1-day-old son, who was very alert at birth, is now sleeping most of the time. The nursing response would be

    1. "Most infants are alert at birth and then require 24–48 hours of deep sleep to recover from the birth experience."
    2. "Your son's behavior is slightly abnormal and bears careful observation."
    3. "Would you like the pediatrician to check him to ease your mind?"
    4. "Your son's behavior is definitely abnormal, and we should keep him in the nursery."

24. During a physical exam of an infant with congenital hip dysplasia, the nurse would observe and report which of the following characteristics?

    1. Symmetrical gluteal folds.
    2. Limited adduction of the affected leg.
    3. Femoral pulse when the hip is flexed and the leg is abducted.
    4. Limited abduction of the affected leg.

25. A neonatal nurse would be aware that small-for-gestational-age (SGA) infants are more likely to develop which of the following neonatal conditions?

    1. Hyperthermia.
    2. Hyperglycemia.
    3. Respiratory distress.
    4. Hypothermia.

26. When the mother of a new baby asks the nurse to feed her baby, the most appropriate response is to say

    1. "I'll feed him today. Maybe tomorrow you can try it."
    2. "It's not difficult at all. He is just like a normal baby, only smaller."
    3. "You can learn to feed him as well as I can; I wasn't good when I first fed a premature infant either."
    4. "It's frightening sometimes to feed an infant this small, but I'll stay with you to help."

27. A client has just delivered her first baby. Hyperbilirubinemia is anticipated because of Rh incompatibility. Hyperbilirubinemia occurs with Rh incompatibility between mother and fetus because

    1. The mother's blood does not contain the Rh factor, so she produces anti-Rh antibodies that cross the placental barrier and cause hemolysis of red blood cells in infants.
    2. The mother's blood contains the Rh factor and the infant's does not, and antibodies that destroy red blood cells are formed in the fetus.
    3. The mother has a history of previous jaundice caused by a blood transfusion, which was passed to the fetus through the placenta.
    4. The infant develops a congenital defect shortly after birth that causes the destruction of red blood cells.

28. The nurse is caring for a mother who requires RhoGAM. What is the condition that must be present for the globulin to be effective after RhoGAM is given?

    1. Mother is Rh positive.
    2. Baby is Rh negative.
    3. Mother has no titer in her blood.
    4. Mother has some titer in her blood.

29. A client in her 36th week of pregnancy is admitted to the maternity unit in an effort to control the further development of eclampsia. She is assigned to a private room. The best rationale for this room assignment is that

    1. The client is financially able to afford it.
    2. The client would be disturbed if placed in a room where another mother was in active labor.
    3. A quiet, darkened room is important to reduce external stimuli.
    4. A rigid regimen is an important aspect of eclamptic care.

30. As part of the prenatal teaching, the nurse instructs the client to immediately report any visual disturbances. The best rationale for this instruction is that the symptom is

    1. A forerunner to preeclampsia.
    2. Indicative of increased intracranial pressure.
    3. A sign of malnutrition.
    4. Indicative of renal failure.

31. Instructing the client about her nutritional needs during pregnancy, the nurse tells her that she will have an increased need for

    1. Simple carbohydrates.
    2. Fat.
    3. High-carbohydrate foods.
    4. Iron.

32. A client delivered a 34-week, 1550-g female infant. The infant demonstrates nasal flaring, intercostal retraction, expiratory grunt, and slight cyanosis. The nurse will place the infant in a heated isolette because

    1. The infant has a small body surface for her weight.
    2. Heat increases flow of oxygen to extremities.
    3. Her temperature control mechanism is immature.
    4. Heat within the isolette facilitates drainage of mucus.

33. The nurses caring for a premature baby use careful hand hygiene techniques because they know premature infants are more susceptible to infection than full-term infants. Which of the following explains why premature infants are more likely to develop infection?

    1. Their liver enzymes are immature.
    2. Premature babies may receive steroid drugs, which affect the immune system.
    3. Premature infants receive few antibodies from the mother, because antibodies pass across the placenta during the last month of pregnancy.
    4. Surfactant is decreased in premature infants.

34. In the delivery room, a client has just delivered a healthy 7-pound baby boy. The physician instructs the nurse to suction the baby. The procedure the nurse would use is to

    1. Suction the nose first.
    2. Suction the mouth first.
    3. Suction neither the nose nor mouth until the physician gives further instructions.
    4. Turn the baby on his side so mucus will drain out before suctioning.

35. While assessing a postpartum client, the nurse observes signs and symptoms of infection. A specific clinical manifestation of infection would be

    1. Dark red lochia.
    2. Bradycardia.
    3. Discomfort and tenderness of the abdomen.
    4. Generalized rash.

36. A 24-year-old client who has just learned she is pregnant tells the nurse that she smokes one pack of cigarettes a day. In counseling, the nurse encourages her to stop smoking because studies show that newborns of mothers who smoke are often

    1. Premature and have respiratory distress syndrome.
    2. Small for gestational age.
    3. Large for gestational age.
    4. Born with congenital abnormalities.

37. The symptoms of respiratory distress syndrome (RDS) are present in a premature baby. The nurse understands that this condition is caused by

    1. Increased amount of vasodilatation in the lungs as a result of decreased oxygenation.
    2. Small surface area of the premature's lungs preventing gas exchange.
    3. Decrease in the production of surfactant in the infant's lungs, leading to alveolar collapse.
    4. Increase in the amount of surfactant in the infant's lungs, preventing alveolar expansion.

38. After a prolonged labor and lack of progress past a dilation of 8 cm, the client had a cesarean delivery. She and her partner express their disappointment that they did not have a natural childbirth. The best response is to say

    1. "Most couples who have an unplanned cesarean birth feel cheated and disappointed."
    2. "You know that at least you have a healthy baby."
    3. "Maybe next time you can have a vaginal delivery."
    4. "You will be able to resume sex sooner than if you had delivered vaginally."

39. Evaluating the mother and her infant's interaction and bonding relationship in the postpartum period is an important nursing function. An indication of an unhealthy mother–infant relationship is when the mother

    1. Identifies infant characteristics that are similar to her husband's.
    2. Refuses to go to a bath demonstration.
    3. Describes only the infant's negative qualities.
    4. Asks to skip a feeding to sleep.

40. A client who is 36 weeks pregnant is having a Contraction Stress Test. After 35 minutes, her uterus begins to contract, and the nurse observes three 40-second-long contractions in a 10-minute period. She has two contractions within 5 minutes, and her

uterus remains contracted after the second contraction. The first nursing action is to

1. Turn off the oxytocin (Pitocin).
2. Administer oxygen by mask.
3. Turn her on her left side.
4. Assess the fetal heart rate.

41. Oxygen and humidity are part of the treatment for premature infants. The statement that best describes the purpose of this treatment is that it

1. Is necessary because premature infants have a depressed Moro reflex.
2. Facilitates perfusion of the kidney to clear blood wastes more quickly.
3. Helps the infant adjust better to the early transition of extrauterine life.
4. Assists the immature respiratory system with systemic oxygenation.

42. A diabetic client who is pregnant asks about breastfeeding. The most accurate response regarding breastfeeding by diabetic mothers is that it is

1. Contraindicated because insulin is passed to the infant through the milk.
2. Not contraindicated, but the diabetic's milk production and mechanism may be faulty.
3. Contraindicated because it puts too much stress on the mother's body.
4. Not contraindicated, but encouraged.

43. A new mother is concerned because her physician said that her baby had jaundice. The nurse understands that jaundice is a (an)

1. Normal condition that appears at 2 to 3 days of life.
2. Normal condition that appears 8 to 24 hours after birth.
3. Abnormal condition that appears within the first 24 hours of life.
4. Abnormal condition that appears at 2 to 3 days of life.

44. A newly pregnant client who is a little overweight asks how much weight she should gain over the 9 months. The most appropriate answer is

1. "For your size, a little heavy, 15–25 pounds would be best."
2. "It really doesn't matter exactly how much weight you gain, as long as your diet is healthy."
3. "A gain of about 25–35 pounds is best for mother and baby."

4. "Because you are a little overweight, it would be best for you not to gain too much weight."

45. The term *dizygotic* refers to twins who have

1. Developed from two ova and two sperms.
2. Been born several hours apart from each other.
3. Developed physically at different rates from each other.
4. Developed in one amnion and have one chorion.

46. A client is 3 days postpartum. Her vital signs are stable; her fundus is three fingerbreadths below the umbilicus, and her lochia rubra is moderate. Her breasts are hard and warm to the touch. The nurse would evaluate that the client

1. Is showing early signs of breast infection.
2. Is normal for 3 days postpartum.
3. Needs ice packs applied to her breasts.
4. Should remove her nursing bra to reduce discomfort.

47. On the first day postpartum for a new mother, the nurse observes that she appears frightened and says, "The baby has been breathing funny, fast and slow, off and on." The most appropriate nursing response would be

1. "That's normal when the baby breast-feeds."
2. "There's nothing to worry about. I'm going to take the baby back to the nursery and we'll check him out."
3. "I'll watch the baby for a while to see if there is something wrong."
4. "Don't be frightened. It's a normal breathing pattern. I'll sit here while you finish feeding him."

48. An amniocentesis is performed for genetic cell analysis. The nurse counsels the client that this test cannot be performed until 14 weeks' gestation because

1. This is when the heartbeat is first heard.
2. The fetus is not mature enough until this time.
3. There is not enough amniotic fluid until this time.
4. The genetic results will not be accurate until this time.

49. A serology test for syphilis is given to pregnant women. The nurse explains to the client that the reason this test is given is because

1. Latent syphilis becomes highly active during pregnancy due to hormonal changes.
2. Syphilis may be passed to the fetus after 4 months of pregnancy.

3. Syphilis is no longer a problem, but the law still requires the serology test.
4. Syphilis may be passed to the infant during delivery.

50. A client is rushed to the emergency room. As she is admitted, her membranes rupture, and the baby's head is crowning. She wants to push. The nursing instructions would be to

1. Go ahead and push to assist delivery.
2. Pant to avoid rapid delivery.
3. Close her eyes and count to 20 before pushing.
4. Breathe naturally and allow the baby to deliver at its own pace.

MATERNAL-NEWBORN NURSING

Answers with Rationale

1. (2) Late decelerations are from decreased blood perfusion to the placenta or compression of the placenta. A position change should increase perfusion or decrease compression. The second action may be to give oxygen (3) as a palliative measure to increase oxygen concentration of whatever blood does get to the placenta. Both are treatments for late deceleration, but the nursing action is to change position first.

NP:I; CN:PH; CL:A

2. (3) High blood pressure is one of the cardinal symptoms of toxemia or eclampsia along with excessive weight gain, edema, and albumin in the urine.

NP:A; CN:H; CL:AN

3. (1) During a normal birth, the fetus passes through the birth canal and pressure on the chest helps rid the fetus of amniotic fluid that has accumulated in the lungs. The baby delivered by cesarean section does not go through this process and therefore may develop respiratory problems.

NP:E; CN:PH; CL:A

4. (2) In a ruptured ectopic pregnancy, there may be signs of shock, excruciating pain, and minimal bleeding. There should be no effect on blood glucose levels (1).

NP:A; CN:PH; CL:C

5. (2) A uterus that is contracted for more than 1 full minute is a sign of tetany, which could lead to uterine rupture. This symptom must be reported to the physician immediately so interventions can be initiated. The other answers are all normal conditions, which occur with labor. The client should be cautioned against bearing down this early as it is not effective and can cause edema of the cervix.

NP:A; CN:H; CL:A

6. (2) The respiratory rate must be maintained at a rate of at least 12 per minute as a precaution against excessive depression of impulses at the myoneural junction. When deep tendon reflexes are absent (1) and the urine output is decreased (3), the medication should be held to prevent complications of depression of the CNS. If the client is complaining of irregular heartbeat (4), she is experiencing a sign of magnesium toxicity.

NP:E; CN:H; CL:A

7. (1) Infants of diabetic mothers are prone to develop hypoglycemia, respiratory distress, and hypocalcemia. The infant of a diabetic mother may develop sepsis (2), but usually from a cause unrelated to the diabetes itself. Hyperbilirubinemia is also fairly common in these infants.

NP:A; CN:H; CL:A

8. (4) This is an example of a congenital abnormality and does not fall into the category of a metabolic or biochemical disorder. Phenylketonuria (1) is an inability to metabolize the amino acid, phenylalanine; maple syrup urine disease (2) is defective metabolism of branched chain keto acids; glutamic-acidemia (3) is an increase in total amino nitrogen.

NP:AN; CN:PH; CL:K

9. (4) Variable deceleration is usually a result of premature rupture of membranes and decreased amniotic fluid. Different accelerations indicate the status of fetal well-being.

NP:E; CN:H; CL:A

10. (2) Changing position will relieve pressure on the umbilical cord which will change the fetal heart rate. Later interventions may include increasing IV fluids and administering oxygen. Doing nothing is not a therapeutic intervention because the underlying cause

---

Coding for Questions/Answers Abbreviations: **Nursing Process: NP,** Assessment: A, Analysis: AN, Planning: P, Implementation: I, Evaluation: E; **Client Needs: CN,** Safe, Effective Care Environment: S, Health Promotion and Maintenance: H, Psychosocial Integrity: PS, Physiological Integrity: PH; **Clinical Area: CA,** Medical Nursing: M, Surgical Nursing: S, Maternal/Newborn Nursing: MA, Pediatric Nursing: P, Psychiatric Nursing: PS; **Cognitive Level: CL,** Knowledge: K, Comprehension: C, Application: A, Analysis: AN.

must be determined. Notifying the healthcare provider would be appropriate for a late deceleration.

NP:I; CN:H; CL:AN

11. (4) The head is at station 0 when it is felt at the level of the ischial spines. Levels above the ischial spines are referred to as minus: −1, −2, −3. Levels below the ischial spines are referred to as plus: +1, +2, +3.

NP:AN; CN:H; CL:C

12. (3) If the head is +3, it is just about crowning, and because the client is a multipara, it would be reasonable to assume delivery is imminent. Answers (1) and (4) are not appropriate nursing actions and answer (2) is wrong because there are no data suggesting a prolapsed cord.

NP:I; CN:H; CL:A

13. (4) Gonorrhea accounts for 65 to 75 percent of all cases of PID. *Streptococcus* (2), *staphylococcus* (3), and *Myobacterium tuberculosis* (1) are less frequent causes.

NP:I; CN:H; CL:K

14. (2) If the infant's temperature is 101°F rectally, the nurse will know this is too high and that the isolette temperature has been set too high. Overheating an infant can lead to an increased need for oxygen and an increased respiratory rate; this, in turn, may lead to hypoglycemia and acidosis.

NP:A; CN:H; CL:A

15. (3) The airway must be cleared before anything else can help. Of the choices, picking the baby up by the feet is the best for clearing the airway by creating a gravity or postural drainage situation.

NP:I; CN:H; CL:AN

16. (3) Although the first trimester is the danger period with German measles, the nurse should first ascertain the client's concerns before she gives any direction. Answer (4) is putting words in the client's mouth.

NP:I; CN:H; CL:A

17. (3) Consultation with a client on the best form of birth control for her is dependent on the frequency of intercourse, number of partners, and her own motivation and reliability. The other responses cut off the client and do not form a therapeutic relationship.

NP:I; CN:H; CL:A

18. (4) Babies that are postmature often look as though they have lost weight. They exhibit long nails, little subcutaneous fat, and the skin is very dry. Often, meconium is stained green or yellow.

NP:A; CN:H; CL:K

19. (4) Oral fluids are usually withheld after surgery until normal conscious levels are reached and bowel sounds are heard. Giving oral fluids before normal consciousness returns can lead to vomiting and aspiration. A cesarean section is also considered a surgical procedure, and normal postop as well as postpartum care should be given.

NP:P; CN:H; CL:A

20. (1) The fetal heart rate needs to be checked first to determine whether the cord is prolapsed. The cord has an increased possibility of prolapsing when the membranes rupture. Following this, the nurse would observe the fluid (2, 3) and notify the physician (4).

NP:I; CN:H; CL:A

21. (4) This answer is more comprehensive than any of the others because it includes them. It is very important to identify postpartum depression to prevent possible injury or suicide. The mother may or may not require medication, but it is necessary to intervene now. The majority of postpartum depression conditions appear around the 4th postpartum week.

NP:I; CN:PS; CL:AN

22. (4) Keeping the nipples moist and soft with hind milk is the best treatment. Massé cream or pure lanolin may be applied sparingly but never harsh agents such as benzoin (1) or alcohol. Teach the mother to use general hygiene practices—wash the breasts once daily; do not use soap as it removes natural oils. To prevent further problems with engorgement, bottles (3) should not be offered.

NP:I; CN:H; CL:A

23. (1) Normally most newborns are alert at birth and then require deep sleep to recover from the birth experience. This should be explained first, and then if the client is still concerned, the nurse could offer to have the pediatrician talk to her.

NP:I; CN:H; CL:A

24. (4) Abduction is limited in the affected leg. The nurse would also find asymmetrical gluteal folds and an absent femoral pulse when the affected leg is abducted.

NP:A; CN:H; CL:A

25. (4) A large proportion of body surface to body weight increases susceptibility to hypothermia. These infants are also more prone to hypoglycemia. Postmature infants are most likely to develop respiratory distress.

NP:AN; CN:H; CL:K

26. (4) The nurse, while recognizing and accepting this mother's apprehension, assures her that she will have assistance and gives her confidence to feed the baby while remaining with her. This is good client teaching.

NP:I; CN:H; CL:A

27. (1) Rh antigens from the fetus enter the bloodstream of the mother, causing the production of anti-Rh antibodies in the mother. These anti-Rh antibodies cross the placenta, enter the fetal circulation, and cause hemolysis. The red blood cells are destroyed and broken down faster than the products of hemolysis, including bilirubin, can be excreted. Serum bilirubin rises quickly.

NP:AN; CN:H; CL:C

28. (3) RhoGAM will not work if there is any titer in the blood; thus it is important to administer it within 72 hours after delivery or abortion if the mother shows no evidence of antibody production. The mother would be Rh negative and the baby Rh positive for RhoGAM to be needed.

NP:AN; CN:PH; CL:A

29. (3) An important aspect of the treatment of pre-eclampsia is absolute quiet, and only a private room could accomplish this objective.

NP:P; CN:H; CL:A

30. (1) Visual disturbance is a symptom of preeclampsia, and the client must immediately be put under a physician's care to prevent further development of eclampsia.

NP:P; CN:H; CL:A

31. (4) During pregnancy, there is an increased need for iron, calories, protein, calcium, and other minerals and vitamins. A high-fat (2), high-carbohydrate diet (3) is not recommended because it may cause excessive weight gain and fat deposits, which are difficult to lose after pregnancy.

NP:I; CN:H; CL:A

32. (3) The premature infant has poor body control of temperature and needs immediate attention to keep from losing heat. Reasons for heat loss include little subcutaneous fat and poor insulation, large body surface for weight, immaturity of temperature control, and lack of activity.

NP:AN; CN:H; CL:A

33. (3) Deficient antibodies can lead to infection in the premature. Immaturity of the liver (1) is responsible for hyperbilirubinemia. White cell count would be related to potential infection. Lack of surfactant (4) occurs in prematures who have RDS.

NP:AN; CN:H; CL:C

34. (2) It is important to suction the mouth first. If the nose were to be suctioned first (1), stimulation of the delicate receptors in the nose could cause the infant to aspirate mucus from the mouth.

NP:P; CN:H; CL:A

35. (3) The major symptoms of infection would be rapid pulse, foul-smelling lochia or discharge, and discomfort and tenderness of the abdomen. A generalized rash (4) would not be a sign of postpartum infection but would indicate a virus infection, such as measles, or an allergic reaction to a medication or food. A rash should never be ignored; rather, it should be charted and its cause investigated.

NP:A; CN:H; CL:A

36. (2) Women who smoke have almost twice the chance of delivering a low-birth-weight infant (less than 2500 g) than nonsmokers.

NP:I; CN:H; CL:K

37. (3) An adequate amount of surfactant is necessary to keep the alveoli expanded. A decrease in the amount of surfactant results in alveolar collapse, atelectasis, and RDS.

NP:E; CN:H; CL:C

38. (1) It is important to recognize their grief and let them know it's normal. They need to work through their grief before they can cope with other information.

NP:I; CN:PS; CL:A

39. (3) An unhealthy relationship may be developing if the mother cannot find any good qualities to describe. Identification of family characteristics (1) is usually a sign of healthy attachment. The mother's need to "take in" in the early postpartum period is seen in her refusal to attend classes (2) and her need for sleep (4) and is normal.

NP:AN; CN:H; CL:C

40. (1) The first action is to turn the Pitocin off. If the fetal heart rate has dropped in response to the prolonged contraction, turning the mother on her side (3) and administering oxygen (2) may be necessary.

    NP:I; CN:PH; CL:AN

41. (4) The premature infant's poorly developed ability to control respirations is a frequent problem. Additional respiratory support with oxygen will decrease potential hypoxemia. The oxygen will also help oxygenate the systemic circulation if the infant has a tendency for hypoventilation.

    NP:AN; CN:H; CL:K

42. (4) Insulin does not cross into the milk (1). The mother's calorie intake needs to be adjusted with increased protein intake. Insulin must be adjusted and care must be exercised during weaning. Breastfeeding may actually have an antidiabetogenic effect and this requires less insulin.

    NP:AN; CN:H; CL:C

43. (1) Jaundice (icterus neonatorum) is a normal newborn condition that appears 48–72 hours after birth and begins to subside on the sixth to seventh day. If the levels go above 13 mg/100 mL, it is considered to be beyond the "safe" physiologic limit. The condition is caused by the breakdown of excess fetal red blood cells after birth.

    NP:AN; CN:H; CL:C

44. (1) The optimum weight gain, if the mother is overweight, for mother's and baby's health is 15–25 pounds. Dieting is contraindicated. There is a lower incidence of prematurity, stillbirths, and low birth-weight infants if the mother gains at least 15 pounds. Normal weight mothers should gain between 15–25 pounds.

    NP:I; CN:H; CL:A

45. (1) About 70 percent of all twins are dizygotic or fraternal. Each fetus remains enclosed in its own amnion and chorion.

    NP:AN; CN:H; CL:K

46. (2) From the assessment findings of the lochia and fundus, the new mother is progressing normally during the postpartum period. The breast signs indicate normal engorgement, which occurs about 3 days after birth. With stable vital signs, infection is not likely to be a problem. Applying warm packs and wearing a nursing bra will reduce discomfort.

    NP:AN; CN:H; CL:A

47. (4) An infant's normal breathing pattern is irregular. Staying with the client helps give her support, and the nurse can reassure her that the infant is all right.

    NP:I; CN:H; CL:A

48. (3) Amniocentesis cannot be done until adequate amniotic fluid is available, which is at about 14 weeks' gestation. It usually is done for genetic counseling purposes before 18 weeks, as the test result requires 2–4 weeks, and elective abortion after 22 weeks is contraindicated. Chorionic Villus Sampling (CVS) may replace this test as diagnostic information is available from 8 to 12 weeks.

    NP:AN; CN:H; CL:C

49. (2) The venereal disease syphilis is again becoming increasingly prevalent. It may cause abortion early in pregnancy and may be passed to the fetus after the fourth month of pregnancy, causing congenital syphilis in the infant. Gonorrhea and herpes virus II may be passed to the infant during delivery, but syphilis is usually passed to the infant in utero.

    NP:I; CN:H; CL:C

50. (2) It is important that the mother pant, not push, to avoid rapid delivery of the head. Closing her eyes and counting will not be sufficient distraction to avoid pushing. Breathing naturally at this point is also not appropriate.

    NP:I; CN:H; CL:A

Pediatric Nursing 113

✦ The icon denotes content of special importance for NCLEX.

Special Topics in Pediatric Nursing

GROWTH AND DEVELOPMENT

GENERAL PRINCIPLES

A. Growth: increasing number and/or size of cells as they divide and synthesize new proteins resulting in increased size and weight of the whole and/or any part.

B. Development: gradual change and advancement from less to more complex; emerging and expanding capacities through growth, maturation, and learning.

C. Maturation: increasing competence and adaptability as in aging; increasing complexity allowing functioning at a higher level.

D. Differentiation: process of developing from simple to more complex activities and functions. Often used in reference to early structures and cells as they are modified from mass to specific to achieve specific characteristics.

E. Growth proceeds in cephalocaudal (head-to-tail) and proximodistal (midline to peripheral) direction.

F. Sensitive periods exist during all phases of prenatal and postnatal growth and development, when the individual interacts with positive or negative environmental influences and is more susceptible to these influences.

G. All individuals develop in a fixed, predictable sequence, but great variation exists in rate of development and age at which milestones are reached.

H. *See* Piaget and Erikson tables in Chapter 3.

PHYSICAL GROWTH

Infants

A. Adjustments are made for premature infants, in corrected gestational age. Guidelines below are for term infants.

✦ B. Birth–6 months.
   1. Birth weight generally should double by 6 months.
   2. Length increases by about 2.5 cm per month (measured supine, head to heel).
   3. Head (OFC) circumference: average newborn head is 33–35.5 cm, increases about 1.5 cm per month.
   4. Anterior fontanel: should be flat and soft (usually closes by 12–14 months).

   5. Posterior fontanel usually closes by 6–8 weeks.
✦ C. 6–12 months.
   1. Birth weight approximately triples at end of 12 months.
   2. Birth length increases approximately 50 percent by 12 months.
   3. OFC approximately equal to chest circumference at 12 months; grow approximately 0.5 cm per month from 6–12 months.

Children (1–6 Years)

✦ A. Toddlers (1–3 years).
   1. Birth weight quadruples by 2½ years; yearly gain 2–3 kg.
   2. Height increases about 12 cm by 24 months, about 6–8 cm from 24–36 months.
   3. Measure height standing at 24 months old; continue measuring OFC until 36 months.
✦ B. Preschoolers (3–6 years).
   1. Weight gain 2–3 kg per year.
   2. Measure height standing; should grow 5–7.5 cm per year.

Middle Childhood to Adolescence

A. School age (6–12 years).
   1. Weight continues to increase 2–3 kg per year.
   2. Height slows to about 5 cm per year.
B. Adolescents (prepubertal 10–13 years; 12–18 years).
   1. Characterized by pubertal growth spurt: 10–14 years in females and 11–16 years in males.
   2. Females gain 7–25 kg (mean 17.5 kg) and 5–25 cm (mean 20.5 cm) during this time. Onset of menses most commonly at 10–13 years.
   3. Males gain 7–30 kg (mean 23.7 kg) and 10–30 cm (mean 27.5 cm) between 11–16 years.

DEVELOPMENTAL MILESTONES

✦ Neonates

A. Physiologic development (transition to extrauterine life).
   ✦ 1. Onset of breathing is the most important task to successfully transition to extrauterine life. Careful monitoring is required. Neonates normally may cough and sneeze to clear fluid present from intrauterine development.
   ✦ 2. Major changes occur in the cardiovascular system with the closure of fetal shunts and increase in pulmonary blood flow.
   ✦ 3. Neurologic function characterized by generalized, reflexive responses to stimuli. Primitive reflexes present include sucking, rooting, gag,

grasp, Babinski, Moro, startle, atonic neck reflex, and stepping.

    a. Adequate functioning of autonomic nervous system important in regulating respiratory and cardiovascular status, maintaining acid–base balance and thermoregulation.

    b. Should be able to focus and follow object, turn toward noises, console to parental comfort. Should have flexed posture.

4. Must be able to ingest, digest, absorb, and metabolize food in order to survive.

    a. Liver must be able to handle by-products and toxins (and conjugate bilirubin).

    b. Meconium should pass in first 24–48 hours after birth, followed by transitional stools. Stools will vary depending on milk ingested (breast milk or formula).

5. Renal functioning—kidneys must be able to cope with changing fluid and electrolyte status and concentrate urine. Structures must be patent to allow adequate urine output; should be approximately 200–300 mL with specific gravity 1.020 by one week.

6. Thermoregulation—newborns subject to heat loss and stress from cold, due to large body surface area and thin subcutaneous fat. Neonates are incapable of shivering. Brown fat stores may help in heat regulation.

B. Behavioral development.

  1. Major developmental task is bonding to parents.

  2. Sleep patterns: average neonate sleeps 16–22 hours per day. Varying "states" evident from birth: sleep, quiet alert, active alert, crying, drowsy, etc.

  3. Developmental theorists.

    a. Erikson: trust versus mistrust.

    b. Piaget: sensorimotor.

    c. Freud: oral.

C. Anticipatory guidance.

  1. Car seats.

  2. Preferred position for sleep is supine, but may be placed supported on side.

  3. Feeding issues and position upright to feed.

  4. Care of umbilicus and circumcision.

  5. Regular well-child exam and immunization schedule.

  6. Thermoregulation.

  7. Prevention of diaper rash.

  8. Bathing (water temperature).

  9. Stress management/prevention of child abuse/shaken baby syndrome.

Infants

A. General concepts.

  1. Rapid period of physical and cognitive development.

  2. Role transition in family structure, important to successfully incorporate infant into family unit.

  3. Interest in auditory stimuli begins by 2 months, turns to sounds by 4–6 months.

  4. "Stranger danger" (anxiety) begins by 6 months.

  5. Responds to own name and begins to play interactive games (peek-a-boo, pat-a-cake) by 9 months.

B. Behavioral development.

  1. Erikson: trust versus mistrust.

  2. Piaget: sensorimotor (primary to secondary circular reactions).

  3. Freud: oral.

C. Moral development: Kohlberg "amoral" stage.

D. Language development.

  1. Cooing stage usually beginning by 2 months.

  2. Reciprocal babbling by 2–6 months. Attentive to voices, smiles, laughs, and squeals at 4 months.

  3. Understands simple commands and may imitate sounds by about 9 months.

  4. By 12 months, usually can say a few words, imitates variety of vocalizations, waves "bye-bye."

E. Motor development.

  1. 2 months: some head control in upright position; when prone can lift head, neck, and upper chest with support on forearms.

  2. 4 months: able to roll from prone to supine; when prone holds head erect and raises body on hands.

    a. Reaches for and bats at objects.

    b. Grasps rattle, opens hands and holds own hands.

  3. 6 months: rolls over; no head lag when pulled to sitting; sits with support; able to stand and bear weight when placed.

    a. Grasps objects and brings to mouth.

    b. Begins to self-feed.

    c. Interested in toys, transfers objects from one hand to another, rakes for small objects.

  4. 9 months: sits independently; crawls, creeps, or scoots to move forward.

    a. May pull to stand; shakes, bangs, or throws objects.

    b. Feeds self with fingers, starts to use cup, uses inferior pincer grasp.

  5. 12 months: pulls to stand, cruises, may take a few steps alone.

    a. Feeds self.

    b. Has precise pincer grasp, bangs two blocks together.

F. Anticipatory guidance.

  1. Birth to 2 months.

✦ a. General safety issues: use of car seats at all times. Continue to put baby to sleep on back or side, turn hot water heater temperature down to 120°F and continue to test water before bathing. Keep home a non-smoking environment; caution when out in sun, fall prevention (never leave baby alone or with young sibling or pet), and smoke detectors in home. Recognition of early signs of illness, immunizations, emergency procedures.

✦ b. Nutrition: ensure adequate nutrition and hydration, do not put infant to bed with a bottle.

✦ c. Breast milk or formula only until 6 months is recommended. Needs 100–108 Kcal/kg.

✦ d. Stress management: never shake baby—may result in "Shaken Baby Syndrome."

  e. Immunizations (*see* schedule): first dose hepatitis B may be given at birth, regular immunization schedule begins at 2 months.

  f. Car seat recommendations: infants should be in a rear-facing car seat, properly installed in the rear seat of the vehicle and properly buckled, until weighing 20 pounds.

✦ 2. 4 months.

  a. General safety issues: above items plus keep sharp objects out of reach. Do not allow infant to play with plastic bags, balloons, or small objects. Keep poisonous objects in a safe place, out of baby's reach and sight.

  b. Nutrition: continue to ensure adequate nutrition. Exclusively breastfed infants need iron supplements.

  c. Play: encourage play with appropriate toys. Establish a bedtime routine. Do not use walkers or rolling wheels.

✦ 3. 6 months.

  a. General safety issues: continue car seats, teach fall prevention, and keep hazardous items up and out of baby's reach. Put plastic plugs in electrical sockets, check floor from baby's eye level for hazards. Keep baby away from tubs and swimming pools, lower crib mattress, avoid dangling cords and install safety locks on cabinets and drawers, begin dental health, establish consistent sleep habits.

✦ b. Nutrition: introduce solids at 6 months starting with single-grain cereals, adding one new food only every 4–7 days in 1 teaspoon to 1–2 tablespoon amounts, then pureed fruits and vegetables, add pureed meats last. Begin offering cup, avoid objects that can be aspirated (hot dogs, peanuts, raw vegetables, whole grapes). Always supervise eating, no bottles in bed, limit juice to 4–6 oz per day. No honey until after 1 year old.

  c. Begin cleaning teeth with eruption—using soft gauze or toothbrush without toothpaste.

  d. Play: provide opportunities for exploration, read to baby, play music. Play interactive games (peek-a-boo and pat-a-cake). Introduce transitional object, play with age-appropriate toys.

✦ 4. 9 months.

  a. General safety issues: car safety and injury prevention as in previous months. Fall prevention—install gates at top and bottom of stairs, safety devices on windows. Learn child CPR. Continue to keep hazardous substances and items out of sight and reach. Vigilance around swimming pools, lakes, ponds, or ocean. Careful selection of caregivers.

  b. Nutrition: continue to supervise meals. Introduce small bite-sized table foods; baby has increased interest in self-feeding. Cup feeding continues. Avoid foods that can be aspirated.

  c. Play: encourage vocalizations, play imitative games, continue talking and reading to baby. Provide age-appropriate toys, avoiding small objects that can be aspirated.

✦ 5. 12 months.

  a. General safety issues: continue car safety, fall prevention, poisons out of reach, water safety, hot water precautions. Keep smokers out of baby's environment. Test smoke detectors yearly. Keep away from cars, lawn mowers, and driveways—keep stairs gated. Begin brushing teeth with tiny amount of toothpaste.

  b. Nutrition: begin to feed at family mealtimes with 2–3 nutritious snacks per day. Allow child to self-feed, amounts eaten will vary. Continue cup training and wean from bottle. Avoid high-sugar drinks; change from formula to whole milk. Avoid foods that may be aspirated (peanuts, popcorn, hard candy, whole grapes).

  c. Play: encourage exploration and initiative. Provide push and pull toys that encourage large motor skills. "Teddy bears" or transitional objects, musical toys, picture books, read to child daily.

  d. Discipline: praise good behavior. Set limits and use distraction, "time out," removal from conflict situation. Discipline geared toward teaching and protection, not punishment.

Toddlers (12–36 Months)

✦ A. General concepts.
1. Time of intense curiosity and exploration of the environment.
2. Often characterized as the "terrible twos"; obstinacy, temper tantrums, and negativism prevail.
3. Physical growth slows after infancy. Senses of vision, hearing, taste, and smell develop well and become coordinated.
4. Respiratory tract continues to mature, increase in size and number of functioning units, and lessen some factors predisposing to frequent illness.
5. Gastric and bladder capacities increase; sphincter control occurs around 24 months (physiological readiness for toilet training).
6. Most children walk well. Stoop and climb stairs by 15 months, throw ball by 18 months.
   a. Refine gross motor skills between 2 and 3 years.
   b. Fine motor control continues to improve; able to stack two blocks and can drop a pellet into narrow bottle at 15 months. Uses a spoon by about 24 months.
7. Separation from mother and differentiation from others begins. Toilet training, sibling rivalry, tantrums, and regression during illness are all common in toddlerhood.
B. Behavioral development.
   ✦ 1. Erikson: autonomy versus shame and doubt.
   ✦ 2. Piaget: sensory motor (tertiary circular reactions) to preconceptual phase (preoperational).
   3. Freud: anal.
   4. Development of spirituality, sexuality, and body image begin.
C. Moral development.
   1. Kohlberg: preconventional (good/bad, right/wrong).
   ✦ 2. Magical thinking begins ("bad" thoughts make "bad" things happen).
D. Language development.
   1. Ability to understand far outweighs words spoken.
   2. By age 2, has vocabulary of around 300 words, uses short sentences, speaks intelligibly to family, and understands simple instructions.
   3. By age 3, has vocabulary of over 900 words and can follow two-step instructions and speaks intelligibly to strangers.
✦ E. Anticipatory guidance.
   ✦ 1. Injury prevention: car seats, in rear seats only in car with air bags. Car seats must also have upper

anchorage devices and locking clips, or Universal Child Safety Seat System (UCSSS). Child should remain in an approved rear-facing car seat until at least one year of age *and* weighs 20 pounds. Water safety, prevention of burns, poisoning prevention, preventing falls, aspiration and choking precautions.
   2. General issues.
      a. Toilet training.
      b. Dental health—first visit to dentist should occur at 12–24 months.
      c. Sleep and activity—total hours of sleep decrease; encourage routines.
F. Nutrition.
   1. Toddlerhood is the phase of "physiological anorexia."
   2. Intake varies daily, may eat large amounts one day and almost nothing the next.
   3. Eating habits established in first 3 years may last whole life—avoid using food as punishment or reward; mealtimes should be enjoyable, give appropriate-size portions, make snacks nutritious.
G. Play.
   1. Increased locomotion skills; beginning tricycles, wagons, balls, low slides—safety should be foremost in toy selection.
   2. Interest in artwork begins—crayons, finger paints, chalk.
   3. Puzzles, blocks—toys that stimulate creativity, freedom of expression.
   4. Limit use of television.
H. Discipline.
   1. Provide limits. Allow choices when possible.
   2. Tell child specifically why discipline is necessary and be consistent.
   3. Avoid power struggles with toddlers.
   4. Use "time out" when needed, teach toddler about disciplinary measures when child is fed, rested, and not angry.

Preschoolers (3–6 Years)

A. General concepts.
   1. Physical growth slows, potbelly of toddlerhood disappears, child becomes taller, more slender, sturdy and agile.
   2. Gross motor skills continue to improve and become more coordinated. Child is able to run well, climb, ride tricycle, balance on one foot, skip; can roller skate by 5 years.
   3. Fine motor skills improve with improved hand–eye coordination. Child can draw recognizable person with three parts by age 4; can dress self without help by age 5, print letters, and copy shapes.

4. Preschoolers are energetic learners and most eagerly anticipate social and educational opportunities at preschool. Enjoy magical thinking and "make believe."

5. Beginning to test limits with adults, but respond well to clearly stated rules and praise.

6. Becoming curious about own bodies, sexual identity, and exploration begins to emerge.

7. Sleep problems common—difficulty falling asleep, nightmares, sleep terrors. Routine bedtime rituals helpful in helping child settle down for sleep. Average preschooler sleeps 12 hours at night with infrequent daytime nap.

B. Behavioral development.
   1. Erikson: stage of initiative versus guilt.
   2. Piaget: preoperational phase—age 2–4 is preconceptual phase; age 4–7 is stage of intuitive thought.
   3. Freud: Oedipal phase.

C. Moral development.
   1. Kohlberg: preconventional stage—from 2 to 4 years, child's moral thinking and behavior is guided by punishment and obedience orientation.
   2. From 4 to 7 years, thinking is more self-centered and concrete sense of justice, characterized as "naive instrumental orientation"; is sensitive to feelings of others.

D. Language development.
   1. Speech and language become more complex. Child speaks intelligibly to strangers. At age 5, able to use the past tense and sentences of four or five words, up to short paragraphs.
   2. From age 3–4, speech is telegraphic (only most essential words used).
   3. At age 4, can remember nursery rhymes, may have some stuttering.
   4. At age 5, able to recite address and phone number, may have vocabulary of > 2100 words, understands opposites.

E. Anticipatory guidance.
   1. Injury prevention.
      a. Children weighing 40–65 pounds should be in a combination booster seat with harness. Child is ready for a properly installed and fitted booster seat when child reaches the top weight or height allowed for infant and toddler car seats, shoulders are above harness slots and ears have reached top of the seat.
      b. Bicycle safety, water safety—swimming lessons feasible, use of sunscreen, smoke detectors and fire drills in home, poisons/toxins out of reach and locked.

2. Parents should be conscious of role-modeling healthy behavior, encouraging regular exercise, limiting television use.
3. Child should be taught about personal hygiene, sexuality, and keeping their own bodies safe.
4. Establish dental hygiene habits.

F. Nutrition.
   1. Preschoolers should have three meals and two snacks at regular times during the day. Encourage healthy breakfast at home or at school.
   2. Calorie requirements approximately 90 cal/kg (1800 cal/day) and 1.2 g/kg protein. Many are "picky" eaters and refuse to try new foods.
   3. By age 5, child may be able to sit through adult meal; important for parents to role-model good eating habits.

G. Play/social development.
   1. Most preschool play is associative; groups involved in similar activities. Play centers on motor skills—running, jumping, riding tricycles and bicycles. Becomes attached to a "favorite" toy, may engage in elaborate fantasy play ("house"), plays interactive games with peers. Can sit still to listen to a story; improving manual dexterity allows interest in drawing, painting, simple carpentry, and sewing. May have imaginary playmate.
   2. Preschoolers more eager to please, can verbalize desires and usually heed warnings of danger.
   3. By 4–5 years, begin to test boundaries.

H. Discipline.
   1. Promote physical activity without aggressiveness. Set developmentally appropriate limits. Use time out, removal of source of conflict for unacceptable behavior, establish consequences for unacceptable behavior.
   2. Help child learn how to get along with peers, teach to respect authority, how to manage anger and resolve conflicts without violence. Parents should be aware of importance of role modeling.

School-Age Children (6–12 Years)

A. General concepts.
   1. Height and weight continue to increase at slower pace. Boys and girls are similar size until pubescent growth spurt. Bodies become slimmer, fat distribution changes and diminishes, legs lengthen, and muscle groups become stronger.
   2. Deciduous teeth are lost and replaced by permanent teeth during middle childhood; "the ugly duckling years"; dental hygiene more important.
   3. Physiologic maturity continues in GI system; fewer GI upsets occur and stomach capacity increases. Immune system continues to become

more competent; child has fewer illnesses normally than during preschool years.

4. Increase in stress-related complaints in older school-age children.
    a. Somaticized as stomach pain, headache, sleep disturbances, changes in eating.
    b. Generally are less fearful than preschoolers, but worry about bodily harm, occasionally about frightening events heard on news (kidnapping, violence).
5. Curiosity increases about bodily functions and sex.
    a. Ideal time for matter-of-fact sex education and information about sexual maturation and reproduction.
    b. Girls need concrete information about menstruation, as age of menarche continues to decline in United States.
6. Neighborhood and friends take on a more important role. Children begin to look outside parents/family for approval.

B. Behavioral development.
    ✦ 1. Erikson: industry versus inferiority.
    2. Piaget: concrete operations; characterized by conservation (age 5–7) and classification skills in later school-age years.
    3. Freud: latency period.
✦ C. Moral development.
    1. Kohlberg: children interpret accidents or mishaps as punishment for bad behavior.
    2. Called "conventional morality" phase; child views rules for the good of all, and by following the rules, he or she is viewed as a "good" child.
D. Language.
    1. Speech becomes progressively more complex, begins to use proper nouns, pronouns, and prepositions. By end of school-age period, has basic mastery of grammar.
    2. Able to write letters by age 6–7.
    3. Reading proficiently by 8–9 years.
✦ E. Anticipatory guidance.
    1. Promote healthy habits, encourage regular exercise/physical activity, limit television to 1 hour/day, personal care, and hygiene.
    2. Car seat recommendations.
        a. Children should ride in back seat *only* until age 13.
        b. Children should stay in a booster seat in rear seat until child reaches about 4 feet 9 inches in height and is 8–12 years of age.
        c. Child is ready to use a lap and shoulder seat belt when belt fits properly.
    3. Bike/skateboard helmets, water safety—swimming lessons, sunscreen, protection from assault.

4. Safety rules in home, ensure guns are locked and unloaded, ensure child has supervision before and after school, teach a family "password" to protect from strangers.
5. Begin smoking, drug, and alcohol education/avoidance.
6. Help child learn to get along with peers and conflict resolution—promote positive interactions between the child, teachers, peers, and adults.
7. Begin sexuality education; prepare girls for menstruation, boys for development and nocturnal emissions.
F. Nutrition.
    1. Encourage three regular meals and healthy snacks. Avoid fad diets or consumption of "junk food."
    2. Parents should model healthy eating and encourage meals together with family.
    3. Calorie needs decrease relative to body size, need approximately 2000 cal/day and 28 g protein.
    4. Monitor for obesity. At risk if BMI for age > 85th percentile.
        a. If present, monitor BP for hypertension, blood glucose (for Type 2 diabetes) and lipid profile.
        b. Risk factors are genetics, psychosocial issues, inactivity, and minority and low-income family.
        c. Dietary counseling, weight loss and exercise programs aimed at children are effective.
    5. Encourage regular activity/exercise.
G. Play/social development.
    1. Trend toward earlier participation in organized competitive sports. Friends become bigger part of life; focus on group activities. Commonly enjoy model or construction kits, swimming, bicycling, skateboarding, video games, swimming, painting, pottery, card and board games.
    2. Children usually can be responsible for designated household chores with financial compensation (allowances).
✦ H. Discipline.
    1. Parents should be encouraged to set limits and establish consequences for bad behavior. Children should be expected to follow family rules for bedtime, TV, and chores.
    2. Reasoning works well with school-age children; allow some choices. Children can help problem solve.
    3. Withholding privileges is generally effective disciplinary consequence—also contracting and imposing penalties.

Adolescents (12–18 Years)

✦ A. General concepts.
1. Major development is onset of puberty and development of primary and secondary sex characteristics; secretion of estrogen and androgens.
2. Physical growth marked by the adolescent growth spurt—begins between 9 and 14 years in girls, and 10 and 16 years in boys.
   a. The final 20–25 percent of height occurs over a 24–36-month period. Amount of growth varies; boys may gain 10–30 cm and 7–30 kg; girls gain 5–20 cm and 7–25 kg.
   b. Growth ceases about 2 years after menarche for girls; at 18–20 years in boys.
3. Physiologic growth in size and strength of muscles, particularly heart, respiratory volume and vital capacity dramatically increase; exercise performance increases dramatically.
4. Parents become less important and influential; peer relationships play major role as adolescents struggle for autonomy and separation from parents.
5. Experimentation in risky behavior is common—sexual activity; alcohol, drug and cigarette use; other risk taking with automobiles and sporting activities.
6. Attitudes and values formulated by late adolescence, which will affect future behavior and quality of life.
7. Stress, depression, and social withdrawal common—parents should be aware of alarming symptoms.
8. Adolescents seek some financial independence—household chores and "allowance"—often obtain part-time employment.
9. Physical exam should include screening for human immunodeficiency virus/sexually transmitted diseases (HIV/STDs), scoliosis, blood pressure, weight, hemoglobin and hematocrit in girls with heavy menses, weight loss, athletic development; screening for diabetes mellitus and hyperlipidemia if positive family history.

B. Behavioral development.
✦ 1. Erikson: identity versus role diffusion.
2. Piaget: formal operations, characterized by formal operations.
3. Freud: genital stage.

✦ C. Moral development.
1. Kohlberg: adolescents begin to substitute their own set of values and beliefs for parents'; phase of "principled morality"—based on what is "universally ethical" on basis of own conscience.
2. Moral conduct is based largely on the desire to avoid the loss of respect of the peer group and a sense of obligation to democratic law.

✦ D. Social development.
1. Primary task is to separate from parents, reestablish relationship with family based on "mutual affection and equality" rather than parental dominance. Separation often difficult for adolescent and parents; conflict is common.
2. Peer group more important, school important as academic and social focus. Groups important, as are best friends and emergence of heterosexual friendships of varying "seriousness."
3. Some adolescents identify as homosexual by late teens; sexual activity encountered by the majority by age 18.

✦ E. Anticipatory guidance.
1. Immunizations: HPV (human papillomavirus vaccine) recommended routinely at age 11–12 before commencing sexual activity. Meningococcal vaccine: MCV4 (Merck) should be given at 11–12 or 15 years.
2. Becoming responsible for own body and health, establishing healthy activities, avoiding risky behavior.
3. Injury prevention: focusing on automobile safety, water safety, respect for firearms, prevention of substance use/abuse. Use of sunscreen, protective sports gear, and helmet use for bicycles and motorcycles.
4. If sexually active, protection from HIV, birth control; self-defense and avoidance of potentially abusive relationships/situations.
5. Mental health issues: stress management, conflict resolution, seeking help if depressed, hopeless, or angry; setting realistic goals; increasing self-confidence; time management for school, friends, family, and employment.
6. Mental health: monitor for depression, suicidal thoughts, aggressive behavior, antisocial activity.

F. Nutrition.
1. High caloric and protein requirements during periods of rapid growth. Protein requirements in males 45–60 g/day (age 11–18), females 44–46 g/day (age 11–18); caloric needs: 2500–3000/day in males (age 11–18) and 2200/day in females.
2. Menstruating girls need extra iron, especially if physically active. Frequent time for girls to diet—observe for continued weight loss.

G. Sleep and activity.
1. Sleep needs are variable—many teens have propensity for staying up late at night, sleeping late in morning whenever possible.
2. Regular patterns of exercise should become established during adolescence and maintained into adulthood.

GENERAL ASSESSMENT OF THE CHILD

GENERAL PRINCIPLES FOR ASSESSING CHILDREN

A. Maturational ability of the child to cooperate with the examiner is of major importance to adequate physical assessment.

B. When planning physical assessment of the child, the following points should be considered:
   ✦ 1. Establish a relationship with the child prior to the examination.
      a. Determine child's developmental level.
      b. Allow the child an opportunity to become accustomed to the examiner, preferably an opportunity to observe the examiner from a distance.
   ✦ 2. Explain in terms appropriate to the child's level of understanding the extent and purpose of the examination.
      3. Realize that the physical examination may be a stressful experience for the child, who depends on others for protection.
      4. Limit the physical examination to what is essential in determining an adequate nursing diagnosis.
      5. Proceed from the least to the most intrusive procedures.
      6. Allow active participation of the child whenever possible.
      7. Allow parents to participate in assessment of younger children. Allow adolescents the option of having parent stay during the exam. (*See* Table 13-1.)
      8. Consider cultural influences and practices—incorporate appropriately into exam.

Assessment of the Infant

A. Accomplish as much of the examination as possible while the infant is sleeping or resting undisturbed.

B. History: gestational age/birth weight, discharge from hospital, weight gain, and sleep patterns.

✦ C. Assess general condition.
   1. Symmetry and location of body parts.
   2. Color and condition of the skin.
   3. State of restlessness and sleeplessness.
   4. Adjustment to feeding regimen.

5. Quality of cry.
6. Interactions with parents/caregivers present.

D. Utilize screening procedures for assessment.
   1. Developmental screening. (Properly administering the Denver II or DDST can take up to 2 hours—by a *skilled* examiner. If indicated, the nurse may refer the child for further screening.)
   2. Vision.
   3. Hearing.
   4. Growth charts: head circumference, weight, length—available on CDC Web site (www.cdc.gov).

E. Provide teaching in the following areas:
   1. Growth and development changes.
   2. Language development.
   3. Anxiety toward strangers.
   4. Separation anxiety.
   5. Transitional objects.

✦ F. Anticipatory guidance.
   1. Accident prevention: use of car seats, fall prevention, poisoning, water heater temperature, prevention of foreign body aspiration.
   2. Immunizations.
   3. Feeding—introduction of solids, weaning from breast or bottle.
   4. Eruption of deciduous teeth and dental hygiene.

G. Assess for nonaccidental trauma.

Assess for Congenital Anomalies

✦ A. Neurological system.
   1. Reflexes: absent or asymmetrical (*see* Neurological section).
   2. Head circumference: microcephaly, hydrocephaly (from growth chart).
   3. Fontanelles: closed or bulging.
   4. Eyes: cataracts, lid folds, spots on iris, pupillary responses.

✦ B. Respiratory system.
   1. History: prematurity, apnea, siblings, previous children with sudden infant death syndrome (SIDS).
   2. Signs of respiratory distress: tachypnea, retractions, nasal flaring, head bobbing, grunting, stridor, cough, asymmetry of chest, crackles, wheezes.

✦ C. Cardiovascular system.
   1. Perfusion: assess pulses in all 4 extremities; temperature of extremities, quality of peripheral pulses (for age), capillary refill time, skin color, color of mucous membranes and nailbeds (pale, mottled or cyanotic).
   2. Auscultation: regularity, tachycardia, bradycardia, relationship to respiratory cycle.
   3. Activity: infant tires and may become cyanotic.
      a. Does infant tire with feeding?
      b. Does skin color change with cry?

◆ **Table 13-1. PEDIATRIC PHYSICAL ASSESSMENT**

Assessment	Normal	Abnormal
MEASUREMENTS		
Measure **height** and **weight** and plot on a standardized growth chart	Height/weight proportional Sequential measurements: pattern follows normal growth curves	Height/weight below fifth percentile Sudden drop in percentile range of height and/or weight: possible sign of disease process or congenital problem (R/O FTT—Failure to Thrive) Sudden and persistent increase (above 95th percentile)
Assess **temperature** (axillary or tympanic until 6 years of age)	Axillary 36.5°–37.5°C (97.7°F) Rectal 36.6°–37.2°C (97.8°F) Elevations following eating or playing not unusual	Temperature of 104°–105°F: corresponds roughly with 101°–102°F in an adult Large daily temperature variations Hypothermia: usually result of chilling, may indicates sepsis in neonates
Measure **circumference of head and chest** Examine or check circumferences when child is less than 2 years old Compare measurements with standardized charts	Head at birth: about 2 cm greater than chest During first year: equalization of head and chest After 2 years: rapid growth of chest; slight increase in size of head	Increase in head circumference greater than 2.5 cm per month: sign of hydrocephalus
Assess **pulse** apically	Birth–1 year: 100–180 1 year: 80–150 2 years: 80–130 3 years: 80–120 Over 3 years: 70–110	Pulse over 180 *at rest* after first month of life: cardiac or respiratory condition Inability to palpate or very weak femoral and pedal pulses: possible coarctation of the aorta
Assess **respirations**	Birth: 30–50 6 years: 20–25 Puberty: 14–16 (Young children have abnormally high respiration rate with even slight excitement)	Consistent tachypnea: usually a sign of respiratory distress Respiratory rate over 100: lower respiratory tract obstruction Slow rate: may be sign of CNS depression
Assess **blood pressure**	Birth: 55–60/80–90 mm Hg systolic 20–60 mm Hg diastolic 1 year: 90–60 Rise in both pressures: 2–3 mm Hg per year of age Adult level reached at puberty	Elevated blood pressure in upper extremities *and* decrease in lower extremities: coarctation of aorta Narrowed pulse pressure (normal or elevated diastolic with lowered systolic; less than 30 mm Hg difference between systolic and diastolic readings): possible sign of aortic or subaortic stenosis or hypothyroidism Widened pulse pressure: possible sign of hyperthyroidism Children and adolescents with elevated BP should be followed and reevaluated for possible hypertension
APPEARANCE		
Observe **general appearance**	Alert, well-nourished, comfortable, responsive	Lethargic, uncomfortable, malnourished, gross anomalies, dull

Continues

◆ **Table 13-1. PEDIATRIC PHYSICAL ASSESSMENT** *(Continued)*

Assessment	Normal	Abnormal
APPEARANCE *(Continued)*		
Listen to **voice and cry**	Strong, lusty cry	Weak cry, low- or high-pitched cry: may indicate neurological problem or chromosomal abnormality
		Stridor: possible upper airway edema or obstruction or hoarse cry
	Facial expression animated	Expressionless, unresponsive
	No indications of pain	Doubling over, rubbing a body part, general fretfulness, irritability
Assess presence of **odor**	No odor	Musty odor: sign of phenylketonuria, diphtheria
		Odor of maple syrup: may be maple syrup urine disease
		Odor of sweaty feet: one type of acidemia
		Fishy odor: may be metabolic disorder
		Acetone odor: acidosis, particularly diabetic ketoacidosis
SKIN ASSESSMENT		
Assess **pigmentation**	Usually even	Multiple cafe au lait spots: possible neurofibromatosis
	Pigmented nevi common	Cyanosis
	Large, flat, black and blue areas over sacrum, buttocks (mongolian spots)	Jaundice
		Pallor
Assess **lesions**	Usually none	Erythematous lesions
	Adolescence: acne	Multiple macules, papules, or vesicles
		Petechiae and ecchymoses: may indicate coagulation disorder
		Hives (allergy)
		Subcutaneous nodules: may indicate juvenile rheumatoid arthritis
Note **consistency of skin**	Good turgor	Poor turgor (tenting)
	Smooth and firm	Dryness
	Check fontanels in infant (should be soft and flat)	Edema or dehydration
		Lack or excess of subcutaneous fat: sign of malnutrition or excess nutrition (obesity)
Assess **nails**	Nailbeds: normally pigmented	Cyanosis
	Good nail growth	Pallor
		Capillary pulsations
		Pitting of the nails: possible sign of fungal disease or psoriasis
		Broad nailbeds: possible sign of Down syndrome or other chromosomal abnormality
Assess **hair** (consistency appropriate to ethnic group)	No excessive breaking	Dry, coarse, brittle hair: possible sign of hypothyroidism
	Consistent growth pattern	Alopecia (loss of hair): may be psychosomatic or due to drug therapy
		Unusual hairiness in places other than scalp, eyebrows, and lashes: may indicate hypothyroidism, vitamin A poisoning, chronic infections, reaction to Dilantin therapy

◆ Table 13-1. PEDIATRIC PHYSICAL ASSESSMENT *(Continued)*		
Assessment	**Normal**	**Abnormal**
SKIN ASSESSMENT *(Continued)*		
		Tufts of hair over spine or sacrum: may indicate site of spina bifida occulta or spina bifida
		Absence of the start of pubic hair during adolescence: possible hypothyroidism, hypopituitarism, gonadal deficiency, or Addison's disease
Assess **lymph nodes**	Nontender, movable, discrete nodes up to 3 mm in diameter in occipital post-auricular, parotid, submaxillary, sublingual, axillary, and epitrochlear nodes	Tender or enlarged nodes: may be sign of systemic infection
	Up to 1 mm in diameter inguinal and cervical nodes	
HEAD AND NECK ASSESSMENT		
Assess **scalp**	Usually without lesions	Ringworm, lice (pediculosis capitus)
Assess frontal and maxillary **sinuses**	Nontender	Tenderness: indicative of inflammatory process
		Seborrheic dermatitis
Assess **face**	Symmetrical movement	Asymmetry: signs of facial paralysis
		Twitching: could be due to psychosomatic causes or Tourette's syndrome, vitamin/mineral deficiency
Evaluate the **eyes**		
Gross screening of vision Snellen chart	With younger child, ability to focus and follow movement and to see objects placed a few feet away	Inability to follow movement or to see objects placed a few feet away
Sclerae	Completely white	Yellow sclera: sign of jaundice
		Blue sclera: may be normal or indicative of osteogenesis imperfecta
Placement in eye socket	Normally placed	Exophthalmos (protrusion of eyeball)
		Enophthalmos (deeply placed eyeball)
Iris	At rest: upper and lower margins of iris visible between the lids	Setting sun sign (iris appears to be beneath lower lid): if marked, may be sign of increased intracranial pressure or hydrocephalus
Movement	In newborn, intermittent strabismus or nystagmus	Fixed strabismus or intermittent strabismus continuing after 6 months of age: indication of muscle paralysis or weakness
		Involuntary, repetitive oscillations of one or both eyes: normal with *extreme* lateral gaze
		Nystagmus: may be cerebellar dysfunction indicative of use of certain drugs (anticonvulsants, barbiturates, alcohol)
Eyelids	Fully covers eye	Ptosis of eyelid: may be an early sign of a neurological disorder
	Fully raised on opening	Sty
Conjunctiva	Clear	Inflammation (conjunctivitis)
		Hemorrhage
		Stimson's lines (small red transverse lines on conjunctiva)

Continues

◆ **Table 13-1. PEDIATRIC PHYSICAL ASSESSMENT** *(Continued)*

Assessment	Normal	Abnormal
HEAD AND NECK ASSESSMENT *(Continued)*		
Cornea	Clear	Opacity: sign of ulceration
		Inflammation
		Redness
Discharge	Tears	Purulent discharges: note amount, color, consistency (bacterial conjunctivitis)
Pupils	Round, regular	Sluggish or asymmetrical reaction to light: indicates intracranial disease
	Clear, equal	
	Brisk reaction to light	Lack of accommodation reflex
	Accommodation reflex (pupil contraction as object is brought near the eye)	
Lens	Clear	Opacities (cataracts)
Evaluate the **ears**		
Sinuses	None present	Small holes or pits anterior to ear: may be superficial but could indicate the presence of a sinus leading into brain
Position	Top of ear above level of eye	Top of ear below level of eye: associated with some congenital defects
Discharge	None	Discharge: note color, odor and amount
Hearing	In infant: turning to sound	Diminished hearing in one or both ears
	In older child: responds to whispered command	
Assess the **nose**	No secretions	Secretions: note characteristics
		Any unusual shape or flaring of nostrils
	Breathing through nose	Breathing through mouth
Assess the **mouth**		Circumoral pallor: possible sign of cyanotic heart disease, scarlet fever, rheumatic fever, hypoglycemia; also seen in other febrile diseases
		Asymmetry of lips: seen in nerve paralysis
	Intact palate	Cleft palate
	Teeth in good condition	Delayed appearance of deciduous teeth: may indicate cretinism, rickets, congenital syphilis, or Down syndrome; may also be normal
	In older child, presence of permanent teeth	
		Poor tooth formation: may be seen with systemic diseases
		Green or black teeth: seen after iron ingestion or death of tooth
		Stained teeth: may be seen after prolonged use of tetracyclines
Assess the **gums**	Retention cysts in newborn	Inflammation, abnormal color, drooling, pus, tenderness (gingivitis)
		Black line along gums: may indicate lead poisoning
Assess the **tongue**	Moves freely	Tremors on protrusion: may indicate chorea, hyperthyroidism, cerebral palsy
		Protruding tongue—Down syndrome
		White spots (thrush)
		Tongue-tie (frenulum)
	Pink, with conical, filiform nontender papillae	Strawberry tongue (scarlet fever)

◆ Table 13-1. PEDIATRIC PHYSICAL ASSESSMENT *(Continued)*

Assessment	Normal	Abnormal
HEAD AND NECK ASSESSMENT *(Continued)*		
Assess the **throat**	Tonsils normally enlarged in childhood	White or gray membrane over tonsils (diphtheria) White pus on sacs, erythema (bacterial pharyngitis), tender: vitamin deficiencies, anemia
Assess the **larynx**	Normal vocal tones	Hoarseness or stridor: possible upper respiratory tract obstruction (laryngotracheobronchitis)
Assess the **neck**	Short in infancy Lengthens at 2–3 years Trachea slightly right of midline	Trachea deviated to left or right: may indicate shift with atelectasis or tension pneumothorax
Thyroid	Not enlarged	Enlarged: may be due to hyperactive thyroid, malignancy, goiter
Motion	Full lateral and upward/downward motion	Limited movement with pain: may indicate meningeal irritation, lymph node enlargement, rheumatoid arthritis, or other diseases
LUNGS AND THORAX ASSESSMENT		
Assess the **lungs**	Normally clear breath sounds bilaterally	Presence of rhonchi, crackles, or wheezes Diminished breath sounds heard over parts of lung
	No retractions	Mild to severe intercostal, supraclavicular or sternal retractions indicative of respiratory distress
	Symmetry of diaphragmatic movement	Asymmetry of movement (phrenic nerve damage)
Assess the **sputum**	None or small amount of clear sputum in morning	Thick, tenacious sputum with foul odor Blood-tinged or green sputum
Assess the **breasts**	Slightly enlarged in infancy Generally slightly asymmetrical at puberty	Discharge or growth in males Masses (especially solid, fixed nonmobile) in older adolescent Premature development (precocious puberty)
HEART ASSESSMENT		
Assess **heart sounds**	S_1, S_2, S_3	S_4 indicates congestive heart failure
Assess **femoral pulses**	Strong	Weak (shock, coarctation of aorta)
Note **edema**	None present	Edema—note location (initially periorbital) and duration, bulging fontanelles—fluid overload, CHF
Note **clubbing** of fingers	None present	Clubbing (congenital cyanotic heart defects)—note location and duration
Note **murmurs**		Murmur grade three or higher is always abnormal No change in quality with positional changes

Continues

✦ **Table 13-1. PEDIATRIC PHYSICAL ASSESSMENT** *(Continued)*

Assessment	Normal	Abnormal
HEART ASSESSMENT *(Continued)*		
Note **cyanosis**	None normally present	Circumoral or peripheral cyanosis: indicates respiratory or cardiac disease (hypoxemia); congenital heart defects
ABDOMEN ASSESSMENT		
Assess **skin condition**	Soft	Hard, rigid, tender
Assess for **peristaltic motion**	Not visible	Visible peristalsis—may indicate pyloric stenosis (olive-shaped mass, palpable, in area of pyloris)
Assess **shape**	"Pot-bellied" toddlers Slightly protuberant in standing adolescent	Large protruding abdomen: may indicate pancreatic fibrosis, hypokalemia, rickets, hypothyroidism, bowel obstruction, constipation, inguinal hernias, unilateral or bilateral: observe for reducibility
	Umbilical protrusion	Umbilical hernia
Assess **hepatic border**	At costal margin or 1–2 cm below	> 3 cm below costal margin (hepatic enlargement)
GENITOURINARY TRACT ASSESSMENT		
Assess **female genitalia**	No signs of sexually transmitted disease (herpes, chlamydia, HPV, or abuse)	Signs of trauma or sexual abuse, pustules or lesions consistent with herpes, HPV, chlamydia, or other STDs
Discharge	Mucoid, no odor	Foul or copious discharge; any bleeding prior to puberty
	Tanner stage consistent with age	Early or delayed pubescent development
Assess **male genitalia**		
Presence of urethral orifice	Orifice on distal end of penis	Hypospadias or epispadias (urethral orifice along inferior or dorsal surface)
Urethral opening	Normal size	Stenosis of urethral opening
Foreskin	Covers glans completely	Foreskin incompletely formed ventrally when hypospadias present
Placement of testes	Descended testes	Undescended testes Enlarged scrotum
	Tanner stage consistent with age	Early or delayed pubescent development
Assess **urine output**	Full, steady stream of urine	Urine with pus, blood, or odor (infection) Excessive urination or nocturia: possible sign of diabetes
Check **anus and rectum**	No masses or fissures present	Hemorrhoids, fissures, prolapse, pinworms Dark ring around rectal mucosa: may be sign of lead poisoning
MUSCULOSKELETAL ASSESSMENT		
Assess **extremities**	Coloration of fingers and toes consistent with rest of body	Cyanosis—indicates respiratory or cardiac disease, or hypothermia in newborn Clubbing of fingers and toes indicates cardiac or respiratory disease
	Quick capillary refill on blanching	Sluggish blood return on blanching indicates poor circulation
	Temperature same as rest of body	Temperature variation between extremities and rest of body indicates neurological or vascular anomalies
	Presence of pedal pulses	Absence of pedal pulses indicates circulatory difficulties

---

◆ Table 13-1. **PEDIATRIC PHYSICAL ASSESSMENT** *(Continued)*

Assessment	Normal	Abnormal
MUSCULOSKELETAL ASSESSMENT *(Continued)*		
	No pain or tenderness	Presence of localized or generalized pain
	Straight legs after 2 years of age	Any bowing after 2 years of age may be hereditary or indicate rickets
	Broad-based gait until 4 years of age; feet straight ahead afterwards	Scissoring gait indicates spastic cerebral palsy
		Persistence of broad-based gait after 4 years of age indicates possible abnormalities of legs and feet or balance disturbance
		Any limp or ataxia
Assess **fine motor movements**	Presence of fine motor activity approximate to age—symmetrical	Continued presence of primitive reflexes after fading of reflex should normally occur may indicate brain damage
Assess **spine**	No dimples	Presence of dimple or tufts of hair indicates possible spina bifida
	Flexible	Limited flexion indicates central nervous system infections
		Hyperextension (opisthotonos) indicates brain stem irritation, hemorrhage, or intracranial infection
Have child bend forward at waist and check level of scapulae (scoliosis screening)	No lateral curvature or excessive anterior posterior curvature	Presence of lordosis (after age 2 years), kyphosis, or scoliosis
	Scapulae at same height	
Assess **hips**		Asymmetrical thigh folds, clicks on adduction—hip dysplasia
Assess **joints**	Full range of motion without pain, edema, or tenderness	Pain, edema, or tenderness indicates tissue injury
Assess **muscles**	Good tone and purposeful movement	Decreased or increased tone
	Ability to perform motor skills approximate to development level	Spasm or tremors may indicate cerebral palsy
		Atrophy or contractures
Signs of **abuse**	No external signs	Bruises, welts, swelling, burns, discharge, bleeding

4. Umbilical vessels: normally two arteries and one vein.

◆ D. Gastrointestinal tract.
 1. History of polyhydramnios.
 2. Patency: coughing, choking, mucus, spitting, cyanosis, ability to pass nasogastric tube to stomach, pass meconium stool?
 3. Mouth: palate and lips intact?
 4. Anus: patent? Stool present? Passage of meconium?
 5. Olive-shaped mass in region of pyloris with history of forceful projectile vomiting and immediate hunger may indicate hypertrophic pyloric stenosis.

◆ E. Genitourinary system.
 1. Urine: stream and position of meatus.
 2. Masses: abdominal (possible Wilms' tumor. DO NOT PALPATE).
 3. Boys: undescended testicles, hernia, urethra— position of testicles, position of urethral meatus on penis, presence of hernia.
 4. Girls: labia mobile, structures identifiable, presence of discharge.
 5. Genitalia: clearly male or female or ambiguous?

◆ F. Skeletal system.
 1. Clavicles: intact or fractured?
 2. Hips: check for dislocation (asymmetric major gluteal or thigh folds, hip click on adduction).
 3. Legs and feet: clubbing, without straight tibial line.
 4. Spine: curved, flexibility, open, presence of masses or dimples.

Common Problems

✦ A. Respiratory infections.
  1. Assess duration and severity of symptoms, medications given.
  2. Look for signs of respiratory distress: wheezing, barking cough, anxiety, restlessness, use of accessory muscles.
  3. Check for white patches on tonsils, unless toxic appearing and drooling.
  4. Feeding difficulties—crying with swallowing, hydration status.
  5. Chronic lung disease in infants with history of prematurity.
✦ B. Ear infections.
  1. Assess for fever, irritability, pulling or rubbing ear(s).
  2. Determine if change in eating habits has occurred recently. (Does infant go to bed with a bottle?)
  3. Previous or recent upper respiratory infections.
  4. Previous ear infections.
C. Rashes.
  1. Assess onset, duration, and location; association with new foods/medications, aggravating or alleviating factors.
  2. Elicit accurate description of rash.
D. Contact dermatitis.
  1. Assess if history of allergies, and family history.
  2. Evaluate diaper area rash: use of lotions, powders, frequency of diaper changes, type of diaper used (cloth vs. paper).
  3. Determine method of cleaning cloth diapers.
  4. Atopic dermatitis: rashes in skin creases and scalp, oozing blisters, or dry scales.
E. Hernias.
  1. For inguinal, assess for lump in groin, reducible—with or without pain.
  2. For umbilical, determine if lump can be pushed back without difficulty or pain.
F. Scalp: "cradle cap" (seborrheic dermatitis).
  1. Assess for scaling or crusted areas.
  2. Determine method of washing hair.
  3. Evaluate lotions or balms applied to hair.
G. Birthmarks.
  1. Assess for change in size, color, or shape.
  2. Look for any bleeding or irritation.
H. Eye symmetry.
  1. Assess position of eyes, presence of doll's eye reflex, ability to focus and follow 180 degrees.
  2. Determine presence of conjunctivitis (redness, discharge).
  3. Evaluate for strabismus/amblyopia; determine if light reflex is symmetrical in both eyes, assess extraocular movements, perform cover/uncover test.

Assessment of the Toddler and the Preschool Child

A. General considerations.
  ✦ 1. Remember that separation anxiety is most acute at toddler age and body integrity fears are most acute at preschool age.
  ✦ 2. Involve the parent in examination as much as possible.
  3. Give simple explanation of each portion of the exam. Proceed in calm and matter-of-fact fashion. Start with least invasive moving to more invasive.
  4. Allow the child to handle the equipment and try out on teaching doll, use play and distraction as needed.
  5. Take into account child's need for autonomy.
  6. Do not disparage imaginary friends.
  7. Allow for rituals and routines, security objects.
B. Utilize screening procedures for assessment.
  1. Developmental landmarks: Denver II data.
  2. Vision.
  3. Hearing.
  4. Growth charts: head circumference, weight, length.
C. Immunization history.
D. Blood pressure measurement, preferably with manual cuff by age 3, or sooner if cardiac or renal disease is suspected.
✦ E. Anticipatory guidance: car seats/seat belts, avoidance of accidental ingestions, hot water heater temp, traffic safety, bicycle helmets, dental hygiene, water safety.

Common Problems

A. Feeding and eating.
  1. Review food intake for last 72 hours, commonly "picky" eaters.
  2. Assess types of food ingested (amount of fat and sweets).
  3. Ensure adequate source of vitamins and minerals, use of supplements.
B. Temper tantrums.
  1. Assess frequency and duration.
  2. Determine precipitating event.
  3. Evaluate response of caretaker.
C. Toilet training.
  1. Ability to ambulate (fine and gross motor capability—neuromuscular maturity).
  2. Determine if child is bothered by wet diapers.
  3. Evaluate child's and parent's interest in toilet training.
D. Respiratory infections.
  1. Assess duration and severity of symptoms.
  2. Look for wheezing, barking cough, anxiety, restlessness, use of accessory muscles.

3. If throat is sore, check for white patches on tonsils, unless toxic appearing and drooling.
E. Communicable diseases.
    1. Assess exposures and onset of symptoms.
    2. Evaluate progression of disease.
    3. Determine treatment of symptoms.
    4. Look for complications.
F. Gastrointestinal infections.
    1. Assess onset and duration.
    2. Evaluate intake and output.
    3. Check for signs of dehydration (dry mucous membranes, tachycardia, tachypnea, decreased urine output).

Assessment of the School-Age Child

A. General considerations.
    ✦ 1. Modesty important, heightened concern for privacy.
    2. Explain all procedures clearly.
    3. Direct questions to child, not to parent.
B. Utilize screening procedures for assessment.
    1. Snellen vision testing.
    2. Sweep check audiometry.
    3. Height and weight measurement.
    4. Inspection of skin and teeth.
    5. Assess for scoliosis.

Common Problems
✦ A. School.
    1. Determine child's attitude toward school, ability and participation.
    2. Assess for signs of school-related problems: procrastination, GI symptoms, depression, anger.
✦ B. Nervous habits.
    1. Assess onset and duration of such habits as stuttering, twitching.
    2. Determine precipitating event.
    3. Evaluate anxiety of child and parent over problem.
✦ C. Anticipatory guidance: seat belts, bicycle helmets, skateboarding gear (helmets and pads), water safety, sports participation (protective gear); diet, nutrition; hazards of cigarette smoking, alcohol, drugs, firearms; dental hygiene—need for orthodontics, cavity prevention.
D. Accidental trauma.
    1. Provide anticipatory guidance.
    2. Assess if physical limitations may have caused accident.
E. Respiratory infections.
    1. Assess duration and severity of symptoms.
    2. Look for wheezing, barking cough, anxiety, restlessness, use of accessory muscles.
    3. If throat is sore, check for white patches on tonsils.
F. Gastrointestinal infections.

1. Assess onset and duration.
2. Evaluate intake and output.
3. Check for signs of dehydration.

Assessment of the Adolescent

A. General considerations.
    ✦ 1. Privacy is important. Give the *adolescent* the choice of having the parent present.
    2. Note signs of puberty (Tanner stages).
    3. Ascertain feelings about body image.
B. Utilize screening procedures for assessment.
    1. Snellen vision testing.
    2. Sweep check audiometry.
    3. Height and weight measurement.
    ✦ 4. Inspection of skin and teeth.
C. Provide anticipatory guidance in the following areas.
    1. Hazards of cigarette smoking, alcohol, drugs, and firearms.
    2. Transmission, symptoms, and prevention of venereal disease, HIV.
    3. Sex education and need for contraception.
    4. Accident prevention, particularly automobile; seat belts and traffic safety.
    5. Principles of nutrition, assess for obesity or excessive dieting, eating disorders (anorexia nervosa, bulimia).
    6. Breast and testicular self-exam.
    7. Sports participation and proper protective equipment.
    8. Dental problems.
    9. Mental health assessment: signs of depression or suicidal thoughts, eating disorders, bipolar disease, schizophrenia, antisocial or sociopathic behavior, substance abuse, sexual or physical abuse.

Common Problems
A. Obesity/eating disorders.
    1. Determine eating patterns, diet "diary."
    2. Evaluate family concern and handling of problem.
    3. Assess amount of exercise.
B. Dysmenorrhea.
    1. Evaluate degree of pain (i.e., absences from school).
    2. Determine use of analgesics.
    3. Assess amount of exercise.
C. Mood changes.
    1. Be alert to signs of depression.
    2. Inquire about outlook for future, attentive to any indication of suicidal thoughts.
    3. Assess anger management strategies.
D. Acne.
    1. Evaluate existing skin care program.
    2. Assess child's personal hygiene.

IMPACT OF HOSPITALIZATION

INFANT

Assessment

A. Obtain history and usual behavior/developmental milestones achieved.

✦ B. Assess psychosocial implications of hospitalization on child.
1. Separation from the parent.
2. Decrease in sensory stimuli.
3. Breakdown in parent–infant relationship due to:
   a. Parental guilt.
   b. Unfamiliar hospital environment.
   c. Feelings of inadequacy in the parenting role.
   d. Subordination of the parents by the staff.

✦ C. Assess behavior of infant in response to illness.
1. Indication of discomfort or pain.
   a. Cries frequently.
   b. Displays excessive irritability.
   c. Appears lethargic or prostrate.
   d. Low-grade fever.
   e. Poor feeding.
   f. Grimaces or cries to touch.
2. Positive reaction behaviors.
   a. Cries loudly.
   b. Appears fussy and irritable.
   c. Rejects everyone except parent.
3. Negative reaction behaviors.
   a. Withdraws from everyone.
   b. Cries monotonously.
   c. Appears completely passive.

Implementation

✦ A. Nursing actions help lessen the detrimental effects of hospitalization.

✦ B. Hold a prehospitalization nursing interview with the parents and give a tour of the pediatric unit when possible.
1. Parents should meet the staff, have procedures and regulations explained to them, and be told the rationale behind the rules.
2. They should be encouraged to visit frequently and/or to room in if possible.

C. Counsel the parents regarding the infant's illness, and elicit their understanding of the disease and its course of action. Correct any misconceptions, and if appropriate, reassure them that they are not the cause of the illness.

✦ D. Encourage the parents to participate in the infant's care.
1. Teach the parents procedures they can perform at appropriate times for learning.
2. Show respect for their superior knowledge of infant's likes, dislikes, and habits.
3. Most institutions now allow/encourage 24-hour visitation. Encourage rooming-in and allow parent to be primary caregiver whenever possible.

TODDLER AND PRESCHOOLER

Assessment

✦ A. Assess psychosocial implications of hospitalization.
1. Hospitalization is a very threatening experience to the child because of the total number of new experiences involved.
2. Because of the threat involved, hospitalization has the potential for disrupting the toddler's new sense of identity and independence.
✦ 3. Separation anxiety—the child mourns the absence of parent through protest, despair, and denial.
   a. Cries loudly, throws tantrums.
   b. Child withdraws and shows no interest in eating, playing, etc.
   c. Behavior often mistaken for happy adjustment; ignores parent and may regress.
   d. Nursing behaviors: reassure the parent, build a relationship with the child, and provide warmth and support to the child during long hospitalization.
✦ 4. The child fears the loss of "body integrity" (prevalence of magical thought). The child also has no realistic perception of how the body functions and may overreact to a simple procedure. Some toddlers believe that drawing blood will leave a hole and that the rest of their blood will leak out.
✦ 5. The child resents the disruption of normal rituals and routines. Toddlers are often very rigid about certain procedures, which allows them a sense of security and control over otherwise frightening circumstances.
6. Loss of mobility is frustrating to the child.
7. Regression—the toddler frequently abandons the most recently acquired behaviors and reverts to safer, less mature patterns.

✦ B. Assess behavior of toddlers and preschoolers in response to illness.
1. Indications of discomfort or pain.
   a. Cries frequently.
   b. Displays excessive irritability.

c. Appears lethargic, withdrawn.
d. Changes eating pattern.
e. Verbalizes discomfort, or becomes stoic.
f. Use pain assessment tool (FACES or Oucher).
2. Positive reaction behaviors.
a. Shows aggressive behavior.
b. Appears occasionally withdrawn.
c. Fantasizes about illness and procedures.
d. Shows regressive behavior.
3. Negative reaction behaviors.
a. Appears completely passive or excessively aggressive.
b. Displays excessive regressive behavior.
c. Withdraws from everyone.

Implementation

✦ A. Suggest that the parent leave a favorite object of his or hers that the child would recognize for the child to "care for" until he or she can return. This procedure assures the child that the parent will return.

✦ B. Encourage the parents to be honest about when they are going and coming (i.e., do not tell the child they will stay all night and then leave when the child is asleep).

✦ C. Use puppet or doll play to explain procedures and to gain an understanding of the child's perception of hospitalization. Use puppets or dolls to work out child's anxiety, anger, and frustration.

✦ D. During developmental history, elicit exact routines and rituals that the child uses; attempt to modify hospital routine to continue these rituals.

E. Consistency among nursing staff in guidelines for behavior that is acceptable; set firm limits.

F. Maintain a schedule that is consistent and as closely resembling the usual routine as possible. (*See* Table 13-2.)

Problem Behaviors

✦ A. Depressed behavior.
1. Encourage child to express himself or herself through play.
2. Talk through a doll or stuffed animal for younger children.
3. Don't avoid child; continue to interact and support.
4. Consult with other professionals.

✦ B. Aggressive behavior.
1. Channel energy positively: older children may enjoy competitive activities; younger children can release tension through pounding boards, large motor activity, or clay projects.
2. Set limits and praise for jobs well done.
3. Help child gain a sense of mastery.

✦ C. Passive behavior.

1. Structure the child's day, provide consistency.
2. Spend more time with the child and attempt to stimulate interest.
3. Provide "win-win" choices.

✦ D. Regressed behavior.
1. Regression is acceptable to a point because it allows child a brief return to a less mature and demanding time.
2. Support independence, mastery of tasks, and self-care.

SCHOOL-AGE CHILD

Assessment

✦ A. Assess psychological implications of hospitalization.
1. The school-age child wants to understand why things are happening.
2. There is a heightened concern for privacy.
3. The child is modest and fears disgrace.
4. Hospitalization means an interruption in the child's busy school life, and the child fears that he or she will be replaced or forgotten by peer group.
5. Absence from peer group means a disruption of close friendships.

B. Assess behavior of school-age children in response to illness.
1. Indications of discomfort or pain.
a. Expresses that something is wrong. ("I feel sick.")
b. Cries easily.
c. Tells adult he or she is ill so adult can do something about it.
2. Use pain assessment tool (e.g., Eland Color Tool) or Visual Analog Scale.
3. Positive reaction behaviors.
a. Shows anger.
b. Feels guilty.
c. Fantasizes and is fearful.
d. Displays increased activity in response to anxiety.
e. Reacts to immobility by becoming depressed or angry or by crying.
f. Cries or aggressively resists treatment.
g. Needs parents and authority.
✦ 4. Negative reaction behaviors.
a. Is excessively guilty and angry and is unable to express feelings.
b. Experiences night terrors.
c. Displays excessive hyperactivity.
d. Will not talk about experience.
e. Is regressive and completely withdrawn.
f. Shows excessive dependency.
g. Has insomnia.

✦ Table 13-2. MANAGING BEHAVIOR THROUGH PLAY

Nursing Goals	Nursing Interventions
To bathe child	Give tub toys such as boats, cups, bottles, bulb syringe Give child something he or she can wash, such as a doll or a car
To administer soaks	Give child something to look at, such as a picture book or kaleidoscope Read a story or have child tell you one Set a timer so that child has the concept of time For hand and foot soaking, give child something to hold down or count
To encourage mobility	Extend environment through use of "fantasy trips," decoration of bed and surrounding area, or imaginative movement Move bed outdoors or to a playroom or a different room Have other children come to visit restricted child Use video games for older children
To ambulate	Give child something to pull or push or ride on Set reasonable distance goal for child to reach Take to visit another child or place Have a parade with hats, horns, etc. Have child walk for a reward, such as a visit to a sibling or the cafeteria
To encourage deep breathing	Give child bubbles, straws, non-latex gloves to blow into Have child blow through straws to race cotton balls Have child play kazoos or harmonicas Give child straws to suck up pieces of paper or cotton balls
To encourage coughing	Put squeaky toy on child's abdomen so toy makes a noise when the child coughs Have child squeeze a pillow or stuffed animal for splinting
To maintain NPO status	Arrange special activities during mealtime, such as a walk, visit to a special place, video or game
To encourage child to eat	Sit child with other children who are eating Encourage family to bring appropriate favorite foods from home Serve familiar and liked food in small portions on a small plate Use a game or story to encourage eating Have child prepare foods that he or she likes
To restrict fluids	Give child a choice of fluids and time when he or she wants to drink them Measure and place in tall narrow container
To encourage child to drink	Give small amounts of liquid frequently over a period of time Use a special decorated cup Let child use syringe instead of straw or cup Give popsicles, jello, or slushes Sit child with other children and have a tea party
To administer medication	Give child a choice of methods to take medication: whole, cut up, with water or apple juice, liquid vs. pill form Let older child give medication to himself Give rewards (stars, stickers) for taking medication Allow parents to administer if desired and able

Implementation

✦ A. Teach the child about his or her illness; take the opportunity to explain the functioning of the body.

B. Explain all procedures completely; allow the child to see special rooms (e.g., intensive care, cardiac cath lab) prior to being sent there for treatments. Whenever possible, provide honest and direct explanations in age-appropriate language.

✦ C. Provide opportunities for the child to socialize with peer group.

1. Allow telephone privileges for calls to home and friends.

2. Provide outlets for anger and frustration (perhaps Velcro or suction dartboard).

D. Give the child the opportunity to make choices and be independent, whenever possible.

E. Protect child's privacy.

F. Continue child's schooling by providing tutors, providing time for schoolwork, providing quiet, needed supplies, turning off television and/or video games.

G. Provide child with the opportunity to master developmental tasks of age group.

ADOLESCENT

Assessment

✦ A. Assess psychological implications of illness.
   1. Disruption of social system and peer group.
   2. Alteration of body image.
   3. Fear of loss of independence or actual loss.
   4. Alteration in plans for future.
   5. Interruption in development of relationships.
   6. Loss of privacy.
   7. The degree to which the young adult is affected is dependent on:
      a. Whether the illness is chronic or acute.
      b. Whether the prognosis necessitates a change in the client's future aspirations.
      c. How many changes must be accepted.

B. Assess behavior of adolescents in response to illness.
   1. Indications of discomfort or pain.
      a. Realizes something is wrong and seeks help.
      b. Shows high anxiety level.
      c. Verbalizes discomfort.
      d. Use pain assessment tool (e.g., Eland or 1–10 Visual Analog Scale).
   2. Positive reaction behaviors.
      a. Shows resistance to accepting illness.
      b. Rebels against authority.
      c. Demands control and independence.
      d. Is fearful.
      e. Temporarily withdraws from social scene.
      f. Verbalizes how illness has affected him or her.
   3. Negative reaction behaviors.
      a. Holds in feelings about illness.
      b. Tries to manipulate staff.
      c. Becomes completely dependent.
      d. Denies illness.
      e. Becomes stoic and doesn't acknowledge pain.

Implementation

✦ A. Adolescents should be in rooms with other adolescents, away from young children.

B. Allow telephone and visitation privileges, with some limit setting.

C. Encourage the feeling of self-worth by allowing as much independence as possible.

D. Allow relationships to develop within reason.

E. Provide for privacy.

F. Assist client in identifying role models.

✦ G. Realistically discuss problems of illness.
   1. Always provide information honestly.
   2. Encourage the adolescent, if possible, to accept some responsibility on the hospital unit.

Table 13-3. ASSESSMENT OF VITAL SIGNS				
Age	Range of Normal Pulse	Average Pulse	Average Blood Pressure	Average Respiration
Newborn	100–180	140	80/55	30–50
1 year	80–150	120	96/60	20–40
2 years	80–130	110	99/65	20–30
4 years	80–120	100	99/65	20–25
6 years	75–115	100	100/56	20–25
8 years	70–110	90	105/56	15–20
10 years	70–110	90	110/58	15–20

NEUROLOGICAL SYSTEM

The central nervous system (brain and spinal cord), the peripheral nervous system (cranial and spinal nerves), and the autonomic nervous system comprise the neurological system; together these provide control functions for the entire body.

System Assessment

A. History.
1. Birth history, developmental milestones, immunizations and exposures.
2. Recent trauma.
3. Current illness.
✦ B. Level of consciousness.
1. Interaction with environment.
2. Glasgow Coma Scale score (infant or adult).
C. Size and shape of head (infants).
1. Size and quality of fontanelles and sutures.
2. Recent acute increase in head circumference.
D. Assessment of motor function.
1. Symmetry of movements.
2. Muscle tone and strength.
3. Tremors or twitching.
4. Seizure activity.
E. Pupil size and reactivity, eye movements.
✦ F. Cranial nerve (CN) assessment.
1. Incorporate into other areas of physical exam when possible.
2. Test CNs II, III, IV, VI (optic, oculomotor, trochlear, and abducens) together by checking pupils and having child follow light.
3. Check CNs V, VII, XII (trigeminal, facial, and hypoglossal) together by having older child bite down, show teeth, and stick out tongue. Test younger infant's ability to root for nipple, and check CN X (vagus) by observing ability to swallow.
4. Test hearing (Rinne and Weber) with tuning fork—CN VIII.
5. Check CNs VII and IX (facial and hypoglossopharyngeal) by tasting sweet, sour, and bitter solutions (older children only).
6. Test CN I (olfactory) in older children only.
G. Reflexes. (*See* Table 13-4.)
1. Infant/persistent.
2. Symmetry.
3. Presence of clonus.

H. Developmental exam.
1. Obtain history from reliable caregiver.
2. Use screening tools to evaluate attainment of major milestones.
3. Communicate concerns/delays to other healthcare providers.
I. Behavioral history and assessment.
1. Assess mood, eating and sleep patterns; any recent changes.
2. Assess ability to concentrate, school progress, and difficulty with relationships.
3. Assess irrational or aggressive behavior (especially with history of head trauma or CNS infection).
4. Family history of behavioral disorders.
J. Respiratory pattern and vital signs.
1. Assess altered respiratory pattern (cluster, ataxic, Cheyne–Stokes, apneustic).
2. Evaluation of fever or signs of infection.
✦ K. Indications of neurological problems.
✦ 1. Meningeal signs.
a. Irritability, nuchal rigidity, opisthonos.
b. Positive Kernig and Brudzinski signs.
✦ 2. Seizures.
a. History.
b. Medications.
c. Duration and assessment of motor involvement.
✦ 3. Signs of increased intracranial pressure (ICP).
a. Altered level of consciousness (LOC).
b. Irritability or lethargy.
c. Headache, nausea, vomiting.
d. Sunset eyes, bulging fontanelles, high-pitched cry, poor feeding in infants.

Diagnostic Procedures

Client and family preparation must precede all procedures unless emergency. Nurses should be available to answer questions concerning the procedure and how the parents can help the client through the procedure.

✦ **Lumbar Puncture (LP)**

A. Withdrawal of cerebrospinal fluid (CSF) by insertion of a hollow needle between lumbar vertebrae L3 and L4 or L4 and L5 into subarachnoid space to identify intracranial pressure, signs of infection, or hemorrhage. Fluid is analyzed for CSF chemistries, cell count, Gram stain, culture.
B. Nursing responsibilities prior to procedure.
1. Maintain baseline record of vital signs.
2. Explain to the parents and child exactly what will happen.
C. Nursing responsibilities during procedure.
1. Place child on side in knee–chest position with head flexed on chest.

✦ Table 13-4, NEWBORN REFLEXES

Reflex	Response	Stimulus	Duration
Babinski's sign	Toes, especially the great toe, hyperextend	Stroke lateral side of the sole of the foot from heel to base of toes	Present at birth; disappears between 12 and 18 months
Neck righting reflex	Shoulder, arms, and legs of opposite side will flex to follow head in turn	Turn infant's head to left or right	Evolving at 4 months; involuntary movement disappears at approx. 9–12 months
Palmar grasp	Grasps and holds adult finger; automatic reflex of full-term newborns	Place finger in infant's palm	Present at birth; disappears at approx. 4 months
Asymmetrical tonic neck reflex	Assumes fencer's position: arm extends on side to which head is turned; opposite arm is flexed	Turn infant's head to one side	Present at birth; disappears at approx. 4 months
Startle reflex	Body stiffens; legs are drawn up; arms are brought up, out, and then in front in an embracing position	Make a loud noise	Present at birth; disappears at approx. 4 months
Reciprocal kicking (stepping)	Steps alternately from one foot to the other	Hold infant upright with feet touching a firm surface	Evolving at birth; disappears at approx. 9 months
Rooting reflex	Turns head to side that has been stimulated	Brush infant's cheek with fingertips	Present at birth; rooting while awake disappears at approx. 3–4 months; rooting while asleep at 7–8 months
Sucking reflex	Makes sucking movements	Touch infant's lips with any object	Present at birth; involuntary sucking disappears at approx. 9 months

2. Help child remain steady in this position and reassure child throughout procedure.

D. Nursing responsibilities following procedure.
   1. Keep child flat in bed.
   2. Encourage fluid intake.
   3. If headache occurs when sitting up, return child to flat position and give analgesic.
   4. Observe neurological status for signs of deterioration.

E. LP should not be performed in clients at high risk for bleeding; extreme caution should be used if elevated ICP is suspected.

✦ Computerized Tomography (CT) Scan

A. Provides visualization of neuroanatomy; differentiates tissue density compared to water.

B. Visualizes brain along vertical or horizontal plane from any axis.

C. Can distinguish hemorrhage, tumors, congenital abnormalities, and inflammatory or hypoxic processes.

D. May use contrast medium for enhanced views.

E. Nursing considerations.
   1. Client/family education about what to expect. Machine may provoke claustrophobia.
   2. Client required to lie still during procedure. May require restraints or sedation.
   3. Assess carefully for allergy or anaphylaxis to contrast (iodine based). Observe IV site carefully to avoid extravasation.
   4. Recent evidence that repeated CT scans in young children *may* increase radiation-related cancers. CT scans should be performed only for clearly delineated purposes.

F. PET scan (positron emission tomography).
   1. Provides a 3D map of functional processes in the body. Used primarily for imaging and staging of suspected tumors or in localizing seizure focus.
   2. Requires IV injection of radioactive tracer isotope, usually fluorodeoxyglucose (FDG) 1 hour before procedure.

3. Teaching: IV is necessary, keep child quiet after injection of FDG until scan; radiation dose is less than used for CT scan; may require NPO status before scan. Scan takes about 1 hour and may require sedation.

✦ **Magnetic Resonance Imaging (MRI)**

A. Allows high-quality imaging of morphology of structures.

B. Distinguishes structures by response to radio frequency pulses in a magnetic field.

C. Tissue differentiation superior to other techniques.

D. Requires immobilization throughout procedure (sedation and respiratory monitoring *required* for young clients).

E. Nursing considerations.
   1. Education of client/family about procedure and what to expect. Reassure older children.
   2. Reinforce medical information as needed.
   3. Follow sedation protocol.
   4. Careful monitoring of vital signs, SaO$_2$, and respiratory status during procedure.
   5. Observe carefully for reaction to contrast medium.

Electroencephalogram (EEG)

A. Provides information about electrical activity of cerebral cortex.

B. Used to assess neuronal functioning and to diagnose seizure activity; shows characteristic abnormalities for seizures.

C. Also may be used in part to determine brain death.

D. May be combined with simultaneous video recording.

✦ E. Nursing responsibilities.
   1. Explain procedure and sensations to expect.
   2. Activities during procedure may include hyperventilation, sleep deprivation, and antiseizure drug withdrawal.
   3. Shampoo head afterward to remove all glue and gel.
   4. Clarify any misconceptions (client does not receive shocks via leads, etc.).

✦ **Electromyelogram**

A. Records electrical activity in muscle fibers.
   1. Nerve conduction velocity is measured by placing needles in muscles and applying electrical current.
   2. May do computed tomographic (CT) myelogram or lumbar myelography. Contrast medium is injected into subarachnoid space to visualize structures around spinal canal.

B. Nursing responsibilities prior to procedure.
   1. Ensure that child is NPO 6–8 hours before procedure (follow sedation protocol).
   2. Maintain baseline record of vital signs and neurological status.

3. Administer sedative as ordered.
4. Educate client and family about sensations to expect (aches or needle pricks).

C. Nursing responsibilities following procedure.
   1. Frequently observe neurological signs and vital signs and compare to baseline.
   2. Assure adequate hydration.
   3. Activity may be restricted.
   4. Watch for signs of infection or hematoma at insertion sites.
   5. Slightly elevate head (30 degrees for at least 8 hours if contrast media is used for CT myelography).

✦ **Angiogram**

A. Radiopaque substance is injected into cerebral vasculature or its extracranial sources to evaluate vascular anomalies, lesions, or tumors.

B. Nursing responsibilities prior to procedure.
   1. Prep area where cannulization is to be made (usually femoral or brachial).
   2. Ensure that child has no solid food for 6–8 hours prior to procedure.
   3. Keep baseline record of neurological and vital signs.
   4. Sedation usually necessary (occasionally anesthesia—follow protocol).
   5. Observe closely for reaction to contrast medium.

C. Nursing responsibilities following procedure.
   1. Observe for changes in level of consciousness, transient hemiplegia, seizures, sensory or motor deterioration, or elevation of blood pressure with widening pulse pressure.
   2. Check CMS in extremity used (adequate pulses, color, sensation, movement, swelling, temperature).
   3. Encourage fluid intake.

System Implementation

For Infants

✦ A. Record head circumferences, and graph results, at least every 24 hours.

✦ B. Observe for changes in fontanelles.

C. Note activity level and interactions with significant others.

D. Observe for the continuous presence of sunset sign, high-pitched cry, feeding problems.

E. Observe for presence of all newborn reflexes. Note the symmetry of movement and the presence of hypertonia or hypotonia.

✦ **For Children**

A. Note activity level and observe for changes in activity.

B. Control and prevent seizure activity. (For specific actions, refer to Seizure Disorders, page 649.)

C. Carefully position child to prevent aspiration if vomiting is an actual or potential problem.

D. Check pupillary responses or movements at least every shift. Note presence of nystagmus or strabismus, abnormal responses.

E. Assess vital signs every 4 hours or more frequently if unstable.

F. Report intake and output (I&O) every 24-hour period.

G. Evaluate the nutritional status of the child if vomiting is present.

H. Provide sterile field for any treatment that involves an area with open entry to the nervous system.

I. Evaluate level of consciousness (*see* Neurological System, Medical–Surgical Nursing).

◆ J. Assess child for presence of meningeal irritation.
1. *Kernig's sign:* Extension of leg causes spasm of the hamstring, pain and resistance when child is in supine position with thigh and knee flexed to right angle.
2. *Brudzinski's sign:* Flexion of head causes flexion of knees and both thighs at the hips.

K. Support the family through accurate reports of the child's condition and by allowing the family to participate in the child's care as much as possible.

L. Explain all procedures in truthful manner to the child. Allow time for questions.

CONGENITAL DEFECTS

Neural Tube Defects (NTD)

Definition: Failure of posterior portion of lamina of bony spine to form, causing an opening in spinal column. Spina bifida and anencephaly are two most common forms. Spina bifida may involve (1) meninges and spinal fluid (meningocele) or (2) meninges, nerves, and spinal fluid (meningomyelocele). NTDs occur in approximately 1 in every 1000 pregnancies in the United States.

Classification

◆ A. *Spina bifida occulta.*
1. Involves a bony defect only and does not involve the spinal cord or the meninges, not visible externally.
2. Generally requires no treatment.

◆ B. *Meningocele.*
1. Meninges of the spinal cord extend through opening in spine.
2. Usually causes no paralysis.
3. Treatment involves closure of sac.

◆ C. *Meningomyelocele.*

1. Nerves, meninges, and CSF protrude through defect in spine.
2. This defect causes neuromuscular involvement, which can vary from flaccidity and lack of bowel and bladder innervation to weakness of lower extremities.

Assessment

A. May be detected prenatally by elevated concentrations of alpha-fetoproteins and by prenatal ultrasonography.

◆ B. Assess for presence of hydrocephalus.

C. Assess neurological involvement.

◆ D. Check urological involvement.
1. Frequent bladder infections.
2. Potential for progressive renal damage.
3. Ileal conduit surgery is frequently required.
4. Credé method of managing urinary retention involves systematic "milking" of the bladder at periodic intervals.

E. Assess for orthopedic involvement.

F. Evaluate bowel function.

Implementation

◆ A. *Prevention:* American Academy of Pediatrics recommends consumption of 400 µg of folic acid daily by all women capable of becoming pregnant.
1. This can prevent 70 percent of NTDs.
2. Folic acid intake should increase to 400 µg per day at least one month before becoming pregnant, and continue throughout the first trimester.

B. Treatment dependent on severity of condition.

◆ C. Neurological interventions.
1. Observe for signs of hydrocephalus; a frequent complication.
2. Measure head circumference at least every 24 hours.
3. Observe for signs of increased intracranial pressure, and signs of CNS infection (meningitis).
4. Surgical closure performed as soon as tolerated. Until closure, the sac should be covered with a sterile, moist, nonadherent dressing (changed every 2–4 hours) and the infant kept in a prone position.

◆ D. Urological interventions.
1. If child is catheterized, use sterile technique.
2. Keep a careful record of intake and output.
3. Teach parents Credé method if treatment is ordered.
4. Observe for signs of urinary tract infection.
   a. Increased temperature.
   b. Foul-smelling urine.
   c. Cloudy urine with possible mucus.

E. Orthopedic interventions.

1. Provide opportunities for the child to exercise and develop unaffected areas, in conjunction with physicians and physical therapists.
2. Prevent contractures through proper positioning.
   a. Provide foot brace to prevent footdrop.
   b. Provide support for legs to prevent external rotation of the hips.
3. Implement range-of-motion exercises.

F. Special considerations.
   1. Children with NTDs are especially prone to developing latex allergies. Exposure to latex should be limited or avoided in infants and throughout all treatment.
   ✦ 2. Use of folic acid supplements in pregnancy has shown to decrease the incidence of NTDs.

Hydrocephalus

✦ *Definition:* A condition in which the normal circulation of the spinal fluid is altered, resulting in pressure on the brain, deformity, and the progressive enlargement of the head. May occur as congenital defect or as the result of trauma, infection, or surgery.

Assessment

✦ A. Assess for gradual enlargement of the head (no more than 2.5 cm per month).
   1. 35 cm at birth.
   2. 40 cm at 3 months.
   3. 45 cm at 9 months.
   4. At birth, the head size is 2 cm larger than the chest. Equals or exceeds chest until 2 years of age.
✦ B. Check for separation of skull sutures.
C. Assess for sunset sign (sclera visible above iris).
D. Check for hyperactive reflexes.
E. Evaluate presence of irritability, failure to thrive, and high-pitched cry.
F. Assess for presence of projectile vomiting.
G. Prepare child and family for CT or MRI.

Implementation

A. Actions depend on the cause of increased pressure.
   1. Removal of part of choroid plexus to decrease production of cerebral spinal fluid.
   2. Shunting of the fluid out of the brain to the heart or to the peritoneal cavity.
   3. Removal of obstruction (mass lesion) to CSF flow.
✦ B. Preoperative care.
   1. Prevent pressure sores on head by changing child's position, placing child's head on gel form or other skin protective device, or by holding the infant.
   2. Provide good head support when the child is sitting in Fowler's position.

3. Promote optimal nutritional status.
4. Keep eyes free of irritation.
✦ C. Postoperative care.
   1. Observe for shunt malfunction and valve patency: watch for progressive increase in head circumference and signs of increased intracranial pressure; evaluate pupils and eye movements carefully.
   2. Observe for infection: increased temperature, rapid pulse, irritability, nausea, or vomiting.
   3. Position child flat on unoperated side.
   4. Prevent postoperative complications: turn every 4 hours, evaluate lung sounds, and assess for signs of infection.
   5. Administer antibiotics as ordered.
   6. Protect the operative site: avoid pressure on the site; ensure sterile dressing changes.
   7. Maintain adequate fluid and nutritional status.

NEUROLOGICAL DISORDERS

Cerebral Palsy

✦ *Definition:* A nonspecific term used to describe a group of disorders characterized by motor and postural impairments due to abnormal muscle tone: cerebral palsy may also involve language, perceptual, and intellectual deficits. The most common permanent physical disability of childhood, occurring in approximately 2 in 1000 live births.

Assessment

A. Etiology is thought to be multifactoral; with prenatal, perinatal, and postnatal causes possible. Prenatal brain abnormalities are probably the most likely cause.
   1. The single most important determinant of cerebral palsy appears to be premature birth.
   2. In roughly one-quarter of cerebral palsy cases, no cause is found.
✦ B. Assess for abnormal movements.
   1. Spasticity.
      a. Voluntary muscles lose normal smooth movements and respond with difficulty to both active and passive movement.
      b. Increased deep tendon reflexes, scissoring.
      c. Contractures of antigravity muscles.
      d. Persistence of primitive reflexes.
      e. Lack of normal postural control.
   2. Athetoid (dyskinetic).
      a. Involuntary muscle action with smooth, writhing movement of extremities.
      b. Reflexes usually normal.
   3. Ataxia: lack of coordination and possibly hypotonia.

C. Assess for seizures which occur in many children with cerebral palsy.

D. Check for vision disturbance which occurs in 20 percent of these children.

✦ E. Assess mental functioning; at least 50 percent function at a subnormal level. Many cerebral palsy children are diagnosed as mentally retarded due to slow motor skills or aphasia, but possess normal or high intellegence.

Implementation

A. Each child requires an individualized program according to the particular manifestations of the disease and the child's capacities.

✦ B. Major focus of interventions is to:
1. Develop motor control.
2. Develop communication skills.
3. Provide adequate nutrition.
4. Prevent orthopedic complications.

Seizure Disorders

✦ *Definition:* A series of seizures that result from focal or diffuse paroxysmal discharges in cortical neurons—symptoms of abnormal brain function. May be congenital or acquired.

Etiology

A. Seizure disorders are idiopathic (cause unknown or acquired) or the result of brain injury caused by trauma, hypoxia, infection, toxins, or other acquired factors.

B. Seizures more common during first 2 years than any other period.

C. Most common cause by age group.
1. Young infants: birth injury, hemorrhage, anoxia, and congenital defects of the brain.
2. Late infancy and early childhood: infections, trauma; middle childhood–onset epilepsy is uncommon.
3. Children older than 3 years: idiopathic epilepsy most common.

Assessment

A. Febrile seizures.
1. Very common; occurs in 3–4 percent of all children, usually in children 6 months to 6 years of age. Usually occurs within 24 hours of onset of fever to > 39°C (but rapidity of rise in fever may be more important than height of fever).
2. Simple febrile seizure—lasts < 15 minutes, generalized may occur once per 24 hours.
3. Compex febrile seizure lasts > 15 minutes, has focal onset, and occurs more than once per 24 hours.

4. Seizure is generally benign, but LP and lab work indicated to locate source of fever. Not usually hospitalized. Risk of developing epileptic syndrome is low.

5. Treatment: rectal diazepam may be offered if seizures are prolonged or multiple, and high risk of recurrent seizures. Long-term prophylaxis (phenobarbital) is generally reserved for children who have other neurological problems.

✦ B. Simple partial seizures.
1. Localized (begins focally in one hemisphere) and does not impair level of consciousness. May involve motor symptoms, accompanied by autonomic or somatosensory symptoms.
2. Localized (confined to a specific area) motor symptoms, accompanied by autonomic or somatosensory symptoms.
✦ 3. Manifestations.
   a. Aversive seizure—most common motor seizure in children. Eye(s) turn away from focus side.
   b. Sylvan seizures—most common during sleep. Tonic–clonic movements involving face.

✦ C. Complex partial (psychomotor) seizures.
1. Jacksonian march—rare in children. Sequential clonic movements.
2. Area of brain most involved is temporal lobe (thus, this type of seizure is called psychomotor).
3. Most common in children from 3 years to adolescence.
4. Characterized by complex sensory phenomena, a period of altered behavior, and amnesia (child is not aware of behavior). Seizure begins focally in one hemisphere and impairs LOC.
5. May perform such mannerisms as lip smacking, chewing, picking at clothes, etc.
6. Seizure lasts several minutes and is accompanied by aura and postictal phase. May have secondary generalization (such as Jacksonian march; spreads to other hemisphere).

✦ D. Generalized seizures.
✦ 1. Tonic–clonic seizures, formerly known as "grand mal."
   a. May begin with an aura, then a tonic phase (lasting 10–20 seconds): stiffening or rigidity of muscles, particularly arms and legs; eyes roll up; followed by loss of consciousness; may be apneic and become cyanotic.
   b. Clonic phase follows (lasts about 30 seconds, but may last as long as 30 minutes): hyperventilation with rhythmic violent jerking of all extremities; may foam at the mouth and become incontinent; full recovery may take several hours.

c. Status epilepticus—a series of seizures that run together and do not allow the child to regain consciousness between attacks.
   (1) A neurological emergency with generalized tonic–clonic seizures.
   (2) Status epilepticus can lead to exhaustion, respiratory failure, and death.
   (3) Usually treated with IV diazepam or lorazepam. Respiratory monitoring is **essential** after administration of benzodiazepines.

✦ 2. Absence seizures, formerly known as "petit mal."
   a. Brief duration, often just 5–10 seconds, brief loss of consciousness; almost no change in muscle tone.
   b. May occur 20–30 times/day.
   c. Common in children; may appear to be "daydreaming," or inattentive.

✦ 3. Myoclonic seizure.
   a. Characterized by a brief, generalized jerking or stiffening of the extremities.
   b. Seizure may throw person to the floor; no loss of consciousness.

✦ 4. Atonic or akinetic seizures, also called "drop attacks."
   a. Onset between 2 and 5 years of age.
   b. Characterized by sudden, brief loss of muscle tone.
   c. Child may fall to ground, momentary loss of consciousness.

✦ 5. Infantile spasms.
   a. Most common in first 6–8 months of life; more common in males; usually associated with low intelligence later in life.
   b. Characterized by sudden, brief, symmetrical contractions; head flexed, legs drawn up, arms extended.
   c. May experience numerous attacks during the day without postictal drowsiness.

Implementation

✦ A. Prevent injury during seizure.
   ✦ 1. Remove any objects that may cause harm.
   2. Remain with child during seizure and provide privacy if possible.
   3. Do not force jaws open during seizure.
   4. Do not restrict limbs or restrain.
   5. Loosen restrictive clothing.
   ✦ 6. Check that airway is open. Do not initiate artificial ventilation during a tonic–clonic seizure without administering appropriate medications.
   7. Apply oxygen by blow-by if available or appropriate.
   8. Following seizure, turn head to side to prevent aspiration and allow secretions to drain; suction as needed.

B. Observe and document seizure pattern.
   1. Note time, LOC, and presence of aura before seizure.
   2. Record type, character, progression of movements.
   3. Note duration of seizure and child's condition throughout.
   4. Observe and record postictal state.

✦ C. Administer and monitor medications—complete control achieved in 50–70 percent of epileptic children.
   1. Medications for simple partial and complex partial seizures: carbamazepine (Tegretol), oxcarbezepine (Trileptal), phenytoin (Dilantin), and phenobarbital; occasionally valproic acid.
   2. Generalized seizures: valproic acid.
   3. New drugs: gabepentin, topiramat, tiagabine, and lamotrigine generally indicated as add-on therapy for partial seizures in children > 12 years old.

✦ D. Administer postseizure procedures—increases speed of recovery.
   1. Reduce stimuli—noise, lights, conversation.
      a. Place sources of light behind client.
      b. Keep away from fluorescent lights.
   2. Remain with child after consciousness returns.
      a. Speak and move slowly.
      b. Use simple phrases—give child time to respond.
   3. Encourage rest following a seizure (child will be exhausted) and maintain privacy.
   ✦ 4. Provide seizure precautions in hospital—keep bed rails raised, pad siderails of bed, suction and oxygen on standby.
   5. At home, child should carry medical identification, wear helmet (if has atonic seizures), and use precaution with hazardous activities.
   6. Ketogenic diet may prove helpful in controlling seizures but remains controversial.

Traumatic Brain Injury

Definition: Any trauma to the scalp, skull, meninges, or brain caused by mechanical force or penetration.

Characteristics

✦ A. Accidental injury is the major single cause of death in the pediatric age group, primarily from head injury sustained in motor vehicle accidents. Approximately 250,000 children are admitted every year for evaluation and treatment of head injury, and approximately 5000 deaths are attributed to traumatic brain injury in children < 19 years old.

B. Causes.
  1. Falls occur most frequently under 1 year of age; 75 percent result in some type of head injury.
      a. More boys than girls are injured by falls.
      b. 8- to 9-year-old age group—result of accidents involving bicycles, skateboarding, or athletics.
  2. Motor vehicle accidents are the most frequent cause in adolescents. Athletic injuries are also common.
C. Types of injuries.
  1. Most head injuries are caused by physical forces that impact on the head through acceleration and deceleration.
      a. *Acceleration:* slower-moving contents of cranium strike bony prominences or dura (coup).
      b. *Deceleration:* moving head strikes fixed object and brain rebounds, striking opposite side of cranium (contrecoup).
  2. Concussion is most common: violent jarring of the brain within the skull; temporary loss of consciousness; seizure activity.
  3. Contusion and laceration: the bruising of the brain and tearing of cerebral tissue.
  4. Closed head injuries: skull is intact.
  5. Open head injuries include deep scalp lacerations that require suturing.
  6. Fractures: the majority of fractures are linear; other types are depressed, compound, and comminuted. A child's skull can withstand a great amount of force before it fractures.
D. Complications.
  1. Epidural hemorrhage: usually the result of skull fracture. Bleeding is usually arterial, and brain compression develops quickly. Blood accumulates between dura and skull and forms a hematoma.
      a. Signs of intracranial compression occur within a few minutes or hours after the injury—significant shock may be present.
      b. Clinical signs include headache, vomiting, hemiparesis, and loss of consciousness.
  2. Subdural hemorrhage: bleeding between dura and cerebrum. (Common in infants due to birth trauma.) Bleeding is usually venous and develops more gradually than epidurals. Much more common than epidurals.
      a. Most common clinical signs are seizures, vomiting, and irritability.
      b. May be evidence of increased intracranial pressure.
  3. Subarachnoid and intracerebral hemorrhages may also occur from head injury.

  4. Cerebral edema (diffuse brain swelling) leads to signs of increased intracranial pressure but no focal signs.

Assessment

A. Assess LOC; changes appear earlier than changes in vital signs.
B. Check for nausea and vomiting.
C. Observe for pupillary changes: pupil dilates on ipsilateral side of injury.
D. Monitor changes in vital signs, reflecting increased intracranial pressure or shock.
E. Observe for seizure activity and describe fully if noted.
F. Observe for changes in position and movement: nuchal rigidity; opisthotonos.
G. Check for headache. (If child is too young to verbalize, he or she may be fussy and irritable.)
H. Observe for vasomotor or sensory losses.
I. Assess for rhinorrhea and otorrhea (infrequent in children).
  1. Bleeding from ear suggests basilar skull fracture.
  2. Drainage from nose should be tested with Dextrostix; if glucose present, it is evidence of cerebrospinal damage.
J. Observe child for any unusual behavior: make interpretation of this behavior in terms of child's normal behavior.
K. Identify any overt scalp or skull trauma.

Implementation

A. Monitor for complications: determine neurological status. (*See* previous section.)
  1. Check for signs of increased intracranial pressure.
      a. LOC: alert and easily aroused or lethargic; in a stupor or coma.
      b. Restless, irritable, crying behavior.
      c. Vital signs: changes in respiratory rate, increased blood pressure, pulse pressure, decreased pulse.
  2. Avoid actions that might increase intracranial pressure.
      a. Sudden changes in position.
      b. Bowel straining.
      c. Confused, noisy environment.
B. Monitor vital signs. Report changes immediately.
C. Maintain adequate respiratory exchange. Increased carbon dioxide levels increase cerebral edema.
D. Protect from injury by using safety measures.
  1. Maintain bedrest.
  2. Keep padded siderails up.
E. Position head to promote fluid drainage, promoting venous return from brain: elevate head of bed 15–30 degrees with head straight.
F. Monitor and protect child if seizure activity.

1. Observe and record type of seizure.
2. Note behavior that preceded seizure.

G. Prevent infection if there is drainage from auditory canal or nose.
   1. Place dry, sterile cotton loosely at orifice.
   2. If drainage from nose is positive for glucose, do not suction nares (risk of secondary infection).
   3. Maintain strict asepsis.

H. Provide adequate nutrition and hydration.
   1. Provide clear liquids as ordered.
   2. Measure intake and output accurately.
   3. Monitor IV if in place.

NEUROLOGICAL INFECTIONS

Meningitis

Definition: An acute inflammation of meninges that is caused by bacteria or viruses and may progress rapidly to neurologic problems, permanent brain damage, or death. Highest incidence is between birth and 2 years, greatest risk immediately following birth and 3–8 months.

Assessment

A. Assess airway, breathing, circulation, and fever; act immediately on abnormalities.
B. Complete neurological examination; assess for nuchal rigidity, positive Kernig's and Brudzinski's signs, headache, irritability, nausea, vomiting, seizure activity, other signs of increased ICP.
C. Often results from sepsis and invasion of the blood–brain barrier; may be caused by direct spread of otitis media or sinusitis, direct inoculation during surgery or trauma.
D. Diagnosis is confirmed by LP and CSF examination.
   1. Usual causes vary with age.
      a. Immediately after birth, cause is usually Group B *Streptococcus*, *E. coli*, or *Listeria*.
      b. After 1 month, usual cause is *Streptococcus pneumoniae*, *Haemophilus influenzae* type B, or *Neisseria meningitidis*.
   2. Viral meningitis is much less serious.
E. Prevention—incidence of meningitis due to *H. influenzae* and *N. meningitidis* should be decreasing with compliance to recommended immunization schedule.

Implementation

A. Evaluate airway, breathing, and circulation—client may present in septic shock.
B. Maintain patent airway; administer oxygen as ordered; respiratory arrest possible with deteriorating neurologic status.
C. Isolate child until the causative agent is identified.

D. Maintain optimal fluid balance, support cardiovascular system, monitor ICP.
E. Monitor neurological signs carefully.
F. Observe for signs of subdural effusion (collection of fluid in the subdural space).
   1. Increasing intracranial pressure.
   2. Irritability.
G. Administer antibiotics on time if bacterial cause.
H. If cause is *N. meningococcus*, contacts should receive antibiotic prophylaxis.
I. Maintain bedrest and position child comfortably; most children prefer a side-lying or flat position; sitting up increases pain. May elevate head of bed with increased ICP.

Encephalitis

Definition: Inflammation of the parenchyma of the brain, resulting from direct viral invasion or hypersensitivity initiated by a virus or another foreign protein.

Assessment

A. Fever, headache, altered LOC, sometimes with seizures and focal neurologic deficits.
B. A GI or respiratory prodrome may precede neurological symptoms.
C. Diagnosis: Requires CSF analysis and neuroimaging.
   1. Most common cause is herpes simplex virus (type 1 or type 2).
   2. Usual mortality rate is around 1 percent, but morbidity is higher.
   3. West Nile encephalitis has spread throughout the United States, with an associated mortality of about 9 percent.

Implementation

A. Mainly supportive, and may include antiviral medications.
B. Monitor for status epilepticus or coma, which suggests severe brain inflammation and poor prognosis.

Poliomyelitis

Definition: An acute viral infection affecting spinal cord and brain stem; may lead to paralysis or death. Polio is no longer a threat in the western hemisphere.

Characteristics

A. A contagious disease caused by three viruses: types 1, 2, and 3.
B. Incubation period is usually 7–14 days, with range of 5–35 days.
C. Communicable: throat holds virus for about 1 week; feces 4–6 weeks.
D. Manifests in three forms: abortive, nonparalytic (most common), and paralytic.

E. The virus is still transmitted in about 10 countries. Outbreaks of vaccine-derived polio have occurred in the Dominican Republic, Haiti and the Philippines.

F. Children are now immunized with 3 doses of inactivated poliovirus (IPV) instead of live oral poliovirus (OPV). Travelers to countries where polio is still transmitted must be fully immunized.

Assessment

◆ A. Assess symptoms of different types.
1. Abortive: fever, sore throat, headache, anorexia, vomiting, abdominal pain. May last few hours to days.
2. Nonparalytic: same as above but more severe, with stiff neck, back, and legs.
3. Paralytic (spinal and bulbar types): similar course as nonparalytic; apparent recovery followed by paralysis.

B. Assess if polio vaccine (OPV) given, and the full course received.

Implementation

A. Preventive: education of public to fully immunize children with IPV series.

◆ B. Maintain complete bedrest during acute period.

C. Provide respiratory support (mechanical ventilation) if respiratory paralysis occurs.

◆ D. Assist with physiotherapy (most important factor in recovery) following acute stage.

E. Evaluate for potential complications.

Reye's Syndrome

◆ *Definition:* Acute encephalopathy with fatty degeneration resulting in marked cerebral edema and enlargement of the liver with marked fatty infiltration.

Characteristics

A. Children from 2 months to adolescence contract illness; ages 6 to 11 years most often affected.

◆ B. Usually follows a viral infection, especially varicella and influenza B.

◆ C. Aspirin (because of links to development of Reye's) is now contraindicated with influenza—acetaminophen is medication of choice.

D. Incidence of Reye's decreased dramatically with decreased use of aspirin in nonspecific viral illness.

Assessment

A. Assess for prodromal symptoms: malaise, cough, rhinorrhea, sore throat.

B. Evaluate LOC.

C. Observe temperature changes.

◆ D. Evaluate clinical stages of the syndrome.
1. Stage 1: vomiting, lethargy, and drowsiness.
2. Stage 2: CNS changes, disorientation, delirium, aggressiveness and combativeness, central neurologic hyperventilation, hyperactive reflexes, and stupor.
3. Stage 3: comatose, hyperventilation, decorticate posturing.
4. Stage 4: increasing comatose state; loss of ocular reflexes; fixed, dilated pupils.
5. Stage 5: seizures, loss of deep tendon reflexes, flaccidity, and respiratory arrest.

E. Evaluate lab findings.
1. Associated with liver dysfunction; serum glutamic oxaloacetic transaminase (SGOT), serum glutamic pyruvic transaminase (SGPT), and lactic dehydrogenase (LDH) are all elevated, dependent clotting factors, decreased prothrombin time (PT), bilirubin and alkaline phosphate unchanged.
2. Associated with renal dysfunction: reduced blood sugar levels to below 50 mg/100 mL, reduced insulin levels and decreased glucagon response.

F. Assess fluid and electrolyte balance; intake and output.

Implementation

◆ A. Most important nursing function is to monitor for signs of increased intracranial pressure; rapidly increasing ICP can result in death.
1. Invasive ICP monitoring usually used.
2. Major effort is toward recognizing and reducing cerebral edema, as this may lead to death.
3. Administer IV Mannitol as ordered to reduce blood osmolarity while increasing urine output, thus reducing cerebral edema.

◆ B. Prepare for tracheal intubation and controlled ventilation (to decrease ICP).

◆ C. Provide respiratory care; suctioning, ventilation, and oxygen as ordered.

D. Monitor vital signs frequently and decrease temperature as needed.

E. Monitor closely for signs of seizure activity, treat promptly, and utilize seizure precautions.

◆ F. Provide nursing care appropriate for semiconscious and unconscious client as neurological status alters.
1. Maintain head elevation at 30 degrees.
2. Monitor reflexes as indicative of clinical stage of syndrome.

◆ G. Provide adequate fluid balance.
1. Ensure adequate urinary output of at least 1 mL/kg/hr.
2. Provide and monitor intravenous fluids.
3. Observe closely for cerebral edema or dehydration.

H. Provide emotional and supportive care for client and family.

CARDIOVASCULAR SYSTEM

The heart is the center of the cardiovascular system, which, by contracting rhythmically, pumps blood through the body to nourish all of the body tissues and cells. This is one of the most essential body systems because failure to function results in death of the client.

System Assessment

A. History.
1. Family history of congenital or acquired heart disease.
2. Perinatal and antenatal course.
3. Gestational age (at birth).
4. Birth weight, hospital stay at birth.
5. Significant illnesses, frequent respiratory infections, family history, rheumatic fever.

✦ B. Inspection.
1. Evaluate skin color (pink, pale, mottled, cyanosis).
2. Evaluate LOC and interaction with caregivers and environment.
3. Observe for signs of respiratory distress (head bobbing, nasal flaring, cough retracting).
4. Assess periorbital area, sacrum, hands, and feet for edema.
5. Observe for clubbing of fingers and toes.

✦ C. Palpation.
1. Palpate peripheral pulses for rate and quality (fullness); be sure to check femoral and pedal pulses.
2. Assess skin temperature, moisture (diaphoresis), and capillary refill time.
3. Palpate liver (should be 1–2 cm below right costal margin).
4. Evaluative precordium for lifts, thrills, or heaves; position of point of maximal impulse.
5. Assess blood pressure (all four extremities if femoral and pedal pulses weak).

D. Percussion.
1. Percuss hepatic margins; spleen if possible.
2. Percuss lung fields if suspect fluid or consolidation.

✦ E. Auscultation.
1. Auscultate heart at aortic, pulmonic, mitral, and tricuspid positions.
2. Assess heart rate for rhythm and regularity, apical–radial deficit.

3. Evaluate S_1 and S_2, note splitting of S_2 on inspiration.
4. Evaluate murmur detected for intensity (grade I–VI), pitch, timing in cardiac cycle, and changes detected with positional change.
5. Evaluate for friction rub, venous hum, clicks in relation to cardiac cycle.
6. Auscultate lung fields for rales, wheezes.

F. Assess growth and development.
1. Feeding patterns or difficulties (tiring easily, sweating, tachypnea).
2. Assess growth patterns (plotted on growth charts—note failure to thrive or obesity).
3. Normal development milestones achieved.

G. Evaluate any other symptoms or history.
1. Chest pain—muscular vs. gastrointestinal versus respiratory, and occurrence at rest or with exercise.
2. Syncope—requires further investigation, family history of sudden death, ECG evaluation, relationship to exercise and illness.
3. Infections—recent streptococcal or rashes on hands and mouth.
4. Blood pressure—screening for hypertension.

Diagnostic Procedures

Fetal Ultrasonography

A. "Routine" scan performed at 18–22 weeks' gestation, if a quality scan and personnel are available. Cardiac, spinal, intracranial, and facial abnormalities can be diagnosed during this time.
B. A Level II ultrasound may be performed, targeting specific anomalies seen on the screening (Level I exam).
C. Proper referral to tertiary medical facility is necessary if further antepartum diagnosis and treatment are advised.

✦ Echocardiography

A. A noninvasive cardiac procedure that records high frequency sound vibrations and reflects mechanical cardiac activity.
B. Usually used to diagnose valvular and other structural anomalies, thickness of septum and ventricular walls, intracardiac defects.
C. May require sedation in young clients—follow institutional protocol.
D. May also be performed via transesophageal route; requires sedation.
E. Nursing responsibilities.
1. Before procedure, assure child that procedure is painless, and prepare child for procedure to help ensure cooperation. Show child and family equipment.

2. After procedure, provide general reassurance; recover from sedation per protocol.

✦ **Electrocardiography**

A. 12-lead ECG used to diagnose arrhythmias as in adults.

B. May need to time with nap schedule in small children unable to hold still for ECG.

✦ **Tilt-Table Testing**

A. Used in definitive diagnosis of syncope in young clients (or adults) after careful history and physical examination in clients experiencing a syncopal event suspected to be of cardiac origin.
   1. Syncope associated with exercise is associated with sudden death.
   2. Most syncope is neurogenic or vasodepressor in origin, and is benign; tilt-table test and monitoring help discern those with potentially lethal cardiac conditions.

B. Tilt test simulates orthostatic stress to provoke a syncopal event while clients are closely monitored with 15-lead ECG monitoring and frequent automatic blood pressure evaluation.

C. Protocols may vary among institutions, but most clients start in supine position, then are tilted up 70–80 degrees for up to 30 minutes to duplicate symptoms, while observing for cardiac changes.

Cardiac Catheterization

✦ A. A procedure in which a catheter is passed into the heart and its major vessels for examination of blood flow, pressures in all chambers and vessels, and oxygen content and saturation. The catheter may be passed through the arterial system into the left side of the heart or through the venous system into the right side of the heart, usually via the femoral artery or vein.

B. Nursing responsibilities before procedure.
   1. Prepare client and/or parents and child for procedure by showing equipment, room, monitors, and pictures.
   2. Establish baseline vital signs.
   3. Assess for evidence of illness. Assure NPO status maintained.

C. Nursing responsibilities during procedure.
   1. Carefully observe vital signs.
   2. Observe for cyanosis or pallor, bradycardia, arrhythmias, and apnea.
   3. Follow sedation protocol.
   4. Assist in comforting the child.

✦ D. Nursing responsibilities following procedure.
   1. Check for peripheral pulses, distal to the site in the extremity used for catheter.
   2. Take and record vital signs every 15 minutes; observe for subnormal temperature.

3. Observe for thrombosis: warmth of extremities, weak arterial pulses, cyanosis, blanching of extremity, skin color.
4. Check for progressive return to normal.
5. Observe for hypotension (internal bleeding) and signs of infection.
6. Check incision site for bleeding or hematoma, maintain pressure dressing as ordered.
7. Observe for reactions to dye used in procedure.
8. Recover from sedation according to protocol (when done via transthoracic route).

✦ **System Implementation— General Principles**

A. Monitor supplemental oxygen concentration to ensure appropriate levels, monitor oxygen saturations (continuously or intermittently).

B. Obtain vital signs at least every 4 hours or more frequently if warranted.

C. Monitor strict I&O and daily weights for changes that may indicate fluid overload.

D. Observe for signs of impending heart failure.
   1. Increase in weight, edema, positive fluid balance.
   2. Increased pulse and respirations.
   3. Presence of adventitious breath sounds, respiratory distress.
   4. Increase in cyanosis.
   5. Liver margin palpable more than 1–2 cm below costal margin.

E. Monitor for signs of polycythemia. Oxygen saturation of arterial blood that is less than 92 percent on 100 percent oxygen may indicate cyanotic heart disease. Hematocrit higher than 52 percent may be a sign of polycythemia.

F. Position cyanotic infants in the knee–chest position during hypercyanotic episodes. The toddler may assume the squatting position by himself.

G. Organize care and feedings to provide sufficient periods of rest.

H. Feed the child by nipple or nasogastric tube. Formula should contain appropriate caloric concentration and fluid volume.

I. Encourage family to participate in infant's care— provide nurturing environment, promote bonding/support child's development.

CONGENITAL HEART CONDITIONS

Fetal Circulation

✦ A. Major structures of fetal circulation. (*See* Table 13-5.)
   1. Ductus venosus: a structure that shunts blood past the portal circulation.

Table 13-5. FETAL TO INFANT CIRCULATION		
	Fetal Circulation	**Infant Circulation**
Ductus venosus	Oxygenized blood from umbilical vein to inferior vena cava; shunts blood past portal circulation	Becomes nonfunctional at birth
Foramen ovale	Opening between right and left atria; shunts blood past lungs	Functional closure by 3 months
Ductus arteriosus	Connects aorta and pulmonary artery; shunts blood past lungs	Contracts and becomes occluded by 4 months
Aorta	Receives mixed blood from heart and pulmonary arteries	Carries oxygenated blood from left ventricle
Pulmonary artery	Carries some mixed blood to lungs	Carries unoxygenated blood to lungs
Ventricles	Ejecting chambers of the heart; pump blood	Ejecting chambers of the heart
Umbilical vein	Carries oxygenated blood from placenta to fetus	Obliterated at birth
Umbilical arteries	Two arteries; carry oxygenated (venous) blood from fetus to placenta	Obliterated at birth
Inferior vena cava	Carries oxygenated blood from umbilical vein and ductus venosus and mixed blood from body	Carries unoxygenated blood back to heart from lower half of body

2. Foramen ovale: an opening between the right and left atria of the heart that shunts blood past the lungs.

3. Ductus arteriosus: a structure between the aorta and the pulmonary artery that shunts blood past the lungs in uterine development.

B. Normal changes in circulation at birth.

1. The umbilical arteries and vein and the ductus venosus become nonfunctional.

2. The lungs expand, reducing pulmonary vascular resistance and greater amounts of blood enter the pulmonary circulation.

3. Increased blood in the pulmonary circulation increases the return of blood to the left atrium, which initiates the closure of the flap of tissue covering the foramen ovale.

4. The ductus arteriosus contracts and the blood flow decreases; eventually, the duct closes. Absence of hypoxemia provides the stimulus for ducts to close.

C. Indications of heart disease in newborns. (*See* Table 13-6.)

1. Congestive heart failure.
   a. Biventricular failure most common in infants (signs of left and right heart failure).
   b. Cyanosis (persistent with administration of 100 percent oxygen).

2. Arrhythmias.

3. Nonductal murmur.

CYANOTIC DEFECTS

Definition: Cyanotic heart defects are a group of congenital heart defects (CHDs) in which the child may appear cyanotic (blue) due to deoxygenated blood bypassing the lungs and entering the systemic circulation. Cyanotic defects account for approximately 25 percent of all CHDs. Causes include transposition of the great arteries (TGA) and defects that involve right-to-left or bidirectional shunting.

Characteristics

A. Causes: No specific cause is known, but may be associated with drug use, chemical exposure, or infections during pregnancy.

B. Types of cyanotic CHD: tetralogy of Fallot, TGA, Ebstiens anomaly, tricuspid atresia, total anomalous pulmonary venous return, pulmonic stenosis, truncus arteriosus, hypoplastic left heart syndrome (HLHS), critical pulmonary valvular stenosis or atresia, severe coarctation of the aorta, interrupted aortic arch.

Assessment

A. Symptoms: Central and peripheral cyanosis, dyspnea (may assume squatting position), hypoxic "spells," syncope, and chest pain. Child may have clubbed fingers, murmur, rales.

B. Diagnostic tests: chest x-ray, CBC, ABG, electrocardiogram, echo-Doppler, TEE, cardiac catheterization and electrophysiologic studies.

◆ Table 13-6. CONGENITAL HEART DEFECTS

Cyanotic Defects	Acyanotic Defects

Conditions that allow unoxygenated blood into the systemic circulation or conditions that result in obstruction of pulmonary blood flow.
A. Signs and symptoms.
  1. Cyanosis.
  2. Retarded growth and failure to thrive.
  3. Lack of energy.
  4. Frequent respiratory infections.
  5. Polycythemia.
  6. Clubbing of fingers and toes.
  7. Squatting.
  8. Cerebral changes—fainting, confusion, CVAs.
B. Diseases in the cyanotic category.
  1. Complete transposition of the great vessels.
  2. Tetralogy of Fallot.
  3. Truncus arteriosus.
  4. Tricuspid atresia.
  5. Total anomalous pulmonary venous connection.
  6. Hypoplastic left heart syndrome.
	Conditions that interfere with normal blood flow through the heart either by slowing it down or by shunting blood from left to the right side of the heart.
	A. Signs and symptoms.
	  1. Audible murmur.
	  2. Discrepancies in pulse pressure in the upper and lower extremities.
	  3. Tendency to develop respiratory infections.
	  4. May develop heart failure with little stress.
	B. Diseases in the acyanotic category.
	  1. Patent ductus arteriosus.
	  2. Atrial septal defect.
	  3. Coarctation of the aorta.
	  4. Pulmonic stenosis.
	  5. Aortic stenosis.
	  6. Atrioventricular canal (endocardial cushion defects).

Implementation

A. General management: Treatment of heart failure, palliative procedures to improve pulmonary blood flow (septostomy, central gortex shunt, Glenn shunt).

B. Monitor polycythemia (hematocrits that are > 50 percent put child at risk for stroke, infectious endocarditis, brain abscess, impaired growth and pulmonary hypertension).

Tetralogy of Fallot

◆ *Definition:* A cardiac malformation characterized by presence of four anatomic abnormalities caused by the underdevelopment of the right ventricular infundibulum.

Characteristics

A. Ventricular septal defect.

B. Dextroposition of aorta so that it overrides the defect.

C. Hypertrophy of the right ventricle.

D. Varying degrees of stenosis of the pulmonary artery.

E. Hemodynamics: a right-to-left shunt arises in this anomaly due to the degree of pulmonary stenosis, position of the aorta, and the hypertrophied right ventricle; thus unoxygenated blood is sent back to the systemic circulation.

F. Cyanosis may not be immediately evident in the newborn due to patent ductus arteriosus, and will be determined by the amount of pulmonary stenosis.

Assessment

◆ A. Observe for symptoms of cyanotic conditions.

B. Assess heart rate; arrhythmias are common.

C. Evaluate fatigue with exercise.

D. Observe for dyspnea and tachypnea.

E. Observe for signs of polycythemia (can lead to clotting problems and cerebral vascular diseases).

F. Assess for hypercyanotic episodes and potential for seizure activity.

Implementation

A. Provide appropriate nursing interventions discussed under general implementation section.

B. Provide postoperative care for child having palliative shunting procedure, increasing blood flow to the lungs.

C. Provide postoperative care for corrective treatment of pulmonary stenosis and ventricular septal defect.

D. Provide support and education to family.

Transposition of the Great Vessels (TGV)

◆ *Definition:* In this condition, the aorta arises from the right ventricle and the pulmonary artery arises from the left ventricle, leading to blood flowing in two parallel circuits. This defect is not compatible with survival unless there is a large defect present in the ventricular or atrial septum, allowing for mixing of oxygenated and unoxygenated blood.

Characteristics

◆ A.   Babies are blue at birth, not responsive to oxygen.
B.   Aorta is anterior to pulmonary artery.
C.   Pulmonary artery ascends parallel to aorta rather than crosses it.
D.   Ventricular septal defect, may or may not be present.
E.   Atrial septal defect must be treated by balloon septostomy (Rashkind procedure) to create mixing of oxygenated and unoxygenated blood.
F.   Patent ductus arteriosus is life preserving in the neonate; allows some oxygened blood to enter the systemic circulation.
G.   Prostaglandin E_1 may be given to prevent PDA from closing until baby can be transferred to a cardiac center.

Assessment

A.   Evaluate for development of subvalvular pulmonic stenosis, decreased pulmonary blood flow, hypoxia, and polycythemia.
B.   Observe for profound cyanosis.
C.   Assess for signs of heart failure.

Implementation

A.   Provide appropriate nursing interventions as listed under general implementation section.
B.   Prostaglandin E_1 (Alprostadil) infusion (0.005–0.1 micrograms/kg/minute) may be used in cyanotic newborns to maintain patency of the ductus arterosus, and improve pulmonary blood flow. Monitor for respiratory distress, seizures, apnea, hypotension, bradycardia and hypoglycemia.
C.   Provide postoperative care for palliative surgery (creation or enlargement of a large septal defect, allowing for greater mix of oxygenated and unoxygenated blood).
D.   Provide postoperative care for palliative surgery (creation of a patent ductus arteriosus or pulmonary artery banding to decrease blood flow through lungs).
◆ E.   Provide postoperative care for corrective surgery: arterial switch procedure.
   1.   In arterial switch procedures, the great arteries are transected and reanastamosed so that the distal aorta arises from the left ventricle and distal pulmonary aorta arises from the right ventricle. Coronary arteries must be reimplanted to the functional aorta and is crucial to survival. This procedure is ideally done in the first few weeks of life.
   2.   Intra-atrial baffle procedure (no longer commonly performed)—creation of an intra-atrial baffle to divert venous blood flow to mitral valve, and pulmonary venous blood to the tri-

cuspid valve using either the child's atrial appendage or prosthetic material. Many clients develop dysrhythmias, heart failure or baffle obstruction, possibly several years after surgery.
F.   Family support and teaching about possible treatments, follow-up, prognosis. Refer to appropriate agencies and support groups.

Truncus Arteriosus

◆ *Definition:* Persistence of a single arterial trunk arising from both ventricles that supplies the systemic, pulmonary, and coronary circulations. Normally, the truncus arteriosus divides at about 34 days of gestation. A ventricular septal defect is usually present, as is a single, defective, semilunar valve.

Assessment

◆ A.   Assess for mottled skin and ashen color; signs of poor cardiac output or hypoxemia.
◆ B.   Evaluate for cyanotic symptoms; if present, provide measures to reduce oxygen demand and increase oxygen supply.
C.   Determine if murmur is present.

Implementation

A.   Provide nursing care as outlined in general intervention section.
B.   Provide postoperative care for palliative treatment or complete repair.

Tricuspid Atresia

◆ *Definition:* Complete obstruction of the tricuspid valve associated with hypoplastic right ventricle, accompanied by atrial septal defect; necessary for survival.

Assessment

◆ A.   Evaluate for a right-to-left shunt through the atrial septal defect. Should hear gurgle S_2 on auscultation; may be variable murmur—often no murmur. Blood mixes with pulmonary venous blood and enters the left ventricle. From the left ventricle, some blood is shunted to the right ventricle and then to the pulmonary artery. The rest passes into the aorta.
B.   Assess for symptoms of cyanotic conditions.
C.   Observe for cyanosis at birth.

Implementation

A.   Provide nursing care as outlined in general intervention section.
B.   Provide postoperative care for palliative surgery designed to increase pulmonary blood flow until corrective surgery may be performed.

INCREASED PULMONARY FLOW (ACYANOTIC) DEFECTS

Patent Ductus Arteriosus (PDA)

✦ *Definition:* A patent ductus arteriosus is present when closure of the fetal shunt after birth fails to occur. The potential for difficulty with this defect is dependent on the amount of blood passing through the defect. PDA occurs often in association with other cardiac defects.

Assessment

✦ A. Assess for loud, continuous machinery-type murmur at left upper sternal border.

B. Palpate for possible thrill.

✦ C. Check for low diastolic blood pressure and for widened pulse pressure.

✦ D. Evaluate for poor feeding habits, diaphoresis, and easy tiring.

E. Check for frequent respiratory infections and distress.

F. Palpate for bounding peripheral pulses.

Implementation

A. Provide appropriate nursing care as listed under general implementation.

✦ B. Closure may be achieved in neonates (especially premies) with indomethocin (IV or orally).

C. Provide appropriate nursing care following occlusion procedure in cardiac cath lab.

D. Provide postoperative care for surgical ligation of ductus and postoperative thoracotomy care.

Atrial Septal Defect (ASD)

✦ *Definition:* A communication between the left and right atria persisting after birth.

Characteristics

✦ A. Patent foramen ovale.

1. In 20 percent of all births, a slit-like opening remains in the atrial septum.

2. This defect usually presents as a functional murmur and requires no surgical intervention, unless symptoms are present.

✦ B. Ostium secundum defects.

1. A defect high in the atrial septum (ostium secundum) in which the foramen ovale fails to close, or the septum fails to fuse.

   a. Frequently asymptomatic.

   b. Murmur in area of pulmonary artery.

   c. May be well tolerated in childhood, as the shunting of blood from the left atrium to the right atrium is under relatively low pressure.

✦ 2. A defect low in the atrial septum (ostium primum) in which there is inadequate development of endocardial cushions. The atrial septum allows a flow of blood from the left high pressure chamber to the right atrial chamber.

   a. May be accompanied by mitral insufficiency.

   b. Asymptomatic if there are no valvular abnormalities.

Assessment

✦ A. Assess for widely split and fixed S_2 heart sound.

B. Auscultate for systolic ejection murmur.

C. Monitor for signs of congestive heart failure (usually not present in infants and children).

Implementation

A. Provide symptomatic care preoperatively.

✦ B. Provide postoperative care (*see* Cardiac Catheterization) following occlusion procedure or following surgical closure (requiring cardiopulmonary bypass).

Ventricular Septal Defect (VSD)

✦ *Definition:* A communication occurring between the left (higher pressure) and right (lower pressure) ventricles allowing oxygenated blood to shunt back into the pulmonary circulation, causing pulmonary volume and/or pressure overload. VSDs account for more than 20 percent of all congenital heart defects and are the most common defect.

Assessment

✦ A. Signs and symptoms depend on size of defect and amount of shunting. Position of defect also impacts severity. Usually children with large defects present with symptomatology.

1. Cardiac enlargement.

2. Pulmonary engorgement.

3. Dyspnea.

4. Frequent respiratory infections.

5. Loud systolic murmur, thrill.

6. Signs may not present until after 4–6 weeks of age and pulmonary vascular resistance falls (creating a pressure gradient across the defect, and shunting of blood through the VSD).

B. Assess for signs of congestive heart failure.

C. Observe for tendency to tire easily.

D. Assess for frequent respiratory infections.

E. Check for poor weight gain, failure to thrive.

F. Evaluate for murmur, may radiate over entire left chest.

Implementation

✦ A. Usually no nursing care needs for child with small asymptomatic defects; up to 50 percent may close spontaneously.

B. Provide symptomatic nursing care for child with large defects as shunting of blood can produce pulmonary dysfunction.

C. Provide preoperative and postoperative care for repair of VSD. Closure of defect is accomplished using a patch, or direct suturing. Requires cardiopulmonary bypass. Closure devices may soon be in use for VSDs.

OBSTRUCTIVE DEFECTS

Pulmonary Stenosis (PS)

◆ *Definition:* Narrowing of the pulmonary artery proximally, at the valve, in the outflow tract or in the branch pulmonary arteries.

◆ **Assessment**
  A. Some children may be asymptomatic.
  B. Evaluate for a decrease in exercise tolerance, evidence of tiring easily, and dyspnea.
  C. Help facilitate diagnostic procedures to evaluate right ventricular pressure, hypertrophy, and degree of severity of PS (echocardiography, ECG, cardiac catheter).
  D. Assess for signs of congestive heart failure.
  E. Oberve for cyanosis in critical pulmonary stenosis.

Implementation
  A. Provide symptomatic nursing care. Children with mild or moderate stenosis may not need intervention.
  B. Monitor drug and oxygen therapy if needed.
  C. Provide preoperative nursing and monitor postop problems: reactive pulmonary hypertension, arrhythmias, and conduction problems.

Aortic Stenosis (AS)

◆ *Definition:* The narrowing or the stricture of the aortic valve. Stenosis may occur in the valve itself, or above or below the annulus.

Assessment
  ◆ A. Infants can be asymptomatic, may present with critical AS and CHF.
  ◆ B. Evaluate child's exercise tolerance.
  ◆ C. Assess older children for chest pain during exercise. Be aware that in rare conditions sudden death may occur after exercise because of inadequate blood flow to the heart muscle.
  D. Observe for episodes of syncope or vertigo, assist in obtaining detailed history of events.
  E. Assist in preparation and obtaining diagnostic evaluations of left ventricular status and degree of AS (echocardiography, ECG, cardiac catheter).

Implementation
  A. Teach children to evaluate their exercise tolerance and to not exceed their limit. Parents may be encouraged to limit child's activity and minimize stress until corrective procedure is performed.
  B. Provide preoperative and postoperative care for surgical intervention; possible prosthetic valve or Ross procedure.

Coarctation of Aorta

◆ *Definition:* The constriction of the lumen of the aorta, usually occurring below the level of the ductus arteriosus, or occasionally above (infantile form or interrupted aortic arch).

Assessment
  ◆ A. Assess for high blood pressure and bounding pulses in areas of the body that receive blood from vessels proximal to the constriction that may result in these conditions (upper extremities).
  B. Evaluate for a diminished blood supply in areas of the body distal to the defect (legs and feet).
  ◆ C. Infant diagnosis: assess for discrepancies in pulses and blood pressure between upper and lower extremities and left-right sides.
  ◆ D. Older child diagnosis: assess for increased cerebral flow—headache, dizziness, epistaxis, fainting.
  E. Evaluate for possible complications (in untreated cases): intracranial hemorrhage, stroke, hypertension, or congestive heart failure.
  F. Assess for leg pain after exertion.

Implementation
  A. Provide symptomatic nursing care as necessary.
  B. Monitor blood pressure and neurological signs in nonsurgical clients.
  ◆ C. May be surgically repaired or some cases may be balloon dilated in cardiac cath lab.
  D. Provide preoperative and postoperative nursing care.
  E. Observe for postsurgical signs of gastrointestinal disturbance and systemic hypertension. (Mesenteric irritation resulting from increased blood flow postop.)

ACQUIRED CARDIAC CONDITIONS

Congestive Heart Failure (CHF)

◆ *Definition:* Cardiac output that is insufficient to meet the metabolic demands of the body, resulting in a series of sympathetic responses. The most common cause of CHF in children is related to congenital anomalies.

Assessment

✦ A. Observe for the following signs of pulmonary and venous congestion:
  1. Tachycardia.
  2. Tachypnea, progressing to respiratory distress.
  3. Intercostal, supraclavicular, substernal retractions.
  4. Rales, wheezing, or rhonchi.
  5. Fluid retention (weight gain), periorbital edema, hand and foot edema.
  6. Hepatic enlargement.

✦ B. Infant signs and symptoms: increased respiratory rate and infections; rales; enlarged liver and spleen, generally little edema, may see periorbital edema; babies do not display distended jugular veins but fontanelles may be full or bulging.

Implementation

✦ A. Increase oxygen supply and reduce oxygen demand.
  1. Ensure that child has secure airway.
  2. Administer oxygen via most appropriate route.
  3. Continuously monitor ventilation, respiratory effort, and SaO_2.

✦ B. Monitor medication administration.
  ✦ 1. Afterload reducing medications (ACE inhibitors, e.g. Captopril and Enalapril).
    a. Drugs inhibit renin-angiotensin system, producing vasodilation in pulmonary and systemic vasculature.
    b. Monitor I&O, HR and observe carefully for hypotension and renal dysfunction.
  ✦ 2. Digoxin.
    a. Monitor vital signs every hour during digitalization. If pulse under 90–100, notify physician; may hold dose.
    b. Observe for digoxin toxicity; nausea, vomiting and diarrhea (early signs seen most often in children); anorexia, dizziness and headaches, arrhythmias, and muscle weakness.
  ✦ 3. Diuretics—important part of treatment.
    a. Observe for electrolyte abnormalities.
    b. Weigh child daily.
    c. Common diuretics: Lasix and Diuril (deplete potassium), and Aldactone (preserves potassium).
  4. Seriously ill children require ICU monitoring and inotropic support.

✦ C. Monitor for signs of complications (other than medications).
  1. Fluid balance—important to keep child adequately hydrated, dehydration may occur from vigorous fluid restriction; maintain strict I&O.
  2. Electrolyte imbalance.
  3. Dysrhythmias.
  4. CNS complications (from poor cardiac output and hypoxemia).
  5. Cardiovascular collapse—pallor, cyanosis, shock.

✦ D. Promote rest for child with heart failure.
  1. Provide outlets such as drawing, doll play, and reading for child with restricted activity.
  2. Organize care to promote child's rest periods.

E. Supervise diet.
  1. Provide small, frequent feedings.
  2. Failure to thrive often present, so meals should be high calorie, attractive, and foods child will eat.

F. Prepare family for home care of infant or child.
  1. Encourage family to participate in care.
    a. Administration of medications.
    b. Signs of medication toxicity.
    c. Techniques for conserving children's energy.
    d. How to contact others for help and guidance.
  2. Support family relationships.
    a. Reinforce positive coping mechanisms.
    b. Assist family to express feelings and fears.
    c. Support as normal a life as possible for child.

Rheumatic Fever

Definition: A systemic inflammatory (collagen) disease that usually follows a group A beta-hemolytic *Streptococcus* infection.

Assessment

✦ A. Jones criteria utilized by healthcare professionals for diagnosis (there is no single clinical pattern).

B. Evaluate supporting evidence.
  1. Recent scarlet fever.
  ✦ 2. Positive throat culture for group A streptococci.
  3. Increased streptococcal antibodies.

JONES CRITERIA

Two major criteria, or one major and two minor criteria, are necessary for a diagnosis.

- **Major criteria.**
  Assess for carditis.
  Check for polyarthritis.
  Evaluate if chorea is present.
  Assess for erythema marginatum.
  Ascertain if subcutaneous nodules are present.
- **Minor criteria.**
  Fever.
  Arthralgia.
  Determine if child has had rheumatic fever or rheumatic heart disease, or if family history is positive.
  Elevated erythrocyte sedimentation rate.
  Positive C-reactive protein.
  Determine if P-R interval is prolonged.

✦ **Implementation**
  A. Provide antibiotic therapy against any remaining streptococci.
  B. Maintain fluid balance.
  C. Ensure sufficient bedrest.
  D. Prevent further infection.
  E. Instruct on use of long-term antibacterial prophylaxis.

Infective (Bacterial) Endocarditis

✦ *Definition:* An infectious disease involving abnormal heart tissue, particularly rheumatic lesions or congenital defects.

✦ **Assessment**
  A. Look for insidious onset of symptoms.
  B. Assess for fever.
  C. Check for lethargic behavior and general malaise.
  D. Assess for anorexia.
  E. Evaluate for splenomegaly.
  F. Assess for retinal hemorrhages.

Implementation
  ✦ A. Current practice for giving antibiotic therapy before surgery or dental procedures: no longer recommended (American Heart Association, 2007) except for clients with the highest risk of adverse outcomes.
  ✦ B. Provide several weeks of IV antibiotic therapy, usually penicillin or cephalosporin, depending on organism.
  C. Monitor aspirin 60–90 mg/kg/day PO; prednisone 0.05–2.0 mg/kg/day for 2–3 weeks (and tapered gradually).
  D. Support cardiovascular function.
  E. Ensure adequate bedrest.
  F. Monitor erythrocyte sedimentation rate (ESR) and increased leukocytes.
  G. Repeat blood cultures as ordered.

Kawasaki Disease

✦ *Definition:* An acute systemic vasculitis—a children's disease, most frequently seen in boys under age 2 of Asian ancestry. It responds like a viral disease of lymph nodes; cause is suspected to be infection with organism or toxin. One in five children with Kawasaki disease develops coronary artery damage.

Assessment
  A. Assess for age, sex, and ancestry to determine if child fits usual profile.
  ✦ B. Assess for acute symptoms: fever, rash, swollen hands and feet, redness of the eyes, swollen lymph glands in the neck, inflammation of mouth, lips, and throat. Subacute phase: fissures on skin, joint pain, thrombocytosis and cardiac disease.
  C. Assess for potential heart involvement (aneurysm, blocked coronary artery leading to a heart attack, myocarditis or pericarditis; arrhythmias, ST segment changes, and enzyme elevations can also occur).
  ✦ D. Lab findings include: elevated ESR, elevated platelet count and elevated C-reactive protein level, elevated liver enzymes.
  E. Thrombocytosis (peaks at 3–4 weeks; may go very high), anemia or leukocytosis.

Implementation
  A. Since cause is unknown, no specific treatment is ordered.
  ✦ B. Intravenous immunoglobulin (IVIG) is administered to prevent coronary artery disease (must be given early).
    1. Commonly given initially in high doses for its anti-inflammatory effect.
    2. Later given in low doses for its anti-aggravation platelet action.
  ✦ C. Monitor high doses of aspirin to reduce fever, pain, and inflammation—high doses may be given to reduce inflammation.
    1. Dose: 80–100 mg/kg/day given when fever is high.
    2. Given until platelet count is normal (to prevent thrombocytosis).
  D. Anticoagulation and thrombolytic therapy may be required.
  E. New research suggests adding corticosteroids—may limit development of coronary artery aneurysms.

CARDIAC SURGERY

Assessment
  A. Preoperative.
    1. Determine if child is physically prepared for surgery.
    2. Determine if child and family is psychologically prepared for surgery.
    3. Assess readiness of child and family to learn postoperative procedures; perform teaching.
    4. Observe for signs of infection and CHF.
    5. Check that all laboratory tests are completed.
  ✦ B. Postoperative.
    1. Observe for patency of the airway, administer appropriate support to reduce respiratory work and maintain oxygenation and ventilation.
    2. Evaluate cardiovascular function, vital signs, quality of pulses, temperature of extremities, and fluid balance. Manage invasive monitoring lines.

3. Evaluate chest tube drainage, clotting, and signs of postoperative bleeding.
4. Monitor cardiac rate and rhythm.
5. Assess need for inotropic support as needed, vigilant monitoring of prescribed fluid balance.
6. Evaluate child's hydration and nutrition status frequently. Advance feedings carefully, when appropriate.
7. Ensure environment provides opportunity for rest.
8. Evaluate pain (efficacy of analgesics and sedation).
9. Observe for postoperative complications and CHF.
10. Promote return to activity as indicated.

Implementation

✦ A. Preoperative.
   1. Evaluate laboratory values for presence of infection or other abnormalities.
   2. Discuss with the parents of the child the extent of preparation that the child has received.
   3. Plan with the parents the approach and timing of preoperative teaching.
   4. Utilize dolls or models to explain the surgery and postoperative treatment.
   5. Conduct a tour of the intensive care unit for the parents and the child and introduce the child to the staff.
   6. Teach the child how to cough and deep-breathe using blow bottles or other devices.
✦ B. Postoperative.
   ✦ 1. Maintain adequate pulmonary function.
      a. Maintain patent airway.
      b. Maintain ventilator if required by child.
      c. Administer oxygen as ordered.
      d. Check rate and depth of respirations.
      e. Suction as necessary.
      f. Instruct child to deep-breathe and cough.
      g. Encourage use of incentive spirometry.
   ✦ 2. Maintain adequate circulatory functioning.
      a. Monitor hemodynamic status and check vital signs.
      b. Monitor rate of IV replacement fluids.
      c. Replace blood when required.
      d. Maintain very accurate hourly intake and output records.
   ✦ 3. Monitor chest tube drainage and patency.
   4. Provide adequate analgesia (and sedation if warranted).
   5. Provide for rest through organized care.
   6. Establish adequate hydration and nutrition.
   7. Encourage ambulation and activity as tolerated.
   8. Observe for complications of cardiac surgery.
      a. Pneumothorax.
      b. Hemothorax.
      c. Shock.
      d. Cardiac failure.
      e. Heart block.
      f. Cardiac tamponade.
      g. Hemorrhage.
      h. Hemolytic anemia.
      i. Postcardiotomy syndrome: sudden fever, carditis, and pleurisy.
      j. Postperfusion syndrome (3–12 weeks after surgery): fever, malaise, and splenomegaly.
      k. Embolism, air or clot.
   9. Observe for late complications.
      a. Respiratory: pneumonia.
      b. Infection: incision area.
      c. Congestive heart failure.
      d. Postpericardiotomy syndrome (assess for symptoms of fever, pericardial friction rub, and pleural effusion).
      e. Postperfusion syndrome (assess for fever, hepatosplenomegaly, leukocytosis, malaise, and maculopapular rash).

Heart Failure (HF)

Definition: HF occurs when cardiac output is insufficient to meet body's metabolic needs or when the heart cannot adequately pump venous return, causing pulmonary congestion (left ventricular failure), systemic edema (right ventricular failure) or both. HF in infants and children has many other causes. Acute severe HF in neonates or infants is a medical emergency.

Assessment

A. In infants, signs of HF include tachycardia, tachypnea, dyspnea with feeding, diaphoresis, restlessness and irritability.
B. Dyspnea causes insufficient caloric intake and poor growth, which may be accentuated by increased metabolic demands in HF and frequent respiratory tract infections.
C. Hepatomegaly is common and easily palpated.
D. Most infants do not have distended neck veins and dependent edema; occasionally have periorbital edema.
E. Findings in older children with HF are similar to those in adults.
F. Children with severe heart failure (cardiogenic shock) appear extremely ill and have cold extremities, diminished pulses, low BP and reduced response to stimuli.
G. Diagnosis: HF is a clinical diagnosis based on auscultation, pulse oximetry, ECG and chest x-ray. Echocardiography usually confirms the diagnosis.

COMMON CAUSES OF HEART FAILURE IN CHILDREN

Age at Onset	Causes
Antenatal (rare)	Chronic anemia (maternal or fetal)
	Myocarditis
	Sustained intrauterine tachycardia
Birth through first few days	Any of the above
	Critical aortic or pulmonic stenosis, or severe cyanotic heart defects (TGA, HLHS)
	Intrauterine or neonatal supraventricular tachycardia
	Large systemic arteriovenous fistulas
	Metabolic disorders (hypoglycemia, hypothermia, severe metabolic acidosis)
	Perinatal asphyxia with myocardial damage
	Severe intrauterine anemia (hydrops fetalis)
Up to 1 month	Any of the above
	Anomalous pulmonary venous drainage, particularly with pulmonary vein obstruction
	Severe coarctation of aorta
	Complete heart block (associated with structural heart anomalies)
	Increased pulmonary flow defects (e.g., patent ductus arteriosus, VSD)
Infancy (especially 6 to 8 weeks)	Anomalous pulmonary venous return
	Bronchopulmonary dysplasia (causing right ventricular failure)
	Rare metabolic disorders (e.g., glycogen storage disease)
	Supraventricular tachycardia
	Defects increasing pulmonary blood flow (VSD, ASD, atrioventricular canal, truncus arteriosus)
Childhood	Acute rheumatic fever with carditis or valvular involvement
	Bacterial endocarditis
	Acute severe hypertension (as with acute glomerulonephritis)
	Dilated cardiomyopathy
	Severe nutritional deficiencies
	Viral myocarditis
	Volume overload in a noncardiac disorder (renal failure, iatrogenic fluid overload)
	Chronic anemia (severe)

Table 13-7. ORAL DIGOXIN DOSAGE IN CHILDREN*

Age	Digitalizing Dose (μg/kg)	Maintenance Dose† (μg/kg BID)
Preterm neonates	20	2.5
Term neonates	30	4–5
1 month to 2 years	40–50	5–6
2–10 years	30–40	4–5
> 10 years	10–15	1.25–2.5

*The IV dose is 75% of the oral dose.

†The maintenance dose is 25% of the digitalizing dose, given in two divided doses.

Notes: All doses based on ideal body weight.

The digitalizing dose is usually necessary only when treating arrhythmias or acute congestive heart failure. The total digitalizing dose is usually given over 24 hours with half the dose given twice separated by 8- to 12-hour intervals with ECG monitoring.

Implementation

A. Medical treatment of HF is similar to that in adults.

B. Treatment may include a diuretic (e.g., furosemide 0.5–1.0 mg/kg PO BID or TID), and ACE inhibitor (e.g., captopril 0.1–0.3 mg/kg PO TID) and/or digoxin.

C. Nursing care.

1. Enhanced caloric content feedings are recommended. Some children require nasogastric or gastrostomy feedings to maintain growth.

2. Surgical repair of the anomaly is indicated if weight gain is not established, with appropriate postoperative nursing care.

3. Cardiac monitoring and meticulous I&O monitoring.

4. Humidified O_2 should be given by mask, or nasal prongs with adequate F_{IO_2} to prevent cyanosis and alleviate respiratory distress.

   a. When possible, F_{IO_2} should be kept < 40 percent to prevent pulmonary epithelial damage in neonates.

   b. Upright position may benefit small infants and children, by reducing pressure in the thorax from abdominal organs and reducing work required for breathing.

RESPIRATORY SYSTEM

The respiratory system accomplishes pulmonary ventilation through the process of inspiration and expiration. The act of breathing involves a complex chemical and osmotic process in which oxygen is taken into the lungs and carbon dioxide, the end product, is given off.

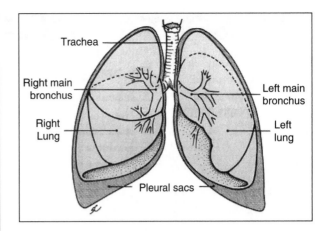

FIGURE 13-1. Anatomy of the lungs.

Pulmonary System Assessment

A. History.
1. Perinatal history—maternal problems, infections, illnesses, smoking.
2. Gestational age—length of hospitalization, pulmonary problems, NICU stay.
3. Respiratory problems since birth—exposures, frequent infections, hospitalizations, chronic diseases, cough, smokers in household.

◆ B. Inspection.
1. Observe respiratory rate and effort (know normal rates for age).
2. Assess skin color—pale, pink, mottled, dusky, cyanotic.
3. Assess level of consciousness and interaction with environment.
4. Observe for drooling, unwillingness to swallow, inspiratory stridor and signs of upper airway obstruction.
5. Evaluate signs of respiratory distress—nasal flaring, head bobbing, tachypnea, cough, audible wheezing, grunting, retractions.
6. Evaluate sputum and secretions from nose and eyes.
7. Assess chest expansion for symmetry, and shape of chest.
8. Observe nailbeds for color and clubbing.

◆ C. Palpation.
1. Evaluate areas of tenderness over chest.
2. Assess lymph nodes.
3. Assess respiratory excursion and tactile fremitus.

D. Percussion.
1. More useful in older children.
2. Should hear resonance over lung surfaces.
3. Note location of any areas of dullness (consolidation); percuss margins.

◆ E. Auscultation.
1. Using diaphragm, systematically evaluate lungs from apices to bases, comparing side to side. (*See* Figure 13-1.)

2. In infants and young children, auscultate in axillae comparing side to side; allow infant/child to sit in lap of caregiver.
3. Note quality of respirations, depth, rate, crackles, or wheezes, any abnormal finding.

F. Hydration.
1. Color and moistness of mucous membranes and secretions.
2. Assess skin turgor.
3. Evaluate for bulging or sunken fontanelles.
4. Assess recent intake and output.

G. Current symptoms.
1. History of illness/onset/recurrences.
2. Medications taken; therapies used.
3. History of asthma/wheezing.
4. Immunization status; recent exposures.

Anatomic Differences in Pediatric Respiratory System

A. Larynx is more cephalad and anterior.
B. Decreased airway size—smaller diameters are more susceptible to change due to swelling and secretions.
C. Narrowest point of the airway is at cricoid cartilage rather than at larynx.
D. Fewer number of airway divisions and alveoli.
E. Ribs are oriented more in horizontal plane.
F. Poorly developed intercostal muscles (thin chest walls).

Physiological Differences in Pediatric Respiratory System

◆ A. Infants are obligate nose breathers until 4–6 weeks of age.
B. Primary muscle of respiration is the diaphragm ("belly breathers").
C. Decreased tidal volume and functional reserve volume.
D. "Stiffer" lungs (with more compliant chest walls).
E. Higher BMR and oxygen consumption relative to body surface area.

✦ Table 13-8. SYMPTOMS OF UPPER AIRWAY AND LOWER RESPIRATORY TRACT OBSTRUCTION	
High Obstruction (Inspiration Problems)	**Low Obstruction (Expiration Problems)**
1. Toxicity	1. Toxicity
2. Fatigue	2. Fatigue
3. Air hunger	3. Air hunger
4. Marked inspiratory stridor with hoarseness	4. Increasingly severe dyspnea
5. Increasing dyspnea	5. Intercostal retractions
6. Severe sternal reactions	6. Prolonged expiratory phase
7. Prolonged inspiratory phase	7. Increased respiratory rate
8. Increased respiratory rate	8. Increased cardiac rate
9. Increased heart rate	9. Harsh cough
10. Barking cough	10. Expiratory wheeze and grunt
	11. Crackles

✦ F. Infants are at high risk for heat and volume loss from high respiratory rates.

✦ G. Increased susceptibility to infective organisms.

System Implementation

✦ A. Monitor for signs of respiratory distress.
  ✦ 1. Early signs.
     a. Increased respiratory rate (tachypnea).
     b. Nasal flaring, head bobbing.
     c. Retractions.
     d. Tachycardia.
     e. Decreasing SaO_2.
  ✦ 2. Late signs.
     a. Cyanosis.
     b. Dyspnea.
     c. Decreased level of consciousness.
     d. Bradycardia.
  B. Ensure patency of airway—administer oxygen as ordered.
     1. Monitor O_2 saturation levels.
     2. Provide postural drainage, coughing, deep-breathing, chest physiotherapy, and suctioning to aid in the removal of secretions.
     3. Provide cool mist for humidifying air.
  C. Maintain IV and/or oral fluid levels.
  D. Administer antibiotic therapy if bacterial infection is present.
  E. Administer antipyretic medication, such as acetaminophen or ibuprofen, tepid sponge baths, or cooling mattress.
  F. Ensure adequate rest and provide a less stressful environment.

G. Organize nursing care to give adequate rest periods.
H. Support family and prepare for discharge.

UPPER AIRWAY OBSTRUCTIVE CONDITIONS

Laryngotracheobronchitis ("Croup")

✦ *Definition:* Viral croup is a syndrome caused by a variety of inflammatory conditions of the upper airway. Viral croup is the most common. More commonly seen in children less than 3 years old. (*See* Table 13-8.)

✦ **Assessment**
  A. Obtain accurate history—ascertain if rhinitis and cough have preceded croup for several days.
  B. Assess for gradual onset, then barking cough and inspiratory stridor—usually for 3–7 days, worse at night.
  C. Assess for mild elevation in temperature (below 102°F).
  D. Observe for hypoxemia, decreasing SaO_2 (resulting in anxiety and restlessness).
  E. Assess for cyanosis, a late sign, which may indicate complete airway obstruction.

Implementation
✦ A. Plan for home treatment if no inspiratory stridor.
     1. Instruct parents in signs of airway obstruction.
        a. Tachypnea.
        b. Increased anxiety.
        c. Pallor, mottling, or cyanosis (circumoral or around eyes).
  ✦ 2. Instruct parents in providing cool mist therapy. Steam from the shower is less desirable, but may be effective.

B. Treatment.
1. For moderate to severe croup that doesn't respond to cool mist and PO fluids, oral or inhaled steroids may be prescribed.
2. For severe croup, a nebulized racemic epinephrine treatment should be administered.
3. Children should be observed in the ED or clinic setting for 1–2 hours after receiving racemic epinephrine because of the risk of "rebound."
✦ C. Provide hospital care for acute onset with inspiratory stridor.
✦ 1. Monitor vital signs every 1–2 hours; check temperature frequently if in cool mist tent.
✦ 2. Check respiratory status at least hourly, depending on severity of distress.
3. Monitor accompanying signs and symptoms.
    a. Respiratory rate.
    b. Grunting, flaring, retracting.
    c. Stridor.
    d. Color.
    e. Auscultation of breath sounds.
    f. Restlessness.
    g. Use of accessory muscles.
    h. Oxygen saturation (pulse oximetry).
4. Obtain baseline ABG/CBG, CBC, and throat culture, if ordered.
✦ 5. Provide cool humidified air or oxygen as ordered.
6. Check oxygen saturations frequently or continuously via pulse oximetry, to keep above 93–94 percent.
✦ 7. Monitor hydration status.
    a. Encourage cool fluid PO intake (cool fluids will help decrease inflammation).
    b. If RR > 60 and NPO, administer adequate intravenous fluids; if RR < 60 and will take fluids, give fluids carefully to maintain hydration, clear liquids as tolerated; supplemental IV.
    c. Maintain patency of IV.
    d. Monitor urinary output, specific gravity, and skin turgor.
8. Treat fever with acetaminophen or ibuprofen.
9. Place on cardiorespiratory monitor if signs of hypoxia or impending respiratory failure.

✦ Epiglottitis

Definition: An acute bacterial infection of the epiglottis, may occasionally be of viral origin. Usually caused by *Haemophilus influenzae* type B or *Streptococcus pneumoniae*. May produce severe upper airway obstruction.

RESPIRATORY SCORING SYSTEM

Inspiratory Stridor
- None (0 points)
- When agitated (1 point)
- On/off at rest (2 points)
- Continuous at rest (3 points)

Retractions
- None (0 points)
- Mild (1 point)
- Moderate (2 points)
- Severe (3 points)

Air Movement/Entry
- Normal (0 points)
- Decreased (1 point)
- Moderately decreased (2 points)
- Severely decreased (3 points)

Cyanosis (Color)
- None (0 points)
- Dusky (1 point)
- Cyanotic on room air (2 points)
- Cyanotic with supplemental oxygen (3 points)

Level of Alertness (Mentation)
- Alert (0 points)
- Restless or anxious (1 point)
- Lethargic/obtunded (2 points)

In general, children with a croup score of less than 4 have mild croup, with a score of 5–6 have mild/moderate croup, with a score of 7–8 have moderate croup, and with a score of greater than 9 have severe croup.

Assessment

✦ A. Observe that illness occurs most frequently in young children, 3–7 years of age.
B. Ascertain if illness was preceded by an upper respiratory infection.
C. Assess for rapid onset with marked inspiratory stridor and retractions, cough, muffled voice.
✦ D. Assess for high temperature (100–104°F).
E. Assess for acute respiratory distress.
F. Evaluate difficulty in swallowing as manifested by excessive drooling and refusal to take liquids.

Implementation

✦ A. Prepare for lateral neck films STAT to confirm diagnosis. Keep child in upright and "sniffing" position. Supine position may cause occlusion of the airway and respiratory arrest.
✦ B. Never use restraints; never use a tongue blade or place *anything* into pharynx.
✦ C. Do not elicit a gag reflex—may cause further spasm of epiglottis and complete airway obstruction.
D. Prepare child for OR if elective intubation is to be done under anesthesia.

E. Maintain tracheostomy set/intubation tray at bedside.

F. Provide cool oxygen mist at all times.

G. Monitor vital signs with respiratory status every hour with continuous close observation.

  1. Monitor respiratory rate, grunting, retracting, stridor, color, restlessness.

  2. Auscultate breath sounds; evaluate use of accessory muscles.

✦ H. Monitor hydration status. Keep child NPO.

  1. Start IV (after airway is secure). Check urinary output, specific gravity, skin turgor, tears.

  2. Maintain patency of IV, administer IV antibiotics (usually ampicillin and cephalosporin until culture and sensitivity back).

✦ I. Monitor temperature every 2 hours—give acetaminophen and ibuprofen for temperature > 100°F as ordered.

J. Place on continuous cardiorespiratory monitor and pulse oximetry.

✦ K. Isolate for 24 hours after start of antibiotic therapy.

✦ L. Maintain endotracheal tube patency once intubated.

  1. Elevate head of bed.

  2. Administer humidified oxygen—assist with CPAP or mechanical ventilation if necessary. Usually child needs only airway and is able to breathe spontaneously.

  3. Evaluate breath sounds every hour.

  4. Restrain child in the same manner as you would for cleft palate repair (prevent bending elbows) to prevent accidental extubation (remains intubated at least 12–48 hours).

✦ M. Monitor signs prior to extubation.

  1. Ability to swallow.

  2. Resolution of sepsis.

  3. Temperature within normal limits for 12 hours.

  4. Resolution of swelling; audible air leak around ET tube.

  5. NPO 4 hours prior to extubation.

Tonsillitis and Adenoiditis

Definition: Infection and inflammation of the palatine tonsils and adenoids. Primary causes are Group A beta-hemolytic *Streptococcus* and viruses.

✦ **Assessment**

A. Assess for difficulty swallowing or breathing.

B. With adenoiditis, child is unable to breathe through nose and must mouth-breathe (may be noisy, snoring at night).

C. Observe for fever, sore throat, and anorexia.

D. Assess for general malaise and dehydration.

E. Assess for pain in ear and recurring otitis media.

F. Evaluate indications for possible surgery.

  1. Surgery is performed only when absolutely necessary because tonsils are thought to have protective immunologic functions.

  2. Assess for difficulty in swallowing, indicating enlargement of tonsils or adenoids.

  3. Assess for repeated episodes of tonsillitis, indicating infection.

  4. Observe for signs of respiratory distress.

  5. Evaluate for hearing, chronic otitis media.

Implementation

PREOPERATIVE INTERVENTIONS

✦ A. Take samples for blood tests (CBC, Hgb, Hct, bleeding and clotting time), serologic tests, and throat culture.

B. Obtain complete health history, including history of allergies.

✦ C. Provide emotional support and preop teaching for the child.

  1. Separation from family

  2. Hospitalization procedure.

  3. Physical layout of surgery room.

  4. Induction of anesthesia.

  5. Recovery room procedure.

  6. Postoperative pain.

  7. Postoperative activity level (play therapy useful).

D. Provide routine preoperative care.

POSTOPERATIVE INTERVENTIONS

✦ A. Maintain in prone or Sims' position until fully awake to facilitate drainage of secretions and prevent aspiration. Then change to semi-Fowler's.

✦ B. Avoid suctioning and coughing to prevent hemorrhage.

✦ C. Observe for signs of postop bleeding and shock.

  1. Restlessness.

  2. Alterations in vital signs (increased pulse, decreased blood pressure, increased respiration).

  3. Frequent swallowing.

  4. Excessive thirst.

  5. Vomiting of blood.

  6. Pallor.

D. Maintain calm, quiet environment to prevent anxiety, which can lead to shock.

✦ E. Provide ice collar.

F. Encourage fluids.

  1. Encourage cold fluids, popsicles, ice chips, or any food or liquid child will take. Avoid red popsicles or fluids; may mask bleeding.

  2. Do not use straws.

G. Administer analgesics for pain as ordered.

H. Discharge teaching.

  1. Avoid highly seasoned or irritating food.

  2. Activity limitations.

3. Use of analgesics.
4. Signs of bleeding or infection.

Acute Otitis Media (AOM)

◆ *Definition:* A common complication of an acute respiratory infection that occurs when edema of the upper respiratory structures trap the infection in the middle ear.

Characteristics

A. Etiology: Viruses such as *Streptococcus pneumoniae* or *Haemophilus influenzae*. Children living with smokers have significant increase in AOM episodes.
B. AOM primarily results from dysfunctional eustachian tubes with retention of secretions.
C. Incidence is greatest from 6 months to 2 years old, more in boys and most often in winter months.

Assessment

◆ A. Assess for high fever, associated upper respiratory infection.
◆ B. Observe for pulling or rubbing of one or both ears.
C. Observe for crying, irritability, restlessness, lethargy, and anorexia.
D. Monitor for language delays in young children with frequent AOM.

Implementation

◆ A. Supervise use of antibiotics, usually amoxicillin, sulfonamides, Omniceph, cefuroxime or azythromycin.
   1. Children under 6 years are usually treated with antibiotics.
      a. AAP recommends that children be treated with amoxicillin, using a high or double the typical dose of 80 or 90 mg/kg/day.
      b. If the amoxicillin doesn't work after 48–72 hours or if the child has a fever at or above 102.2°F, then high-dose Augmentin or Augmentin ES should be used.
   2. Due to drug-resistant antimicrobials, current guidelines are to delay Rx for 48–72 hours after diagnosis for children 6 months to 2 years with nonsevere illness.
B. Administer analgesics and/or analgesic ear drops for pain, and acetaminophen or ibuprofen for fever.
C. Advise parents that during the course of the infection the child may have a conductive hearing loss.
D. Maintain adequate diet and fluid intake.
E. Provide education and support if myringotomy and/or insertion of tympanostomy (PE) tubes is necessary for chronic infection and hearing loss.
◆ F. Parents of infants should be taught to never put child in bed with a bottle, and to feed infants in upright position.
G. Strongly encourage family members to keep child's environment smoke free.

LOWER RESPIRATORY OBSTRUCTIVE CONDITIONS

Bronchitis

◆ *Definition:* Inflammation of the large airways, usually associated with a URI. (*See* Table 13-8.)

◆ Assessment
A. Assess for "hacking" and moderately productive cough.
B. Examine for crackles and wheezes.
C. Assess for acute respiratory distress with acute bronchitis.
D. Evaluate fever and hydration.

◆ Implementation
A. Perform chest physiotherapy and postural drainage as ordered.
   1. Focus on timing—never after meals.
   2. Complete according to client's tolerance.
B. Administer humidified air or oxygen as necessary.
C. Increase and monitor fluid intake.
D. Instruct child how to cough and breathe deeply.
E. Administer cough suppressants and expectorant as ordered.

Bronchiolitis/Respiratory Syncytial Virus Bronchiolitis

◆ *Definition:* An acute infection characterized by thick production of mucus causing spasm and occlusion of the bronchioles and small bronchi. It occurs most frequently in winter and spring in infants and children under age 2, and is usually preceded by a viral upper respiratory infection. RSV is responsible for over half of all bronchiolitis. Adenoviruses and parainfluenza virus may also cause bronchiolitis.

◆ Assessment
◆ A. Assess for abrupt onset of accelerated respiratory rate, nasal flaring, and intercostal retractions with prolonged expiratory phase.
B. Evaluate cough; generally is paroxysmal, nonproductive.
C. Check for tachycardia and hydration status. Intervene if dehydrated.
D. Evaluate for expiratory wheeze, grunt, or emphysema.
E. Assess oxygenation via pulse oximetry.
F. Infants may present with apnea episodes.

◆ Implementation
◆ A. Place upright, "sniffing position" to facilitate breathing.
◆ B. Administer cool, humidified oxygen by delivery mode best tolerated.

SIGNS OF DEHYDRATION

- Sunken fontanelle.
- Poor skin turgor.
- Dry mucous membranes.
- Decreased and concentrated urinary output.

C. Maintain adequate hydration. IV is necessary if marked respiratory distress and unable to tolerate PO feedings.

D. Conserve energy, allow to rest.

E. Monitor cardiac, respiratory, and oxygen saturation carefully.

F. Administer ordered medications.

1. Aerosolized ribavirin may be used to treat high-risk infants, immunosuppressed infants, or those with multiple disease processes. Extreme caution should be used to protect pregnant or potentially pregnant healthcare personnel from contacting ribavirin because of its high teratogenic potential.

2. RespiGam (hyper immune gamma globulin) may be given prophylactically to lessen severity of the disease.

3. Recommended use of palivizumab (Synagis) to prevent RSV infection.

   a. Give to children < 2 years old with chronic lung disease (CLD) who required medical therapy for CLD in 6 months preceding RSV "season."

   b. Give 15 mg IM 1×/month during months with highest incidence (usually Oct–Dec onset through March–May).

4. RSV-IVIG (RE9839) given 750 mg/kg once a month to high-risk infants. Contraindicated in those with cyanotic congenital heart disease.

5. Use of palivizumab and RSV-IVIG is controversial in infants born between 32–35 weeks—requires individual evaluation.

Pneumonia

Definition: Inflammation of the pulmonary parenchyma caused by bacteria, viruses, mycoplasma organisms, aspiration, or inhalation. May be lobar, lobular, or interstitial in location.

✦ Pneumococcal Pneumonia

✦ Assessment

A. Symptoms may appear suddenly.

B. Assess for high fever, often accompanies illness.

C. Evaluate for increased respiratory rate; retractions, crackles, and grunting are present.

D. Assess for tachycardia.

E. Evaluate abdominal pain, nausea and/or vomiting.

F. Check for cough and evaluate secretions.

G. Assess for signs of dehydration.

H. Monitor nausea.

✦ Implementation

A. Administer oxygen as ordered or required.

B. Supervise antibiotic therapy.

C. Monitor fluid balance.

D. Measure intake and output.

E. Reduce body temperature with antipyretic medication, cool water mattress, or sponge baths.

F. Maintain isolation for protection, if necessary.

G. Conserve child's energy.

H. Support and educate family, discharge planning.

I. Investigate use of pneumococcal polysaccharide vaccine for children or families at risk.

Staphylococcal Pneumonia

Definition: *S. aureus* pneumonia is a potentially catastrophic, often community-acquired infection. It is often a complication of influenza, with a mortality rate between 26 and 33 percent. Community-acquired staphylococcal pneumonia is often caused by MRSA.

✦ Assessment

A. Onset of the disease may be rapid, and severe.

B. Assess for high fever, cough, and respiratory distress.

C. Check for possible severe dyspnea and cyanosis.

D. Assess for tension pneumothorax or empyema (caused by lesions on the periphery of the lungs that eroded into the pleural space; this development occurs late in disease course).

✦ Implementation

✦ A. Maintain strict isolation, clients often require PICU care.

B. Supervise administration of medications (frequently methicillin or cephalosporins) and watch for side effects (hematuria and proteinuria).

C. Provide oxygen therapy as ordered.

D. Monitor patency of chest tubes and drainage if needed to manage empyema or pneumothorax.

E. Monitor fluid balance.

F. Maintain accurate I&O records.

G. Teaching and support for families, prepare for discharge.

Viral Pneumonia

✦ Assessment

A. Note that illness usually follows an upper respiratory infection.

B. Assess for low-grade fever, nonproductive cough, and tachypnea.

C. Evaluate breath sounds for crackles and diminished air exchange.

✦ Implementation

A. Administer therapy similar to that for bacterial pneumonia (without antibiotics).
   1. Humidified oxygen.
   2. Chest physiotherapy.
B. Observe for signs of complications.
   1. Atelectasis.
   2. Bronchiectasis.

ASSOCIATED CONDITIONS

Asthma

Definition: A pulmonary disorder that has physical, chemical, or psychological influences causing the release of histamine and other substances resulting in edema of the bronchial walls, excess secretion of mucus by the bronchial glands, and constriction of the bronchioles (bronchial irritability).

✦ Assessment

A. Classification. (*See* Table 13-9.)
   1. Mild intermittent (no daily medication needed).
   2. Mild persistent (meds used > 2/week but < 1/day). Preferred treatment: low med dose, inhaled corticosteroids with MDI.
   3. Moderate persistent (daily meds—low-dose inhaled corticosteroids and long-acting inhaled beta$_2$ agonists).
   4. Severe persistent—continual/frequent meds needed. Prefer high-dose inhaled corticosteroids AND long-acting inhaled beta$_2$ agonists AND systemic corticosteroids if needed.
B. Obtain history of conditions that led to asthmatic attack: exposure to certain foods, infections, vigorous activity, or emotional factors.
C. Assess for spasms of bronchiolar musculature, increased wheezing and air trapping.
D. Observe for thick, tenacious mucus that accumulates and causes obstruction of air passages.
E. Look for obstructive emphysema caused by trapping of air.
F. Assess for wheezing and crackles.
G. Assess cough, paroxysmal and nonproductive.
H. Assess for cyanosis, especially in lips and nailbeds.
I. Evaluate psychological state of child who may be anxious and upset; degree of distress the illness causes.

J. Constantly monitor symptoms, which may become rapidly worse resulting in acute respiratory failure with cyanosis and acidosis.

✦ Implementation

A. 2007 recommendations by National Heart Lung and Blood Institute aimed at four components:
   1. Assess and monitor severity and control.
   2. Education of parents and child.
   3. Control of environmental factors and comorbid conditions.
   4. Medications.
✦ B. Relieve bronchospasm.
C. Identify and remove suspected allergen or trigger ("allergy-proof" the home), or treat underlying infection.
✦ D. Supervise medication administration.
   1. Beta$_2$ agonists: albuterol, metaproterenol and terbutaline; sympathomimetics causing bronchodilation given in aerosolized form. May be continuous in seriously ill children.
   2. Corticosteroids: reduce inflammation. May be given aerosolized, PO or IV.
   3. Methylxanthines: aminophylline, usually best used in exercise-induced or nocturnal asthma.
   4. Cromolyn: preventive only.
   5. Newer medications—leukotriene modulators (zafirlukast–Accolyte and montelukast–Singulair) most used for severe persistent asthma.
   6. Teach child to use peak expiratory flow meter before and after using medications.
E. Ensure removal and control of secretions.
   1. Encourage large fluid intake: liquefies secretions and maintains electrolyte balance.
   2. Provide humidified air or oxygen as needed.
   3. Perform chest physiotherapy and postural drainage with lower airway congestion.
F. Provide emotional support for parents and child to reduce anxiety, and drive toward common therapeutic goals.
G. Educate child to live optimally with chronic problem, encourage independence with medications.

Cystic Fibrosis

✦ *Definition:* Cystic fibrosis is a genetic disorder in which the mucus-producing exocrine glands, particularly those of the lungs and pancreas, are abnormal. They produce thick and viscous mucus. Abnormal mucus production in the pancreas leads to pancreatic insufficiency and, in the lungs, to emphysematous changes. CF affects approximately 30,000 children and adults in the United States; approximately 10 million are carriers.

Table 13-9. CLASSIFYING SEVERITY OF ASTHMA EXACERBATIONS

	Symptoms and Signs	Initial PEF (or FEV$_1$)	Clinical Course
Mild	Dyspnea only with activity (assess tachypnea in young children)	PEF ≥ 70% predicted or personal best	• Usually cared for at home • Prompt relief with inhaled, short-acting beta$_2$ agonists (SABA) • Possible short course of oral systemic corticosteroids
Moderate	Dyspnea interferes with or limits usual activity	PEF 40–69% predicted or personal best	• Usually requires office or ED visit • Relief from frequent inhaled SABA • Oral systemic corticosteroids; some symptoms last for 1–2 days after treatment is begun
Severe	Dyspnea at rest; interferes with conversation	PEF < 40% predicted or personal best	• Usually requires ED visit and likely hospitalization • Partial relief from frequent inhaled SABA • Oral systemic corticosteroids; some symptoms last for > 3 days after treatment is begun • Adjunctive therapies are helpful
Subset: Life-threatening	Too dyspneic to speak; perspiring	PEF < 25% predicted or personal best	• Requires ED/hospitalization; possible ICU • Minimal or no relief from frequent inhaled SABA • Intravenous corticosteroids • Adjunctive therapies are helpful

ED, emergency department; FEV$_1$, forced expiratory volume in 1 second; ICU, intensive care unit; PEF, peak expiratory flow; SABA, short-acting beta$_2$ agonist.

Assessment

A. Assess neonates with meconium ileus—often presenting sign.

B. Assess weight gain because infants with high caloric intake do not gain weight.

C. Evaluate for recurrent, severe respiratory infections caused by thick mucus and bronchial plugs, which can cause atelectasis and chronic infections.

D. Assess for mild diarrhea with frothy, malodorous stools caused by malabsorption of fats and proteins, secondary to pancreatic "plugs."

E. Clients frequently also have GERD (gastro-esophageal reflux disease) and hyperacid stomach.

F. Evaluate diagnostic tests, including the sweat test for elevated chloride content and trypsin test. (> 60 mEq/L chloride in sweat is considered diagnostic of CF. Trypsin is absent in cystic fibrosis.)

Implementation

A. Provide adequate nutritional maintenance. Clients with CF require 130 percent more than normal daily requirements.
   1. Pancreatic enzymes, Viokase and Cotazym, *prior* to meals.
   2. Water-soluble vitamins and fat-soluble vitamins (A, D, and E in water-miscible form) as well as mineral supplements should be given daily.
   3. Diet high in calories, protein and fat.

B. Provide for adequate pulmonary toilet. Major objective is to keep lungs clear of mucus.
   1. Dornase alfa (Pulmozyme) improves lung function by
      a. Breaking down extracellular DNA in thick sputum.
      b. Administration via inhalation through a special nebulizer device helps liquefy secretions.
   2. Aerosolized Mucomyst.
   3. Cool mist at night to help liquefy secretions.
   4. Postural drainage, TID, following breathing treatments.
   5. Breathing exercises. (Children tend to breathe shallowly.)

C. Administer antibiotics as ordered to treat infection.
   1. Inhaled antibiotics (tobramycin) useful in children with chronic *Pseudomonas aerugenosa* infection.
   2. IV antibiotics may include piperacillin, ticarcillin, cephalexin, cefrazidine or ciprofloxacin.

D. Provide parental education and support.
   1. Information about the disease and its long-term effects—median age of survival now approximately 35 years.
   2. Genetic counseling.
   3. New drugs: most target gene therapy attempting to replace gene causing CF, adding normal

genes to airways to correct defective cells. Many clinical trials underway.

4. Resource centers such as Cystic Fibrosis Foundation (www.cff.org) and local organizations.
5. Care of the child at home.
    a. Normal family routine.
    b. Children are irritable, frightened, and insecure.
    c. Children need attention, discipline, and reassurance.

Bronchopulmonary Dysplasia (BPD)

✦ *Definition:* Chronic lung disease seen in infants who were born prematurely, managed with mechanical ventilation, requiring high inspiratory pressures and oxygen concentrations. Alveolar damage ensues, with hyperinflation, atelectasis, pulmonary edema, inflammation and hypertension, and chronic oxygen dependence.

✦ **Assessment**

A. Infant is barrel chested and oxygen dependent.
B. Infants exhibit failure to thrive, and are difficult feeders.
    1. Obtain history, and feeding habits.
    2. Assess ability to feed in conjunction with respiratory exam.
C. Assess respiratory effort.
    1. Tachypnea, retractions, respiratory acidosis, and wheezing are characteristic.
    2. Chest x-ray shows lung disease, scattered areas of hyperinflation, and patchy infiltrates.
D. Evaluate lab studies: chronic respiratory acidosis develops with retention of bicarbonate.
E. Infants often require frequent hospitalizations for infections, acute respiratory distress or failure, and congestive heart failure.
    1. Assess family functioning and parental bonding.
    2. Evaluate degree of developmental delay present, related to gestational age.

Implementation

✦ A. Goal is to maintain adequate oxygenation and ventilation.
✦ B. Usual therapy includes oxygen, bronchodilators, steroids, diuretics, and caloric support.
C. Monitor pulse oximetry carefully to adjust oxygen requirements. Need for supplemental oxygen will vary according to activity.
    1. Assist family in preparing for discharge with home oxygen therapy.
    2. Teach family members methods of monitoring oxygen needs and administration.
D. Monitor electrolytes carefully if on diuretic therapy (metabolic alkalosis is common).
E. Administer and teach families to administer inhaled bronchodilators (e.g., albuterol) and steroids.
✦ F. Nutritional support is a key component of management.
    1. High-calorie diet should be administered in low volumes.
    2. Infants frequently are "difficult feeders" and families may require extensive teaching.
    3. Observe for gastroesophageal reflux and treat accordingly.
✦ G. Families require *extensive* support.
    1. If hospitalized, involve parents in daily care and teach to do as much of care as possible.
    2. Prepare for home care: skilled nursing care may be required, or respite care may need to be arranged.
    3. Educate families on signs of deterioration and need for medical evaluation/intervention.
    4. Support infant's development and provide appropriate stimulation.
    5. BPD is a *chronic* condition, requiring multidisciplinary planning and teamwork, but infants can recover and develop to optimal capabilities with adequate support.

GASTROINTESTINAL SYSTEM

The primary function of the alimentary tract is to provide the body with a continual supply of nutrients, fluids and electrolytes for tissue nourishment. This system has three components: a tract for ingestion and movement of food and fluids; secretion of digestive juices for breaking down the nutrients; and absorption mechanisms for the utilization of foods, water, and electrolytes for continued growth and repair of body tissues.

System Assessment

A. History: family history, perinatal events, prior feeding or stooling disorders, anorexia, emesis, pain, fever, allergies, usual bowel and bladder patterns.
B. Inspection.
   1. Assess symmetry and contour standing and lying ("pot-belly" is normal until puberty).
   2. Observe umbilicus for evidence of hernia.
   3. Observe for visible peristaltic waves (often indicates obstruction).
   4. Inspect area around anus for fissures or polyps. Inspect skin for diaper rash.
C. Auscultation (be sure to do *before* palpation).
   1. Listen to all four quadrants.
   2. High-pitched, "tinkling" sounds indicative of diarrhea or gastroenteritis.
   3. Children's bowel sounds often "hyperactive."
D. Percussion.
   1. Tympany normally heard throughout abdomen.
   2. Dullness usually along right costal margin to 1–3 cm below.
   3. Dullness around symphysis pubis indicative of full bladder and is normal.
E. Palpation.
   1. Palpate last any areas identified as painful.
   2. Ticklish children can place their hand under examiner's to palpate.
   3. Spleen tip can be felt 1–2 cm below left costal margin during inspiration in infants and young children.
   4. Kidneys may be palpable in neonates, rarely in any other age group.
   5. Sigmoid colon may be felt as a tender, sausage-shaped mass.
   6. Palpate for inguinal and femoral hernias.
F. Assess hydration status.
   1. Skin color, temperature, turgor, fontanelles.
   2. Recent intake and output history.
G. Nutritional status.
   1. Failure to gain weight—evaluate growth patterns on chart.
   2. Abnormal stools, pattern, recent changes.
   3. Usual diet.

Diagnostic Procedures

For additional GI tests, please refer to Chapter 11.

Oropharyngeal Motility (Swallowing) Study
A. Child is given small amounts of a liquid containing barium to drink with a bottle, spoon, or cup.
B. A series of x-rays are taken to evaluate what happens as child swallows the liquid.

Ultrasound.
A. High-frequency sound waves create computer-generated images of blood vessels, tissues, and organs; used to view internal organs as they function.
B. Helpful in diagnosing appendicitis and structural abnormalities.

Colonoscopy
A. Colonoscope is through the rectum up into the colon.
B. The colonoscope allows physician to see the lining of the colon, remove tissue for further examination, and possibly treat some problems that are discovered.
C. Client may require conscious sedation.

Endoscopic Retrograde Cholangiopancreatography (ERCP)
A. Procedure allows the physician to diagnose and treat problems in liver, gallbladder, bile ducts, and pancreas.
B. Combines x-ray and use of an endoscope—guided through the mouth and throat, esophagus, stomach, and duodenum.
C. Tube is then passed through scope and a dye is injected that allows internal organs to appear on x-ray.

Esophagogastroduodenoscopy (EGD; Upper Endoscopy)
A. EGD allows physician to look at inside of the esophagus, stomach, and duodenum.
B. Endoscope allows physician to view inside of this area of the body and to insert instruments through a scope for removal of a sample of tissue for biopsy (if necessary).

Esophageal pH Monitoring
A. Measure acidity inside of esophagus—helpful in evaluating gastroesophageal reflux disease (GERD).

B. A think plastic tube is placed into a nostril, guided down the throat and then into esophagus. The tube stops just above lower esophageal sphincter.

C. At end of the tube inside the esophagus is a sensor that measures pH or acidity.

D. The other end of the tube (outside body) is connected to a monitor that records the pH levels for a 12- to 24-hour period.
   1. Normal activity is encouraged during the study, and a diary is kept of symptoms experienced or activity that might be suspicious for reflux, such as gagging or coughing.
   2. The pH readings are evaluated and compared to child's activity for that time period.

Anorectal Manometry

A. Helps determine strength of muscles in rectum and anus and is helpful in evaluating anorectal malformations and Hirschsprung's disease, among other problems.

B. A small tube is placed into rectum, and pressures inside the anus and rectum are measured.

Esophageal Manometry

A. Helps determine strength of the muscles in the esophagus.

B. Useful in evaluating gastroesophageal reflux and swallowing abnormalities.
   1. Small tube is guided into the nostril, then into the esophagus.
   2. The pressure that esophageal muscles produce at rest is then measured.

✦ Barium Enema

A. A procedure in which a barium mixture is placed in the large intestine via a rectal catheter for x-ray visualization of the entire large intestine.

B. Nursing responsibilities prior to procedure.
   1. Cleanse the bowel through enemas.
   2. Restrict diet (clear fluids for 24 hours).
   3. Prepare child and family through teaching.

C. Nursing responsibilities following procedure.
   1. Avoid impaction from barium.
      a. Provide child with large fluid intake.
      b. Administer laxative or cleansing enemas.
   2. Advise parents and child that stools will be white for 24–72 hours following procedure.

✦ Upper Gastrointestinal Radiography

A. Radiographic study of esophagus, stomach, and small bowel using barium contrast.

B. Client must be NPO before procedure.

C. Children often are resistant to swallowing barium.

✦ Small Bowel Follow-Through

A. Radiographic study of lower small intestine using sequential films as barium contrast progresses.

B. Test may take up to 90 minutes depending on intestinal transit time, sequential films taken.

✦ Liver Biopsy

A. Many liver diseases are diagnosable only by direct biopsy.

B. Sample of liver tissue is obtained with large-bore needle.

C. Requires sedation per institutional protocol.

D. Child must have normal coagulation studies or receive vitamin K or fresh frozen plasma with procedure.

✦ Cholangiography

A. Variety of tests to examine gallbladder and biliary tree.

B. Contrast medium may be administered orally and/or IV, or pushed into biliary tree from duodenal endoscope or directly injected into liver.

System Implementation

A. Evaluate vital signs.
   1. Increased temperature and pulse are signs of infection.
   2. If significant dehydration has occurred, respirations and heart rate may be rapid.

B. Maintain hydration status.

C. Isolate child with vomiting or diarrhea until the causative organism is identified.

D. Maintain nutritional status.
   1. Compare child's growth with standardized growth chart.
   2. Evaluate food intake and meal pattern; vomiting pattern.
   3. Record stooling pattern and reaction to feedings. (If fatty, bulky stools, assess for malabsorption problem.)
   4. Evaluate laboratory results of stool culture.
   5. Determine child's likes and dislikes and orient diet accordingly.
   6. Allow bottle if child regresses and is comforted by sucking.
   7. Allow between-meal snacks that are both nutritious and fun (popsicles, fruit bars).

E. Provide meticulous skin care, especially if diapered.

ANATOMIC DEFECTS

Cleft Lip

✦ *Definition:* A congenital defect that involves a fissure resulting from incomplete merging of embryonic processes that normally form the face or jaws. The development of a cleft lip is usually considered to be of multifactoral origin, but may be familial. More common in males than females. Incidence of isolated CL is about 1 in 800, may occur with cleft palate.

Assessment

A. Assess respiratory status.
B. Assess for adequate nutrition.
C. Assess vital signs for baseline data.

Implementation

✦ A. Preoperative care for surgical repair.
  ✦ 1. Use soft or regular nipple with crosscut. May use Lamb's nipple, "gravity flow" nipple (from Ross Laboratories), flanged nipple, or syringe with tubing to administer feeding; may breast-feed, also.
   2. Place nipple on opposite side from cleft.
   3. Burp frequently.
   4. Advise parents that babies will be "noisy eaters."
   5. Mouth should be rinsed with water after feeding.
✦ B. Postoperative care. (Surgery usually done at 6–12 weeks of age.)
   1. Observe for respiratory distress and swelling of tongue, nostrils, and mouth.
   2. Avoid circumstances that will cause crying.
   3. Watch for hemorrhage.
   4. Use elbow restraints and provide supervised rest periods to exercise arms.
   5. Secure lip protecting device used to prevent trauma to suture site.
   6. Modify feeding technique to adapt to surgical site, feeding upright, and teaching parents in preparation for home care.
   7. After feeding, keep infant upright to decrease chance of aspiration; clean suture line with half-strength hydrogen peroxide.
   8. Prevent crust formation on suture line.
   9. Lay infant on unoperated side or back with support; goal is to prevent rubbing suture site on the sheet.
 C. Support family and promote bonding.
   1. Provide education and support to families of neonates.
   2. Prepare for discharge needs.

Cleft Palate

✦ *Definition:* A birth defect in which the primary and secondary palatine plates—openings between nose and roof of mouth—fail to close properly. It is usually considered hereditary. Types include clefted soft palate, clefted hard palate, and a cleft that infrequently involves the nose. Incidence of CP (without CL) is approximately 1 in 2000.

Assessment

✦ A. Assess for difficulty in sucking.
 B. Assess for increase in upper respiratory infections.
 C. Evaluate mother–child relationship (i.e., mother feels frustrated and baby is fussy).

✦ ### Treatment

A. Surgical repairs: some surgeons prefer to wait until the palate has had the opportunity to grow or child is 9–18 months old. Most prefer to operate prior to the onset of speech.
B. Repair in stages: may be required with extensive defects.
C. Surgical repair usually needs to be followed by treatment from an orthodontist, a speech therapist, and a plastic surgeon.

Implementation

A. Preoperative care.
   1. Observe for respiratory infections.
   2. Ensure that child is sitting up when fed.
   3. Provide frequent mouth care.
  ✦ 4. Introduce the method of postoperative feeding; for example, have the child drink from a cup, or feeder to be used after surgery.
   5. Practice arm restraints on the child, so that child becomes familiar with them.
   6. Prepare parents and give them support.
B. Postoperative care.
  ✦ 1. Immediate postoperative period.
    a. Place child on abdomen to prevent aspiration of mucus or blood.
    b. Observe for signs of airway obstruction, and have suction apparatus at the bedside.
    c. Observe for shock or hemorrhage.
    d. Utilize elbow restraints but release frequently.
    e. Irrigate suture line frequently.
    f. Provide a mist tent if indicated.
    g. Oral packing may be in place for 2–3 days.
  ✦ 2. Second postoperative day prior to discharge.
    a. Start introducing fluids by paper cup; avoid straws and glasses or spoons.
    b. Advance diet as tolerated. Usually child is discharged on blenderized diet.
    c. Irrigate sutures following feedings.
   3. Provide support and education to families.

Esophageal Atresia with Tracheoesophageal Fistula (TEF)

✦ *Definition:* Failure of the esophagus to be continuous from the pharynx to the stomach. TEF is an abnormal connection between the trachea and the esophagus. Defects may occur separately or in combination, and are rapidly fatal if not detected.

Characteristics

A. Anomaly occurs during embryonic development. Cause is unknown. (Occurs in about 1 in 3000 births.)

✦ B. There are several different types of esophageal atresia.
   1. The most simple type involves the narrowing of the esophagus.
   2. The second type involves the upper and lower segments of the esophagus that are not attached to each other, creating two blind pouches.
   3. Other types involve fistulas between the upper and/or lower segments of the esophagus and trachea.

C. Fistulas may be present when the esophagus is patent, when it is narrowed, or when it is not joined to its distal portion.

D. Infants at risk for TEF: premature infants and those with polyhydramnios.

Assessment

✦ A. Assess for excessive amounts of mucus with much drooling.

✦ B. Assess for coughing, choking, and cyanosis when fed (the three Cs of TEF).

✦ C. Assess infant status to ingest formula.
   1. Early recognition of the defect is imperative to prevent aspiration.
   2. Inability to pass NG tube at birth indicates esophageal atresia.

D. Check to see if food is expelled through the nose immediately following feeding.
   1. Assess severe coughing and choking.
   2. Assess struggling with resulting cyanosis.

E. Evaluate frequent respiratory problems; apnea may occur.

F. Check for abdominal distention caused by inspired air going into the stomach.

Implementation

✦ A. Maintain patent airway; observe for signs of respiratory distress.

✦ B. Prevent aspiration pneumonia.
   1. Discontinue oral fluids immediately.
   2. Position infant at 30-degree head elevation to decrease potential of aspiration. Infant seat works well for positioning.
   3. Change position every 2 hours.
   4. Suction accumulated secretions frequently.

✦ C. Initiate and monitor IV fluids as ordered to prevent dehydration.

✦ D. Prepare for gastrostomy tube insertion (decompresses stomach and prevents aspiration of gastric contents from fistula).
   1. Administer gastrostomy tube feedings.
   2. Observe for patency of all tubes. Do not clamp gastrostomy tube.

   3. Use gentle suctioning of the upper pouch to minimize aspiration of saliva.
   4. Monitor the gastrostomy tube in place until total repair is performed.

POSTOPERATIVE IMPLEMENTATION

✦ A. Maintain patent airway.
   1. Suction secretions as necessary.
   2. Position for optimal ventilation.
   3. Administer oxygen as needed.
   4. Maintain care of chest tubes.

✦ B. Prevent infection.
   1. Provide meticulous care of operative site.
   2. Observe for signs of inflammation or infection.

C. Maintain fluid and electrolyte balance.
   1. Monitor IV fluids; record intake and output.
   2. Record weight daily.
   3. Measure specific gravity of urine.

D. Maintain infant in radiant warmer with nebulized humidity.

✦ E. Provide adequate nutrition.
   1. Administer gastrostomy feedings (usually after third postoperative day).
   2. Continue until infant tolerates oral feedings, 10–14 days postoperatively (based on condition of child and degree of healing).
   3. Monitor gradual increase in feedings and elevation of gastrostomy tube.
      a. Feed slowly to allow for swallowing and to provide infant rest.
      b. Position upright to prevent aspiration.
      c. Burp frequently.

F. Meet sucking needs by providing a pacifier (if approved by physician).

G. Prepare parents for discharge.
   1. Teach techniques parents will need for home care: tube feedings, suctioning, etc.
   2. Educate parents to look for signs of complications such as esophageal constriction: difficulty in swallowing, choking, and breathing difficulties.
   3. Provide support and preparation for future procedures.

Imperforate Anus

✦ *Definition:* A congenital abnormality in the formation of the anorectal canal or in the location of the anus, resulting in the rectum ending blindly. A fistula or a severe narrowing of the anal canal.

Assessment

✦ A. Assess patency of anal opening with small finger or soft catheter if the following symptoms are present.
   1. No meconium stool within 24 hours.

 2. Green-tinged urine.
 3. Progressive abdominal distention.
B. Assess for presence of other anomalies if imperforate anus is present.
C. Observe for signs of abdominal distress.

Implementation

◆ A. Maintain NPO status when anomaly is diagnosed, monitor IVs.
B. Check vital signs frequently and hydration.
C. Maintain temperature by using isolette or radiant warmer.
◆ D. Provide postoperative care.
 1. Prevent infection of operative site.
 2. Provide colostomy care if colostomy is performed and prevent skin breakdown.
 3. Check for return of peristalsis so that oral feedings may be started.
E. Provide supportive care to parents before and after surgery.
F. Provide education and appropriate referrals for follow-up.

OBSTRUCTIVE DISORDERS

Obstruction of the Bowel

◆ *Definition:* Cause of the obstruction of the bowel could be mechanical or muscular. If congenital intestinal obstruction occurs, may be life-threatening.

Assessment

A. Absent or abnormal stools.
B. Presence of vomiting—may be projectile.
◆ C. Distended abdomen.
 1. Presence of slightly protuberant abdomen is normal.
 2. If abdomen is distended or excessively hard, evaluate for possible obstruction.
 3. Monitor respiratory status carefully as abdominal distention impinges on ability to expand diaphragm.
◆ D. Hyperactive bowel sounds above level of obstruction, hypoactive or absent below.

Implementation

◆ A. Passage of meconium should occur during first 3 days after birth.
 1. If not, assess the child for abdominal distention.
 2. If more than 20 mL of gastric contents is aspirated through nasogastric tube, assess for lower intestinal obstruction.
 3. Meconium ileus highly associated with cystic fibrosis.

◆ B. Attempt to insert a nasogastric tube into stomach and aspirate contents as ordered.
C. Evaluate for excessive mucus and choking.
D. Observe for presence of cyanosis and choking on first feeding.
◆ E. Check for projectile vomiting following feedings.
 1. Evaluate infant's diet. (Overfeeding can cause projectile vomiting.)
 2. If vomiting occurs, evaluate for signs of infection or increased intracranial pressure.
 3. If these conditions are not present, vomiting may be a sign of an obstruction.
F. Document evidence of abdominal pain.
◆ G. Evaluate for absent or abnormal stooling cycle.
 1. If the child has very harsh intermittent crying or continual crying, evaluate the stool cycle for normal or abnormal stools.
 2. Ribbon-shaped stools; bulky, foul-smelling stools; or other abnormalities can be signs of a gastrointestinal abnormality.

Hypertrophic Pyloric Stenosis (HPS)

◆ *Definition:* The pyloric canal, which is at the distal end of the stomach and connects with the duodenum, is greatly narrowed. This narrowing is believed to be caused by a combination of muscular hypertrophy, spasms, and edema of the mucous membrane. Occurs in about 5 in 1000 males and 1 in 1000 females.

Assessment

◆ A. Assess for vomiting in newborn. Vomiting usually begins 30–60 minutes after feedings.
 1. Progressively increases in frequency and force; usually begins at around 1 week of age.
 ◆ 2. Projectile vomitus may contain mucus and blood, but usually not bile.
 3. May progress to complete obstruction.
◆ B. Check for constant hunger, fussiness, frequent crying, colicky abdominal pain, and abdominal distention.
◆ C. Palpate epigastrium just right of umbilicus for classic "olive"-shaped mass.
D. Evaluate stools for decrease in size and number, and assess for constipation.
◆ E. Observe for peristaltic waves: frequently noted passing from left to right during or immediately following a feeding.
F. Assess for later symptoms, which may include malnutrition, dehydration, electrolyte imbalance, and alkalosis.
G. Evaluate growth since birth for failure to thrive.

Implementation

◆ A. Monitor infant for metabolic alkalosis from vomiting.

B. Provide preoperative care.
1. Ensure accurate regulation of IV to prevent dehydration and correct electrolytes.
2. Accurately record intake and output.
3. Observe feeding behavior for definitive diagnosis.
4. Prepare for possible diagnostic procedures (upper GI or abdominal ultrasound).
5. Support mother and infant.
C. Maintain proper insertion and observation of gastric tube for gastric decompression.
1. Measure length of tube externally on infant from bridge of nose to ear to stomach.
2. Check position of the tube. Infant should show no sign of respiratory difficulty with external end of tube occluded.
3. Aspirate gastric contents and check pH. If < 3 (acidic) tube is in stomach.
4. Keep head of bed flat or slightly elevated.
D. Perform nursing care following surgery. Follow standard postoperative procedures for pyloromyotomy.
1. Maintain patent airway.
2. After anesthesia has worn off, place in semi-Fowler's position.
3. Begin feedings 4–6 hours after surgery and progress slowly.
4. Keep a careful record of feeding behavior to assist physician in determining progress of feedings. (Most infants may vomit in first 24–48 hours after surgery.)
5. Do not handle infant excessively after feeding.
6. Observe for bleeding at wound site or signs of shock.

Intussusception

◆ *Definition:* A segment of the bowel telescopes into the portion of bowel immediately distal to it. Probably results from hyperactive peristalsis in the proximal portion of the bowel, with inactive peristalsis in the distal segment. Usually occurs at the junction of the ileum with the colon, generally in children between 3 and 12 months old, or before age 2. Common in children with cystic fibrosis and celiac disease, but usual cause is unknown.

Assessment

A. Assess for sudden onset of acute abdominal pain.
B. Evaluate for sudden onset of vomiting, abdominal pain and distention; and later, infrequent stools with blood and mucus (appears like currant jelly).
C. Child frequently pulls knees to chest, indicating pain; may appear normal between painful episodes.
D. Assess level of hydration.
E. Abdomen is distended and tender.
F. Sausage-shaped mass palpable in upper right quadrant.
G. Right lower quadrant "empty."

H. Passage of "normal" brown stool indicates intussusception has reduced.

Implementation

A. Prepare child for barium enema x-ray, which frequently reduces the bowel; making surgery unnecessary if successful.
B. Observe and monitor for recurrence of symptoms. Surgery may need to be performed for bowel reduction.
C. Observe and maintain IV fluid and electrolyte replacement.
D. Perform nasogastric suction to deflate the stomach to prevent vomiting.
E. Gradually reintroduce fluids and foods.
F. Maintain care of operative site following surgery.
G. Prepare family for discharge.

DISORDERS OF MOTILITY

Acute Diarrhea (Acute Gastroenteritis)

◆ *Definition:* Diarrhea occurs when there is a disturbance of the intestinal tract that alters motility and absorption, and accelerates the excretion of intestinal contents (3–30 stools per day). Fluids and electrolytes that are normally absorbed are excreted, causing electrolyte imbalances. Most infectious diarrheas in the United States are caused by a virus (usually rotavirus). Bacterial causes include Salmonella groups, Shigella, Yersinia, campylobacter and clostridium difficile. Diarrhea can be a separate disease, or it may be a symptom of another disease. Acute diarrhea becomes chronic if it lasts more than 2 weeks.

Assessment

A. Obtain history; ascertain exposures to allergens, new foods; infectious agents or current medications, exposure to rotavirus.
B. Assess child's general state: LOC, activity, and vital signs.
C. Assess quantity and quality of stools.
1. Assess for increased rate of peristalsis carrying intestinal contents (include base bicarbonates).
   a. Blood, pus, or mucus in stools, which are often green in color.
   b. Increase in frequency of stools of watery consistency.
D. Lab tests ordered when child is moderately to severely dehydrated.
1. Stool cultures indicated if blood is present.
2. Stools examined for ova and parasites if cultures are negative.
3. CBC, electrolytes, hemoglobin and hematocrit, BUN and creatinine indicated if admission is required.
E. Assess amount of dehydration.

Implementation

✦ A. Intravenous fluids begun immediately with severe diarrhea and dehydration. Admission to hospital is usually warranted to replace fluid deficit and correct electrolytes.

B. Provide small, frequent offerings of oral rehydration solutions (ORS) throughout course, unless vomiting is severe.

✦ C. Breast-feeding should be continued throughout the disease and ORS given to replace ongoing losses.

D. Early reintroduction of the normal diet is becoming common and beneficial in reducing the number of stools and decreasing weight loss.
  1. Discourage the administration of juices, broth, gelatins, or BRAT diet (*see* page 731).
  2. Cow's milk and milk-based formulas are usually included unless clearly not tolerated.

✦ E. Maintain isolation until causal organism or other factors are determined.
  1. Encourage careful handwashing at home.
  2. Dispose of stools and diapers in proper containers.

F. Maintain careful ongoing assessment and management of dehydration level and acidosis.

G. Complete accurate recording of the number and consistency of stools.

H. Maintain excellent skin care to prevent excoriation caused by alkaline stools; apply appropriate skin protectants (such as zinc oxide).

Dehydration

Definition: Loss of water with resulting sodium excess. (Fluid volume deficit occurs when water and sodium losses are proportional.)

Assessment

✦ A. Check for increased heart rate and respiratory rate.

B. Assess for increased irritability and fussiness.

✦ C. Assess for depressed fontanelles and eyes that appear sunken.

D. Assess for dry mucous membranes—become dried and cracked.

E. Note dry skin with loss of normal elasticity.

✦ F. Assess for decreased urine.
  1. Urine may be dark in color (concentrated).
  2. Increase in urine specific gravity.
  3. Acidosis is a common result.

Implementation

A. Maintain strict recording of I&O.

✦ B. Administer oral rehydration therapy (ORT).
  1. Usually 60–80 mL/kg over 2 hours of solution containing 75–90 mEq per liter sodium; then give 40–50 mL/kg over next 4 hours; then move to maintenance solutions containing 40–60 mEq/L sodium.
  2. Additional fluids should include low-salt fluids (breast milk or water).
  3. Approximately 10 mL ORS per kg body weight per each diarrheal stool.

C. Continue regular diet while rehydrating.

D. Vomiting children should be given ORS in frequent, small amounts.

✦ E. Severe dehydration (loss of 15 percent circulating volume) must be treated urgently (shock). Treatment is guided by the serum sodium levels—dehydration is classified as isotonic, hypotonic, or hypertonic.

F. Continue to closely monitor electrolytes.

G. Maintain skin integrity; monitor for diaper rash.

H. Family teaching (handwashing, avoiding high-sugar containing fluids to rehydrate, avoid BRAT diet).

Constipation

Definition: The infrequent passage of stools associated with difficulty in passing stool, abdominal pain, passage of small, hard stools sometimes streaked with blood. May be associated with a variety of abnormalities.

Assessment

A. Obtain history of usual bowel habits and characteristics.

✦ B. Assess diet habits, over-the-counter and prescription medications taken recently and any used for constipation.

✦ C. Observe for passage of meconium in newborns (possible meconium ileus or Hirschsprung's).

D. Closely evaluate diet in constipated infants and older children.

E. Investigate bowel patterns and timing of stools with older children.

Implementation

✦ A. Dietary counseling appropriate to age. May refer to dietitian.
  1. Encourage fluid intake and diet higher in fiber.
  2. Eliminate any foods known to be constipating.

✦ B. Establish regular time for bowel movements.
  1. Encourage child to *take time* to have bowel movement daily (may use times for child to practice sitting longer).
  2. Establish a routine time for bowel movements (e.g., 10–15 minutes after a meal).

C. Discourage regular use of laxatives.
  1. May become dependent.
  2. Use of stool softeners or enemas may be necessary to empty bowel, thereafter focus on preventing constipation.

Hirschsprung's Disease (Congenital Aganglionic Megacolon)

Definition: A disease caused by the congenital absence of parasympathetic nerve ganglion cells in the distal bowel.

Characteristics

◆ A. The distal portion of the bowel is unable to transmit regular peristaltic waves, which are coordinated with the proximal portion of the bowel.

◆ B. When a stool reaches the diseased area, it is not transmitted down the colon, but accumulates in the segment just proximal to this area, forming a functional obstruction.

C. The bowel above the obstructed portion eventually becomes hypertrophied in its attempts to transmit the stool.

Assessment

◆ A. Assess for failure to pass meconium in newborn; may not be diagnosed until later in infancy or childhood.

B. Assess for symptoms of bile-stained vomiting and reluctance to feed.

◆ C. Evaluate for signs of intestinal obstruction.

D. Evaluate for signs of constipation and abdominal distention.

E. Assess for foul odor of breath and stool.

F. Note that in older child symptoms of constipation, offensive odor, and ribbonlike stools may be present.

◆ Treatment

A. The majority of children require surgical rather than medical treatment. Children beyond the newborn phase may require bowel emptying with enemas and antibiotics to reduce colonic flora preoperatively.

B. The first stage of treatment is usually a transverse or sigmoid colostomy.

C. The child is then brought back to optimal health and nutritional status.

D. The final procedure consists of dissection and removal of the nonfunctional bowel and anastomosis.

E. Final treatment is closure of temporary colostomy.

Implementation

A. Prior to diagnosis, observe carefully for all gastrointestinal manifestations of the disease and report them accurately.

◆ B. Prior to the colostomy procedure.
1. Cleanse bowel.
   a. Oral antibiotics.
   b. Liquid diet.
   c. Colonic irrigation—saline.
   d. Measure abdominal girth when taking vital signs.
2. Prepare parents for the procedure.
   a. Clarify the surgical technique.
   b. Describe stoma.
   c. Prepare for care of the child with a colostomy.
   d. Give parents the opportunity to express their feelings about the procedure.

◆ C. Postoperative care.
1. Maintain optimal nutrition.
2. Closely observe stools for reestablishment of normal elimination pattern.
3. Maintain skin care of colostomy and anal areas.
4. Involve older children in care of ostomy—provide support and referrals to parents in discharge preparations.

Gastroesophageal Reflux Disease (GERD)

◆ *Definition:* The transfer of gastric contents into the esophagus. A significant problem in approximately 1/300 to 1/1000 children. Occurs as result of relaxation of lower esophageal sphincter.

Assessment

A. Begins in infancy, but only a small percentage continue to have GERD later in childhood.

B. History.
1. Previous TEF surgery, CNS disease, asthma, CF, scoliosis.
2. Frequent respiratory symptoms from aspiration.

◆ C. Symptoms.
1. Stomach contents in esophagus damage the esophageal lining. In some children, the stomach contents go up to the mouth and are swallowed (or potentially aspirated) again.
2. When refluxed material passes into back of the mouth or enters airway, child may become hoarse, have a raspy voice, or have a chronic cough.
3. Other symptoms include recurrent pneumonia, wheezing, irritability, choking during feedings, apnea in newborns, difficult or painful swallowing, vomiting, sore throat, weight loss or poor weight gain, heartburn (in older children).

D. Diagnosed by pH probe test of esophageal acidity, upper GI, endoscopy, and swallowing studies.

Implementation

◆ A. Modify feedings to small and frequent feedings—may use thickening agents.

◆ B. Infants generally positioned prone with head elevated (exception to recommended supine position to prevent SIDS).

◆ C. Pharmacologic therapy.
1. Famotodine, cimetidine, or ranitidine may prevent esophagitis.

2. Proton-pump inhibitors (PPIs) often used to block production of stomach acid (esomeprazole, omeprazole, lansoprazole, rabeprazole, pantoprazole).

3. Prokinetic agents may also be used to make the LES close tighter so stomach acid cannot reflux into the esophagus; often used in combination with acid reducers. Prokinetic agents include metoclopramide, erythromycin, bethanechol.

D. Surgery indicated for severe cases (Nissen fundoplication).
   1. Often combined with pyloroplasty.
   2. Numerous potential complications.

E. Most infants improve by one year of age.

F. Support and education for family.
   1. Feeding techniques.
      a. Have child eat more frequent smaller meals; avoid eating 2–3 hours before bed.
      b. Raise head of child's bed 6–8 inches by putting blocks of wood under bedposts. Just using extra pillows will not help.
      c. Children should avoid carbonated drinks, chocolate, caffeine, and foods that are high in fat or contain a lot of acid (citrus fruits) or spices.
   2. Positioning.
   3. Respite care and support for parents.
   4. Continued reinforcement of therapeutic regimen; teach importance of administering prokinetic medications before feedings and regular timing (2–3 times/day) for antacids.
   5. Discharge planning and appropriate referrals.

INFLAMMATORY DISEASES

Appendicitis

See Chapter 8.

Inflammatory Bowel Disease (Encompasses Ulcerative Colitis and Crohn's Disease)

✦ *Definition:* An inflammatory disease of the colon and the rectum in which the mucous membrane becomes hyperemic, bleeds easily, and tends to ulcerate. The exact etiology is unknown; however, the incidence is highest in young adults and middle-age groups.

✦ **Assessment**
✦ A. Assess for diarrhea.
   B. Evaluate for weight loss—can be moderate to severe.
   C. Assess for rectal bleeding.
   D. Evaluate for abdominal pain, nausea, and vomiting.
   E. Assess for presence of anemia.
   F. Assess for fever and dehydration.

G. Evaluate personality and attachments; children with the disease tend to be passive, pessimistic, fearful, and strongly—though ambivalently—attached to a parent.

Implementation
A. Assist with diagnostic procedures.
   1. Barium enema.
   2. Mucosal biopsy.
   3. Stool examination, blood tests (CBC, total protein, albumin, ESR).
✦ B. Control inflammation.
   1. Supervise medication regimen (sulfasalazine, cyclosporine, corticosteroids, 5-ASA and azothioprine).
   2. Provide adequate hydration with intravenous therapy and oral fluids as indicated.
✦ C. Provide rest to intestinal tract.
   1. Observe for amount of bowel activity and symptoms of bleeding and hyperactive peristalsis.
   2. Administer sedatives sparingly; observe for side effects.
✦ D. Support nutrition.
   1. Encourage well-balanced, high-protein, high-calorie diet.
   2. May require special formulas, continuous NG feedings at night, especially successful with elemental formulas.
   3. TPN may be necessary for complete bowel rest.
   4. Record I&O.
   5. Institute vitamin therapy, monitor Hgb, Hct, iron levels, folic acid.
   6. Avoid cold foods because they increase gastric motility.
   7. Arrange for attractive environment with opportunities for socialization at mealtimes.
   8. Avoid sharp cheeses, highly spiced foods, smoked or salted meats, fried foods, raw fruits, and vegetables.
E. Surgical treatment.
   1. Colectomy may be needed in severe cases, is curative in Crohn's disease.
   2. Variety of procedures possible, some preserve normal defecation.
F. Provide counseling and education to client and family.
   1. Educate child about diet, medication, and symptoms of bleeding, management of chronic disease.
   2. Observe for signs of psychological problems; adaptation to chronic disease; initiate appropriate referral if necessary.

INTESTINAL PARASITES

Definition: Worms affect not only the gastrointestinal system, but also are found in the lungs, heart, and other body systems. As parasites, they feed off the host, which leads to a variety of symptoms.

Roundworms

Characteristics

✦ A. Eggs are laid by the worm in the gastrointestinal tract of any host and passed out of the body in feces.

B. After the worms have been ingested, egg batches are laid.

C. Larvae in the host invade lymphatics and venules of the mesentery and migrate to the liver, the lungs, and the heart.

D. Larvae from lungs reach the host's epiglottis and are swallowed; once in the gastrointestinal tract, the cycle is repeated—larvae mature and mate, and the female lays eggs.

Assessment

✦ A. Assess for atypical pneumonia.

✦ B. Assess for gastrointestinal symptoms: nausea, vomiting, anorexia, and weight loss, stooling patterns.

C. Determine if insomnia is present.

D. Evaluate for signs of irritability.

E. Assess for presence of intestinal obstruction, vomiting and dehydration.

Implementation

A. Prevent infection through the use of a sanitary toilet.

B. Provide hygiene education of the family.

C. Dispose of infected stools carefully.

✦ D. Administer piperazine citrate.

Pinworms (Enterobiasis)

Characteristics

✦ A. A common parasite infection in United States, especially in warm climates.

B. Eggs are ingested or inhaled.

C. Eggs mature in cecum, then migrate to anus.

✦ D. Worms exit at night and lay eggs on host's skin.

Assessment

A. Assess for acute or subacute appendicitis.

B. Evaluate for eczematous areas of skin.

C. Determine if irritability is present.

D. Ascertain loss of weight and anorexia.

E. Determine if child suffers from insomnia.

✦ F. Diagnose condition by tape test: place transparent adhesive tape over anus and examine tape for evidence of worms.

Implementation

✦ A. During treatment, maintain meticulous cleansing of skin, particularly anal region, hands, and nails.

B. Ensure that bed linens and clothing are boiled.

C. Use ointment to relieve itching.

D. Teach careful hygiene as a preventative measure.

E. Instruct all infected persons living communally that they must be treated simultaneously.

✦ F. Drugs available: piperazine citrate, pyrantel pamoate; drug of choice is mebendazole.

Giardiasis

✦ *Definition:* The most common intestinal parasitic pathogen in the United States, this condition is caused by the protozoan, *Giardia lambia*.

Characteristics

A. Often occurs in children in day-care centers (estimates are 9–38 percent).

✦ B. Major mode of transmission is person-to-person, water (especially mountain lakes and streams), food, and animals.

C. Adults may be asymptomatic, but children usually manifest symptoms.

Assessment

✦ A. Infants and young children.
1. Diarrhea.
2. Vomiting and anorexia.
3. Failure to thrive.

✦ B. Children over 5 years of age.
1. Abdominal cramps.
2. Loose stools may be intermittent.
3. Stools may be watery, pale, and smelly.

C. Assess condition through stool specimens—may need six or more over several weeks.

Implementation

✦ A. The most important nursing measure is to teach prevention—meticulous sanitary practices during diaper changes and cleaning of children.
1. Inform parents of importance of hand-washing.
2. Drink water that is purified, especially when near potentially contaminated streams.

✦ B. Administer drugs available for treatment: quinacrine, furazolidone (drug of choice), and metronidazole.
1. If cost is a factor, quinacrine is usually given; administer with or after meals and crush tablets into jam or syrup.
2. Quinacrine's side effects: nausea and vomiting.

HEPATIC DISORDERS

Hepatitis

See adult section on hepatitis, Chapter 8. Hepatitis B is included in vaccination schedule. Hepatitis A is recommended for all children aged 1 year.

Biliary Atresia

✦ *Definition:* The atresia or absence of bile ducts outside the liver. A progressive inflammatory process causing intrahepatic and extrahepatic bile duct inflammation and obstruction. Affects between 1 in 10,000 and 1 in 25,000 infants without preference to race or sex.

Assessment

A. Diagnosis based on history, physical exam, and diagnostic evaluation.

✦ B. Early signs: jaundice (may be present at birth—generally evident by 2–3 weeks), dark urine, light-colored stools, hepatomegaly, pruritus, irritability, failure to thrive.

C. Etiology is poorly understood; possibly viral injury or immune mechanism.

D. Gradual deterioration of liver function, loss of intralobular ducts and developing cholestasis, and buildup of bile acids and toxins.

Implementation

✦ A. Early surgery yields highest successes (hepatoportoenterostomy—Kasai procedure); segment of small bowel is anastomosed to resected porta hepatis to facilitate bile drainage.

B. Bile drainage achieved in most clients undergoing surgery in first 2 months of life.

C. Large number still have progressive liver failure and go on to require transplantation.

✦ D. Dietary management: high-calorie diet (Pregestamil) plus low-salt diet and diuretics.

E. Prophylactic antibiotics.

F. Support and education for family.
1. Multidisciplinary process.
2. Appropriate community and support group referrals.

GENERAL DISORDERS

Celiac Disease (Gluten-Induced Enteropathy)

✦ *Definition:* A chronic disease of intestinal malabsorption precipitated by ingestion of gluten or protein portions of wheat or rye flour.

Characteristics

✦ A. A major cause of malabsorption in children, second only to cystic fibrosis. Appears in children from 1–5 years of age.

B. Highest incidence occurs in Caucasians.

✦ C. Major problem is an intolerance to gluten, a protein found in most grains.

✦ D. Basic defect is believed to be an inborn error of metabolism or an autoimmune response.

✦ E. Primary physiological effect is inadequate fat absorption; as disease progresses, it affects absorption of all ingested elements.

F. Long-term effects can be anemia, poor blood coagulation, osteoporosis, and lymphoma.

Assessment

A. Assess age disease occurs: usually when child begins to ingest grains.

✦ B. Assess for diarrhea or loose stools: foul-smelling, pale, and frothy.

✦ C. Check for failure to gain weight after a bout of diarrhea.

D. Check for abdominal distention.

E. Assess for anorexia.

F. Evaluate behavioral changes: irritability and restlessness.

G. Observe for celiac crisis.
1. Vomiting and diarrhea (acute and severe).
2. Acidosis and dehydration.
3. May be precipitated by respiratory infection, fluid and electrolyte imbalance, emotional upset.
4. Excessive perspiration.
5. Cold extremities.

Implementation

✦ A. Monitor appropriate diet; "gluten-free" diet necessary.
1. Wheat and rye gluten, as well as barley and oats, are eliminated. Corn, rice, and millet are substituted grain sources.
2. Consultation with a nutritionist.
3. Supplemental vitamins and iron.

✦ B. Instruct parents and child how to recognize impending celiac crisis, how to manage diet at home and deal with school lunches and meals away from home.
1. Teach primary symptoms of crisis.
2. Institute medical intervention to correct dehydration and metabolic acidosis.

✦ C. Prevent infection and precipitating events.

D. Provide support and education for child and family.
1. Teach diet.
2. Provide for follow-up by home care nurse and nutritionist for continued teaching and assistance. Assess financial strain on family of special diet.
3. Explain prognosis: clinical symptoms decrease with increasing age.
4. Refer to American Celiac Society; other appropriate community agencies and support groups.

Obesity

+ *Definition:* The accumulation of body fat resulting from an excess of caloric intake over caloric output, usually from overeating. Often defined as body weight over 120 percent ideal weight for height, taking into account lean body weight relative to body fat.

Characteristics

A. Obesity is twice as common in adolescents as it was 30 years ago. In the United States, 17 percent of children and teens are overweight or obese.

B. Most complications of obesity occur in adulthood, but obese school-age and adolescent children are twice as likely to have high blood pressure and Type 2 diabetes.

C. Familial tendencies exist, but most childhood and adolescent obesity is attributed to eating too much and exercising too little.

D. Psychosocial causes of overeating should be identified and treated with counseling. Group counseling for overweight children and adolescents is effective, along with dietary and exercise programs. (*See* anticipatory guidance.)

+ E. The impact of childhood obesity becomes most obvious at adolescence, when body image and peer approval become important.

Assessment

A. Assess height and weight according to standard growth and development scale.

B. Risk factors: diet (amount and type of food), inactivity, genetics (other family member are overweight), psychosocial factors, poverty.

C. Screening: BMI > 85th–95th percentile, diabetes (Type 2), eating and exercise habits and looking for other health conditions the child may have.

D. Identify possible hormonal or genetic factors related to the child.

E. Evaluate eating patterns and habits, and food types.

F. Assess length of time child has been obese.

G. Evaluate child's and family's feelings and attitudes about obesity.

H. Considerable cultural implications of body size and usual diet.

Implementation

+ A. Provide a balanced diet with limited calories.
   1. Slow and steady weight loss of 1 pound per week to 1 pound per month.
   2. Set achievable goals and plan for long-term lifestyle and eating changes.
   3. Encourage healthy diet (for the entire family), limiting snacks, fast food, and concentrated sweets, while providing a wide assortment of healthy choices.

B. Set up a routine of daily exercise; frequently, groups for after-school exercise programs can be organized by school nurses.

C. Help the young person work through underlying problems causing or caused by obesity.

+ D. Provide family counseling—family-centered programs have higher success rates.
   1. Examine the eating patterns of the family. Some cultures have a high proportion of starches; others associate large meals with prosperity.
   2. Suggest the use of positive reinforcement for the adolescent rather than shaming the child.
   3. Have family support child by removing high-calorie food from their meals.
   4. Child and family must be motivated for weight loss to occur.
   5. Incorporate cultural values and diet considerations into nutritional plan.

E. Complications: Type 2 diabetes, metabolic syndrome, high blood pressure, asthma, sleep disorders, liver disease, early puberty, skin infections.

F. Monitor and treat hypertension if dietary and exercise modifications do not result in decreased blood pressure. Obese children shold be monitored for Type 2 diabetes and treated with oral antihyperglycemic agents if indicated.

RENAL SYSTEM

The genitourinary system—the kidneys and their drainage channels—is essential for the maintenance of life. This system is responsible for excreting the end products of metabolism as well as regulating water and electrolyte concentrations of body fluids.

System Assessment

A. History.
1. Assess perinatal history, family history of renal disease.
2. Normal feeding patterns, diet, number of wet diapers/voidings per day, growth patterns, fever, straining or pain with voiding, irritability.
✦ 3. Recent infections (especially streptococcal), illnesses.
B. Inspection.
1. Assess male genitalia for urethral orifice and inspect shaft of penis for abnormalities (hypospadias).
2. Assess scrotum for edema (normally present for several days after birth).
3. Assess female urethral orifice for redness, swelling, discharge, normal anatomy.
4. Observe for edema, evaluate periorbital area, sacral region, hands, and feet in infants. Also evaluate fontanelles.
5. Observe character of urine for cloudiness, casts, or blood. Evaluate with bedside dip test if available.
6. Evaluate intake and output, weights.
C. Palpation.
1. Kidneys rarely palpable past the neonatal period.
2. Bladder often palpable above symphysis pubis.
3. Palpate infant's fontanelles for fullness if edema suspected.
4. Assess quality of pulses and blood pressure.
5. Palpate for descended testes bilaterally in scrotal sac.

Diagnostic Procedures

Evaluation of Blood

A. CBC with differential.
B. Blood Urea Nitrogen.
C. Creatinine.
D. Uric Acid.

Evaluation of Urine

A. pH.
B. Protein.
C. Specific gravity.
D. Presence of glucose and ketones.

✦ Cystoscopy

A. Direct visualization of bladder and urethra done under general anesthesia.
B. Nursing responsibilities.
1. Prior to procedure—NPO 6–8 hours.
2. Following procedure—check I&O, observe for urinary retention and hematuria.
3. Sedation per institutional protocol.

✦ Intravenous Pyelogram (IVP)

A. A radiographic study of kidneys, bladder and other structures via contrast media injection.
B. Nursing responsibilities.
1. Prior to IVP—NPO 6–8 hours; bowels cleaned with cathartic; have child void.
2. Following procedure—evaluate for dye reaction; assess child's alertness and gag reflex; check for signs of perforation (intense pain in stomach).

✦ Renal/Bladder Ultrasound

A. Transmission of ultrasound through renal parenchyma, along ureters and over bladder.
B. Noninvasive and without radiation.
C. Useful in assessment of structural abnormalities and masses.

✦ Urodynamic Evaluation

A. Includes voiding cystourethrogram, uroflowmetry, cystometrogram, voiding pressure studies.
B. Provides graphic view of bladder, with volume changes.
C. Valuable for assessing ureters and urethra, voiding dysfunction related to urinary infections, retention, or bladder dysfunction.

✦ CT/MRI

A. Accurate views of cross-sections of kidneys from different axes.
B. Most valuable in viewing masses and differentiating tumors and cysts.

Renal Biopsy

A. May be open or via percutaneous technique.
B. Differentiates between types of nephrotic syndromes.

System Implementation

A. Monitor laboratory results of serum electrolytes. (Refer to Chapter 11 for major electrolyte disorders.)

B. Provide excellent skin care.

C. Monitor IV solutions for appropriate electrolytes depending on the disorder.

✦ D. Monitor urine.
   1. Utilize urine dip-stick testing for each voiding. Check for presence of blood, protein, and ketones.
   2. Describe the appearance of urine: dark, light, cloudy, pink, mucus present.
   3. Evaluate the specific gravity of the urine.
   4. Monitor for possible urinary tract infection.

E. Monitor edema through daily weights and qualitative assessment.

F. Measure intake and output.

G. Monitor vital signs (especially BP) every 4 hours or more frequently if warranted.

H. Administer medications—antihypertensives.

I. Evaluate for rapid respirations associated with acidosis.

J. Isolate children who have an increased susceptibility to infection.

K. Control infection, if present, with appropriate medications.

L. Collect urine specimens from children suspected of having urinary tract infections.

M. Provide diet for degree of renal dysfunction.

Monitoring Urine in Renal Disorders

✦ A. Intake and output.
   1. Significant drop in output could signal worsening renal failure.
   2. Output should not drop below 1 mL/kg/hr.
   3. For severe renal disease, child must be catheterized for accurate assessment of output.

✦ B. Measure intake and output and observe for signs of diuresis following the initiation of medical intervention.
   ✦ 1. Normal output dependent on ages and sizes. Generally, 1 mL/kg/hr is accepted as *minimum* urine output.
   2. Always evaluate output in relation to input and insensible water losses (through fever, respiration, and diaphoresis).

C. Urine should be clear and yellow with no ketones, protein, blood, or sugar—use Hemastix and Clinitest if available.

✦ D. Specific gravity.
   1. Morning specimen usually concentrated around 1.020–1.030 is normal.
   2. Diluted urine around 1.001 may be found in normal infants or in children going through diuresis.

Monitoring Diet for Renal Conditions

✦ A. If there is a high protein loss in urine, a high protein intake is important.

   1. Restrict foods rich in potassium and sodium as prescribed.
   2. Allow parents to bring in appropriate foods from home.
   3. Sit with child during meals and talk about subjects other than food.
   4. Provide nutritious snacks between meals.

✦ B. Provide appropriate diet for degree of renal dysfunction.
   1. Glomerulonephritis: low-sodium, regular diet.
      a. Evidence of renal failure: restrict protein and potassium.
      b. Edema, hypertension, or congestive heart failure: restrict fluids.
   2. Nephrosis: low sodium, high potassium. Fluids may be restricted if severe edema is present.

RENAL/URINARY DISORDERS

Urinary Tract Infections

✦ *Definition:* *Urinary tract infection* (UTI) is a term that refers to a wide variety of conditions affecting the urinary tract in which the common denominator is the presence of a significant number of microorganisms.

Characteristics

✦ A. *Escherichia coli* most frequent organism (80 percent of cases).

✦ B. The most important factor influencing ascending infection is obstruction of free urine flow.
   1. Free flow, large urine output, and pH are antibacterial defenses.
   2. If defenses break down, the result may be an invasion of the tract by bacteria.

C. More common in girls than in boys.

D. Urinary stasis is usually the most important factor.

Assessment

✦ A. Obtain urine for culture (clean catch no more beneficial than midstream specimen). Aseptic catheterization provides most accurate specimen for culture. Specimen should be taken to lab immediately.

✦ B. Assess symptoms of urinary tract infection: burning on urination, cloudy, foul-smelling urine, fever.
   1. In children under 2 years of age, symptoms are nonspecific, and include vomiting, poor feeding, failure to gain weight, pallor, diaper rash, and excessive thirst.
   2. Incontinence in a toilet-trained child may signal UTI.
   3. More serious infections signaled by jaundice, seizures, dehydration, abdominal or back pain, blood in urine, edema, hypertension, tachycardia and tachypnea.

C. Perform chemical tests to determine presence of bacteria for screening for UTI.

D. Evaluate microscopic examination for detailed identification of the organism (especially important in chronic infections).

✦ E. Note that usually a colony count of over 100,000/mL of a single organism from a midstream specimen (or over 1000/mL from suprapubic tap; 10,000/mL from a sterile catheterization) is the most important lab finding and indicates infection.

F. Urosepsis may be present (more commonly in females and young infants), characterized by systemic evidence of bacterial infection with UTI and blood cultures positive for urinary pathogen.

G. Recurrent UTIs should warrant further diagnostic procedures to evaluate structural defects.

Implementation

✦ A. Encourage fluids (after cultures are obtained) to amount appropriate for age.

✦ B. Administer antibiotics as indicated by culture and sensitivity results.
1. Specific for causative bacteria (given 1–2 weeks).
2. Common drugs—penicillins, sulfonamide, aminoglycosides, trimethoprim-sulfamethoxazole, or cefixime.
3. Monitor side effects: nausea, vomiting, vertigo, diarrhea, rash, pruritus, urticaria.

✦ C. Teach mother and child to wipe child front to back, especially for females.

D. If stool in diaper, clean immediately, wiping front to back.

E. Teach early signs of UTI and when to seek medical care.

Vesicoureteral Reflux (VUR)

✦ *Definition:* The retrograde flow of urine from bladder up into ureters.

Assessment

✦ A. Frequently a cause for recurrent UTIs in children.

B. Obtain history of recent illness, previous UTIs.

C. May result from congenital abnormality or from an acquired disorder.

Implementation

A. Prepare family and child for diagnostic procedures (ultrasound, voiding cystogram).

✦ B. Tests will reveal anatomic abnormality in ureteral insertion into bladder (primary reflux).

C. VUR also results from acquired condition as with recurrent UTI (secondary reflux).

✦ D. Treatment is with antibiotics initially, in lower doses, with frequent cultures.

E. Family and nurses should closely monitor urine output (check diaper every 30 minutes).

F. Surgery indicated if anatomic defects are significant, UTIs continue, family is noncompliant, or VUR persisting after puberty.

G. Education and family support essential.

H. Routine preoperative care if surgery indicated.

I. Postoperative management: care of wound, possible management of stents, pain management, and discharge planning.

Acute Glomerulonephritis (AGN)

✦ *Definition:* Acute glomerulonephritis is believed to be an antigen–antibody reaction usually secondary to an infection from group A beta-hemolytic streptococci originating elsewhere in the body. The disease can range from minimal to severe, even though the preceding infection may be minimal. It is most common in children 4–7 years of age.

Assessment

✦ A. Assess renal system.
1. Protein and blood cells present in urine.
2. Oliguria and occasional anuria.
3. Mild edema—facial (periorbital). Worse in mornings.
4. Tea- or cola-colored urine.
5. Elevated BUN and serum creatinine.

B. Assess cardiovascular system.
1. Possible hypertension, slowed pulse, and generalized edema.
2. Possible congestive heart failure or circulatory congestion.

C. Assess for preceding infection and fever, symptoms usually appear approximately 10 days after streptococcal infection.

D. Assess for anorexia and fatigue, irritability, headaches, lethargy.

Implementation

✦ A. Maintain rest during acute stage. Bedrest is not necessarily needed once the gross hematuria, edema, azotemia and hypertension have subsided.

B. Monitor antibiotic treatment if there are positive bacterial cultures.

✦ C. Monitor diet and fluid intake.
1. Elevated BUN and oliguria—protein moderately restricted only if oliguria is prolonged and azotemia is severe.
2. Liberal carbohydrates and fats for energy.
3. Restrict sodium (moderately) if edema or hypertension present.

✦ D. Give antihypertensive drugs (e.g., hydralazine or nifedipine if moderate; nitroglycerin or nitroprusside if severe).

✦ E. Prevent fluid overload—replace fluid loss only.
    1. Weigh daily, same time, same scale.
    2. Measure intake and output, calculate insensible losses.
   F. Prevent complications.
    1. Observe for signs of cerebral edema: headache, dizziness, vomiting.
    2. Monitor for renal failure: nausea, vomiting, oliguria.
    3. Prevent skin breakdown.
    4. Antibiotics used only if streptococcal infection is indicated.
   G. Support of family and discharge teaching.

Nephrotic Syndrome

Definition: The most common form of glomerular injury in children. A symptom complex with multiple and varied pathological manifestations; usually massive hyperlipidemia, edema, proteinuria, and hypoalbuminemia, the etiology of which is unknown. Nephrotic syndrome occurs primarily in preschool age groups (2–3 years of age). Overall prognosis is good, but relapses common.

Assessment

✦ A. Assess for generalized edema from fluid overload.
    1. Periorbital and facial (may be severe) edema.
    2. Abdominal edema (ascites); may lead to respiratory distress.
    3. Respiratory difficulty with pleural effusion.
    4. Diarrhea, vomiting, and malabsorption from edema of gastrointestinal tract.
✦ B. Assess for marked proteinuria.
   C. Assess for malnutrition.
   D. Assess for potential hypertension.

Implementation

✦ A. Administer corticosteroid therapy as ordered, generally oral doses of 2 mg/kg/day.
✦ B. Monitor edema formation through daily weights and abdominal circumferences; accurate recording of intake and output.
    1. Measure abdominal girth at umbilicus.
    2. If ascites present, evaluate for respiratory embarrassment from pressure on the diaphragm.
    3. Place child in semi-Fowler's position if massive edema is present.
✦ C. Provide meticulous skin care.
    1. Bathe body surfaces frequently.
    2. Turn and position client frequently to prevent skin breakdown.
    3. Support edematous areas such as the scrotum.
   D. Monitor use of diuretics.
✦ E. Monitor use of steroids. Prednisone, which reduces edema and proteinuria, is drug of choice.

    1. Diuresis usually occurs in 7–21 days.
    2. Dosage is usually tapered after urine is free of protein and remains normal.
    3. Prepare child and family for side effects: Cushing's syndrome, weight gain, acne, hirsutism.
    4. Protect from infection.
✦ F. Provide appropriate diet.
    1. Protein not usually restricted; may encourage foods rich in protein.
    2. Moderate sodium restrictions.
    3. High-calorie diet.
   G. Teaching principles.
    1. Emphasize diagnosis and treatment regimen, skin care, diet, monitoring urine at home.
    2. Support of family and child.

Hemolytic Uremic Syndrome (HUS)

✦ *Definition:* Among the most frequent causes of acute renal failure in children. Etiology is unclear but most likely bacterial toxins, chemicals, or viruses, particularly *E. coli*, *Rickettsia*, pneumococci, *Shigella*, or *Salmonella*. Clinically produces hemolytic anemia, thrombocytopenia, renal injury, and CNS symptoms. Occurs mainly in young children (younger than 5 years), predominantly in Caucasians.

✦ Assessment

   A. Obtain thorough history.
    1. Possible exposures to known causative organisms.
    2. Prodromal illness (gastroenteritis or URI).
    3. Sudden-onset renal failure.
   B. Assess CNS status for seizures, irritability, or lethargy.
   C. Assist in obtaining lab tests; triad of anemia, thrombocytopenia, and renal failure is diagnostic.
   D. Assess renal function.
    1. May be oliguric or anuric.
    2. Elevated BUN and serum creatinine.
    3. Urine has protein, blood, and casts.
    4. Monitor electrolytes.
   E. Evaluate for hypertension or arrhythmias.

Implementation

   A. Early diagnosis and management of renal failure most important.
✦ B. Dialysis (peritoneal or hemo) generally begun if anuric for 24 hours or if seizures or severe hypertension develop.
✦ C. Monitor respiratory status.
    1. Assure airway is protected (CNS status).
    2. Support ventilation and oxygenation as needed.
✦ D. Careful monitoring of cardiovascular status.
    1. Maintain optimal fluid and electrolyte status.

2. Monitor blood pressure carefully, administer appropriate medications.
3. Continuous ECG monitoring if arrhythmias likely.
4. Treat anemia—PRBCs may be given cautiously.
E. Support family and child.
1. Long-term sequelae develop in 10–50 percent of cases (chronic renal failure, hypertension, CNS disorders).
2. Provide teaching and emotional support—teach families to avoid meat cooked < 160°F (risk of *E. coli* contamination, especially in ground beef).
3. Discharge planning.

Enuresis

✦ *Definition:* Involuntary urination in a child who is of age to have bladder control, or previously had control. Frequently occurs at night (nocturnal enuresis), may be due to organic causes and occurs more often in boys after 4–5 years old. Sometimes associated with sleep disorders.

Assessment

✦ A. Obtain accurate history (toilet training, prior habits).
B. Assess for UTI, diabetes, pelvic mass.
✦ C. Assess for signs of child abuse or sexual abuse.
D. Evaluate developmental milestones (delays may occur).
E. Assess family response to enuresis.

Implementation

✦ A. Assist with and help prepare child for diagnostic procedures (ultrasound, voiding cystourethrogram, UA, developmental assessment).
✦ B. Administer and instruct about appropriate medications (antibiotics if UTI is cause, possibly anticholinergics or tricyclic antidepressants).
C. Emotional care.
1. Promote child's self-esteem. Give reassurance that bed-wetting is common.
2. Support and teaching to family.
D. Teaching.
1. Limit fluids at bedtime; urinate just before bedtime.
2. Establish bladder routine.
3. Medications (imipramine).
4. Potential complications.

STRUCTURAL DEFECTS

Extrophy of the Bladder

Definition: A rare defect in which the bladder wall fails to close during development and a portion of the bladder wall extrudes through the abdominal wall; the upper urinary tract is normal.

Assessment

A. A mass of bright red tissue in the lower abdomen where the abdominal wall has not closed.
B. Assess for continual leaking from an open urethra.

Treatment and Implementation

A. Surgical reconstruction in several stages; the initial stage is completed shortly after birth.
B. Some children require permanent urinary diversion because it is impossible to reconstruct a functional bladder.
C. Nursing management.
✦ 1. Position infant side-lying to promote drainage and help reduce risk of infection.
2. Prevent trauma to exposed bladder; avoid abduction of the legs.
✦ 3. Clean exposed area daily using meticulous skin care to protect from urine leakage and infection.
4. Observe for obstruction in drainage tubes (decreased urine output, blood drainage from urethra, bladder spasms).
5. Complete discharge teaching.
a. Dressing change protocol.
b. Prevention of infection.
c. Observe for changes in urinary function.

Hypospadias/Epispadias

✦ *Definition:* Hypospadias is the malposition of the external urethral opening behind the glans penis, along the ventral surface. Epispadias is a condition in which the urethra is located on the upper surface of the penis. Hypospadias is more common and has familial tendencies.

Assessment

A. Assess location of urethral opening on penis and ability to void in a normal elevated position.
B. Check for presence of fistulas, chordee.
C. Assess child's understanding of procedure (word for penis, urine).
D. Evaluate parents' understanding of surgery and fears.

Implementation

A. Preoperative care.
1. Use drawings or dolls to reinforce physician's explanation.
2. Prepare child for presence of urinary catheter(s).
3. Prepare child for the possibility of postop bladder spasms.
4. Prepare child for nursing and medical personnel looking at his bandages frequently.
✦ B. Postoperative care.
1. Maintain adequate hydration.

a. Measure urine specific gravity.

b. Encourage fluid as needed.

◆ 2. Expect a Foley catheter that may be sutured in place; urine should be rose-colored immediately postop, gradually becoming clear.

3. If staged repair, may have a suprapubic catheter for urinary diversion and a Foley catheter.

4. Tape catheters in place securely. (Do not adjust position or remove catheter.)

5. Administer analgesics as needed.

6. Remove Foley and clamp suprapubic intermittently to allow child to void through the meatus.

7. After Foley is removed, note presence of fistula (should not be present).

8. Chart when the child voids through the meatus; report to physician:

a. Character of flow, presence of spray, dribbling, leaking, pain.

b. Expect pain on the first voids, should decrease in subsequent voids.

9. Discharge teaching and support of family and child.

Cryptorchidism (Undescended Testes)

◆ *Definition:* The failure of one or both testes to descend into the scrotal sac. Occurs more in premature infants and approximately 80 percent resolve spontaneously.

Assessment

A. Palpate for presence of testis in scrotal sac.

B. Assess for presence of accompanying hernia (present in 50 percent of clients).

C. Evaluate normal development of secondary sex characteristics.

D. May lead to sterility if persists into adolescence.

Implementation

◆ A. Support child and family during surgery. Orchiopexy usually performed before 5 years of age.

B. Provide postoperative care: maintain traction which anchors testes to scrotum (5–7 days); prevent contamination of incision.

C. Provide adequate postoperative analgesics.

D. Support family and child.

E. Discharge teaching.

DISORDERS OF THE BLOOD

The circulatory system, a continuous circuit, is the mechanical conveyor of the body constituent called blood. Blood, composed of cells and plasma, circulates through the body and is the means by which oxygen and nutrients are transported to the tissues.

System Assessment

A. History.
   1. Perinatal and birth history, significant family history.
   2. Recent illnesses or appearance of bleeding or bruising, dietary history.
✦ B. Inspection.
   1. Assess skin color for general pallor (especially mucous membranes).
   2. Observe for bruising or petechiae.
   3. Evaluate activity level and general level of energy.
   4. Plot growth on curve, noting delays.
✦ C. Palpation.
   1. Palpate liver and spleen margins, noting enlargement.
   2. Palpate peripheral pulses for quality and rate.
   3. Note any enlarged lymph nodes.
D. Percussion—may percuss liver and spleen.
E. Auscultation.
   1. Note heart rate and respiratory rate.
   2. Evaluate cardiac murmur.
   3. Assess blood pressure.
F. Evaluate the CBC.

RED BLOOD CELL DISORDERS

Anemia

Definition: A deficit of red blood cells or hemoglobin caused by impairment of red blood cell production or increased erythrocyte destruction. A reduced oxygen-carrying capacity results, with decreased oxygen available to the tissues.

Assessment

✦ A. Classifications of anemia.
   1. Etiology/pathology: RBC hemolysis, decreased RBC production or from acute or chronic blood loss.
   2. Morphology: based on RBC size, shape, or color.

✦ B. Assess for general changes in behavior: listlessness, fatigue, poor suck, pica, pallor, tachypnea, tachycardia or shortness of breath, cardiac murmur.
✦ C. Assess for central nervous system manifestations: headache, dizziness, irritability, decreased attention span, apathy, or depression.
D. Observe for signs of shock (poor peripheral perfusion; cool, clammy skin; tachycardia and decreased blood pressure) in severe cases.
✦ E. Determine if nutritional deficiency is present; iron, folic acid, vitamin B_6 or B_{12}.
F. Evaluate tests for impairment of red blood cell production: red cell, aplastic, or hemolytic anemia or leukemia.
G. Look for sources of blood loss (GI tract) with stool hemoccult exam.
H. Consider racial/ethnic background.

Implementation

A. Prepare child for blood draws.
✦ B. Decrease oxygen demands (providing rest, quiet activities).
✦ C. Support RBC production by maintaining nutritious diet with vitamin and iron supplements, excellent hygiene, adequate rest, and avoidance of exposure to infections.
D. Teach parents that stools will be dark with iron supplements. Vomiting and diarrhea can occur.
E. Monitor blood transfusions and observe for signs of transfusion reactions.
✦ F. Administer iron preparations or injections by special method (Z-track if severe iron deficiency is present) and take special precautions.
G. Support family, make appropriate consults/referrals, support growth and development, prepare for discharge.

Sickle Cell Anemia

✦ *Definition:* An autosomal disorder in which red blood cells sickle when under low-oxygen tension (hemoglobin A is partly or completely replaced by hemoglobin S). Sickled erythrocytes hemolyze or cause poor blood flow through capillaries and decrease oxygen delivery to tissues. Usually confined to African Americans, but may be present in people from Mediterranean areas.

Assessment

✦ A. Assess major symptoms.
   1. Usually asymptomatic until under stress (illness, exercise, high altitude).
   2. Severe chronic anemia—pallor.
   3. Periodic crises with abdominal and joint pain.
   4. Lethargy and listlessness.
   5. Irritability.

6. High fever.
7. Enlarged spleen from increased activity.
8. Jaundice from excessive blood cell destruction.
9. Widening of the marrow spaces of the bones.
10. Renal dysfunction.
11. Decreased growth.

✦ B. Thrombotic crises.
1. Most frequent type.
2. Caused by occlusion of the small blood vessels producing distal ischemia and infarction.
3. Beginning of crises may be characterized by the swelling of the hands and feet or decreased appetite, irritability, or fever.
4. May experience pain and swelling in abdomen.
5. CVA possible at any age.

✦ C. Sequestration crises.
1. Occurs usually in children under 5 years of age.
2. Caused by pooling of blood in spleen.
3. Enlargement of spleen and circulatory collapse.

Implementation

A. Alleviate pain with analgesics.
✦ B. Prevent dehydration with intravenous infusion, if necessary, and increased fluid intake; hydration can reduce sickling.
✦ C. Supplemental oxygen may be administered to optimize tissue oxygenation.
✦ D. Keep child warm.
E. Offer parents genetic counseling.
F. During sequestration crises, supervise blood transfusions.
✦ G. Teaching: emphasizing preventing crises, signs of crises, emotional support, prescribed activity, supporting development, safe activities for child to participate in, Medic-Alert® bracelet.
H. Discharge planning with appropriate referrals.
I. Genetic counseling for families and young adults considering childrearing.

Thalassemias

✦ *Definition:* An inherited group of hemolytic anemias caused by too few hemoglobin polypeptide chains. A chronic condition. Most often seen in individuals of Mediterranean descent.

Assessment

✦ A. Assess for skin breakdown, especially leg ulcers.
✦ B. Observe for jaundice; serum bilirubin elevated.
✦ C. Check for intolerance to fatty foods and abdominal discomfort.
D. Check blood studies; fetal hemoglobin as high as 90 percent.

Implementation

✦ A. Supportive: rest, decreased activity, heat lamp to open wounds, excellent skin care.
✦ B. Administer packed red cells or chelating agent for excess iron, deferoxamine with vitamin C; may also treat with folic acid.
C. Prepare for splenectomy if transfused cells are rapidly destroyed by spleen.
D. Monitor HIV status appropriately.
✦ E. Teaching: explain prognosis and treatment regimen to parents and child, need for frequent transfusions, genetic counseling, support in adapting to chronic illness, appropriate referrals.

BLOOD DISORDERS

Infectious Mononucleosis

✦ *Definition:* An acute, self-limited infectious disease, caused primarily by the Epstein–Barr virus, that causes an increase in the mononuclear elements of the blood, most common in individuals < 25 y.o.

Assessment

✦ A. Evaluate length of incubation period: around 11 days. (Usually a 2–5-day prodromal phase with fatigue and malaise with or without fever.)
B. Blood test ("monospot") used to make diagnosis, with clinical signs.
✦ C. Assess for specific symptoms.
1. Malaise.
2. Sore throat with pharyngitis (may be severe).
3. Prolonged fever (may last 2 weeks), may be high.
4. Enlargement of the lymph nodes.
5. Splenomegaly.
6. Skin rashes.

Implementation

✦ A. Provide symptomatic and supportive measures—no specific treatment.
1. Initially bedrest is indicated, promote rest.
2. Encourage high fluid intake.
3. Increase in activity should be gradual.
4. Acetaminophen is given for fever, chills, and muscle pain.
5. Prevent secondary infections by limiting contacts while acutely ill.
B. Acyclovir may be administered to immunosuppressed clients.

Hemophilia

✦ *Definition:* A sex-linked disorder in which certain factors necessary for coagulation of the blood are missing.

Sex-linked traits are passed from unaffected carrier females to affected males along with the X chromosome.

Characteristics

✦ A. Hemophilia A—Factor VIII deficiency: treated with monoclonal factor VIII concentrate and often DDAVP.

✦ B. Hemophilia B—Factor IX deficiency (Christmas disease): treated with purified, concentrated Factor IX.

Assessment

✦ A. Assess for type A or B.
   1. Possible bleeding tendency in neonatal period because factors are not passed through the placenta.
   2. Excessive bruising.
   3. Large hematomas from minor trauma.
   4. Persistent bleeding from minor injuries.
   5. Hemarthrosis with joint pain, swelling, and limited movement.
   ✦ 6. Abnormalities in clotting studies (PT, PTT, fibrinogen, Factor VIII or IX assay).
   7. Possible progressive degenerative changes with osteoporosis, muscle atrophy, and fixed joints.
B. Assess for type C.
   1. Usually appears as a mild bleeding disorder.
   2. Autosomal dominant trait with both sexes affected.

Implementation

✦ A. Prevent bleeding.
   1. Protect child from environment by padding crib and playpen.
   2. Supervise child carefully when child is learning to walk.
✦ B. Treatment if bleeding occurs:
   1. Apply cold compresses and pressure.
   2. Hemarthrosis (effusion of blood into joint).
      a. Immobilize joint initially.
      b. Initiate passive range of motion within 48 hours to prevent stiffness.
      c. Manage pain adequately.
   3. Immobilize site of bleeding.
   ✦ 4. Administer needed factors or blood products, monitor for transfusion reaction.
   5. Monitor HIV status appropriately. (Many were inadvertently infected before blood was routinely screened.)
   6. Multidisciplinary education program—genetic counseling, home management, support growth and development, family needs and assistance, appropriate referrals.

HIV and Children

Definition: Considered to have AIDS when at least one complicating illness develops or when CD4 drops below 200.

Characteristics

A. About 2 percent of the people infected with HIV in the United States are children or adolescents.
B. Symptoms and complications of HIV and death result from opportunistic infections from viruses, parasites and (unlike adults) bacteria.
C. Transmission.
   1. HIV infection is almost always acquired from mother. Fewer than 7 percent of children with AIDS acquire infection from blood transfusions or sexual abuse.
   2. Risk is highest from mothers acquiring the infection during pregnancy (who have more virus in their bodies or who are severely ill).
   3. Transmission usually takes place during labor and delivery.
   4. Transmission can also be via breastmilk.

Implementation

A. If an infected woman conceives, anti-HIV drugs are fairly effective.
B. Drug treatment.
   1. Woman may receive zidovudine (ZDV, also called AZT) by mouth during the second and third trimesters (last 6 months) of pregnancy.
   2. ZDV given IV during labor and delivery.
   3. ZDV given daily to the newborn for 6 weeks.
   4. Transmission rates decrease by about 30 percent with ZDV.
C. Cesarean delivery decreases baby's risk of acquiring HIV infection.
D. Drugs given (trimethoprim–sulfamethoxazole) to prevent opportunistic infections.
   1. Children with a significantly impaired immune system may also be given azithromycin to prevent *Mycobacterium avium* complex infection.
   2. Transmission of infections, such as chickenpox, to the HIV-infected child is a danger.
E. Social issues.
   1. A child with HIV and open skin sores, or who engages in potentially dangerous behavior, such as biting, should not attend child care.
   2. HIV-infected children should participate in as many routine childhood activities as their physical condition allows.
   3. Interaction with other children enhances social development and self-esteem.
F. Standard Precautions should be practiced.

BLOOD TRANSFUSIONS

Assessment

A. Identify type of therapy to be administered.
   1. Whole blood.
   2. Packed red blood cells.
   3. Platelets.
B. Check that type and cross-match are correct before administering blood.
C. Assess baseline vital signs.
D. Review institution policy about blood products.

✦ Implementation

A. Check identification of child with blood slip and Identaband before administering blood.
B. Obtain baseline vital signs.
C. Ensure that proper IV tubing and filter are used for blood administration (per institution policy).
D. Use infusion pump; monitor vital signs every 15 minutes for the first hour of infusion, then every 30 minutes until transfusion is complete.
E. Never give medications in blood, and never hang blood with dextrose and water (use only normal saline).
F. Observe for transfusion reaction: backache, generalized discomfort, chilly sensations, distention of neck veins, tachycardia, tachypnea, and fall in blood pressure.
G. Observe for allergic reactions: wheezing, laryngeal edema, hives, itching and rash, and flushed appearance.
H. If either reaction occurs, stop transfusion, assess symptoms, and call physician.
I. Never use blood that is discolored or cloudy or that has been unrefrigerated for more than 30 minutes.

MUSCULOSKELETAL SYSTEM

The musculoskeletal system comprises the bones, joints, and muscles. In order to effectively assess and treat disorders associated with this system, it is necessary to consider the effects of the blood vessels, skin, nerves, and tendons.

System Assessment

A. History.
1. Pertinent perinatal and birth history.
2. Family history of musculoskeletal disorders.
3. Previous injuries, fractures, surgeries, or other musculoskeletal problems.
4. Any pain, swelling, or current problems.
♦ B. Inspection.
1. Observe gait (or crawling) for limping, toe-walking, equal movement, and balance.
2. Inspect spine and curvature of spine. Have child bend forward at waist and observe level of scapulae, ribs, and hips.
3. Assess shape of back; toddlers normally have lumbar lordosis, older children may have kyphosis from chronic slouching.
4. Observe strength and size of muscles.
5. Evaluate length and shape of extremeties.
6. Observe gluteal skin folds for symmetry.
C. Palpation.
1. Assess strength of upper extremities by having child squeeze examiner's fingers.
2. Palpate hips of neonate by performing Barlow and Ortolani maneuvers to check for hip dysplasia.
3. Palpate joints for swelling or pain, evaluate ROM.

System Implementation

♦ A. Identify abnormality of musculoskeletal structure.
1. Evaluate newborn for congenital abnormality of the musculoskeletal system.
2. Check for adequate range of motion and strength in all extremities.
3. Check for normal hip joints in newborn.
4. Check for abnormal spinal curvature (usually most noticeable in the school-age child.)
♦ B. Prevent abnormal movement.
1. Limit movement if developing abnormal patterns.
2. Establish program of teaching ambulation with a physical therapist.

C. Prevent limitation of movement.
1. Position body parts in proper alignment.
2. Complete appropriate active and passive range of motion.
D. Control pain.
1. Schedule painful procedures around analgesic schedule.
2. Implement measures to reduce pain (i.e., massage, heat and/or cold compresses, relaxation techniques).
E. Promote adequate circulation.
1. Remove any restrictive garments or bandages.
2. Check circulation of extremities at frequent intervals.
a. Capillary filling.
b. Temperature.
c. Color.
d. Peripheral pulses.
e. Edema.
F. Promote alignment through traction.
1. Check the vascular status of the extremity.
2. Check the neurological status of the extremity.
a. Level of sensation.
b. Motion.
3. Observe traction for intactness in both skeletal and skin traction.
G. Promote healing through proper casting and cast care.
1. Check the vascular status of the extremity.
2. Examine the cast for signs of bleeding. If bleeding is present, draw a circle around the site, indicating time and date.
3. Examine the cast for any pressure areas.
4. Pull stockinette over cast edges and secure with tape (prevents cast crumbs from falling inside cast).
5. Keep the cast clean and dry.
6. If appropriate, keep the level of the cast above the heart to prevent edema formation.

CONGENITAL DEFECTS

Developmental Dysplasia of the Hip (DDH)

♦ *Definition:* Abnormalities of the hip present at birth, usually accompanied by abnormalities of the acetabulum, subluxation, or dislocation. Occurs in 1 or 2 per 1000 live births, and 6 times more often in females.

Assessment

♦ A. Check for unequal major gluteal folds in infants, or varying heights of bent knees as viewed distally with infant supine.
♦ B. Assess for presence of a hip "click" on abduction as femur slips over acetabulum.

C.   Assess for femur that may appear shortened, or limp in older child.

◆ D.   Assess degree of dysplasia.
1.   Preluxation (acetabular dysplasia): mildest form, femoral head remains in acetabulum but delayed acetabular development occurs.
2.   Subluxation: most common form. Femoral head remains in contact with acetabulum, but is partially displaced.
3.   Dislocation: femoral head loses acetabulum contact.

Implementation

A.   Referral and complete evaluation by orthopedic specialist.
B.   Teach parents importance of splinting, application of splint, and maintaining alignment.
C.   Protect skin under the splint.
D.   Bring environment to child: surround with age-appropriate toys, support development.
◆ E.   Maintain hip in flexion and abduction.
◆ F.   Continue double diapering, if advised.
G.   Monitor traction if hospitalized.
◆ H.   Correction of DDH in older children may require operative reduction; osteotomy usually required and tenotomy of contracted muscles. Casting is necessary after surgery (hip spica).
1.   Cast care teaching essential: diapering, keeping cast clean, checking skin frequently.
2.   Feeding more challenging if casted—head must be elevated—may require modified chair.
3.   Assist in discharge planning/teaching; focusing on daily activities; bathing, play, car seat adaptations, mobility (wagon, stroller, or scooter).

Congenital Clubfoot

Definition: Congenital deformity in which the foot is twisted out of its normal position. The deformity is described according to the position of the foot and ankle. The most common type is talipes equinovarus (95 percent) in which the foot is pointed downward and inward. Other forms include talipes varus (foot bends inward), talipes valgus (foot bends outward), talipes equinus (plantar flexion with toes lower than heel), or talipes calcaneus (dorsiflexion with toes higher than heel).

Assessment

◆ A.   Assess whether foot deformity is accompanied by other problems such as neurological defects or spina bifida.
B.   Assess general health status of infant in preparation for treatment.
C.   Determine aspects of treatment: occurs in three stages and includes exercises, manipulation, casting, and splinting.

Implementation

◆ A.   Treatment plan consists of correction, maintenance, and follow-up.
1.   Correction usually starts with manipulation followed by serial casting (shortly after birth).
2.   Casts are changed every few days, as needed due to rapid growth of infant.
3.   More severe forms may require surgery.
4.   Occasionally, splinting may be used.
◆ B.   Assist in passive exercises (manipulation) of the foot following a demonstration by physician: hold position to count of 10 and continue for 10 minutes several times a day.
C.   Instruct parents in cast and/or splint care.
D.   Provide emotional support and encourage bonding and infant development.

Osteogenesis Imperfecta

◆ *Definition:* A congenital defect (most commonly autosomal dominant, but may also occur as autosomal recessive inheritance) resulting in severely brittle and fragile bones. Affected individuals appear to have abnormal precollagen preventing the formation of collagen; classified into four grades of severity. Tendency to fracture may not occur until later in childhood, but may occur at early ages.

Assessment

A.   Refer for genetic counseling.
B.   Assess skin—often is thin, easily injured, excessive diaphoresis.
C.   Assess bleeding tendencies—frequently bruise, frequent epistaxis.
D.   Radiographs show thin bone shafts; possibly multiple old, healed fractures (must rule out child abuse).
E.   Assess ROM, activity, limitations in ADLs, level of comfort.

Implementation

◆ A.   Careful handling of infant to prevent fractures, especially when diapering.
B.   Teaching and support in use of casts, braces, or splints utilized.
C.   Assist with physical therapy plan.
D.   Surgery may be necessary to correct deformities.
E.   Support growth and development of infant and child.
F.   Teaching principles.
1.   Emphasize safety and prevention of fractures.
2.   Reinforce medical therapeutic plan and prognosis.
3.   Refer to appropriate community agencies and support groups.
4.   Teach other healthcare professionals about defect. Families may be wrongfully accused of non-accidental trauma.

Muscular Dystrophy

Definition: Gradual degeneration of muscle fibers with progressive weakness of symmetric groups of the skeletal muscles.

Characteristics

◆ A. Duchenne's muscular dystrophy is the most common type and the most severe.

◆ B. Genetic pattern is an X-linked recessive; 30–50 percent have no family history.

C. Usually this disease appears at 3–5 years of age; rare in infancy or at birth; ambulation usually impossible after about 12 years.

D. Death usually occurs from pneumonia or cardiac failure; some live into their 20s or 30s.

Assessment

◆ A. Assess for delay in motor development: clumsiness, walking on toes, waddling gait.

B. Assess for abnormal fatigue when walking or running.

◆ C. Check for presence of Gower's maneuver: climbing up on legs from supine position, marked lordosis when upright.

D. Assess for progressive muscle weakness: axial and proximal before distal, in symmetric muscle groups.

Implementation

◆ A. Provide support so that child can maintain independence as long as possible.
   1. Assist parents to develop physical therapy program.
   2. Support use of wheelchair when necessary to maintain mobility.

◆ B. Counsel parents to prevent respiratory infection.
   1. Teach deep-breathing exercises.
   2. Maintain adequate diet to promote healthy status.

C. Counsel parents to monitor child's weight to promote mobility and health.

D. Assist parents to obtain emotional support to deal with child more adequately at home.
   1. Identify community resources that will support family.
   2. Refer for genetic counseling.
   3. Counsel family to deal with chronic illness and with eventual death of the child.

ACQUIRED DEFECTS

Fracture

See Fractures, Chapter 8.

Legg–Calvé–Perthes Disease

◆ *Definition:* A self-limiting disease in which aseptic necrosis of the femoral head produces hip deformation and dysfunction.

Characteristics

◆ A. Usually affects children 3–12 years of age and males 4–8 years of age; usually unilateral and self-limited.

◆ B. Phases.
   1. Phase I—septic necrosis or infarction of the femoral capital epiphysis—the avascular stage.
   2. Phase II—gradual revascularization takes place and necrotic bone is replaced with connective tissue.
   3. Phase III—connective tissue ossifies, which results in healing.

Assessment

◆ A. Assess for pain in hip or knee most evident on rising or at end of the day.

B. Assess for limp or joint dysfunction on the affected side—may be intermittent.

C. Assess for stiffness and tenderness over hip capsule.

Implementation

◆ A. Goal of treatment is to keep the head of the femur contained in the acetabulum.
   ◆ 1. Initial therapy is rest to reduce inflammation and restore motion.
      a. Active motion is encouraged during this phase.
      b. Traction may be applied to stretch tight adductor muscles.
   ◆ 2. Containment accomplished by several measures.
      a. Non–weight-bearing devices such as abduction brace, leg cast, or leather harness sling that prevents weight bearing on affected limb.
      b. Weight-bearing appliances such as abduction–ambulation brace or cast.
   3. Conservative treatment may be continued for 2–4 years; surgical correction allows the child to resume normal activities in 3–4 months.
   ◆ 4. Disease is self-limiting, but early treatment is essential to avoid permanent damage.

◆ B. Most care is outpatient, so nursing emphasis is on teaching.
   1. Teach family use of corrective device selected for therapy.
   2. Stress importance of compliance for resolution of disease.
   3. Provide support for inactivity forced upon child.

   4. Support normal growth and development and school progress.

Slipped Femoral Capital Epiphysis

+ *Definition:* The spontaneous displacement of the proximal femoral epiphysis in a posterior and inferior direction. Most often occurs around puberty in obese children (slightly more often in boys).

Assessment

A. Obtain growth history and correct height and weight, recent injury/trauma.
+ B. X-rays demonstrate widening of growth plate; slipping produces deformity of femoral head and stretching of blood vessels.
C. Assess gait for limping.
D. Evaluate pain (may be hip or knee pain) and ROM of hip.

Implementation

+ A. Usually requires fixation with pins, osteotomy, or bone graft.
+ B. Routine postop cast care, and pain management.
C. Support family, reinforce diagnosis with child and parents.
D. Teach activity limitations and traction/crutch walking.
E. Discharge planning/teaching; emphasize ADLs and support growth and development.

Scoliosis

+ *Definition:* Scoliosis is a lateral curvature of the spine and may be "C-shaped" or "S-shaped." The "S-shaped" curve has a secondary or compensatory curve.

Characteristics

+ A. Age of onset—the younger the child, the greater the chances for deformity.
    1. Deformity increases during growth periods.
    2. Usually not noticed until adolescence.
    3. Affects more girls than boys.
+ B. Size of curve—curves between 20 and 50 degrees usually treated nonsurgically. Curves more than 50 degrees or causing respiratory compromise warrant surgical intervention.
C. Pattern of curve—when the primary curve is thoracic, there is a greater likelihood that deformity will occur.
D. Can be detected in 2–3 percent of children aged 10–16 years; 60–80 percent are girls. One shoulder seems higher than the other or clothes do not hang straight, usually detected during routine physical exam.

TREATMENT

Nonsurgical correction of curvature.
1. Exercise.
2. Plastic braces (orthoses).
3. TLSO (thoracolumbosacral) or Milwaukee brace (usually when curve is 20–40 degrees)—worn 16–23 hours per day.
4. Casting.

+ **Surgical correction options.**
1. Considerations: any client with a curve of 40 degrees is considered to be a candidate for surgery—after growth stops, a lateral curve can continue to progress at about 1 degree a year. Surgery is necessary in < 10 percent of cases.
2. Spinal fusion: prevents progression of scoliosis and is done by inserting bone chips to achieve fusion of the vertebrae.
3. Harrington instrumentation: straightens the spine; acts as a splint to allow solid fusion of bony parts. Steel rods are placed along the spine and attached by wires at the cephalic and caudal ends of the spine.
4. Dwyer and Zielke instrumentation: anterior spinal fusion and instrumentation; used as first part of two-part surgery with Harrington rods (posterior).
5. Luque segmental spinal instrumentation: rigid internal fixation of the spine; a method of internal segmental spinal instrumentation by wiring each vertebra to steel rods.
6. Kaneda and CD fixation systems: use surgically placed hooks, rods and screws to correct curvature.
7. USS hardware: screws and rods are surgically placed to create a frame to correct.
8. Video-assisted thoracoscopy is currently being performed for anterior fusion and stabilization with promising results.

E. Scoliosis and its treatment often interfere with an adolescent's self-image and self-esteem. Counseling or psychotherapy may be needed.
+ F. Types.
    1. *Kyphosis:* flexion deformity usually at thoracic spine.
    2. *Lordosis:* fixed extension deformity usually occurring to compensate for other abnormalities.
    3. *Scoliosis:* lateral curvature of the spine.
        a. Nonstructural: caused by changes outside the spine; treated with exercises.
        b. Structural: the spine itself has rotated; treated by bracing, exercise, insertion of the Harrington rod or Luque procedure.

Assessment

+ A. Assess fatigue in the lumbar region after prolonged sitting or standing. Muscular backaches in areas of strain (e.g., in the lumbosacral angle) or dyspnea may be reported.
B. Question client about ability to breathe and when client usually has difficulty breathing.

✦ C. Assess physical status—expose back and check for deviations. Have client bend forward at waist—check level of scapulae.
   1. Difference in shoulder height, elbow level, and height of iliac crests.
   2. The in-folding of one flank and flattening of another.
D. Assess range of motion of the spine.
E. Observe for deviations of the hips, rib cage, shoulders, and iliac crest.
F. Assess for mild pain and/or discomfort.

Implementation

✦ A. Instruct on use of braces.
   1. Teach adolescent to wear the brace correctly and remove it only to bathe or as prescribed by the physician.
   2. Explain necessity for good skin care where brace touches.
   3. Assist adolescent to understand the need for the brace, and help the client deal with the altered body image.
✦ B. Provide care when child undergoes surgery.
   1. Harrington instrumentation.
      a. Decortication of the bone over the laminas and spinous processes.
      b. Bone grafts from iliac crest are inserted to achieve fusion of the vertebrae.
      c. Rods are inserted along the vertebrae and attached by Harrington hooks and wires to achieve tension along the spine.
      d. Casting is required postoperatively to protect the spinal fusion and to add stability.
   ✦ 2. Luque procedure.
      a. Placement of wire loops under the lamina at each vertebral level.
      b. Steel rods aligned along the curvatures of the spine are fixated to the spine by the wires.
   ✦ 3. Cotrel–Dubousset (CD) system.
      a. Consists of two rods, multiple hooks, and a transverse coupling device.
      b. Advantage—requires no postop immobilization.
   4. USS Hardware.
   5. Video-assisted thoracoscopy for anterior fixation and stabilization.

✦ Preoperative Nursing Interventions

A. Evaluate child's level of understanding regarding condition and development progression.
B. Check preop lab work to ensure all values are within normal limits.
✦ C. Assist child with pulmonary function tests.

   1. Teach child to do tri-flows, cough, and deep-breathe.
   2. Explain the importance of doing this postoperatively.
D. Evaluate child's and parents' understanding of surgical procedure.
   1. Explain to their level of understanding.
   2. Discuss postoperative course with child and parents to help them know what to expect.
   3. Answer questions they may have.
E. Visit the ICU, when appropriate, with family and child to familiarize them with the surroundings.

✦ Postoperative Nursing Interventions

✦ A. Check vital signs every 15 minutes until stable, then every hour.
✦ B. Watch for signs and symptoms of hypovolemia, tachycardia, BP. (Blood loss in the OR can be considerable.)
C. Assess respiratory function: BS, RR, chest excursion, color, grunting, flaring, retractions.
   ✦ 1. Continual assessment of respiration function with vital signs is essential; pneumothorax or punctured lung is a risk after surgery.
   2. Start tri-flows as soon as awake after 1 hour. Encourage to cough and deep-breathe between use of tri-flows.
D. Check ABGs.
E. Monitor hydration status.
   1. Maintain strict I&O.
   ✦ 2. Monitor urine output hourly. Urine output must be adequate (at least 1 mL/kg/hr). Assess for clinical signs of hypovolemia.
   3. Check specific gravity to assess hydration status.
✦ F. Check CMS (circulation–color, movement, sensation) of lower extremities and feet qh × 8 hrs, q2h × 24 hrs, then q4h.
✦ G. Turn after 1 or 2 hours by logrolling only. Maintain alignment of spine.
H. Medicate child prior to turning or doing procedures (per orders).
   1. It is important to keep child comfortable and administer narcotics in appropriate doses—preferably by continuous IV infusion.
   2. Observe vital sign changes as indicative of pain.
I. Maintain NPO until child has positive bowel sounds, is passing flatus, or has had a stool.
✦ J. Start diet with ice chips only. (Paralytic ileus is a common side effect.)
K. Check skin and dressing hourly to assess for skin breakdown and bleeding.
L. Instruct child to flex feet to improve circulation and maintain muscle tone.
✦ M. Rehabilitation postoperatively.

1. Harrington instrumentation.
   a. Most children are casted after recovery from surgery; they can be out of bed 1 to 2 weeks after the cast has been applied.
   b. Cast stays on 6 months.
   c. After cast is removed, a Milwaukee brace or thoracolumbar support is worn approximately 3 months—removed only at night.
2. Luque, CD and thoracoscopic procedures:
   a. After the wound is stable and child recovered from anesthesia, child may sit at the side of the bed.
   b. Progresses to ambulation. No postop immobilization is required.

N. Discharge planning and teaching specific to surgical intervention performed; support of family and growth and development.

INFLAMMATORY DISEASES

Osteomyelitis

✦ *Definition:* Infection usually of the long bones caused most frequently by *Staphylococcus aureus*. In younger children, *Haemophilus influenzae* or *Salmonella* may cause osteomyelitis. Occurs most frequently in children between 5 and 14 years of age. It is twice as common in boys. The infection can result from exogenous causes (direct bacterial invasion from the outside) or hematogenous spread from a preexisting infection.

✦ **Assessment**
A. Assess for abrupt onset or trauma to affected bone.
B. Assess for recent infection or injury anywhere else in child's body.
C. Evaluate for fever, malaise, and pain.
D. Assess for localized tenderness in the bone at the metaphysis.
E. Evaluate for swelling and redness over affected bone.
F. Observe for fever, irritability, GI symptoms (vomiting or diarrhea).

Implementation
✦ A. Control infection.
1. Supervision of antibacterial therapy, usually a combination of penicillinase-resistant synthetic penicillin and a third-generation cephalosporin, but is specific to organism cultured. Monitor for side effects.
2. Careful handling of drainage.
B. Control pain.
1. Immobilization of affected limb; casting may be necessary.
2. Analgesics as needed.
C. Surgical drainage of area may be necessary.

D. Monitor hydration and nutrition.
1. Child should be encouraged to drink fluids (supplement with IVs when necessary).
2. Encourage high-calorie foods and supplements; offer frequent snacks.
E. Prepare for discharge—support family and child's growth and development.

Juvenile Rheumatoid Arthritis

✦ *Definition:* This is a systemic autoimmune disorder with multiple manifestations, arthritis being the most characteristic. Etiology is unknown. Incidence is about 1 in 2000 children, more in Caucasians. Generally, onset is seen between 2 and 16 years of age.

Assessment
✦ A. Assess for inflammation of joints.
B. Assess for edema and congestion of synovial tissues. (As the disease progresses, synovial material fills the joint, causing narrowing, fibrous ankylosis, and bony fusion.)
C. Assess for premature closure or accelerated epiphyseal growth.
D. Assess joint involvement.
1. Arthritis may start slowly with gradual development of joint stiffness, swelling, and loss of motion.
2. Most frequently affects knees, ankles, feet, wrists, and fingers—although any joint may be involved.
3. Affected joints are swollen, warm, painful, and stiff.
4. Young children appear irritable and anxious, guarding their joints.
5. Weakness and atrophy of muscles appear around affected joints.
6. Chronically affected joints may become deformed, dislocated or fused.
E. Assess systemic involvement.
1. Frequently occurs.
2. Irritability, anorexia, and malaise.
3. Fever.
4. Intermittent macular rash is occasionally seen.
5. Hepatosplenomegaly and generalized lymphadenopathy in 20 percent of clients.
6. Anemia is common with active cases of the disease.
7. Inflammation of eye: redness, pain, photophobia, decreased visual acuity, and nonreactive pupil.

Implementation
✦ A. Supervise medication administration—major goal is to relieve pain, while maintaining function.

1. Primary drugs are nonsteroidal anti-inflammatory drugs (NSAIDs).
2. Monitor levels carefully.
✦ 3. Observe for gastric irritation. (Give drug in four doses daily, with meals and at bedtime.)
✦ 4. Slower-acting antirheumatic drugs (SAARDs). Added when one or two NSAIDs are ineffective.
   a. Injectable gold is the first SAARD added; usually given in weekly injections.
   b. Side effects.
      (1) Dermatitis.
      (2) Stomatitis.
      (3) Nephritis with hematuria or albuminuria.
      (4) Thrombocytopenia.
      (5) Bone marrow depression.
   c. Weekly blood and urine tests.
5. Cytotoxic drugs.
   a. Cyclophosphamide, azathioprine, methotrexate, or chlorambucil.
   b. May be given to clients not responding to NSAIDs or SAARDs, with continuing severe symptoms.
✦ 6. Corticosteroids—to reduce inflammation and prevent joint damage. Usually given in low doses and every other day to decrease undesirable side effects.
   a. Side effects and toxicity.
      (1) Masked infection.
      (2) Hypertension.
      (3) Vascular disorders.
      (4) Mental disturbances.
      (5) Edema and weight gain.
      (6) Increased appetite.
      (7) Peptic ulcer.
   b. Regular observation of vital signs.
   c. Careful supervision during initiation and tapering off of drug.
7. Immunologic modulators—to decrease inflammation and alter the immune response (example: etanercept).

B. Maintain joint function.
   1. Exercise joints.
   2. Provide night splints, provide heat, and encourage proper positioning at rest.
   3. Educate parents in how child should perform exercises and impress upon them the child's need for physical therapy and splints.

C. Prevent eye damage—encourage parents to report any signs of eye problems in the child immediately to the physician. Iridocyclitis carries a good prognosis if treated early.

D. Counsel family. Encourage compliance with the treatment plan.
   1. Explain physiology and unpredictable nature of the disease to the parents and the child.
   2. Provide emotional support to the parents for dealing with a chronically ill child or adolescent.
   3. Refer to appropriate support groups.
   4. Encourage independence in the child and in ADLs.
   5. Encourage mastery of developmental tasks appropriate to the age group of the child; encourage participation in school and school activities.

INTEGUMENTARY SYSTEM

The integumentary system comprises the skin, including the epidermis and the dermis, as well as all the derivatives of the epidermis, such as hair, nails, and various glands. It forms a barrier against the external environment and participates in many vital body functions.

System Assessment

A. History of previous skin conditions, allergies.
B. Inspection.
1. Observe skin odor (indicative of poor hygiene or infection).
2. Assess color and pigmentation of skin as normal within ethnicity; especially in areas less exposed to sunlight, and nailbeds, sclera, conjunctiva, lips and mouth (note cyanosis, pallor, jaundice, yellow or brown discoloration).
3. Observe moistness of skin and mucous membranes.
4. Inspect and palpate skin texture for scar tissue, turgor, edema, temperature, and lesions.
✦ C. Note types of abnormal lesions.
1. *Macule:* small, flat, colored lesion.
2. *Papule:* small, solid, elevated lesion.
3. *Vesicle:* elevated lesion filled with fluid.
4. *Nodule:* larger solid form of papule.
5. *Petechia:* pinpoint hemorrhage in the skin.
6. *Ecchymosis:* bruise of variable size initially purple, fades to green and brown.
7. *Tumor:* abnormal mass.
8. *Hives:* eruption of itching wheals.
✦ D. Observe for variations on skin, "birthmarks" in infants.
1. Mongolian spot (hyperpigmented nevi): large, flat, blue, black, or slate-colored area found on buttocks and lumbosacral area, more often in Asian children.
2. Salmon patch or "stork beak mark": common in all races; flat, pink mark found on eyelids, nasolabial area, or at nape of neck. Most disappear by 1 year.
3. Strawberry nevus: begins as defined grayish, white area, becomes red, raised, well defined. May not be obvious at birth. Most resolve spontaneously by 9 years old.
E. Note distribution of lesions with other symptoms that occur simultaneously, assist with diagnosis.

System Implementation

✦ A. Identify and treat cause of skin disorder.
1. Record the size, shape, and distribution of skin lesions.
2. Note all other concurrent symptoms.
3. Evaluate child's recent history, particularly medications, new foods, and exposure to communicable diseases.
4. Isolate possible allergens and remove from environment.
B. Assist in reducing pruritus.
1. Apply lotion (i.e., calamine lotion) to reduce itching, or cool compresses.
2. Administer antihistamine if ordered.
3. Apply topical medication if ordered (steroid creams or antibiotic, antifungal preparations).
C. Note abnormal change in skin lesions.
1. Describe accurately the placement, size, shape, and distinguishing characteristics of all lesions.
2. Evaluate for changes on a routine basis.
3. Teach family to notify physician if any skin lesions such as birthmarks or moles change shape or color or start to bleed.
✦ D. Observe and record any abnormal coloring.
1. Describe cyanosis if present. Include location and under what conditions (i.e., during feeding) it occurred.
2. Check the child for other signs of cardiac or respiratory disease.
3. Evaluate child's laboratory values if pallor is present to determine presence of anemia. Ask for a 24-hour accounting of diet.
4. Monitor jaundice for change.
E. Correct any abnormal texture.
1. For poor skin turgor:
   a. Increase the fluid intake.
   b. Monitor intake and output.
   c. Monitor specific gravity.
2. For edema:
   a. Establish and treat the underlying cause.
   b. Give meticulous skin care.
   c. Monitor intake and output.
F. Prevent secondary infections.
1. Encourage the child not to scratch the lesions.
2. Apply mittens to hands of neonates.
3. Keep child's hands and nails clean with the nails trimmed.
4. Keep infant clean and dry. Change diapers frequently, apply appropriate protection from diaper rash.
G. Prevent allergic responses.
1. Assist in obtaining an accurate environmental history including exposure to common household allergens, food, and medications.

2. Educate the family on changes in the environment that are necessary.

H. Provide teaching and anticipatory guidance, especially in avoiding preventable skin conditions.
1. Use of sunblock and minimizing exposure to sun.
2. Signs of skin cancers.
3. Avoidance of known irritants, maintaining good hygiene and overall health.

SKIN DISORDERS

Acne Vulgaris

Definition: The presence of blackheads, whiteheads, and pustules usually found on face, chest, and back; due to plugging of sebaceous glands. Most commonly occurs in adolescence when sebaceous gland activity increases.

Assessment

A. Assess areas of inflammation and secondary infection.
B. Assess current treatment practices.
C. Evaluate impact of acne on body image and self-esteem.

Implementation

A. Instruct adolescent to use gentle cleansing products. Benzoyl peroxide kills P. acnes organisms.
B. Advise adolescent that improvement may take several weeks.
C. Provide teaching on prescribed regimen; medications used much more frequently than systemic treatment. Topical medications used include ketolytic (Tretinoin), antibiotic (Clendamycin), and/or retinoid (accutane) therapy.
D. Provide support and reassurance that condition improves with age; promote self-esteem.

Impetigo

✦ *Definition:* A skin infection usually caused by *Staphylococcus*. Usually begins as a scratch or scrape that becomes infected.

Assessment

✦ A. Assess for multiple macular-papular rash seen at various stages of healing.
B. Check rupture of papules, which produce honey-colored serous exudate and form a crust, or scab.
C. Assess location: usually found on face, head, and neck, but may spread over any part of the body.
D. May be superimposed on eczema.

Implementation

✦ A. Frequent cleansing with mild soap, may remove crusts.
✦ B. Monitor topical (usually mupirocin ointment) and/or systemic antibiotic therapy (cephalosporins or penicillins if severe).
C. Cut nails to avoid scratching in infants and small children.
D. Document size and appearance of lesions.
E. Emphasize communicability of infection, maintaining thorough handwashing (child and caregiver) and overall good hygiene to avoid spread of infection.

Eczema (Atopic Dermatitis)

✦ *Definition:* A superficial dermatitis generally seen in children with allergic tendencies. It usually begins with pruritic, erythematous, papulovesicular lesions and progresses to crusty, thickened areas.

Assessment

A. Assess for erythema, papules, vesicles, often in creases of skin, on cheeks.
B. Check drainage if crusting is present.
C. Assess for intense itching.
D. Look for symptoms in children 2 months to 5 years, but may be present in any age group.
✦ E. Assess when symptoms appear: often commences with the introduction of new foods, particularly eggs and cow's milk, and the cessation of breast-feeding.
F. Stress can exacerbate outbreaks.
G. Evaluate family history.

Implementation

✦ A. Interventions aimed at reducing inflammation, pruritis and hydrate the skin.
B. Remove dust-carrying objects in environment (stuffed animals), eliminate molds and cigarettes.
C. Eliminate strong soaps, in laundry and on skin.
✦ D. Provide symptomatic treatment of lesions: administer topical steroids, and maintain skin hydration. May teach parents to apply lanolin-based or oil-in-water–based emulsions immediately following bathing to seal in moisture to skin.
E. Prevent scratching, secondary infections.
F. Teach parents about prescribed therapy (drug dose, route, and side effects).
G. May use antihistamines if pruritus is intense.
H. Many children outgrow atopic dermatitis by adolescence.

Seborrheic Dermatitis

✦ *Definition:* A chronic, recurrent dermatitis due to excessive sebaceous discharge, usually found on the scalp in infants ("cradle cap") or eyebrows. Commonly occurs in infants, may be found in adolescents.

Assessment

A. Appears as patchy lesions covered by yellowish, oily scales.
B. Observe for signs of secondary infection.

Implementation

A. Prevent occurrence with improved hygiene.
✦ B. When scales are present, shampoo with an antiseborrheic shampoo containing sulphur and salicyclic acid.
   1. Shampoo is applied to crusts and allowed to penetrate.
   2. After thorough rinsing, remove crusts gently with soft brush or fine-toothed comb.
C. More severe cases may require topical steroids and/or antibiotic therapy.
D. Teach parents or adolescents the importance of good hygiene and frequent use of mild shampoos. Reassure that generally cases resolve easily with simple treatment.

Diaper Dermatitis (Diaper Rash)

Definition: Erythematous lesions and maceration in the diaper area caused by prolonged contact with urine or feces, chemical irritants, bacteria or fungi, or reactions to foods. Incidence peaks at 9–12 months of age; more common in bottle-fed infants.

Assessment

✦ A. Observe for reddened, macerated skin, with sharply demarcated edges.
✦ B. Evaluate for signs of candidal infection, characterized by "beefy red" central erythema with satellite lesions.
C. Observe for secondary infection.
D. Assess current diapering habits and history.

Implementation

✦ A. Treatment focuses on teaching.
   1. Discuss necessity of keeping area clean and dry. Change diapers as soon as soiled.
   2. Avoid alcohol-based wipes and perfumed soaps.
   3. Expose skin to air (not heat) for several minutes each day.
   4. Apply barrier-type ointment when skin is dry.
   5. If using cloth diapers, avoid plastic pants—use overwraps allowing air to circulate.
   6. If candidiasis is present, apply anti-fungal creams as prescribed.
B. Reassure parents that baby will become less irritable as rash clears.

Cellulitis

✦ *Definition:* An infection in the subcutaneous tissue or dermis, usually caused by *Staphylococcus aureus, Haemophilus influenzae,* or group A beta-hemolytic streptococci.

Assessment

✦ A. Observe for redness, swelling, and tenderness in area.
✦ B. Evaluate systemic symptoms; fever, malaise, or enlarged lymph nodes.
C. X-ray evaluation to rule out osteomyelitis; blood cultures; CBC may be done.
D. Obtain vital signs, evaluate for fever; weight and height; aspiration and culture of inflamed area.
E. Obtain history of injury and previous treatment.

Implementation

✦ A. Administer or supervise antibiotics.
B. Provide pain relief.
C. Apply warm compresses/soaks as ordered.
D. Administer IV antibiotics and monitor carefully if infection extensive or around eye.
E. Provide family support and discharge teaching.

Burns

See also Chapter 8.

✦ ### Assessment

A. Assess degree and extent of burn.
B. Assess prescribed treatment for burn.
C. Assess for complications associated with burns.
   1. Fluid and electrolyte imbalances.
      a. In deeper wounds, edema appears around the wound from damage to capillaries.
      b. Loss of fluid at the burn area.
      c. On the second day, large loss of potassium.
      d. Objective of fluid therapy is to maintain adequate tissue perfusion.
   2. Circulatory changes.
      a. Drop in cardiac output, initially.
      b. A decrease in blood volume occurs from loss of plasma protein into extravascular and extracellular spaces.
      c. Moderate amount of hemolysis of red blood cells.
   3. Pulmonary changes—inhalation injury.
      a. Pulmonary edema.
      b. Obstruction of the air passages from edema of the face, neck, trachea, and larynx.
      c. Restriction of lung mobility from eschar on chest wall.
   4. Renal changes.
      a. Renal insufficiency caused by reaction to hypovolemic shock.

b.   A decreased blood supply to kidneys results in decreased renal perfusion.

c.   In burns of 15–20 percent of the body surface, there is a decreased urinary output that must be avoided or reversed.

d.   Urinary tract infections are frequent.

5.   Gastrointestinal changes.

a.   Acute gastric dilation.

b.   Paralytic ileus.

c.   Curling's ulcer—producing "coffee ground" aspirant.

d.   Hemorrhagic gastritis—bleeding from congested capillaries in gastric mucosa.

Implementation

✦ A.   *See* Interventions for Burns in Chapter 8.

B.   Maintain optimum circulating fluid volume.

C.   Relieve pain.

1.   Reduce anxiety and fear.

2.   Medicate appropriately before dressing changes or procedures.

D.   Maintain pulmonary function.

E.   Provide adequate nutrition.

1.   Give twice the normal amount of calories.

2.   Give three to four times the normal requirement for protein.

3.   Provide small, frequent, and attractive meals.

4.   Encourage child, who is frequently anorexic, to eat. Have parents bring foods from home.

✦ F.   Support ability to cope with lifelong disfigurement.

1.   Support use of appliances to minimize scarring.

2.   Seek referrals for psychological problems associated with disfigurement.

3.   Prepare child and family for common issues encountered with long-term plastic surgery.

4.   Minimize distortion of self-image and lowering of self-esteem due to disfigurement, encourage participation in group activities.

✦ G.   Design activities for the burned child while child is hospitalized.

1.   Actively involve the child (e.g., acting out part of a story verbally).

2.   Provide television, books, and games.

3.   Allow the child to associate with friends.

4.   Reduce risk for impaired mobility—adhere to physical therapy schedule.

H.   Counsel parents.

1.   Parents and child have difficulty dealing with disfigurement and need assessment and interventions.

2.   Parents frequently feel guilty, although they are usually not at fault and need assistance working out these feelings.

3.   Refer to appropriate support groups.

4.   Anticipatory guidance.

ENDOCRINE SYSTEM

The endocrine system consists of a series of glands that function individually or conjointly to integrate and control innumerable metabolic activities of the body. These glands automatically regulate various body processes by releasing chemical signals called hormones, which produce specialized effects on their specific target tissues.

System Assessment

A. History: family history, significant perinatal history and events. Assess for history of endocrine disorders, Marfan's syndrome, and adult size of relatives.

✦ B. Assess growth patterns: evaluate patterns plotted on growth charts.
  1. Excessive growth; sudden spurts or consistently > 95th percentile.
     a. Pituitary or hypothalamic disorders.
     b. Excess adrenal, ovarian, or testicular hormone.
  2. Retarded growth; consistent pattern < 5th percentile or sudden dropoff.
     a. Endocrine and metabolic disorders; difficult to distinguish from dwarfism.
     b. Hypothyroidism or hypopituitarism possible.

C. Obesity.
  1. Sudden onset suggests hypothalamic lesion (rare); assess dietary practices.
  2. Cushing's syndrome (with characteristic buffalo hump); evaluate medications used (chronic steroid use).

D. Abnormal skin pigmentation.

E. Abnormal hirsutism.
  1. Normal variations in body occur on nonendocrine basis.
  2. May be first sign of neoplastic disease.
  3. Indicates change in adrenal status.

✦ F. Evaluate appetite changes.
  1. Polyphagia is a common sign of uncontrolled diabetes.
  2. Indicates thyrotoxicosis.
  3. Nausea and weight loss may indicate Addisonian crisis or diabetic acidosis.

✦ G. Presence of polyuria and polydipsia.
  1. Symptoms usually of nonendocrine etiology.
  2. If sudden onset, suggest diabetes mellitus or insipidus.
  3. May be present with hyperparathyroidism or hyperaldosteronism.

✦ H. Noticeable mental changes.
  1. Though often subtle, may be indicative of underlying endocrine disorder.
     a. Nervousness and excitability may indicate hyperthyroidism.
     b. Mental confusion may indicate hypopituitarism, Addison's disease, or myxedema.
  2. Mental deterioration is observed in untreated hypoparathyroidism and hypothyroidism.
  3. Mental retardation is present in some endocrine gland disorders.

System Implementation

A. Give medications on schedule to maintain accurate blood level.

B. Instruct the child and parent on signs and symptoms and side effects of medications.

C. Instruct the child and parent on methods to decrease infection.

D. Provide appropriate nutrition and education.

THYROID GLAND DISORDERS

Hypothyroidism

✦ *Definition:* Hypothyroidism is a condition caused by low production of thyroid hormones. It can be congenital or acquired, acute or chronic. Screening is routinely done on neonates. Beyond the first 2 years of life, primary hypothyroidism can be caused by many defects, and the effects are generally less severe than the congenital form.

Assessment

✦ A. Assess for severe retardation of physical development, resulting in decelerated growth, sexual development retardation.

✦ B. Evaluate severe mental retardation, apathy in older children.

✦ C. Assess for dry skin; coarse, dry, sparse brittle hair, puffiness around eyes (myxedematous skin changes).

D. Evaluate constipation.

E. Assess teething pattern (usually slow).

F. Assess for poor appetite.

G. Examine tongue (usually large).

H. Check for pot belly with umbilical hernia.

I. Assess for sensitivity to cold.

J. Evaluate laboratory values to confirm diagnosis.
  1. T_4 levels decreased, elevated TSH.
  2. Elevated serum cholesterol.
  3. Low radioactive iodine uptake.

Implementation

✦ A. Monitor administration of drugs; must be started immediately in infants to avoid mental deficiencies.

1. Levothyroxine.
2. Dosage is based on age, weight, and response to treatment.
B. Involve older children in treatment plan.
C. Support and education of family and child; make appropriate referrals.

Hyperthyroidism (Graves' Disease)

Definition: The oversecretion of thyroid hormone, occurring more commonly in adolescents. The etiology is unknown, but the disease is more common in girls and has familial tendencies.

Assessment

A. Obtain family history.
B. Assist with diagnostic evaluation.
   1. Increased levels of T_3 and T_4.
   2. Decreased levels of TS_4.
✦ C. Weight loss with excellent appetite.
✦ D. Nervousness; irritability, difficulty sleeping, heat intolerance, excessive sweating, tachycardia.
E. Characteristic exophthalmos.
F. Vomiting/diarrhea.
G. Occasionally palpable goiter.
H. Heat intolerance.
I. Warm, moist skin.

Implementation

✦ A. Oral administration of propylthiouracil (antithyroid medicine), iodine, and a beta blocker.
   1. Teaching about medications and side effects.
   2. Administer iodine preoperatively as ordered.
B. Surgery may be necessary (thyroidectomy).
✦ C. Monitor for thyroid storm—teach child and parents signs of and management.
D. Support child and family—discharge teaching.

PITUITARY GLAND DISORDERS

Hypopituitarism (Growth Hormone Deficiency)

Definition: Hyposecretion of growth hormone (growth hormone deficiency—GHD) by the anterior pituitary. Growth is symmetrical but decreased. Most causes are idiopathic, but may be related to previous trauma to pituitary area (infection, tumor, radiation therapy).

Assessment

✦ A. Assess for retarded linear physical growth with normal weight; review family history.
✦ B. Assess for delay of body-aging processes, delay in appearance of permanent teeth, delayed sexual development.

C. May have premature aging.
D. Examine pale, dry, smooth skin; thin hair.
E. Assess for poor development of secondary sex characteristics and external genitalia.
F. Assess for slow intellectual development.

Implementation

✦ A. Assist with diagnostic studies (x-rays, blood tests, CT scan, MRI) and support child and family.
B. Monitor administration of human growth hormone (HGH) injections; if the imbalance is diagnosed and treated in early stage, 80 percent of children respond to growth hormone and increase their growth.
C. Monitor response to medication; plotting growth chart and evaluating development of secondary sex characteristics.
D. Support family and refer to social services if condition continues.
E. Support and teaching to client and family (most children responding to HGH will reach adult height but puberty may be delayed). Teach families to give injections, monitor for complications.

Pituitary Hyperfunction

Definition: Hypersecretion of growth hormone by the anterior pituitary (termed *acromegaly* if occurring after epiphyseal plates close), which occurs in childhood prior to closure of the epiphyses of the long bones.

Assessment

✦ A. Evaluate growth trends—patterns of height and weight overgrowth. Assess for symmetrical overgrowth of the long bones, increased development of muscles and viscera.
✦ B. Assess for increased height in early adulthood (may reach height of 8 feet or more).
C. Evaluate deterioration of mental and physical processes, which may occur in early adulthood if condition untreated.
D. Early diagnosis and intervention is essential.

Implementation

A. Care for client as irradiation or surgical intervention of pituitary program is instituted.
B. Administer care for hypophysectomy.
C. Provide emotional support to child and family.

Phenylketonuria (PKU)

✦ *Definition:* An inborn error of metabolism, inheritance is via autosomal recessive transmission with an absence of the enzyme converting phenylalanine to tyrosine. Byproducts accumulate and are toxic to the CNS. Phenylalanine is present in almost all foods.

Assessment

✦ A. Neonatal screening done on all newborns (Guthrie blood test) before leaving hospital.
1. Phenylalanine levels greater than 4 mg/dL along with serum tyrosine level 3 mg/dL confirms diagnosis.
2. Questionable results may be rescreened or child is given phenylalanine challenge.
B. Infant/child generally is fair skinned, with light hair and eyes (decreased melanin production from inability to generate melanin precursor, tyrosine).

Implementation

✦ A. Treatment is dietary, restricting phenylalanine intake to 20–30 mg/kg body weight.
1. Keep phenylalanine serum levels 2–8 mg/dL.
2. Use Lofenalac formula for infants and later.
3. Monitor serum phenylalanine; significant brain damage occurs when levels are 10–15 mg/dL.
B. Family and child need comprehensive multidisciplinary teaching program about diet and nutrition.

Diabetes Mellitus

Definition: A total or partial deficiency of insulin. The most common childhood endocrine disorder, incidence peaks in adolescence. (*See* Diabetes in Chapter 8, Endocrine section.)

Characteristics

A. Until the 1990s, more than 95 percent of children with diabetes had Type 1, usually from genetic predispositions and environmental triggers.
1. The number of children, especially adolescents, with Type 2 diabetes has increased dramatically.
2. Between 10 and 50 percent of newly diagnosed children with diabetes have Type 2.
B. Rates are highest in Native Americans, blacks and Hispanics.
C. Family history and obesity are major contributors.

Classification

A. Type 1. An absolute deficiency of insulin and clients are insulin dependent. Often diagnosed in early childhood or adolescence. Requires replacement of insulin.
B. Type 2. The body fails to use insulin properly and may also have deficient insulin levels. Type 2 diabetes has increased dramatically in children.

Assessment

A. Type 1. Obvious symptoms develop quickly in Type 1, usually over 2–3 weeks or less.
1. High blood sugar levels cause the child to urinate excessively, causing an increase in thirst and desire to consume fluids.

2. Some become dehydrated, resulting in weakness, lethargy, and tachycardia.
3. Diabetic ketoacidosis occurs at onset of the disease and is diagnosed in about one-third of children with Type 1 diabetes.
a. Ketoacidosis causes nausea, vomiting, fatigue, and abdominal pain.
b. Acetone-smelling breath, Kussmaul respirations, headaches, and changes in LOC may be present; in extreme cases, condition progresses to coma or death.
B. Type 2. Symptoms are milder in children with Type 2 diabetes, than those with Type 1 and develop more slowly—over weeks or even a few months.
1. Parents may notice a mild or moderate increase in child's thirst and urination or only vague symptoms, such as fatigue.
2. Usually children with Type 2 diabetes do not develop ketoacidosis or severe dehydration.
C. As with adults; random blood glucose levels > 200 mg/dL or fasting glucose level > 130 mg/dL.
D. Clinical signs: polyphagia, polyuria, polydipsia, weight loss, enuresis, decreased attention span, glycosuria and ketonuria.

Implementation

A. When Type 1 diabetes is initially diagnosed, children are usually hospitalized, and those with diabetic ketoacidosis are usually managed in a PICU and given fluids (to treat dehydration) and insulin (often intravenously) for a brief time.
1. Those without ketoacidosis typically receive two or more daily injections of insulin or continuously by a small infusion pump.
2. Frequent blood glucose monitoring is necessary.
B. Children with Type 2 diabetes do not usually need to receive treatment in the hospital.
1. They do require treatment with drugs to lower blood sugar levels (antihyperglycemic drugs), which are taken by mouth.
2. Drugs used for adults with Type 2 diabetes are also used in children; some of the side effects (diarrhea) cause more problems in children.
3. Occasionally some children with Type 2 diabetes need insulin.
4. Children who lose weight, improve their diet, and exercise regularly can be tapered off drugs.
C. Nutritional management and education are important for all children with diabetes.
1. Parents and older children are taught how to gauge carbohydrate content of food and adjust what children eat to maintain a consistent daily intake of carbohydrates.
2. Children of all ages may find it difficult to consistently follow a properly balanced meal plan

(consumed at regular intervals) and avoid high-sugar snacks.

D. Infants and preschool-aged children are difficult to manage because of the need to support growth and avoid hypoglycemia.

E. Adolescents may have particular problems controlling glucose levels.

  ✦ 1. Hormonal changes during puberty affect how the body responds to insulin, and higher doses are usually required.

    2. Adolescent lifestyle: peer pressure, increased activities, erratic schedules, body image, or eating disorders may interfere with prescribed treatment regimen, especially meal plan compliance.

3. Alcohol, cigarettes, and illicit drug use—experimentation with these substances may cause adolescents to neglect their treatment regimen.

4. Conflicts with parents and other authority figures impact compliance and interfere with management.

5. Adolescents need adults to recognize issues and give them the opportunity to discuss problems with a healthcare practitioner and participate in a group setting with other adolescent diabetics.

    a. The focus should remain on keeping their blood sugar levels under control.

    b. Adolescents also need to check their blood sugar levels frequently.

PEDIATRIC ONCOLOGY

The signs and symptoms of pediatric malignancy may be subtle and not easily recognized. In addition, the causal factors associated with cancer in children are not clearly defined. Current research supports the theory of a genetic cause, allowing the uncontrolled proliferation of abnormal cells from previously normal ones. Current treatment focuses on chemotherapy and radiation therapy; combinations of the two; and surgical intervention. The specialty area of pediatric oncology is becoming more prominent as the incidence increases and the etiology remains somewhat a mystery.

TREATMENT MODALITIES

Chemotherapy

✦ **Characteristics**

A. Chemotherapeutic agents work on rapidly dividing cells.
B. Tumor's location and cell type affect choice of drugs.
C. Most antineoplastic drugs are metabolized in the liver and excreted by the kidneys so they must be adequately functioning to prevent toxicity.

Assessment

A. Assess if more than one chemotherapeutic agent is being administered.
B. Identify potential side effects of medications (specific to medications used).
   1. GI disturbance.
   2. Loss of hair.
   3. Bone marrow suppression.
C. Assess for fluid and electrolyte imbalances associated with drug therapy.
D. Assess for adequate urine output.
E. Monitor laboratory values.
F. Assess oral cavity for irritation and bleeding gums.

✦ **Implementation**

A. Establish baseline data.
   1. Nutritional status.
   2. Oral condition.
   3. Skin condition.
   4. Degree of mobility.
   5. Psychological status.
   6. Neurological condition.
B. Observe for side effects of cell breakdown.

✦ **CARDINAL SYMPTOMS OF MALIGNANCY**

- Unusual mass or swelling.
- Unexplained paleness, weakness.
- Sudden tendency to bruise.
- Persistent, localized pain or limp.
- Prolonged, unexplained fever.
- Frequent headaches, often with vomiting.
- Sudden eye or vision changes.
- Excessive, rapid weight loss.

✦ 1. Signs of acute tumor lysis syndrome (ATLS): tumor degradation rapidly releases intracellular components causing rapid rise in uric acid, phosphate, and potassium. Kidneys are unable to clear substances quickly enough and renal failure may develop. Observe for
   a. Rising serum potassium, phosphates, BUN and creatinine.
   b. Serum calcium may fall.
   c. Anticipate initiation of dialysis (peritoneal, or hemodialysis, continuous venovenous hemofiltration).
✦ 2. Stone formation in urinary tract, cystitis.
C. Maintain chemotherapy flow sheet, per institutional protocols.
D. Observe for side effects on rapidly dividing cells.
   ✦ 1. Gastrointestinal mucosa: diarrhea, nausea, vomiting.
      a. Administer antiemetics.
      b. Provide mouth care with normal saline every 4 hours. Do not use toothbrush or glycerin.
      c. Administer anesthetic spray to mouth prior to meals.
      d. Provide frequent cold, high-calorie beverages.
   2. Hair follicles: loss of hair.
      a. Prepare client for loss (i.e., suggest wig, hats, scarves).
      b. Reassure client that hair will begin to grow back 6–8 weeks after chemotherapy ends.
✦ E. Monitor administration of common drugs according to protocol.
   ✦ 1. Corticosteroids: prednisone used most frequently.
      a. Monitor side effects, which may include ravenous appetite, change in fat distribution, retention of fluid, hirsutism, occasional hypertension, growth disturbances, and psychological disturbance.
      b. Monitor serum blood sugar levels.
      c. Monitor tapering of medication if prolonged use.

✦ 2. Mercaptopurine (6MP): interrupts the synthesis of purines essential to the structure and function of nucleic acids.
   a. Monitor side effects: anorexia, dermatitis, stomatitis; very little toxicity in children but the kidneys must excrete increased amount of uric acid—may be hepatotoxic.
   b. Observe kidney function and possible increase in fluid intake.
✦ 3. Methotrexate: folic acid antagonist (antimetabolite) that suppresses the growth of abnormal cells enough to permit regeneration of normal cells.
   a. Monitor side effects: ulceration of oral mucosa and nausea, vomiting, diarrhea, and abdominal pain.
   b. Toxic effects: hepatitis, nephropathy, pneumonitis, osteoporosis.
   c. Observe for ulcerations. Discontinue drug temporarily at the appearance of ulcers.
   d. Observe renal function (e.g., drug is excreted through kidneys).
   e. High dose methotrexate often followed with citrovorum rescue.
✦ 4. Cyclophosphamide, Ifosfamide: alkylating agent that suppresses cellular proliferation; has greater effect on abnormal than normal cells.
   a. Monitor side effects: hemorrhagic cystitis, severe immunosuppression.
   b. Provide large quantities of fluids preceding and immediately following drug administration to help prevent side effects (usually three times normal maintenance).
✦ 5. Vincristine: alkylating agent used to rapidly induce remissions.
   a. Monitor side effects: insomnia, severe constipation and peripheral neuritis or weaknesses, SIADH.
   b. Once disease is in remission, maintain client on another less toxic drug as ordered.
F. Observe for tumor mass effects.
   1. Leukostasis (peripheral WBC > 100,000).
      a. High number blast cells causes capillary obstruction, microinfarction, and end-organ dysfunction (primary lungs and brain).
      b. Thorough and frequent CNS and respiratory assessment necessary.
   2. Superior vena cava syndrome (obstruction to venous return from upper body due to tumor or enlarged lymph nodes).
      a. Assess swelling or discoloration of face, tachypnea, wheezing, lethargy, headache or visual disturbances.
      b. Assist with diagnostic procedures: x-ray, CT scan, MRI.

   c. Maintain patent airway, support ventilation and oxygenation, CNS status and cardiac output until tumor can be reduced.
   3. Spinal cord compression—arising from primary tumor or metastases.
      a. Assess motor weakness, back pain, sensory loss, respiratory compromise (high lesion).
      b. Assist with diagnosis (usually MRI).
      c. Provide pain relief, measures to assist with bowel or bladder dysfunction, ROM if motor impairment.

Radiation

Characteristics

A. Radiation affects all cells but is particularly lethal to rapidly developing cells.
B. Radiation is often utilized in conjunction with chemotherapy and surgery, or as primary therapy.
C. Radiation may be used to eradicate or shrink tumors or to relieve pressure.
D. Total body irradiation used in preparation for bone marrow transplant.
E. Side effects usually dependent on irradiated area.

Assessment

A. Assess for easy fatigability.
B. Assess fluid and electrolyte imbalances due to vomiting, diarrhea, and urinary frequency associated with radiation therapy.
C. Monitor hemoglobin and hematocrit for anemia.
D. Assess skin condition in radiated area.
E. Assess for dental caries, gum disease, and ulcerations.
F. Assess condition of hair.

Implementation

A. Treat radiation sickness.
   1. Monitor symptoms: nausea, vomiting, malaise.
   2. Offer frequent high-calorie feedings (milkshakes with extra protein and vitamins).
   3. Make food trays attractive and palatable.
B. Observe side effects of cell breakdown: signs of ATLS and renal compromise, rising potassium, phosphate, creatinine, and BUN; accumulation of uric acid; and stone formation in urinary tract.
C. Treat side effects of cell breakdown.
   1. Increase fluid intake if adequate renal function.
   2. Monitor intake and output.
D. Treat skin breakdown.
   1. Check client regularly for any redness or irritation at radiation site.
   2. Notify physician immediately.
   3. Apply lotion to area following termination of radiation therapy.

4. Avoid any irritation to area from clothing, soap, or weather extremes.
E. Treat bone marrow depression.
 1. Watch lab values carefully.
 2. Isolate client if WBC dangerously low.
 3. Avoid injections (low platelets), bruising.
 4. Administer antibiotics.
 5. Meticulous handwashing, limit contacts, keep those with any illness away from client.

Surgery

A. Goal is to remove all traces of the malignancy and restore normal functioning. May be palliative or curative (if tumor is encapsulated and localized—and detected early).
B. Current trend is toward more conservative excision (e.g., resections rather than complete amputations).
C. Surgery is generally combined with chemotherapy and/or radiation in treatment of many pediatric cancers.

✦ Biologic Response Modifiers (BRMs)

A. Change in reaction to tumor cells—most agents are monoclonal antibodies.
 1. Influence the immune response by affecting numerous cellular activities.
 2. Particularly useful in T cell suppression in anti-rejection therapy for transplant recipients (cyclosporine, OKT-3, etc.).
 3. Also used to deplete T cells to reduce graft versus host disease in bone marrow transplant.
 4. Some BMRs have direct antitumor effects.
 5. Major categories include interferons, interleukins, and colony-stimulating factors.
B. Method being tested in leukemia diagnosis; therapy is the center of much research.

✦ Bone Marrow Transplantation

A. Often in cancers that don't respond to conventional therapy, but is high-risk and expensive.
B. May be considered earlier in treatment in children with acute myeloblastic leukemia (AML).
C. Marrow may be retrieved from living relative or unrelated with histocompatibility.
D. High-dose chemotherapy and total-body irradiation are given first in attempt to destroy all malignant cells, and transplanted marrow should then produce normally functioning cells.
E. Post-transplant care involves prolonged stay in protected environment to monitor marrow function and protect from infection.

F. Most serious complication is graft-versus-host disease (GVHD).
G. Child and family require *extensive* multidisciplinary support throughout process.

MALIGNANT DISEASES

Leukemia

Definition: The most common childhood cancer. A potentially fatal malignant disease caused by the unrestricted proliferation of leukocytes and their precursors. Average life expectancy was 3–4 years in the 1940s, but new therapies have extended life expectancy and long-term disease-free survival rates. Types include acute lymphocytic leukemia, which is responsible for about 80 percent of all childhood cases, and chronic myelocytic leukemia, which affects young adults. Long-term survival in *all* types treated at major research centers is now around 80 percent, and a majority are cured. The annual incidence is around 4–5 per 100,000 in Caucasian children less than 15 years old and less in black children under age 15.

Assessment

A. Obtain complete history of symptoms, previous illnesses, cancers, or therapies.
B. Assess for early manifestations, usually vague, non-specific complaints.
 1. Bone and abdominal pain.
 2. Fever.
 3. Bruising, epistaxis.
 4. Lethargy, pallor, anorexia, or malaise.
 5. Lymph node enlargement.
 6. Night sweats.
 7. Lingering illness (usually a cold or "flu").
C. Assess for late manifestations.
 1. Oral and rectal ulcers.
 2. Hemorrhage.
 3. Infection, overwhelming sepsis.
 4. Increased intracranial pressure, ventricular enlargement.
 5. Invasion of bone, weakened periosteum.
 6. Muscle wasting, weight loss.

Treatment

A. Clinical course.
 1. Untreated: rapid deterioration and death.
 2. Treated: with chemotherapy, 90 percent of those treated experience at least an initial remission.
B. Initial remission usually occurs following the commencement of induction therapy, the chemotherapy lasting 4–6 weeks. The goal is complete eradication of leukemic cells.

C. Induction is followed by CNS prophylactic therapy and maintenance/intensification therapy.

✦ D. Drugs most commonly used for induction and maintenance of remissions in acute lymphocytic leukemia.
1. Corticosteroids.
2. L-asparaginase.
3. Doxorubicin.
4. Vincristine.
5. Daunorubicin.
6. Cytosine arabinoside.

E. Methotrexate, hydrocortisone, and cytarabine administered by intrathecal injection soon after start of remission to prevent central nervous system involvement in high-risk children or those with CNS involvement.

F. Induction therapies differ with AML and CML.

G. Maintenance therapy begins after induction is complete.

Implementation

A. Counsel parents, child, and siblings.
1. Prepare for diagnostic procedures (bone marrow aspiration, biopsy, LP, and MRI).
2. Provide support and education throughout therapy: reinforcement of medical information, preparation for procedures.
3. During periods of remission, encourage normal activity, support growth and development.
4. Provide support for occurrence of complications or recurrences.
5. Refer to parents' support group.
6. Provide for continuing follow-up of family.

✦ B. Prevent infection.
1. Meticulous hand hygiene in *all* contacts.
2. Avoid contact with communicable diseases.
3. Do not give regular immunizations while in treatment.
4. Provide oral hygiene and frequent peri-care.
5. Prevent and/or treat candida oral infections.
6. Change intravenous tubing daily, as institutional protocol; monitor IV site closely.
7. If WBC very low, reverse isolation.
8. Monitor fever, CBC, and vital signs closely for early signs of infection.

✦ C. Prevent hemorrhage.
1. Handle infants carefully.
2. Pad beds: head, feet, and sides.
3. Follow platelet count closely, other clotting studies.
4. Avoid all unnecessary intramuscular and intravenous injections.
5. Gentle tooth cleaning and oral care.
6. Monitor for GI bleeding; avoid rectal temps.

7. Platelet transfusions if actively bleeding.

✦ D. Promote nutrition.
1. Administer antiemetic 30 minutes before meals (ondansetron most effective) and as needed.
2. Use anesthetic mouthwash before meals.
3. Avoid toothbrushes, use soft swabs.
4. Offer cold liquids high in calories, frequently and in small amounts (popsicles, ice cream, milkshakes) or any food child will eat.

E. Monitor renal status.
1. Observe for hemorrhagic cystitis (related to cyclophosphamide).
2. Monitor for acute tubular disease.
3. Meticulous I&O daily weights.

F. Provide ongoing education and support as therapy progresses.
1. Management of complications.
2. Alopecia.
3. Mood changes.
4. Altered body image.

Wilms' Tumor (Nephroblastoma)

Definition: A cancerous unilateral tumor of the kidney. The most common type of renal cancer in children; peak age of occurrence is 3 years. Multimodal therapy can give 90 percent cure in localized tumors (stage I or II).

Assessment

A. Evaluate family history, previous symptoms and illnesses, usual voiding patterns.

✦ B. Carefully assess child's abdomen (*see* Implementation B).

C. Assess for presence of fever or abdominal pains.

D. Assist with diagnostic evaluation; ultrasound, CT scan, blood studies, urine evaluation, venogram, bone marrow, aspiration if metastases are suspected.

E. Evaluate abdominal girth, anemia, hypertension.

F. Assess for other congenital abnormalities of genitourinary system.

Implementation

✦ A. Avoid palpation of the tumor preoperatively. (Although tumor is generally well encapsulated, seeding is possible. If a mass is present, defer palpation of abdomen to physicians ONLY.)

B. Treatment is surgical removal of affected kidney and adrenal gland, combined with chemotherapy and possible radiation.
1. Chemotherapy is indicated for all stages of tumor, usually vincristine, dactinomycin, and doxorubicin, from 6–15 months.
2. Radiation may be added if tumor is large, not completely resectable or with metastasis or recurrence.

C. Provide appropriate nursing care aimed at routine post-abdominal surgery management, minimizing complications of chemotherapy and radiation therapy (as previously discussed).

D. Support growth and development of child, provide family support and appropriate referrals.

Hodgkin's Disease

✦ *Definition:* A malignancy of the lymph system characterized by painless enlargement of lymph nodes—large, primitive, reticulum-like, malignant cell. Prognosis is greatly improved due to recent staging and treatment protocols. The long-term survival rates are as high as 90 percent in early-stage disease; 65–75 percent in advanced stages.

Assessment

A. Assess age. Symptoms usually peak between 15 and 29 years of age.

B. Evaluate enlarged, painless lymph nodes (i.e., nodes are firm and movable).

C. Assess for frequent infections.

✦ D. Assess for stage of disease (CBC, liver function tests; UA, ESR; CT scan of chest, liver, and spleen; bone scans all useful in staging).
   1. Stage I: disease is restricted to single anatomic site or is localized in a group of lymph nodes; asymptomatic.
   2. Stage II(a): two or three adjacent lymph nodes in the area on the same side of the diaphragm are affected.
   3. Stage II(b): symptoms appear.
   4. Stage III: disease is widely disseminated into the lymph areas and one or more extralymphatic site (spleen, liver, bone marrow, or lungs).

Implementation

A. Provide symptomatic relief of the side effects of radiation and chemotherapy.
   ✦ 1. Radiation and chemotherapy used in combination is usual treatment of choice.
      a. Combination drugs commonly used: doxorubin, bleomifin, vinblastinone, decarbazine (ABVD) regimen.
      b. Extensive follow-up is mandatory.
   ✦ 2. Radiation is used for stages I, II, and III in an effort to eradicate the disease. May be used in involved areas only or to include adjacent nodes.

B. Counsel client and family.
   1. Enlist participation of client and family in treatment plan.
   2. Provide reinforcement of medical teaching, make appropriate multidisciplinary referrals.
   3. Encourage independence where possible.

C. Observe for pressure from enlargement of the lymph glands on vital organs, particularly for respiratory problems from the compression of the airway. Observe for other complications of therapy.

D. Appropriate discharge planning and teaching.

Brain Tumors

✦ *Definition:* The second most common childhood cancer. Two-thirds of brain tumors arise in the infratentorial region of the brain compared with those in adults, which are usually supratentorial. The most common types are cerebellar astrocytoma, medulloblastoma, and brain stem glioma.

Characteristics

A. Stereotactic surgery and procedures using lasers and brain mapping have greatly increased the numbers of tumors that can be resected. Many childhood brain tumors, however, are impossible to remove, or are so situated as to cause damage if completely removed.

B. Tumors occur most frequently in the 5–7 age group.

✦ C. Location: most tumors occur in the posterior fossa.

✦ D. Types most frequently seen in children:
   ✦ 1. Astrocytoma (most common pediatric brain tumor).
      a. Located in the cerebellum.
      b. Insidious onset and slowly progressive course.
      c. Surgical removal usually possible.
   ✦ 2. Medulloblastoma (about 15 percent of pediatric brain tumors).
      a. Located in the cerebellum.
      b. Highly malignant, fast growing.
      c. Prognosis poor.
   ✦ 3. Brain stem gliomas (about 15 percent of pediatric brain tumors).
      a. Surgical excision difficult. Poor long-term prognosis.
      b. Develops slowly with initial symptoms of cranial nerve palsies.
   4. Ependymoma.
      a. Usually, a ventricular blockage, which leads to signs of increased intracranial pressure.
      b. Treated with incomplete internal compression and radiation therapy.
   5. Neuroblastoma.
      a. A malignant, solid tumor primarily occurring in infants and young children.
      b. The tumor generally arises in the adrenal gland, but may originate in any part of the sympathetic chain.
      c. Growth is by extension and invasion; prognosis is guarded.

    d. Chemotherapy (vincristine and cyclophosphamide) can be successful, especially under 1 year of age.

Assessment

✦ A. Assess for increased intracranial pressure.
1. Vomiting without nausea, or projectile.
2. Headache (especially one that awakens from sleep).
3. Irritability/lethargy (changes in LOC).
4. Seizures.
B. Measure OFC in children under 4 years old.
✦ C. Neuromuscular changes (motor weakness, clumsiness, poor fine-motor control).
D. Vital sign disturbances.
E. Papilledema, cranial nerve neuropathy.

Implementation

A. Control and relieve symptoms.
✦ B. Institute seizure precautions.
C. Frequent, thorough neuro assessment—report any changes promptly.
✦ D. Administer postoperative care—prevent postoperative complications.
1. Maintain child flat in bed on unaffected side if infratentorial procedure. Elevate head of bed with supratentorial procedure.
2. Logroll for change of position.
3. Control fever with hypothermia mattress.
4. Frequently observe vital signs until stable, every 15–30 minutes, with neuro checks. Be alert to signs of CNS infection.
5. Reinforce a wet dressing with sterile gauze.
6. Notify physician of increased wetness of dressing and test for possible cerebral spinal fluid leakage.
7. Minimize increases in ICP: prevent vomiting, coughing, straining with stool, keep lights dim and noise to minimum.
8. Child may have drain in place postoperatively; handle as ordered and with aseptic technique.
✦ E. Surgery may be followed by chemotherapy and/or radiation therapy.
1. Radiation therapy is detrimental to brain growth and development in children less than 3 years old.
2. Chemotherapy may be used after surgery in children under age 3, and radiation postponed.
3. Many clinical trials are currently underway.
F. Educate and counsel family.
1. Counsel family and child through the stages of acceptance of the disease.
2. Instruct on the use of medications and dosage.
3. Alert family to signs of increased intracranial pressure.

4. Suggest the use of a wig, a hat, or a scarf to cover the child's shaved head.
5. Encourage return of the independence of the child.

BONE TUMORS

Osteogenic Sarcoma

✦ *Definition:* The most common malignant bone tumor in children, originating from osteoblasts (bone-forming cells). Occurs twice as frequently in boys as in girls, most occurring between 4 and 25 years of age. The usual location is in the metaphysis of long bones, near growth plates, especially in lower extremities.

Assessment

✦ A. Assess for tumor. Usually located at the end of the long bones (metaphysis). Most frequently seen at the distal end of the femur or the proximal end of the tibia or humerus. Other sites include the pelvis, jaw, or phalanges.
B. Assist with diagnostic procedures; CT scan, biopsy, bone scan.
✦ C. Assess for pain at site, swelling, and limitation of movement. Tumors are usually painless—pain indicative of metastasis from other cancer, or non-cancer trauma.
D. Evaluate lungs, kidneys, thyroid; common sites of metastasis.

Implementation

✦ A. Therapy is aimed at salvaging the limb whenever possible, limb-sparing tumor resection, followed by adjuvant irradiation and/or chemotherapy.
B. Provide postoperative care and pain relief appropriate to procedure.
C. Assist with irradiation and chemotherapy as needed.
✦ D. Administer and monitor frequently used chemotherapy.
1. Doxorubicin, bleomycin (antibiotics).
2. High-dose methotrexate (antimetabolite).
3. Cyclophosphamide, ifosfamide (alkylating agents).
4. Vincristin (plant alkaloid).
5. Cisplatin (synthetic agent).
E. Monitor and manage side effects of chemotherapy and irradiation.
F. Provide education and support to child and family. Involve child immediately with plan of care, therapeutic regimen, and decision making. Make appropriate referrals to community agencies, other healthcare professionals, and support groups. Educate child and family about long-term activities/prognosis and signs of treatment complications and side effects. Support growth and development.

Ewing's Sarcoma

+ *Definition:* A malignant tumor of the bone originating from myeloblasts with early metastases to lung, lymph nodes, and other bones. Occurs predominantly in individuals 4–25 years old.

Assessment

A. Assist in obtaining history of tumor development.
+ B. Palpate tumor. Usually located on the shaft of the long bones. Femur, tibia, and humerus are common sites. Lesions at distal ends of extremities have highest cure rate.
+ C. Assess for swelling and tenderness.
+ D. Check elevation in temperature, other signs of metastases (enlarged lymph nodes, cough, CNS symptoms).
E. Assess for side effects of therapy.

Implementation

A. Assist with diagnostic procedures; MRI, x-rays, CT scans, biopsy.
+ B. Treatment is generally limb-sparing surgery with adjuvant irradiation and/or chemotherapy.
C. Rarely, amputation may be necessary.
D. Encourage inclusion of child in discussions of treatment, options, risks, and prognosis.
E. Monitor for side effects of radiation.
+ F. Administer chemotherapy to treat tumor and prevent metastases.
  1. Doxorubicin, bleomycin.
  2. Methotrexate.
  3. Cyclophosphamide, ifosfamide.
  4. Vincristine.
  5. Cisplatin.
G. Treat the side effects of chemotherapy and radiation, relieve pain.
H. Listen to parents, child, and siblings as they work through denial, anger, acceptance; allow them their grieving process.
I. Promote age-appropriate activities and group discussions with peers.
J. Assist parents in avoiding overprotection, promoting normal growth and development, encouraging safe activities, interactions with friends and family.

SPECIAL TOPICS IN PEDIATRIC NURSING

Special topics in pediatric nursing include a broad category of subjects relevant to pediatrics but which do not fit in the system format. This section encompasses venereal diseases, the mentally retarded child, accidents, the battered child syndrome, and, finally, death and children.

THE CHILD WITH COGNITIVE IMPAIRMENT

General Concepts

✦ A. Cognitive impairment is synonymous with mental retardation; a condition defined as significantly below average intelligence that occurs in association with developmental delays (motor, language, and adaptive behavior). (*See* Table 13-10.)

B. Mental retardation may result from genetic, familial, birth-related factors, and acquired conditions.
1. Genetic conditions: inborn errors of metabolism, chromosomal abnormalities (Down syndrome).
2. Fetal or birth-related factors: fetal alcohol syndrome, maternal infections, asphyxia, prematurity, hyperbilirubinemia.
3. Familial factors: low parental intelligence or environmental deprivation.
4. Acquired conditions: CNS infections, lead poisoning, hydrocephalus (untreated), tumors or post-traumatic injury.

Caring for Children with Cognitive Impairment

✦ A. Treat the child according to developmental age rather than chronological age.

✦ B. Give the child as much stimulation and love as a child with normal cognitive abilities.

C. Behavioral modification therapy works well with children.

✦ D. Support parents' reaction to the birth of a child with cognitive impairment.
1. Birth presents a threat to the parents' marital relationship and family dynamics.
2. Stages of reactions.
   a. Denial: initial reaction of defense, which protects the parents from admitting that this child, this extension of themselves, is not normal.
   b. Self-awareness: recognition of difference between their child and other children.
   c. Recognition of problem: active search for information on their child's problem and for professional advice.

✦ E. Assess developmental delay—may be first indication of impairment (almost 75 percent have no physical abnormality).

F. Diagnosis is difficult and should be done by skilled team to ensure no child is mislabeled.

Down Syndrome

Etiology

✦ A. Caused by the presence of an extra chromosome, number 21.

B. Usually the result of nondisjunction in division of gametes. Incidence increases dramatically with increasing maternal age.

✦ Table 13-10. CLASSIFICATION OF COGNITIVE IMPAIRMENT			
Type I	**Type II**	**IQ**	**Description**
Mild	Educable	50–75	Can develop social and sensorimotor skills. Can be self-supporting with vocational skills.
Moderate	Trainable— delays in motor development	35–50–55	Can communicate. Minimal learning ability. Poor social interaction skills, but can be independent with supervision.
Severe	Minimally trainable—marked delay in motor development	20–35–40	Poor communicative, social, and sensorimotor skills. Needs supervision and protective environment. Can benefit from habit training.
Profound	Custodial	Below 20–25	Gross retardation. Minimal capacity to function. Requires custodial care.

Assessment

✦ A. Assess facial characteristics: almond-shaped eyes, round face, protruding tongue, flattened posterior and anterior surfaces of the skull, epicanthus, and flat nose.

✦ B. Assess musculoskeletal system: muscles are flaccid and joints are loose.

✦ C. Assess extremities: broad hands, abnormal palmar crease, in-curved fifth finger, first and second toe widely spaced.

D. Assess mental capacity: ranges from slightly incapacitated (educable) to severely retarded.

Implementation

A. Refer parents for genetic counseling.

B. Following discharge from hospital, provide follow-up for the family for counseling and child guidance.

C. Refer to the community health agency for follow-up.

D. Alert the parents to the child's increased susceptibility to infections and the need for extra precautions to prevent illness.

E. Assist the parents in developing a program for the child by identifying for them signs of neurological development in the child that indicates readiness for developmental tasks such as sitting, self-feeding, and crawling.

IMMUNIZATIONS

A. Refer to schedule (Appendix 13-2).

B. The main change to schedule format is the division of recommendation into two schedules.
1. One schedule for persons aged 0–6 years and another for persons aged 7–18 years.
2. Special populations are represented with bars.

C. The new rotavirus vaccine (Rota) is recommended in a three-dose schedule at ages 2, 4, and 6 months.
1. The first dose should be administered at ages 6 weeks through 12 weeks with subsequent doses administered at 4- to 10-week intervals.
2. Rotavirus vaccination should not be initiated for infants aged > 12 weeks and should not be administered after age 32 weeks.

D. The influenza vaccine is now recommended for all children aged 6–59 months.

E. Varicella vaccine recommendations are updated. The first dose should be administered at age 12–15 months, and a newly recommended second dose should be administered at age 4–6 years.

F. The new human papillomavirus vaccine (HPV) is recommended in a three-dose schedule, with the second and third doses administered at 2 and 6 months after the first dose.
1. Routine vaccination with HPV is recommended for females aged 11–12 years.

2. Vaccination series can be started in females as young as age 9 years.

3. Catch-up vaccination is recommended for females aged 13–26 years who have not been vaccinated previously or who have not completed the full vaccine series. Caution should be used as several deaths have been reported after the vaccination (2008).

G. Educating parents.
1. Need for immunizations.
2. Minimizing pain and psychological trauma—most well-child visits at 12 scheduled dates will still include at least 3 injections (or as many as 5, if no combination vaccines are used).
3. Studies have found no link between vaccines and autism (but this remains a controversial issue).
4. Parents do have the choice of requesting individual vaccines (thus MMR would be separated into three injections).
5. Thimerosal has been essentially eliminated from pediatric vaccines. Studies have not demonstrated any cognitive and behavioral problems in babies who might have received these thimerosal-containing vaccines in the past.
6. If doses of vaccines are switched to combination vaccines, no harm has yet been demonstrated.
7. Educate parents about possible side effects (fever, fussiness, local reaction) to immunizations—and management (acetaminophen/ibuprofen to manage fever and pain, massage and warm compresses to local reactions).

POISONING

Definition: Ingestion of toxic substances, which may result in death or severe illness.

Characteristics

✦ A. The most common age group affected is 2-year-olds because of their exploration of the environment through tasting.

✦ B. The major cause of poisoning is improper storage of toxic agents.
1. Legislation has mandated childproof tops on prescription drugs, but many children can still remove the tops.
2. Some new forms of drugs, such as transdermal patches or lozenges, are packaged so that they present a danger.

✦ C. Interventions for poisoning.
✦ 1. Identify the toxic substance and retrieve the poison and its container.

◆ 2. Consult local poison control telephone number and inform them of the toxic substance.

3. Reverse the effect of the poison.

◆ 4. Vomiting is contraindicated with some substances.

D. Poison control center should always be consulted before treatment is initiated.

E. As of 2008, syrup of ipecac is no longer recommended or available.

Types of Poisoning

◆ A. Acetaminophen poisoning (a substance commonly ingested by children).
1. Toxic at 150 mg/kg body weight.
2. Symptoms: diaphoresis; nausea and vomiting; lethargy; weakness; slow, weak pulse; depressed respirations; decreased urine; coma; liver failure.
3. Intervention: call poison control center and follow directions; lavage; antidote—acetylcysteine (Mucomyst) binds with acetaminophen.

◆ B. Salicylate poisoning.
1. Toxic dose is 4–7 gr/kg body weight.
2. Symptoms: hyperventilation (from severe acidosis); diaphoresis; nausea and vomiting; diarrhea; delirium; dizziness; confusion; bleeding.
3. Intervention: induce vomiting; lavage; activated charcoal; IV fluids; dialysis in severe cases; vitamin K if bleeding present.

◆ C. Chemical poisoning.
1. Toxic dose: any corrosive chemical is toxic.
2. Symptoms: respiratory problems, burns.
3. Interventions: avoid emesis, which could cause further damage; dilute with water if ordered; maintain patent airway; give steroids if ordered.

Lead Poisoning

◆ *Definition:* An environmental disease caused by the ingestion of lead-based materials, such as paint. Death results in 25 percent of the cases of lead encephalopathy, and there are many neurologic and intellectual residual problems in survivors.

Assessment

A. Standard blood levels indicating toxicity have been lowered from < 25 mg/dL to < 10 mg/dL. This level aids in early detection and treatment, before severe symptoms appear.

B. Assess age of child: usually 12–36 months old, usually those in age group of oral exploration.

◆ C. Assess gastrointestinal symptoms.
1. Unexplained, repeated vomiting; loss of weight.
2. Vague chronic abdominal pain.
3. Pallor, listlessness, fatigue due to anemia caused by interference with the biosynthesis of heme.

◆ D. Assess central nervous system symptoms.
1. Irritability.
2. Drowsiness.
3. Ataxia.
4. Convulsive seizures.

Implementation

◆ A. Institute preventive measures.
1. Inspect buildings 25 years old or older in which lead-based paint was used.
2. Change old lead pipes now corroded.
3. Cover areas painted with lead paint with plywood or linoleum.
4. Educate parents.

◆ B. Treat condition.
1. Acute: gastric lavage followed by magnesium sulfate.
◆ 2. Chronic: medications that aid in removal of lead are calcium disodium edetate (EDTA) and dimercaprol (BAL)—given IM only.
◆ 3. Method: IV preferable because IM injections are very painful.
   a. Prepare child for IV or IM procedures.
   b. Inject slowly.
   c. Rotate injection sites.
   ◆ d. With EDTA observe for signs of hypocalcemia: tetany and convulsions.
   e. Provide for seizure precautions.
   f. Record accurate intake and output to evaluate kidney response to chelating agents.

Treatment of Poisoning at Home

A. *See* Poisoning section, page 719.

B. At a well-child visit, give parent the telephone number of the local poison control center.

◆ C. Keep poison control telephone number immediately available.

◆ D. Instructions to the family.
1. When poisoning occurs, telephone the control number. Be sure to know the brand name of the poison and the approximate amount ingested.
2. Institute the program suggested by poison control.
3. If no telephone number is available, call a physician and take the child to the emergency room; bring the bottle of poison and have a neighbor or a friend drive.

E. Diagnostic information the physician will need.
1. What infant ingested.
2. The amount ingested.
3. Odor on breath.
4. Pupil changes.
5. Presence of abdominal pain, nausea, or vomiting.
6. Convulsions.

ACCIDENTAL INJURY

Definition: Unexpected events that lead to recognizable injury or metabolic changes.

General Categories of Injuries

A. Incidence: unintentional injuries are the leading cause of death from 1 to 24 years of age.
B. Each year, 20–25 percent of all children sustain an injury severe enough to require medical attention and missed school.
    1. For every childhood death from injury, there are 34 hospitalizations and 1000 ER visits.
    2. Lower socioeconomic status and male sex have higher incidence of accidental death.
C. The top three causes of death by age group (CDC statistics).
    1. 0–1 years.
        a. Developmental and genetic conditions that were present at birth.
        b. Sudden infant death syndrome (SIDS).
        c. All conditions associated with prematurity and low birth weight.
        d. Accidents (suffocation, MVA, drowning, and burns).
    2. 1–4 years.
        a. Accidents—MVA, drowning, fire/burns, suffocation, pedestrian, falls.
        b. Congenital abnormalities present at birth.
        c. Cancer.
        d. Homicide.
    3. 5–9 years.
        a. Accidents—MVA, fires/burns, drowning, suffocation, other land transport (bicycles, skateboards, etc.), pedestrian, firearms.
        b. Cancer.
        c. Congenital abnormalities present at birth.
        d. Homicide.
    4. 10–14 years.
        a. Accidents—MVA, drownings, fires/burns, other land transport, suffocation, poisoning, firearms.
        b. Cancer.
        c. Suicide.
        d. Homicide.
    5. 15–24 years.
        a. Accidents—MVA, poisonings, drowning, other land transport, falls, fires/burns, firearms.
        b. Homicide.
        c. Suicide.
        d. Cancer.

D. There are almost twice as many deaths in the first year of life than there are in the next 13 years total (due to congenital defects and SIDS).
    1. The death rate rises rapidly following puberty due to the large number of deadly accidents (MVAs), homicides, and suicides in the 15- to 24-year age group.
    2. The top three causes of death in teens should all be preventable.
    3. Other top causes of accidental death are drowning, fire, falls, and poisoning.

Accident Prevention

A. Control of agent when possible.
    ✦ 1. Education of parents as to what substances are hazardous and how to "safety-proof " a home.
    ✦ 2. Use of car seats and seat belts, use of bicycle helmets.
    3. Smoke detectors in home.
    4. Decrease temperature on hot water heater to 120°F.
    ✦ 5. Safe storage of poisons and prescriptions (with safety caps).
    6. Pools should have 5-foot-tall circumferencial fence, vigilant observation of children around water.
    7. Firearms kept unloaded and with trigger locks and locked up where child cannot obtain access.
B. Recognition of risk.
    1. Provide accident prevention education appropriate to the age of the child.
    2. For children with a history of accidents, take special care to make the environment safe.
    3. Encourage parents and siblings to take CPR course.
C. Control of the environment; during crisis periods in families, suggest help for child care and supervision.
D. Encourage families to make "disaster plans."

Car Restraints

A. Educate parents about car seats.
    1. After even a minor accident, replace car seat.
    2. Car seat faces rear until child is both 1 year old and weighs 20 pounds.
    3. At 40 pounds, use a booster seat and be sure seat belt is positioned correctly.
B. Do not place child in front of air bag because child could be thrown into air bag after braking.
C. All children under 12 are safest in back seat because of air bags.
D. Children should be in protected car or booster seats until adult belt fits them properly.

BEHAVIORAL AND MENTAL HEALTH PROBLEMS

Failure to Thrive

✦ *Definition:* A syndrome characterized by an infant's failure to grow and develop with or without characteristic posturing or "body language." Etiology is nonspecific. May be organic or nonorganic.

Assessment

✦ A. Assess history of infant: feeding problems, vomiting, sleep disturbance, irritability, sucking ability, aversion to formula, and irregularity in daily activities.

B. Assess general physical–physiological status to assist in ruling out organic cause of disorder.

✦ C. Assess normal nutritional intake to help determine if cause is related to deficient intake, malabsorption, or poor assimilation.
1. Assess number of calories, quality of calories, and feeding patterns.
2. Check weight daily and observe reaction to nutritional program.

D. Assess nature of mother–child relationship.
1. Relationship patterns.
2. Ability of mother to perceive infant's needs.

Implementation

✦ A. Priority—provide sufficient nutrients so that infant will grow.
1. Develop a structured feeding routine.
2. Weigh daily to assess weight gain.
3. Foster parent–infant attachment.

✦ B. Provide nurturing to infant.
1. Ensure a warm, loving environment through holding, cuddling, and physical contact.
2. Limit number of persons interacting with infant; primary nursing preferred.
3. Spend time talking to infant and building a trusting relationship.
4. Maintain as much eye-to-eye contact as possible.

C. Provide a positive, quiet, nonstimulating environment to promote psychosocial growth.

D. Assist parents to develop a positive relationship with infant.
1. Do not be judgmental in evaluating parent–infant relationship.
2. Support parent as she/he attempts to cope with situation.
3. Encourage parent to express feelings.
4. Include parent in plan of care.
5. Evaluate continuing parent–infant relationship.

E. Document feeding behaviors and evaluate infant progress.

F. Coordinate referral services for family when infant discharged.

Child Abuse

✦ *Definition:* Child maltreatment is any nonaccidental physical abuse resulting from an absence of reasonable standards of care by the parents or the child's caretaker.

Epidemiology

✦ A. Incidence.
1. An estimated 2.8 million incidents of child abuse or neglect occurred in 2000 in children age 3–17 years.
2. One study reports incidence of maltreatment as high as 42 per 1000. Children less than 1 year old accounted for 44 percent of child maltreatment fatalities.
✦ 3. Neglect is the most common form of maltreatment, according to CPS reports (34 percent). Physical abuse occurred in 28 percent of reported cases, 10 percent suffer from sexual abuse, and 8 percent from emotional abuse.
✦ 4. In the hospital emergency room it is estimated that 10 percent of the injuries seen in children under 5 are actually caused by parents or are the result of negligence.

B. *Shaken baby syndrome* has been documented in children up to five years old.
1. In 2000, 60 percent of perpetrators were female.
2. Children who have experienced neglect or abuse are at higher risk for smoking, drug abuse, obesity and some chronic illnesses as adults.

C. Victims.
✦ 1. Premature infants have a three times greater risk of becoming battered children than full-term infants.
2. Stepchildren have an increased risk.

D. Environment.
✦ 1. Abused child often has characteristics that make him or her demanding or "difficult."
✦ 2. Abuse usually occurs on the same day as a crisis or stressful event.
3. Abuse usually occurs in anger after the parent (or perpetrator) is provoked.

Clinical Indications of Abuse

A. History of the problem.
✦ 1. The cause given for the condition is implausible, e.g., punishment is inappropriate for the age of the child.
✦ 2. There are discrepancies in the history from neighbors or various members of the family.
✦ 3. There is a delay in seeking medical help for the child.

◆ B. Physical examination and indications for diagnosis.
   1. Bruises, welts, and scars in multiple stages of healing.
   2. Fingermark pattern of bruises.
   3. Bite, rope, or choke marks.
   4. Cigarette and/or hot water burns.
   5. Eye damage, subdural hematoma, failure to thrive, and/or intra-abdominal injuries.
   6. Radiographic findings of multiple bone injuries at different stages of healing.
   7. Passive, noncommunicative, and/or withdrawn child.

Characteristics of Perpetrators

A. Majority of perpetrators are parents, relatives; approximately only 2 percent are caregivers.
◆ B. Parents were usually abused as children.
◆ C. Abusers are unable to utilize outside help (neighbors, friends, or professionals) when angry at their child.
D. Abusers usually are under age 40 and two-thirds are female.
E. Spouse of abuser frequently does not know how to prevent the occurrence or recurrence of the abuse.
◆ F. Abusive parents frequently have unreasonable expectations of their children—they expect a baby to meet their needs, cannot cope with demands of infant (or protracted crying).
G. Personality characteristics.
   1. Dependent personality.
   2. Low self-esteem and poor self-image.
   3. Immature personality.
   4. Low impulse control and inability to handle feelings.

Legal Responsibility

◆ A. Both nurse and doctor are legally responsible to report a suspected battered child to the proper authorities.
B. The designated community authorities are responsible for determining placement of the abused child.
C. Support prevention educational programs.

◆ Attention Deficit–Hyperactivity Disorder (ADD/ADHD)

◆ *Definition:* A developmental disorder that involves a group of behavioral symptoms such as hyperactivity, hyperkinesis, or overactivity. Affects 3–10 percent of school-age children. Etiology is unclear but recent studies suggest mother's intake of essential fatty acids during pregnancy is below normal.

Assessment

◆ A. Identify child with this disorder by assessing presence of diagnostic criteria (modified from American Psychiatric Association *DSM-IV*). Behavior must be inconsistent with developmental level, persist for at least 6 months, and demonstrate at least six of the following behaviors for diagnosis of ADHD.
   ◆ 1. Inattention.
      a. Does not complete things, often loses things, is forgetful in daily activities.
      b. Fails to give close attention to details or makes careless mistakes.
      c. Demonstrates difficulty in concentrating.
      d. Easily distractible by external stimuli, has difficulty organizing tasks.
      e. Cannot stick to a play activity.
   ◆ 2. Impulsivity.
      a. Often acts before thinking.
      b. Moves rapidly from one activity to another.
      c. Cannot organize work effectively.
      d. Requires close supervision.
      e. Interrupts in class.
      f. Cannot wait to take turns; has difficulty in group activities.
   ◆ 3. Hyperactivity.
      a. Runs around, jumps, and climbs constantly, excessively.
      b. Cannot sit still or stay seated for very long, interrupts, blurts out answers in school, has difficulty waiting turn and staying in seat.
      c. Moves around during sleep.
      d. Seems to be always active, fidgets or squirms.
   4. Onset before 7 years of age.
   5. Duration of at least 6 months.
   6. Cause is not identified as schizophrenia, affective disorder, or mental retardation.
B. Observe for additional traits.
   1. Negativistic.
   2. Emotional lability.
   3. Easily frustrated.
   4. Nonlocalizing neurological signs, learning disabilities, and abnormal EEG may or may not be present.

Implementation

A. Coordinate treatment plan with physician, family and educational counselor.
   1. Behavioral therapy with medications has mixed results.
   2. Behavior therapy alone has lesser results.
◆ B. Provide safe environment with minimal stimulation.
   1. Decrease number of stimuli; reduce extraneous stimuli.
   2. Set limits on behavior.
   3. Structure activities.

4. Provide for energy outlets: allow large muscle movements.
5. Provide for quiet area and time.

C. Establish primary relationship, if possible, with short contact times.

D. May establish behavior modification program; encourage positive behavior. Assist to build self-esteem, which is usually low.

E. Assist client to establish own controls and behavior.

F. Coordinate diet: limit sugar, additives, and artificial colors.

G. Administer medication if ordered: Ritalin, a mild nervous-system stimulant, is controversial at present, especially in young children.
   1. Medications most widely used: melhyolphenidate or dextroamphetamine.
   2. Atomoxetine or antidepressants may also be tried.

Learning Disorders

Definition: Described as the inability to acquire, retain, or broadly use specific skills or information, which affects how a person understands, remembers and responds to new information.

Characteristics

A. Result from deficiencies in attention, memory, or reasoning and can cause difficulty in listening or paying attention, speaking, reading or writing, and in math performance.

B. Include disorders such as dyslexia, dysgraphia, dyscalculia, dyspraxia and information-processing disorders.

Assessment (Warning signs)

A. Delays in language development: children are unable to put sentences together by age 2½.

B. Speech difficulty: parents and others cannot understand what children say more than half of the time at age 3 years.

C. Coordination difficulty: children are unable to tie shoes, button, hop, and cut by around age 5.

D. Short attention span: between 3 and 5 years old, children are unable to sit still while being read a short story. (Attention span should increase with age during this period.)

E. Eye, ear, speech, and psychological evaluations are helpful; early diagnosis is critical.

Implementation

A. No evidence that special diets, vitamins or visual programs provide quick fixes.

B. Children need individualized approach, specific to identified learning disability, and help in developing lifelong strategies to accommodate the disorder.

Autism

Definition: A disorder where a young child cannot develop normal social relationships, has language delays or uses abnormal language, may fail to develop normal intelligence and engages in ritualistic or compulsive behavior. Also referred to as pervasive developmental disorder syndrome (PDDS).

Characteristics

A. Signs usually appear before age 3 years.

B. Previously occured in about 5 out of 10,000 children.

C. As of 2007, statistics show it is 1 out of 150 children.

Assessment

A. Abnormal development seen in language (about 50 percent may never speak). Echolalia or reverse pronouns, unusual pitch and rhythm are common, and children rarely are able to carry an interactive dialogue.

B. Social relationships abnormal.
   1. Infants avoid eye contact, do not cuddle, lack of attachment to parents, prefer to play alone rather than with other children; older children are unable to interpret expressions or moods of others.
   2. Behavior involves repetitive movements (such as hand flapping, rocking, or self-injury), excessive attachment to particular inanimate objects.

C. Majority have intellectual delays.
   1. Unpredictable performance on IQ tests.
   2. Some have ability to perform complex mental or musical skills, but are unable to use the skills in a socially productive or interactive manner.

D. Diagnosis: made by close observation and standardized tests. Metabolic, chromosomal or genetic abnormalities must be ruled out before diagnosis is made.

Implementation

A. Prognosis influenced by language skills at age 7, and those with severe intelligence deficits may require institutional care.

B. Behavioral modification and special education including physical, occupational, and speech therapy may be helpful.

C. Drug therapy ineffective for underlying disorder, but may help reduce ritualistic behaviors. Antipsychotics may alleviate self-injurious behavior.

D. Special diets, immunologic therapies and GI therapies are still unproven.

See Pervasive Development Disorders in Chapter 14, Psychiatric Nursing.

Asperger's Syndrome (Pervasive Developmental Disorder Not Otherwise Specified [PDD-NOS])

Definition: Children have impaired social interactions and repetitive behaviors similar to children with autism. Language skills and IQ are normal or above average.

Characteristics
A. Children tend to function at higher levels than children with autism, and may be able to function independently.
B. Psychotherapy may also be helpful.

Depression

Definition: Intense sadness, often following a recent loss or sad event, but persists and becomes out of proportion to the event.

Characteristics
A. May affect 1 to 2 percent of children and around 8 percent of adolescents, and familial tendencies are noted.
B. Physiological causes, such as hypothyroidism, must be investigated.
C. Other behavioral/psychiatric problems, such as schizophrenia, must also be ruled out.

D. History from parents and teachers, and structured questionnaires aid in diagnosis.
E. Risk factors.
  1. Stressful life events (death, divorce).
  2. Developmental conflict in families, reaction to traumatic or disturbing event.
  3. Substance abuse.
  4. Child abuse.
  5. Family history of depression.
  6. Unstable relationships with friends, unstable caregiving.
  7. Chronic illness.

Assessment
A. Signs include irritability, faltering school performance, relationship problems with friends and family, sleep disturbances (excessive sleeping or difficulty), concentration or memory problems, change in eating habits, preoccupation with death or suicidal ideation/threats.
B. Any talk of suicide should be taken seriously.

Implementation
A. Rule out physical causes, bipolar disorder, schizophrenia, or other psychiatric disorders.
B. Combination psychotherapy and antidepressant therapy is needed.
C. Use caution with SSRI medications as some "activation" of suicidal thoughts and efforts is reported.

DEATH AND CHILDREN

Assessment
A. Assess child's understanding of death.
  ✦ 1. Young child's concerns.
    a. Views death as temporary separation from parents, sometimes viewed synonymously with sleep.
    b. May express fear of pain and wish to avoid it.
    c. Child's awareness is lessened by physical symptoms if death comes suddenly.

d. Gradual terminal illness may simulate the adult process: depression, withdrawal, fearfulness and anxiety.

✦ 2. Older children's concerns.
   a. May identify death as a "person" to be avoided.
   b. May ask directly if they are going to die.
   c. Concerns center around fear of pain, fear of being left alone and leaving parents and friends.

3. Adolescent concerns.
   a. Recognize death as irreversible and inevitable.
   b. Often avoids talking about impending death and staff may enter into this "conspiracy of silence."
   c. Adolescents have more understanding of death than adults tend to realize.

B. Assess impact of death on child.
C. Assess parent's ability to cope with death of child.

Implementation

✦ A. Always elicit child's understanding of death before discussing it with him or her.

✦ B. Before discussing death with child, discuss it with child's parents.

C. Parental reactions include the continuum of grief process and stages of dying.
   1. Reactions depend on previous loss experience.
   2. Reactions also depend on relationship with the child and circumstances of illness or injury.
   3. Reactions depend on degree of parental guilt.

D. Assist parents in expressing their fears, concerns, and grief so that they may be more supportive of the child.

E. Assist parents in understanding siblings' possible reactions to a terminally ill child.
   1. Guilt: belief that they caused the problem or illness.
   2. Jealousy: desire for equal attention from parents.
   3. Anger: feelings of being left behind.

F. Enlist multidisciplinary support.

Sudden Infant Death Syndrome (SIDS)

✦ *Definition:* The sudden, unexplainable death of an infant during sleep.

Characteristics

A. SIDS was the third leading cause of death in infants in 2000.

✦ B. Peak incidence from 2–4 months of age. Less danger during first month; rare after 12 months.

✦ C. Higher incidence in winter, June and July, and low-income groups.

D. On autopsy, inflammation of upper respiratory tract is found, often pulmonary edema.

E. Maternal factors: SIDS more common in unwed mothers, younger mothers, multiparous mothers with shorter between-pregnancy intervals, cigarette-smoking mothers, and mothers who do not fully utilize healthcare facilities or use them later in pregnancy.

✦ F. Infant factors: SIDS more common in prematures and small-for-gestational-age infants; infant's growth after birth is slower than average.

G. Sleep: most deaths are unobserved; death during sleep is common although not universal.

H. Feeding: bottle-feeding more prevalent in SIDS, but breast-fed infants are not immune.

I. Familial recurrence: greater than normal population but only 1–2 percent risk. No evidence of genetic link.

J. Specificity: occurrence rate of SIDS parallels the rate for general infant mortality.

K. Etiology unknown and controversial. Current research into etiology includes carbon dioxide sensitivity, massive virus, allergic reaction, poor response to stimulus, deficiency of one or more nutrients, long QTC syndrome, use of pacifiers, gastroesophageal reflux, group B *streptococci* from mother.

Assessment

A. Assess age of infant and remaining epidemiologic findings.

B. Assess for prematurity/low-birth-weight infant.

C. Check for respiratory pauses, sleep apnea.

D. Check for gastroesophageal reflux/apnea associated with regurgitation after feeding, or tiring during feeding.

E. Assess for past history of oxygen administration.

F. Assess for history of allergic response.

Implementation

✦ A. Recent research suggests that there is a correlation between SIDS and infants sleeping on abdomen. Incidence of SIDS has reportedly decreased more than 40 percent since encouragement of "Back-to-Sleep" program in 1994. Teach mothers to place infant on side or back for sleep.

✦ B. Apneic episode discovered: infant responds when stimulated (near-miss SIDS). Instruct parents in care.
   1. Shake/stimulate infant. If no response, immediately begin rescue breathing and CPR.
   2. Take infant to physician or nearest emergency room.
      a. Record accurate history from parents: time of discovery of infant, color of infant, skin temperature, spontaneous respirations after stimulation.

    b.   Ask relevant questions: Was CPR begun? How long after? How long was it continued? Did infant respond? Did there appear to be regurgitation of formula when infant was discovered? When did infant last eat?

3.   Assist physician in a complete neurological, developmental and physical exam of infant, including lab work.

4.   Teach parents CPR.

5.   Instruct parents about care of a child on a home monitor.

6.   Give parents phone numbers for respite care and support groups.

7.   Suggest to parents that infant join sleep study program (polygraph monitoring of near-miss SIDS infants).

C.   Infant dies; upon autopsy, SIDS is diagnosed.

1.   Support parents through loss and grieving process. Reassure parents that they did everything right for the child. Emphasize blamelessness of parents and siblings.

2.   Inform parents of result of autopsy as soon as possible so grieving process may begin.

3.   Refer parents to National Foundation for SIDS, other local support groups.

4.   If other infants in home, suggest they be tested for possible sleep apnea.

◆ Appendix 13-1. DENTAL DEVELOPMENT

Part 1. DENTITION PRINCIPLES

A.   Age at eruption of deciduous teeth is variable. Generally lower central incisors erupt first at approximately 6–10 months, followed by upper central incisors between 8–12 months, then lower lateral incisors at 10–16 months and upper lateral incisors between 9–13 months.

B.   First molars: generally appear between 13–19 months (upper and lower)—somewhat earlier in males.

C.   Second molars usually erupt between 23–33 months, sometimes slightly earlier in males.

D.   Eruption of teeth often accompanied by drooling, irritability, biting, and decreased sucking, and sometimes low-grade temperature and sleep disturbances.

E.   Parents need reassurance and teaching. Cold objects (frozen teething rings), topical gels, or acetaminophen in proper doses may be helpful.

F.   Loss of deciduous teeth and eruption of permanent teeth is usually in the same order as eruption, usually starting at 6–7 years old.

G.   At age 6–7, the first permanent molars erupt.

H.   By age 11–12, children have 28 of 32 permanent teeth.

I.   Anticipatory guidance.
   1.   Regular brushing of deciduous teeth from eruption of first tooth.
   2.   Children up to 8–9 years old need help flossing.
   3.   Fluoride supplements may be given, considering fluoridation of water supply.
   4.   Regular visits to a dentist start early. Schedule varies depending on the child's general health and compliance with dental health practices.

Part 2. DENTAL DEVELOPMENT STAGES

Deciduous Teeth	Age at Eruption		Age at Shedding	
	Maxillary	Mandibular	Maxillary	Mandibular
Central incisors	6–8 months	5–7 months	7–8 years	6–7 years
Lateral incisors	8–11	7–10	8–9	7–8
Cuspids	16–20	16–20	11–12	9–11
First molars	10–16	10–16	10–11	10–12
Second molars	20–30	20–30	10–12	11–13

Permanent Teeth	Age at Eruption	
	Maxillary	Mandibular
Central incisors	7–8 years	6–7 years
Lateral incisors	8–9	7–8
Cuspids	11–12	9–11
First molars	6–7	6–7
Second molars	12–13	12–13
First premolars	10–11	10–11
Second premolars	10–12	11–13
Third molars	17–22	17–22

✦ Appendix 13-2. IMMUNIZATION SCHEDULES

Vaccines are listed under routinely recommended ages for administration.

Vaccine ▼ Age ▶	Birth	1 month	2 months	4 months	6 months	12 months	15 months	18 months	19–23 months	2–3 years	4–6 years
Hepatitis B	HepB	HepB			HepB						
Rotavirus			Rota	Rota	Rota						
Diphtheria, Tetanus, Pertussis			DTaP	DTaP	DTaP		DTaP				DTaP
Haemophilus influenzae type b			Hib	Hib	*Hib*	Hib					
Pneumococcal			PCV	PCV	PCV	PCV				PPV	
Inactivated Poliovirus			IPV	IPV	IPV						IPV
Influenza					Influenza (Yearly)						
Measles, Mumps, Rubella						MMR					MMR
Varicella						Varicella					Varicella
Hepatitis A						HepA (2 doses)				HepA Series	
Meningococcal										MCV4	

Legend: Range of recommended ages; Certain high-risk groups

FIGURE A-1. Recommended Immunization Schedule for Persons Aged 0–6 Years, 2008. (*Source:* CDC.)

Vaccine ▼ Age ▶	7–10 years	11–12 years	13–18 years
Diphtheria, Tetanus, Pertussis		Tdap	Tdap
Human Papillomavirus		HPV (3 doses)	HPV Series
Meningococcal	MCV4	MCV4	MCV4
Pneumococcal	PPV		
Influenza	Influenza (Yearly)		
Hepatitis A	HepA Series		
Hepatitis B	HepB Series		
Inactivated Poliovirus	IPV Series		
Measles, Mumps, Rubella	MMR Series		
Varicella	Varicella Series		

Legend: Range of recommended ages; Catch-up immunization; Certain high-risk groups

FIGURE A-2. Recommended Immunization Schedule for Persons Aged 7–18 Years, 2008. (*Source:* CDC.)

Immunizations

A. Refer to schedules above.
B. Providers need to adjust administration when combination vaccine (combine DTaP, IVP and Hep B) series are begun, but not completed.
C. Generally vaccines are interchangeable, but care must be taken to assure series is completed and record keeping is accurate.
D. Educating parents.
   1. Need for immunizations.
   2. Minimizing pain and psychological trauma—most well-child visits at 12 scheduled dates will still include at least 3 injections (or as many as 5, if no combination vaccines are used).

Continues

✦ Appendix 13-2. IMMUNIZATION SCHEDULES (*Continued*)

3. Independent studies have refuted claims that MMR causes autism.
4. Multiple immunizations given simultaneously do NOT overwhelm immune system—thought to use about 0.1% of immune system capacity.
5. If extra doses of vaccines are given or if switched to combination vaccines, no harm has been demonstrated.
6. Educate parents about possible side effects (fever, fussiness, local reaction) to immunizations—and management (acetaminophen/ibuprofen to manage fever and pain, massage and warm compresses to local reactions).

Approved by Advisory Committee on Immunization Practices (ACIP), the American Academy of Pediatrics (AAP), and the American Academy of Family Physicians (AAFP).

Note: These schedules are reviewed and subject to change every 6 months. To be up-to-date, check current schedules on CDC or ACIP Web site.

Appendix 13-3. DRUG ADMINISTRATION FOR CHILDREN

A. Clark's weight rule

$$\text{child's dose} = \frac{\text{child's weight in pounds}}{150} \times \text{adult dose}$$

Convert from kilograms to pounds: multiply by 2.2 (1 kg = 2.2 lb).

B. Majority of drugs are calculated on a per-kilogram (or BSA) basis.

C. Intravenous microdrip has 60 drops/mL. ALL pediatric IV therapy should be infused using reliable infusion pumps.

D. Conversion of administration units:
    1 tsp = 5 mL
    1 tbl = 15 mL
    1 mL = 16 minims
    1 grain = 60 mg
    1 gm = 1000 mg
    1 oz = 30 mL
    1 dram = 4 mL

✦ Appendix 13-4. FLUID REQUIREMENTS IN CHILDREN

Part 1. CALCULATION OF MAINTENANCE FLUID REQUIREMENTS IN CHILDREN

0–10 kg (body weight):	100 mL/kg/24 hr
11–20 kg:	1000 mL + 50 mL/kg/24 hr
21–40 kg:	1500 mL + 20 mL/kg/24 hr

Divide total fluid requirement by 24 to obtain hourly fluid rate.

Part 2. ORAL REHYDRATION THERAPY (ORT) FOR MILD–MODERATE DEHYDRATION

A. Fluids available: Pedialyte, Infalyte and Rehydrate.

B. Rehydration: 40–50 mL/kg of rehydration fluid over 4 hours (rehydration fluids should contain 75–90 mEq of sodium per liter).

C. Maintenance: Fluids should contain 40–60 mEq/L sodium. Examples: breastmilk, lactose-free formulas or half-strength lactose-containing fluids.

D. Approx. 10 mL/kg replacement with rehydrating solution should be used for each diarrheal stool after rehydration therapy is complete.

◆ **Appendix 13-5. PEDIATRIC INFECTIOUS AND COMMUNICABLE DISEASES**

Disease	Characteristics	Transmission	Nursing Care
Diphtheria	Local and systemic manifestations Malaise, fever, cough with stridor Toxin has affinity for renal, nervous, and cardiac tissue Adherent white or gray pharyngeal membrane Incubation: 2–6 days or longer	Spread by droplets from respiratory tract or carrier	Maintain strict isolation in hospitalized children Antitoxin and antibiotic therapy to kill toxin Strict bedrest, prevent exertion Liquid or soft diet Observe for myocarditis and neuritis Monitor carefully for respiratory depression or obstruction Suctioning, humidified oxygen, and emergency tracheotomy may be necessary Assure child is fully vaccinated to prevent
Erythema Infectiosum (Fifth Disease)	Rash in 3 stages: I—Facial Erythema ("slapped cheek" appearance) Lasts 1–4 days II—Symmetrically distributed maculopapular red spots on upper and lower extremities Progresses from proximal to distal locations, may last > 7 days III—Rash subsides but *can* reappear Caused by human parvovirus B19 (HPV) Incubation: usually 4–14 days, can be up to 21 days	Unknown Possibly respiratory secretions and/or blood	Standard precautions Isolation of hospitalized child only necessary if immunosuppressed or if in aplastic crisis May precipitate aplastic crisis in clients with chronic hemolytic disorders
Lyme Disease	First sign generally a ring-shaped rash (erythema migrans), fever, headache, red eyes, arthralgia, lymphadenopathy and general malaise Complications: meningitis, facial palsy, pericarditis Incubation: between 3–30 days	Caused by *Borrelia burgdorferi,* transmitted by infected ticks	Oral antibiotic administered (tetracycline) in early localized infection—educate parents Promote rest and fluid intake Anticipatory guidance to families in areas known to have ticks (bug repellant use, clothing covering legs)
Mumps	Acute viral disease, characterized by fever, swelling, and tenderness of one or more parotid glands Caused by paramyxovirus Potential complications including meningoencephalitis Complications: deafness, orchitis, arthritis, hepatitis Incubation: 14–21 days	Spread by droplet and direct and indirect contact with saliva of infected person Most infectious 48 hours prior to swelling	Prevent by vaccination (MMR) Isolate (respiratory precautions) in hospital Treat symptoms Warm or cool compresses to neck Encourage fluids and soft, bland food Fever and pain control Watch for symptoms of neurological involvement, fever, headache, vomiting, stiff neck

Continues

◆ Appendix 13-5. PEDIATRIC INFECTIOUS AND COMMUNICABLE DISEASES (*Continued*)

Disease	Characteristics	Transmission	Nursing Care
Pertussis (whooping cough)	Dry cough occurring in paroxysms Dyspnea and fever may be present Lymphocytosis Incubation: 5–21 days	Direct contact or droplet from infected person Infants at risk until DPT series is complete	Child is symptomatic: rest, keep warm, humidify air Bedrest until afebrile Antimicrobial therapy (erythromycin) Maintain nutritional status, encourage fluids Protect from secondary infections May be devastating to young infants who may not be fully immunized
Rubella (German measles)	Viral infection Slight fever, mid coryza, and headache Discrete pink-red maculopapules that last about 3 days Incubation: 14–21 days	Spread by direct and indirect contact with droplets Fetus may contract measles in utero if mother has the disease	Basically a benign disease unless contracted by pregnant female (highly associated with congenital anomalies in fetus) Symptomatic: bedrest until fever subsides Preventable by vaccine (MMR)
Rubeola (Measles)	Acute viral disease, characterized by conjunctivitis, bronchitis, Koplik's spots on buccal mucosa Dusky red and splotchy rash 3–4 days Usually photophobia Complications can be severe in respiratory tract, eye, ear, and nervous system Incubation: 10–12 days	Spread by droplet or direct contact	Symptomatic: bedrest until cough and fever subside; force fluids, dim lights in room; tepid baths and lotion to relieve itching Cool mist humidifier Observe for signs of neurological involvement Preventable by vaccine (MMR)
Scarlet Fever	Usually seen in children age 6–12 Manifested by sore throat, headache, abrupt, high fever, vomiting, then "beefy red" tonsils and "strawberry tongue." Sandpaper-like erythematous rash, spreads from chest and arms to abdomen, groin and buttocks Complications: sinusitis, arthritis, glomerulonephritis, retropharyngeal or peritonsillar abscess Incubation: 1–7 days	Caused by *Streptococcus pyogenes* (group A β-hemolytic *streptococci*—GAS) Transmitted by droplets, direct contact with infected person, or indirectly by contact with contaminated articles or food	Treat fever, sore throat Administer antibiotics (penicillin) Respiratory precautions until 24 hours of antibiotics completed Encourage fluids
Tetanus	Acute or gradual onset Muscle rigidity and spasms, headache, fever, and convulsions Death may result from aspiration, pneumonia, or exhaustion Incubation: 3–21 days	Organisms in soil Enter body through wound Not communicable through person-to-person contact	Toxins must be neutralized Bedrest during illness in quiet, darkened room Avoid stimulation, which can cause spasms Observe for complications of laryngospasm and respiratory failure Assure child is fully vaccinated to prevent
Varicella (Chickenpox)	Acute viral disease; onset is sudden with high fever; maculopapular rash and vesicular scabs in multiple stages of healing Incubation: 10–21 days	Spread by droplet or airborne secretions; scabs not infectious	Isolate Treat symptoms: fluids for fever, acetaminophen Prevent scratching Observe for signs of complications, which can be fatal in immuno-compromised children Preventable by varicella vaccine

◆ Appendix 13-6. NUTRITIONAL GUIDELINES FOR INFANTS AND CHILDREN

Nutrition for the Infant

A. Caloric requirements
1. Birth–6 months
2. Infants require 100–108 kcal/kg/day and 2.2 g/kg/day protein.

B. Fluids.
1. First six months—120–150 mL/kg/24 hours.
2. Requirements increase in hot weather.

C. Number of feedings per 24 hours.
1. First week—6 to 10 per day.
2. One week to one month—six to eight per day (4–5 oz/feeding).
3. One to three months—five to six per day (5–7 oz/feeding).
4. Three to six months—four to five per day (6–7 oz/feeding).
5. Six to twelve months—three per day (6–8 oz/feeding).

D. Vitamins.
1. Breast-fed infants—if mother's source adequate, infant adequate.
2. Formula-fed infants—vitamin supplements depend on type of formula and what vitamins are already included in it.
3. Mixing cereal with vitamin-C–containing juices will aid iron absorption.
4. Vitamin supplements: may be added at 3–6 mo if advised by healthcare provider.
5. Teaching.
   a. No cow or goat milk until 12 months old.
   b. Never prop bottles—feed infant in upright position.
   c. Don't put infant to bed with a bottle (development of dental caries).
   d. No cereal should be routinely added to bottles (unless prescribed for GERD).

E. Solid foods—introduce solid foods at four to six months of age.
1. Cereal—infants are least allergic to rice; fortified cereal is a good source of iron and should be given until 18 months.
2. Fruits and vegetables.
   a. Introduce new foods once a day in small amounts until the child becomes accustomed to them.
   b. Introduce only one new food per week.
   c. Bananas and applesauce are well tolerated.
   d. Orange juice is usually not well tolerated, initially. It can be introduced, diluted with water, when the child is six months old.
   e. Green and yellow vegetables can be introduced at about four months of age.

3. Eggs.
   a. Introduce yolks after child is six months old.
   b. Usually yolks are well tolerated, but sometimes there are allergic reactions to egg whites; introduction of whites should be delayed until 12 mo.
4. Meat.
   a. May be introduced at six months.
   b. Usually more palatable if mixed with fruits or vegetables.
5. Starchy foods.
   a. May be introduced during the second six months.
   b. Should not be given in place of green vegetables or fruit.
   c. Chief value is caloric.
   d. Zwieback and other crackers are good for the teething infant.
6. Whole milk should not be given until *after* 1 year of age.

F. Diarrhea—temporary.
1. Usually caused by viral infection or incorrect formula preparation.
2. Review feeding preparation and storage of formula with caretaker.
3. Usually corrected with oral rehydration therapy (ORT).
   a. Solution containing 75–90 mEq Na$^+$/L.
   b. Give 40–50 mL/kg over 4 hours.
   c. Reevaluate need for further therapy.
4. Avoid intake of fluids high in carbohydrates and osmolality and low in electrolytes.
5. BRAT (bananas, rice, applesauce and toast) diet is *NOT* recommended.

G. Constipation.
1. Increase fluid intake.
2. In child three months old or older, increase cereal, fruit, and vegetable intake.
3. On occasion, prune juice (half an ounce) may be given.

H. Avoid honey until at least 1 year old (risk of infantile botulism).

Nutrition for the Second Year

A. Rate of growth is slowing down; thus there is a decreased caloric need.
B. Self-selection children usually, over a period of several days, select a diet that is balanced.
1. Serve small amount of food so child can finish it.
2. Don't mix food on plate.
C. Child should be feeding himself or herself, with some assistance.

Continues

D. Assess food intake by associated findings.
   1. Weight, growth normal for age.
   2. Level of activity.
   3. Assess condition of skin, eyes, hair.
   4. Assess elimination problems.
   5. Assess emotional state: Is child happy and content, fussy or unhappy?
E. Avoid baby bottle syndrome or "sippy" cup: juice, formula or milk bottle at night leads to dental caries.

Nutrition for the Preschooler

A. Child begins to imitate family's likes and dislikes.
B. Finger foods are popular.
C. Single foods are preferable to a combination.
D. Counsel mothers—they express concerns about poor eating habits, which are common at this age.

Nutrition for the School-Age Child

A. Patterns of good eating habits are established at this time.
B. Avoid snacks–except fruits.
C. Appetite increases due to increased calorie needs for growth.
D. Child's appetite at a meal is influenced by the day's activity level.
E. Boys require more calories than girls.
F. Both boys and girls need more iron in prepuberty than in seven- to ten-year-old age group.
G. Tendency toward obesity at this age.
H. Every child needs daily exercise.

Adolescent Eating Patterns

A. Period of rapid growth and appetite increases.
B. Adolescents frequently gain weight easily and use fad diets.

C. Girls adapt themselves to fashionable weight goals, which may be unhealthy.
D. There is social eating of non-nutritious foods.
E. One form of rebellion against parents is to refuse to eat "healthy" foods.
F. Adolescent girls are often deficient in iron, calcium, vitamins C and A.
G. Important teaching for adolescents is that they must not just fill stomachs with food, but nutritious food necessary for growth.

Malnutrition Disorders

A. Kwashiorkor—caused by a lack of protein; frequently seen in ages one to three, when high protein intake is necessary.
B. Nutritional marasmus—a disease caused by a deficiency of food intake. It is a form of starvation.
C. Vitamin A deficiency—night blindness may progress to xerophthalmia and, finally, keratomalacia.
D. Vitamin C deficiency: scurvy—symptoms begin with muscle tenderness as walls of capillaries become fragile. Hemorrhage of vessels results.
E. Vitamin D deficiency: rickets—caused because vitamin D is necessary for adequate calcium absorption by the bones.
F. Thiamine deficiency: beriberi—primarily a disease of rice-eating people; symptoms include numbness in extremities and exhaustion.
G. Niacin deficiency: pellagra—symptoms include dermatitis, diarrhea, dementia, and, finally, death.
H. Iodine deficiency—leads to hyperplasia of the thyroid gland, or goiter.

PEDIATRIC NURSING REVIEW QUESTIONS

1. A 7-month-old infant is tentatively diagnosed with mental retardation. The parents have come into the hospital for further assessment and counseling. During the nursing assessment, the observation that will assist in diagnosing mental retardation is that the infant

   1. Is unable to sit unsupported for brief periods.
   2. Is able to approach a toy and grasp it.
   3. Frequently rolls from back to stomach.
   4. Can grasp a spoon and bring it to his mouth.

2. Following a child's treatment in the emergency room for poisoning, the nurse notes many bruises on the child and asks the mother (who is there with her boyfriend) how this happened. She replies that the child often falls down and hurts himself. The next action the nurse should take is to

   1. Report this suspected child abuse case to the authorities.
   2. Continue evaluating the circumstances.
   3. Ask the psychiatrist to talk with the mother.
   4. Ask the mother to bring her boyfriend into the room for a conference.

3. When two types of insulin are being administered, the intermediate-acting insulin is drawn into the syringe _____ the regular insulin. (Place the correct number in the blank space.)

   1. Before.
   2. After.

4. An infant was born with spina bifida and has remained on the pediatric unit for observation. The priority assessment would be to

   1. Measure head circumference daily.
   2. Monitor for contractures.
   3. Observe for signs of infection.
   4. Observe intake and output.

5. A 5-year-old child with suspected epiglottitis has just been admitted to the pediatric unit. His temperature is 102°F, he has difficulty swallowing, and he has inspiratory stridor. The most important immediate intervention is to

   1. Check the mouth for a gag reflex.
   2. Sit the child in an upright position.

3. Monitor vital signs.
4. Give the child sips of ice water.

6. A medication order for a child is for one fluid dram of liquid. The medication cup is measured in milliliters. The number of milliliters that will be administered is _____ mL.

7. The most accurate area to check the pulse of an infant is at the

   1. Carotid artery.
   2. Apex of the heart.
   3. Brachial artery.
   4. Temporal artery.

8. A female child, age 8, is admitted with a diagnosis of seizure disorder. A priority in protecting the child against injury during a seizure is to

   1. Restrain her arms so that she won't hit herself.
   2. Use a padded tongue blade so that she won't injure her tongue.
   3. Keep her on her back to facilitate breathing.
   4. Position her on her side to facilitate drainage.

9. A 6-month-old infant is admitted with a diagnosis of severe diarrhea. The priority nursing assessment is the

   1. Child's dehydration status.
   2. Number of the child's stools.
   3. Method of disposal of the stools.
   4. Electrolyte lab results.

10. A young child with severe diarrhea is to be fed via intravenous hyperalimentation. A complication related to the implanted catheter that the nurse will assess for is

    1. Plugging or dislodging of the catheter.
    2. Air embolism.
    3. Insertion in the superior vena cava.
    4. Generalized infection.

11. When providing diversional activities for a child in isolation, the nurse will remember that

    1. Any articles brought into the unit should be washable.
    2. These children are always on bedrest.

3. The room is usually darkened to protect the child's eyes.
4. Most children are satisfied with books.

12. A 15-year-old client has been admitted to the adolescent unit with scoliosis and will be having surgery for insertion of a Harrington rod. Considering the course of therapy with a Harrington rod insertion, the nurse will anticipate a problem with

   1. Identity crisis.
   2. Body image changes.
   3. Feelings of displacement.
   4. Loss of privacy.

13. Which of the following procedures is contraindicated for a child with infantile eczema?

   1. Have the child vaccinated to prevent childhood diseases.
   2. Cover the child's hands and feet with cotton materials.
   3. Apply open wet dressings or corn starch.
   4. Adhere strictly to an elimination diet.

14. Which one of the following therapeutic approaches would be appropriate in the nursing/medical management of a 12-year-old client with juvenile rheumatoid arthritis?

   1. Encourage prolonged periods of complete joint immobilization.
   2. Apply warm compresses and night splints to the affected joint.
   3. Discourage the child's active participation in his care in the initial phases of the disease.
   4. Allow unlimited salicylates as necessary for control of pain.

15. Considering a 17-month-old child's developmental level, the most effective technique to reestablish nutritional status after an immediate postoperative period would be

   1. Semisoft foods QID.
   2. Finger foods at frequent intervals.
   3. Regular diet put into a blender and given in liquid state.
   4. A high-roughage diet.

16. A 2-year-old toddler was diagnosed with iron-deficiency anemia. Which one of the following statements best describes the anemias of childhood?

   1. The clinical manifestations of anemia are directly related to the decrease in the oxygen-carrying capacity of the blood.

2. Significant deficiencies of all vitamins will result in reduced production of red blood cells.
3. A 2-year-old child with a hemoglobin of 5 g/100 mL will not manifest signs and symptoms of the disorder.
4. All anemias in childhood are potentially terminal.

17. A child is brought to the emergency room with a leg fracture involving the epiphyseal plate. Fractures of this type are serious in children because

   1. The blood supply to the bone is disrupted.
   2. Normal bone growth can be affected.
   3. Bone marrow can be lost through the fracture.
   4. Healing in this area is very difficult.

18. When determining if a child has Down syndrome characteristics, which of the following would be present? List all that apply _____ .

   1. Abnormal palmar creases.
   2. Protruding tongue.
   3. Low-set ears.
   4. Loose joints and flaccid muscles.
   5. Almond-shaped eyes.
   6. Low birth weight.

19. A special, controlled diet instituted relatively early after birth may prevent or limit mental retardation in children with the condition of

   1. Cretinism.
   2. Down syndrome.
   3. Phenylketonuria (PKU).
   4. Tay–Sachs disease.

20. A mother with a 4-month-old infant comes to the clinic for a well-baby examination. The nurse advises the mother to change the formula she is feeding the baby to one that contains iron. The nurse explains the reason for this is that

   1. Iron is required by the infant's eyes as they begin to focus and develop.
   2. The infant requires extra iron to grow.
   3. The infant's iron source from the mother is depleted.
   4. The infant requires more iron for the breakdown of bilirubin.

21. A 1-month-old child manifests all of the following signs and symptoms. Which of these is most suggestive of a complication of a central nervous system infection?

   1. Separation of cranial sutures.
   2. Depressed anterior fontanel.

3. Oliguria.

4. Photophobia.

22. During a routine physical examination, the following reflexes are noted in a 9-month-old child. Which of the following is an abnormal finding?

1. Parachute reflex.
2. Neck righting reflex.
3. Rooting and sucking reflex.
4. Moro reflex.

23. A 3-month-old is admitted to the hospital with a diagnosis of chalasia. He has had severe weight loss because of frequent vomiting. To minimize vomiting, the nurse would place the infant

1. In a prone position after feeding.
2. On his abdomen with his head to one side.
3. On his left side with his head elevated.
4. On his right side with his head elevated.

24. During the hospitalization of a 14-month-old toddler, his parents tried to spend time at his bedside. One day, however, after his parents left his room and returned home, he began screaming and throwing things out of his crib. In this situation, the most therapeutic nursing action is to

1. Turn on TV as a distractor.
2. Ignore the crying and wait until he wears himself out.
3. Stay in his room, talking and trying to comfort him.
4. Call his parents and ask them to return.

25. What anatomic condition must be present for an infant with complete transposition of the great vessels to survive at birth?

1. Coarctation of the aorta.
2. Large septal defect.
3. Pulmonic stenosis.
4. Mitral stenosis.

26. In addition to assessing for hemorrhage, the most important objective in client care following a tonsillectomy is prevention of

1. Coughing.
2. Swallowing blood.
3. Aspiration of mucus.
4. Airway constriction.

27. A mother calls the emergency hotline and asks how she should cope with a 7-year-old child just diagnosed with mumps. She has 3 other children at home and none has been vaccinated. What precautions should the nurse tell her about?

1. No precautions; just symptomatic care for the child.
2. Isolation precautions, especially respiratory.
3. Airborne precautions.
4. Indirect precautions.

28. A child is admitted to the pediatric unit with a diagnosis of dehydration. The child weighs 10 kg. Oral rehydration therapy is ordered, 40 mL/kg over 4 hours. The child will receive _____ milliliters per hour.

29. When assessing a child with a possible cardiac condition, the nurse would expect a child with a large patent ductus arteriosus to exhibit which of the following symptoms?

1. Often assuming a squatting position.
2. Becoming cyanotic on exertion.
3. Being acyanotic but having difficulty breathing after physical activity.
4. Having breathing difficulty and becoming cyanotic with slight activity.

30. A 4-week-old infant was admitted to the Infant Surgical Unit for correction of pyloric stenosis. In assessing the infant, which one of the following clinical manifestations is *not* consistent with the diagnosis of pyloric stenosis?

1. Palpable olive-size mass in the upper right quadrant.
2. Visible peristaltic waves passing left to right during and after feeding.
3. Severe projectile vomiting after each feeding.
4. Fluid overload, demonstrated by bulging fontanels, widely separated cranial sutures, and urine specific gravity of 1.002.

31. Which of the following clinical profiles present in a 2-week-old neonate would alert the nurse to assess for a possible renal disorder?

1. Low-set ears, periorbital edema, hypertension, palpable abdominal mass.
2. Tachycardia, urine specific gravity of 1.005, polyuria.
3. Hypotension, dyspnea, dependent edema.
4. Lethargy, depressed fontanels, mongolian spots.

32. The nurse is caring for a hospitalized toddler who was toilet trained at home. He wets his pants. The best response to this situation is to say

1. "It's okay; try not to wet your pants next time."

2. "That's okay; now let's get you cleaned up."
3. "I know you understand how to use the toilet; what happened?"
4. "Your mom told me you don't wet anymore; what's wrong?"

33. A client gave birth to a baby who weighed only 5 pounds and is considered premature. The infant will be on formula. One of the most important principles in providing nutrition is to use a

    1. Regular nipple with a large hole.
    2. Regular nipple.
    3. Premie nipple for bottle feeding.
    4. Pacifier between feedings.

34. Which of the following behaviors would a normal 18-month-old child be likely to exhibit during the first few hours of hospitalization?

    1. Crying loudly when the parents leave.
    2. Readily accepting the nurse caring for him.
    3. Showing considerable interest in new toys.
    4. Sitting quietly in the corner of the crib, showing little or no interest in his surroundings.

35. A 4-month-old infant has been spitting up his feedings and the mother asks for advice. What initial instructions will the nurse give to the mother?

    1. Carefully feed the infant the correct amount of formula for his age.
    2. Reduce the amount of formula given at one time.
    3. Feed the infant slowly with a small-holed nipple.
    4. Change the infant before feeding, but not after.

36. When obtaining an infant's respiratory rate, the nurse should count his respirations for 1 full minute because

    1. Young infants are abdominal breathers.
    2. Infants do not expand their lungs fully with each respiration.
    3. Activity will increase the respiratory rate.
    4. The rhythm of respiratory rate is irregular in infants.

37. An 8-year-old child with an acute asthma attack is admitted to the hospital. Epinephrine is administered. The nursing assessment of the child will probably reveal

    1. Noisy, hoarse inspirations.
    2. Wheezing on expiration.
    3. Labored abdominal breathing.
    4. Flail chest with inspiratory wheeze.

38. A 10-year-old child in respiratory difficulty is admitted to the emergency department and given a β-adrenergic drug with nebulized albuterol. The nurse observes that he is short of breath with circumoral cyanosis and sweating. The nursing action will be to

    1. Notify the physician immediately.
    2. Encourage the child to lie down and administer oxygen.
    3. Reassure the child that the medication will begin working soon.
    4. Encourage the child to sit upright, and reassure the child to reduce fear and stress.

39. A definitive diagnosis to determine if a child has bacterial meningitis is based on the

    1. Clinical manifestations and history of exposure.
    2. Blood culture.
    3. Lumbar puncture.
    4. Serum white blood cell count.

40. Once a child has had one poison ingestion, statistically he is nine times more likely to have another poisoning episode within the year. To prevent further poisoning incidents, the most important information the nurse should give to the child's mother is to

    1. Keep purses out of the child's reach.
    2. Never give medications to others in front of the child.
    3. Keep all cabinets locked at all times.
    4. Keep medicine only in high cupboards.

41. A 9-year-old child is hospitalized to undergo evaluation. Her history indicates that she has frequent severe respiratory infections. The tentative diagnosis is cystic fibrosis. The nurse anticipates that the child will have a test used in the diagnosis of cystic fibrosis called

    1. Sweat chloride test.
    2. Blood glucose analysis.
    3. Sputum culture.
    4. Stool analysis for fat content.

42. An infant warmer is used in the newborn nursery to ensure maintenance of adequate body temperature. The major safety factor involved with the use of the warmer is for the nurse to

    1. Ensure the warmer is on manual control.
    2. Tape the thermometer skin probe in place.
    3. Inspect the skin under the temperature probe at routine intervals.
    4. Adjust the temperature of the warmer each day to ensure it is set at 102°F.

43. The nurse makes a home visit and observes that one of the young children has red marks across his cheeks. How will the nurse continue to assess the situation?

    1. Ask the mother if the child has been slapped across the cheeks.
    2. Assume the child has a little rash and continue with the original purpose for the visit.
    3. Ask questions necessary to determine child abuse.
    4. Ask how long the facial erythema has been there and check the child's upper and lower extremities for a rash.

44. The nurse explains to the mother of a 1-year-old girl that the child is more likely to have otitis media than her 13-year-old brother because

    1. Her hands are often contaminated when she crawls on the floor.
    2. She is still "cutting" new teeth.
    3. The angle of the child's eustachian tube is straighter than her brother's.
    4. She is not old enough to have learned how to "clear" her nasal passages.

45. At the age of 18 months, a child returns to the hospital for a cleft palate repair. An important intervention to prepare the child for this experience is to

    1. Always allow her a choice.
    2. Never leave her with strangers.
    3. Give her affection and a feeling of security.
    4. Remind her of her previous hospital experience.

46. With a diagnosis of hemophilia B, part of the teaching plan for a child's parents will include treatment measures to control minor bleeding episodes. These will include

    1. Topical coagulants, cold packs, and constant pressure to affected areas.
    2. Elevation of the affected area, oral anticoagulants, and warm compresses.
    3. Gentian violet, ice packs, and pressure dressings.
    4. Bedrest, topical coagulants, and cold compresses.

47. A mother of a 3-month-old infant asks the nurse if her baby can eat solid food now so she can sleep through the night. The appropriate response is to say

    1. "Infants obtain all the nutrients they need from the formula and they really can't digest foods well at that early age."
    2. "Infants at age 3 months do not usually sleep through the night, so solid food probably will not help this problem."
    3. "It would be best to give the baby her bath at night to relax her and then she might sleep through the night."
    4. "It sounds like she's not getting enough food to satisfy her, so it is probably a good idea to start introducing solid food."

48. Evaluating a 1-month-old infant's social developmental skills, the nurse should observe that the infant

    1. Actively follows movements of familiar persons with her eyes.
    2. Responds to "No, No."
    3. Turns her head to a familiar noise.
    4. Discriminates between family and strangers.

49. As the nurse enters the room of a 7-year-old autistic child, she sees him banging his head against the wall. The first action is to

    1. Call the attendant to hold the child so that he cannot hurt himself.
    2. Go to him and immediately get between the child and the wall.
    3. Move slowly toward him talking softly but making sure to get his attention.
    4. Immediately call an attendant to put a helmet on the child.

50. While a 1-year-old child is hospitalized with bronchitis, she is receiving care for the respiratory condition. An appropriate toy for her would be a

    1. Book with pop-up pages.
    2. Set of blocks.
    3. Mobile hanging from the crib.
    4. Terry-cloth teddy bear.

PEDIATRIC NURSING

Answers with Rationale

1. (1) At 7 months, a child should be sitting with minimal support. Often, with retarded children, their flaccid muscles and loose joints prevent the attainment of simple developmental milestones. The ability to sit is one of the most important milestones in development.

   NP:A; CN:H; CL:A

2. (2) The nurse does not have enough data or information to report this as child abuse, so she should continue the assessment. When she has sufficient data to suspect child abuse, then the nurse will notify the designated authorities so that they may investigate the case fully. The nurse is legally responsible to report any suspected case of child abuse.

   NP:I; CN:H; CL:AN

3. The answer is (2), *after.* You would first draw the regular insulin into the syringe to prevent inadvertent injection of intermediate-acting insulin into the regular insulin bottle, which would inactivate its rapid action.

   NP:P; CN:S; CL:A

4. (1) While all of the assessments would be done, the most important is to measure head circumference daily. An increase in size would indicate a neurological condition developing (hydrocephalus is a frequent complication). Infection (3) might occur in the urinary tract; I&O (4) is also related to the possible urological complications. Contractures (2) could be prevented through proper positioning.

   NP:A; CN:PH; CL:A

5. (2) The most important intervention is to keep the child upright; the supine position could occlude the airway and cause respiratory arrest. The nurse would never check the gag reflex (1) because it could cause further spasms of the epiglottis. The child should be NPO and the hydration status frequently monitored. Vital signs (3) are important, but positioning to facilitate breathing takes precedence.

   NP:I; CN:PH; CL:A

6. The answer is 4 mL because 4 mL is equal to one dram of fluid. (Some textbooks use 5 cc equals 1 dram.)

   NP:P; CN:PH; CL:A

7. (2) The apical pulse at the apex of the heart, using a stethoscope, is the most reliable way to take a pulse in an infant. The brachial artery can be used in checking the pulse of an infant but is difficult to locate. The carotid arteries (1) are difficult to locate in an infant.

   NP:P; CN:PH; CL:C

8. (4) The major goal in protecting the seizing child against injury is to always maintain an adequate airway. Placing the child on her side assists in preventing aspiration. Current treatment of seizures no longer advocates the use of a padded tongue blade (2) during a seizure because of possible injury to teeth. Restraints (1) may also cause injury.

   NP:I; CN:S; CL:A

9. (1) All objectives are important, but assessing for dehydration level and acidosis is the most critical (priority) because this condition can be life-threatening.

   NP:A; CN:S; CL:AN

10. (1) If the catheter becomes plugged or dislodged, it is a complication. Air embolism can occur during a tube change, not during infusion. A local skin infection, not generalized, may occur.

    NP:A; CN:S; CL:A

11. (1) Things that go into the room will have to be disinfected when they are removed, so they should be

---

Coding for Questions/Answers Abbreviations: **Nursing Process: NP,** Assessment: A, Analysis: AN, Planning: P, Implementation: I, Evaluation: E; **Client Needs: CN,** Safe, Effective Care Environment: S, Health Promotion and Maintenance: H, Psychosocial Integrity: PS, Physiological Integrity: PH; **Clinical Area: CA,** Medical Nursing: M, Surgical Nursing: S, Maternal/Newborn Nursing: MA, Pediatric Nursing: P, Psychiatric Nursing: PS; **Cognitive Level: CL,** Knowledge: K, Comprehension: C, Application: A, Analysis: AN.

washable. The children are not always on bedrest (2), nor does the room necessarily have to be dark (3).

NP:P; CN:S; CL:C

12. (2) A change in body image is the most likely problem. Identity crisis occurs in adolescence, but will probably not be related to the surgery. The body casting that follows the rod insertion creates some privacy problems; however, a changed body image will cause more difficulty.

NP:AN; CN:PS; CL:A

13. (1) The vaccine can cause vaccinia, which can superimpose the pustular eruptions of the viral infection on the eczema. Eliminating foods that exacerbate the problem is helpful, but not using any specific diet (4). Either soaks with Burow's solution or normal saline is the treatment of choice.

NP:P; CN:H; CL:C

14. (2) Warm compresses will help relieve the pain, and night splints are important. During an exacerbation of this childhood disorder, hospitalization is usually required; however, affected joints should *not* be immobilized for extended periods of time (1) because residual effects (joint atrophy) will ensue. Active participation in care (3) should be encouraged in all stages of the disease. Unlimited salicylates (4) could be dangerous to the child.

NP:P; CN:PH; CL:A

15. (2) The developmental period is the autonomy stage. The child wants to do things for himself and will respond well to finger foods offered frequently. If the child will eat a variety of nutritious finger foods, the nutritional status will be reestablished more effectively.

NP:P; CN:PH; CL:A

16. (1) Clinical manifestations of fatigability, anorexia, weakness, and tachycardia are a result of vitamin B_{12} and folic acid deficiency. This results in reduced production of red blood cells, and a 2-year-old child will manifest symptoms of this disorder.

NP:AN; CN:PH; CL:K

17. (2) The epiphysis is the child's growth plate, and fractures here can cause growth disturbances. Bone marrow (3) is not affected, but healing (4) is generally rapid in children because they are still growing. The medical and surgical management of epiphyseal fractures is different from fractures of the bone shaft.

NP:AN; CN:PH; CL:C

18. (3) The answer is *1 2 4 5*. Although low-set ears are a sign of congenital defects, they are usually associated with a kidney problem. Low birth weight is not a characteristic of Down syndrome. The other characteristics will be present with Down syndrome.

NP:A; CN:H; CL:C

19. (3) A strictly controlled diet, eliminating protein because the infant cannot metabolize the amino acid phenylalanine, will prevent or limit mental retardation. A special formula is used for the infant, and a special diet must be followed until adulthood.

NP:P; CN:H; CL:A

20. (3) Between 3 and 5 months of age, the infant has used up the iron provided by the mother and requires further supplementation if bottle feeding.

NP:P; CN:PH; CL:A

21. (1) Meningitis is a common CNS infection of infancy and early childhood. Increased intracranial pressure, which can accompany meningitis, accounts for separation of the cranial sutures, bulging fontanels, and/or projectile vomiting. Oliguria (3) and photophobia (4) are not symptoms common to CNS infection.

NP:AN; CN:PH; CL:A

22. (4) The Moro reflex begins to fade at the third or fourth month. Thus, if found in a 9-month-old child, it would be abnormal. The remaining reflexes would be normal development.

NP:AN; CN:H; CL:C

23. (4) The greater curvature of the stomach is toward the left side, so the right side position affords less pressure. Elevation of the head would lessen the tendency to vomit.

NP:I; CN:PH; CL:A

24. (3) This will help promote a nurse–client relationship and provide the child with comfort. While the nurse cannot take the place of his parents, the nurse can be comforting. The more time the nurse is with the child, the more trust develops.

NP:I; CN:PS; CL:A

25. (2) Because complete transposition results in two closed blood systems, the child can survive only if a large septal defect is present.

NP:AN; CN:PH; CL:K

26. (4) Trauma to the airway may cause a severe inflammatory response resulting in blockage. Therefore, the goal is to prevent airway constriction. Application of an ice collar, maintaining a semi-Fowler's position, and encouraging fluids would be the treatment of choice.

    NP:P; CN:PH; CL:C

27. (2) The child should be isolated from the other children because mumps is spread by droplet, through direct and indirect contact via the respiratory tract as well as saliva. Options (3) and (4) are incomplete.

    NP:I; CN:S; CL:A

28. The answer is 100 mL/hour. Dehydration formula is usually 40–50 mL/kg over 4 hours. In this case, the child would receive 400 mL every 4 hours or 100 mL/hour.

    NP:AN; CN:S; CL:A

29. (3) PDA is acyanotic. If the ductus is large and much blood is shunted into the pulmonary circulation, there may be growth retardation and limitation of physical activity. Squatting (1) occurs with cyanotic disorders.

    NP:A; CN:PH; CL:C

30. (4) Pyloric stenosis presents in early infancy with projectile vomiting after feeding. Dehydration and electrolyte imbalances are possible complications if therapy is not performed; thus fluid overload is not a symptom.

    NP:A; CN:PH; CL:C

31. (1) Embryologically, the ears and kidneys are formed at the same time; therefore, if a child presents with low-set ears or any defect in the ears, renal disease is also suspected. In addition, certain syndromes are characterized by both renal and ear malformations. Periorbital edema is seen in neonates with renal and/or cardiac disease. A palpable abdominal mass in a neonate could indicate Wilms' tumor, a malignant tumor.

    NP:AN; CN:PH; CL:AN

32. (2) The nurse knows that children tend to regress when under the stress of hospitalization, so it is important not to make a judgment or imply that the child should know better. The best approach: Be matter-of-fact, not blaming.

    NP:I; CN:H; CL:A

33. (3) A regular nipple is too hard and will make it difficult for the infant to suck, even with a large hole in it, causing unnecessary fatigue. Use a premie soft nipple. A pacifier may be useful but does not take the place of a bottle with nipple.

    NP:P; CN:PH; CL:A

34. (1) When a toddler is hospitalized, he or she may suffer from separation anxiety syndrome. The behavior that would indicate the first stage, protest, would be loud crying or even throwing a tantrum when the parent leaves. Answer (4) would indicate the final stage, denial.

    NP:A; CN:PS; CL:C

35. (2) Regurgitation or spitting up can be caused by feeding too much formula at one time, or the need for more burping. It usually diminishes by the age of 5 or 6 months. Reducing the amount of each feeding may be sufficient to stop the problem. A nipple with a large opening, not a small one, can cause regurgitation, so changing the nipple can be tried next.

    NP:I; CN:H; CL:C

36. (4) Infants breathe in an irregular pattern with varying depth and rate so that a 1-minute count is appropriate. Answers (1), (2), and (3) are true statements, but not the correct answer.

    NP:P; CN:PH; CL:C

37. (2) The hallmark of asthma is wheezing. Wheezing is an expiratory sound. There is no vocal cord involvement so "hoarse" (1) is unlikely. Abdominal breathing (3) does not occur with asthma.

    NP:A; CN:PH; CL:A

38. (4) The child's immediate situation needs to be addressed before calling the physician. Nebulized albuterol and medication are usually effective immediately. Breathing is more effective in an upright position; reassuring the child will help to improve breathing.

    NP:I; CN:PH; CL:AN

39. (3) Examination of the cerebrospinal fluid is the only definitive way to verify bacterial meningitis.

    NP:AN; CN:PH; CL:K

40. (3) The other answers are also necessary information but keeping cabinets locked is critical. It is not enough to keep medicine only in high cupboards (4) because other products, such as cleaning materials, can be poison. The child's mother should also be given the telephone number of a poison control center.

    NP:I; CN:H; CL:A

41. (1) Children with cystic fibrosis produce abnormally high levels of sodium chloride in their sweat. Although answers (3) and (4) might be used during the diagnostic work up, they do not definitively diagnose the disease.

   NP:AN; CN:PH; CL:C

42. (3) The probe can cause irritation. If this occurs, the probe is placed in a different location. An infant's skin is very delicate and becomes irritated easily. The warmer should be on automatic, not manual. The thermometer is not taped in place and the temperature should not exceed 102°F.

   NP:P; CN:S; CL:A

43. (4) The correct assessment is to continue to focus on the rash to confirm or eliminate fifth disease or erythema infectiosum. Questions about child abuse are inappropriate initially (1 and 3). Not exploring further is also inappropriate (2) because if fifth disease is present, standard precautions should be implemented.

   NP:A; CN:S; CL:AN

44. (3) It is easier for infectious agents to travel from the nasopharyngeal area to the middle ear in younger than in older children because the eustachian tube is straighter when they are younger.

   NP:I; CN:H; CL:C

45. (3) A child needs extra assurance at this age. Children suffer separation anxiety and need to feel that someone is close to protect them.

   NP:I; CN:PS; CL:A

46. (1) Local measures that sometimes help control minor bleeding episodes are topical coagulants, constant pressure, and cold packs (which cause vasoconstriction) to the bleeding areas.

   NP:P; CN:PH; CL:C

47. (1) Studies have indicated that breast milk or formula will provide sufficient nutrition to infants up to 6 months and even 1 year. Many pediatricians begin introducing solid food at about 6 months of age, as infants cannot easily digest food before this time. Sleeping patterns for infants vary on an individual basis and the introduction of solid food does not ensure a full night's sleep.

   NP:I; CN:H; CL:A

48. (1) Actively following movements would occur at 1 month. Responding to "No" (2) and turning the head in response to a noise (3) begins at 4 months, and discrimination between family and strangers (4) appears at 5 months of age.

   NP:A; CN:H; CL:C

49. (3) It is crucial to establish a relationship with the child, so talking is important. It is also necessary to get the attention of autistic children, for without their attention, they continue the maladaptive behavior. The other three responses are nontherapeutic and may be perceived as threatening by the child, so it is better to move in slowly as a first action.

   NP:I; CN:S; CL:AN

50. (4) Because the child is in a mist tent, she will need a toy that can get wet, then dry out. A book (1) might not last in this misty environment. The blocks (2) would be difficult to play with and the mobile (3) is for a younger child.

   NP:P; CN:H; CL:A

Psychiatric Nursing 14

✦ The icon denotes content of special importance for NCLEX.

MENTAL STATUS ASSESSMENT

The mental assessment is completed throughout the physical assessment and history-taking time frame. It is not generally considered a separate entity. Mood, memory, orientation, and thought processes can be evaluated while obtaining the health history.

The purpose of a mental status assessment is to evaluate the present state of psychological functioning and to determine if there is an immediate risk of harm to self or others. It is not designed to make a diagnosis; rather, it should yield objective data that will contribute to the total picture of the client as he or she is functioning at the time the assessment is made. (*See* Table 14-1.)

The initial factors that the nurse must consider in completing a mental status assessment are to correctly identify the client, the reason for admission, record of previous mental illness, present complaint, any personal history that is relevant (living arrangements, role in family, interactional experience), family history if appropriate, significant others and available support systems, assets, and interests.

A spiritual assessment can be obtained as a part of the health history, although specific sociocultural beliefs may need to be ascertained separately. The purpose of a spiritual assessment is to facilitate the client adapting to the hospital environment and help the staff understand stressors the client may be experiencing as a result of belief systems.

The actual assessment process begins with an initial evaluation of the appropriateness of the client's behavior and orientation to reality. The assessment continues by noting any abnormal behavior and ascertaining the client's chief verbalized complaint. Finally, the evaluation determines if the client is in contact with reality enough to answer particular questions that will further assess the client's condition.

THE NURSE–CLIENT RELATIONSHIP

✦ *Definition:* The nurse–client relationship is a dynamic, therapeutic, professional relationship in which interaction occurs between two persons—the nurse, who possesses the skills, abilities, and resources to relieve another's discomfort, and the client, who is seeking assistance for alleviation of some existing problem or need.

Principles Underlying Relationship Therapy
A. The client's value as a unique individual with physical and psychosocial needs must be acknowledged.
B. The nurse's level of self-awareness, motivation, and needs enhances the development of the therapeutic relationship.

RATIONALE FOR COMPLETING A MENTAL STATUS ASSESSMENT
- To collect baseline data to aid in establishing the etiology, diagnosis, and prognosis.
- To evaluate the present state of psychological functioning.
- To evaluate changes in the individual's emotional, intellectual, motor, and perceptual responses.
- To determine the guidelines of the treatment plan.
- To ascertain if some seemingly psychopathological response is, in fact, a disorder of a sensory organ (i.e., a deaf person appearing hostile, depressed, or suspicious).
- To document altered mental status for legal records.

C. Some degree of emotional involvement is required, but objectivity on the part of the nurse must be maintained.
D. Appropriate limits must be set, and consistency must be maintained.
E. Empathic understanding is therapeutic; sympathy is nontherapeutic.
F. Honest, open, genuine, and respectful communication is basic to the therapeutic process.
G. Expression of feelings, within safe limits, should be encouraged.

✦ **Phases in Nurse–Client Relationship Therapy**

A. Initiation or orientation phase.
   1. Establish boundaries of relationship.
   2. Assess anxiety levels of self and client.
   3. Identify expectations/needs of client.
   4. Identify problems; set goals of the relationship.
   5. Responsibilities of client and nurse are defined.
   6. Confidentiality is stressed.
B. Continuation or active working phase.
   1. Promote attitude of acceptance of each other to maintain therapeutic relationship.
   2. Use specific therapeutic and problem-solving techniques to develop working relationship.
   3. Continually assess and evaluate problems.
   4. Focus on increasing client's independence and promoting the client's problem-solving skills.
   5. Maintain the goal of client's confronting and working through identified problems to facilitate change.
C. Termination phase.
   1. Plan for the conclusion of therapy early in the development of relationship.
   2. Maintain initially defined boundaries.
   3. Anticipate problems of termination.
      a. Client may become too dependent on the nurse. Encourage client to become independent.

◆ Table 14-1. MENTAL STATUS ASSESSMENT

Assessment	Normal	Abnormal
GENERAL APPEARANCE, MANNER, AND ATTITUDE		
Assess **physical appearance, sleep patterns**	General body characteristics, energy level, sleep patterns	Inappropriate physical appearance, high or low extremes of energy, poor sleep patterns
Note **grooming,** mode of dress, and **personal hygiene**	Grooming and dress appropriate to situation, client's age, and social circumstance Clean	Poor grooming Inappropriate or bizarre dress or combination of clothes Unclean
Note **posture**	Upright, straight, and appropriate	Slumped, tipped, or stooped Tremors
Note speed, pressure, pace, quantity, volume, and diction of **speech**	Moderated speed, volume, and quantity Appropriate diction	Accelerated or retarded speech and high quantity Poor or inappropriate diction
Note relevance, content, and organization of **responses**	Questions answered directly, accurately, and with relevance	Inappropriate responses, unorganized pattern of speech Tangential, circumstantial, or out-of-context replies
EXPRESSIVE ASPECTS OF BEHAVIOR		
Note **general motor activity**	Calm, ordered movement appropriate to situation	Overactive (e.g., restless, agitated, impulsive) Underactive (e.g., slow to initiate or execute actions)
Assess **purposeful movements** and **gestures**	Reasonably responsive with purposeful movements, appropriate gestures	Repetitious activities (e.g., rituals or compulsions) Command automation Parkinsonian movements
Assess style of **gait**		Ataxic, shuffling, off-balance gait
Mutism	Verbal response to questions	No verbal response
CONSCIOUSNESS		
Assess **level of consciousness**	Alert, attentive, and responsive Knowledgeable about time, place, and person	Disordered attention; distracted, cloudy consciousness Delirious Stuporous Disoriented in time, place, and person
THOUGHT PROCESSES AND PERCEPTION		
Assess **coherency, logic,** and **relevance** of thought processes by asking questions about personal history (e.g., "Where were you born?" "What kind of work do you do?")	Clear, understandable responses to questions Attentiveness	Disordered thought processes Autistic (detachment from reality when self-preoccupation and involvement are predominant) or dereistic (absorbed with self and withdrawn); abstract (absent-mindedness); concrete thinking (being definitive and specific rather than abstract)
Assess **reality orientation:** time, place, and person awareness	Orderly progression of thoughts based in reality Awareness of time, place, and person	Disorders of progression of thought: looseness, circumstantial, incoherent, irrelevant conversation, blocking (a gap or interruption in speech that is related to distracted or absent thoughts)

◆ Table 14-1. MENTAL STATUS ASSESSMENT (*Continued*)

Assessment	Normal	Abnormal
		Delusions of grandeur or persecution: neologisms (use of words whose meaning is known only to the client) Echolalia (automatic repeating of words or questions) Echopraxia (mimicking of behavior or actions) No awareness of day, time, place, or person
Assess **perceptions** and reactions to personal experiences by asking questions such as "How do you see yourself now that you are in the hospital?" "What do you think about when you're in a situation like this?"	Thoughtful, clear responses expressed with understanding of self	Altered, narrowed, or expanded perception Illusions (distorted perceptual experience where the individual misinterprets actual data from the environment) Depersonalization (feeling or subjective experience of separateness or alienation from oneself; the state in which the client cannot distinguish self from others)

THOUGHT CONTENT AND MENTAL TREND

Assessment	Normal	Abnormal
Ask questions to determine general themes that identify **degree of anxiety** (e.g., "How are you feeling right now?" "What kinds of things make you afraid?")	Mild or 1+ level of anxiety in which individual is alert, motivated, and attentive	Moderate to severe (2+ to 4+) levels of anxiety
Assess **ideation** and **concentration**	Ideas based in reality Able to concentrate	Ideas of reference (a distortion of reality in which a person believes that activities of others have a personal reference to him or her) Hypochondria (abnormal concerns about health) Obsessional Phobias (irrational fears) Poor or shortened concentration

MOOD OR AFFECT

Assessment	Normal	Abnormal
Assess prevailing or **variability in mood** by observing behavior and asking questions such as "How are you feeling right now?"	Appropriate, even mood without wide variations high to low	Cyclothymic mood swings (alterations in mood from euphoria, elation, and ecstasy to depressed and withdrawn)
Check for presence of abnormal **euphoria** (flight of ideas)		
If you suspect **depression,** continue questioning to determine depth and significance of mood (e.g., "How badly do you feel?" "Have you ever thought of suicide?")	May be sad or grieving but mood does not persist indefinitely	Flat or dampened responses Inappropriate responses Ambivalence (the simultaneous existence of contradictory or contrasting emotions toward a person or object—that is, love and hate feelings existing together)

MEMORY

Assessment	Normal	Abnormal
Assess **past and present memory** and **retention** (ability to listen and respond with understanding or knowledge); ask client to repeat a phrase, such as an address	Alert, accurate responses Able to complete digit span Past and present memory appropriate	Hyperamnesia (excessive loss of memory); amnesia (loss of memory caused by physical or emotional trauma); paramnesia (belief in events that never occurred) Preoccupied Unable to follow directions

Continues

◆ Table 14-1. MENTAL STATUS ASSESSMENT (*Continued*)		
Assessment	**Normal**	**Abnormal**
Assess **recall** (recent and remote) by asking questions such as "When is your birthday?" "What year were you born?" "How old are you?"	Good recall of immediate and past events	Poor recall of immediate or past events
JUDGMENT		
Assess **judgment, decision-making ability,** and interpretations by asking questions such as "What should you do if you hear a siren while you're driving?" "If you lost a library book, what would you do?"	Ability to make accurate decisions Realistic interpretation of events	Poor judgment, poor decision-making ability, poor choices Inappropriate interpretation of events or situations
AWARENESS		
Assess **insight** (the ability to understand the inner nature of events or problems) by asking questions such as "If you saw someone dressed in a fur coat on a hot day, what would you think?"	Thoughtful responses indicating an understanding of the inner nature of an event or problem	Lack of insight or understanding of the problems or situations Distorted view of situation
INTELLIGENCE		
Assess **intelligence** by asking client to define or use words in sentences (e.g., recede, join, plural)	Correct responses to majority of questions	Incorrect responses to majority of questions indicates possible severe disorders
Assess **fund of information** by asking questions such as "Who is President of the United States?" "Who was the President before him?" "When is Memorial Day?" "What is a thermometer?" (Consider client's cultural and educational background)	Correct responses to majority of questions	Deteriorated or impaired cognitive processes

b. Termination may cause client to recall previous separation experiences, feelings of abandonment, rejection, and depression.

c. Discuss client's previous experiences and help work through any negative ones.

4. Discuss client's feelings about termination.

5. Summarize the goals and objectives achieved.

Assessment

A. Determine purpose of establishing a nurse–client relationship.

◆ B. Assess the overall condition of the client to determine what benefits will be derived from a nurse–client relationship.

C. Observe what is happening with the client here and now.

◆ D. Identify developmental level of client so relationship goals will be realistic.

◆ E. Determine whether client exhibits verbal or nonverbal communication patterns so the nurse can respond therapeutically.

F. Assess anxiety level of client.

G. Identify client expectations of a therapeutic relationship and describe parameters of the relationship.

H. Examine your own feelings and expectations that may potentially impact the development of a therapeutic relationship.

Implementation

◆ A. Assume the role of facilitator in the relationship.

◆ B. Accept client as having value and worth as a unique individual.

◆ C. Maintain relationship on a professional, therapeutic level.

◆ **Table 14-1. MENTAL STATUS ASSESSMENT** (*Continued*)

Assessment	Normal	Abnormal
SENSORY ABILITY		
Assess the **five senses**—vision, hearing, tasting, feeling, and smelling abilities	Able to perceive, hear, feel, touch appropriate to stimulus	Lack of response Suspicious, hostile, depressed Kinesthetic imbalance
DEVELOPMENTAL LEVEL		
Assess client's **developmental level** as compared to normal	Behavior and thought processes appropriate to age level	Wide span between chronological and developmental age Mentally retarded
LIFESTYLE PATTERNS		
Identify **addictive patterns** and effect on individual's overall health	Normal amount of alcohol ingested Smoking habits Prescriptive medications Adequate food intake for physical characteristics	High quantity of alcohol taken frequently Heavy smoker Addicted to illegal drugs Habituative medication; user of over-the-counter or legal medications Anorexic eating patterns Obese or overindulgence of food
COPING DEVICES		
Identify **defense-coping mechanisms** and their effect on individual	Conscious coping mechanisms used appropriately such as compensation, fantasy, rationalization, suppression, sublimation, or displacement Mechanisms effective, appropriate, and useful	Unconscious mechanisms used frequently such as repression, regression (reverting to types of behavior characteristic of an earlier level of development), projection (defense mechanism by which one transfers to another person impulses, thoughts, or wishes that actually belong to oneself), reaction-formation, insulation, or denial Mechanisms inappropriate, ineffective, and not useful

D. Provide an environment conducive to client's experiencing corrective emotional experiences.

◆ E. Keep interaction reality oriented—that is, in the here and now.

F. Listen actively, reflect feelings.

G. Use nonverbal communication to support and encourage client.
1. Recognize meaning and purpose of nonverbal communication.
2. Keep verbal and nonverbal communication congruent by identifying and exploring incongruent messages.

H. Focus content and direction of conversation on client.

I. Interact on client's intellectual, developmental, and emotional level.

◆ J. Focus on "how, what, when, where, and who" rather than on "why."

◆ K. Teach client problem-solving skills to correct maladaptive patterns.

L. Help client to identify, express, and cope with feelings; assist client to express thoughts *and* feelings that result in an emotional release (catharsis).

M. Help client develop alternative, adaptive coping mechanisms.

N. Recognize a high level of anxiety and assist client to deal with it.

◆ O. Use therapeutic communication techniques.
1. Use techniques to increase effective communication. (*See* Therapeutic Communication Techniques, Table 14-2.)
2. Recognize blocks to communication and work to remove them. (*See* Blocks to Communication, Table 14-3.)

◆ **Table 14-2. THERAPEUTIC COMMUNICATION TECHNIQUES**

Listening	The process of consciously receiving another person's message. Includes listening eagerly, actively, responsively, and seriously.
Acknowledgment	Recognizing the other person without inserting your own values or judgments. Acknowledgment may be simple and with or without understanding. For example, in the response "I hear what you're saying," the person acknowledges a statement without agreeing with it. Acknowledgment may be verbal or nonverbal.
Feedback	The process the receiver uses to relay to the sender the effect the message has had, which either helps keep the sender on course or alters his or her course. It involves acknowledging, validating, clarifying, extending, and altering. *Nurse to client:* "You did that well." Involves giving constructive information to clients about how the nurse perceives and hears them.
Mutual fit or congruence	Harmony of verbal and nonverbal messages. For example, a client is crying and says, "I feel okay." The nurse says, "You say you feel okay, but you are crying. Let's talk about what's going on."
Clarification	The process of checking out or making clear either the intent or hidden meaning of the message, or of determining if the message sent was the message received. *Nurse:* "You said you feel funny. Can you describe what "funny" means?"
Focusing or refocusing	Picking up on central topics or "cues" given by the individual; concentrates attention on a single point. *Nurse:* "You were telling me how hard it was to talk to your mother."
Validation	The process of verifying the accuracy of the sender's message. *Nurse:* "Yes, it is confusing with so many people around."
Reflection	Identifying and sending back a message acknowledging the feeling expressed or reflecting back last few words of the message; directs questions, feelings, and ideas back to the client (conveys acceptance and great understanding). *Nurse:* "You feel depressed?" or "Depressed?"
Open-ended questions	Asking questions that cannot be answered "Yes" or "No" or "Maybe," generally requiring an answer of several words to broaden conversational opportunities and to help the client communicate. Do not ask, "Did you have a good time on your pass?" Rather, ask, "How did your pass go?"
Nonverbal encouragement	Using body language to communicate interest, attention, understanding, support, caring, and/or listening so as to promote data gathering. *Nurse:* Nods appropriately as someone talks.
Restatement	Restating what the client says; repeats the main idea expressed. *Nurse:* "You said that you hear voices."
Paraphrase	Summarizing or rewording what has been said. *Nurse:* "What I hear you saying is that you can't live comfortably at home."
Neutral response	Showing interest and involvement without saying anything else. *Nurse:* "Yes . . ." "Uh hmm . . ."
Incomplete sentences	Encouraging client to continue. *Nurse:* "Then your life is . . ."
Minimum verbal activity	Keeping your own verbalization minimal and letting the client lead the conversation. *Nurse:* "You feel . . .?"
Broad opening statements	Opening the communication by allowing the client freedom to talk and to focus on himself or herself. *Nurse:* "How have you been feeling?" "What would you like to talk about today?"
Confrontation	Pointing out a discrepancy in behavior, negative result of behavior or incongruence in behavior. If done in a positive, caring way, may lead to positive change. An example may be, "You say you have no self-confidence, yet you take over every meeting and won't let others talk."

THERAPEUTIC COMMUNICATION PROCESS

◆ *Definition:* Communication is a continuous, dynamic process of sending and receiving messages by means of symbols, words, signs, gestures, or other action. It is a multilevel process consisting of the content or informa-tion of the message and the part that defines the mean-ing of the message. Messages sent and received define the relationship between people. *Therapeutic communica-tion utilizes the principles of communication in a goal-directed professional framework.*

Characteristics

A.   A person cannot *not* communicate.

✦ Table 14-3. BLOCKS TO COMMUNICATION

Internal validation	Making an assumption about the meaning of someone else's behavior that is not validated by the other person (jumping to conclusions). The nurse finds the suicidal client smiling and tells the staff he's in a cheerful mood.
Giving advice	Telling the client what to do. Giving your opinion, or making decisions for the client, implies client cannot handle his or her own life decisions and that you are accepting responsibility for the client. *Nurse:* "If I were you, . . ."
Changing the subject	Introducing new topics inappropriately, a pattern that may indicate anxiety. The client is crying and discussing her fear of surgery, when the nurse asks, "How many children do you have?"
Social response	Responding in a way that focuses attention on the nurse instead of the client. *Nurse:* "This sunshine is good for my roses. I have a beautiful rose garden."
Invalidation	Ignoring or denying another's presence, thoughts, or feelings. *Client:* "Hi, how are you?" *Nurse:* "I can't talk now. I'm on my way to lunch."
False reassurance/agreement	Using clichés, pat answers, "cheery" words, advice, and "comforting" statements as an attempt to reassure client. Most of what is called "reassurance" is really false reassurance. *Nurse:* "It's going to be all right."
Overloading	Talking rapidly, changing subjects, or asking for more information than can be absorbed at one time. *Nurse:* "What's your name? I see you're 48 years old and that you like sports. Where do you come from?"
Underloading	Remaining silent and unresponsive, not picking up cues, and failing to give feedback. *Client:* "What's your name?" *Nurse:* Smiles and walks away.
Incongruence	Sending verbal and nonverbal messages that contradict one another; two or more messages, sent via different levels, seriously contradicting one another. The contradiction may be between the content, verbal message or nonverbal message. This contradiction is labeled a double message. Nurse says, "I'd like to spend time with you," then turns and walks away.
Value judgments	Giving one's own opinion, evaluating, moralizing, or implying one's own values by using words such as "nice," "good," "bad," "right," "wrong," "should," and "ought." *Nurse:* "You shouldn't do that—it's not right." "That's good."

B. Communication is a basic human need.

C. Communication includes verbal and nonverbal expression (includes tone and quality of speech, manner of dress, use of space).

D. Successful communication includes
1. Appropriateness.
2. Efficiency.
3. Flexibility.
4. Feedback.

✦ E. Communication skills are learned as the individual grows and develops.

F. The foundation of the person's perception of him- or herself and the world is the result of communicated messages received from significant others.

✦ G. High anxiety in both nurse and client impedes communication.

H. Self-awareness during the interview facilitates honest communication.

I. Factors that affect communication:
1. Intrapersonal framework of the person.
2. Relationship between the participants.
3. Purpose of the sender.
4. Content of the message.
5. Context of the message.
6. Manner in which the message is sent.
7. Effect on the receiver.
8. Environment in which the interaction takes place.

J. Purpose of communication.
1. To transfer ideas from one person to another.
2. To create meaning through the communication process.
3. To reduce uncertainty, to act effectively, and to defend or strengthen one's ego.
4. To affect or influence others, one's physical environment, and oneself.

The Interview Process

Assessment

A. Determine purpose of the interview.

B. As the first step in therapeutic interviewing, assess the client's total condition—physical, emotional, spiritual, and social.

C. Observe accurately what is happening with client in the here and now.

D. Be aware of your own feelings, reactions, and level of anxiety.

E. Assess client's communication patterns, behavior, and general demeanor.

F. Determine life situation of client.

G. Assess environmental conditions that may affect nurse–client interaction.

Implementation

✦ COMPONENTS OF INTERVIEW PROCESS

A. Provide a safe, private, comfortable setting if possible.

B. Encourage client to describe perceptions and feelings.
1. Focus on communication; offer leads.
2. Speak briefly.
3. Encourage spontaneity, expression of feelings.

C. Assist client to clarify feelings and events and place them in time sequence.
1. Focus on emotionally charged area(s).
2. Maintain accepting, nonjudgmental attitude.

D. Give broad openings and ask open-ended questions to enable client to describe what is happening with him or her.

E. Use body language to convey empathy, interest, and encouragement to facilitate communication.

F. Use silence as a therapeutic tool; it enables client to pace and direct his or her own communications. Long periods of silence, however, may increase client's anxiety level and should be avoided.

G. Define the limits of the interview: determine the purpose and structure the time and interaction patterns accordingly.

H. Never employ interviewing techniques as stereotyped responses during an interview.
1. Use of such responses negates open and honest communication.
2. Use of structured responses is counterproductive, as it presents nurse as a nonempathic communicator.
3. Interaction must be alive and responsive, not dependent on a technique for continuance.
4. Use "I" messages rather than "you" messages. (For example, "I feel uncomfortable," not "You make me feel uncomfortable.")

I. Watch for transference reaction from client (unconscious process of attributing feelings toward the therapist that originally belonged to a significant person in client's previous experience).

J. Assist client to build more effective coping mechanisms:
1. Gather pertinent data.
2. Define the problem.
3. Mutually agree on working toward a solution.
4. Mutually set goals.
5. Select alternatives.
6. Activate problem-solving behavior for identified problems.

ANXIETY

✦ *Definition:* Anxiety is an affective response subjectively experienced as a response to an internal or external threat(s), real or imagined. Anxiety is experienced as a painful, vague uneasiness or diffuse apprehension. It is a form of energy whose presence is inferred from its effect on attention, behavior, learning, and perception.

Characteristics

A. Anxiety is perceived subjectively by the conscious mind of the person experiencing it.

✦ B. Anxiety is a result of conflicts between the personality and the environment or between different forces within the personality.

C. Anxiety may be a reaction to threats of deprivation from something biologically or emotionally vital to the person.

D. The causative conflicts and/or threats are not in the awareness or in the conscious mind of the person.

✦ E. The amount or level of anxiety is related to the following factors:
1. Degree of threat to the self.
2. Degree to which behavior reduces anxiety.

F. Varying degrees of anxiety are common to all human beings at one time or another.

G. Anxiety is always found in emotional disorders.

H. Anxiety is easily transmitted from one individual to another.

✦ I. Constructive use of low-to-moderate levels of anxiety is healthy; it is often an incentive for growth.

J. The more capacity to manage anxiety, the more control an individual has over his or her environment.

K. Anxiety may be acute (precipitated by an event or threat) or chronic (caused by various sources) present for a long period of time.

Assessment

✦ A. A major assessment criterion for measuring the degree of anxiety is the person's ability to focus on what is happening to him or her in a situation.

✦ B. Physiological reaction present in client.
1. Increased heart rate.
2. Increased or decreased appetite.
3. Hyperventilation.
4. Tendency to void and defecate.
5. Dry mouth.

STAGES OF ANXIETY

- *Mild anxiety:* Client is able to focus realistically on most of what is happening within and to him or her.
- *Moderate anxiety:* Client is able to partially focus on what is happening; focus is limited.
- *Severe anxiety:* Client cannot focus on what is happening to him or her; focus is on scattered details.

---

6. Butterflies in stomach, nausea, vomiting, cramps, diarrhea.
7. "Fight or flight" response.
8. Tremors.
9. Dyspnea.
10. Palpitations.
11. Tachycardia.
12. Numbness of extremities.
13. Perspiration.

C. Psychological reactions present in client.
1. Lack of concentration on work.
2. Feelings of depression and guilt.
3. Harbored fear of sudden death or insanity.
4. Dread of being alone.
5. Confusion.
6. Tension.
7. Agitation and restlessness.

✦ D. States of anxiety vary in degree and can be assessed as follows:
1. Ataraxia (absence of anxiety).
   a. State is uncommon.
   b. Can be seen in persons who take drugs.
   c. Indicates low motivation.
2. Mild.
   a. Senses are alert.
   b. Attentiveness is increased.
   c. Motivation is increased.
3. Moderate.
   a. Peripheral field is narrowed, and attention is selective.
   b. Degree of pathology depends on the individual.
   c. May be detected in complaining, arguing, teasing behaviors.
   d. Can be converted to physical symptoms such as headaches, low back pain, nausea, diarrhea.
4. Severe.
   a. All senses are gravely affected.
   b. Perceptual field greatly reduced.
   c. Behavior becomes automatic toward immediate relief.
   d. Energy is drained.
   e. Defense mechanisms are used to control severe levels of anxiety.

f. Cannot be used constructively by person.
g. Psychologically extremely painful.
h. Learning and problem solving not possible.
i. Nursing action always indicated for this state.

✦ 5. Panic.
   a. Individual is overwhelmed and feels helpless.
   b. Personality may disintegrate producing hallucinations or delusions.
   c. Wild, desperate, ineffective behavior may be observed, including sense of awe, dread, terror, uncanniness.
   d. Detail previously focused on is exaggerated.
   e. Client may do bodily harm to self and others.
   f. Panic state cannot be tolerated very long.
   g. Condition is pathological.
   h. Immediate intervention is needed.

Implementation

A. Identify anxious behavior and the level of anxiety that determines degree of intervention.
✦ B. Remain with an anxious client.
C. Recognize anxiety in self may escalate client's anxiety.
✦ D. Maintain appropriate attitudes toward client.
1. Acceptance.
2. Calm, matter-of-fact approach.
3. Willingness to listen and help.
4. Emotional support.
E. Recognize if additional help is required for intervention.
F. Provide activities that decrease anxiety and provide an outlet for energy.
G. Establish person-to-person relationship.
1. Allow client to express his or her feelings.
2. Proceed at client's pace.
3. Avoid forcing client to verbalize feelings.
4. Assist client in identifying anxiety.
5. Assist client in learning new ways of dealing with anxiety.
✦ H. Provide appropriate physical environment.
1. Nonstimulating.
2. Structured.
3. Designed to prevent physical exhaustion or self-harm.
I. Administer medication as directed and needed.

Defense Mechanisms

Definition: Defense mechanisms are automatic, psychological processes caused by internal or external perceived dangers or stressors that threaten self-esteem and disrupt ego function.

✦ Table 14-4. DEFENSE MECHANISMS	
Compensation	Covering up a lack or weakness by emphasizing a desirable trait, or making up for a frustration in one area by overemphasis in another area. This is learned early in childhood and may be easily recognized in adult behavior; for example, the physically handicapped individual who is an outstanding scholar.
Denial	Refusal to face reality. The ego protects itself from unpleasant pain or conflict by rejecting reality. Denial of illness is a common example; people wait to see a doctor because they don't want to know the truth. A more subtle example is the individual who avoids reality by getting "sick."
Displacement	Discharging pent-up feelings from one object to a less dangerous object. A fairly common mechanism; for example, your supervisor yells at you, you yell at your husband.
Dissociation	Emotional conflict is handled by altering consciousness, identity, memory or perception of the environment. An example is amnesia for an event (such as a car accident) that was traumatic.
Fantasy	Gratification by imaginary achievements and wishful thinking; for example, children's play. Sometimes, to satisfy a need, one relieves the tension by anticipating the pleasure of gratification.
Fixation	The persistence in later life of interests and behavior patterns appropriate to an earlier developmental age.
Identification	The process of taking on the desirable attributes in personalities of people one admires. Identification plays an important role in the development of a child's personality; for example, the child who mimics mother or father. A kind of satisfaction can be derived from sharing the success or the experience of others, such as the nurse who feels sick watching a traumatic procedure on a client.
Insulation	Withdrawal into passivity, becoming inaccessible to avoid further threatening circumstances. Sometimes the individual appears cold and indifferent to his or her surroundings. Insulation may be used harmlessly at times but becomes very serious if used so much it interferes with interaction with others.
Isolation	Excluding certain ideas, attitudes, or feelings from awareness. Isolation is separating the feelings from the intellect by putting emotions concerning a specific traumatic event into a lock-tight compartment; for example, the individual talks about a significant situation such as an accident or death without a display of feelings. This pattern can be positive if used temporarily to protect the ego from being overwhelmed.
Introjection	A type of identification in which there is a symbolic incorporation of a loved or hated object, belief system, or value into the individual's own ego structure; there is no absolute assimilation as in identification.
Projection	Placing blame for difficulties on others or attributing one's own undesirable traits to someone else; for example, the child who says to a parent, "You hate me," after the parent has spanked the child. In an adult, this mechanism is a predominant indicator of paranoia. The paranoid client projects hate for others by saying that others are out to get the client.

Characteristics

✦ A. The purpose of defense mechanisms is to attempt to reduce anxiety and to reestablish equilibrium.

B. Adjustment depends on one's ability to vary responses so that anxiety is decreased.

✦ C. Use of defense mechanisms may be a conscious process but usually takes place at the unconscious level.

D. Defense mechanisms are compromise solutions and include those listed in Table 14-4.

E. Defenses may be pathological as well as adaptive.

Assessment

A. Assess whether client evidences healthy adjustment in the way he or she uses defense mechanisms.

✦ 1. Healthy adjustment is characterized by
   a. Infrequent use of defense mechanisms.
   b. Ability to form new responses.
   c. Ability to change the external environment.
   d. Ability to modify one's needs.
   e. Use of defense mechanisms to lower anxiety to achieve goals in acceptable ways.

2. Healthy adjustment patterns may include mechanisms such as rationalization, sublimation, compensation, and suppression.

✦ B. Assess whether client evidences unhealthy adjustment in the way he or she uses defense mechanisms.

1. Unhealthy adjustment is characterized by
   a. Undeveloped ability or loss of ability to vary responses.
   b. Retreat from the problem or reality.
   c. Frequent use of defense mechanisms, which may interfere with maintenance of self-image and interfere with individual growth and interpersonal satisfaction.

✦ **Table 14-4. DEFENSE MECHANISMS** (*Continued*)	
Rationalization	The mechanism that is almost universally employed to prove or justify behavior. It is face saving to give a reason that is acceptable rather than the real reason, as in remarks such as "It wasn't worth it anyway," "It's all for the best." This mechanism relieves anxiety temporarily and helps the person avoid facing reality.
Reaction-formation	Prevention of dangerous feelings and desires from being expressed by exaggerating the opposite attitude—a kind of denial. The overly neat, polite, conscientious individual may have an unconscious desire to be untidy and carefree. The behavior becomes pathological when it interferes with tasks or produces anxiety and frustration.
Regression	Resorting to an earlier developmental level to deal with reality. Regression is an immature way of responding, and it is frequently seen during a physical illness. It is sometimes used to an extreme degree by the mentally ill, who may regress all the way back to infancy.
Repression	The unconscious process whereby one keeps undesirable and unacceptable thoughts from entering the conscious. This repressed material may be the motivation for some behavior. The superego is largely responsible for repression; the stronger, more punitive the superego, the more emotion will be repressed. The child who is frustrated and downtrodden by a parent may rebel against authority in later life.
Sublimation	The mechanism by which a primitive or unacceptable tendency is redirected into socially constructive channels. This adjustment is at least partly responsible for many artistic and cultural achievements, such as painting and poetry.
Substitution	The replacement of a highly valued unacceptable object with an object that is more acceptable to the ego.
Suppression	The act of keeping unpleasant feelings and experiences from awareness.
Symbolization	Use of an idea or object by the conscious mind to represent another actual event or object. Sometimes the meaning is not clear because the symbol may be representative of something unconscious. Children use symbolization in this way and have to learn to distinguish between the symbol and the object being symbolized. Examples include obsessive thoughts or behavior (handwashing, cleansing) and the incoherent speech of the schizophrenic (by the time the painful thoughts reach the surface, they are so jumbled that they lose their painfulness).
Undoing	Closely related to reaction-formation—performance of a specific action that is considered to be the opposite of a previous unacceptable action. This action is felt to neutralize or "undo" the original action; for example, when Lady Macbeth washed her hands over and over.

2. Unhealthy adjustment patterns may include mechanisms such as regression, repression, denial, projection, and dissociation.

Implementation

A. Facilitate more appropriate use of defense mechanisms.

✦ B. Remember that defense mechanisms serve a purpose and cannot be arbitrarily eliminated without being replaced by more adaptive coping mechanisms.

C. Avoid criticizing client's behavior and use of defense mechanisms.

D. Help client explore the underlying source of the anxiety that gives rise to an unhealthy response.

✦ E. Assist the client in learning new or alternative coping mechanisms for healthier adaptation.

F. Use techniques to alleviate client's anxiety.

✦ G. Use a firm supportive approach to explore any maladaptive use of defense mechanisms.

ANXIETY DISORDERS

✦ *Definition:* Anxiety disorders are those disorders in which the predominant disturbance is one of anxiety. The individual with an anxiety disorder uses rigid, repetitive, and maladaptive behaviors to try to control anxiety. Anxiety may be manifested as panic, generalized anxiety, phobias, or obsessive–compulsive behavior.

Characteristics

A. Repression and projection are common defense mechanisms.

✦ B. Patterns of behavior are used in a rather stereotyped and rigid way.

C. Client becomes more dependent and disabled as times goes on.

✦ D. Client is almost always unaware of his or her maladaptive behavior patterns.

E. The disorder that manifests is the client's attempt to deal with anxiety.

✦ F. Secondary gains become associated problems.
1. Secondary gains are social and psychological advantages (fringe benefits) that the client may derive from his or her symptoms.
2. Client does not understand unconscious motivation for secondary gains.
3. Secondary gains reinforce neurotic behavior.

G. Client has little difficulty talking, but conversation may be vague and unrevealing.

H. Low self-esteem is often observable in disorder.

I. Reality is not grossly distorted.

J. Personality is not grossly disorganized.

K. Attitude of martyrdom is common.

L. Client is highly amenable to suggestion.

Generalized Anxiety Disorder (GAD)

Assessment

✦ A. Client has unrealistic, diffuse persistent anxiety about two or more life experiences.

B. Client cannot control anxiety by defense mechanisms.

C. The individual's worry is out of proportion to the true impact of the worried event or situation.

✦ D. Psychological symptoms.
1. Lack of concentration on work.
2. Feelings of depression and guilt.
3. Harbored fear of sudden death or insanity.
4. Dread of being alone.
5. Confusion.
6. Rumination.
7. Agitation and restlessness—motor tension.
8. Impatience.
9. Difficulty making decisions.

✦ E. Physiological symptoms.
1. Tremors.
2. Dyspnea.
3. Palpitations.
4. Tachycardia.
5. Numbness of extremities.
6. Sleep disturbance.

Implementation

A. Recognize behavior in client that denotes anxiety.

B. Maintain calm, serene approach because nurse's anxiety reinforces client's anxiety.

✦ C. Help client to develop conscious awareness of anxiety.

D. Help client identify and describe feelings and source of anxiety.

✦ E. Provide physical outlet for anxiety.

F. Remain with client.

G. Decrease environmental stimuli.

H. Avoid reinforcing secondary gains (attention, sympathy).

Panic Disorder

A. Panic attacks are characterized by recurrent attacks of severe anxiety lasting minutes to a few hours.
1. Intense physical symptoms of palpitations, sweating, shaking, dyspnea.
2. Fear of losing control, choking, fear of losing their mind or dying are also present.
3. People with panic disorder have a significantly higher incidence of mitral valve disorder (57 percent, versus 5–7 percent in the general population). The exact relationship between the two is unclear.

B. Attacks appear suddenly with no warning. May become associated with specific situations.

C. Interventions: implement actions as you would for generalized anxiety disorder.

Phobic Disorders

Assessment

✦ A. Fear is recognized by individual as excessive or unreasonable in proportion to reality.

B. A compelling desire exists to avoid subject or situation.

✦ C. Client has unrealistic, irrational fear of object or situation that presents no actual danger.

D. Client uses projection, displacement, repression, and sublimation.

E. Client transfers anxiety or fear from its source to a symbolic idea or situation.

✦ F. Phobic disorders are classified into many diffferent types. Examples are
1. Agoraphobia—intense, excessive anxiety or fear about being in places or situations from which escape might be difficult or embarassing.
2. Acrophobia—fear of high places.
3. Social phobia—desire to avoid social situations in which individuals fear they will behave in an embarassing way.
4. Simple phobia—persistent or irrational fear of simple objects or situations.
5. Claustrophobia—fear of enclosed spaces (elevators).

Implementation

✦ A. Draw client's attention away from phobia.

B. Have client focus on awareness of self.

C. Do not force client into situation feared.

D. Slowly develop sound, therapeutic relationship with client.

◆ E. Assist client to go through desensitizing process.
1. New studies indicate that high-tech virtual reality programs enable the client to become desensitized to the phobia.
2. Fear of elevators and flying are programs currently available as examples of in vivo densensitization.

Obsessive–Compulsive Disorder

Assessment

◆ A. Client has anxiety associated with persistent, undesired ideas, thoughts, or images that are experienced as senseless or repugnant.
◆ B. Client releases anxiety through repetitive, ritualistic, stereotyped acts.
C. Personality characteristics.
1. Insecure, guilt-ridden.
2. Sensitive, shy.
3. Straight-laced.
4. Fussy and meticulous.
D. Client uses repression, isolation, and undoing to reduce anxiety.
E. Client is unable to control feelings of hostility and aggression.
F. Behavior interferes with social or role functioning.
G. Symptoms are distressing to client.
H. Most common obsessions are thoughts of violence, contamination, and doubt.
◆ I. Most common compulsions involve handwashing, counting, checking, and touching.

Implementation

A. Avoid punishment or criticism.
◆ B. Allow episodes of compulsive acts, setting limits only to prevent harmful acts.
◆ C. Engage in alternative activities with client.
D. Limit decision making for client.
E. Provide for client's physical needs.
F. Convey acceptance of client regardless of behavior.
G. Establish routine to avoid anxiety-producing changes.
◆ H. Gear assignments to those which are routine and can be done with perfection, such as straightening linen or cleaning.
I. Plan therapy, any change in routine, or one-to-one contact after completion of a compulsive episode.

POST-TRAUMATIC STRESS DISORDER

◆ *Definition:* Condition follows a traumatic event that is outside the range of common experience (military combat, rape, assault, etc.).

Characteristics

◆ A. Traumatic event is consistently reexperienced in dream state, as flashbacks, connected to events that trigger memory.
◆ B. As event is reexperienced, client suffers behavioral and emotional symptoms. (Abreaction occurs: vivid recall of painful experience with emotion appropriate to the original situation.)
C. Individual is not able to adjust to the event.
D. Persistent avoidance of stimuli associated with trauma occurs.
E. Persistent symptoms of increased arousal, such as difficulty falling/staying asleep and irritability, exist.

Assessment

A. Assess for symptoms of anxiety and depression.
1. Emotional instability.
2. Feelings of detachment or guilt.
3. Nightmares, difficulty sleeping.
4. Withdrawal and isolation.
5. Self-destructive behavior.
B. Aggressive or acting-out behavior.
1. Explosive or unpredictable behavior.
2. Impulsive behavior; change in lifestyle.

Implementation

A. Implement treatment protocol for anxiety disorders.
B. Assist client to go through recovery process.
1. Deal with conscious awareness of traumatic experience.
2. Adjust to acceptance of experience.
C. Protect client from self-destructive behaviors or acting-out behaviors.
◆ D. Recovery process follows four stages.
1. *Recovery*—reassure client that he or she is safe following experience of the traumatic event.
2. *Avoidance*—client will avoid thinking about traumatic event; support client.
3. *Reconsideration*—client deals with event by confronting it, talking about it, and working through feelings.
4. *Adjustments*—client rehabilitates and adjusts to environment following event; functions and is able to view future positively.

SOMATOFORM DISORDERS

◆ *Definition:* Somatoform behaviors are physical symptoms that may involve any organ system, and whose etiologies are in part precipitated by psychological factors. There are three main types: psychosomatic, conversion disorder, and hypochondriasis.

Characteristics

A. An individual must adapt and adjust to stresses in life.

1. The way a person adapts depends on the individual's characteristics.
2. Emotional stress may exacerbate or precipitate an illness.

B. Psychosocial stress is an important factor in symptom formation.

Psychosomatic Disorders

Assessment

◆ A. Assess which body system is involved that resulted in somatoform disorder.
   1. Gastrointestinal system.
      a. Peptic ulcer.
      b. Colic.
      c. Ulcerative colitis.
   2. Cardiovascular system.
      a. Hypertension.
      b. Tachycardia.
      c. Migraine headaches.
   3. Respiratory system.
      a. Asthma.
      b. Hay fever.
      c. Hiccoughs.
      d. Common cold.
      e. Hyperventilation.
   4. Skin—most expressive organ of emotion.
      a. Blushing.
      b. Flushing, perspiring.
      c. Dermatitis.
   5. Nervous system.
      a. Chronic general fatigue.
      b. Exhaustion.
   6. Endocrine.
      a. Dysmenorrhea.
      b. Hyperthyroidism.
   7. Musculoskeletal system.
      a. Cramps.
      b. Rheumatoid arthritis.
   8. Other.
      a. Diabetes mellitus.
      b. Obesity.
      c. Sexual dysfunctions.
      d. Hyperemesis gravidarum.
      e. Accident proneness.

B. Evaluate history for physical symptoms of several years' duration.
C. Observe closely and assess client's present condition.
   1. Collect data about physical illness—symptoms (multiple sources).
   2. Psychosocial adjustment.
   3. Life situation.
   4. Coping mechanisms that work for client.
   5. Strengths of client.
   6. Problem-solving abilities.

D. Note if symptoms are intermittent.
E. Assess what kinds of things aggravate or relieve symptoms.

Implementation

A. Provide restful, supportive environment.
   1. Balance therapy and recreation.
   2. Decrease stimuli.
   3. Provide activities that deemphasize the client's physical symptoms.
B. Care for the "total" person—physical and emotional.
◆ C. Realize physical symptoms are real and that person is not faking.
◆ D. Recognize that treatment of physical problems does not relieve emotional problems.
E. Reduce demands on client.
F. Develop nurse–client relationship.
   1. Respect the person and the person's problems.
   2. Help client to express his or her feelings.
   3. Help client to express anxiety and explore new coping mechanisms.
   4. Allow client to meet dependency needs.
   5. Allow client to feel in control.
◆ G. Help client to work through problems and learn new methods of responding to stress.

Conversion Disorder

Assessment

A. Establish psychosomatic origin by assessing physical condition and ruling out any organic basis for symptoms (i.e., neurological examinations, laboratory tests).
◆ B. Identify conversion behavior/symptoms. Conversion behavior is the development of a physical symptom (blindness, paralysis, deafness) with no physical etiology identified.
◆ C. Evaluate client's attitude toward condition: "la belle indifference" (French term describing client's lack of concern or indifference toward physical symptom—a definite clue that condition is a conversion disorder).
◆ D. Identify primary gain.
   1. Keeps internal conflict or need out of awareness (repression).
   2. Symptom has symbolic value to client.
◆ E. Identify secondary gain.
   1. Provides additional advantages that result from particular behaviors that are not connected to the primary gain, such as avoidance, attention, or sympathy.
   2. Reinforces maladjusted behavior.
F. Assess whether symptoms disappear under hypnosis.

Implementation

◆ A. Establish therapeutic nurse–client relationship.

B. Reduce pressure on client.

C. Control environment.

D. Provide recreational and social activities.

✦ E. Do not confront client with his or her illness.

F. Divert client's attention from symptom.

G. Do not feed into secondary gains through anticipating client needs.

Hypochondriasis

Assessment

✦ A. Preoccupation with an imagined illness for which no observable symptoms or organic changes exist.

B. Evaluate severe, morbid preoccupation with body functions or fear of serious disease.

C. Assess whether client shows lack of interest in environment.

D. Assess whether client shows severe regression.

E. Determine if client goes from doctor to doctor to find cure or enjoys recounting medical history.

✦ F. Differentiate from malingering—deliberately making up illness to prolong hospitalization.

Implementation

✦ A. Accept client; recognize and understand that physiological complaints are not in client's conscious awareness.

B. Provide diversionary activities in which client can succeed in building self-esteem.

✦ C. Use friendly, supportive approach but do not focus on physical condition (i.e., avoid asking, "How are you today?").

D. Help client to refocus interest on topics other than physical complaints.

E. Provide for client's physical needs; give accurate information and correct any misinformation.

F. Assist client to understand how he or she uses illness to avoid dealing with life's problems.

G. Be aware of staff's negativity, as it may lead to exacerbation of client's symptoms.

EATING DISORDERS

Anorexia Nervosa

✦ *Definition:* A potentially life-threatening (results in death 10 percent of the time) eating disorder characterized by an intense fear of gaining weight or becoming fat. The psychological aversion to food results in emaciation, physical problems, and possible death.

Characteristics

✦ A. Almost exclusively female—90 to 95 percent.

B. Most common in adolescent girls and young adults (age 12 to mid-30s).

C. Often unnoticed in early stages; female "goes on diet to lose weight."

✦ D. Dynamics of disorder.

1. History of a "model child"—extreme perfectionism.

2. Overprotected by parents in rigid, enmeshed family structure.

3. Conflict erupts at adolescence between poor involvement and family loyalty.

4. Becomes negative due to power struggles with family over pressure to eat.

5. Intense fear of obesity leads anorectic to report feeling fat.

6. Not a disturbance in appetite but distorted body image perceptions; related to disturbance in sense of self, identity, and autonomy.

7. Hormones altered—whether cause or effect is yet to be determined.

8. Anorectics do not want treatment. Potentially lethal disease: mortality 5–18 percent.

9. Many anorectics have a single episode, then recover. Factors associated with positive prognosis include onset of problem before age 15 and weight gain within 2 years.

Assessment

✦ A. Assess weight: refusal to maintain body weight at or above a normal weight for age and height (loss of 15 percent or greater average body weight).

✦ B. No menstrual period for 3 months.

✦ C. Assess for physical symptoms.

1. Malnutrition.

2. Fractures—calcium leaked from bones.

3. Teeth enamel eroded and poor gums.

4. Hypotension, hypothermia.

5. Anemia and decreased white blood cells.

6. Hypoproteinemia.

7. Sleep disturbances.

8. Cold intolerance (cyanosis and numbness of extremities).

D. Monitor for potential complications.

1. Severe electrolyte imbalance (decreased K, kidney failure).

2. Heart failure and coma, possible death.

Implementation

✦ A. Actions to improve nutritional status (to stabilize medical condition).

1. Diet.

   a. High protein, high carbohydrate, especially amino acids.

   b. Identify foods client prefers.

   c. Small, nutritious, attractive feedings.

2. Nasogastric feedings: if client refuses to eat, administer tube feedings as ordered.

B. Psychological care.
1. Care plan.
❖ a. Formulate plan that all staff agree on. Do not allow manipulation. Do not engage in power struggle.
❖ b. Do not focus on food, taste, recipes, etc.
c. Remain with client when eating or monitor when client eats with others.
d. Do not accept excuses to leave eating area (to vomit).
e. Set limits on amount client must eat. Reward when client adheres to plan.
f. Ensure that weight is taken same time every day with client dressed in only a hospital gown.
g. Be warm and caring in approach to client, both verbally and physically.
2. Therapy.
❖ a. Medications: antidepressants—selective serotonin reuptake inhibitor (SSRI).
❖ b. Focused on behavior therapy.
(1) Set limits with positive and negative reinforcement.
(2) Establish contract that specifies weight gain or loss correlated with privileges/restrictions.
c. Insight-oriented therapy: correcting client's body perceptions and misconceptions about feelings, needs, self-worth, autonomy.
d. Family therapy: important focus as issues of control and autonomy are connected to eating.

Bulimia

❖ *Definition:* Eating disorder characterized by loss of control during binge eating, frequently followed by self-induced vomiting.

Characteristics

❖ A. Etiology is unknown but this disorder is often accompanied by an underlying psychopathology.
B. More common in women than men.
C. Begins in adolescence or early adulthood and often follows a chronic course over many years.
D. Generally aware that eating patterns are abnormal (in contrast to anorectics).
E. Typically evidences impaired impulse control, low self-esteem, and depression.

Assessment

A. Assess degree of disruption in life caused by eating disorder.
❖ B. Assess degree of depression: often due to guilt over eating binges. (New studies suggest link between bulimia and affective disorder.)

C. Assess weight fluctuation and potential danger of weight loss.
❖ D. Assess for physical symptoms.
1. Enlarged parotid glands.
2. Dental erosion and caries.
3. Electrolyte imbalance (hypokalemia).
4. Fluid retention.

Implementation

A. Client is usually not hospitalized but does require therapy.
B. Behavior-modification and insight-oriented therapy used with limited success.
C. Care plan is similar to anorexia nervosa with focus on interrupting binge/purge cycle and altering attitudes toward food and self.
❖ D. Combination of cognitive-behavioral therapy and psychopharmacology (SSRI antidepressants) more effective.

SLEEP DISORDERS

Definition: Sleep disorders or sleep pattern disturbance can be categorized into 4 different groups: primary sleep disorders (dyssomnias and parasomnias), sleep disorders related to mental conditions, a medical condition, or substance-induced disorder.

Assessment

A. Dyssomnias.
1. Primary insomnia.
a. Assess difficulty falling asleep or continuing sleep.
b. Assess problems with nonrestorative sleep.
2. Primary hypersomnia.
a. Assess for prolonged sleep and excessive sleepiness that interferes with daily functioning.
b. Excessive sleepiness is not caused by insomnia and is not accounted for by inadequate sleep.
3. Breathing-related sleep disorders.
a. Assess for sleep apnea, obstructive type (upper airway partially collapses and opening it involves at least partial arousal).
b. Assess for predisposing factors: obese, middle-aged men with a history of snoring.
4. Narcolepsy.
a. Assess for a pattern of brief episodes of deep sleep, occurring daily.
b. May be accompanied by cataplexy (sudden collapse of muscle tone or recurrent episodes of rapid eye movement).
5. Circadian rhythm sleep disorders.

a. Assess for a recurrent pattern of sleep disruption due to mismatched sleep–wake schedules.
   (1) Disturbance causes stress or impairment of functioning.
   (2) Disturbance is not connected to other sleep disorders or a substance abuse.
b. Assess for specific types: delayed sleep phase, jet lag, shift work phase or unspecified.

B. Parasomnias.
   1. Somnambulism—sleep walking, nightmares, sleep terrors.
   2. Bruxism—teeth grinding.
   3. Enuresis—bed-wetting.

Implementation

A. Intervention is based on thorough identification of the type of sleep disturbance.
   1. Diagnostic sleep tests (polysomnography) assists in confirming the diagnosis.
   2. Treatment is based on subjective analysis unless specific symptoms suggest other disorders.
B. Interventions may include principles of sleep hygiene, coping mechanisms, medication, reduction or removal of an obstruction (sleep apnea), CPAP by nasal mask; in general, treatment is specific to each individual's problem.

DISSOCIATIVE DISORDERS

◆ *Definition:* These disorders involve disruptions in the usually integrated functions of consciousness, identity, memory, or perception of the environment.

Characteristics

◆ A. Client attempts to deal with anxiety through various disturbances or by blocking certain areas out of the mind from conscious awareness.
B. Client has a psychological retreat from reality.
C. Repression is used to block awareness of traumatic event.
◆ D. Manifestations.
   ◆ 1. *Amnesia*—circumscribed, selective or generalized, and continuous loss of memory.
   ◆ 2. *Fugue*—condition experienced as a transient disorientation—client is unaware he or she has traveled to another location. Client does not remember period of fugue.
   ◆ 3. *Dissociative identity disorder (DID)*—dominated by two or more personalities, each of which controls the behavior while in the consciousness.
   ◆ 4. *Depersonalization*—alteration in perception or experience of self; sense of detachment from self.

Assessment

◆ A. Determine that symptoms are not of organic origin.
B. Assess in which form the dissociative disorder is manifesting.
C. Evaluate degree of interference in lifestyle and interpersonal relationships.
D. Assess presence of accompanying symptoms such as depression, suicide ideation, use of alcohol and drugs, etc.
E. Note inconsistencies in elapsed time.
F. Note complaints of voices "inside" the head talking to one another, as opposed to hallucinations that are "outside" the head.

Implementation

A. Support therapeutic modality as established by treatment team.
B. Reduce anxiety-producing stimuli.
C. Redirect client's attention away from self.
D. Avoid sympathizing with client.
E. Increase socialization activities.
◆ F. Therapy.
   1. Hypnosis.
   2. Abreaction (assisting client to recall past, painful experiences).
   3. Cognitive restructuring.
   4. Behavioral therapy.
   5. Psychopharmacology (antianxiety and antidepressants).

PERSONALITY DISORDERS

◆ *Definition:* Disorders in which individual exhibits inflexible and maladaptive responses to stress, which produce dysfunctional behavioral problems.

Characteristics

A. Three major categories referred to as clusters: odd–eccentric, dramatic–emotional, and fearful–anxious.
B. Several traits are common to all 3 clusters.
   1. Lacks understanding of how his or her behavior affects others; lacks insight.
   2. Cannot take responsibility for own behavior.
   3. When threatened, cannot change own behavior, but attempts to change environment.
C. Other general traits common to personality disorders:
   ◆ 1. Experiences inadequate interactions with society and individuals.
      a. Difficulty in forming loving and lasting interpersonal relationships.
      b. Difficulty with authority, laws, and rules.
   ◆ 2. Assets may be social skills—intelligence, charm, and manipulation.

3. Experiences low tolerance for anxiety and inability to tolerate frustration—will go to great lengths to avoid increased intellectual and emotional demands that raise anxiety.

✦ 4. A common characteristic is manipulation—influencing others or events to meet own needs without regard for others' needs.

D. For specific personality types, *see* Table 14-5.

Nursing Interventions for Manipulative Behavior

✦ A. Recognize characteristics of manipulative behavior—pervasive in all personality disorders.
   1. Uses bargains, threats, demands, or intimidation to get own way.
   2. Shows ability to identify and use other people's weaknesses for own benefit.
   3. Makes continuous, unrealistic demands.
   4. Pits one individual against another (e.g., clients against staff) and primitive defense mechanism of splitting.
   5. Pretends to be helpless and sorry for behavior.
   6. Lies to gain sympathy of staff or other clients.
   7. Acts out even when given acceptable behavioral alternatives.
   8. Keeps all relationships on a superficial level.
   9. Uses flattery, charm, and excessive compliments to have needs met.
   10. Exploits the generosity of others.
   11. Identifies with staff or authority figure and acts as if he or she is not incarcerated.
   12. Finds a way around the unit rules and expectations.
   13. Uses sexuality to gain control over others—may even approach the staff sexually.

✦ B. Interventions for manipulative behavior.
   ✦ 1. Set clear and realistic limits with appropriate consequences. Be consistent and firm in setting behavioral expectations and limits.
   ✦ 2. Confront client about the manipulative behavior. Do not try to outmanipulate—client is a master at it.
   3. Reinforce adaptive behavior through positive feedback and realistic praise.
   ✦ 4. Do not be influenced by client's charming ways—all directed toward manipulating you.
   5. Do not be intimidated by client's behavior.
   6. Clearly and consistently communicate care plans and client's behavior to other staff. Present a united front.
   7. Accept no flattery, gifts, or favors.

C. Impulsiveness and not taking responsibility for behavior are common with these disorders.

1. Assist client to identify consequences of behavior.
2. Begin a behavior modification plan in which all staff consistently implement consequences of behavior.

D. Poor social/interpersonal relationships.
   1. Form a therapeutic nurse–client relationship in which positive behavior is reinforced.
   2. Help to develop trust in relationship by being consistent and doing what you promise to do.
   3. Point out unrealistic expectations in relationships.

E. Low self-esteem, which may lead to self-destructive behavior.
   1. Work with client to see assets and strengths and positive attributes—group feedback is useful for this intervention.
   2. Use of cognitive behavior techniques (stopping negative thoughts) is useful.
   3. Self-destructive behavior may necessitate a stable, safe, secure environment with clear expectations of behavior, firm limits and strict consequences.

F. Aggressive behavior.
   1. Safe environment with strict limits for any unacceptable behavior.
   2. Anger management so client can differentiate feeling angry from behavioral expression of anger.

Nursing Interventions for Paranoid Personality Disorder

A. Determine client's degree of suspiciousness and mistrust of others.
   1. Assess client's hostility toward others.
   ✦ 2. Determine if delusions are present. Delusions include persecution, grandeur, and/or hypochondriasis.
      a. *Delusions of grandeur:* false belief that one is in a position of power, wealth, and prominence.
      b. *Delusions of persecution:* false belief that one is being pursued, followed, or intimidated by an opposing power.
   3. Evaluate client's degree of insecurity, inadequate self-concept, and low self-esteem.
   4. Assess anxiety level and its impact on disorder.

✦ B. Establish a trusting relationship.
   1. Be consistent and friendly despite client's hostility.
   2. Avoid talking and laughing when client can see you but not hear you.
   3. If client is very suspicious, use a one-to-one relationship, not a group situation.

Table 14-5. PERSONALITY DISORDERS

Personality Types	Profile Characteristics
CLUSTER A (ODD–ECCENTRIC)	
Paranoid personality	Pervasive, unwarranted suspiciousness, and mistrust of people
	Guarded, secretive, devious, and scheming
	Puts blame on others for problems
	Argumentative and exaggerates difficulties
	Affectively restricted and cold
	Lacks soft, sentimental, or tender feelings
Schizoid personality	Loners, lack of social relationships, pervasive pattern of detachment
	No warmth or tender feelings toward others—appears cold and aloof
	Prefers to be alone and has few friends—seclusive
	Appears reserved, withdrawn, and seclusive
	Flat affect—humorless and dull, emotionally cold
	Takes pleasure in few activities
Schizotypal personality	Peculiar ways of thinking, behavior and looking
	Related to schizophrenia but not severe enough to be labeled as such
	Inappropriate affect, speech, and ideation
	Under periods of severe stress, symptoms of schizophrenia may develop
CLUSTER B (DRAMATIC–EMOTIONAL)	
Histrionic personality	Overly reactive, dramatic, and intense
	Disruptive relationships with others
	Seeks attention and tends to exaggerate
	May exhibit angry outbursts or tantrums
	Immature, self-centered and dependent
	Seductive and flirty with others
Narcissistic personality	Grandiose sense of self-importance and entitlement
	Preoccupation with fantasies of power, beauty, etc.
	Exhibitionistic, with indifference or rage in response to criticism
	Lack of empathy and exploits others
	Arrogant and haughty
Borderline personality	Efforts to avoid abandonment
	Impulsiveness that is self-damaging (e.g., gambling, sex, spending)
	Pattern of unstable relationships and affect
	Explosive temper, affective lability, suicide gestures, and acts of self-mutilation
	Lack of self-identity
	Chronic feeling of boredom and emptiness
Antisocial personality	Intelligent, charming, self-centered, "con artist"
	Inability to feel guilt or learn from past experience
	Repeated lying and cheating, steals—diagnosis common in prisons
	Emotionally immature—lack of impulse control and low frustration tolerance
	Manipulation of others to fulfill wants and needs
	Resists authority, rules, and laws
	Impulsive, lacks judgment
	Excessive use of drugs, alcohol, and sex
	Uses rationalization to justify behavior
CLUSTER C (FEARFUL–ANXIOUS)	
Dependent personality	Passive, little sense of self-responsibility
	Low self-esteem
	Sees self as stupid and helpless
	Dependent on others to meet needs
	Inability to make decisions

Continues

Table 14-5. PERSONALITY DISORDERS *(Continued)*	
Personality Types	**Profile Characteristics**
Obsessive–compulsive personality	Restricted ability to express warmth toward others—cold, rigid
	Perfectionistic preoccupation with rules, orders, etc.; inflexible and stubborn
	Excessive devotion to work
	Indecisiveness but often high achiever
Avoidant personality	Fears of not being liked or being shamed or ridiculed
	Procrastinates, dawdles, and forgets; avoids interpersonal contact
	Reluctant to take personal risks
	Pervasive pattern of social inhibition, feelings of inadequacy, fear of negative evaluation

PERSONALITY DISORDERS—NOT SPECIFIED

Passive–aggressive disorder	Behavior that is hostile, covered up by passivity and submissiveness
	Manifested by procrastination, forgetfulness, inefficiency, lateness, and deniability
Repressive personality disorder	Unhappy, gloomy people who get no joy out of life
	Pessimistic about the future
	Low self-esteem

4. Involve client in the treatment plan.
5. Give support by being nonpunitive.

C. Reduce client's anxiety associated with interpersonal interactions.
 ✦ 1. Avoid power struggles—do not argue with the client; arguing increases anxiety and hostility.
 2. Do not proceed too quickly with one-to-one nurse–client relationship. Remember that a paranoid client is suspicious and mistrustful of others.
 3. Be consistent and honest in approaches to client.
✦ D. Help differentiate delusion from reality (refer to section on delusions).
 1. Do not explain away false ideas. Ideas are real to the client.
 2. Avoid any attempt to disagree with delusion, as this action may reinforce it.
 3. Use reality testing when possible.
 4. Focus on reality situations in the environment.
 5. Attempt to engage in activities that require concentration.

MOOD (AFFECTIVE) DISORDERS

Bipolar Affective Disorders

Definition: A group of mood disorders that include manic, hypomanic and mixed episodes as well as depressed and cyclothymic episodes.

Manic Episode of Bipolar Affective Disorder
 ✦ *Definition:* One manifestation of an affective disorder that involves mood swings of elation, euphoria, and grandiose behavior.

Characteristics
A. Specific etiology is unknown. May be related to a genetic predisposition to illness or to increased levels of dopamine and norepinephrine in the brain. Attempts are now being made to discover why lithium is therapeutic in hopes of solving the mystery of manic illness.
B. Women experience this illness slightly more frequently than men. The lifetime risk of developing this illness is 1 to 2 percent of the population.
C. The first manic episode usually occurs before age 30 and, interestingly, is more common in the higher socioeconomic group.

Cyclothymic Disorder
A. Category of bipolar disorder but a milder form—no severe manic or major depressive episodes.
B. Diagnosis is after client has evidenced chronic mood swings from hypomanic to depressive episodes for 2 years.

Hypomanic Disorder—Bipolar II: one or more hypomanic episodes and a number of depressive episodes
 ✦ A. Mild elation, euphoria, "high"—a less extreme form of mania.
B. Mood swings are not severe enough to require hospitalization.
C. Therapeutic intervention and medication usually not necessary—unless mood swings interfere with lifestyle.

Mixed Disorder (Manic–Depressive)—Bipolar I: one or more manic episodes and one or more depressive episodes
A. Both manic and depressive episodes are experienced almost every day for a 3-week period.
B. Episodes are severe and require hospitalization.

Assessment: Manic Episode

✦ A. Assess which stage of mania client is experiencing.
  1. *Mild elation:* difficult to detect, as it may not progress. Persons are often referred to as "hypo-manics."
     a. Affect: feelings of happiness, freedom from worry, confidence, and noninhibition.
     b. Thought: rapid association of ideas but with little evidence of introspection.
     c. Behavior: increased motor activity (person always "on the go") and increased sexual drive.
  ✦ 2. *Acute manic episode:* symptoms more intensified and observable. Client usually requires hospitalization.
     ✦ a. Mood disturbance and lability: mood is one of excessive euphoria. Expansive toward others, enthusiastic, and intrusive. Mood may change to one of irritability, annoyance, and even rage and violence. Mood swings may last for hours or days.
     ✦ b. Hyperactivity: motor restlessness and overindulgence in recreational, sexual, and other activities. Engages in sexual indiscretions and poor money management. Client uses poor judgment in planning and starting projects and is overoptimistic and unrealistic. Evidences disturbed sleep patterns, often going without sleep for days.
     ✦ c. Flight of ideas and pressured speech: manic clients jump from one idea to another, using puns, jokes, and nuances in a continuous flow of loose and accelerated speech. Often, speech is loud, rapid, and inappropriate.
     ✦ d. Distractibility: manic clients overly respond to environmental stimuli, switching focus rapidly from one stimulus to another.
     e. Distortion of self-esteem: grandiose perceptions of one's importance is common with an inflated self-esteem. Often this characteristic is manifested in delusions of grandeur (special relationship with God or the president).
  3. *Delirium:* state of extreme excitement. Person is disoriented, incoherent, agitated, and frenetic.
     a. May experience visual or olfactory hallucinations.
     b. Exhaustion, dehydration, injury, and death are real dangers and must be prevented by the nurse.
 B. Determine if client requires hospitalization (depends on range of symptoms).
 C. Assess physical health.

  1. Poor sleep habits and no apparent fatigue.
  2. Poor nutrition.
  3. Poor or even bizarre habits of grooming.

Implementation

✦ A. Maintain a safe environment.
  1. Reduce external stimuli: noise, people, and motion.
  2. Avoid competitive activities. (Mild exercise, group singing, and swimming are examples of therapeutic activities.)
  3. Redirect energy into short, useful activities.
✦ B. Establish a nurse–client relationship.
  1. Maintain accepting, nonjudgmental attitude and create conditions where trust can develop in the relationship.
  2. Avoid entering into client's playful, joking activity.
  3. Allow client to verbalize feelings, especially hostility.
✦ C. Set realistic limits on behavior.
  1. Provide scope and limitations to behavior for a sense of security.
  2. Anticipate destructive behavior and set limits.
  3. Be firm and consistent.
  4. Involve client in setting own limits.
     a. Gives client sense of control.
     b. Client fears inability to control own behavior.
 D. Give attention to physical needs.
  1. Provide a high-calorie diet with vitamin supplements.
  2. Ensure adequate rest and sleep.
 E. Limit decision making during acute phase.

Depressive Episode of Bipolar Disorder
See Depressive Disorders below.

Schizoaffective Disorder
See page 781.

Depressive Disorders

✦ *Definition:* Another manifestation of affective disorder; symptoms range from a dysphoric, down mood that is mild and only slightly debilitating to a pathological condition of overwhelming intensity and long duration. This disorder may be chronic or episodic but it involves no episodes of elation.

Characteristics

✦ A. The most common of all psychiatric illnesses, 10 times more common than bipolar disorder. Depression is a symptom probably experienced by 15 out of 100 adults in our society.

B. Most common age for adult onset is between ages 25 and 44.

C. One cause is now thought to involve a genetic link; other possible causes are personality traits such as low self-esteem, neurochemical imbalances, and other biological factors.

✦ D. Most acute depressive episodes are self-limiting and last from a few weeks (with treatment) to a few months.

E. More than half of those persons who experience a first episode go on to suffer a recurrence.

F. About 20 to 25 percent never return to their premorbid state of mental health.

Major Depression/Unipolar Disorder

A. General characteristics.
   1. May be a single episode or recurrent (2 or more) episodes.
   ✦ 2. Symptoms of a major depressive episode usually develop over a period of days to weeks and represent a change in previous functioning.
   3. Episode may begin at any age and is twice as common in women.
   4. The clinical picture of depression varies considerably, with no single symptom present in all clinical profiles.

✦ B. Affective symptoms.
   ✦ 1. Distinguished from grief reactions: normal, self-limited reaction to obvious loss is labeled grief. Grief reactions are usually brief and milder than pathological depression.
   ✦ 2. Majority of depressed people experience prolonged periods of sadness, feeling down, gloomy, or unhappy. This depressed mood tends to color the whole of a person's life; it is pervasive and dominant.
   ✦ 3. Loss of motivation: loss of interest in life and activities, feelings of hopelessness and helplessness, and suicidal thoughts.
      a. Suicide is the most serious complication.
      b. One percent kill themselves within 1 year. In recurrent depression, 15 percent eventually commit suicide.
      c. The highest risk is the 6- to 9-month period after some improvement.
   ✦ 4. Vegetative behavior: related to physical problems that include loss of energy, loss of libido, psychomotor retardation, or agitation. Individual experiences sleep problems (insomnia is more common) and appetite disturbance, usually anorexia.
   ✦ 5. Cognitive problems: persistent low self-esteem is present, difficulty in concentrating, poor memory, and apparent occupation with inner

thoughts. A pervasive sense of guilt and worthlessness is also present.

   6. Physical complaints: a series of bodily complaints often accompany this illness, ranging from headaches and backaches to constipation and chest pain.

Dysthymic Disorder

✦ A. Characterized by a chronic depressive syndrome (mild to moderate in degree) that is usually present for most of the day:
   1. Symptoms are present for at least 2 years.
   2. Depression may be episodic or constant.

B. Psychosis is not present.

C. Significant distress in social and occupational functioning.

D. Several of the following symptoms are usually present with this diagnosis.
   1. Low energy level.
   2. Loss of interest in pleasurable activities.
   3. Pessimistic attitude toward the future; thoughts of suicide.
   4. Tearful, crying demeanor.
   5. Feelings of low self-esteem.
   6. Decreased ability to concentrate.

Assessment-Depression Episode

✦ A. Assess mood level (affect is sad, gloomy, or unhappy), and establish diagnosis of depression.

✦ B. Evaluate behavior (slowed actions, diminished purposeful movement, and neglect of personal appearance).

✦ C. Assess thought processes (slowed down until there is a paucity of thinking).

✦ D. Evaluate attitudes (pessimistic and self-denigrating; focus is on the problems and uselessness of life).

E. Assess physical symptoms.
   1. Usually a preoccupation with body and poor health.
   2. Weight loss.
   3. Insomnia.
   4. General malaise.

F. Determine social interaction patterns, which are reduced and inappropriate.
   1. Feelings of isolation.
   2. No contribution to interpersonal relationships.

G. Evaluate potential for suicide and perform suicide lethality assessment.

Implementation

✦ A. Provide a safe milieu and protect the client from self-injury (prevent suicide).

✦ B. Provide a structured environment to mobilize the client.
   1. Allow time for daily activities.

2. Stimulate recreational activity.
3. Reactivate interests outside of the client's concerns.
4. Motivate client for treatment.
5. Introduce psychotherapy and occupational therapy.

✦ C. Build trust through a one-to-one relationship.
  1. Employ a supportive, unchallenging approach.
  2. Use accepting, nonjudgmental attitude and behavior.
  3. Show interest; listen and give positive reinforcement.
  4. Redirect the client's monologue away from painful depressing thoughts.
  5. Focus on the client's underlying anger and encourage expression of it.

D. Build the client's ego assets to increase his or her self-esteem.
  1. Lower standards to create successful experiences.
  2. Limit decision making with the severely depressed.
  3. Support use of defenses to alleviate suffering.

E. Be attentive to the client's physical needs: provide adequate nutrition, sleep, and exercise.

F. Monitor ECT treatments if ordered. *See* page 785.

For Alternative Therapies (e.g., St. John's wort for depression), *see* Herb–Drug Interaction Table in Chapter 5, Pharmacology, Table 5-1.

Suicide

Definition: Suicide is an act or instance of intentionally killing oneself. Fifteen percent of client with mood disorder commit suicide.

Characteristics

✦ A. Suicide is the seventh most common cause of death for all ages in the United States today and the second cause of death among college students.

✦ B. Suicide statistics are probably low because of unknown cases such as car accidents.

  1. Suicide ranks fourth as the cause of death in the 15 to 40 age group.
  2. For every successful suicide, it is believed that there are five to ten attempted suicides.
  3. Women make more suicide attempts than men. Four times as many men as women actually commit suicide.
  4. Suicide is increasing in the adolescent and elderly age groups.

C. Factors that contribute to suicide attempts.
  ✦ 1. The single most common cause is depression; alcohol is the second most common cause.
  2. Another common cause is that individuals feel overwhelmed by problems in living.
  3. A final cause may be the attempt to control others.

✦ D. Depressed clients, when severely ill, rarely commit suicide.
  1. They do not have the drive and energy to make a plan and follow it through when severely depressed.
  2. Danger period occurs when depression begins to lift.

✦ E. Eight out of ten known cases give warnings or messages through direct or indirect means.

F. Accompanying symptoms range from depression, disorientation and defiance to intense dependence on another.

Assessment

✦ A. Recognize level of depression and potential for suicide (when depression begins to lift).

✦ B. Determine presence of suicide ideation.

C. Observe behavior closely as clues to potential suicide.

D. Listen to verbalization to determine what is meaningful for client.

E. Observe physical status so you can intervene if necessary (if client is not eating, sleeping, etc.).

F. Recognize ambivalence when client is considering suicide.

Implementation

✦ A. Client safety is the first priority—provide a safe environment to protect client from self-destruction.

✦ B. Observe client closely at all times, especially when depression is lifting.

✦ C. Establish a supportive relationship, letting client know you are concerned for his or her welfare.

D. Encourage expression of feelings, especially anger.

✦ E. Ask relevant questions that relate to potential suicide ideation (ideas): "Do you wish you were dead?" "Did you think you might do something about it? What?" "Have you taken any steps to prepare? What are they?"

F. Evaluate the lethality of a suicide plan (specificity of details, lethality of proposed method, and availability of means).

G. Recognize a continued desire to commit suicide by the client.

H. Focus on client's strengths and successful experiences to increase client's self-esteem.

I. Provide a structured schedule and involve client in activities with others.

J. Structure a plan for client to use as a means of coping when next confronted with suicide ideation.

K. Help client plan for continued professional support after discharge.

SUBSTANCE-RELATED DISORDERS

Definition: Substance dependence includes any process by which an individual ingests any mind-altering, non-prescribed chemical that produces physiological and/or psychological dependence. Withdrawal symptoms are usually manifested when the substance is not taken.

Characteristics

A. Psychological dependence: emotional dependence, desire, or compulsion to continue taking the substance or drug to experience "normal" functioning.

B. Tolerance: the need for greatly increased amounts of the substance to achieve the desired effect.

C. Physiological dependence: physical need for the substance manifested by appearance of withdrawal symptoms when the substance is withheld.

D. Withdrawal from substance causes substance-specific syndrome—leads to impairment in areas of functioning.

Alcohol Abuse

Definition: The abuse of any alcoholic substance combined with physical and psychological addiction.

Characteristics

A. Alcohol consumption is permitted by law and supported by most people in our society as a recreational activity.

B. A fine line exists between the social drinker and the addicted or problem drinker.

C. The greatest difference involves the degree of compulsion to drink and the inability to survive the trials of everyday living without the ingestion of alcohol.

D. Alcoholism, the third largest health problem in the United States (heart disease and cancer rank first and second), affects 10 million people.

E. Alcoholism is involved in about 30,000 deaths and one-half million injuries (auto accidents) every year.

F. The legal definition of intoxication in most states is 0.10 percent or more blood alcohol level (in California, it is 0.08 percent).

G. Alcoholism decreases life span 10 to 12 years.

H. Fifteen percent of alcoholics commit suicide compared to 1 percent of the general population.

I. Loss to industry caused by alcoholism is estimated at $15 billion a year (affecting primarily the 35 to 55 age group) and overall costs of alcohol-related problems is estimated to be over $70 billion per year.

J. Major U.S. social concern is the dramatic rise in teenage alcoholism (estimated to affect 3 million adolescents).

Dynamics of Alcoholism

A. Alcoholic disease implies the consumption of alcohol to the point where it interferes with the individual's physical, emotional, and social functioning.
   1. The syndrome consists of two phases: problem drinking and alcohol addiction.
   2. Dependence on other drugs is very common.

B. A genetic or familial predisposition to dependence may exist. Genetically determined genes determine the type of dependence an individual may develop.
   1. Genetic influences are the same for both men and women.
   2. Children of alcoholics have a four times higher risk of becoming alcoholic.

C. Alcohol blocks synaptic transmission, depresses the central nervous system (CNS), and releases inhibitions. It acts initially as a stimulant but is actually a depressant.
   1. Chronic excessive use can lead to brain damage (sedative effect on CNS).
   2. High blood levels may cause malfunctions in cardiovascular and respiratory systems.

D. Psychological effects of alcohol appear to be the gratification of oral impulses and the reduction of superego forces; abuse leads to shame and guilt and impaired ego formation.

E. Alcohol may be said to be a defense against overwhelming psychological needs and conflicts; therefore, the client needs to work on problems causing his or her distress.

F. Illnesses associated with chronic alcoholism.
   1. Wernicke-Korsakoff's syndrome (related to thiamine deficiency).
   2. Delirium tremens.
   3. Chronic gastritis.
   4. Malnutrition resulting in beriberi, pellagra, cerebellar degeneration, and anemia.
   5. Laënnec's cirrhosis, hepatitis, and fatty liver.

6. Peripheral neuropathy (related to vitamin B deficiency).
7. Osteoporosis.
8. Individual is prone to infection.
9. Blood dyscrasias.
10. Sexual dysfunction.

Personality Characteristics of an Alcoholic

✦ A. Dependent personality with resentment toward authority.
B. High self-expectations and low frustration tolerance.
C. Life usually characterized by patterns of failure.
D. False sense of success, power, and confidence from use of alcohol.
E. Apparent need to ease suffering, reduce anxiety, and cope with life stresses through use of alcohol.
F. Decreased ability to function intellectually, emotionally, and socially as need for alcohol increases.
G. Difficulty in interpersonal relationships.
H. Tendency to work, play, and engage in sex more than is normal.
I. Risk-taking propensity.

Assessment

✦ A. Assess inability to control alcohol consumption.
1. Episodic drinking.
2. Continuous excessive drinking.
3. Sneaking drinks.
4. Morning drinking.
5. Blackouts.
6. Arguments about drinking.
7. Absence at work or school due to hangovers and drinking episodes.
8. Difficulty with interpersonal relationships due to drinking habits.
9. Alcohol-related police record.
B. Recognize physical condition due to improper nutrition.
1. Cirrhosis.
2. Anemia.
3. Peripheral neuropathy.
4. Brain damage.
5. Delirium tremens.
C. Evaluate accidents or physical injuries caused by intoxication.
D. Determine level of acute intoxication.
1. Drowsiness, ataxia, nystagmus.
2. Respiratory depression, stupor, possible coma, and death.

Alcohol Withdrawal Symptoms

A. Hangover: mild alcohol withdrawal (usually the day after); symptoms include headache, nausea, vomiting, restlessness, irritability and the "shakes."

B. General withdrawal symptoms from heavy drinking.
1. Nausea and vomiting.
2. Insomnia.
3. Anorexia.
4. Anxiety.
5. Hyperalertness and irritablity.
6. Restlessness.
7. Chronic tremors of hands, tongue, and eyelids.
8. Malaise and weakness.
9. Sweating.
10. Elevated temperature.
11. Depressed mood.
12. Headache.
C. Delirium tremens: an acute condition usually manifested within 24 to 72 hours after the last ingestion of alcohol. May appear 7 to 10 days later during drinking periods when no food is ingested.
1. Marked tremors/seizures.
2. Hallucinations/illusions.
3. Paranoia.
4. Disorientation and severe agitation.
5. Tachycardia.
6. Tachypnea.
7. Diaphoresis.
8. Diarrhea and vomiting.
9. Convulsions (grand mal).
10. Death (10 to 15 percent from cardiac failure).

Implementation

✦ A. Nursing attitudes.
1. Maintain a nonjudgmental attitude toward the alcoholic.
2. Be firm and consistent in approach.
3. Be accepting toward the individual, not his or her deviant behavior.
4. Be supportive of attempts to change life patterns.
✦ B. Acute treatment phase.
1. Provide adequate diet and fluid intake.
2. Provide vitamin therapy, especially vitamin B_6 and B complex.
3. Administer some type of tranquilizers as ordered, usually Valium.
4. Institute measures to control nausea and insomnia.
5. Observe signs of infection or physiological problems.
6. Promote rest.
7. Control environment to decrease stimuli.
8. Observe vital signs.
C. Long-term treatment phase.
✦ 1. Set up a controlled and structured environment until client is able to manage his or her own circumstances.

    a.   Set behavior limits and confront the client who is manipulative.

    b.   Suggest group involvement for the client who experiences loneliness.

    c.   Remember that client needs support, firmness, and a reality-oriented approach.

✦ 2.   Treatment techniques.

    a.   Client must first go through detoxification—acute nursing care to cope with toxic state and return to a nonalcoholic state.

    b.   Help client accept the fact that alcoholism is an illness.

    c.   Help client accept that life must be managed without the support of alcohol.

    d.   Provide psychotherapy techniques such as group and family therapy and nurse–client relationship therapy.

       (1) Focus on the underlying emotional problems.

       (2) Offer assistance in handling anxiety.

       (3) Focus on relieving feelings of inferiority and low self-esteem.

    e.   Provide for rehabilitation or long-term supportive care.

       (1) Have client continue psychotherapy on an outpatient basis.

       (2) Refer client to Alcoholics Anonymous.

       (3) Encourage client to continue taking prescribed medication such as Antabuse (alcohol-sensitizing drug that causes vomiting and cardiovascular symptoms if the person drinks alcohol).

       (4) Suggest social or vocational rehabilitation community programs that are available.

Substance Dependence

Definition: Substance dependence is a state of dependency on drugs other than alcohol or tobacco that involves alteration of perception or mood and is produced by repeated consumption of the drug, causing tolerance to the substance and withdrawal symptoms.

Generalized Personality Characteristics

A. Difficulty forming intimate relationships.

B. Feelings of insecurity and inadequacy.

C. Rebellious toward authority.

D. Self-centered.

E. Copes through escapism.

F. Difficulty with sexuality and sexual identification.

Specific Drug Addictions

✦ A. Opioid addiction.

    1. The most common types of opioids are heroin, morphine and OxyContin.

    2. Emotional dependence on the drug (to alter mood) occurs first, followed by physical dependence on the drug.

    3. Opioids (narcotics) have a sedative effect on the CNS.

    4. Tolerance level increases, so greater amounts of the drug are necessary to produce pleasurable effects.

    5. Addiction tends to be chronic, with a high rate of relapse.

    6. Withdrawal symptoms.

       a. Anxiety.

       b. Nausea and vomiting.

       c. Sneezing, yawning, watery eyes, and runny nose.

       d. Tremor and profuse perspiration.

       e. Stomach cramps and dehydration.

       f. Convulsions and coma.

✦ B. Sedative–hypnotics addiction.

    1. Common drugs include Librium, Valium, Quaalude, Seconal, Nembutal, and sodium amytal.

    2. Barbiturates have CNS sedative effect—danger of death from overdose and withdrawal.

    3. Psychological dependence occurs, followed by tolerance and physical dependence.

    4. Drug may have been prescribed for relief of chronic pain or sleeplessness.

    5. Individual usually has emotional problems and an anxious temperament.

    6. Sudden withdrawal of barbiturates may result in acute psychosis, seizures, and death.

    7. Overdoses and acute withdrawal from barbiturates are medical emergencies and require hospitalization.

✦ C. Amphetamines, benzedrine, and dexedrine.

    1. All produce a "high."

    2. All are CNS stimulants, so overuse may result in brain damage, capillary bleeding, and death.

    3. Large doses produce a hyperactive and agitated state.

    4. Amphetamines are emotionally addictive, especially for persons with insecure, inadequate personalities.

    5. Amphetamines affect individual's physical condition as the drug reduces appetite and awareness of body needs.

D. Lysergic acid diethylamide (LSD)—"acid."

    1. LSD is a hallucinogenic drug and mimics hallucinations seen in psychoses.

2. LSD produces changes in perception and logical thought processes.

3. Drug not considered addictive per se, but individuals may become emotionally dependent on it.

4. Experiences with LSD range from ecstasy to terror, and the results are unpredictable.

E. Cannabis (marijuana).

1. Marijuana was considered to have low abuse potential but now most professionals agree that this is not the case.

2. It produces a "dreamy" state and feelings of euphoria, hilarity, and well-being.

3. Moods vary according to environmental stimuli.

4. Marijuana changes perception of space and time, which seem distorted and extendible.

5. High dosage may produce hallucinations and delusions.

◆ F. Cocaine.

1. Cocaine is classified as a stimulant.

2. Usual method of ingestion is by sniffing, IV, or smoking.

3. Use may cause strong psychological dependence.

4. Most professionals believe use does develop physical dependence or tolerance.

5. Chronic users often abuse or are dependent on a narcotic, alcohol, or antianxiety drug to lessen the withdrawal symptoms of cocaine.

G. Crack.

1. The most addictive drug known; a form of hydrochloride cocaine.

2. It is smoked in cigarettes or glass water pipes.

3. Crack is cheap and rapidly addictive because there is a rapid high, then a "downer" that makes the person desire more crack.

4. Symptoms include paranoia, depression, and physical symptoms.

H. Phencyclidine (PCP)—"crystal," "elephant tranquilizer," "angel dust."

1. PCP is usually smoked with marijuana. It may also be ingested, injected, taken intravenously, or sniffed.

2. Reactions vary from a sense of well-being to acute anxiety to total disorientation and hallucinations.

3. PCP is considered an extremely dangerous "street" drug.

4. Psychological dependence may occur.

5. Cardinal signs of PCP use are blank stare, ataxia, muscle rigidity, nystagmus, and tendency toward violence.

6. Cerebral cellular destruction and atrophy occur with even small amounts.

7. Overdoses or "bad trips" are characterized by erratic, unpredictable behavior; withdrawal symptoms; disorientation; self-mutilation; or self-destructive behavior.

8. Overdoses are treated with sedatives, decreased environmental stimuli, and protecting client from harming self and others. Cannot be "talked down."

Assessment

A. Establish name and action of drug used.

B. Assess when addiction or abuse began in client's life.

C. Determine amount of drug used.

D. Determine other drugs used.

E. Assess physical condition of client by physical exam and blood and urine lab work.

F. Assess psychological network in which client lives.

G. Evaluate rehabilitative potential and support systems.

Implementation

◆ A. Support client during heroin withdrawal, which is the first step in treatment and may be accomplished abruptly ("cold turkey") or gradually over a period of days.

◆ B. Administer substitute drug (methadone, a synthetic nacotic) for heroin addiction, if ordered, to reduce the physical reaction to withdrawal.

C. Provide prolonged medical and psychiatric treatment for physical and emotional deterioration as part of convalescence.

D. Encourage client to take advantage of resocialization programs by professional or community resources.

E. Provide client with information concerning rehabilitation programs designed to help client reenter the mainstream of society.

1. Various self-help groups offer aid in rehabilitation.

2. Therapeutic communities and group therapy programs also provide rehabilitation.

◆ F. Provide support to client during "bad trips," acute anxiety, and panic reactions to drug experience.

1. Place client in a quiet, safe environment with a person to "talk them through" the experience for LSD.

2. Reassure client that this reaction is drug caused and of short duration.

3. Provide careful reality orientation by nurse.

4. Use nonthreatening, supportive approach.

5. Reassure client that he or she will not be allowed to harm himself or herself.

6. Refer client to drug counseling when the experience is over.

COGNITIVE IMPAIRMENT DISORDERS

◆ *Definition:* Cognitive disorders are psychiatric disorders with organic etiology that may be reversible (delirium) or irreversible (dementia), and include clinically significant deficits in cognition or memory that result in significant changes in a client's level of functioning and disturbed behavior.

Delirium

Characteristics

◆ A. Characterized by a disturbance or fluctuation of consciousness and a change in cognition that develops over a short period.
 B. Approximately 10 percent of all hospitalized elderly have delirium.
 C. Global intellectual impairment with rapid onset.
 D. Thinking, memory, attention, and perception are disturbed and impaired, but may vary—is not stable.
◆ E. Condition may last hours or weeks; usually resolves in a few days.
◆ F. Etiology.
   1. Any acute disease or injury that interferes with cerebral function and often is temporary and reversible.
   2. Includes infections, circulatory disturbances, metabolic and endocrine disorders, neoplasms, and tumors.
   3. Injuries include brain trauma, invasive trauma.
   4. Other causes are toxic exposure, drugs, or systemic intoxication.

Assessment

 A. Assess for clouding of consciousness—a cardinal symptom.
◆ B. Assess for intellectual deficits and changes.
   1. Recent memory loss.
   2. Poor abstract thinking.
   3. Poor problem-solving ability.
◆ C. Assess for presence of hallucinations (visual most common), delusions, and confusion.
◆ D. Assess for loss of contact with reality.
   1. Inattentive and distractible.
   2. Disorientation to time and place, but not usually to person.
 E. Check for increased motor activity with no defined purpose (groping, sudden movements).
 F. Assess emotional stability.
   1. Reactions are blunted.
   2. Fearful.
   3. Apathetic.
   4. Anxious.
   5. Euphoric.

 G. Assess alterations in adjustment: tend to be worse at night, more fearful, moaning and calling out.

Implementation

 A. Provide adequate nutritional and fluid intake as ordered by treatment plan.
◆ B. Keep client in a quiet, structured environment.
 C. Observe and monitor vital signs as necessary.
◆ D. Keep siderails up and use restraints as necessary to protect client.
 E. Implement treatment plan for elimination of causative factors.
 F. Provide reality orientation approach with client.
 G. Set limits on inappropriate behavior.
◆ H. Express directions in a simple and concrete manner.
 I. Observe client for signs of fever, shock, and increased intracranial pressure such as restlessness, acute anxiety, pain, and changes in vital signs.
 J. Reassure and involve family as is appropriate.
 K. Involve client in rehabilitation program as necessary.

Dementia

Characteristics

◆ A. Organic condition characterized by development of multiple cognitive deficits.
◆ B. Common cognitive disturbances include at least one of the following: aphasia, apraxia (impaired ability to carry out motor activities, despite intact motor function), agnosia (loss of sensory ability to recognize objects), or a disturbance in executive functioning.
   1. Finds it difficult to think abstractly and to plan, initiate, sequence, and monitor complex behavior.
   2. Causes difficulties in social and occupational functioning.
◆ C. Insidious onset but slow, progressive deterioration occurs.
 D. Etiology is specifically unknown: results from wide variety of sources.
   1. *Prenatal causes:* congenital cranial anomaly, congenital spastic paraplegia.
   2. *Infection:* central nervous system, syphilis, meningoencephalitis, human immunodeficiency virus (HIV).
   3. *Intoxication:* drug or poison, alcohol.
   4. *Trauma:* brain trauma by gross force, brain surgery.
   5. *Circulatory disorder:* cerebral arteriosclerosis.
   6. *Disturbance of innervation:* convulsions.
   7. *Disturbances of metabolism, growth, or nutrition.*
      a. Senile brain disease: dementia.
      b. Glandular problems.
      c. Pellagra.
   8. *New growths:* brain neoplasm.

Table 14-6. DELIRIUM VERSUS DEMENTIA		
	Delirium	**Dementia**
Onset	Acute, rapid onset of impairment	Insidious onset—slow deterioration
Etiology	Interference with cerebral function Could be caused by injury, infection, metabolic, chemical or toxic exposure	Unknown, but may result from a variety of sources (prenatal, infection, circulatory, trauma, growth, etc.)
Progression	Reversible—lasts hours or weeks, usually resolves in few days	Irreversible—slow, progressive deterioration
Primary Characteristics	Cloudy state of consciousness	Multiple cognitive deficits

Types of Degenerative Conditions

Dementia, Alzheimer's Type (DAT)

✦ A. Most common form of dementia: accounts for almost 50 percent of known cases (about 4 million in the United States).
  1. One in 10 persons over age 65 has Alzheimer's disease.
  2. By 2050, over 14 million will develop this disease.
✦ B. Unknown etiology but diffuse atrophy of cerebral cortex occurs.
  C. Usually begins after age 60 but can be observed at age 40. DAT average course is 5 to 10 years.
  D. Symptoms gradually and progressively worsen.
  E. Clients may live for 10 years but will eventually progress to requiring total care.
  F. Three clinical stages of DAT.
  1. Early stage: client is forgetful, confused, irritable; family begins to notice changes.
  2. Middle stage: increased memory loss, recall of recent events diminishes, ADLs become difficult to accomplish. Aggressiveness and social inappropriateness present. Wandering increases.
  3. Late state: severely disoriented, delusional and paranoid. Client may not speak, forgets family members and soon becomes helpless.

Pick's Disease

✦ A. Rare heredodegenerative process of frontal lobe not associated with normal aging.
  B. Becomes well advanced in 2 to 3 years.
✦ C. Characterized by changes in personality early in course of illness.
  D. Similar to Alzheimer's disease but involvement spares parietal lobes.
  E. These clients act dull and lack initiative; otherwise, their disease resembles Alzheimer's disease.

Huntington's Chorea

✦ A. Genetically transmitted disorder caused by a single autosomal dominant gene.
  B. Onset of symptoms—age 40 to 50 years.

  C. Progressive mental and physical deterioration inevitable.
  D. Characterized by personality changes with psychotic behavior, intellectual impairment, and, finally, total dementia.

Korsakoff's Syndrome

✦ A. A disorder that occurs in chronic alcoholism and is often associated with Wernicke's encephalopathy.
  ✦ 1. Wernicke's encephalopathy.
    a. Acute, life-threatening neurologic condition that can occur as a result of chronic alcoholism (inadequate diet leading to thiamine deficiency).
    b. Usual symptoms are cloudy consciousness, impaired mentation, ataxia, peripheral neuropathy.
    c. Treatment is oral vitamin B complex and thiamine 100 mg IM STAT if client presents with the above symptoms and has a history of alcohol abuse.
  2. Korsakoff's syndrome is a chronic condition that remains after Wernicke's encephalopathy is treated.
✦ B. Most important feature is recent memory impairment, especially in learning new information.
  1. Confabulation (making up stories) accompanies memory impairment.
  2. Memories for past events are not usually affected.
✦ C. Syndrome improves with adequate diet (especially including vitamin B complex and thiamine) but only 25 percent recover fully.

Vascular Dementia

  A. Type of dementia involving intermittent emboli or infarcts that destroy brain tissue. (Also called ischemic vascular dementia.)
  B. This form accounts for about 19% of dementias.
  C. Characteristics include abrupt onset with numerous remissions and exacerbations; client may also have a history of diseases affecting other organs.

Creutzfeldt–Jakob Disease (CJD)

A. Suspected to be caused by an infection of a prion spread after transplant (cornea) or injection of human growth hormone.
B. A new variant of this disease known as mad cow disease (bovine spongiform encephalopathy [BSE]) was identified in 1996 and may be linked to eating contaminated beef.

Dementia with Lewy Bodies (DLB)

A. This form of dementia is named for the development of Lewy bodies in the cerebral cortex.
   1. The appearance of Parkinsonism symptoms caused by effects on the extrapyramidal tract of the CNS.
   2. Symptoms include intermittent confusion, lapses of consciousness and psychiatric problems.
B. Clients may have this form of dementia alone (less common) or concurrent with DAT (20 to 30 percent).

Dementia Due to HIV Disease

A. Presence of a dementia that is a direct consequence of HIV disease.
B. Involves diffuse, multifocal destruction of white matter and subcortical structures.
C. Characterized by forgetfulness, slowness, poor concentration, difficulties with problem solving, and hallucinations.

Assessment

A. Assess onset, which is generally slow.
B. Evaluate if illness is stabilized or in remission.
C. Assess for increasing deterioration.
D. Look for the following symptoms:
   ✦ 1. Cognitive impairment.
      a. Disorientation.
      b. Severe loss of memory.
      c. Judgment impairment.
      d. Loss of capacity to learn.
      e. Perceptual disturbances.
      f. Decreased attention span.
      g. Paranoid ideation.
   ✦ 2. Cognitive impairment.
      a. Decreased motivation, interests, and self-concern.
      b. Loss of normal inhibitions.
      c. Loss of insight.
   ✦ 3. Affective impairment.
      a. Labile mood, irritableness, and explosiveness.
      b. Depression.
      c. Withdrawal.
      d. Anxiety.
   ✦ 4. Behavioral impairment.
      ✦ a. *Sundowning*—a syndrome of restlessness, confusion and disorientation that typi-cally begins in late afternoon and gradually worsens. Clients wander or exhibit other aberrant motor activities (such as pacing).
      b. Ritualistic, stereotyped behavior to deal with environment.
      c. Possible combativeness.
      d. Possible inappropriate and regressive behavior.
      e. Alterations in sexual drives and activity.
      f. Neurotic or psychotic behavior as client's defenses break down.
E. Assess psychological reactions to organic brain disorder.
   1. Change in self-concept.
   2. Anger and frustration as reactions to forced change in life role.
   3. Denial used as defense.
   4. Depression.
   5. Acceptance of limitations.
   6. Assumption of "sick" role by dependency and lack of motivation.

Implementation

✦ A. Meet client's physical needs.
   1. Avoid fostering dependence.
   2. Establish routine for activities of daily living.
✦ B. Help client maintain contact with reality.
   1. Give feedback.
   2. Avoid small chatter.
   3. Personalize interaction.
   4. Supply stimulation to motivate client.
   5. Keep client from becoming bored and distracted.
C. Assist client in accepting the diagnosis.
   1. Be supportive.
   2. Maintain therapeutic communication.
   3. During denial phase, listen and accept; do not argue.
   4. Assist development of awareness.
   5. Help client develop the ability to cope with his or her altered identity.
✦ D. Focus interactions with client and establish consistent contact.
   1. Have short, frequent contacts with client.
   2. Use concrete ideas in communicating with client.
   ✦ 3. Maintain reality orientation by allowing client to talk about his or her past and to *confabulate*—filling in memory gap with a made-up response (lie) to protect one's self-esteem.
   4. Acknowledge client as an individual.
✦ E. Provide activities that increase success of client.
   1. Social groups.

2. Occupational therapy.
3. Allow client, as interested, to do small chores around unit.

F. Monitor medications for dementia management.
   1. Acetylcholinesterase inhibitors.
      a. Inhibits the enzyme acetylcholinesterase, which slows the breakdown of acetylcholine, thereby allowing more information to be transmitted from one cell to another.
      b. Memory and general cognitive activity increases, thus slowing the progression of dementia, especially early in the process of the disease.
      c. Commonly used drugs in the category are donepezil (Aricept), which slows breakdown of brain chemical acetylcholine vital for transmission of nerve signals, revastigmine (Exelon), and galantamine (Reminyl).
      d. These drugs have both positive and negative results and must be individualized for the client.
   2. Depressive symptoms for dementia.
      a. SSRIs appear to be more efficacious (Celexa, Prozac, Paxil and Zoloft).
      b. Evidence fewer side effects than other antidepressants.
   3. Psychosis and dementia.
      a. If psychotic thoughts are a problem for clients, drugs are required.
      b. When psychosis is associated with violence or dangerous behavior, Haldol (0.5 mg or more) is indicated.
      c. For chronic aggressive behavior, Risperdal (2–6 mg) is effective.
      d. Seroquel is also effective and does not worsen cognition.
   4. Anger and aggression.
      a. For an acute episode, Haldol may be recommended.
      b. For gradually evolving tendencies, Depakote (125 mg BID increasing to 1500 mg daily) may be administered.

✦ G. Provide supportive environment.
   1. Ensure a consistent staff and environmental structure.
   2. Do not change schedule suddenly.
   3. Provide handrails, walkers, wheelchairs, etc., as necessary.
   4. Ensure that the floor is not slippery and that the environment is well lighted.

H. Assess client's disabilities and develop a nursing plan to deal with them.

1. Update conferences with treatment team.
2. Involve client in treatment planning as able.
3. Communicate client needs to rehabilitation team.

I. Involve family and community in treatment and rehabilitation program.
   1. Plan visits by client to social community events.
   2. Encourage family involvement.
   3. Establish communication with family by using a friendly, warm approach.
   4. Encourage and arrange community groups (church groups, volunteer societies, and school groups) to visit on units.
   5. Refer family to support services.

J. Assist client to function at the highest level possible.
   1. Increase self-esteem.
   2. Avoid dependency.
   3. Allow and encourage personalization of client's room and environment.
   4. Dress client in his or her own clothing.
   5. Maintain client's cleanliness: clothes, hair, and person.
   6. Do not isolate client from others on the unit.

SCHIZOPHRENIC DISORDERS

Definition: Schizophrenia is a psychiatric syndrome characterized by thought disturbance, impairment in reality testing, regressive behavior, ineffective communication, and severely impaired interpersonal relationships.

✦ **Characteristics**

A. Schizophrenia may result from many possible factors: genetic constellation and abnormalities in levels of neurotransmitters (the most current theory), individual adaptive patterns, lack of ego development, a deficit in cognitive development, or a biological origin.

B. Ego boundaries are weak and ego is unable to function as mediator between the self and external reality.

C. Regression and repression are considered to be the primary mechanisms of schizophrenia.

D. Major maladaptive disturbances include impaired interpersonal relationships, inappropriate mental and emotional processes, and disturbances in overt behavior patterns.

E. Manifestations of the illness include acute psychosis involving the total personality or a group of symptoms circumscribed to one area of the personality. (*See* Table 14-7.)

F. Schizophrenia is classified into positive and negative symptoms and thought disorganization.

Table 14-7. PROFILE DIFFERENTIATION	
Schizophrenic	**Nonschizophrenic (Anxiety Disorders)**
Major ego impairment. Includes faulty reality testing, delusions, hallucinations (especially auditory)	No grave impairment of reality testing. No hallucinations or delusions
Serious impairment of client's life, including social, vocational, and sexual	Difficulty in relating, but interaction with others is present. Personality usually remains organized
Little insight into problems and behavior. Client generally does not recognize he or she is ill	Some awareness into problems. Keenly feels subjective suffering. Often unconsciously fights any changes in status (getting well)
Severe personality disorganization (e.g., poor judgment, memory, and perceptions)	Less severe disorganization. Can function but with decreased efficiency
May be caused by both physiological or psychological factors	Always a functional disorder; not organic in origin
Usually requires hospitalization and long-term treatment	Usually does not require hospitalization. May require long-term treatment
Maladaptive adjustment mechanisms used in rigid, fixed way. May be seen as severe regression	Suppression and repression used to handle internal conflicts; defenses are largely symbolic
No secondary gain received	Symptoms generally exploited for secondary gain

SCHIZOPHRENIA—POSITIVE AND NEGATIVE SYMPTOMS (DSM-IV-TR)

- Positive symptoms.
  a. Hallucinations.
  b. Delusions.
  c. Disordered speech; loose associations—when one thought does not connect to another or does not make any logical sense.
  d. Bizarre, disordered or hyperactive behavior.
  e. Inappropriate affect.
  f. Suspiciousness.
  g. Hostility.
- Negative symptoms.
  a. Poverty of speech or alogia.
  b. Affective blunting.
  c. Social withdrawal, isolation.
  d. Apathy.
  e. Lack of motivation (avolition).
  f. Anhedonia (inability to experience pleasure)
  g. Attention impairment.
  h. Memory deficit.

Positive Symptoms

Definition: Excessive symptoms not normally present in healthy adults.

A. *Delusions*—fixed misinterpretation of reality; false beliefs maintained despite evidence to the contrary (somatic delusions are false beliefs that something is wrong with the body).

B. *Hallucinations*—unwilled sensory perceptions with no basis in reality; auditory, visual, olfactory, tactile, gustatory.

C. *Disordered speech and behavior.*
  1. Disordered speech includes frequent derailment or incoherence.
  2. Behavior is disorganized—catatonic or random, purposeless.

D. Terms associated with disordered speech or behavior.
  1. *Withdrawal*—adoption of more satisfying regressive behavior; focus on internal world (autism).
  2. *Depersonalization*—feelings of estrangement or unconnectedness of body parts.
  3. *Echolalia*—a condition in which the individual consistently repeats what is heard.
  4. *Echopraxia*—a condition in which the individual mimics what is done.
  5. *Neologism*—term that refers to the coining of a new word.
  6. *Word salad*—communication characterized by jumbled words with no coherent message.

Negative Symptoms

Definition: Loss of normal function normally present in healthy adults.

A. Flat affect—feelings or emotions minimal (i.e., flat, blunted, or inappropriate).

B. Alogia or poverty of speech. Client answers questions with one word, which may signify lack of thoughts.

C. Avolition is when the client is unable to follow goal-directed behavior; this is not the same as laziness.

D. Anhedonia is the inability to experience joy or pleasure in any aspect of life.

E. The previous 4 symptoms can be remembered by the "four As": Affect flattened, Alogia, Avolition, and Anhedonia.

✦ **Schizophrenic Subtypes**
✦ A. *Paranoid type.*
  1. Persecutory or grandiose delusions are prominent; often delusions are part of a system where several delusions fit together.
  2. Extreme suspiciousness and withdrawal are common manifestations.
✦ B. *Catatonic type.*
  1. Secondary symptoms of motor involvement are present.
     a. Underactivity results in bizarre posturing; labeled *waxy flexibility*.
     b. Overactivity leads to agitation.
  2. Negativism: doing the opposite of what is asked.
     a. Rigidity is the simplest form of negativism.
     b. Mute behavior is another form of negativism.
  3. Catatonic excitement—the opposite of mute, withdrawn behavior when client is agitated and out of control.
✦ C. *Disorganized type.*
  1. Flat or inappropriate affect: giggling and silly laughter (formerly labeled *hebephrenia*).
  2. Disorganization of speech.
  3. Disorganized behavior.
  4. Absence of systematized delusions.
✦ D. *Undifferentiated type.*
  1. This type is characterized by a combination of symptoms, none of which discriminates a specific type of disorder.
  2. Flat affect and/or autism is usually present.
  3. Association disorders and thought disturbance, such as delusions or hallucinations, are usually present.
  4. This condition includes other behavioral maladaptations that cannot be otherwise classified.
E. *Residual type.*
  1. A subtype that refers to a client who has had one episode of schizophrenia but now has no positive symptoms.
  2. Negative symptoms are present.

Assessment
✦ A. Assess any disturbance in thought processes.
  1. Client's thoughts are confused and disorganized, and ability to communicate clearly is limited.
  2. Client manifests tangential (off target or off the original point) or circumstantial speech and has problems with symbolic meaning of certain words.
     a. May be very concrete in thinking and demonstrate an inability to think in abstract terms.
     b. May live in a fantasy world, responding to reality in a bizarre or autistic manner, thereby having great difficulty in testing reality.
✦ B. Assess any disturbance in affect.
  1. Client has difficulty expressing emotions appropriately, and subjective emotional experience may be blunted or flattened.
  2. Client has difficulty expressing positive or warm emotions; when they are expressed, it is often in an inappropriate manner.
  3. While client's feelings may seem inappropriate to the thoughts expressed, they are appropriate to the client's inner experience and are meaningful to him.
  4. Client's inappropriate affect makes it difficult to establish close relationships with others.
✦ C. Assess any disordered behavior.
  1. Client's behavior is often disorganized and inappropriate and apparently lacks a purposeful activity.
  2. Client typically lacks motivation or drive to change his or her circumstances; general condition is one of apathy and listlessness.
  3. Client's behavior may appear to be bizarre and extremely inappropriate to the circumstances.
✦ D. Assess any disturbance in interpersonal relationships.
  1. Client typically has great difficulty in relating to others.
     a. Cannot build close relationships; probably has not experienced close, meaningful relationships in the past.
     b. Has difficulty trusting others and experiences fear, ambivalence, and dependency that influence client's relationships with others.
     c. Often learns to protect self from further hurt by maintaining distance, thus experiences lack of warmth, trust, and intimacy.
  2. Client's relationships are impaired by the inability to communicate clearly and to react in an appropriate and empathic manner.

Implementation
✦ A. General approaches.
  1. Establish a nurse–client relationship.
     a. Gradually increase client's social contacts with others.
     b. Build a positive and trusting relationship with client.

c. Provide client with a safe and secure environment.

✦ 2. Stress reality, help client to reality test, to leave his or her fantasy world.
   a. Involve client in reality-oriented activities.
   b. Help client find satisfaction in the external environment.

3. Accept client as he or she is.
   a. Do not invalidate disturbed thoughts or fantasies.
   b. Do not invalidate client by inappropriate responses.

✦ 4. Use therapeutic communication techniques.
   a. Encourage expression of emotions, negative or positive.
   b. Encourage expression of thoughts, fears, and problems.
   c. Attempt to have nonverbal behavior become congruent with verbal communications.
   d. Focus on clear communications with the client.

5. Avoid fostering dependency relationship.

6. Avoid stressful situations or increasing client's anxiety.

7. Use real objects or activities (singing, for example) to distract or redirect delusional client.

8. Decrease client's anxiety level.

9. Use warm, honest, matter-of-fact approach.

10. Recognize that the nurse and others influence client even if client appears unresponsive, remote, and detached at times.

B. Approaches to specific symptoms.
   ✦ 1. *Delusions.*
      a. Encourage client to recognize distorted views of reality.
      b. Focus on client's ego assets, strengths, etc.
      c. Provide a safe, nonthreatening milieu.
      ✦ d. Divert focus from delusional material to reality; involve in games, tasks, simple activities.
      e. Provide experiences in which client can feel success.
      ✦ f. Utilize specific nursing responses:
         (1) Avoid confirming or feeding into delusion.
         (2) Stress reality by denying you believe the client's delusion, but do not invalidate client by saying delusion is not true—for the client, it is true.
         (3) Respond to feelings underlying the content of the delusion. For example, validate the feelings of client by asking, "I sense you are afraid. Is this true?"

✦ 2. *Hallucinations.*
   ✦ a. Provide a safe, structured environment with routine activities.
   b. Protect client from self-injury or hurting others prompted by "voices."
   c. Initiate short, frequent interactions.
      ✦ (1) Respond verbally to anything real that client talks about.
      ✦ (2) Avoid denying or arguing with client about the hallucinations he or she is experiencing.
      ✦ (3) Involve the client in reality-based tasks or activities (i.e., a person cannot sing and hallucinate at the same time).
      (4) Increase client's social interaction gradually from interaction with one person to interaction with small groups as tolerated by client.

✦ 3. *Withdrawn behavior.*
   ✦ a. Assist client to develop satisfying relationships with others.
      ✦ (1) Initiate interaction; do not expect a withdrawn client to seek you out.
      (2) Build a trusting relationship by being consistent in keeping appointments, in attitudes, and in nursing practice.
      (3) Be honest and direct in what you say and do.
      (4) Deal with your own feelings in relation to client's hostility or rejection.
   b. Help client to modify perception of self.
      ✦ (1) Do not structure situation in which client will fail.
      (2) Increase client's self-esteem by focusing on genuine assets or strengths.
      (3) Relieve client from decision making until client is able to make decisions.
   c. Teach client renewal of social skills.
      ✦ (1) Gradually increase social contacts with staff and other clients.
      (2) Increase social contacts with significant others when appropriate.
   d. Focus on reality situations.
      (1) Use a nonthreatening approach.
      (2) Provide safe, nonthreatening milieu.
   e. Attend to physical needs (e.g., nutrition, sleep, exercise, occupational therapy).

C. Approaches to dealing with aggressive or combative behavior.
   ✦ 1. Observe client acutely for clues that client is getting out of control.
      a. Note rising anger—verbal and nonverbal behavior.

b. Note erratic or unpredictable response to staff or other clients.

2. Intervene immediately when loss of control is imminent.

3. Use a nonthreatening approach to client.

4. Set firm limits on unacceptable behavior.

5. Maintain calm manner and do not show fear.

6. Avoid engaging in an argument or provoking client.

7. Summon assistance only when indicated; sudden involvement of many people will increase client's agitation.

8. Remove client from the situation as soon as possible.

9. Use seclusion and/or restraints *only* if necessary.

10. Attempt to calm client so that he or she may regain control.

11. Be supportive and stay with client.

12. Use problem-solving focus following outburst of aggressive or combative behavior.
    a. Encourage discussion of feelings surrounding incident.
    b. Attempt to look at causal factors of the behavior.
    c. Examine client's response to stimulus and alternative responses.
    d. Point out consequences of aggressive behavior.
    e. Discuss client's role of taking responsibility for his or her aggressive behavior.

D. Approaches to dealing with verbally abusive behavior.
1. Do not respond in kind to abusive comments.
2. Do not take abuse personally.
3. Interact with client on a therapeutic basis.
    a. Help client examine his or her feelings.
    b. Do not reject client despite abuse.
    c. Give client feedback concerning your reactions to abusive comments.
    d. Teach alternative ways for client to express his or her feelings.
4. Maintain a calm, accepting approach to client.

E. Approaches to dealing with demanding behavior.
1. Do not ignore demands; they will only increase in intensity. Respond to realistic demands.
2. Attempt to determine causal factors of behavior (e.g., high anxiety level).
3. Set limits when client is demanding.
4. Control own feelings of anger and irritation.
5. Teach alternative means to getting needs met.
6. Plan nursing care to include frequent contacts initiated by the nurse.
7. Alert the staff to try to give client the reassurance he or she needs.

Schizoaffective Disorder

◆ *Definition:* Condition that does not directly fit either schizophrenia or a mood disorder and, thus, is a mixture of symptoms. Illness is characterized by episodes of depression, mania, or both, concurrent with symptoms of schizophrenia.

Charactertistics

A. Client may experience depression, manic or mixed symptoms.

B. Symptoms may include delusions, hallucination, disorganized speech and behavior.

C. Clients often have difficulty functioning in their lives.

Assessment

A. Assess thought processes as similar to schizophrenic disorder.

B. Observe for bizarre behavior and mood disorders ranging from depression to elation (bipolar disorder).

Implementation

◆ A. Clients will be treated according to symptoms manifested—schizophrenic and/or mood disorder.

B. Drug therapy may be either antipsychotic (usually prescribed) or antidepressant drugs.

C. Check implementation section for both schizophrenic and mood disorders.

CHILD PSYCHIATRIC CONDITIONS

Definition: Emotional disturbance in childhood encompassing markedly abnormal or impaired development in social interaction and communication and a marked restricted repertoire of activity and interests.

Pervasive Development Disorders

◆ Characteristics

◆ A. Severe and pervasive impairment in reciprocal social interaction and communication skills.

B. Prevalence rate is 2 to 5 in 10,000; more common in males.

C. In most cases, there is an associated diagnosis of mental retardation.

D. Situational crises such as separation anxiety and developmental deviations are considered in Chapter 13, Pediatric Nursing.

Assessment

A. Assess for presence of somatic manifestations: enuresis or eating or sleeping difficulties.

B. Evaluate for evidence of withdrawn behavior.

✦ C. Assess for presence of autistic behavior.
  1. Assess for bizarre responses, such as rocking, hand movements in the air, fecal smearing.
  2. Evaluate absent or inappropriate language skills.
  3. Evaluate flat or inappropriate affect.
  4. Assess for tantrums or self-destructive behavior, such as head banging.
  5. Identify aggressive behavior toward persons or objects.
  6. Assess for absence of "self" image (e.g., inability to identify parts of the body).

Characteristics

✦ A. Autism is complete self-involvement—withdrawal to an "inner world."
B. It occurs in infancy. While the etiology is not known at this time, a physiological cause is suspected.
C. The Gesell Institute believes inherited cognitive abnormalities or brain damage at birth are possible causes.
D. It is generally thought that the autistic child manifests weak ego boundaries and fails to develop a separate concept of the "self."
E. The autistic child can neither distinguish himself or herself from the world nor distinguish internal from external stimuli.
F. Autism is differentiated from childhood schizophrenia, in which the child has more sense of self and views self as separate from mother.

Implementation

✦ A. Establish a method of relating to the child, either verbal or nonverbal.
  1. Communication is essential for the development of a relationship.
  2. An effective relationship with a mute and/or withdrawn child may be difficult unless the nurse has mastered his or her own feelings.
  3. Genuine concern, warmth, and acceptance must be felt by the nurse toward the child for any interaction to be effective.
✦ B. Teach and support the child to master beginning developmental tasks that were never completed.
C. Give good physical care and protect the child from self-destructive behavior.
D. Set firm limits and be consistent to provide a secure milieu.
E. Provide activities for participation, fun, and re-education according to the developmental level of the child.

Attention Deficit–Hyperactivity Disorder (ADHD)

Definition: Emotional disorder characterized by a persistent pattern of inattention and/or hyperactivity–impulsivity.

Characteristics

✦ A. More common in males; prevalence rates for school children are boys, 17 percent, and girls, 8 percent.
B. Children with this disorder represent 40 to 50 percent of child disorders as inpatients and an even higher percentage as outpatients.
C. Fundamental cognitive deficit responsible for ADHD remains unclear but may involve reduced blood flow to certain areas of the brain.

Assessment

✦ A. Assess for symptoms of inattention that are maladaptive.
  1. Makes careless mistakes.
  2. Difficulty sustaining attention in tasks or play.
  3. Does not listen when spoken to directly.
  4. Has difficulty organizing tasks.
  5. Is easily distracted.
  6. Forgetful in daily activities.
✦ B. Assess for symptoms of hyperactivity–impulsivity.
  1. Fidgets with hands or feet.
  2. Leaves seat when expected to stay seated.
  3. Runs/climbs excessively.
  4. Has difficulty playing quietly.
  5. Constantly "on the go."
  6. Talks excessively.
C. Assess symptoms of impulsivity.
  1. Blurts out answers before question is completed.
  2. Has difficulty waiting for turn.
  3. Intrudes/interrupts others' conversations and games.
D. Assess for symptoms of conduct disorder.
  1. Persistent disregard for rights of others—aggression, destruction of property, theft or violation of rules.
  2. Two subtypes—childhood disorder onset (at least 1 symptom prior to 10 years) and adolescent onset.

Implementation

✦ A. Develop therapeutic relationship with child.
B. Refer to special education programs for attention difficulties.
C. Conduct relationship therapy and play therapy with child for emotional problems related to disorder.
D. Work with parents to set up home environment that promotes successful completion of developmental tasks.

Adolescent Adjustment Problems

Definition: Adolescent emotional disturbances occur in adolescents when their behavior becomes maladaptive and they cease to function effectively.

Table 14-8. ADOLESCENT BEHAVIOR CHART

Normal Behavior	Dysfunctional Behavior
Tends to be secretive and demands privacy from rest of family. Uses friends to ventilate feelings and concerns	Secretive about experiencing severe emotional distress. Has no friends with whom he or she can communicate
Varying degrees of loneliness; may feel loved but not understood	Profound loneliness; feels total lack of loving; has no meaningful relationships. Danger of suicide
Experiences need for peer involvement; is very conscious of peer pressure	May be friendless and does not socialize well; may act indifferent to making friendships
Varying levels of depression	Long-standing depression may show as excessive passivity or agitation (agitated depression is seen as restless, hyperactive, bored, reckless, acting-out behavior). Danger of suicide
Usually has at least one person who provides loving, supportive parenting	Absence of parent or parents from home because of work or divorce Emotional abandonment by parents Conflict with stepparents Alcoholic or abusive parents
Families have varying degrees of conflict, overt or covert	Adolescent views family as having severe, long-term conflict
Family may move several times while child is growing up; usually location is stable	Very frequent moves with little internal stability; may be accompanied by breakup of family
Usually has infrequent school changes; school achievement varies	May have frequent school changes; poor school achievement
Parental discipline varies	Extremes of parental discipline: too harsh or too permissive; inconsistent discipline
Usually has few, infrequent major losses while growing up	Many losses (parental love, frequent moves, etc.)
Impulse control varies; usually has had consistent parental help to control behavior	Poor impulse control, usually from lack of positive role model; can lead to drug abuse, violence, criminal behavior, suicide
Usually feels safe and cared for at home	May feel unsafe and unwanted at home (child abuse, conflict with stepparent, sexual abuse in home)
Self-esteem varies; struggles to find own identity; uses conflict with family as a vehicle to work out internal struggles	Poor self-esteem; extreme difficulty in working out self-identity; cannot use conflict with family to work out internal struggles
Develops personal goals	Unable to develop personal goals
May have vague physical ailments that come and go, especially when going through a high-growth period	May present physical symptoms of chronic stress: frequent headaches, panic attacks, stomach ulcers, etc.

Characteristics

✦ A. Adolescence is a period of ambivalence—dependence versus independence.

✦ B. Influenced by peer group pressures, the adolescent may experience an identity crisis because his or her own identity has not yet been resolved.

C. The adolescent evidences an inability to resolve conflicts and to master developmental tasks (identity versus role diffusion). For a full discussion of Erikson's stages of development, *see* Chapter 3.

✦ D. Tasks of this stage of growth.
1. Emotional separation from the parents.

2. Foundations for an adult sense of self. One of the most difficult situations parents must face is the arguing and the testing of limits in which their child engages to develop this sense of self.

3. Sense of personal identity. Teenagers continue to need love, support, and consistency from the adults around them.

4. Resolution of dependency and control issues.

E. Normal adolescent behavior can be bizarre at times, so abnormal behavior may not be so blatant. Families may become desensitized to abnormal behavior. (*See* Table 14-8.)

Assessment

✦ A. Assess degree of maladaptation or adjustment problems.

B. Assess presence of confusion that may result in anxiety, depression, acting out, or antisocial behavior.

✦ C. Observe for specific behaviors in adolescent maladjustment.

    1. Defiance and hostility, especially toward authority figures.

    2. Sullenness and withdrawal.

    3. Sexual deviations.

    4. Addiction to drugs or alcohol.

    5. Depression and self-destructive impulses.

    6. Acting out or testing.

D. Assess developmental level at which adolescent is functioning.

E. Assess skills in problem solving, motivation, and general attitude.

F. Assess if the client is in touch with his or her feelings; how does client see relationship with parents, other adults, own-age peers?

G. Determine if client is in treatment willingly or because of a court order, parental insistence, etc.

H. Evaluate client's general communication skills and level of self-esteem.

I. Assess how client uses the problem behavior to meet needs.

J. Evaluate family structure.

    1. Determine whether the parents will join in treatment program.

    2. Ask parents how they believe the client's problems can be resolved.

    3. Determine the communication skills of each parent.

    4. Observe how the client's behavior meets the parents' needs.

    5. Assess other problems in the family (marital problems, other children with behavioral problems, financial worries, etc.).

K. Family behaviors that foster adolescent dysfunction.

    1. Scapegoating.

    2. Child or sexual abuse.

    3. Marital disharmony.

    4. Parental indifference.

    5. Unhealthy communication patterns—use of double messages.

Implementation

✦ A. Provide the experience of a positive relationship.

    1. Encourage open interaction so that adolescent can share fears, problems, concerns.

    2. Reinforce authentic behavior from client.

    3. Encourage group interaction with peers.

✦ B. Use behavioral approach to therapy.

    1. Set firm limits and be consistent in approach.

    2. Confront maladaptive behavior and reinforce efforts to change it.

    3. Avoid being manipulated or supportive of acting-out behavior.

    4. Give verbal positive reinforcement for appropriate behaviors.

    5. Help client create alternate activities to use as substitutes for destructive behaviors.

    6. Assist client to notice when he or she returns to old patterns of destructive behavior.

C. Use clear, open communication.

    1. Role model effective communication skills.

    2. Assist client to practice new styles of communicating; make use of role-playing, etc.

    3. Encourage exploration of feelings; provide safe environment for expression of feelings.

D. Assist adolescent to develop personal goals.

    1. Encourage client to set up personal goals, and provide encouragement and feedback.

    2. Assist client to identify steps in obtaining goal.

    3. Encourage client to examine his or her family's rules and develop alternate rules for living.

    4. Support client in sharing alternate rules with family and explore areas of negotiation.

TREATMENT MODALITIES

Energetic Psychotherapies

A. New emerging therapies are dealing with psychological issues that traditional therapies took years to resolve.

B. Several forms of new style therapies are being used.

    1. EMDR: Eye Movement Desensitization and Reprocessing is the most popular and well known.

    2. TFT: Thought Field Therapy.

    3. EFT: Emotional Freedom Technique.

    4. WHEE: Wholistic Hybrid EMDR, a combination of EFT and EMDR.

C. Types of populations treated with energetic therapies.

    1. Post-traumatic stress syndrome (especially combat veterans).

    2. Phobias and panic disorders.

    3. Crime victims.

    4. Excessive grief.

    5. Children with traumas of assault or natural disaster.

    6. Sexual assault or sexual dysfunction.

    7 Dissociative disorders.

    8. Chemical dependence.

D. Advantages of therapies.

1. Remarkable results for resolution of problems (high efficacy). Almost 1 million people treated with these techniques.
2. Takes only a few sessions; previously, it could take years to resolve these problems.
3. Results show
   a. Decrease in subjective distress (traumatic memories).
   b. Significant increase in confidence and positive beliefs.
   c. Increase in insight and cognitive changes.

Electroconvulsive Therapy (ECT)

✦ *Definition:* Use of electronically induced seizures for the safe and effective treatment of severe depression, psychotic depression and mania.

A. Shock therapy has been negatively perceived by general public; in fact, it is one of the most useful treatments for major depression, and does not cause tissue damage or brain damage. Current studies have proved its short-term efficacy.

B. Involves induction of grand mal seizure via an electric pulse through the brain—may resynchronize circadian rhythms or restore equilibrium between right and left brain hemispheres.

C. Usually given for a series of 6–12 treatments several times/week.

✦ D. Advantages.
   1. Works more quickly than antidepressants; used when imminent risk of suicide requires quicker results.
   2. Safer for elderly with history of cardiac illness than antidepressant medication therapy.
   3. Major depressive episode with vegetative aspects improvement rate of 80 percent.

✦ E. Administration.
   1. Three types of medication administered: an *anticholinergic* (*atropine, Robinul*) to block vagal stimulation so secretions are reduced; a short-acting *general anesthesia* administered IV, to make the client more comfortable; and a *muscle relaxant* (such as Anectine), to reduce complications from the convulsion itself.
   2. Pre-oxygenation of the brain reduces risk of anoxia.
   3. EEG monitoring monitors the seizure to ensure a therapeutic effect.
   4. New shock waveforms are being used that require one-third as much power—reduces amnesia, confusion, and EEG abnormalities.
   5. Have emergency care available.
   6. Preparation: informed consent, medical history, and physical exam; lab work-up and education of client and family.

7. Side effects: memory loss for recent events and difficulty learning new information—effects resolve in 6–9 months; headaches, muscle aches, weight gain, hypertension, and, occasionally, cardiac arrhythmias.

✦ F. Nursing considerations.
   1. Prior to procedure.
      a. Explain to client and family about the procedure and how client will react upon awakening: confusion, disorientation.
      b. Keep NPO after midnight or for at least 4 hours.
      c. Have client void and remove lenses, dentures and jewelry prior to treatment.
      d. Check to see if consent form is signed.
   2. Following procedure.
      a. Place client in lateral, recumbent position for drainage.
      b. Remain with client until alert.
      c. Monitor vital signs after general anesthesia.
      d. Reorient to unit.
      e. Reassure regarding memory loss and confusion.
      f. Assist to eat breakfast.

Behavior Modification

✦ *Definition:* Behavior modification is a process for dealing with problematic, maladaptive human behavior through planned, systematic interventions. It is a three-stage process involving behavior assessment, intervention, and evaluation.

Characteristics

✦ A. Behavior modification assumes that maladaptive behaviors have been learned or acquired through life's experiences.

B. The process draws on learning theory as an approach to the modification of behavior.
   1. It involves stimulus–response type learning.
   2. Techniques are drawn from Pavlov, Skinner, or stimulus–response theory.
   3. It has been labeled *behavior conditioning;* the older term was *operant conditioning.*
   4. It assumes that learned behavior is specifically connected with environmental reinforcers (e.g., U.S. eating patterns).
   5. The appropriate location for behavioral intervention and change is the individual's environment.

C. Behavior cannot be thoroughly understood independent of events that precede or follow it.

D. The concept of contingency relationships is basic.
   1. Relationships occur between behavior and reinforcing events.

✦ 2.   Positive reinforcer is a desirable reward produced by a specific behavior; for example, salary is contingent on work: no work, no salary.

✦ 3.   Negative reinforcer is a negative consequence of behavior; for example, a mother spanks a child for playing with matches.

4.   Removal of a positive reinforcer; for example, a student is not allowed to watch TV until his or her homework is finished.

5.   Removal of a negative reinforcer; for example, a mother threatens a child until the child cleans up his room. Removal produces avoidance behaviors.

✦ 6.   Principle of extinction.
   a.   Reduces the frequency of a behavior by disrupting its contingency with the reinforcement.
   b.   Arranges conditions so that the reinforcing event, which has been maintaining the behavior, no longer occurs.

E.   Goal is to arrange and manage reinforcement contingencies so that desired behaviors are increased in frequency and undesirable behaviors are decreased in frequency or removed.

F.   Specific terminology.
   1.   *Behavior problem:* condemned, excessive, or deficient behavior.
   2.   *Operant behavior:* voluntary activities that are strongly influenced by events that follow them.
   3.   *Reinforcer:* a reward that positively or negatively influences and strengthens desired behavior.
      a.   A primary reinforcer is inborn.
      b.   An acquired reinforcer is not inborn.
   4.   *Stimulus:* any event impinging on, or affecting, an individual.
   5.   *Accelerating behavior:* increase in frequency of a desired behavior.
   6.   *Decelerating behavior:* decrease in frequency of an undesirable behavior.
   7.   *Target behavior:* particular activities that the nurse wants to accelerate.

Principles of Implementation

A.   The nurse can be the major treatment agent because he or she has the most significant number of contacts with the client and his or her environment.

B.   The nurse may be in charge of designing and implementing the program.

C.   The nurse may be in charge of supervising a program that another staff member is putting into effect.

D.   Proximity to the client enables the nurse to identify any specifically maladaptive behavior.

Domestic Violence

Definition: In a domestic or family setting, the abuser becomes destructive and abusive; threatens or attacks the victim.

Characteristics

A.   The abuser (the majority are males) makes demands and threats against the victim who attempts to appease the abuser.

B.   The abuser loses control and hurts the victim and then tries to make up for this behavior by becoming loving and apologetic.

C.   Most often other family members or outsiders do not know what is happening inside the family.

D.   Often the victim hides the abuse and will not seek help from their family or the outside.

E.   Abusers evidence certain characteristics similar to sociopathic personalities.
   1.   Poor self-esteem.
   2.   Suspicious and dependent.
   3.   History of sexual abuse or violent abuse during childhood.

F.   Victims also have low self-esteem, are dependent and often depressed; they feel helpless and without power to change the situation.

Assessment

A.   Recognize and assess for abuse in the victim (bruises, cuts, broken bones, etc.).

B.   Assess the family situation.

C.   Report suspected cases of domestic abuse.

Implementation

A.   Assure privacy for the victim during examination; remind victim that information is confidential to allay fears.

B.   Establish a nurse–client relationship to provide climate for the victim to feel safe in discussing family situation.

C.   Encourage therapy for both victim and abuser; suggest group therapy, family counseling and support groups.

D.   Suggest therapy for the victim that focuses on building self-esteem, self-protective abilities and problem-solving ability.

Crisis Intervention

✦ *Definition:* Crisis intervention is a form of therapy aimed at immediate intervention in an acute episode or crisis in which the individual is unable to cope alone.

Crisis Situation

A.   An individual is typically in a state of equilibrium or homeostatic balance.

B. This state is maintained by behavioral patterns involving interchange between the person and his or her environment.

C. When problems arise, the individual uses learned coping mechanisms to deal with them.

◆ D. When a problem becomes too great to be handled by previously learned coping techniques, a crisis situation develops.
1. Result is major disorganization in functioning.
2. In circumstances of inability to resolve crisis, the individual is more amenable to intervention, and the potential for growth increases.

E. Precipitant factors in a crisis.
1. Threat to individual security, which may be loss or threat of loss.
   a. Situational crisis: actual or potential loss (job, friend, mate, etc.).
   b. Developmental or maturational crisis: any change (i.e., marriage, new baby).
   c. Adventitious crisis: crisis of disaster.
   d. Two or more severe problems arising concurrently.
2. Precipitants typically occur within 2 weeks of onset of disorganization.

Stages of Crisis Development

A. Initial perception of problem occurs first.

B. Tension and anxiety rises; usual coping mechanisms are tried.

C. Usual situational supports are consulted.

D. Known methods prove unsuccessful and tension increases.

E. If new problem-solving methods are unsuccessful, the problem remains and cannot be avoided.
1. Person's functioning becomes disorganized.
2. Extreme anxiety is likely to be experienced.
3. Perception is narrowed.
4. Coping ability is further reduced.

F. Resolution usually occurs within 6 weeks with or without intervention.

Characteristics

◆ A. Crisis is self-limiting, acute, and lasts 1–6 weeks.

◆ B. Crisis is initiated by a triggering event (death, loss, etc.); usual coping mechanisms are inadequate for the situation.

C. Situation is dangerous to the person; he or she may harm self or others.

◆ D. Individual will return to a state that is better, worse, or the same as before the crisis; therefore, intervention by the therapist is important.

E. Person is totally involved—hurts all over.

◆ F. At this time the individual is most open for intervention; therefore, major changes can take place and the crisis can be the turning point for the person.

Assessment

A. Examine period of disorganization.
1. Assess degree of disorganization.
2. Assess length of time situation has existed.
3. Determine level of functioning.

◆ B. Determine precipitant event.
1. Determine problem that triggered crisis.
2. Evaluate significance of the event to the individual.

◆ C. Assess past coping mechanisms.
1. Check history of occurrence of similar situations in past.
2. Assess past history of coping with similar situations.

D. Evaluate situational supports.
1. Ask about significant others in individual's life.
2. Check available agencies and resources.

E. Determine alternative coping mechanisms.
1. Assess new coping alternatives.
2. Assess uses of situational supports.

◆ Implementation

A. Focus on immediate problem.

B. Use reality-oriented approach.

C. Stay with "here and now" focus.

D. Set limits.

E. Stay with client or have significant persons available if necessary.

F. Explore available coping mechanisms.
1. Develop strengths and capitalize on them.
2. Do not focus on weakness or pathology.
3. Help explore the available situational supports.

G. Clarify the problem and help the individual understand the problem and integrate the events in his life.

H. When the above steps are completed, some plans for future support should be worked out by the therapist and the client.

Rape Trauma Syndrome

◆ *Definition:* Rape is a nonconsensual sexual assault on a person (93% of victims are female and 90% of perpetrators are male) that is basically an act of violence; only secondarily considered a sex act.

Assessment

A. Before assessment, inform victim of his or her rights.
1. Use of a rape crisis advocate.
2. Notify victim's personal physician.
3. Privacy rights during assessment.
4. Confidentiality is maintained by staff.
5. Client gives consent for all tests and procedures.

B. Physical data gathered.

1. Assist with a complete physical examination.
2. Carefully assess and document all physical damage.
   a. Injuries.
   b. Signs of physical entry.
C. Emotional data.
   1. Degree of emotional trauma.
   2. Presence of symptoms.
✦ D. Crisis response phases.
   1. *Impact or acute phase:* shock, crying, high anxiety, hysterical, incoherent, agitated, fearful, volatile, poor problem-solving ability.
   2. *Reconstitution phase:* denial, appears calm and controlled, withdrawn, fearful, begins to talk about feelings, expresses anger, makes decisions.
   3. *Resolution phase:* realistic attitudes, able to express feelings, controlled anger, acceptance of facts.

Implementation

✦ A. Treatment focus for rape trauma syndrome.
   1. *Emotional:* crisis counseling and call Women Against Rape; rape advocate.
   2. *Medical:* immediate medical care; assess assault and degree of trauma.
   3. *Legal:* do not bathe, douche, or change clothes; gather evidence.
B. Guidelines for care.
   ✦ 1. Recognize that the assault of rape is a humiliating and violent experience and that the victim is experiencing severe psychological trauma.
   2. Accept the fact that the victim was indeed raped and that the victim is to be supported, not treated as the "accused."
   3. Understand that the victim's behavior might vary from hysterical crying and/or laughing to very calm and controlled.
   4. Victims may need encouragement and support to report rape to the authorities.
✦ C. Interventions.
   ✦ 1. Provide immediate privacy for examination.
   2. Choose a staff member of the same sex to be with the victim.
   3. Remain with the victim.
   4. Administer physical care.
      a. Do not allow client to wash genital area or void before examination; these actions will remove any existing evidence such as semen.
      b. Keep client warm.
      ✦ c. Prepare client for complete physical examination to be completed by physician (same sex as client if possible).
      d. Physical exam includes
         (1) Head-to-toe exam.
         (2) Pap smear.
         (3) Saline suspension to test for presence of sperm.
         (4) Acid-phosphatase to determine how recently the attack occurred.
      e. Physical treatment may include
         (1) Prophylactic antibiotics.
         (2) Tranquilizers.
   ✦ 5. Provide emotional support.
      a. Demonstrate a nonjudgmental and supportive attitude.
      b. Express warmth, support, and empathy in relating to the victim.
      c. Listen to what the victim says and document all information.
      d. Encourage the victim to relate what happened, having client tell you in his or her own words if it appears that client would like to talk about the experience.
      e. Do not insist if client chooses not to talk; allow the victim to cope in his or her own way.
      f. During the interview, continue to be sensitive to the victim's feelings and degree of control. If in relating the attack client becomes hysterical, do not continue questioning at this time.
   6. Provide beginning follow-up care.
      a. Assess ability to cope when client leaves hospital (suicide potential).
      b. Explore support system and resources.
      c. Encourage victim to arrange follow-up visits with a counselor.
      d. Involve in planning and support decisions.
   ✦ 7. Termination of crisis relationship.
      a. Counsel client to receive repeat test for sexually transmitted diseases in 3 weeks and HIV in several months, or sooner if symptoms appear.
      b. Help reestablish contact with significant people.
      c. Refer to appropriate community resource for follow-up care.
         (1) Sexual assault can have a long-term impact on the victim.
         (2) Many communties have a "hotline" that offers crisis counseling to victims.
      d. Keep accurate records, as they may be important in future legal proceedings.

Environmental Therapy

Definition: Environmental therapy is a broad term that encompasses several forms and mechanisms for treating the mentally ill.

Community Mental Health Act

✦ A. The Community Mental Health Act of 1964 provides for the establishment of mental health centers to serve communities across the country.

B. Each community must provide full service for its population.

C. Services include in- and outpatient treatment services, long-term hospitalization if necessary, emergency services, and consultation and educational services.

✦ Characteristics

A. Hospitalization may be provided by private or public psychiatric hospitals or in psychiatric units of general hospitals.

B. Day–night hospitals provide structured treatment programs for a specified part of each day, after which the client returns to his or her family.

C. Halfway houses provide live-in facilities with guidance and treatment available for clients who are not quite ready to return to the community and function independently.

D. Therapeutic communities provide milieu therapy, a therapy involving the total community (or unit). The staff formulates and, together with the clients, implements the treatment program. Emphasis is often on group therapies and group techniques.

Group Therapy

✦ *Definition:* Group therapy refers to the psychotherapeutic processes that occur in formally organized groups designed to improve symptoms or change behavior through group interactions.

Types of Groups

A. Structured group: group has predetermined goals and leader retains control. Group has directed focus, factual material is presented, and format is clear and specific.

B. Unstructured group: responsibility for goals is shared by group and leader; leader is nondirective. Topics are not preselected, and discussion flows according to concerns of group members. Often, emphasis is more on feelings than facts, and decision making is part of the group process.

Phases of Group Therapy

A. *Initial phase:* group is formed; goals are clarified and expectations expressed; members become acquainted; superficial interactions take place.

B. *Working phase:* problems are identified; confrontation between members occur; problem-solving process begins; group cohesiveness emerges.

C. *Termination phase:* evaluation occurs; fulfillment of goals is explored; support for leave-taking is undertaken.

✦ Principles Underlying Group Work

A. *Support:* members gain support from others in group via sharing and interaction.

B. *Verbalization:* members express feelings, and group reinforces appropriate (versus inappropriate) communication.

C. *Activity:* verbalization and expression of feelings and problems are stimulated by activity.

D. *Change:* members have opportunity to try out new, more adaptive behaviors in group setting.

✦ Methods of Focusing Group Therapy

A. Focus on here and now versus there and then. Group members are helped to express inner experiences occurring in the present rather than in the past. The past cannot be altered; the person can only report on it.

B. Focus on feelings versus ideas. Abstract or cognitive focus directs group away from dealing with here-and-now feelings and experiences, and allows no opportunity for exploring and coping with feelings.

C. Focus on telling versus questioning. Focus on the individual's reporting about self rather than on questioning of others, which is artificial and a defensive posture.

D. Focus on experience versus "ought" or "should." Avoid "should" systems, which focus on judgmental and critical content rather than on supportiveness.

Leader Functions and Roles

A. Determine structure and format of group sessions.

B. Determine goals and work toward helping group achieve these goals.

C. Establish the psychological climate of group (e.g., acceptance, sharing, and nonpunitive interactions).

D. Set limits for the group and interpret group rules.

E. Facilitate group process to promote flow of clear communication.

F. Encourage participation from silent members and limit participation of monopolizers.

G. Exert leadership when group flounders; always maintain a degree of control.

H. Act as resource person and role model.

Advantages of Group Therapy

A. Economy in use of staff is possible.

B. Increased socialization potential in group setting leads to increased interaction between clients.

✦ C. Feedback from group members occurs.

1. Increases reality-testing mechanisms.

2. Builds self-confidence and self-image.

3. Can correct distortions of problem, situation, or feelings by group pressure.
4. Gives information about how one's personality and actions appear to others.

D. Reduction in feelings of being alone with problem and being the only one experiencing despair—universality.

✦ E. Opportunity for practicing new alternative methods for coping with feelings such as anger and anxiety.

F. Increased feelings of closeness with others, thus reducing loneliness.

G. Potential development of insight into one's problems by expressing own experiences and listening to others in group.

H. Therapeutic effect from attention to reality, from focus on the here and now rather than on own inner world.

Family Therapy

✦ *Definition:* Family therapy is a form of group therapy based on the premise that it is the total family, rather than the identified client, that is dysfunctional.

Basic Assumptions

✦ A. An identified client is not ill; rather, the total family is in need of and will benefit from treatment.

B. An identified client reflects disequilibrium in the family structure.

C. Family therapy focuses on exploration of patterns of interaction within the family rather than on individual pathology.

D. Conjoint family therapy (Virginia Satir) treats the family as a group. Method was originally developed for treatment for schizophrenics.

Therapist Behaviors

A. Models role of clear communicator.
1. Clarifies and validates communication.
2. Points out dysfunctional communication.
3. Sets limits for inappropriate behavior.

✦ B. Acts as resource person.

✦ C. Observes and reports on congruent and incongruent communications and behaviors.

D. Supports entire family as members attempt to change inappropriate patterns of relating and communicating with one another.

E. In general, follows the same therapeutic approaches as in nurse–client relationship therapy.

PSYCHOTROPIC DRUGS

Definition: Psychotropic drugs are those used in psychiatry in conjunction with other forms of therapy that affect psychic functioning, mood, behavior, or experience; and are used to treat symptoms of psychiatric disorders. (*See* Table 14-9.)

Characteristics

A. Psychotropic drugs affect both the central and autonomic nervous systems.

✦ B. These drugs affect behavior indirectly by chemically interacting with other chemicals, enzymes, or enzyme substrates.
1. Changes in cellular, tissue and organ functions occur.
2. Drug effects vary from cellular activity to psychosocial interaction.

C. Most psychotropic medications affect biological imbalances in the brain.

Antipsychotic Drugs

A. Drugs also known as ataractic or neuroleptic; introduced about 1953.

B. Action: to block the dopamine receptors in the CNS.

✦ C. Antipsychotic drugs relieve positive psychotic symptoms and assist in controlling behavior—medication can calm an excited client without producing marked impairment of motor function or sleep.

✦ D. Most common are phenothiazine derivatives (typical: Thorazine, Stelazine, Trilafon, and the long-acting phenothiazine, Prolixin).

E. Another common antipsychotic drug (classification—butyrophenones) is haloperidol (Haldol).
1. Less sedative than phenothiazines.
2. Indicated for use with psychosis, Tourette's disorder, and as an antiemetic.
3. Incidence of severe extrapyramidal reactions.
4. Other side effects include leukocytosis, blurred vision, dry mouth, and urinary retention.
5. Avoid alcohol and other CNS depressants.

✦ F. Clozapine (Clozaril) and loxapine (Loxitane) are antipsychotics for management of psychotic symptoms in clients who do not respond to other antipsychotics.
1. Rare or lowest incidence of extrapyramidal effects and tardive dyskinesia.
2. Side effects similar to other antipsychotics; be aware of blood dyscrasias (leukopenia, neutropenia, agranulocytosis, eosinophilia).

✦ 3. Requires weekly WBC count to determine potential for agranulocytosis. (Drug is discontinued if WBC < 2000 µL or granulocytes < 1000 µL.)
4. Monitor monthly bilirubin, liver function studies.

G. Other classes of drugs are thioxanthenes (Taractan and Navane).

H. Other classes of drugs, formerly called "atypical antipsychotics," such as Risperdal, Seroquel, Zyprexa and Geodon.

  1. These drugs appear to have few or no extrapyramidal symptoms.

  2. The "atypical antipsychotics" have been found to be no more effective and no safer than the older and cheaper drugs (*New England Journal of Medicine*, 2006).

  3. Higher risk of adverse drug reaction in elderly.

  4. Increase in liver enzymes.

✦ I. Side effects.

  ✦ 1. Blood dyscrasias.

    a. Agranulocytosis occurs in first 4–18 weeks of treatment. *Symptoms:* fever, sore throat, malaise, infection.

    b. Leukopenia, preceded by altered white blood cell count.

  ✦ 2. Extrapyramidal side effects (EPSEs) occur in 30 percent of clients, affecting the voluntary movements and skeletal muscles.

    a. *Drug-induced Parkinsonism:* symptoms occur in 1–4 weeks; *signs* are similar to classic Parkinsonism: rigidity, shuffling gait, pill-rolling hand movement, tremors, dyskinesia, and masklike face.

    b. *Akathisia:* very common; occurs in 1–6 weeks; *signs:* uncontrolled motor restlessness, foot-tapping, agitation, pacing.

    c. *Dystonia:* occurs early, 1–2 days; *signs:* limb and neck spasms; uncoordinated, jerky movements; difficulty in speaking and swallowing; and rigidity and spasms of muscles.

    d. *Tardive dyskinesia:* develops late in treatment; estimated to occur in more than 25 percent of elderly and in up to 50 percent of chronic schizophrenics. Antiparkinson drugs are of no help in decreasing symptoms. This is a permanent side effect; *signs:* shuffling gait, drooling, and general dystonic symptoms. Intervention is to stop all medications.

  ✦ 3. Hypotension: orthostatic hypotension may occur. Monitor closely when client is elderly. Keep client supine for 1 hour and advise to change positions slowly.

  ✦ 4. Anticholinergic effects: dry mouth, blurred vision, tachycardia, nasal congestion, and constipation. Treat symptomatically.

  ✦ 5. Neuroleptic malignant syndrome—a rare complication caused by an antipsychotic—a medical emergency (20 percent mortality rate) and must be recognized and treated immediately.

    ✦ a. *Signs and symptoms:* muscle rigidity, irregular vital signs, hyperpyrexia, altered mental status, autonomic instability, elevated creatine phosphokinase, and possibly acute renal failure.

    ✦ b. *Treatment:* immediate discontinuation of drug, medical monitoring, administration of a dopamine-enhancing drug and/or Dantrium.

Antiparkinson Drugs (Antidyskinetics)

A. The term *extrapyramidal disease* refers to a motor disorder often associated with pathologic dysfunction in the basal ganglia. Antiparkinson drugs block the extrapyramidal symptoms.

  1. Clinical symptoms of the disease include abnormal involuntary movement, change in tone of the skeletal muscles, and a reduction of automatic associated movements.

  2. Reversible extrapyramidal reactions may follow the use of certain drugs—the most common are the phenothiazine derivatives.

✦ B. Antiparkinson drugs act on the extrapyramidal system to reduce disturbing symptoms experienced from antipsychotic medications.

  1. They are usually given in conjunction with antipsychotic drugs.

  ✦ 2. The most common drugs are anticholinergics: Artane, Cogentin, Kemadrin, and Akineton.

  3. Side effects are dizziness, gastrointestinal disturbance, headaches, urinary hesitancy, and memory impairment.

✦ C. Benadryl, an antihistamine, is often given in place of Artane or Cogentin.

  1. Controls the extrapyramidal side effects of phenothiazines.

  2. Preferred because it does not cause as many untoward side effects as the other antiparkinson drugs.

D. Other drugs occasionally ordered in this category are amantadine, benzodiazepines, propranolol, clonidine, nifedipine (Procardia), verapamil, and dantrolene (Dantrium) used for treating *neuroleptic malignant syndrome.*

Anxiolytic (Antianxiety) Drugs

✦ A. Drugs induce sedation, relax muscles, and inhibit convulsions; major use to reduce anxiety.

B. These drugs are the most frequently prescribed drugs in medicine; demand is great for relief from anxiety and they are safer than sedative–hypnotics.

✦ C. Potentiate drug abuse. Greatest harm occurs when combined with alcohol.

D. Prescribed for neuroses, psychosomatic disorders, or functional psychiatric disorders, but do not modify psychotic behavior.

✦ E. Drugs from two major classes.
1. *Benzodiazepines:* safer and more common (Librium, Valium, Ativan, Restoril, Centrax, Versed, Serax, and Xanax—being tested for use in depression, panic, and obsessive–compulsive disorders).
2. New benzodiazepines have shorter onset and half-lives (triazolam, Doral) and Klonopin (with usual onset and half-life).
3. *Nonbenzodiazepines:* BuSpar, Sonata, Ambien, and Equanil—more effective in managing GAD than benzodiazepines.
4. Antihistamines are sometimes used to treat anxiety but are not as effective (Vistaril, Atarax and Benadryl).

✦ F. Side effects.
1. Drowsiness (avoid driving or working around equipment).
2. Blurred vision, constipation, dermatitis, mental confusion, anorexia, polyuria, menstrual irregularities, and edema.
3. Habituation and increased tolerance.
4. Pancytopenia, thrombocytopenia, and agranulocytopenia.
5. Withdrawal symptoms occur with prolonged use (6+ months) and high doses.

Antidepressant Drugs

✦ A. Tricyclics, one of the most commonly used classes of antidepressants; include Elavil, Norpramin, Tofranil, Aventyl, Vivactil, and Pamelor.
1. Block uptake of norepinephrine and serotonin.
✦ 2. A lag period of 1 to 6 weeks between starting the medication and experiencing symptom relief exists.
3. Anticholinergic effect—produces antagonism of the parasympathetic system.
4. Clients with morbid fantasies do not respond well to these drugs.
✦ 5. Side effects.
   a. Anticholinergic effects: dry mouth, blurred vision, constipation, postural hypotension.
   b. CNS effects: tremor, agitation, angry states, mania, seizures.
   c. Cardiovascular and cardiotoxic effects; changes in the electrical conduction, so assess any client with history of cardiovascular disease, especially heart block.

d. Elderly clients should have ECG.
e. Alterations in sexual functioning
f. Orthostatic hypotension.
g. Sedation.
h. Weight gain.
i. Most side effects appear in first 1 to 2 weeks and diminish over a period of a few weeks or months.

✦ 6. If client is switched from a tricyclic drug to a monoamine oxidase (MAO) inhibitor, a period of 1 to 3 weeks must elapse between drugs.

✦ 7. Blood level assays provide therapeutic levels of tricyclic antidepressants.

✦ B. The MAO inhibitors include Marplan (most effective), Nardil, and Parnate.
1. MAO inhibitors are toxic, potent, and produce many side effects.
2. They should not be the first antidepressant drug used; effect is at best equal to a tricyclic and side effects more dangerous.
✦ 3. Side effects.
   ✦ a. Most dangerous is hypertensive crisis.
   b. Drug interactions (sympathomimetic medications) can cause severe hypertension, hypotension, or CNS depression.
   c. Postural hypotension, headaches, constipation, anorexia, diarrhea, and chills.
   d. Tachycardia, edema, impotence, dizziness, insomnia, and restlessness.
   e. Manic episodes and anxiety.
✦ 4. All clients must be warned not to eat foods with high tyramine content (aged cheese, pickled fish, meat extracts, red wine, beer, chicken liver, yeast); certain vegetables (pea pods, fava beans); bananas; combination foods such as pizza, lasagna, quiche, liver pate; soy sauce; sauerkraut; drink alcohol; or take other drugs, especially sympathomimetic drugs (amphetamines, L-dopa, epinephrine).
5. MAO inhibitors must not be used in combination with tricyclics.

✦ C. Hypertensive crisis, due to elevated tyramine levels.
1. Severe symptoms: throbbing, occipital headache, confusion, drowsiness, vomiting, stiff neck, chills, chest pain.
2. Monitor for potential complications: encephalopathy, heart failure.
3. Treatment.
   a. Drug of choice: Regitine, IV 5 mg with close monitoring; antihypertensive.
   b. Monitor vital signs, electrocardiogram (ECG), and neurological signs; BP q 5 min.
   c. Norepinephrine is administered for severe hypotension.

D. Selective inhibitors of the uptake of serotonin (SSRIs).

1. Studies suggest that increased serotonin in critical areas of the brain modifies certain affective behavior. Results in the increased concentration of active serotonin in critical synaptic areas in the brain.

2. A number of neurochemical pathways can be affected by existing antidepressants.

3. Drugs are highly selective for the serotonin pathway and exert little or no effect on the uptake of the other neurotransmitters or receptor sites.

4. Examples of SSRIs are Prozac, Zoloft, Paxil, Celexa and Lexapro.

5. Exhibit fewer side effects than other antidepressant drugs.

 a. Anticholingeric side effects such as dry mouth, constipation are fewer.

 b. Side effects observed are nausea (the most common), anxiety/nervousness, insomnia, drowsiness, and headache.

 c. Coadministration of alcohol and drugs is not recommended.

6. Important to know that Prozac and other SSRIs together could be fatal.

 a. Must be 5-week space between drugs due to half-life of Prozac.

 b. Other SSRIs have a shorter half-life, so 1- to 2-week gap is necessary.

7. Note danger of giving SSRIs to children.

E. New-generation antidepressants.

1. Trazodone HCl (Desyrel) is a member of a class of antidepressant drugs unrelated to the tricyclics.

 a. Inhibits the reuptake of serotonin.

 b. Well tolerated, with minimal side effects (sedation and orthostatic hypotension).

 c. *Warning*: this drug has been associated with priapism—persistent, abnormal erection. If symptom occurs, immediately discontinue drug.

2. Netazodene (Serzene) is a newer antidepressant with few to no side effects.

3. Venlafaxine (Effexor) blocks uptake of both norepinephrine and serotonin; first in a new class called phenethylamine antidepressants.

4. Serotonin.

 a. Relatively free of side effects.

 b. Useful in treatment of severely depressed and melancholic clients.

 c. Some clients experience heightened anxiety, nausea, vomiting, and dizziness.

 d. Some clients experience abnormal ejaculation and male impotence.

F. A significant number of clients improve when 600 mg of lithium is added to antidepressant therapy.

Mood Stabilizers (Antimanic Drugs)

A. These drugs control mood disorders, especially the manic phase.

B. Elevate mood when client is depressed; dampen mood when client is in manic episode.

C. Before lithium therapy is begun, baseline studies of renal, cardiac, and thyroid status obtained.

D. The most common form of drug is lithium carbonate, a naturally occurring metallic salt; other forms: lithium citrate, Tegretol, Klonopin, valproic acid.

E. Drug must reach a certain blood level before it is effective—1.0 to 1.5 mEq/L.

1. Stabilizing concentration occurs in 5 to 7 days; therapeutic effect 7 to 28 days or more.

2. Drug dose is lowered after 10 days to 900–1200 mg/day with serum level maintained in range of 0.6–1.2 mEq/L.

F. Lithium is metabolized by the kidney.

1. Deficiency of sodium results in more lithium being reabsorbed (lithium substitutes for sodium ion), thus increasing risk of toxicity.

2. Excessive sodium causes more lithium to be excreted and may lower level to a nontherapeutic range.

3. Normal dietary intake of sodium with adequate fluids to prevent dehydration is necessary.

4. Diuretics will increase absorption of lithium leading to toxic effects.

5. Serum levels measured 2 to 3 times weekly (12 hours after last dose) in beginning of therapy; for long-term maintenance therapy, every 2 to 3 months.

G. Drug concentration and side effects.

1. Therapeutic range of serum levels is 0.6–1.2 mEq/L; for acute manic state, 1.0–1.5 mEq/L.

2. Side effects occur at upper ranges, usually above 1.5 mEq/L.

3. Gastrointestinal disturbances, metallic taste in mouth, muscle weakness, fatigue, thirst, polyuria, and fine hand tremors are common side effects.

4. Hypothyroidism is a long-term side effect of lithum therapy.

H. For acute manic episodes, Zyprexa (olanzopine) has been approved.

I. Risperdal (risperidone) combined with lithium provides more rapid mood stabilization than lithium alone.

Table 14-9. DRUG CLASSIFICATION CHART					
Trade Name	**Daily Dose**	**Trade Name**	**Daily Dose**	**Trade Name**	**Daily Dose**
Antipsychotics		Xanax	0.25–0.5 mg	Zoloft	25–150 mg
Thorazine	150–1500 mg	Ativan	2–6 mg	Prozac	10–40 mg
Mellaril	100–800 mg	Restoril	15–30 mg	Celexa	20–40 mg
Serentil	30–400 mg	BuSpar	15–30 mg	Lexapro	10–20 mg
Trilafon	6–64 mg	Klonopin	5–20 mg	Luvox	50–300 mg
Prolixin Decanoate	12.5–25 mg	Tranxene	15–60 mg		
Prolixin Permitil	3–45 mg	Trancopal	300–800 mg	**Antimanic Drugs**	
Stelazine	10–60 mg			Depakote	125–500 mg
Taractan	30–600 mg	**Antidepressants (Mood Elevators)**		Lithium carbonate, citrate (Lithane, Lithonate)	300–1800 mg
Navane	10–60 mg	*MAO Inhibitors*			
Haldol	2–40 mg	Nardil	15–90 mg		
Haldol Decanoate	50 mg/mL	Parnate	10–30 mg	Tegretol	200–1200 mg
Loxitane	10–100 mg	Marplan	10–30 mg	**Antipanic Agents**	
Clozaril	12.5–900 mg	Eldepryl	patch	Klonopin	0.5–20 mg
"Atypical" Antipsychotics				Paxil	10–40 mg
Risperdal	0.5–6 mg	*Tricyclics*		Xanax	0.25–1 mg
Seroquel	300–400 mg	Pamelor	50–100 mg	Zoloft	25–100 mg
Zyprexa	5–20 mg	Tofranil	75–300 mg		
Geodon	20–40 mg	Elavil	75–300 mg	**Antiparkinson Drugs**	
Abilita	15–20 mg	Norpramin	75–300 mg	Cogentin	8 mg
Antianxiety Drugs		Aventyl	40–200 mg	Artane	15 mg
Atarax	200–400 mg	Vivactil	20–60 mg	Akineton	8 mg
Vistaril	200–400 mg	Sinequan	75–300 mg	Kemadrin	15 mg
Librium, Librax	10–100 mg	Ludiomil	100–225 mg	Symmetrel	300 mg
Valium	4–30 mg	Welbutrin	100–300 mg	Benadryl	100 mg
Serax	30–60 mg	*Selective Serotonin Reuptake Inhibitors (SSRIs)*		Parsidol	50–200 mg
Centrax	20 mg	Paxil	10–40 mg	Disipal	50–300 mg

J. For clients who cannot take lithium, seizure medications may be prescribed (carbamazepine and Depakote).

✦ K. Lithium toxicity.
1. Appears when blood level exceeds 1.5 to 2.0 mEq/L. May appear sooner depending on individual client.
2. Central nervous system is the chief target.
3. Initial symptoms include nausea, vomiting, drowsiness, tremors, slurred speech, blurred vision, muscle twitching, oliguria.
4. If drug is continued, coma, convulsions, and death may result.
5. Treatment for toxicity: gastric lavage, correction of fluid balance, administration of Mannitol to increase urine excretion.

✦ **General Nursing Responsibilities for Administering Psychoactive Drugs**

A. Give correct *drug* and *dose* at correct *time* to correct *client*.
B. Know specific actions and uses of drugs.
C. Be familiar with the side effects and precautions of major drug groups.
D. Observe client carefully for side effects.
E. Be aware that certain drug groups are not compatible—know half-lives and drug interactions.
F. Notify doctor of extrapyramidal side effects and lithium toxicity, and immediately implement nursing intervention.

PSYCHIATRIC NURSING REVIEW QUESTIONS

NURSE–CLIENT RELATIONSHIP/ THERAPEUTIC COMMUNICATION

1. Trust may develop in the nurse–client relationship when the nurse

   1. Avoids limit setting.
   2. Encourages the client to use "testing" behaviors.
   3. Tells the client how he or she should behave.
   4. Uses consistency in approaching the client.

2. A client has just begun to discuss important feelings when the time of the interview is up. The next day, when the nurse meets with the client at the agreed-upon time, the initial intervention would be to say

   1. "Good morning, how are you today?"
   2. "Yesterday you were talking about some very important feelings. Let's continue."
   3. "What would you like to talk about today?"
   4. Nothing and wait for the client to introduce a topic.

3. A new staff nurse is on an orientation tour with the head nurse. A client approaches her and says, "I don't belong here. Please try to get me out." The staff nurse's best response would be

   1. "What would you do if you were out of the hospital?"
   2. "I am a new staff member, and I'm on a tour. I'll come back and talk with you later."
   3. "I think you should talk with the head nurse about that."
   4. "I can't do anything about that."

4. The nurse is in the day room with a group of clients when a client who has been quietly watching TV suddenly jumps up screaming and runs out of the room. The nurse's priority intervention would be to

   1. Turn off the TV, and ask the group what they think about the client's behavior.
   2. Follow after the client to see what has happened.
   3. Ignore the incident because these outbreaks are frequent.
   4. Send another client out of the room to check on the agitated client.

5. A nurse observes a client sitting alone in her room crying. As the nurse approaches her, the client states, "I'm feeling sad. I don't want to talk now." The nurse's best response would be

   1. "It will help you feel better if you talk about it."
   2. "I'll come back when you feel like talking."
   3. "I'll stay with you a few minutes."
   4. "Sometimes it helps to talk."

ANXIETY AND STRESS DISORDERS/ DEFENSE MECHANISMS

6. A student failed her psychology final exam and spent the entire evening berating the teacher and the course. This behavior would be an example of which defense mechanism?

   1. Reaction-formation.
   2. Compensation.
   3. Projection.
   4. Acting out.

7. The most effective nursing intervention for a severely anxious client who is pacing vigorously would be to

   1. Instruct her to sit down and quit pacing.
   2. Place her in bed to reduce stimuli and allow rest.
   3. Allow her to walk until she becomes physically tired.
   4. Give her PRN medication and walk with her at a gradually slowing pace.

8. A client is experiencing a high degree of anxiety. It is important to recognize if additional help is required because

   1. If the client is out of control, another person will help to decrease his anxiety level.
   2. Being alone with an anxious client is dangerous.
   3. It will take another person to direct the client into activities to relieve anxiety.
   4. Hospital protocol for handling anxious clients requires at least two people.

9. A client with a diagnosis of obsessive–compulsive disorder constantly does repetitive cleaning. The nurse knows that this behavior is probably most basically an attempt to

1. Decrease the anxiety to a tolerable level.
2. Focus attention on nonthreatening tasks.
3. Control others.
4. Decrease the time available for interaction with people.

10. A client is suffering from post-traumatic stress disorder following a rape by an unknown assailant. One of the primary goals of nursing care for this client would be to

   1. Establish a safe, supportive environment.
   2. Control aggressive behavior.
   3. Deal with the client's anxiety.
   4. Discuss the client's nightmares and reactions.

11. A client's deafness has been diagnosed as conversion disorder. Nursing interventions should be guided by which one of the following?

   1. The client will probably express much anxiety about her deafness and require much reassurance.
   2. The client will have little or no awareness of the psychogenic cause of her deafness.
   3. The client's need for the symptom should be respected; thus, secondary gains should be allowed.
   4. The defense mechanisms of suppression and rationalization are involved in creating the symptom.

12. A female client has just received the diagnosis of hypochondriasis. This client continually focuses on gastrointestinal problems and constantly rings for a nurse to meet her every demand. The best nursing approach is to

   1. Ignore the demands because the nurse knows it is not necessary to respond.
   2. Assign various staff members to work with the client so no staff member will become negative.
   3. Anticipate the client's demands and spend time with her even though she does not demand it.
   4. Provide for the client's basic needs, but do not respond to her every demand, which reinforces secondary gains.

13. Persons with personality disorders tend to be manipulators. In planning the care of a person with this diagnosis, the nurse would

   1. Allow manipulation so as to not raise the client's anxiety.
   2. Appeal to the client's sense of loyalty in adhering to the rules of the community.
   3. Know that when the client's manipulations are not successful, anxiety will increase.

4. Establish a nurse–client relationship to decrease the client's manipulations.

14. A male client on the psychiatric unit becomes upset and breaks a chair when a visitor does not show up. The first nursing intervention should be to

   1. Stay with the client during the stressful time.
   2. Ask direct questions about the client's behavior.
   3. Set limits and restrict the client's behavior.
   4. Plan with the client for how he can better handle frustration.

15. The nurse has been interviewing a client who has not been able to discuss any feelings. This day, 5 minutes before the time is over, the client begins to talk about important feelings. The intervention is to

   1. Go over the agreed-upon time, as the client is finally able to discuss important feelings.
   2. Tell the client that it is time to end the session now, but another nurse will discuss his feelings with him.
   3. Set an extra meeting time a little later to discuss these feelings.
   4. End just as agreed, but tell the client these are very important feelings and he can continue tomorrow.

MOOD (AFFECTIVE) DISORDERS/SUICIDE

16. In working with a depressed client, the nurse should understand that depression is most directly related to a person's

   1. Experiencing poor interpersonal relationships with others.
   2. Remembering a traumatic childhood.
   3. Having experienced a sense of loss.
   4. Stage in life.

17. A 45-year-old female client has been in the hospital for 3 days with a diagnosis of depression. During this time, she has not put on a clean dress, washed her hair, or participated in any of the unit activities. On this day, the nurse observes that she is wearing a clean dress and has combed her hair. The appropriate statement to the client is

   1. "Oh, I'm so pleased that you finally put on a clean dress."
   2. "Something is different about you today. What is it?"
   3. "That's good. You have on a clean dress and have combed your hair."

4. "I see that you have on a clean dress and have combed your hair."

18. A depressed client refuses to get out of bed, go to activities, or participate in any of the unit's programs. The most appropriate nursing action is to

1. Tell her the rules of the unit are that no client can remain in bed.
2. Suggest she better get out of bed or she will go hungry later.
3. Tell her that the nurse will assist her out of bed and help her to dress.
4. Allow her to remain in bed until she feels ready to join the other clients.

19. When encouraged to join an activity, a depressed client on the psychiatric unit refuses and says, "What's the use?" The approach by the nurse that would be most effective is to

1. Sit down beside her and ask her how she is feeling.
2. Tell her it is time for the activity, help her out of the chair, and go with her to the activity.
3. Convince her how helpful it will be to engage in the activity.
4. Tell her that this is a self-defeating attitude and it will only make her feel worse.

20. A 60-year-old male client has been admitted to the psychiatric unit, with symptoms ranging from fatigue, an inability to concentrate, an inability to complete everyday tasks, to refusal to care for himself and preferring to sleep all day. One of the first interventions should be aimed at

1. Developing a good nursing care plan.
2. Talking to his wife for cues to help him.
3. Encouraging him to join activities on the unit.
4. Developing a structured routine for him to follow.

21. Three days after admission for depression, a 54-year-old female client approaches the nurse and says, "I know I have cancer of the uterus. Can't you let me stay in bed and have some peace before I die?" In responding, the nurse must keep in mind that

1. The client must be postmenopausal.
2. Thoughts of disease are common in depressed clients.
3. Clients suffering from depression can be demanding, making many requests of the nurse.
4. Antidepressant medications frequently cause vaginal spotting.

22. When a depressed client becomes more active and there is evidence that her mood has lifted, an appropriate goal to add to the nursing care plan is to

1. Encourage her to go home for the weekend.
2. Move her to a room with three other clients.
3. Monitor her whereabouts at all times.
4. Begin to explore the reasons she became depressed.

23. The nurse is assigned a client who is potentially suicidal. Of the following nursing objectives, which one is the most important?

1. Observe the client closely at all times.
2. Recognize a continued desire to commit suicide.
3. Involve the client in activities with others to mobilize him.
4. Provide a safe environment to protect the client.

24. A client makes a suicide attempt on the evening shift. The staff intervenes in time to prevent harm. In assessing the situation, the most important rationale for the staff to discuss the incident is that

1. They need to reenact the attempt so that they understand exactly what happened.
2. The staff needs to file an incident report so that the hospital administration is kept informed.
3. The staff needs to discuss the client's behavior to determine what cues in his behavior might have warned them that he was contemplating suicide.
4. Because the client made one suicide attempt, there is high probability he will make a second attempt in the immediate future.

25. When assessing a client for possible suicide, an important clue would be if the client

1. Is hostile and sarcastic to the staff.
2. Identifies with problems expressed by other clients.
3. Seems satisfied and detached.
4. Begins to talk about leaving the hospital.

26. A client with the diagnosis of manic episode is racing around the psychiatric unit trying to organize games with the clients. An appropriate nursing intervention is to

1. Have the client play Ping-Pong.
2. Suggest video exercises with the other clients.
3. Take the client outside for a walk.
4. Do nothing, as organizing a game is considered therapeutic.

27. A client has the diagnosis of manic episode. Her disruptive behavior on the unit has been increasingly an-

noying to the other clients. One intervention by the nurse might be to

1. Tell the client she is annoying others and confine her to her room.
2. Ignore the client's behavior, realizing it is consistent with her illness.
3. Set limits on the client's behavior and be consistent in approach.
4. Make a rigid, structured plan that the client will have to follow.

SUBSTANCE ABUSE

28. While working with an alcoholic client, the most important approach by the nurse would be to

1. Maintain a nonjudgmental attitude toward the client.
2. Establish strict guidelines of behavior.
3. Explicitly outline expectations of the client.
4. Set up a working nurse–client relationship.

29. A client is admitted with the diagnosis of delirium tremens. He is exhibiting marked tremors, hallucinations, and tachycardia, and is perspiring profusely. The first nursing intervention is to

1. Establish an IV of D$_5$W with vitamin B complex supplement (standard orders).
2. Administer Valium IM (standard orders).
3. Control the environment with a quiet, single room, siderails, and soft lights.
4. Establish baseline vital signs.

30. A client is admitted with Wernicke's encephalopathy. The nurse anticipates that the first physician's orders will include

1. Ordering an MRI.
2. Administering a steroid medication, such as Decadron.
3. Giving thiamine 100 mg IM STAT.
4. Ordering an EEG.

COGNITIVE DISORDERS

31. A client has the diagnosis of cognitive disorder— Alzheimer's disease. The client is constantly making up stories that are untrue. This charateristic of the disease is called

1. Senility.
2. Confabulation.
3. Lability.
4. Memory loss.

32. A client in a long-term care facility has the diagnosis of dementia—Alzheimer's disease. His care plan should include the goal of assisting him to participate in activities that provide him a chance to

1. Interact with other clients.
2. Compete with others.
3. Succeed at something.
4. Get a sense of continuity.

33. A 70-year-old client is admitted with the diagnosis of cognitive disorder, dementia type. In discharge planning with the family, the nurse would take into account that his prognosis is

1. Good, because the condition tends to be reversible.
2. Unpredictable, because the condition may reverse.
3. Poor, because symptoms are reduced intellectual capacity, emotional stability, memory, and judgment.
4. Poor, because the condition will rapidly progress.

34. A 56-year-old client is tentatively diagnosed as having Korsakoff's syndrome. In developing a strategy to care for this client, the nurse knows that this condition is a(n)

1. Neurological condition common with alcohol poisoning.
2. Neurological degeneration caused by vitamin deficiency.
3. Organic brain lesion brought on by repeated hepatitis attacks.
4. State resulting from severe, long-term psychosis.

SCHIZOPHRENIC DISORDERS

35. The most appropriate short-term nursing goal for schizophrenic clients is to

1. Set limits on bizarre behavior.
2. Establish a trusting, nonthreatening relationship.
3. Quickly establish a warm, close relationship.
4. Protect client from inappropriate impulses.

36. When the nurse is talking with a schizophrenic client, she suddenly says, "I'm frightened. Do you hear that? Terrible things." Which initial response by the nurse would be most appropriate?

1. "I don't hear anything."
2. "Who is saying terrible things to you."
3. "I don't hear anything, but you do seem frightened."
4. "What is someone saying to you?"

37. One day the nurse overhears a client with the diagnosis of schizophrenia talking to herself. She is saying, "The mazukas are coming. The mazukas are coming." Her use of the word *mazuka* is most likely

    1. An example of associative looseness.
    2. Flight of ideas.
    3. A neologism.
    4. A manifestation of dyslexia.

38. A young schizophrenic meets with the nurse regularly. On one occasion, with no apparent connection to the topic being discussed, he blurts out, "I am the devil! I am God! Open the gate for me!" The most *nontherapeutic* response would be to say

    1. "Tell me your thoughts about religion and God."
    2. "I don't understand. Can you tell me what that means?"
    3. "Are you saying that you are both good and bad?"
    4. "Most people have good thoughts and ones that they fear are bad."

39. The best explanation for the term "depersonalization," as seen in schizophrenics, is

    1. The client cannot tolerate personal relationships.
    2. The client personalizes all threats and uses projection.
    3. A flight from reality related to oneself or the environment.
    4. A mechanism seen in chronic schizophrenia.

40. A client with the diagnosis of schizophrenia has improved and is now able to attend group therapy meetings. One day, she jumps up and runs out after the group has been laughing at a story one of the clients told. She states, "You are all making fun of me." This client is displaying

    1. Symbolic rejection.
    2. Hallucinations.
    3. Depersonalization.
    4. Ideas of reference.

41. A 20-year-old male client is admitted to the psychiatric unit with a diagnosis of schizophrenia, acute episode. He is having auditory hallucinations and seems disoriented to time and place. The nurse knows that a hallucination can be explained as a(n)

    1. Sensory experience without foundation in reality.
    2. Distortion of real auditory or visual perception.
    3. Voice that is heard by the client but is not really there.
    4. Idea without foundation in reality.

42. A client with the diagnosis of paranoid personality disorder is admitted to the psychiatric unit. As the nurse approaches the client with medication, he refuses it, accusing the nurse of trying to kill him. The nurse's best strategy would be to tell him that

    1. "It is not poison and you must take the medication."
    2. "I will give you an injection if necessary."
    3. "You may decide if you want to take the medication by mouth or injection, but you must take it."
    4. "It's all right if you don't take the medication right now."

43. A 16-year-old client is hospitalized for adolescent adjustment problems. After assessing her, the nurse's first objective is to establish a nurse–client relationship. The next day, the nurse is late for the appointment. Knowing that the client has difficulty assuming responsibility for her own behavior, the nurse would like to use this situation as an opportunity for role modeling. The most appropriate statement the nurse could make is

    1. "I'm late. I apologize."
    2. "Thank goodness you are still here; I just had a flat tire."
    3. "Oh, you are here. I thought we'd be arriving at the same time."
    4. "What do you mean you are angry with me? I bet you keep people waiting."

44. The nurse is assigned to work on a unit that has a group of autistic children as inpatients. They have all been on the unit for at least 6 months and exhibit self-destructive and withdrawn behavior as well as bizarre responses. As a new member of the health team, the nurse knows that the first goal is to

    1. Set limits on their behavior so the children will perceive the nurse as an authority figure.
    2. Assess each child's individual developmental level so the nurse will have the data for realistic care plans.
    3. Understand that the children must be protected from self-destructive behavior.
    4. Establish some method of relating to the children, either verbal or nonverbal.

45. A newly admitted client to the psychiatric unit will receive electroconvulsive therapy (ECT). ECT is considered most effective in treating

    1. Young clients with depressive reactions.
    2. Elderly clients with depressive reactions.
    3. Any age client with schizophrenia.
    4. Young clients with paranoid reactions.

46. The treatment in crisis intervention centers is specifically intended to help clients

    1. Return to prior levels of functioning.
    2. Understand the dynamics underlying symptoms.
    3. Make long-range plans for the future.
    4. Accept their illness.

PSYCHOTROPIC DRUGS

47. A client comes to the emergency room with complaints of headache and vomiting. Upon questioning, the client says she is taking the drug Parnate. The nurse would continue the assessment by first asking

    1. The dose of Parnate she is taking.
    2. If she has recently had flu symptoms.
    3. What foods she has been ingesting.
    4. What other medication she is taking.

48. A client is to take lithium regularly after he is discharged from the hospital. The nursing care plan includes discharge planning. The most important information to impart to the client and his family is that the client should

    1. Have an adequate intake of sodium.
    2. Limit his fluid intake.
    3. Have a limited intake of sodium.
    4. Not eat foods that have a high tyramine content (e.g., cheese, wine, liver, yeast) or drink alcohol.

49. A 50-year-old male client has a history of many hospitalizations for schizophrenic disorder. He has been on long-term phenothiazines (Thorazine), 400 mg/day. The nurse assessing this client observes that he demonstrates jerky choreiform movements, lip smacking, and neck and back tonic contractions. From these symptoms and his history, the nurse concludes that the client has developed

    1. Tardive dyskinesia.
    2. Parkinsonism.
    3. Dystonia.
    4. Akathisia.

50. A client with the diagnosis of schizophrenia has orders for clozapine (Clozaril). The nurse will evaluate the drug's effect as positive if the

    1. Client develops leukopenia.
    2. Monthly liver function studies change moderately.
    3. Psychotic symptoms, such as hearing voices, are reduced.
    4. Client's energy level and involvement in activities goes up.

PSYCHIATRIC NURSING

Answers with Rationale

NURSE-CLIENT RELATIONSHIP/ THERAPEUTIC COMMUNICATION

1. (4) One of the most important elements of trust is consistency. The client learns to trust that the nurse will follow through and do what is promised. Avoiding limit setting will not instill trust, nor will encouraging testing behaviors or telling the client how he should behave.

   NP:P; CN:PS; CL:C

2. (3) This is a broad opening statement and the nurse is giving the client the opportunity to bring up the same topic or not. The nurse should not make the assumption that what was most important to the client yesterday is still most important today. Answer (2) has the nurse directing the focus, not the client. The other two responses are not as therapeutic as (3).

   NP:I; CN:H; CL:AN

3. (2) As a new staff member, the nurse should clarify who she is and why she is there. She also should acknowledge the client's attempt to initiate interaction by offering to talk at a more appropriate time. Answer (1) might be used in a later interaction, but is not appropriate at this time.

   NP:I; CN:S; CL:A

4. (2) The immediate priority is to find the client and assess what further intervention may be needed. Whether the behavior has happened frequently in the past is irrelevant, because the behavior exhibited now is significant and should be followed up. Sending another client is inappropriate because an immediate intervention may be necessary.

   NP:I; CN:S; CL:A

5. (3) Simply offering comfort by staying with the client and being open for communication is the most therapeutic. The other responses place an additional burden on the client if she does not wish to talk.

   NP:I; CN:PS; CL:A

ANXIETY AND STRESS DISORDERS/DEFENSE MECHANISMS

6. (3) The client is placing blame on others and not taking responsibility for her own behavior. The nurse needs to interpret the behavior in terms of the defense mechanism to understand the client. Reaction-formation is preventing "dangerous" feelings from being expressed by exaggerating the opposite attitude. Compensation is covering up a weakness by emphasizing a desirable trait. Acting out is not a defense mechanism.

   NP:AN; CN:PS; CL:AN

7. (4) This client is in severe anxiety heading for a panic level. She requires immediate medication, constant attention, and a gradual lessening of activity according to her expressed level of energy. With moderate anxiety, directed activity helps to reduce the level.

   NP:I; CN:PS; CL:A

8. (1) If the client and/or the situation gets out of control, anxiety will only increase. Additional help may prevent this from occurring.

   NP:AN; CN:PS; CL:AN

9. (1) The primary reason for the compulsive activity is to decrease the anxiety caused by obsessive thoughts. The client is not trying to focus her atten-

---

Coding for Questions/Answers Abbreviations: **Nursing Process: NP,** Assessment: A, Analysis: AN, Planning: P, Implementation: I, Evaluation: E; **Client Needs: CN,** Safe, Effective Care Environment: S, Health Promotion and Maintenance: H, Psychosocial Integrity: PS, Physiological Integrity: PH; **Clinical Area: CA,** Medical Nursing: M, Surgical Nursing: S, Maternal/Newborn Nursing: MA, Pediatric Nursing: P, Psychiatric Nursing: PS; **Cognitive Level: CL,** Knowledge: K, Comprehension: C, Application: A, Analysis: AN.

tion on tasks, control others, or lessen interaction with others.

NP:AN; CN:PS; CL:C

10. (1) A goal for this disorder should be broad-based and general, like establishing a safe, supportive environment. Other answers would more directly refer to implementation of the goal strategies.

NP:P; CN:PS; CL:C

11. (2) This disorder has an unconscious mechanism in place; thus, there is a relative lack of distress or anxiety regarding the symptom. The client is likely to demonstrate "la belle indifference," an unconcerned, indifferent attitude toward the loss of function with no awareness of the psychogenic cause. Answer (3) is incorrect because secondary gains should be minimized. Answer (4) is incorrect because repression and displacement are the operating mechanisms.

NP:AN; CN:PS; CL:A

12. (3) Anticipating demands (rather than ignoring them) from a hypochondriacal client will break the pattern of demanding behavior. These clients are usually fearful and anxious. Spending time with the client will be reassuring and therapeutic. Assigning various staff members (2) may be useful so no one will become overwhelmed, but it is not the primary approach.

NP:I; CN:PS; CL:A

13. (3) Because a person with this disorder tends to manage his or her life through manipulation of others, when it doesn't work, the anxiety level goes up. The nurse should never allow the client to manipulate him or her. Answers (2) and (4) are not true.

NP:P; CN:PS; CL:A

14. (3) The first intervention is to set firm, clear limits on his behavior. The nurse would also remain with the client until he calms down and then encourage him to discuss his feelings rather than act out.

NP:I; CN:S; CL:A

15. (4) Because he may be trying to manipulate the nurse, it is important to end the interview at the agreed-upon time. Also, because the feelings are important, the nurse would need to encourage the client to bring them up again. Going over the agreed-upon time (1) is nontherapeutic because it allows manipulation. Answers (2) and (3) are also nontherapeutic.

NP:I; CN:PS; CL:AN

MOOD (AFFECTIVE) DISORDERS/SUICIDE

16. (3) Depressed people often suffer from a sense of loss—loss of status, relationships, significant other, etc. While depression is more common in the middle-age to older adult group, it is not necessarily related to stage of life (4). Neither poor interpersonal relationships (1) nor a traumatic childhood (2) is relevant as a cause of depression.

NP:AN; CN:PS; CL:C

17. (4) The correct answer does not place a value judgment on the change by stating that it is good or that the nurse is pleased. It simply acknowledges that change, which is a positive reinforcement of the behavior. Answer (1) implies that the client needs to please the nurse. The opposing conclusion may be that if she does not continue this behavior, the nurse will be displeased. Answer (2) implies that the nurse does not care enough about the client to really notice what is different. This conclusion would contribute to the client's already lowered self-esteem. Answer (3) places a definite value judgment on the change in behavior. It may be interpreted as being "bad" if she does not continue to wear a clean dress.

NP:I; CN:PS; CL:AN

18. (3) Be positive, definite, and specific about expectations. Do not give depressed clients a choice or try to convince them to get out of bed. Physically assist the client to get up and dressed to mobilize her. Do not allow her to remain in bed (4) or try to convince her by quoting the rules of the unit (1).

NP:I; CN:PS; CL:A

19. (2) The nursing intervention is directed toward mobilizing the client without asking her to make a decision or trying to convince her to go. The nurse must be direct, specific, and not take no for an answer.

NP:I; CN:S; CL:A

20. (4) While a good nursing care plan is important, the priority would be to get the client mobilized. Even without a specific diagnosis, the nurse will realize that part of what is happening with the client is a depressed mood. Providing a structured plan of activities for the client to follow will help his mood to lift and provide a focus so that he will not be centered on internal suffering.

NP:I; CN:PS; CL:C

21. (2) Concern with having a life-threatening disease is a common issue with depressed clients. While demanding behavior (3) may be a symptom, it is not the issue here. Whether the client is postmenopausal (1) is not relevant.

    NP:AN; CN:PS; CL:C

22. (3) The goal is to implement suicide precautions because the danger of suicide is when the depression lifts and the client has the energy to formulate a plan. The nurse would not encourage her to go home (1) where she could not be observed constantly. She could be moved into a room with other clients (2), but this is not the priority concern.

    NP:P; CN:S; CL:A

23. (4) Because it is unrealistic to observe a client every minute (1), the environment must be kept safe for client protection. Answer (2) is important, but not the most critical objective. Involving the client in activities (3) does not address the problem of safety with a client who is potentially suicidal.

    NP:P; CN:S; CL:A

24. (3) Even though all of the reasons are important and should not be ignored, the most important task for the staff is to assess the client's behavior and to identify cues that might indicate another impending suicide attempt.

    NP:A; CN:PS; CL:AN

25. (3) Most suggestible of suicide is the sudden sense of satisfaction or relief (perhaps from finally making the decision to commit suicide) and detachment. Hostility (1), identifying with others (2), or thinking of the future (4) do not as clearly suggest suicidal thinking.

    NP:E; CN:S; CL:A

26. (3) Engaging the client in a large-muscle activity, such as walking with the nurse, will direct the client's energy but not be too stimulating, as would a competitive game such as Ping-Pong (1) or group exercise (2). Answer (4) is nontherapeutic because it is too stimulating for a manic client.

    NP:I; CN:PS; CL:A

27. (3) Setting limits is important to avoid rejection of the other clients with subsequent lowering of self-esteem. Confronting the client (1) will not be productive and may just increase the annoying activity. Ignoring the behavior (2) will also be nontherapeutic, and the other clients on the unit will become even more hostile. This client will not be able to follow a rigid plan.

    NP:I; CN:PS; CL:A

SUBSTANCE ABUSE

28. (1) The most important nursing attitude, which underlies all interactions with this client, including a nurse–client relationship, would be to maintain a nonjudgmental approach. If a nurse carries any judgments about alcoholism, it will negate a working relationship with the client.

    NP:P; CN:PS; CL:A

29. (3) The first intervention is to place the client in a single room so stimuli are decreased and the siderails are up for safety. This client could begin convulsing. Lights should be on, especially if the client is hallucinating, because seeing shadows might be very scary (and this client could die of heart failure). The next interventions would be to establish an IV (1), take vital signs (4), and then administer a tranquilizer (2).

    NP:I; CN:PS; CL:AN

30. (3) With Wernicke's encephalopathy, the critical and often life-saving intervention is to give vitamin B (thiamine) STAT. This acute condition occurs in relation to chronic alcoholism (Korsakoff's syndrome) with an inadequate intake of basic nutrients. The syndrome improves with an adequate diet, but only 25 percent fully recover. Korsakoff's condition remains after Wernicke's encephalopathy is treated. The other answers would not be implemented.

    NP:P; CN:S; CL:C

COGNITIVE DISORDERS

31. (2) When clients make up stories or lies, it is called *confabulation*. This is an attempt to fill in memory gaps caused by the destruction of the neurons. This process protects their self-esteem and should not be discouraged or confronted.

    NP:AN; CN:PS; CL:K

32. (3) It is essential that the client participate in activities that provide him with immediate success and increase his self-esteem. Interaction with others is important but is secondary to improving his self-esteem. Competition may cause anxiety and would be nontherapeutic. Continuity in personnel is important, but not in activities.

    NP:P; CN:PS; CL:A

33. (3) Dementia has a poor prognosis and is usually progressive and irreversible; the symptoms are closely related to the client's basic personality. All of the char-

acteristics in (3) fit the picture of cognitive disorder. The condition may or may not progress rapidly, but will generally deteriorate and is irreversible.

NP:A; CN:PH; CL:C

34. (2) Korsakoff's syndrome (also called polyneuritic psychosis) is a form of cognitive disorder that is associated with long-term alcohol abuse and a deficiency of vitamin B complex, especially thiamine. Answer (2) is more specific than answer (1). This condition is not caused from a lesion, hepatitis (3), or psychosis (4).

NP:A; CN:PH; CL:C

SCHIZOPHRENIC DISORDERS

35. (2) The most important goal with a schizophrenic is to establish a trusting relationship, but not a warm, close one, which would be too threatening (3). It is not a short-term goal to set limits on behavior or protect the client from deviant impulses—inappropriate behavior will diminish as medication takes hold and the client becomes less disturbed (1).

NP:P; CN:PS; CL:K

36. (3) The best response when a client has the diagnosis of schizophrenia is to validate reality by saying the nurse doesn't hear anything and then to explore real feelings, like fear. Answer (1) is not enough to be therapeutic; answers (2) and (4) give validity to the voices if, in fact, the client is hallucinating.

NP:I; CN:PS; CL:A

37. (3) Mazuka is a made-up word, called a neologism. This characteristic is frequently present with the disorder and is a part of associative looseness. Answer (1) is not incorrect, but answer (3) is more specific. Flight of ideas is observed with a manic episode.

NP:AN; CN:PS; CL:C

38. (1) This response asks the client to discuss religion and God; this subject is very confusing for schizophrenics because they have difficulty knowing what is real. It is considered a nontherapeutic topic to discuss. The other three responses are acceptable. Answer (2) is the most therapeutic.

NP:I; CN:PS; CL:AN

39. (3) Depersonalization is the feeling or subjective experience of separating oneself or alienation; it is also the state in which the client cannot distinguish the self from others and involves disintegration of the ego—often observed in schizophrenics as a flight from reality.

NP:AN; CN:PS; CL:K

40. (4) Ideas of reference or misinterpretation occur when the client believes that an incident has a personal reference to oneself when, in fact, it is not at all related. Symbolic rejection does not apply to this situation and is not a term used in psychiatric theory (1). Hallucinations are false perceptions with no basis in reality (2). Depersonalization is alienation from oneself (3).

NP:AN; CN:PS; CL:A

41. (1) Hallucinations may involve any sense, and they have no basis in reality. The most common are auditory. Answer (3) is an example of an auditory hallucination. Answer (2) is an illusion; answer (4) is a delusion.

NP:AN; CN:PS; CL:K

42. (3) Giving the client a choice of how he would like to take his medication, while being firm that he must take it, gives the client a sense of control and helps to reduce the power struggle. Telling the client that the medication is not poison will do little to persuade him to comply. Answer (2) would represent a punishment. The client must take his medication; therefore, answer (4) is not appropriate.

NP:I; CN:PS; CL:A

43. (1) Assuming responsibility for one's behavior includes acknowledging the behavior and may include a statement of one's current status. It does not include making excuses, focusing outside of oneself, or blaming another.

NP:I; CN:PS; CL:AN

44. (4) Before the nurse can implement any care plan that might include setting limits or integrating the child into the group, the nurse would need to establish a relationship, either through verbal or nonverbal communication. After establishing a relationship, the nurse will assess each child.

NP:P; CN:S; CL:A

45. (2) Depression is more successfully treated by ECT than are the other conditions listed. It is a treatment of choice for elderly clients who experience depression with vegetative aspects. A dramatic lift of the depression may be seen after only a few treatments. None of the other disorders have been found to be successfully treated with ECT.

NP:P; CN:PS; CL:K

46. (1) The major goal in crisis treatment centers is to have the client return to a prior level of functioning. At this time in a crisis, it is not therapeutic to work on the dynamics underlying the symptom (2) or make long-range plans (3). Accepting the illness (4) may be a part of returning to a prior level of functioning.

    NP:P; CN:PS; CL:C

PSYCHOTROPIC DRUGS

47. (3) The nurse must first recognize that the drug Parnate is an MAO inhibitor. The assessment for the side effects of Parnate should include ascertaining whether the client has ingested foods containing tyramine (cheese, wine, etc.), which could lead to hypertensive crisis, which the presenting symptoms suggest.

    NP:A; CN:S; CL:AN

48. (1) The most important teaching is to maintain an adequate sodium intake to maintain fluid level. Low Na$^+$ or limited fluids can lead to lithium toxicity. (4)

    This instruction refers to an MAO-inhibiting drug that is given for depression.

    NP:P; CN:H; CL:A

49. (1) Tardive dyskinesia usually develops late in treatment and may occur in up to 50 percent of chronic schizophrenics with the long-term use of phenothiazine drugs. Antiparkinson drugs such as Artane and Cogentin are of no help in decreasing the symptoms. Parkinsonism (2), dystonia (3), and akathisia (4) are also extrapyramidal side effects of phenothiazine use, but these conditions are reversible with drugs.

    NP:AN; CN:PH; CL:A

50. (3) This new drug (similar to a phenothiazine) manages psychotic symptoms such as hallucinations, and the incidence of these symptoms should be reduced. Leukopenia (agranulocytosis) (1) is a side effect, and altered liver function studies (2) would be negative. This medication should not affect the client's energy level (4).

    NP:E; CN:PS; CL:A

Gerontological Nursing 15

✦ The icon denotes content of special importance for NCLEX.

GENERAL CONCEPTS OF AGING

General Concepts

A. Aging is an *individual* process.
B. Most older persons view their health as a positive state.
C. Coping with life has been successful because the person has "survived" to be old.
D. "Normal" aging may be confused with disease process in aging persons.
   1. Illness is frequently misdiagnosed as "normal" aging.
   2. Because of "decline" due to "normal" aging, symptoms are neglected by family and medical personnel.
   3. Older persons underreport symptoms of illness because they interpret symptoms as "growing older."
E. Most older persons have more than one chronic disease.
F. Chronological age is simply the number of years a person has lived.
G. Functional age refers to the person's ability to function effectively within society.

Definitions Relating to Older Adults

A. *Gerontology:* Scientific study of the process of aging; examining the changes that occur as a person ages; study of the needs of the older adult.
B. *Aging:* Process of growing older; physiological changes in body systems as the person grows older; a biological/physiological process influenced by emotional state and social context.
C. *Life span:* Maximum potential for survival of a species.
D. *Life expectancy:* Amount of time lived from birth to death.
E. *Frail old:* Person 75 years of age or older with some impairment in ability to provide functional self-care.
F. *Gerontological nursing:* Use of the nursing process in caring for the physiological, psychological, and sociological needs of the aging person.

Demographics

✦ A. In 2030, the U.S. population will include > 35 million persons, 21 percent of the total over the age of 65 years.
   1. The post–World War II "baby boom" babies will reach senior status around the year 2010.
   2. The number of persons over 65 years of age is projected to grow from 34 to 40 million between 1995 and 2010, an increase of nearly 20 percent.
✦ B. Average life expectancy in the United States hit a new high of 77.6 years in 2003, up from 77 years in

---

> ### CLASSIFICATION OF AGING
>
> *Middle age:* 40–64 years of age.
> *Young old:* 65–74 years of age.
> *Old:* 75–84 years of age.
> *Old old:* 85–100 years of age.
> *Elite old:* Over 100.

2000. Life expectancy increased for both men and women and for whites and blacks.
   1. For men, life expectancy increased from 74.3 years in 2000 to 75.1 years in 2002.
   2. For women, life expectancy increased from 79.7 years to 80.3 years in 2002.
   3. The age-adjusted death rate hit an all-time low in 2002, at 855 deaths per 100,000 people, compared to 869 deaths per 100,000 in 2000.
   4. White females live approximately 5.2 years longer than white males.
   5. African American females live approximately 9 years longer than African American males.
   6. White females live approximately 5.2 years longer than African American females.
C. Human potential life span is estimated to be 115 years.
D. Increased life expectancy due to
   1. Advanced health care.
   2. Decreased infant/child mortality.
   3. Improved nutrition and sanitation.
   4. Increased infectious disease control.
E. Five to ten percent of older adults are alcohol abusers.

Healthcare Costs

A. Government spending for health care of older adults has doubled in the last 20 years.
   1. Healthcare services are used more by the aged person.
   2. The older the age of the person, the longer the stay in the hospital.
   3. Older persons personally pay just over 50 percent of the cost of their health care. The remainder is paid by Medicare, Medicaid, and insurance.
B. The percentage of aged who live in nursing homes is 4–6 percent.
   1. Twenty-two percent over age 85 are in nursing homes.
   2. Before death, 20–27 percent of the aged use institutional care.
✦ C. Nursing home residents have an average of 3.9 diseases.
   1. Over 40 percent have more than one illness.
   2. Diseases may be multiple and chronic.

3. In 2002 and 2004, nursing home population was 1.5 million. An upward trend is expected to continue for the next several decades.
D. Eighteen percent of older adults die at home.
E. Institutional placement most often results from a lack of social support as families become exhausted with caregiving.

Morbidity and Mortality

A. In 2001, there were decreases in several leading causes of death. Stroke was down by almost 5 percent, heart disease 4 percent, cancer 2 percent, and accidents 2 percent.
✦ B. Leading causes of death (in order of frequency): heart disease, cancer, stroke, chronic obstructive pulmonary disease (COPD), pneumonia/flu, diabetes, accidents, suicide.
✦ C. Three out of four older adults die of heart disease, cancer, or stroke.
   1. Heart disease is leading cause of death in the United States, although it has declined since 1968.
   2. Death rates from cancer continue to rise, especially lung cancer.
   3. Death statistics for people in the 65 to 74 age group:
      a. Heart disease accounted for 38 percent of deaths.
      b. Cancer accounted for 30 percent of deaths.
✦ D. Leading chronic conditions for older adults.
   1. Arthritis.
   2. Hypertensive disease.
   3. Heart conditions.
   4. Hearing impairments.
   5. Visual impairments.
   6. Dementia.
E. Objectives are to maintain vitality and independence of people age 65 and older.

Theories on Aging

A. Biological.
   ✦ 1. *Cellular.* As cells are damaged, there is instability in the body.
      ✦ a. Free radicals—oxidation releases chemicals that affect the cell membrane and DNA replication.
      b. Cross-link—chemical bondage of elements that are generally separated.
      c. Doubling/biological clock—a cell has a genetically predetermined number of replications (Hayflick's theory).
      d. Stress—homeostatic imbalance causes wear and tear on the organism.

   e. Error catastrophic—transcription errors in the RNA and DNA, leading to cell mutation, which is perpetuated.
   2. *Immunity.* The thymus and bone marrow become less functional, so the body is less protected.
✦ B. Psychological.
   1. Adaptation to stress—genetic makeup and personal learning to deal with life crises.
   2. Life experience.
      a. Disengagement—the person and society let go of each other.
      b. Dependence—reliance on others for satisfaction of physical and emotional needs.
C. Sociological.
   1. Cultural and role expectation—relates to adaptation/dependence when defining level of activity/behavior/wellness.
   2. Environment—toxins and pollutants.

NURSING PROCESS IN CARING FOR THE AGED PERSON

System Assessment

✦ A. Priority—determine individual's capacity for safe, functional self-care.
✦ B. Utilize multidimensional approach to provide basis for individualized care plan.
   1. Physiological.
      a. Structural changes, normal and abnormal.
      b. Signs of chronic illness.
      c. Signs of medication effects.
   2. Psychological.
      a. Mentation.
      b. Motivation.
      c. Needs.
   3. Sociological.
      a. Usual and preferred living arrangements.
      b. Status of social network and caregiving.
C. Assess altered presentation of data.
   1. Complex interrelationship between aging and chronic and acute illness.
   2. Signs and symptoms of illness—atypical or lacking.

System Implementation

A. Perform and/or supervise needed care.
B. Support level of self-functioning to maintain independence.
✦ C. Maintain safety precautions.
   1. Siderails when in bed but have been found *not* to prevent injury.

a. Watch for disorientation when client awakens.

b. Prevent falls due to decreased muscle mass and decreased balance.

c. Prevent orthostatic hypotension.

2. Bed in low position when not giving direct client care.

3. Handrails in bathrooms and halls.

4. Uncluttered rooms and floors.

5. Adequate, nonglare lighting.

6. Restraints when necessary.

✦ D. Provide psychosocial care.

1. Encourage psychological activity to aid sense of normality.

2. Encourage verbalization about the past.

3. Assist in selecting and attending activities.

4. Foster touching, which is a very useful tool in establishing trust.

5. Provide dignity and the feeling of worth.

6. Foster the wellness approach to life.

7. Care plans should be collaborative with client.

E. Teach family how to help/cope.

THE AGING BODY

Physiological Implications

✦ A. Physical changes.

1. Decrease in physical strength and endurance.

2. Decrease in muscular coordination.

3. Tendency to gain weight; redistribution of fat, decreased subcutaneous tissue.

4. Loss of pigment in hair and skin.

5. Increased brittleness of the bones.

6. Greater sensitivity to temperature changes with low tolerance to cold.

7. Degenerative changes in the cardiovascular system.

8. Decreased sensory faculties.

9. Decreased resistance to infection, disease, and accidents.

B. Intellectual impairment may be present.

1. Delirium impairment caused by medication and secondary-cause infection.

2. Drugs and poor nutrition contribute to this deterioration (delirium).

Psychological Implications

A. Fears about losing job—focus for living.

B. Competition with younger generation.

C. Relationships change.

1. Loss of nurturing functions within family.

2. Role change within and outside of family.

D. Loss of spouse, particularly females.

E. Realization that person is not going to accomplish some of the things that he or she wanted to do may lead to depression.

F. Physiological changes in body.

G. Changes in body image.

H. Illness.

I. Fears of approaching old age and death.

Developmental Tasks of Older Adults

✦ A. Maintains ego integrity versus despair (Erikson).

1. Integrity results when an individual is satisfied with his or her own actions and lifestyle, feels life is meaningful, remains optimistic, and continues to grow.

2. Despair results from the feeling that he or she has failed and that it is too late to change.

B. Continues a meaningful life after retirement.

C. Adjusts to income level.

D. Makes satisfactory living arrangements with spouse.

1. Adjusts to loss of spouse.

2. Maintains social contact and responsibilities.

E. Faces death realistically.

F. Provides knowledge and wisdom to assist those at other developmental levels to grow and learn.

G. Developmental process retrogresses.

1. Increasing dependency.

2. Concerns focus increasingly on self.

3. Interests may narrow.

4. Needs tangible evidence of affection.

Sociological Implications

✦ A. Major fears of the aged.

1. Physical and economic dependency.

2. Chronic illness—high percentage of older adults have chronic problems.

3. Loneliness.

4. Boredom resulting from not being needed.

✦ B. Major problems of the aged.

1. Economic deprivation.

a. Increased cost of living while income remains fixed.

b. Increased need for costly medical care.

c. Increased poverty rate for persons age 65 and older.

(1) Women, African Americans, Hispanics, and those who live alone are poorest.

(2) Major source of income is Social Security (35 percent).

2. Chronic disease and disability.

3. Loneliness and social isolation.

a. Suffer losses of friends.

b. Men die earlier, so many women are on their own.
    (1) Five times more women than men are widowed.
    (2) Half of older women are widows.
4. Visual impairment.
5. Organic brain changes.
    a. Most people have memory impairment.
    b. The change is gradual.
C. Death in the life cycle.
    1. In U.S. culture, death is not considered a positive process.
    2. Older adults may see death as an end to suffering and loneliness.
    3. Death is not feared if the person has lived a long and fulfilled life, having completed all developmental tasks.
    4. Religious beliefs and/or philosophy of life are important.
D. Older adults may provide knowledge and wisdom from their vast experiences, which can assist those at other developmental levels to grow and learn.

Elder Abuse and Neglect

Characteristics

A. Over 1 million older adults are estimated to be abused or neglected.
B. Seldom reported to authorities even though there is often a pattern of repetition.
C. Typical victim.
    1. Older women with limitation in one ADL.
    2. Most are widowed.
    3. Caucasian.
    4. Low income.
    5. Dependent on abuser for some aspect of care.
D. Abused is associated with
    1. Substance abuse.
    2. Caregiver strain.
    3. Depression.
✦ E. Forms of elder abuse.
    1. Physical: intentionally inflicting injury or pain.
    2. Emotional: verbal harassment, intimidation, denigration, or isolation.
    3. Sexual abuse: any nonconsensual touching or sexual contact.
    4. Neglect: deteriorating health, dehydration, malnutrition, failure to provide food or services or care necessary to maintain health and safety; pressure ulcers, dirt, body odor, over- or undermedication.
    5. Financial: improper or unauthorized use of funds or property or power of attorney.
F. Suspect abuse if client has unexplained injuries or conflicting stories from client and caregiver.

G. All states have enacted elder abuse laws designed to protect older or vulnerable adults from abuse.
✦ H. Majority of states require nurses and other healthcare providers to report cases of suspected elder abuse.
    1. Standard for reporting is "reasonable" belief.
    2. Most states provide immunity from civil and criminal liability.
    3. Support suspicions with documentation and witnesses.

✦ Assessment

A. Ask client and caregiver to explain injury.
    1. If client appears to be a victim, separate from caregiver and question.
    2. Follow up by documenting and report according to facility policy.
B. Assess physical injuries for abuse.
    1. Multiple injuries or fractures.
    2. Bruises or burns.
    3. Sprains or dislocations (frequent falls).
C. Assess for neglect (a form of abuse).
    1. Deteriorating health, failure to thrive.
    2. Dehydration or malnutrition.
    3. Pressure ulcers or contractures.
    4. Over- or undermedication.
    5. Excessive dirt or body odor.
D. Question client about emotional or financial abuse.

Implementation

✦ A. Report all cases of suspected elder abuse even if there is no direct evidence—just a "reasonable" belief that abuse is present.
B. Promote family problem-solving actions to resolve situation.

General Physiological Changes

A. Cells.
    1. Fewer in number.
    2. Larger in size.
    3. Decreased total body fluid due to decreased intracellular fluid.
B. Ear.
    1. Age-related changes can result in hearing loss.
    ✦ 2. Presbycusis (sensorineural hearing loss).
        a. Progressive hearing loss in inner ear.
        b. High-frequency tones are lost first.
        c. Sounds are distorted; difficulty understanding words when other noises are in the background.
        d. Present in 30–40 percent of those over age 65.
        e. No clear-cut cause.
        f. May be due to insults from

      (1)   Noise exposures.
      (2)   Systemic or vascular disease.
      (3)   Nutrition.
      (4)   Ototoxic drugs.
      (5)   Pollution exposure.
   3.   Tympanic membrane atrophic, sclerotic.
   4.   Cerumen accumulates; may become impacted due to increased amount of keratin.

C. Eye.
   ✦ 1.   Presbyopia—vision impairment caused by diminished power of accommodation from loss of elasticity of lens.
   2.   Pupil sphincter sclerosis with loss of light responsiveness.
   3.   Cornea more spherical.
   4.   Lens more opaque.
   5.   Increased light perception threshold.
      a.   Adapt to darkness more slowly.
      b.   Difficulty seeing in dim light.
   6.   Loss of accommodation.
   7.   Decreased visual field; less peripheral vision.
   8.   Decreased color discrimination on blue/green end of scale.
   9.   Distorted depth perception.
  10. Glare intolerance.
  11. Reduced lacrimation.

✦ D. Vital signs.
   1.   Blood pressure increases with age; there is a higher incidence in men than women up to age 70.
   2.   Heart rate remains unchanged.
   3.   Respiratory rate unchanged.
   4.   Core temperature unchanged.
   5.   Prone to hypothermia.

E. Mood.
   1.   Suffer multiple losses.
   2.   Neurological changes.
   3.   Loss of environment and interpersonal stimuli.
   4.   Defense mechanisms are less effective.

Baseline Admission Assessment

A. Temperature.
   1.   May be as low as 95°F.
   2.   Sublingual most accurate.
   3.   Easily dehydrated with increased temperature.

B. Pulse.
   1.   Rate, rhythm, volume.
   2.   Apical, radial, pedal, other sites as indicated by disorder.

C. Respirations.
   1.   Rate, rhythm, depth.
   2.   Irregularity common.

D. Arterial blood pressure.
   1.   Lying, sitting, standing.

   2.   Postural hypotension is common.
   3.   Hypertension (160/95 mm Hg or greater).

E. Weight—gradual loss in late years.
F. Orientation level.
G. Memory.
H. Sleep pattern.
I. Psychosocial adjustment.
   1.   Depression.
   2.   Paranoia.
   3.   Loneliness.
   4.   Increasing dependency.
   5.   Concerns focus increasingly on self.
   6.   Displays narrower interests.

J. Immunization history.
K. General appearance.
   1.   Gray and thinning hair.
   2.   Wrinkled, pigmented, and thin skin.
   3.   Eyes slightly sunken.
   4.   Ears/nose appear slightly larger.
   5.   Responds more slowly to questions and directions.
   6.   Normal aging—intake of new information and abstract reasoning is prolonged.
   7.   Trunk thicker; thinner arms and legs.
   8.   Gait slower and less steady.
   9.   Slower movements.
  10. Possible slight tremor.
  11. Flexion of spine/limbs.

Neurological System

✦ **Physiological Age Changes**

A. Decreased speed of nerve conduction.
B. Delay in response and reaction time, especially with stress.
C. Diminution of sensory faculties.
   1.   Decreased vision.
   2.   Loss of hearing.
   3.   Diminished sense of smell and taste.
   4.   Greater sensitivity to temperature changes with low tolerance to cold.

Assessment

A. Facial symmetry.
B. Poor reflex reactions; slowed reaction time.
✦ C. Level of alertness—presence of organic brain changes.
   1.   Not all persons become confused.
   2.   Most people have some memory impairment; learning takes longer.
   3.   Change is gradual.
   4.   Potential for accidents, falls.
✦ D. Malnutrition—dehydration.
✦ E. Eyes: movement, clarity, presence of cataracts.
   1.   Level of visual impairment.

2. Pupils: equality, dilation, constriction.
3. Visual acuity—decreases with age.
   a. Do not test vision while client is facing window.
   b. Use handheld chart.
   c. Check condition of glasses.
4. Dry eyes—tearing is decreased.
F. Sensory deprivation—understimulation or sensory overload.
G. Hypothermia.
H. Hearing acuity.
   1. Hearing aid.
   2. Tinnitus.
   3. Cerumen in outer ear—refer to specialist.
I. Presence of pain.
J. Sleep distrubances.
K. Depression.

Implementation
A. Maintain safety precautions.
   1. Evaluate reflex reactions to protect against accidents.
   2. Evaluate level of alertness.
B. Monitor dietary intake and fluid intake.
C. Provide adequate lighting to prevent falls.
   1. Natural lighting best.
   2. Avoid glare.
   3. Night-light at all times in bathrooms, halls.
D. Encourage sensory stimulation.
   1. Large-print books.
   2. Changes in environment.
   3. Colors client can see.
E. Maintain reality orientation.
   1. Calendars.
   2. Clocks.
   3. One-to-one visits.
F. Keep client warm—prevent hypothermia.
G. Check sedative or hypnotic abuse for poor sleep patterns.
H. Check for antidepressant drugs.

Cardiovascular System

Physiological Age Changes
A. Structural changes.
   1. Mitral and aortic valves become sclerotic and calcified.
   2. Decreased baroreceptor sensitivity.
   3. Mild fibrosis and calcification of valves.
B. Cardiac output.
   1. Decreases 1% per year after age 20 due to decreased heart rate and decreased stroke volume.
   2. Force of contraction decreased.
   3. Ventricular wall thickens.
   4. Heart muscle decreased.

C. Vessels lose elasticity.
   1. Less effective peripheral oxygenation.
   2. Position change from lying to sitting or sitting to standing can cause blood pressure to drop as much as 65 mm Hg.
D. Increased peripheral vessel resistance.
   1. Blood pressure increases: systolic may normally be 170 mm Hg, diastolic may normally be 95 mm Hg.
   2. Smooth muscle in arteries is less responsive.
E. Blood clotting increases.

Assessment
A. Peripheral circulation, pulses, color, warmth.
   1. Widened pulse pressure.
   2. Jugular vein distention.
B. Circulatory status; orthostatic hypotension; hypertension.
   1. Dizziness; fainting.
   2. Auscultate heart sounds.
C. Premature beats and dysrhythmias.
D. Edema—decreased venous return.
E. Activity intolerance.
   1. Weakness.
   2. Fatigue.
F. Dyspnea.
G. Transient ischemic attacks (TIAs).
H. Anemia.

Implementation
A. Monitor vital signs—pulse, blood pressure.
   1. Apical pulse for 1 minute so premature beats are not missed.
   2. Take blood pressure in both arms.
B. Monitor medications—digitalis, diuretics, etc.
C. Maintain dietary restrictions (low salt).
D. Change position slowly, especially from horizontal to vertical, to prevent hypotensive reaction.
E. Maintain circulatory homeostasis.
   1. Encourage activity to increase circulatory stimulation; leg exercises, leg elevation while sitting.
   2. Provide warmth by applying blankets and clothing.
   3. Use gentle friction during bath.
   4. Avoid tight/restrictive clothing.

Respiratory System

Physiological Age Changes
A. Respiratory muscles lose strength and become rigid.
B. Ciliary activity decreases.
C. Lungs lose elasticity (decreased breath sounds at base).
   1. Residual capacity increases.
   2. Larger on inspiration.

3. Maximum breathing capacity decreases; depth of respirations decreases.
D. Alveoli increase in size, reduce in number.
    1. Fewer capillaries at alveoli.
    2. Dilated and less elastic alveoli.
✦ E. Gas exchange is reduced.
    1. Arterial blood oxygen PaO_2 decreases to 75 mm Hg at age 70.
    2. Arterial blood carbon dioxide $PaCO_2$ unchanged.
F. Coughing ability is reduced—less sensitive mechanism.
G. Decline in immune response.
H. More dependent on the diaphragm for breathing.
I. System less responsive to hypoxia and hypercardia.
J. Ability to maintain acid–base balance decreased.

✦ **Assessment**

A. Chest excursion.
B. Auscultate lung/breath sounds.
C. Quality of cough, if present; sputum.
D. Rib cage deformity.
E. Dyspnea, hypoxia, and hypercarbia.
F. Need for oxygen therapy.
G. Activity intolerance.
H. Anxiety.
I. Rate and rhythm.

Implementation

✦ A. Manage airway clearance.
    1. Clean nares if nasal passages are clogged.
    2. Postural drainage, if necessary.
B. Monitor hydration status.
✦ C. Promote respiratory activity with exercises.
    1. Teach deep-breathing exercises.
    2. Forced expiration.
    3. Coughing.
D. Monitor oxygen therapy.
    1. *Caution:* check for carbon dioxide narcosis.
    2. *Symptoms:* confusion, profuse perspiration, visual disturbance, muscle twitching, hypotension, cerebral dysfunction.

Gastrointestinal System

Physiological Age Changes

A. Tooth loss.
    1. Periodontal disease is major cause of loss after 30 years of age.
    2. Other causes include poor dental health, poor nutrition.
    3. Dentine decreased.
    4. Gingival retraction.
B. Taste sensation and thirst decrease.
    ✦ 1. When there is diminished sense of thirst, less water is consumed and dehydration may result.

2. Atrophy of up to 80 percent of taste buds.
3. Less sensitivity of those on tip of tongue first: sweet and salt.
4. Less sensitivity of those on sides of tongue later: salt, sour, bitter.
C. Esophagus dilates, decreased motility, lower sphincter pressure decreases. Increased risk for aspiration.
D. Stomach.
    1. Hunger sensations decrease.
    2. Secretion of hydrochloric acid decreases.
    3. Emptying time decreases.
E. Peristalsis decreases and constipation is common.
✦ F. Absorption function is impaired.
    1. Body absorbs less nutrients due to reduced intestinal blood flow and atrophy of cells on absorbing surfaces.
    2. Decrease in gastric and pancreatic enzymes affects absorption.
G. Hiatal hernia common (40 to 60 percent of elderly).
H. Diverticulitis (40 percent over age 70).
I. Liver.
    1. Fewer cells with decreased storage capacity.
    2. Decreased blood flow.
    3. Enzymes decrease.
    4. Ability to regenerate decreases.
    5. Hepatic protein synthesis is impaired.
J. Pancreas.
    1. Impaired pancreatic reserve.
    2. Ducts become distended.
    3. Lipase production decreased.
K. Decreased glucose tolerance.

Assessment

A. Tooth loss—poor dentition, inadequate chewing, poor swallowing reflex.
B. Condition of teeth, gums, buccal cavity.
✦ C. Dietary intake—malnutrition.
    1. Anorexia; nausea and vomiting.
    2. Regurgitation.
    3. Anemia.
D. Indigestion, heartburn, pain, indications of possible hiatal hernia.
✦ E. Bowel problems.
    1. Constipation, fecal impaction.
    2. Fecal incontinence.
    3. Diarrhea.
F. Drug toxicity.

Implementation

A. Monitor for adequate nutrition; stimulate appetite.
    1. Small, frequent feedings of high quality.
    2. Attractive meals, wine if allowed.
    3. Female, 1600 calories; male, 2200 calories.
    4. Preferred foods if possible; ethnic choices.
B. Lessen/prevent indigestion.

1. Fowler's position for meals and keep upright 30 minutes after meals.
2. Antacids contraindicated.
3. Plan meals.
   a. Smaller meals without gas formers.
   b. Low fat.
   c. Avoid foods that cause distress.
4. Adequate fluids; monitor for dehydration.

✦ C. Prevent constipation.
1. Ensure adequate bulk (fiber) and fluid in diet.
2. Encourage activity.
3. Ensure regular and adequate time for bowel movement.
4. Provide privacy and normal positioning.
5. Administer laxative or suppository if above not effective. Note that laxatives are often abused—use with caution.

Genitourinary System

Physiological Age Changes

A. Kidneys.
1. Smaller due to nephron atrophy.
2. Renal blood flow decreases 50 percent.
3. Glomerular filtration rate decreases 50 percent.
   ✦ 4. Tubular function diminishes.
   a. Less able to concentrate urine; lower specific gravity.
   b. Proteinuria 1+ is common.
   c. Blood urea nitrogen (BUN) increases to 21 mg/%.
5. Renal threshold for glucose increases.
6. Potential for dehydration increases.
7. Excretion of toxins and drugs decreases.
8. Nocturia, frequency and urgency increase.

✦ B. Bladder.
1. Muscle weakens.
2. Capacity decreases to 200 mL or less, causing frequency.
3. Emptying is more difficult, causing increased retention.
4. Decreased sphincter control.
5. Less control, increased stress incontinence.

C. Age-related changes and associated clinical manifestations in male reproductive system.
   ✦ 1. Prostate enlarges to some degree in 75 percent of men over age 65.
   a. Enlarges with age—hypertrophy.
   b. Difficulty initiating urine stream.
2. Testicular volume decreases.
3. Sperm count decreases.
4. Seminal vesicles atrophy.
5. Serum testosterone constant.
6. Estrogen levels increase.
7. Sexual response less intense.
8. Longer to achieve erection.
9. Erection maintained without ejaculation.
10. Force of ejaculation decreased.

D. Age-related changes and associated clinical manifestations in female reproductive system.
1. Menopause occurs by mean age of 50.
2. Perineal muscle weakens.
3. Vulva atrophies.
4. Vagina.
   a. Mucous membrane becomes dryer.
   b. Elasticity of tissue decreases, so surface is smooth.
   c. Secretions become reduced, more alkaline.
   d. Flora changes.
5. Estradiol, prolactin, progesterone diminish.
6. Size of ovaries, uterus, cervix, fallopian tubes, labia decreases.
7. Elasticity of the pelvic area decreases.
8. Breast tissue decreases.
9. Intensity of sexual response decreases.
10. Potential for vaginal infection increases.
11. Potential for vaginal and uterine prolapse increases.

E. Sexuality.
1. Older people continue to be sexual beings with sexual needs.
2. No particular age at which a person's sexual functioning ceases.
3. Frequency of genital sexual behavior (intercourse) may tend to decline gradually in later years, but capacity for expression and enjoyment continue far into old age.
4. Risk of STDs and AIDS continues with age.

✦ **Assessment**

A. Dehydration, fluid intake and output (I&O).
B. Drug toxicity.
C. Urine: appearance, color, odor.
D. Bladder: frequency, urgency, hesitancy.
1. Distention; incontinence.
2. Males: difficulty initiating urine stream.
E. Nonspecific signs: fever, vomiting, dysuria, lower abdominal discomfort, hematuria for possible asymptomatic urinary tract infection.
F. Sexuality—females.
1. Vaginal irritation.
2. Painful coitus.

Implementation

✦ A. Adequate fluid intake: 1500 mL minimum to 2500 mL daily.
B. Incontinence prevention.
1. Offer opportunity to void every 2 hours.
2. Provide easy access to bathroom.
3. Keep night-light in bathroom to prevent falls.

4. Schedule diuretics for maximum effect during daylight hours.
5. Limit fluids near and at bedtime.
6. Teach female clients Kegel exercises to strengthen perineal muscles.
7. Avoid caffeine.

C. Sexuality.
1. Provide counseling if desired.
2. Provide opportunity for desired sexual expression.
3. Encourage touching and companionship, which are important for older people.

Musculoskeletal System

Physiological Age Changes

A. Contractures.
1. Muscle mass decreases; regenerates slowly.
2. Tendons shrink and sclerose.
B. Range of motion of joints decreases.
1. Lack of adequate joint motion, ankylosis.
2. Slight flexion of joints.
✦ C. Mobility level.
1. Ambulate with or without assistance or devices.
2. Limitations to movement.
3. Muscle strength lessens.
4. Gait becomes unsteady.
D. Kyphosis, such as postural changes with forward bend.
E. Intervertebral discs narrow, height diminishes by 1–4 inches (2.5–10 cm).
F. Trunk length decreases.
G. Redistribution of subcutaneous fat to abdomen/hips.
H. Bone changes.
1. Loss of trabecular and cortical bone.
2. Decreased density.
3. Become brittle.
I. Degeneration of the extrapyramidal tract.

✦ Assessment

A. Backward tilt of head (kyphosis).
B. Hips, knees, and wrists more flexed.
C. Decreased height (thinning discs).
D. Decreased movement; impaired mobility.
E. Muscle cramps and/or tremors.
F. Pain.
G. Decreased flexibility; stiff and enlarged joints.
H. Frequent falls.

Implementation

A. Ambulate within limitations.
✦ B. Alter position every 2 hours; align correctly.
C. Prevent osteoporosis of long bones by providing exercises against resistance; calcium, vitamin D supplements.
D. Provide active and passive exercises.

1. Rest periods necessary.
2. Paced throughout the day.
E. Provide range-of-motion exercises to all joints three times a day.
F. Educate family that allowing the client to be sedentary is not helpful.
G. Encourage walking, which is best single exercise for the elderly, and swimming.
H. Use assistive devices as needed.

Integumentary System

Physiological Age Changes

A. Skin is less effective as a barrier.
1. Decreased protection from trauma.
2. Less ability to retain water.
3. Decreased temperature regulation.
4. Decreased sensory receptors.
B. Skin composition changes.
1. Dryness (osteotosis) due to decreased endocrine secretion.
2. Loss of elastin.
3. Increased vascular fragility.
4. Thicker and more wrinkled on sun-exposed areas.
5. Melanocyte cluster pigmentation.
C. Sweat glands.
1. Decreased number and size.
2. Decreased function of sebaceous glands.
D. Hair.
1. General hair loss.
2. Decreased melanin production.
3. Facial hair increases in women, decreases in men, except in nose and ears—impacts sensory perception.
E. Nails are more brittle and thick.

Assessment

A. Skin.
1. Temperature, degree of moisture, dryness.
2. Intactness, open lesions, tears, pressure ulcers.
3. Turgor, dehydration.
4. Pigmentation alterations, potential cancer.
5. Pruritus—dry skin most common cause.
B. Bruises, scars.
C. Condition of nails (hard and brittle).
1. Presence of fungus.
2. Overgrown or horny toenails; ingrown.
D. Condition of hair.
E. Infestations (scabies, lice).

Implementation

A. Bathing can minimize dryness.
1. Have client take complete bath only twice a week.

2. Use superfatted soap or lotions to aid in moisturizing.
3. Use tepid, not hot, water.
4. Apply emollient (lanolin) to skin after bathing.

B. Clip facial hairs for female clients if desired.

C. Handle client gently to prevent skin tears.

✦ D. Monitor for skin tears, bruising, and pressure ulcers.

E. Cut toenails unless contraindicated.
   1. Mycosis of nails.
   2. Certain medical/surgical conditions, such as diabetes, may require special order.

Endocrine System

Physiological Age Changes

A. Production of most hormones is reduced.

B. Parathyroid function and secretion are unchanged.

C. Pituitary decreases in weight and changes in cell type proportion. Significance is undetermined.
   1. Growth hormone present, but in lower blood levels.
   2. Reduced ACTH, TSH, FSH, LH production.

D. Reduced thyroid activity.
   1. Decreased basal metabolic rate.
   2. Reduced ^{131}I uptake.

E. Reduced aldosterone production.

F. Reduced gonadal secretion of progesterone, estrogen, testosterone.

COMMON CONDITIONS IN THE AGED

Delirium

Definition: A cognitive disorder that may be reversible as opposed to dementia, which is irreversible.

CAUSES OF FALSE DELIRIUM

- Drug side effects: most common are lithium, barbiturates, atropine, bromides.
- Depression.
- Nutritional deficiency.
- Toxins: air pollution and alcohol.
- Heavy metals: lead and mercury.
- Diseases (e.g., metabolic disorders, multiple sclerosis, hyperthyroidism, anemia, hypoglycemia).

Dementia*

Definition: An organic condition resulting in an impairment of cognitive function manifested by long- and short-term memory loss with impaired judgment, abstract thinking, and behavior, resulting in self-care deficit.

* *See* Dementia in Chapter 14, Psychiatric Nursing.

Characteristics

A. Etiology is unknown.

B. Incidence is 5 million in the United States over age 65 (10 to 20 percent of the population).

✦ C. Leading cause of institutionalization in older people. Of 1.3 million nursing home residents, one-half to two-thirds have some form of cognitive impairment.

D. A leading cause of death (120,000 annually).

E. Cost to society is $30 billion annually.

F. Ten to 21 percent of dementias are pseudodementia—reversible—may be related to depression.

✦ G. Determine if false delirium is present.

H. Irreversible dementia: gradual onset with a progressive course.
   1. Fifty to 70 percent are Alzheimer type (most common).
   2. Fifteen to 25 percent are multi-infarct or vascular type.
   3. Other types include Parkinson's disease, alcohol abuse, Huntington's chorea, intracranial mass.

Diagnosis

✦ A. Diagnostic criteria—must meet one criterion listed below.
   1. Sufficiently severe loss of intellectual abilities that interferes with social or occupational functioning.
   2. Memory impairment, usually of short-term memory.
   3. Impairment of abstract thinking or impaired judgment; disturbance of higher cortical function or personality change.
   4. Presence of a specific organic etiology or presumed presence.

B. Onset slow, insidious, unrelated to specific situation.

C. Gradual degeneration.

D. Mental status examination shows poor reality orientation, confusion, lack of understanding, etc.

✦ E. History reveals symptoms.
   1. Onset slow; progressive decline.
   2. Personality changes, withdrawn.
   3. Confusion noted by others but not by client.
   4. Early in the disease will attempt to find the right answer; later will not understand question.
   5. Unaware of memory loss.
      a. Begins with recent memory loss.
      b. Later, there are problems with coding and retrieving information.
   6. Oblivious to failures.

F. Possible predisposing factors: genetic, familial history of Down syndrome, enzyme deficiency, immune system deficiency, aluminum toxicity, acetylcholine (a neurotransmitter) deficiency.

Assessment

A. Adequate physical health; usually not affected.

B. Intellectual impairment; complete a mini-mental assessment tool.
   1. Alertness.
   2. Orientation.
   3. Appropriate responses to questions.
   4. Aphasia, may produce words but not sentences.
   5. Does not recognize staff or family.
C. Behavior.
   1. Performance of grooming and hygiene tasks gradually diminishes.
   2. Cooperative.
   3. Distracted.
   4. Agitated.
   5. Paranoid, delusions.
   6. Restless.
   7. Wandering behavior (frequently at sundown).
D. Motor responses.
   1. Stability of gait (motor ability declines).
   2. Functional position of limbs/joints.
E. Condition of skin.
F. Bowel and bladder function—incontinent.

Implementation

A. Provide safe environment to prevent falls, unsafe wandering.
B. Monitor medications.
   1. Give lowest dose of antipsychotic (one-fourth the dose of a middle-aged adult).
   2. Evaluate effect of antipsychotic, antidepressant, antianxiety medication.
C. Use clear, verbal communication techniques.
   1. Short words, simple sentences, verbs, and nouns.
   2. Call client by name and identify yourself.
   3. Speak slowly, clearly; wait for response.
   4. Ask only one question, give one direction at a time.
   5. Repeat, do not rephrase.
D. Use nonverbal communication.
   1. Approach in a calm, friendly manner.
   2. Use gestures, move slowly.
   3. Stand directly in front of client; maintain eye contact.
   4. Move or walk with client; do not try to stop.
   5. Listen actively; show interest.
   6. Chart all phrases and nonverbal techniques used and use those that "work."
E. Monitor activities of daily living.
   1. Orient to environment and activity on a "here and now" basis.
   2. Provide consistent routine with activities.
   3. Remind how to perform self-care activities as dressing, eating, toileting.
   4. Avoid activities that tax the memory.
   5. Give tasks that distract and occupy, such as listening to music, coloring, watching TV.

F. Assess suicide risk in early stages.
G. Maintain the client's physical activity within limits of safety.
   1. Walk outside if grounds are wander protected (fenced, alarmed) or if accompanied.
   2. Dance.
   3. Exercises with simple commands.
   4. Active games.
   5. Balance activities.
   6. Activities of daily living.
H. Provide mental stimulation.
   1. Simple hobbies.
   2. One-to-one contact.
   3. Reality orientation.
   4. Play word or number games.
I. Use consistent staff to provide care; change is frightening.
J. Encourage self-care; give cues. Pantomime brushing teeth instead of brushing client's teeth.
K. Put families in touch with support groups such as Alzheimer's Disease and Related Disorders Association, Inc. (ADRDA), chapters.

Depression

Definition: A mood disorder dominated by sadness, gloomy attitude, hopelessness, and a lack of pleasure in life.

Characteristics

A. Seven to 11 percent of community-based older adults are depressed; 1 to 2 percent suffer from major depression.
B. Most commonly treated disorder in older adults.
C. Fifteen percent of all older adults suffer from this problem (double the normal population).
D. Often mistaken for "hardening of the arteries" or other type of dementia.
E. Depression leads to other major problems, increasing the susceptibility to disease.
   1. Undernourishment.
   2. Dehydration.
   3. Inactivity.
   4. Self-neglect.
   5. Isolation.

Assessment

A. History of depression.
   1. Loss of interest in life.
   2. Sense of hopelessness and sadness.
   3. Difficulty sleeping.
   4. Weight loss due to loss of interest in food.
   5. Fatigue.
   6. Reduced sexual desire.
B. History of multiple losses.

1. Death of a spouse, friends.
2. Loss of job-related challenges and focus.
3. Loss of normal physical functioning.
4. Loss of social interaction and contacts; isolation.
5. Loss of self-esteem.

C. Complaints of memory loss.
D. Complaints of physical pain.
E. Drug side effects.
✦ F. Potential suicide risk—high incidence in the older population.
   1. With depression comes high risk for suicide.
   2. The suicide rate for 75- to 85-year-old white males is 53 per 100,000.
   3. Most significant risk factor is recent loss of major relationship.
   4. Assess for specific cues related to suicide.
      a. Hopeless talk about the future.
      b. Hints: "Things will change soon."
      c. Relates plan for ending life.
      d. Gives away belongings.

Implementation

✦ A. Implement safety precautions for suicide risk (*see* the section on suicide in Chapter 14, Psychiatric Nursing).
B. Establish daily activities to reinforce positive experiences.
   1. Give some area of control or power to person.
   2. Provide variation in daily schedule but not too many changes, as change is anxiety-producing for the elderly.
C. *See* specific nursing interventions for depression in Chapter 14, Psychiatric Nursing.

Hip (Femoral Neck) Fracture

Definition: Fracture at femoral neck can result in avascular necrosis: death of the bone due to insufficient blood supply. Occurs most frequently in elderly women.

Characteristics

A. Usually results from a fall.
B. Directly related to loss of bone strength due to osteoporosis.
✦ C. People over age 65 account for 87 percent of hip fracture cases.
   1. More than 250,000 occur each year.
   2. Most are women.
D. Fourteen to 36 percent of older clients with complications die.
E. More than 25 percent of survivors lose their ability to walk independently.
F. Sixty percent do not regain their pre-injury level of ambulation.
G. Personal and social consequences for older adults.

1. Restriction of daily activities can result in depression, complications, etc.
2. Hospitalization adds financial burden, dependence.

Assessment

A. Assess for pain, tenderness, or muscle spasm over fracture site or in groin.
B. Assess for lateral rotation and shortening of leg with minimal deformity.
C. Degree of disability.
D. Elimination problems.
E. Nutritional status.
F. Emotional reaction to immobility.
G. Degree of support from family.

Implementation

A. Operative procedure.
   1. Femoral head replacement—surgical fixation with nails, pins, or screws.
   2. Occasional total hip replacement.
B. Preoperative care.
   ✦ 1. Provide care such as that given to clients in skin traction.
      a. Buck's extension may be applied to relieve muscle spasm at the fracture site.
      b. Movement of fracture fragments will increase muscle spasms and pain.
   2. Observe for elimination regularity.
   ✦ 3. Teach coughing and deep-breathing. Encourage isometric exercises and use of overhead trapeze.
   4. Maintain proper positioning—splinting injured leg with pillows on unaffected side.
   5. Assist client with eating; nourishing diet is essential for healing process.
✦ C. Postoperative care.
   1. Turn client from unaffected side to back as routine, turn every 2 hours; a physician's order is required to turn from side to side.
   2. Turn client with hip prosthesis by always placing pillows between legs to avoid adduction.
   3. Elevate head; may be limited to 30 to 40 degrees to avoid acute hip flexion.
   4. Introduce quadricep and gluteal setting muscle exercises; encourage use of overhead trapeze for assistance in moving.
   5. Take measures to protect client when moving from bed to chair (client not to bear weight on affected leg).
   6. Provide routine postoperative measures to ensure client's comfort.
   7. Take measures as necessary to prevent complications.
      a. Avascular necrosis of femoral head.
      b. Nonunion.

c. Pin complications.

d. Dislocation of prosthesis.

e. Infection.

Urinary Incontinence

Definition: Involuntary release of urine of such severity as to have social and/or hygienic consequences.

Characteristics

A. Ten million adults are incontinent—over half the residents of nursing homes and one-third of elderly living at home are affected.

B. Prevalence rises with age.

C. This condition is not a normal consequence of aging; it is a symptom signaling the presence of other problems.

✦ D. Types.

   1. *Stress incontinence:* result of sudden increase in intra-abdominal pressure that pushes urine out of the bladder.

   2. *Urge incontinence:* leakage of urine before one reaches the toilet usually caused by uncontrolled contraction of the bladder.

   3. *Overflow incontinence:* constant dribble of urine results when bladder is not completely emptied during voiding.

   4. *Functional incontinence:* nonorganic; impaired mobility, depression, and dementia can prevent client from reaching bathroom.

Assessment

A. Assess pattern of problem—*see* types of incontinence as noted above.

   1. Decreased bladder tone/volume.

   2. Muscle tone—urgency and frequency.

B. Presence of other problems, disease states, or change in physical health.

   1. Congestive heart failure.

   2. Urinary tract infection.

   3. Pneumonia.

   4. Stool impaction.

C. Effects of medication(s).

D. Smoking.

E. Environmental problems.

   1. Access to toilet.

   2. Restraints.

   3. Privacy.

   4. Response of staff/family.

F. Skin condition.

G. Emotional coping in relation to the problem.

Implementation

✦ A. Monitor medical treatment.

   1. Pelvic floor muscle exercises (Kegel exercises) and behavioral training (biofeedback).

   2. Drug therapy.

      a. Anticholinergic drugs (Pro-Banthine).

      b. Antispasmodic drugs (Ditropan) inhibit bladder contractions.

   3. Perform surgery to strengthen pelvic muscles, repair a damaged urethra, remove an obstruction.

B. Provide appropriate skin care.

C. Establish toileting schedule.

   1. Easy access.

   2. Appropriate clothing—client's own, if possible.

✦ D. Assist client to learn Kegel exercises.

   1. Will help to control stress and urge for incontinence.

   2. Steps are to contract pubococcygeus muscle, hold contraction for 10 seconds, relax for 10 seconds. Work up to 25 repetitions 3 times per day.

E. Provide protection plan for accidents.

   1. Accidents are embarrassing and often limit excursions and social activities.

   2. Prevent problems and avoid disrupting client's life.

F. Devise ways to build client's self-esteem.

   1. Positive reinforcement.

   2. Plan activities that client can enjoy.

Impaired Mobility/Disability

Definition: Older adults can suffer impaired mobility and disability due to decreased physical function and/or accidents.

Characteristics

A. Nearly 23 percent of older people living in the community have some degree of disability.

   1. Those 85 and older constitute a disproportionate share of those who are dependent in physical functioning.

   2. Those 85 and older constitute 27 percent of those who have impaired mobility.

✦ B. Impaired mobility can lead to many subsequent problems: depression, negative self-image, dependent behavior, loss of independence, etc.

C. Effects of disability.

   1. Impact on the individual's body image.

      a. Physical appearance.

      b. Bodily sensations.

   2. Behavior during reaction period.

      a. Appears confused and disorganized.

      b. Denies disability exists.

      c. Overreacts to situations and physical condition.

      d. Assumes false-positive attitude.

      e. Becomes self-centered.

      f. Becomes depressed.

g.   Mourns loss of function or body part.

3.   Adaptation and adjustment.

    a.   Revises body image by modifying former picture of self.

    b.   Reorganizes values.

    c.   Accepts degree of dependency.

    d.   Accepts limitations imposed by disability.

    e.   Begins to develop realistic goals.

Assessment

A.   Specific source of disability or impaired mobility.

B.   Presence of accompanying disease state: arthritis, stroke, dementia, diabetes, congestive heart failure (CHF), COPD.

C.   Strength and function of limbs and joints.

D.   Stability of gait.

E.   Presence of pain.

F.   Condition of skin.

G.   Drug effects—sedation, incontinence, orthostatic hypotension.

H.   Motivation for rehabilitation.

I.   Nutritional status.

J.   History of falls.

Implementation

A.   Develop nursing care plan to meet client's needs.

B.   Focus on disability or impaired mobility.

C.   Establish supportive relationship.

✦ D.   Teach activities of daily living.

    1.   Activities that must be accomplished each day for the individual to care for own needs and be as independent as possible.

    2.   Ascertain best assistive aid for client.

    3.   Demonstrate and encourage individual to practice.

    4.   Increase activities as individual progresses and is able to assume activity.

    5.   Give positive reinforcement for all effort expended.

E.   Prevent deformities and complications.

✦   1.   Turn and position in good alignment.

    a.   Prevent contractures.

    b.   Stimulate circulation.

    c.   Prevent thrombophlebitis.

    d.   Prevent pressure ulcers.

    2.   Prevent edema of extremities.

    3.   Promote lung expansion.

✦ Types of Exercise for Rehabilitation

A.   Passive.

    1.   Carried out by the therapist or nurse without assistance from client.

    2.   Purpose—retain as much joint range of motion as possible, and maintain circulation.

B.   Active assistive.

    1.   Carried out by the client with assistance of therapist or nurse.

    2.   Purpose—encourage normal muscle function.

C.   Active.

    1.   Accomplished by the individual without assistance.

    2.   Purpose—increase muscle strength.

D.   Resistive.

    1.   Active exercise carried out by the individual working against resistance produced by manual or mechanical means.

    2.   Purpose—provide resistance to increase muscle power.

E.   Isometric or muscle setting.

    1.   Performed by the individual without assistance.

    2.   Purpose—maintain strength in a muscle when a joint is immobilized.

F.   Range of motion (ROM).

    1.   Movement of a joint through its full range in all appropriate planes.

    2.   Purpose—maintain joint mobility and increase maximal motion of a joint.

    3.   Nursing care.

       a.   Assess general condition of client.

       b.   Establish extent of ROM before present condition.

       c.   Discontinue ROM at point of pain.

    4.   Deterrents to ROM exercises: fear and pain.

Use of Aids/Devices

✦ A.   Cane.

    1.   Purpose.

       a.   Provide greater stability and speed when walking.

       b.   Relieve pressure on weight-bearing joints.

       c.   Provide force to push or pull body forward.

✦   2.   Safety factors.

       a.   Handle at level of greater trochanter.

       b.   Elbow flexed at 25- to 30-degree angle.

       c.   Lightweight material.

       d.   Rubber suction tip.

✦   3.   Techniques for walking with cane.

       a.   Hold cane close to the body.

       b.   Hold in hand on unaffected side.

       c.   Move cane at same time as affected leg.

B.   Crutches.

    1.   Purpose—provide support during ambulating when lower extremities unable to support body weight.

✦   2.   Safety factors.

       a.   Measure 1½ to 2 inches from axillary fold to floor (4 inches in front and 6 inches to side of toes).

       b.   Hand piece adjusted to allow 30-degree elbow flexion.

c. Rubber suction tips on crutches.

d. Well-fitting shoes with nonslip soles.

✦ 3. *See* gait sequence on page 372.

C. Prosthesis—artificial replacement for a missing body part.

D. Brace—support that protects or supports weakened muscles.

Infections in Older Adults

A. Older clients are more susceptible to infection—diminished resistance.

B. Important to recognize high-risk clients.

C. Diseases that contribute to high risk.

1. Diabetes mellitus.

2. CHF.

3. Malignancy—double risk due to chemotherapy depressing the immune system.

4. Renal failure.

✦ D. Conditions that make clients prone to infection.

1. Dehydration.

a. Fluid depletion—skin more penetrable by pathogens.

b. Thick mucosal secretions—coughing more difficult.

2. Increased urinary retention.

a. Monitor fluid intake.

b. 1500 to 2500 mL daily.

3. Bed confinement.

a. Increases risk of renal infection by causing urine backflow through ureters up into kidneys.

b. Voiding while bedridden increases pressure on bladder, adds to risk of urinary tract infection.

c. To minimize risk, assist client to sit when voiding, if possible.

4. Poor skin turgor; less effective as barrier to trauma.

a. Less resistance to friction increases risk of pressure ulcers.

b. Maintaining nutrition and fluid intake lessens risk.

5. Bowel problems lower resistance.

a. Constipation may lead to intestinal obstruction and perforation.

b. Prevention—fiber-rich fruits and vegetables, whole-grain breads and cereals.

E. When infection develops.

✦ 1. Older person may not show a fever (baseline may be low so slight increase is not noted).

a. Take baseline temperature.

b. Lower temperature only when it goes above 102°F to 104°F. (Fever inhibits bacterial and viral growth.)

c. Evaluation of antibiotic therapy (fever decreases) is more accurate without antipyretic.

2. Older clients are more susceptible to adverse effects of antibiotics.

a. Hearing loss—especially with isoniazid and aminoglycosides.

b. Vertigo with aminoglycosides.

c. Monitor BUN and creatinine levels to check for nephrotoxicity.

d. Diarrhea (ampicillin, tetracycline, chloramphenicol)—leads to electrolyte imbalance.

e. Increased risk of yeast infection.

COMMON PROBLEMS FROM IMMOBILITY

Pressure Ulcers

Definition: Localized areas of necrosis of skin and subcutaneous tissue due to pressure.

Characteristics

A. Cause—pressure exerted on skin and subcutaneous tissue by bony prominence and the object on which body rests.

B. Predisposing factors.

1. Malnutrition.

2. Anemia.

3. Hypoproteinemia.

4. Vitamin deficiency.

5. Edema.

✦ C. Common sites: bony prominences of body such as sacrum, greater trochanter, heels, elbows, etc.

Assessment

A. Stage of ulcer.

B. Identify if infection is associated with pressure ulcer.

C. Effectiveness of ulcer treatment.

D. Healing process of the ulcer.

E. Other bony prominences for potential formation of pressure ulcer.

F. Presence of conditions that inhibit wound healing.

Implementation

✦ A. Prevention.

1. Relieve or remove pressure.

2. Stimulate circulation.

3. Keep skin dry.

✦ B. Positioning.

1. Encourage client to remain active.

2. Change position frequently—every 1–2 hours.

C. Maintain good skin hygiene; inspect frequently.

D. Provide for active and/or passive exercises.

E. Use alternating-air-pressure mattress, etc.
F. Avoid massaging bony prominences.
G. Provide for adequate nutritional and fluid intake.

External Rotation of Hip

Definition: Outward rotation of hip joint.

Characteristics
A. Cause—lying for long periods of time on back without support to hips.
B. Incorrect positioning in bed.

Implementation
✦ A. Trochanter roll extending from crest of ileum to midthigh when positioned on back.
B. Frequent change of position.
C. Proper positioning.

Footdrop

Definition: Tendency for foot to plantar flex.

Characteristics
✦ A. Causes.
   1. Prolonged bedrest.
   2. Lack of exercise.
   3. Weight of bed clothing forcing toes into plantar flexion.
B. Complications.
   1. Individual walks on his or her toes without touching heel on ground.
   2. Unable to walk.

Implementation
✦ A. Prevention.
   1. Position feet against footboard.
   2. Use footcradle to keep weight of top linen off toes.
   3. Provide ROM exercises.
B. Check that soles of feet are against footboard to prevent permanent footdrop.

Contractures

Definition: Abnormal shortening of muscle, tendon, or ligament so joint cannot function properly.

Characteristics
A. Cause—improper alignment, lack of movement.
B. Result is decrease in mobility and joint movement.

Implementation
✦ A. Proper alignment at all times.
   1. Use pillows.
   2. Provide supportive splints.
B. Provide for ROM exercises.

Bladder Dysfunction

Definition: When an individual is unable to void and the reflex act of micturition (urination) cannot occur.

Characteristics
A. Causes.
   1. Disease process (urinary tract infection).
   2. Lack of innervation.
   3. Lack of motivation.
B. Treatment involves bladder retraining, surgery, drugs.

Implementation
A. Bladder training—purpose.
   1. Prevent urinary tract infection and preserve renal function.
   2. Keep individual dry and odor free.
   3. Help individual maintain social acceptance.
✦ B. Procedure.
   1. Set up specific time to empty bladder.
   2. Give measured amounts of fluids.
   3. Position in normal voiding position.
   4. Instruct client on how to Credé bladder.
   5. Keep record of amount and time of intake and output.
   6. Encourage client to wear own clothing, particularly underwear.
   7. Provide protective underwear when needed.

Bowel Dysfunction

Definition: Normal elimination does not occur due to a structural problem or disease state.

Characteristics
A. Cause.
   1. Disease process.
   2. Inadequate intake.
   3. Poor prior habits.
B. Treatment involves surgery, dietary modifications, or drugs.

Implementation
A. Identify purpose of bowel training.
   1. Develop regular bowel habits.
   2. Prevent fecal incontinence, impaction, and/or irregularity.
✦ B. Implement nursing procedure.
   1. Establish specific time.
   2. Provide for adequate roughage and fluid intake.
   3. Use normal posture.
   4. Instruct to bear down and contract abdominal muscles.
   5. Provide privacy and time.
   6. Provide exercise.
   7. Provide protective underwear when needed.

Hypostatic Pneumonia

Definition: Inflammatory process in the lungs in which alveoli fill with exudate.

Characteristics

A. Incidence.
    1. Very young, very old.
    2. Debilitated.
    3. Immobile.
B. Cause—stasis of secretions in lungs.

Implementation

✦ A. Prevention.
    1. Assess lung function.
    2. Encourage deep-breathing, coughing.
    3. Turn every 2 hours.
    4. Ensure adequate hydration.
B. Provide for postural drainage, if indicated.
C. Administer oxygen, as ordered.
D. Monitor antibiotic therapy.

PROBLEM AREAS FOR OLDER ADULT CLIENTS

Sensory Impairment

A. Elderly experience loss of function in the senses.
    1. Ability to taste declines after age 40; taste buds are fewer in number and there is less saliva flow.
    2. Ability to smell declines.
    3. Hearing fades, especially in high-frequency ranges.
    4. Regulation of body temperature is less efficient.
B. Major diseases or degeneration of organs occurs.
    ✦ 1. Vision loss—*see* sections on page 812 for nursing implications.
        a. Glaucoma—increased pressure causes damage to optic nerve, leading to blindness.
        b. Cataracts—clouding of the lens leading to blurred vision.
        c. Retinal detachment.
        d. Macular degeneration—loss of central vision due to degeneration of macula.
    ✦ 2. Hearing loss—*see* sections on page 811 for nursing implications.
        a. Otosclerosis requiring a stapedectomy.
        b. Hearing loss due to accumulation of earwax—requires periodic irrigation of auditory canal.

Nutrition

A. Physiological requirements do change (decrease) with age.

✦ 1. Nutrition intake must meet two major demands.
    a. Normal structural repair.
    b. Energy production for functional needs.
2. Met by protein and amino acids and adequate calorie intake.
✦ B. Many older adults are deficient in nutrients, especially protein, B vitamins, vitamins A and C, iron, and calcium.
    1. Change in diet is often responsible.
        a. Senses of taste and smell decrease, thus less conscious of hunger.
        b. Teeth in poor condition or dentures don't work properly.
        c. Physical disabilities or lack of mobility; unable to buy groceries.
        d. Loss of interest in eating.
        e. Limited income affects buying nutritious food.
    2. System cannot assimilate nutrients as well as when younger.
        a. Reduced hydrochloric acid, reduced stomach activity.
        b. Decreased salivary flow.
C. Health status affects nutritional state.
    1. Chronic diseases: heart disease, cancer, diabetes, gastrointestinal problems, etc.
    2. Drugs: antacids, antidepressants, anticonvulsants, cathartics, diuretics, antimicrobials, etc.
D. Decreased physical activity and metabolic changes reduce caloric needs.
E. Financial resources, emotional, and physical state affect nutritional status.

✦ Assessment

A. Hydration status, body weight, edema.
B. Anemia.
C. Appetite.
D. Ability to feed self—physical and mental.
    1. Dentition.
    2. Mastication.
    3. Swallowing.
    4. Desire to eat.
E. Fatigue, energy reserve.
F. Constipation.
G. Compliance to special diets.
H. Effects of drugs on nutrition.
    1. Gastrointestinal irritation.
    2. Food–drug interactions.
    3. Some drug side effects are nausea and vomiting.
I. Skin and mucous membrane condition.

Implementation

A. Offer/give oral fluids in small amounts every hour.
B. Plan diet to be high in nutrients.

1. Give foods with high fiber content.
2. Balance of vitamins and minerals.
3. Use lemon, vinegar, herbs on foods (rather than salt) to stimulate appetite.

C. Devise tools and plates that assist self-feeding.
D. Serve meals with others present to reduce isolation.

Medications

A. Thirty percent of all prescriptive drugs are used by older adults, and this does not include over-the-counter drugs.
B. Eighty percent of people age 65 and over have at least one chronic medical problem that requires medications (one-third have three or more chronic problems).
C. The typical older adult in the United States takes 4–7 prescription drugs each day in addition to over-the-counter drugs.
D. Often older adults have several medical problems for which they have different doctors, each prescribing different drugs.
E. "Polypharmacy" is responsible for 28 percent of hospital admissions.
✦ F. Older adults (13 percent of the population) suffer 50 percent of all drug side effects (estimated 17 per 100,000 population).
  ✦ 1. Increased risk for drug toxicity.
    a. Renal excretion altered—kidneys cannot process drugs as well.
    b. Liver enzymes altered.
    c. Diminished blood circulation to liver.
    d. May take multiple drugs that compete with each other.
    e. CNS more sensitive to drugs.
      (1) Drugs interfere with neurotransmitters (chemicals) that regulate brain function.
      (2) Side effects result in confusion.
    f. Lean body mass replaced by fat, so aging affects how much of the drug reaches bloodstream (e.g., Coumadin and digitalis distributions in lean tissue may reach higher levels in older adults).
  2. Iatrogenic illness can be caused by drug therapy.
  ✦ 3. Most commonly abused drugs by older adults.
    a. Alcohol.
    b. Tranquilizers most frequently abused.
    c. Sleeping pills.
    d. Medications to control pain.
    e. Laxatives.
✦ G. Major problems with prescriptive drugs in older adults.
  1. Drug interactions—people who use multiple physicians and pharmacies run the risk of taking drugs that interact to cause adverse reactions.

> ### GUIDELINES FOR ANALGESIC MEDICATION ADMINISTRATION
>
> - Older adult clients often receive less analgesic medications than younger adults, thus leading to inadequate pain relief.
> - Safe analgesic administration is complicated by interactions with multiple chronic disorders and multiple drugs to treat these disorders.
> - Older adults experience greater peak and longer duration of action from analgesics than younger individuals.
> - Drug interactions occur more frequently in older adults.
> - NSAID complications are common and must be carefully monitored.

    a. Some drugs use the same metabolic pathway and can result in hazardous blood levels.
    b. The combined effects of some drugs can be more potent than the physician intended.
  2. Medication errors—the more medications a person takes, the greater the risk of medication error (people over age 75 take an average of 17 prescriptions annually).
  3. Opioids—produce greater analgesic effect in older adults.
    a. Opioid therapy should be initiated with 25 to 50 percent lower dose than that given to adults.
    b. Monitor for respiratory depression and reduced arterial O_2 saturation.
    c. Monitor for other side effects: sedation, hypotension, urinary retention, constipation, etc.
  4. Noncompliance—not taking right dose at right time or discontinuing drug without consultation; common due to lack of understanding about reason to take drug and general knowledge base of drug action.
  5. Unpredictable drug action—physiological changes associated with age and disease may alter effects of the drugs.
    a. Beta blockers—may increase respiratory or heart disease in clients with asthma, COPD or heart failure.
    b. NSAIDs—may increase GI bleeding or worsen disease states.
    c. Psychotropic drugs—aggravate glaucoma or worsen heart block.
  6. Drug side effects not recognized—older adults not aware or do not understand potential dangerous side effects of drugs.
  7. Inadequate monitoring—older adult is often alone or not monitored consistently so drug problems are not identified.

8. Cost of drugs—multiple medications are costly for many older adults, so they stop taking drugs.

H. Preventing problems with drugs in older adults.
  1. Keep an up-to-date list of all drugs taken, including herbs, with dose and dosing schedule.
  2. Take the list to every doctor seen, and to the pharmacy.
  3. Order all prescriptions from same pharmacy.
  4. Know the expected side effects of all drugs.

Administration of Medications

A. Oral route.
  1. Check for mouth dryness.
    a. Drug may stick and dissolve in mouth.
    b. Drug may irritate mucous membranes.
  2. Place client in sitting position.
  3. Crush tablets if they are very large.
  4. Do not open capsules.
  5. Do not crush enteric-coated tablets.
  6. Check with pharmacy for liquid preparations if client has difficulty swallowing tablets.

B. Topical medications will be absorbed more slowly.

C. Suppository.
  1. Position for comfort.
  2. May take longer to dissolve due to decreased body core temperature.
  3. Do not insert suppository immediately after removing from refrigerator.

D. Parenteral.
  1. Site may ooze medication or bleed due to decreased tissue elasticity.
  2. Do not use immobile limb.
  3. Danger of overhydration with IV.
  4. Decreased muscle mass may determine length of needle for injections.

E. Self-administration.
  1. Check compliance with amounts and times.
  2. Color code to facilitate proper administration.

Assessment

A. Changes in mental status.
B. Vital signs.
  1. Orthostatic blood pressure.
  2. Apical pulse.
C. Urine production, retention.
D. Hydration and appetite.
E. Visual disturbances.
F. Swallowing ability.
G. Evaluate effects of drug.
  1. Laboratory studies.
  2. Signs and symptoms for toxic/interaction effects of drugs.
H. Bowel function.
I. Effects of nutrition and foods on drug response.

Implementation

✦ A. No alcohol or alcohol-based elixirs when receiving benzodiazepines or antihistamines.

B. Method of administering drugs.
  1. Deep-breathing and relaxation to reduce use of analgesic drugs.
  2. Position client sitting with head slightly flexed to reduce chance of aspiration.

C. Administering tablets.
  ✦ 1. Do not crush time-released or enteric-coated tablets.
  2. Crush large tablets if not contraindicated.
  3. Give with textured foods (nectar, applesauce) if not contraindicated.

D. Stroke victim—give drug on functional side of mouth.

Pain in Older Adults

Characteristics

A. More than 80 percent of all older adults suffer pain from chronic diseases.

✦ B. Pain management is different with older adults.
  1. Underreported by older clients—may feel pain is a normal part of growing older.
  2. Physiology of the body affects absorption and metabolism of medication—pain drugs may have altered pharmacodynamics.

C. Important to recognize and assess pain in older adults or the results may affect the ability to function.

Assessment

✦ A. Nonverbal cues to pain.
  1. Moaning or groaning.
  2. Restlessness or agitation.
  3. Crying.

B. Verbal cues to pain.
  1. Reporting pain—try to establish a method of calibrating degree of pain (use pain scale that client understands).
  2. Assessing if pain medication is working.

✦ ### Implementation

A. Monitor pain cues closely, especially nonverbal ones.

B. Judge impact of pain on client—how much the pain contributes to poor functioning in activities of daily living.

C. Monitor pain relief methods.
  1. Medications: *see* Medications section on preceding pages.
  2. Provide pain relief through alternative methods (massage, acupuncture, relaxation, visualization, etc.).

3. Listen to client's reports of pain relief and adjust care plan accordingly (if pain medication is not working, ask physician to change drug).

D. *See* Joint Commission Pain Standards on page 47.

Drug–Food–Herb Interactions in Older Adults

A. Certain foods, vitamins/minerals, and "natural" remedies can interfere with therapeutic effects of drugs.
    1. Reduce absorption of drug.
    2. Interfere with cellular action.
B. Medication regimen affected by nutrition may put client at risk.
    1. Important to assess client's diet.
    2. Monitor potential vitamin–drug interactions.
    3. Certain drugs deplete essential nutrients; monitor client for low vitamin B complex, B_{12}, etc.
C. Review client's prescriptive and over-the-counter drugs.
    1. Review in relation to normal dietary intake.
    2. Consider vitamin/mineral intake and supplements in terms of decreasing effect of medications.
    3. Check lab values for problems.
D. Review herbs client is taking because interaction with medications may be dangerous. (*See* Herb–Drug Interactions on page 96.)
E. Document findings so healthcare team is informed of diet/drug plan.
✦ F. Food sources of vitamins and minerals.
    1. Folic acid sources: liver, kidney, fresh vegetables.
    2. Niacin sources: yeast, meat, fish, milk, eggs, green vegetables, and cereal grains.
    3. Pantothenic acid sources: meat, vegetables, cereal grains, legumes, eggs, milk, fish, and fruit.
    4. Pyridoxine hydrochloride (vitamin B_6) sources: cereal grains, legumes, vegetables, liver, meat, and eggs.
    5. Cyanocobalamin (vitamin B_{12}) sources: animal foods, liver, kidney, fish, shellfish, meat, and dairy foods.
    6. Ascorbic acid (vitamin C) sources: fresh fruits and vegetables.
    7. Vitamin A sources: eggs, milk, cream, butter, organ meats, fish.
    8. Vitamin D source: activated in body by sunlight.
    9. Vitamin E sources: vegetable oils, whole grains, animal fats, eggs, and green vegetables.
    10. Vitamin K sources: green leafy vegetables, spinach, broccoli, cabbage, and liver.

Lab Values in Older Adults

✦ **Urinalysis**

A. Protein.
    1. Normal 0–5 mg/100 mL—rises slightly.
    2. May reflect changes in kidney or subclinical urinary tract infection.
B. Glucose.
    1. Normal 0–15 mg/100 mL—declines slightly.
    2. May reflect changes in kidney.
C. Specific gravity.
    1. 1.010; changes to 1.024 by age 80 (which means older adults have more concentrated urine).
    2. Thirty to 50 percent decline in number of nephrons affects ability to concentrate urine.

✦ **Hematology**

A. Hemoglobin.
    1. Men, 13–18 g/100 mL—drops 10–17 g/100 mL.
    2. Women, 12–16 g/100 mL—no change.
B. Hematocrit.
    1. Men, 40–54 percent—no change.
    2. Women, 37–48 percent—no change.
C. Leukocytes.
    1. 4300–10,800/mm³—drops to 3100–9000/mm³.
    2. As bone marrow diminishes, hematopoiesis declines.
D. Lymphocytes—1500–4500/mm³.
    1. T lymphocytes fall.
    2. B lymphocytes fall.
E. Platelets, prothrombin time (PT), and partial thromboplastin time (PTT)—no change.

✦ **Blood Chemistry Tests That Change with Age**

A. BUN.
    1. Men, 10–20 mg/100 mL—increases, may be as high as 69 mg/100 mL.
    2. Women, 8–20 mg/100 mL—increases.
    3. Renal function decreased due to decline in cardiac output, renal blood flow, and glomerular filtration rate.
B. Creatinine.
    1. 0.6–1.2 mg/100 mL—increases as high as 1.9 mg/100 mL in men and women.
    2. Endogenous creatinine is produced as lean body mass shrinks.
    3. Drugs excreted by urinary system may cause toxicity if creatinine level is too high.
C. Creatinine clearance.
    1. 104–132 mL/min (females); 110–150 mL/min (males).
    2. Referenced interval: men's formula for age: $140 - \text{age} \times \text{kg body weight}$ divided by $72 \times$ serum creatinine.

✦ 3. Reduced levels result in older adults more likely to develop toxicity to drugs excreted by kidneys.
D. Albumin.
   1. Decreases within the normal range—3.5 to 5.0 g/dL.
   2. Increases with dehydration.
E. Glucose tolerance.
   1. One hour: 160–170 mg/100 mL.
      Two hours: 115–125 mg/100 mL.
      Three hours: 70–110 mg/100 mL.
   2. With age, results rise more quickly in first 2 hours, then drop to baseline more slowly.
   3. Alcohol, MAO inhibitors, and beta blockers can all cause a rapid fall in glucose.
F. Fasting serum glucose.
   1. 70–115 mg/dL increases with age.
   2. Older adults are more prone to glucose intolerance and diabetes.
G. Thyroxine (T_4) 4.5–13.5 μg/dL and triiodothyronine (T_3) 90–220 μm/dL—both decrease by 25 percent.

Prescription for Long Life and Good Health

A. Regular exercise—older adults must continue to exercise regularly to maintain health (can increase function by 50 percent through exercise).
✦ B. Nutritious diet—intake of adequate nutrients and calories to maintain body.
   1. Malnutrition contributes to high incidence of chronic disease.
   2. Obesity contributes to increased health risks (heart disease, hypertension).
   3. Diet adequate to maintain normal body weight, low fat, and include all four food groups for minimal nutrients, vitamins, and minerals.
C. No smoking—smokers die earlier than non-smokers and have a higher incidence of heart disease, heart attack, cancer, and chronic lung disease.
D. Moderate alcohol intake; high alcohol intake is a health risk that leads to liver disease, nervous system damage, gastrointestinal problems.
✦ E. Prevention of health problems—yearly physical examinations are important for older adults to diagnose an early disease process.
   1. Check warning signs of cancer, heart disease (hypertension).
   2. Pap smear and mammogram for women as precaution against cancer.
   3. Men should have PSA, along with exams for colon, prostate cancer.
F. Managing stress—stress is associated with increased incidence of heart disease, hypertension, cancer, and other diseases.
G. Maintain contact with friends for support; studies show that isolated older adults have more health problems and die earlier than people who have close attachments.
H. Smile more and give thanks daily.
I. Involvement in a community of faith indicates better health and outcomes in older adults.

GERONTOLOGICAL NURSING REVIEW QUESTIONS

1. List by numbers all of the client characteristics that would influence the client's adaptation to the hospital _____.

   1. Age.
   2. Sense of humor.
   3. Level of consciousness.
   4. English language ability.
   5. Nationality.
   6. Disease state.

2. An older adult client is in a long-term care facility. She had a left-sided CVA 4 weeks ago and has been bedridden since that time. A sign or symptom indicating a possible complication of immobility is

   1. A reddened area over the sacrum.
   2. Stiffness in the left leg.
   3. Difficulty moving her left arm.
   4. Difficulty hearing low voices.

3. The visiting home health nurse is assigned to a client who just had cataract surgery. A care plan would include instructions to

   1. Maintain bedrest for at least 2 days with bathroom privileges only.
   2. Keep the head up and straight and not to look down.
   3. Deep-breathe and cough four times a day.
   4. Lie only on the affected side when in bed.

4. A client has been admitted to the orthopedic unit with an intracapsular fracture of the right hip sustained after a fall on the ice. Buck's extension is applied and arrangements are being made for hip prosthesis surgery in the morning. The purpose for the application of Buck's extension at this time is to

   1. Reduce the fracture.
   2. Relieve muscle spasm.
   3. Keep the knee extended.
   4. Stabilize the fractured hip.

5. After a Foley catheter had been inserted for 2 days, it was removed by the nurse. The nurse should assess for an expected outcome of

   1. Dribbling after the first several voidings.
   2. Urgency and frequency for several days.

3. Frequent voidings in small amounts.
4. Retention of urine for 10- to 12-hour periods.

6. A client is being discharged in the morning to an extended care nursing facility. He asks the nurse why he has to go to "that place." The best response is

   1. "The physician has determined that this is the best place for you right now."
   2. "You will need to ask the physician that question when he comes in to see you."
   3. "Did the physician or anyone else talk to you about going to the nursing home?"
   4. "Your family can't take care of you at home so you will need to go there."

7. Among older adults, the leading cause of death is

   1. Heart disease.
   2. Cancer.
   3. Stroke.
   4. Pneumonia.

8. When an older adult client is in the hospital, an important safety consideration is to

   1. Restrain the client when in bed.
   2. Assign the client to a double room with another client.
   3. Keep the bed in high position.
   4. Place upper siderails in up position when the client is alone.

9. Which of the following changes is not considered a normal process of aging?

   1. Renal function diminishes.
   2. Short-term memory diminishes.
   3. Intelligence diminishes.
   4. Secretions decrease or change in composition.

10. A 68-year-old client comes to the clinic with complaints of pain in her joints. She is given the diagnosis of rheumatoid arthritis, and the physician orders ASA therapy, 20 tabs/day. Before discharge, the nurse teaches the client that possible side effects of ASA therapy are

    1. Bleeding, nausea, and constipation.
    2. Gastritis, nausea and vomiting, and bleeding.

3. Blurred vision and nausea and vomiting.
4. Blurred vision and tinnitus.

11. When instructing a 60-year-old client with long-term diabetes on preventing chronic complications of retinopathy or nephropathy, an important principle to teach would be to

1. Visit the physician frequently for check-ups.
2. Obtain frequent lab values of BUN and creatinine.
3. Complete frequent fasting plasma glucose testing.
4. Maintain stable blood glucose levels.

12. The signs of pacemaker malfunction that the nurse would include in discharge teaching for a client with a new pacemaker are

1. Increased urine output and headache.
2. Irregular, rapid pulse.
3. Weakness and fatigue.
4. Disorientation and confusion.

13. A client with increased right atrial pressure has a central venous line in place. The nurse expects that his central venous pressure (CVP) reading will be

1. 0–2 mm Hg.
2. 5–10 cm H_2O.
3. 8–10 mm Hg.
4. 15–20 cm H_2O.

14. As the nurse develops a care plan for a client who sustained an intertrochanteric fracture of the left hip, she knows that initial care includes

1. Abductor splints in place until edema is reduced.
2. Pelvic traction until edema is reduced.
3. Buck's extension until edema is reduced.
4. Balanced suspension traction until surgery is completed.

15. An elderly client has received radiation for cancer. Based on an understanding of blood changes associated with radiotherapy, the nurse will focus the assessment on

1. Checking lab tests for low hemoglobin.
2. Observing for signs of infection.
3. Checking the need for subcutaneous vitamin K.
4. Monitoring for prophylactic antibiotics.

16. A 63-year-old male client with a history of alcohol abuse has been admitted with a diagnosis of acute pancreatitis. After completing an assessment on the client, the priority nursing diagnosis is

1. Fluid volume deficit due to fluid losses into body spaces.
2. Impaired oxygenation due to rapid respirations.
3. Potential for infection due to decreased immune response.
4. Alteration in nutrition, less than requirements, due to decreased intake.

17. When assessing a client for possible dehydration, which of the following clinical manifestations would indicate this state?

1. Taut, shiny skin.
2. Firm eyeballs.
3. Bounding pulse.
4. Dry, flaking skin.

18. The nurse is assessing a 75-year-old client who is taking digitalis. The initial clinical symptoms indicating digitalis toxicity would include

1. Anorexia, nausea, and vomiting.
2. Diarrhea, headache, and vertigo.
3. Nausea, vomiting, and diarrhea.
4. Vomiting, diarrhea, and vertigo.

19. An 81-year-old male client has begun Cheyne–Stokes respirations. The nurse understands that this respiratory pattern involves

1. Periods of hyperpnea alternating with periods of apnea.
2. Periods of tachypnea alternating with periods of apnea.
3. Respirations characteristically increased in both rate and depth.
4. Deep, regular, sighing respirations.

20. A client has been given the diagnosis of Alzheimer's disease. The nurse observes that he has been incontinent and soiled his clothes for the second time on this shift. The most appropriate nursing intervention is to

1. Put the client in adult diapers to protect him from embarrassment.
2. Scold the client and tell him not to wet his pants again.
3. Tell the client you will change his pants and establish a 2-hour schedule of taking him to the bathroom.
4. Tell the client to ask you for assistance the next time he has to go to the bathroom.

21. The client's physician orders 20 mEq of KCl. The label on the KCl is 10 mEq/5 mL. The nurse will give the client

1. 10 mL.
2. 2 mL.
3. 5 mL.
4. 20 mL.

22. A 78-year-old client who suffered a cerebrovascular accident (CVA) is in a long-term facility. She has developed a pressure ulcer. The nurse is applying a wet-to-moist dressing. The rationale for using this type of dressing is to

    1. Prevent the dressing from leaking on the bed clothes.
    2. Prevent damage to granulating tissue when removing the dressing.
    3. Enable the dressing to almost dry on the ulcer to promote healing.
    4. Assist in debriding the wound.

23. After the client has recovered from coronary bypass surgery, her physician has advised a low-cholesterol diet. The nurse will know that the client understands this diet when she includes foods such as

    1. Meats, especially organ meats, and dairy products.
    2. Eggs, cheese, fruits, and vegetables.
    3. Vegetables, fruits, lean meats, and vegetable oils.
    4. Raw or cooked vegetables, fruits, and red meat.

24. An 87-year-old client is admitted to the hospital complaining of weakness and shortness of breath. Her diagnosis is congestive heart failure. As the nurse is assessing the client's condition, which of the following signs will indicate that she is in left-sided heart failure?

    1. Fatigue, dyspnea, and wheezing.
    2. Hepatomegaly and oliguria.
    3. Decreased pulmonary artery pressure.
    4. Peripheral edema such as sacral edema.

25. A 70-year-old client with organic brain syndrome, dementia type, is frequently incontinent, even when he is fully dressed. An initial plan to deal with this behavior is to

    1. Remind the client to tell the nurse when he has to urinate.
    2. Put the client in diapers.
    3. Take the client to the bathroom on a 2-hour schedule.
    4. Tell the client that he must remember to go to the bathroom before he wets his pants.

GERONTOLOGICAL NURSING

Answers with Rationale

1. There are several answers to this question—*1 3 4 6.* While sense of humor may help adaptation, it is not a major influence. Nationality is also not important; rather, it is the ability to communicate with personnel that influences how a client adapts.

   NP:A; CN:H; CA:M; CL:C

2. (1) A reddened area over the sacrum may be the first sign of a pressure ulcer. If it is recognized at this stage and nursing actions are taken to avoid additional pressure (frequent turning, massaging the skin, etc.), the ulcer may be avoided. Answers (2) and (3) can be expected with left-sided CVA, and (4) is usually an expected development with an elderly person.

   NP:A; CN:PH; CA:M; CL:C

3. (2) Keeping the head straight and avoiding looking down will prevent intraocular pressure. The nurse would practice breathing exercises with the client but will not encourage coughing, as this could cause an increase in intraocular pressure in the operative eye.

   NP:P; CN:PH; CA:S; CL:A

4. (2) The purpose of Buck's extension application following hip fracture is immobilization to relieve muscle spasm at the fracture site and thereby relieve pain. Any movement of fracture fragments will aggravate severe muscle spasm and pain. Skin traction such as this is not used to reduce a fracture (1), and it is not important to keep the knee extended (3). Bryant's or Russell's traction will stablize a fractured femur, not the hip.

   NP:AN; CN:PH; CA:S; CL:K

5. (1) Dribbling may be normal until the sphincter muscles regain their tone. If the catheter had been in place for several weeks, frequent voidings in small amounts (3) might have been the most appropriate response. Urgency and frequency (2) are symptoms of a bladder infection.

   NP:E; CN:PH; CA:S; CL:A

6. (3) is the most appropriate response. It is important to identify what the client thinks he has heard about his discharge. Clarification of information can proceed after this. The other answers do not allow the client to verbalize his fears or concerns.

   NP:I; CN:PS; CA:M; CL:A

7. (1) The leading cause of death is heart disease, even though the incidence has declined since 1968. Cancer (2) is second, stroke (3) third, and respiratory diseases (4) last as the cause of death.

   NP:AN; CN:H; CA:M; CL:K

8. (4) Upper siderails in the up position is the most important safety intervention to prevent the client from falling out of bed. Clients should be restrained (1) only as a last resort; restraints require a physician's order. The bed should be in low position to prevent the client from falling from a greater height. Placing the client in a double room (2) would not be considered a safety intervention.

   NP:I; CN:S; CA:M; CL:A

9. (3) Intelligence is not affected. Long-term memory usually is not affected. Short- or intermediate-memory changes are affected by the aging process.

   NP:AN; CN:H; CA:M; CL:K

10. (2) Gastritis, nausea, vomiting, and bleeding are the most common side effects of ASA therapy. Blurred vision is not a side effect of ASA therapy, and tinnitus would indicate that the toxic level of the drug had been reached.

    NP:I; CN:PH; CA:M; CL:C

Coding for Questions/Answers Abbreviations: **Nursing Process: NP,** Assessment: A, Analysis: AN, Planning: P, Implementation: I, Evaluation: E; **Client Needs: CN,** Safe, Effective Care Environment: S, Health Promotion and Maintenance: H, Psychosocial Integrity: PS, Physiological Integrity: PH; **Clinical Area: CA,** Medical Nursing: M, Surgical Nursing: S, Maternal/Newborn Nursing: MA, Pediatric Nursing: P, Psychiatric Nursing: PS; **Cognitive Level: CL,** Knowledge: K, Comprehension: C, Application: A, Analysis: AN.

11. (4) The most important principle to teach the client is the necessity of maintaining stable blood glucose levels. Frequent testing (1, 2, 3) is part of the picture, but unless the levels are stabilized, testing itself is not enough.

NP:I; CN:H; CA:M; CL:C

12. (3) Weakness and fatigue are symptoms that indicate hypoxia to the tissues. The client should be taught to recognize these as symptoms of pacemaker malfunction.

NP:I; CN:H; CA:M; CL:A

13. (4) An elevated CVP is expected in this client due to the increased right atrial pressure. The normal reading is 5 to 10 cm of water pressure.

NP:AN; CN:PH; CA:M; CL:A

14. (4) The client is usually placed in balanced suspension traction until surgery can be completed. This type of traction allows the client to move up and down in bed without interfering with the alignment of the bones. It also prevents muscle spasms. The surgical intervention is done early in elderly clients to prevent complications of immobilization.

NP:P; CN:PH; CA:S; CL:A

15. (2) Clients undergoing radiotherapy may have a decreased white blood cell count and should be observed closely for infections. They will probably not have a low hemoglobin (1) and will not need vitamin K (3). These clients do not usually receive prophylactic antibiotics (4).

NP:A; CN:PH; CA:M; CL:AN

16. (1) Because of the autodigestion of pancreatic and surrounding tissue, there is interstitial hemorrhage, local vascular drainage, increased vascular permeability, and vasodilation. Fluid loss will lead to fluid volume deficit. The client will be placed on bedrest, a nasogastric tube will be inserted, and analgesics will be used liberally for extreme pain.

NP:P; CN:PH; CA:M; CL:C

17. (4) Dry, flaking skin is present when a client is dehydrated. All of the other responses are indicative of an overhydrated state.

NP:A; CN:PH; CA:M; CL:C

18. (1) Anorexia is the initial symptom associated with digitalis toxicity. Nausea and vomiting are also very common symptoms.

NP:A; CN:PH; CA:M; CL:C

19. (1) Cheyne–Stokes respirations are found in clients with increased intracranial pressure and heart conditions. There is a pattern of deep respirations followed by progressively shallow respirations and then apnea.

NP:AN; CN:PH; CA:M; CL:C

20. (3) Even though the nurse may eventually have to place diapers on the client, this is not the first intervention. An every-two-hour bathroom schedule may solve the problem because he will not remember to say when he needs to urinate.

NP:I; CN:PS; CA:PS; CL:A

21. (1) 10 mL. To calculate the KCl, you would use the equation: $20 \text{ mEq} = x \text{ mL}$; thus, $10 \text{ mEq} = 5 \text{ mL}$; $10x = 100$; $x = 10 \text{ mL}$.

NP:I; CN:PH; CA:M; CL:A

22. (2) Wet-to-moist dressings prevent damage to new tissue when dressing is removed. Wet-to-dry dressing debrides the wound (4). This dressing is not to prevent leaking (1), and allowing the dressing to almost dry (3) will not support new tissue.

NP:AN; CN:PH; CA:M; CL:A

23. (3) These food choices will provide the lowest cholesterol content. Whole milk, dairy products, and fatty meats (1) are all high in cholesterol.

NP:E; CN:PH; CA:S; CL:A

24. (1) In left-sided heart failure, congestion occurs mainly in the lungs. It is caused by inadequate ejection of the blood into the systemic circulation. Dyspnea, sneezing, coughing, rales, and fatigue are common symptoms. The other answers refer to right-sided failure.

NP:A; CN:PH; CA:M; CL:AN

25. (3) Because the client cannot remember to tell the nurse or remember to go himself to the bathroom, the best plan is to take him on a schedule. This is preferable to dressing him in diapers (2), even though this may eventually have to be done.

NP:P; CN:S; CA:PS; CL:A

Simulated NCLEX-RN CAT Tests

COMPREHENSIVE TEST I QUESTIONS

1. You are making a home visit to a client who has the diagnosis of heart failure and is on daily diuretics. Considering the possibility of potassium deficiency, you will assess for

   1. Pitting edema and excessive weight gain.
   2. Muscle weakness, leg cramps, nausea and fatigue.
   3. Increased blood pressure and dyspnea.
   4. Oliguria, restlessness, weakness and hyperpnea.

2. You are assigned to care for a bedridden client and one of your nursing goals is to prevent pressure ulcers from developing. The priority nursing action would be to

   1. Massage bony prominences that are reddened.
   2. Provide for active and passive exercises.
   3. Reposition the client every 2 hours.
   4. Keep the skin moist and supple.

3. You are caring for a cardiac client and you observe the ECG rhythm strip presented below. You identify it as

   1. Multifocal PVCs.
   2. Ventricular tachycardia.
   3. Third-degree heart block.
   4. Normal sinus rhythm.

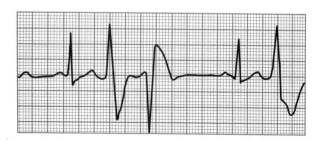

4. A male client has just been told his blood work indicates that he has a high iron level in his blood. An example of the foods he should eliminate from his diet is

   1. Fish.
   2. Beef.
   3. Egg yolks.
   4. Shellfish.

5. A client has a subtotal thyroidectomy and is returned from the recovery room. Immediate postoperative care would include correct positioning. The safe position for the client is

   1. Semi-Fowler's with neck erect.
   2. High-Fowler's with neck extended.
   3. Semi-Fowler's with neck flexed.
   4. Sims' with neck extended.

6. A young man, age 25, fell from a ladder and broke his leg. He is placed in skeletal traction to reduce the fracture prior to surgery. 24 hours after admission, he complains of shortness of breath and pain in his chest. In completing your nursing assessment of the client, you will particularly observe for

   1. Developing pneumonia.
   2. Developing fat embolus.
   3. Cardiac complications.
   4. Hypoxic condition.

7. You are caring for a client who requires telemetry monitoring. When placing a telemetry electrode for Lead I, looking at the heart's left lateral wall, would you place the negative and positive electrodes in position 1 or 2? _____ (Fill in the blank with 1 or 2.)

   1.

   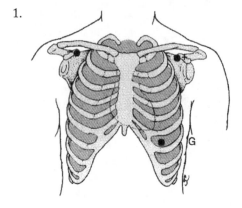

   2.

   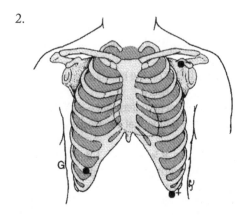

8. You are admitting a client for abdominal surgery the next day, and you observe that he appears very anxious. A priority intervention is to

   1. Tell him there is nothing to worry about.
   2. Suggest that he talk to his doctor.
   3. Ask what he expects will happen tomorrow.
   4. Ask if he is feeling anxious.

9. A 64-year-old client has been admitted to the Coronary Care Unit. He is diagnosed with an anterior septal myocardial infarction (MI) with lateral ischemia and potential for infarct extension. His orders include nitroprusside drip and dobutamine. The nurse understands that the rationale for ordering dobutamine is to

   1. Dilate veins and arteries.
   2. Improve cardiac output.
   3. Reduce hypertension.
   4. Reduce heart rate.

10. A priority nursing intervention for a client with a suspected myocardial infarction who has just been admitted is to

    1. Monitor his intake and output.
    2. Explain to the client the relationship between heart work and need for O_2.
    3. Intervene for anxiety management.
    4. Insist on complete bedrest.

11. You are assigned a client with the diagnosis of intracranial pressure. Physician's orders include an IV of hypertonic solution, dextrose 10% in saline. What is the rationale for using this solution?

    1. It reduces edema of the brain.
    2. It provides needed fluid to maintain adequate intake and output balance.
    3. This solution causes cells to expand or increase in size.
    4. It expands extracellular volume.

12. Defibrillation is usually attempted first using _____ watt-seconds.

13. A female client has a cesium needle implanted in her cervix. She asks the nurse if she may get out of bed to go to the bathroom. The appropriate response is to tell her

    1. She may not get out of bed while the needle is implanted.
    2. She may get out of bed with the nurse's help.
    3. The nurse will have to get a physician's order for her to get out of bed.

    4. She must stay in bed, but she can move around to be more comfortable while the needle is implanted.

14. A 60-year-old female client has received the diagnosis of hypertension. Her blood pressure is 160/100. Which of the following symptoms would the nurse be likely to find in the assessment?

    1. Dizziness and flushed face.
    2. Drowsiness and confusion.
    3. Faintness when getting out of bed.
    4. Ataxia and tachycardia.

15. A mother calls the pediatric hotline and tells the nurse that her 3-year-old child has a virus and a fever. She asks how much aspirin she should give the child. The best response is

    1. "You'll have to call your physician."
    2. "Give her no more than three baby aspirin every four hours."
    3. "Give her Tylenol, not aspirin."
    4. "Follow directions on the aspirin bottle for her age and weight."

16. Clients with hepatitis may have a regular diet ordered, unless they become increasingly symptomatic. The diet will then be modified to decrease the amount of

    1. Carbohydrates.
    2. Fats.
    3. Fluids.
    4. Protein.

17. Place in sequence from 1 to 4 the protocol for leaving an isolation room.

    _____   1. Take off foot socks.
    _____   2. Wash hands.
    _____   3. Remove gown.
    _____   4. Take off gloves.
    _____   5. Untie gown at waist.
    _____   6. Untie gown at neck.

18. In evaluating the condition of a child who has been treated for lead poisoning, the nurse will assess for the complication of

    1. Glomerulonephritis.
    2. Reye's syndrome.
    3. Multiple sclerosis.
    4. Tetany.

19. A client with a gunshot wound to the chest had a right-sided pneumothorax. The physician inserted

two chest tubes into the pleural cavity, and connected the water-seal drainage system to a walled-in suction. To assist in chest drainage, the nurse will place the client in the position of

1. High-Fowler's.
2. Supine.
3. Right-side, low-Fowler's.
4. Left-side, semi-Fowler's.

20. The nurse knows that the client understands the principles of managing Type 1 diabetes when he says that he maintains his health status with

    1. Oral hypoglycemics.
    2. A diabetic diet (ADA) regimen.
    3. Weight reduction.
    4. Insulin injections.

21. A 6-month-old child is brought to the clinic with a suspected diagnosis of cerebral palsy. In the initial assessment of his developmental status, the nurse would be likely to find that he

    1. Tracks an object with his eyes.
    2. Needs to be propped to sit up.
    3. Smiles when he sees his mother.
    4. Exhibits a pincer grasp.

22. A 41-year-old client has had recurrent dull flank pain, nausea, and vomiting for 24 hours. He is admitted to the hospital for a genitourinary work-up. Which of the following orders written by his physician would be considered a priority and thus carried out promptly?

    1. Keep accurate intake and output records.
    2. Strain all urine.
    3. Record temperature every 4 hours.
    4. Administer an antiemetic every 4 hours.

23. When a person is experiencing severe stress, the nurse would recognize behaviors such as

    1. Restlessness and anxiety.
    2. Crying and upset demeanor.
    3. Laughing and amusement.
    4. Assertiveness and determination.

24. A 60-year-old male client with chronic osteoarthritis is severely debilitated. Betamethasone (Celestone) therapy has been ordered for him. The nurse will advise the client to take a single, daily dose of the drug

    1. At bedtime with a glass of milk.
    2. With orange juice at bedtime.
    3. With milk in the morning.
    4. On an empty stomach in the morning.

25. In completing a full assessment on a client, it is important to identify breathing patterns. The abnormal breathing pattern depicted in the drawing is

    1. Bradypnea.
    2. Apnea.
    3. Kussmaul's.
    4. Hyperpnea.

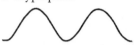

26. In the preoperative period for correction of pyloric stenosis, nursing care for the baby will include placing him in

    1. A prone position.
    2. Semi-Fowler's position on his left side.
    3. Fowler's position or on his right side.
    4. Sims' position.

27. An elderly client with heart disease has orders for Diuril. Serum potassium levels should be evaluated for a client on diuretics. To determine if the potassium level is low, the nurse would assess for

    1. Dyspnea.
    2. Skeletal muscle weakness.
    3. Hypertension.
    4. Headache.

28. The first postoperative day following surgery for a detached retina, the nursing care plan will include the intervention to

    1. Turn, cough, and deep-breathe every 2 hours.
    2. Allow the client up out of bed ad lib.
    3. Allow the eye patch to be removed during the day.
    4. Give the client a complete bed bath.

29. A 43-year-old male is brought to the mental health unit by the police for vandalizing his neighbor's car, but says that it was his neighbor's fault. The client seems bright, articulate, and oriented upon admission and is diagnosed with paranoid disorder. A person with a paranoid disorder can be described as exhibiting

    1. Delusions that are less firmly established than those of schizophrenia.
    2. None of the other classical symptoms of schizophrenia.
    3. Delusions that are usually more bizarre than schizophrenic delusions.
    4. Emotions and behavior not appropriate to the content of the delusional system.

30. A client the nurse is assessing appears to be having respiratory difficulty. The condition that leads the nurse to determine he is hypoxic is

   1. Bradycardia.
   2. Agitation.
   3. Mucosal cyanosis.
   4. Decreased blood pressure.

31. A client with a partial colectomy was returned to the unit at 1:30 PM. During a 6:00 PM assessment, the nurse observes the following data. Which sign or symptom would require the earliest intervention?

   1. Dressing that is moderately saturated with serosanguineous drainage.
   2. Warm and reddened area on the client's left calf.
   3. Distended bladder that is firm to palpation.
   4. Decrease in breath sounds on the right side.

32. A 48-year-old female has been experiencing irregular menstrual periods, hot flashes, and mood swings for the last 15 months. She has come to the clinic for her yearly checkup and says she has a number of questions. Her first question is, "When can I stop using birth control methods?" The most appropriate reply for the nurse to give her is

   1. "Anytime now because your periods have been irregular for more than 12 months."
   2. "You should use a birth control method until your 50th birthday."
   3. "It depends on whether you have regular menses."
   4. "You should use a birth control method until you have missed your period for 24 consecutive months."

33. The nurse will know that the client understands how to maintain an acid urinary pH by dietary means when he says he should avoid

   1. Prunes and figs.
   2. Cereals and breads.
   3. Meat, fish, and poultry.
   4. Milk.

34. A client's physician orders an aminophylline IV infusion at 2 mg per minute. A safety intervention for administering this medication is to

   1. Use an IV controller.
   2. Protect the IV bottle from sunlight.
   3. Give the client a test dose of aminophylline first.
   4. Run the IV at 1 mg per minute for 1 hour before increasing the dose.

35. Charting is one of the nurse's most important functions. Which of the following statements identifies the most important purpose of charting?

   1. To communicate to other members of the client's healthcare team.
   2. To evaluate the staff's performance.
   3. To provide information for a nursing audit.
   4. To enable physicians to monitor nursing care.

36. When moving the client up in bed, the nurse would remove the pillow and place it at the head of the bed. The rationale for this action is to

   1. Get it out of the way.
   2. Prevent the client from striking his head.
   3. Facilitate completing the procedure.
   4. Enable the client to push from his knees.

37. A client on the unit is observed to have severe anxiety. The priority nursing action is to

   1. Remain with the client while she is anxious.
   2. Provide an activity to get the client's mind off feeling anxious.
   3. Encourage the client to identify, discuss and find the cause of her anxiety.
   4. Establish a nurse–client relationship.

38. An elderly client on bedrest has developed a pressure ulcer. The priority nursing diagnosis is

   1. Altered Health Maintenance.
   2. Altered Tissue Perfusion.
   3. Dysfunctional Grieving.
   4. Self-Care Deficit.

39. A client with AIDS is being discharged to home. Client teaching for home care should include which one of the following concepts?

   1. Good household cleaning practices will prevent the spread of infection.
   2. Any equipment that comes in contact with blood or body fluids needs to be disinfected for 24 hours.
   3. AIDS clients should not be responsible for food preparation.
   4. Soiled dressings should be burned, not placed in a trash container.

40. Percussion, vibration and postural drainage are ordered for a 15-year-old client hospitalized for pneumonia. Prior to providing this intervention, the priority action is to

   1. Instruct the client in diaphragmatic breathing.
   2. Assess vital signs.

3. Auscultate lung fields.

4. Assess characteristics of her sputum.

41. To prevent venous stasis, a client is to be measured for knee-high elastic hose. The nursing intervention is to measure

1. Leg length from heel to buttocks and calf circumference while he is standing.

2. Ankle and calf circumference while he is standing.

3. Leg length to the knee when he is lying down.

4. Calf circumference and leg length from bottom of heel to bend of knee.

42. During the first 10 minutes of a blood transfusion, the nurse will infuse the blood at how many drops per minute?

1. 10 gtts/min.

2. 20 gtts/min.

3. 40 gtts/min.

4. According to physician's orders.

43. The nurse explains to the client that the major difference between a plaster of Paris and a synthetic cast is that the

1. Drying time is prolonged with a synthetic cast.

2. A synthetic cast is less restrictive.

3. A plaster cast requires expensive equipment for application.

4. A synthetic cast is more effective for immobilizing severely displaced bones.

44. If a client were suspected to have developed atelectasis, a major postoperative complication, which of the following assessment findings would be most conclusive?

1. Bradycardia.

2. Temperature of 102°F.

3. Dullness to breath sound percussion.

4. Restlessness.

45. What is the most significant factor in identifying a normal ECG strip?

1. P-R interval falls before the QRS complex on the strip.

2. T wave is in the inverted position on the strip.

3. P-R interval is no longer than 0.12 second.

4. QRS interval is no longer than 0.20 second.

46. A 25-year-old client has been admitted to the psychiatric unit with a diagnosis of acute schizophrenic disorder. He is unkempt and speaks in unclear sentences. In the first nurse–client interaction, the client says, "Yester-

noon the sunmoon went over the rover to see the lawnmower." The nurse knows that the client is manifesting

1. A delusion.

2. Disordered speech.

3. A hallucination.

4. Disturbance of affect.

47. A client is to receive codeine for pain with her diagnosis of head injury. The nurse would also expect the physician to order a stool softener. The reason for this order is to

1. Prevent paralytic ileus.

2. Prevent bowel stasis.

3. Avoid straining during evacuation.

4. Prevent complications from the codeine.

48. A client was hospitalized briefly with an episode of urolithiasis until a stone was passed. She has now been readmitted with complaints of low back pain, nausea and diarrhea. Formulating a care plan for this client, the nurse knows that a priority goal is to

1. Record intake and output.

2. Provide appropriate diet therapy.

3. Limit fluid intake initially.

4. Encourage fluids to 3000 mL per day.

49. An 18-year-old client was hospitalized for anorexia nervosa. After 1 week of treatment, the nursing team met to evaluate the client's progress and improvement. Signs of improvement would be indicated by

1. Talking about going home.

2. Attending all groups.

3. Gaining 4 pounds.

4. Expressing a desire to "get into shape" again.

50. A client with peptic ulcer disease has had a subtotal gastric resection. His postoperative pain can most effectively be controlled by

1. Medicating for pain before the previous dose totally wears off.

2. Medicating for pain at least every 6 hours.

3. Waiting until the client requests pain medication.

4. Alternating a maximum dose with a minimum dose.

51. An 18-year-old client is hospitalized after an accident in which she lost the use of her legs. The nurse observes her sitting in a wheelchair crying and she says, "Go away; no one can help me." The nurse's best response is to say

1. "It will help to talk about it."

2. "I'll go away, but I'll come back in 30 minutes and perhaps we can talk."

3. "I'd like to help. Can you tell me about what's wrong?"

4. "Crying doesn't help; perhaps talking will make you feel better."

52. A 52-year-old male client has an admitting diagnosis of rheumatoid arthritis. He is started on indomethacin, an anti-inflammatory medication. Part of the care plan is to assess side effects of the drug. The nurse would assess for

1. Hypertension.
2. Tinnitus.
3. Joint stiffness.
4. GI disturbance.

53. Transmission-based respiratory precautions indicate that when the disease is airborne, the precaution(s) that must be used is (are)

1. Gloves.
2. A mask.
3. A gown.
4. Full isolation gear.

54. The severity of a burn is the combination of the depth of the burn and the extent of body surface area (BSA) involved. Which of the following factors is the first priority when assessing the severity of the burn?

1. Age of the client.
2. Associated medical problems.
3. Location of the burn.
4. Cause of the burn.

55. A female client is admitted to the hospital with an obstruction just proximal to her old ileostomy stoma from surgery six months ago. For a client with an ileostomy, which one of the following foods should be eliminated in the diet because it could cause obstruction?

1. Cabbage.
2. Corn.
3. Red meat.
4. Radishes.

56. The priority nursing care to administer to a client in prehepatic coma is to

1. Maintain protein intake at a moderate or normal level.
2. Administer neomycin and lactulose to reduce bacterial production and ammonia.

3. Maintain a mildly sedative state to reduce stress.
4. Offer the client adequate fluids by mouth to maintain fluid and electrolyte balance.

57. An important initial goal for a client just admitted to the psychiatric unit because he attacked a friend is to

1. Establish a relationship and set behavioral limits.
2. Explain to the client that his behavior was unacceptable and dangerous.
3. Explore the truth of the client's statements.
4. Set behavioral limits on the client.

58. A client has just returned from surgery for evacuation of a subdural hematoma. Immediately after the evacuation, the priority intervention is to

1. Observe for CSF leaks around the evacuation site.
2. Assess for an increase in temperature, indicating infection.
3. Establish and maintain a patent airway.
4. Observe for signs of increasing intracranial pressure.

59. The nurse is assisting a 9-year-old child's mother to plan her care at home following discharge after an acute asthma attack. In the discharge planning, the growth and development stage according to Erikson that would be important to take into account is

1. Autonomy versus shame and doubt.
2. Initiative versus guilt.
3. Industry versus inferiority.
4. Identity versus role confusion.

60. You are tabulating a client's intake and output record for your shift. 1 cup is 6 ounces. 1 bowl is 8 ounces.

INTAKE	IV	= 1000 mL normal saline
	Coffee	= 1 cup
	Water	= 6 ounces
	Soup	= 1 bowl
	Jello	= 3 ounces
	Ice cream	= 3 ounces

How many milliliters will you document as the client's intake? _____ mL.

61. Assessing urine of a client with suspected cholecystitis, the nurse expects that the color will most likely be

1. Pale yellow.
2. Greenish-brown.
3. Red.
4. Yellow-orange.

62. An 18-year-old client has been in a motorcycle accident and sustained a head injury. The nurse admitting

him notices that his IV is infusing at 125 mL/hour. Until there are orders for the IV rate, the nursing intervention is to

1. Slow the rate to 20 mL/hour.
2. Continue the rate at 125 mL/hour.
3. Slow the rate to 50 mL/hour.
4. Increase the rate to 150 mL/hour.

63. An 11-year-old client with cystic fibrosis will take pancreatic enzymes three times per day. The nurse will know that the child's mother needs more education on the purpose and timing of these enzymes if she says

1. "They should be taken at mealtimes, three times a day."
2. "They should be given following breakfast, lunch and dinner."
3. "The purpose of the enzymes is to help digest the fat in foods."
4. "My daughter should take them prior to meals."

64. For a 38-year-old client with chronic lymphocytic leukemia, a priority nursing diagnosis is

1. Risk for Infection.
2. Impaired Skin Integrity.
3. Altered Issue Perfusion.
4. Fluid Volume Deficit.

65. A client, age 60, has been admitted to the hospital with a diagnosis of right ventricular failure. With a central venous line in place, the nurse would assess the CVP reading. Considering the diagnosis, the CVP reading would be expected to be

1. 0 to 2 mm Hg.
2. 5 to 20 cm H_2O
3. 8 to 10 mm Hg.
4. 15 to 20 cm H_2O.

66. A client is brought into the emergency room bleeding profusely from a deep laceration on his left lower forearm. After observing standard precautions, the initial nursing action should be to

1. Apply a tourniquet just below the elbow.
2. Apply pressure directly over the wound.
3. Cleanse the wound to determine the extent of damage.
4. Elevate the limb and apply ice to decrease blood flow.

67. A client is admitted to the psychiatric unit with a diagnosis of anxiety disorder. Effective nursing measures to help this client cope with anxiety would include

1. Giving her some responsibility for manipulating the environment.
2. Removing all disturbing factors in the environment.
3. Encouraging her to read to provide distraction.
4. Remaining close by her and allowing her to express her feelings.

68. A client is brought into the emergency room with an admitting diagnosis of delirium tremens (DTs). After admitting the client to a private room, the priority intervention is to

1. Administer the standing order of Valium.
2. Put up the siderails of the bed.
3. Attempt to get a history to validate if he really is experiencing DTs.
4. Keep the room very quiet with lights down to minimize stimulation.

69. A client is admitted to the labor room. She tells the nurse that contractions started 2 hours ago, and she has soaked a perineal pad with bright-red blood in the past 10 minutes. The nurse suspects a placenta previa. The first nursing action is to

1. Perform a vaginal examination to determine cervical dilatation.
2. Notify the physician immediately.
3. Order blood to be typed and cross-matched.
4. Apply an external fetal monitor.

70. You are discharging a client with the diagnosis of angina. The physician is sending the client home with a prescription for Verapamil. Teaching will include telling the client that the main use of this medication is to

1. Increase the pumping ability of the heart.
2. Cause coronary vasodilation and increase myocardial oxygenation.
3. Increase the heart rate.
4. Lower low-density lipoprotein (LDL) levels.

71. A 3-year-old child is brought to the hospital by his mother, who explains that the child has been sick for several days and has had a "barklike" cough. The nurse assesses nasal flaring. The nursing action is to

1. Tell him to cough.
2. Give 4 back blows.
3. Ask him to speak.
4. Obtain an immediate order for oxygen.

72. If a child has impetigo contagiosa, to prevent further spread of the disease the nurse should instruct the mother to

1. Strictly isolate this child from others in his family.
2. Wash toys and other objects the child uses with soap and very hot water.
3. Take all other children in the family to the physician to be vaccinated for this disease.
4. Not take any special precautions.

73. A client is admitted to the maternity unit 2 weeks before her actual delivery date. She is there for evaluation because she is experiencing polyhydramnios. The nurse understands that this diagnosis means that

1. There is the normal amount of amniotic fluid, thinner in volume.
2. A less-than-normal amount of amniotic fluid is present.
3. An excessive amount of amniotic fluid is present.
4. A leak is causing fluid to accumulate outside the amniotic sac.

74. A client is unable to sleep. He is pacing the floor, head down, and wringing his hands. Recognizing that he is anxious, the nurse's most appropriate intervention is to

1. Encourage him to go back to bed.
2. Give him his PRN sleeping medication.
3. Let him know that the nurse is interested and willing to listen.
4. Explore with him the alternatives to pacing the floor.

75. A 32-year-old client in active labor was admitted through the emergency room. She is having contractions every 2 minutes, lasting 50 to 60 seconds. A vaginal exam shows she is 6 cm dilated and 100 percent effaced. After the exam, the FHR is 140 and regular and her blood pressure 80/40. The first nursing action would be to

1. Place the client in knee–chest position.
2. Take the blood pressure again to check accuracy.
3. Call the physician immediately.
4. Turn the client on her side and check her blood pressure.

COMPREHENSIVE TEST I

Answers with Rationale

1. (2) Thiazide diuretics are potent antihypertensives but may lead to the electrolyte imbalance and loss of potassium. The symptoms you would assess for are muscle weakness, leg cramps, hypotension and even arrhythmias. Options (1) and (3) are sodium excess symptoms and option (4) is potassium excess.

   NP:A; CN:PH; CA:M; CL:A

2. (3) The most important intervention to stimulate circulation and prevent ulcers is to change the client's position every two hours. It is no longer accepted practice to massage bony prominences because it can lead to deep tissue trauma (1). Option (2) is important, but not the priority intervention. The skin should be kept dry and free of drainage (4).

   NP:I; CN:S; CA:M; CL:A

3. (1) The rhythm strip is showing *multifocal PVCs*. The client could be hypoxic or in acidosis with a diagnosis of COPD or diabetes mellitus. Lidocaine may be administered to decrease automaticity and increase the electrical stimulation threshold of the ventricles.

   NP:A; CN:PH; CA:M; CL:AN

4. (3) The client should eliminate egg yolks, which are high in iron. Beef is high in protein and cholesterol; fish is also high in protein, and shellfish is high in sodium and iodine.

   NP:AN; CN:H; CA:M; CL:C

5. (1) Semi-Fowler's with the neck erect is the position of choice to maintain respiratory status. The objective is to decrease pressure on the suture line and prevent edema formation, which could cause respiratory distress.

   NP:I; CN:PH; CA:S; CL:A

6. (2) The priority assessment is for a fat embolus, which can occur from 24 to 96 hours after fracture of a long bone. The first symptoms may be pulmonary, including dyspnea and respiratory depression. It is critical that this diagnosis be made early to stabilize the client. ABGs will help to confirm the diagnosis.

   NP:A; CN:PH; CA:M; CL:A

7. (1) The answer is *1* because this position is where the lead records activity between a negative electrode (below the right clavicle) and a positive electrode (below the left clavicle). This lead records activity at (looks at) the heart's left lateral wall. Illustration 2 shows Lead III, which records activity at (looks at) the left inferior wall.

   NP:P; CN:PH; CA:M; CL:A

8. (3) Determining what the client knows about the surgical procedure and expects to happen will give you data about how to intervene. Fear of the unknown increases anxiety and stress. The first two interventions will close off communication, and answer (4) is too direct and may result in a negative response.

   NP:I; CN:PS; CA:S; CL:A

9. (2) The primary objective in giving dobutamine, a sympathomimetic agent, is to improve cardiac output. It does not cause an excessive increase in heart rate as a side effect. Nitroprusside is an arterial dilator and a venodilator. Diuretics would reduce preload and lower hypertension, and beta blockers would reduce heart rate.

   NP:AN; CN:PH; CA:M; CL:C

10. (3) The priority intervention in this situation is to perform anxiety management, because anxiety (as well as pain) will stimulate sympathetic cardiac responses, which in turn will increase heart work, a risk for more

---

Coding for Questions/Answers Abbreviations: **Nursing Process: NP,** Assessment: A, Analysis: AN, Planning: P, Implementation: I, Evaluation: E; **Client Needs: CN,** Safe, Effective Care Environment: S, Health Promotion and Maintenance: H, Psychosocial Integrity: PS, Physiological Integrity: PH; **Clinical Area: CA,** Medical Nursing: M, Surgical Nursing: S, Maternal/Newborn Nursing: MA, Pediatric Nursing: P, Psychiatric Nursing: PS; **Cognitive Level: CL,** Knowledge: K, Comprehension: C, Application: A, Analysis: AN.

cardiac damage. Answers (1) and (2) may be important, but are not the priority. Activity should be minimized, but complete bedrest is not usually ordered.

NP:I; CN:PS; CA:M; CL:AN

11. (1) A hypertonic solution is a solution with higher osmotic pressure than blood serum. It is used for intracranial pressure because it reduces edema by rapid movement of fluid out of the ventricles into the bloodstream. Option (2) describes effects of a hypotonic solution, which causes cells to expand or increase in size (3). Isotonic solutions expand excellular volume.

NP:P; CN:PH; CA:M; CL:C

12. The answer is *200*. 200 watt-seconds is the point at which defibrillation should be started, because electric shock is damaging to the myocardium. You would proceed, if necessary, to 300 J, then to 360 J (one joule [J] = one watt-second).

NP:I; CN:S; CA:M; CL:A

13. (1) While the sealed source is implanted, the client must remain on bedrest, and movement is restricted to prevent dislodging the radiation source. The client must remain on her back and should not turn or move in bed.

NP:I; CN:PH; CA:S; CL:A

14. (1) Cardinal symptoms are dizziness and flushed face as well as headache, tinnitus, and epistaxis. Drowsiness and confusion (2) occur in hypertensive crisis, and faintness (3) would occur in hypotension.

NP:A; CN:PH; CA:M; CL:C

15. (3) Children from 2 months to adolescence are advised not to take aspirin for a virus infection due to the connection to Reye's syndrome, an acute encephalopathy condition. Tylenol is the treatment of choice for any virus infection.

NP:I; CN:PH; CA:P; CL:A

16. (4) With liver cell damage, the liver cannot break down and eliminate the protein. Protein needs to be decreased until symptoms dissipate.

NP:P; CN:PH; CA:M; CL:C

17. The answers are *5 4 6 3*. You first untie the gown at waist, take off gloves, untie gown at neck (which is clean) and remove gown. Washing hands would be the last step.

NP:I; CN:H; CA:M; CL:A

18. (4) Following therapy, children can develop tetany because the chelating agent, EDTA, will take out calcium along with the lead. Therefore, the nurse will monitor for hypocalcemia.

NP:A; CN:PH; CA:P; CL:AN

19. (4) Positioning a client on the left side will assist in drainage, and semi-Fowler's will assist in breathing. The client can usually be turned to both sides and back.

NP:I; CN:PH; CA:M; CL:A

20. (4) The insulin dosage is generally given once or twice daily. It is either intermediate-acting insulin alone or in conjunction with a short-acting insulin. With Type 1 diabetes, the pancreatic beta cells are not producing insulin, so insulin must be given. Diet is also important for both Types 1 and 2; frequently Type 2 diabetes can be controlled with a diabetic diet (2) or with a combination of oral hypoglycemics (1) and diet.

NP:E; CN:H; CA:M; CL:C

21. (2) At 6 months of age, the child should be able to sit by himself. This delayed developmental milestone is frequently seen in children with cerebral palsy. A neat pincer grasp (4) is not expected until 10 to 11 months of age. The other two abilities would be present before 6 months of age.

NP:A; CN:H; CA:P; CL:C

22. (2) The client has symptoms indicative of a urinary calculus; therefore, it is important to strain all the urine to detect whether the stone has passed and confirm the diagnosis.

NP:P; CN:PH; CA:M; CL:A

23. (2) Crying and being upset are typical behaviors experienced when a person is under stress. Restlessness and anxiety (1) might be present, but they are not typical responses. Laughing and humor (3) relieve stress. Assertiveness and determination (4) are not responses to stress.

NP:AN; CN:H; CA:PS; CL:C

24. (3) A single dose in the morning promotes better results and less toxicity. It is given with milk to reduce GI irritation.

NP:I; CN:PH; CA:M; CL:A

25. (1) Bradypnea—slow, regular respirations; rate is below 10/minute. Tachypnea is increased rate, above 24/minute. Biot's are abrupt interruptions between a

faster, deeper rate. Kussmaul's respirations are deep, gasping breaths.

NP:A; CN:PH; CA:M; CL:A

Abnormal Breathing Patterns

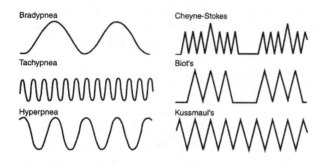

26. (3) Many infants are fed in a semi-Fowler's or Fowler's position with either thick formula or small frequent feedings. They are best maintained in a Fowler's position or lying on their right side to facilitate gastric emptying following feeding.

NP:P; CN:H; CA:P; CL:C

27. (2) Skeletal muscle weakness is a result of low potassium levels in the blood; potassium is required for normal muscle function. Hypotension may occur later, as well as cardiac arrhythmias and tachycardia. Dyspnea (1) and headache (4) are specific indications of hypokalemia.

NP:E; CN:PH; CA:M; CL:A

28. (4) A complete bath in bed is the most likely choice, as the client will still have patches on both eyes and be on bedrest. Coughing could increase intraocular pressure, which could lead to hemorrhage.

NP:P; CN:PH; CA:S; CL:C

29. (2) Paranoid disorders are characterized by delusions of persecution but not by the other classic symptoms of schizophrenia, such as associative looseness, affective disturbance, autism, and ambivalence. Clients with this disorder have emotional behaviors that are appropriate to the content of the delusional system.

NP:AN; CN:PS; CA:PS; CL:C

30. (3) Hypoxia is defined as inadequate oxygenation of the tissues. The quantity of oxygen delivered to the tissues depends on the flow of blood to the tissues and the oxygen content of the blood. Mucosal cyanosis is an indication of hypoxia. The client would be likely to also exhibit tachycardia, hypertension, and restlessness.

NP:AN; CN:PH; CA:M; CL:A

31. (3) Inability to void after surgery is a common problem. It is important to be aware of the client's output for several reasons: to ensure adequate intake, to detect renal problems, and to assess for blood pressure problems. Solution to this problem is catheterization (with a physician's order). The dressing should be closely observed but is not presently a problem. The area on the calf is probably thrombophlebitis and should be reported to the physician immediately. The breath sounds are due to potential lung problems and can be improved by turning, coughing and deep-breathing.

NP:I; CN:S; CA:S; CL:AN

32. (4) Usually 24 months after menstruation ceases is advised as the length of time a woman should continue using birth control to avoid pregnancy. It is important to reinforce the possibility of pregnancy in the presence of irregular menses.

NP:I; CN:H; CA:MA; CL:A

33. (4) Of the listed foods, milk has alkaline ash. All of the other foods could be included in the diet to maintain an acid urine.

NP:E; CN:PH; CA:M; CL:C

34. (1) The infusion of all IV drugs that affect the CNS should be carefully monitored and an IV controller is essential for accurate monitoring. Toxic levels of aminophylline, a bronchodilator, could cause arrhythmias or seizures.

NP:I; CN:S; CA:M; CL:A

35. (1) All the answers except (4) are purposes of charting. Answer (1) is the most inclusive and, therefore, the best answer.

NP:AN; CN:S; CA:M; CL:C

36. (2) With no cushion, the client may hit his head as he is moved up in bed. With the pillow there, his head will be protected.

NP:AN; CN:S; CA:M; CL:A

37. (1) Staying with a client is the most effective way to reduce anxiety. A nurse–client relationship is important, but it will take time to establish. The nurse should proceed at the client's pace and not push her to deal directly with the source of her anxiety.

NP:P; CN:PS; CA:PS; CL:A

38. (2) Blood supply may be altered to the wound area leading to an alteration in tissue perfusion. While Health Maintenance and Self-Care Deficit are appro-

priate areas of concern, the highest priority nursing diagnosis would be Altered Tissue Perfusion.

NP:AN; CN:PH; CA:M; CL:A

39. (1) Clean surfaces, including floors, showers, and kitchens, prevent contact with the HIV virus. Therefore, good cleaning practices will prevent the spread of viruses and bacteria. Equipment does not require being disinfected for 24 hours.

NP:P; CN:PH; CA:M; CL:C

40. (3) Auscultating lung fields provides knowledge of which lung areas are most affected. These areas should be treated first, as many clients cannot tolerate a 30-minute procedure. Assessing vital signs will be done on every shift, but does not need to be done before PVD.

NP:A; CN:PH; CA:M; CL:A

41. (4) The client should be in dorsal recumbent position with the bed elevated. For knee-high hose, measurement is taken from the Achilles tendon to the popliteal fold and the mid-calf circumference.

NP:I; CN:PH; CA:M; CL:A

42. (2) Infusing blood at 20 gtts/minute allows adequate time to observe for possible transfusion reactions. A faster flow rate would allow too much blood into the system before noting the reaction.

NP:I; CN:PH; CA:M; CL:AN

43. (2) A synthetic cast is less restrictive, is lighter in weight and requires less drying time than a plaster of Paris cast.

NP:AN; CN:PH; CA:S; CL:C

44. (2) The temperature usually reaches 102°F within the first 48 hours postoperatively. Restlessness and dullness to percussion might be present but the increase in temperature is the most significant finding. Tachypnea, not bradycardia, occurs in atelectasis.

NP:E; CN:PH; CA:M; CL:AN

45. (1) The P-R interval indicates atrial contraction; therefore, it should precede the QRS complex, which is indicative of ventricular contraction.

NP:A; CN:PH; CA:M; CL:A

46. (2) This is an example of disordered speech where the ideas do not connect to each other and are expressed in garbled language. A delusion is a false belief. This example represents disturbed thoughts. A hallucination is an unwilled sensory perception with

no basis in reality. Affect refers to feelings that are flat or inappropriate; a disturbance in this area is typical of this disorder.

NP:A; CN:PS; CA:PS; CL:C

47. (3) Codeine is constipating and it is important to avoid straining during evacuation so that the ICP is not increased. Bowel stasis is not the issue. A complication of codeine ingestion is constipation and this may increase ICP, but answer (3) is more specific than (4).

NP:AN; CN:PH; CA:M; CL:AN

48. (4) Fluids are essential to flush the kidneys and urinary system. The other goals such as intake and output are important, but not the top priority. Diet consultation will be a later goal to be implemented before discharge and after the chemical composition of the stones has been determined.

NP:P; CN:PH; CA:M; CL:A

49. (3) Gaining 4 pounds is concrete evaluation criteria for her positive progress. She may talk about going home and continue to not deal with her problem. The client may attend all groups and never deal with her problem. Answer (4) is incorrect because it may indicate the client's continual obsession with her altered body image.

NP:E; CN:PS; CA:PS; CL:A

50. (1) Immediate postoperative pain can best be controlled by medicating before pain becomes severe—usually every 4 hours. Waiting until the effect of the medication wears off is not therapeutic, nor is alternating doses.

NP:P; CN:PH; CA:S; CL:C

51. (2) The nurse is responding to the client's wishes, but coming back lets her know the nurse is concerned and open to talk about her feelings. Asking the client to talk right now is putting an extra demand on her. Telling her that crying doesn't help is denying her feelings.

NP:I; CN:PS; CA:PS; CL:A

52. (4) An expected side effect of the anti-inflammatory medication, indomethacin, is GI disturbance. Hypertension is not an expected side effect of this drug. Tinnitus is a side effect of salicylates.

NP:E; CN:PH; CA:M; CL:C

53. (2) A mask must be used for respiratory precautions when the disease is airborne; for droplet precautions, a mask is indicated when working within 3 feet of the

client. Contact precautions do not indicate a mask, but require gloves.

NP:P; CN:S; CA:M; CL:A

54. (3) The location of the burn requires priority assessment, as burns surrounding the face, neck, and upper extremities can lead to respiratory involvement.

NP:A; CN:PH; CA:M; CL:A

55. (2) Corn can cause obstruction of the ileostomy and thus should be avoided. Answers (1) and (4) cause flatus and usually are avoided by clients as well.

NP:A; CN:H; CA:S; CL:A

56. (2) Neomycin exerts a powerful effect on intestinal bacteria and lactulose decreases ammonia by pulling ammonia into the bowel. Protein should be reduced in the diet, sedatives restricted, and intravenous intake started to maintain fluid and electrolyte balance.

NP:I; CN:PH; CA:M; CL:A

57. (1) Initiating a relationship that includes limit setting is the first priority. To do any interacting with a client requires a beginning relationship before explaining, exploring the truth, or setting limits.

NP:P; CN:PS; CA:PS; CL:C

58. (3) A patent airway will establish adequate oxygenation and prevent carbon dioxide buildup. All of the nursing interventions listed would be carried out for the client; however, the most important one is to prevent cerebral hypoxia, which contributes to cerebral edema. The acid–base imbalance and hypoxia are often mistaken for signs of increased intracranial pressure, leading to unnecessary surgical intervention.

NP:I; CN:PH; CA:S; CL:AN

59. (3) According to Erikson's developmental stages, a school-age child is working on developing industry versus inferiority. This is the stage where children need to engage in tasks and activities that they can carry through to completion. Autonomy is the stage for the toddler; initiative is found in the preschooler, and identity is the stage for puberty and adolescence.

NP:AN; CN:PS; CA:P; CL:C

60. The total intake is *1780* mL. The nurse would change the ounces to milliliters and add: 1000 mL IV; 1 cup coffee = 180 mL; 6 ounces water = 180 mL; 1 bowl soup = 240 mL; 3 ounces Jello = 90 mL; and 3 ounces ice cream = 90 mL.

NP:I; CN:PH; CA:M; CL:A

61. (4) The presence of bile in the urine would lead to a yellow-orange or brown-colored urine. Red-colored urine may indicate the presence of blood or a disease in the body.

NP:AN; CN:PH; CA:M; CL:C

62. (3) Because of the potential of increased cerebral fluid, fluids will be given very sparingly at approximately 50 mL/hour before the nurse has a physician's order. 20 mL/hour is barely a "keep open" rate.

NP:I; CN:PH; CA:M; CL:AN

63. (2) The purpose of the pancreatic enzymes is to replace the enzymes unavailable in the child's system that assist with the digestion of fats. Therefore, they should be taken at or prior to—not following—the ingestion of food.

NP:E; CN:PH; CA:P; CL:A

64. (1) Immature white blood cells predispose the client to infections, so this nursing diagnosis is a priority. Fluid volume deficit may also be an important nursing diagnosis, because the client may be prone to bleeding. It does not, however, have as high a priority as (1).

NP:AN; CN:PH; CA:M; CL:C

65. (4) An elevated central venous pressure is expected in this client due to the increased right atrial pressure. The normal reading is 5 to 10 cm of water pressure.

NP:E; CN:PH; CA:M; CL:AN

66. (2) The initial nursing action is to stop the bleeding with direct pressure over the wound unless there is glass in the wound. If that is not successful, the nurse then has the option of using elevation, pressure on the supplying arteries, and, as a last resort, a tourniquet.

NP:I; CN:PH; CA:S; CL:AN

67. (4) Once anxiety has risen to a high level, staying near the client and allowing her to ventilate will help decrease anxiety. If the client chooses to pace around the unit, the nurse might walk with her. Answers (1) and (3) will not be effective in reducing anxiety. Answer (2) is unrealistic.

NP:P; CN:PS; CA:PS; CL:C

68. (2) The first intervention is a safety issue. Because the client may respond to illusions or hallucinations or he may experience a seizure due to the DTs, siderails need to be in place. The lights should be on so that they do not create shadows on the walls. After these

actions, an IV will be started and a tranquilizer administered.

NP:I; CN:PS; CA:PS; CL:A

69. (2) The nurse would first notify the physician so that he is present to prepare for an emergency cesarean section. Vaginal examinations are never performed when there is heavy vaginal bleeding and the possibility of a placenta previa. Massive hemorrhage can result when a placenta is touched by an examining finger.

NP:I; CN:PH; CA:MA; CL:AN

70. (2) This calcium-channel blocker causes vasodilation and is especially appropriate for vasospastic angina. Digitalis increases the pumping ability of the heart (1). A sympathomimetic agent, such as epinephrine HCl, increases the heart rate (3). Drugs such as Zocor are antihyperlipidemic agents that lower cholesterol (4).

NP:P; CN:PH; CA:M; CL:A

71. (4) The child may be suffering from either croup or epiglottitis. From the symptoms, the nurse knows that he does not have a foreign object in his airway. Attempting to have him cough to open his airway could lead to laryngospasm. Administering high-flow O_2 and keeping him calm is the appropriate nursing care.

NP:I; CN:PH; CA:P; CL:A

72. (2) Impetigo is a bacterial infection. Washing with soap and hot water keeps the objects relatively free of streptococci and lessens the danger of spreading the disease.

NP:I; CN:S; CA:P; CL:A

73. (3) Polyhydramnios is a condition where an excessive amount of amniotic fluid is present. The normal amount is 500 to 1000 mL. While the actual cause of this condition is unknown, it occurs more frequently in mothers with diabetes and eclampsia.

NP:AN; CN:H; CA:MA; CL:K

74. (3) This is the most comprehensive answer, although (4) is also appropriate. Sleeping medication should be avoided if at all possible or unless absolutely necessary, because it helps suppress the client's feelings only temporarily. Encouraging the client to go back to bed closes off communication.

NP:I; CN:PS; CA:PS; CL:A

75. (4) The low blood pressure is likely due to supine hypotensive syndrome. Turning the client on her side will relieve the pressure from the inferior vena cava. After this action, the nurse will repeat the blood pressure reading.

NP:I; CN:H; CA:MA; CL:AN

COMPREHENSIVE TEST 2 QUESTIONS

1. The physician orders an intravenous infusion of rito-drine for a client in premature labor in an attempt to stop the contractions. Because ritodrine is a beta-sympathomimetic agent that causes muscle relaxation, the nurse will monitor closely for

   1. Hypertension and tachycardia.
   2. Hypotension and tachycardia.
   3. Tachycardia with irregular pulse.
   4. Bradycardia with regular pulse.

2. A 70-year-old male client was on extracorporeal circu-lation (heart–lung machine) for an extended length of time due to intraoperative complications during heart surgery. He is considered at risk for disseminated in-travascular coagulopathy (DIC). Which of the follow-ing lab values would be most critical for the nurse to assess and report to the physician?

   1. Hemoglobin of 13.
   2. Prothrombin time (PT) of 14 seconds.
   3. Partial thromboplastin time (PTT) of 75 seconds.
   4. Fibrinogen level of 85 mg/dL.

3. After 5 days of delirium tremens, the client has no further hallucinations, tremors, diaphoresis, or illu-sions. He seeks permission from the nurse before un-dertaking his own personal care, such as bathing and eating, and he sometimes asks the nurse where the bathroom and dining room are located. These requests indicate that this client

   1. Is ready for discharge, because he is out of bed and ready to do these things for himself.
   2. May be starting to have a recurrence of delirium tremens.
   3. Is somewhat disoriented but functioning very inde-pendently because he is feeding and bathing himself.
   4. Is exhibiting dependency and is somewhat disori-ented.

4. A nursing measure to prevent the complication of deep vein thrombophlebitis following surgery would include

   1. Placing pillows under the affected limb.
   2. Wearing elastic hose at all times.
   3. Having the client sit up TID.
   4. Elevating the foot of the bed.

5. Evaluating the condition of a client who has just re-ceived Lasix, the nurse would observe for which major side effect of the drug?

   1. Dyspnea.
   2. Tachycardia.
   3. Muscular weakness.
   4. Headache.

6. While conducting a cardiac assessment, the two best positions to hear S_2 heart sounds are indicated at _____ (insert numbers).

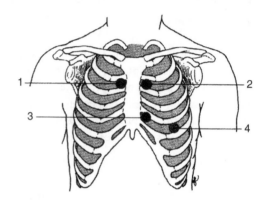

7. Which of the following complications of acute bacter-ial (infective) endocarditis would the nurse constantly observe for in an acutely ill client?

   1. Presence of a heart murmur.
   2. Emboli.
   3. Fever.
   4. Heart failure.

8. While bathing a 1-year-old client, the nurse feels a large mass in the abdominal area and notices that his diaper is soiled with pinkish-tinged urine. The initial nursing action is to

   1. Assess if the tumor has spread to the lymph nodes.
   2. Immediately notify the physician.
   3. Continue the assessment by observing his behavior indicating pain on palpation.
   4. Gently palpate the abdominal mass to determine if it is a Wilms' tumor.

9. Considering the physical developmental period of a 1-year-old child, hospitalization may affect or delay his progression with

1. Crawling.
2. Running.
3. Walking.
4. Sitting.

10. A 21-year-old client was injured in a motorcycle accident yesterday. As a treatment for his fractured right femur, Kirschner wires were inserted and he was placed in balanced suspension traction. The position that will best promote healing is

1. Supine and flat to keep the traction in place.
2. With his right leg flat on the bed to promote the effectiveness of the traction.
3. In semi-Fowler's to prevent the traction from slipping.
4. With his right leg positioned at a 20-degree angle to maintain traction pull.

11. It is the nurse's responsibility to monitor the oxygen level in an incubator of a premature infant. The highest safe level of oxygen the nurse will administer to premature infants is

1. 25 percent.
2. 40 percent.
3. 55 percent.
4. 70 percent.

12. Respiratory acidosis, a serious complication of respiratory distress syndrome (RDS) occurring in infants, occurs as a result of

1. Retention of carbon dioxide due to inadequate ventilation.
2. Retention of oxygen due to inadequate ventilation.
3. Poor exchange of oxygen and carbon dioxide in the lungs.
4. Pulmonary hyperperfusion.

13. The nurse explains to a new mother that the condition of small for gestational age (SGA) is caused by

1. Placental insufficiency.
2. Maternal obesity.
3. Primipara.
4. Genetic predisposition.

14. You are admitting a client for abdominal surgery the next day, and you observe that he appears very anxious. A priority intervention is to

1. Tell him there is nothing to worry about.
2. Suggest that he talk to his doctor.
3. Ask what he expects to happen tomorrow.
4. Ask if he is feeling anxious.

15. A client has had a cystectomy and ureteroileostomy (ileal conduit). The nurse observes this client for complications in the postoperative period. Which of the following symptoms indicates an unexpected outcome and requires priority care?

1. Edema of the stoma.
2. Mucus in the drainage appliance.
3. Redness of the stoma.
4. Feces in the drainage appliance.

16. For a client with a detached retina, the preoperative nursing care plan will include

1. Bathroom privileges with assistance.
2. Turn, cough, and deep-breathe.
3. Keep both eyes bandaged.
4. Turn to the left side only.

17. Calculate the following drug dosage: If you were to give a client one half of a grain ¼ tablet, the client would receive _____ grain(s) of medication.

18. A 48-year-old client admitted with a diagnosis of depression quietly sits by herself, gazing out the window and occasionally crying. Her husband says that her personal neglect is recent and really started after their last child left home for college. This client's personality prior to the illness probably resembled a woman who

1. Had a very organized household and often put her husband's and children's wishes ahead of her own.
2. Kept a neat house and was indecisive most of the time.
3. Was not inclined toward much recreation and who often thought of suicide.
4. Focused her activity exclusively around her children and who lived with an unresolved relationship with her parents.

19. A client took a medication overdose soon after admission to the hospital. She has now been returned from ICU to a room on the psychiatric unit. Upon seeing the nurse who admitted her, the client looks down at the floor and mumbles, "Hello." The nurse's best initial statement is

1. "You have been transferred back to this unit. This is your new room."
2. "Hello. I see that in ICU you've been getting a light diet. How does your stomach feel now?"
3. "I was upset when I found you had tried to kill yourself."
4. "Would you like to talk about what happened?"

20. A female client who is 37 weeks pregnant presents to the labor room with vaginal bleeding and abdominal pain. A tentative diagnosis of abruptio placentae is made. Following a nursing assessment, the priority intervention is to

    1. Immediately call the physician.
    2. Prepare for an emergency cesarean section.
    3. Place the client on bedrest.
    4. Complete a pelvic exam to determine progress of labor.

21. A physician ordered a half-strength nasogastric dilution of the formula. Evaluating that this formula is effective for the client, the client will report that it

    1. Decreases constipation.
    2. Decreases diarrhea.
    3. Increases the pain in his liver.
    4. Makes him feel less bloated.

22. A 20-year-old male client sustained a head injury in an automobile accident. He is admitted to a medical–surgical unit. During the initial assessment, the nurse observes fluid draining from the client's left ear. The nurse will immediately position the client with the head of his bed

    1. Elevated and his head turned to the left.
    2. Flat and his head turned to the right.
    3. Flat and his head turned to the left.
    4. Elevated and his head turned to the right.

23. Monitoring a burned client's fluid replacement, the fluid that is commonly used for the first 24 hours is

    1. 5% dextrose in water.
    2. 5% dextrose in normal saline.
    3. Normal saline.
    4. Ringer's lactate.

24. There are two basic types of respiratory tract injuries associated with burns: smoke inhalation and upper airway injuries. In a client with an upper airway burn, the nurse would expect to assess

    1. Hoarseness and stridor.
    2. Pulmonary parenchymal dysfunction.
    3. Sootlike secretions.
    4. Cherry-red lips.

25. The RN observes the nursing assistant (NA) regulating the IV of an oncology client receiving morphine sulfate for pain. An LVN on the RN's team is responsible for the client and has assigned the client to the NA. The RN's intervention is to

    1. Inform the LVN so that he or she intervenes to instruct the NA that this action is not within the realm of responsibility of an NA.
    2. Immediately inform the charge nurse and fill out an incident report.
    3. Call a staff meeting and confront the LVN and the NA.
    4. Ask the LVN and the NA to meet with the RN to discuss the responsibility parameters each of them has.

26. The complication that the nurse will evaluate for following a transurethral resection (TUR) is

    1. Hemorrhage.
    2. Infection.
    3. Urinary retention.
    4. Adhesions of the neck of the bladder.

27. Instructions given to clients following cataract surgery include the information that

    1. The eye patch will be removed in 3 to 4 days, and the eye may be used without difficulty.
    2. They must use only one eye at a time to prevent double vision.
    3. They will be able to judge distances without difficulty.
    4. Contact lenses will be fitted before discharge from the hospital.

28. Of the following, the nursing intervention most important in the postoperative nursing care for a 2-month-old child with a repair of cleft lip is

    1. Feeding her with a rubber-tipped syringe.
    2. Suctioning the nasopharynx frequently.
    3. Keeping the suture area clean.
    4. Removing elbow restraints frequently.

29. Following abdominal surgery several days ago for removal of a benign tumor, the home care nurse observes that the client's dressing is wet with serosanguineous drainage. After changing the dressing, the nurse learns that the client changed the dressing 4 hours previously and the same drainage was charted. The appropriate conclusion is that

    1. This kind and amount of drainage are to be expected after abdominal surgery.
    2. This amount of drainage is frequently a sign of impending dehiscence.
    3. The serosanguineous drainage means that he is losing too much blood.
    4. The dressing should be changed more frequently than every 4 hours.

30. You are working with an LVN reviewing the latest CPR guidelines from the American Heart Association. You know the LVN is using current information when she tells you to

    1. Retrieve the AED first, before doing anything else.
    2. Give rescue breaths, then do chest compression at a 15:1 ratio.
    3. Institute CPR within 5 minutes to avoid brain damage.
    4. Give 2 rescue breaths, then provide chest compressions at a 30:2 ratio.

31. A 2-year-old child has eaten half a bottle of his grandmother's ferrous sulfate tablets. They live 30 miles from the hospital. The first action is to tell the mother to

    1. Take the child to the hospital immediately.
    2. Give the child syrup of ipecac.
    3. Contact the poison control center by phone.
    4. Do nothing because vitamins are nonpoisonous.

32. The diet regimen usually prescribed for a child with noncomplicated acute glomerulonephritis is a

    1. Low-sodium, high-protein diet.
    2. Regular diet, no added salt.
    3. Low-sodium, low-protein diet.
    4. Low-protein, low-potassium diet.

33. The nurse realizes that the mother does not fully understand the significance of the effect the Rh factor will have on her future pregnancies. The nurse explains that the purpose of administering RhoGAM is to prevent erythroblastosis fetalis in the next pregnancy, which could result in

    1. Hydrops fetalis.
    2. Hypobilirubinemia.
    3. Congenital hypothermia.
    4. Transient clotting difficulties.

34. A male client is admitted to the hospital and is diagnosed with kidney failure. The physician orders hemodialysis treatments. Immediately following hemodialysis, which of the following signs and symptoms would indicate the need to administer Dilantin, a PRN medication?

    1. Decreased blood pressure, rapid pulse.
    2. Nausea, vomiting, twitching.
    3. Pain and tingling at the access site.
    4. Muscle cramps, headache.

35. A client has a Swan–Ganz catheter inserted before undergoing spinal fusion surgery. The nurse will use this catheter to monitor the client's

    1. Intracranial pressure.
    2. Spinal cord perfusion.
    3. Renal function.
    4. Hemodynamic status.

36. Assessing the psychosocial development of a toddler, the nurse is aware that it is characterized by

    1. Imaginary playmates.
    2. Erikson's stage of initiative versus guilt.
    3. Demonstrations of sexual curiosity.
    4. Extreme negative behavior resulting from the child's assertion of autonomy.

37. The significance of hearing the S_3 heart sound ("Ken-tuc-ky") at the apex of the heart is

    1. Cardiac disease.
    2. Cardiac decompensation.
    3. Closure of the aortic valve.
    4. Closure of pulmonic valve.

38. A female client is admitted to the therapeutic community with a diagnosis of conversion disorder with symptoms of aphasia. The nurse understands which of the following statements is true about conversion disorder?

    1. Conversion disorders are consciously triggered.
    2. A high level of anxiety underlies the symptom of aphasia.
    3. The client's aphasia is always symbolic of a basic problem.
    4. The client will exhibit increased affect proportionate to the severity of her symptoms.

39. A young man who accidentally came in contact with a high-tension electrical wire has a small injury on his right hand and on his left calf. When his family arrives at the hospital, they are understandably distraught and want to know exactly how he is and what will happen to him. The most therapeutic response is to say,

    1. "He is doing well, although he may be in the hospital for some time."
    2. "He has received an electrical burn. His condition is stable, and we will keep you informed of any change."
    3. "He has received an electrical burn, which caused coagulation of some tissues."
    4. "He does not appear to have much damage and should be fine soon."

40. A client who has a subclavian central venous catheter (CVC) develops acute shortness of breath. The nurse finds that the CVC has become disconnected from the IV tubing. The initial nursing action should be to

1. Cap all ports on the CVC and closely monitor the client.
2. Position the client in Trendelenburg position on the left side.
3. Call the physician and request an order for oxygen.
4. Place the client in high-Fowler's position, leaning on the overbed table.

41. A 58-year-old female client is in the hospital for the second time, diagnosed with myxedema. Considering the diagnosis, the initial assessment should reveal symptoms that include

1. Bradycardia, heart failure, weight loss, diarrhea.
2. Lethargy, weight gain, slow speech, decreased respiratory rate.
3. Tachycardia, constipation, exophthalmos.
4. Hypothermia, weight loss, increased respiratory rate.

42. The RN observes two team members putting the bedclothes they have taken off a client's bed on the floor. The appropriate intervention is to

1. Bring them a clothes basket and tell them to use it next time.
2. Explain the principles of medical asepsis to both team members.
3. Tell them this is unacceptable and the RN will counsel both of them later.
4. Do nothing because the bedclothes are on their way to the laundry to be disinfected.

43. The nurse is assigned to work on a unit that has a group of autistic children as inpatients. They have all been on the unit for at least 6 months and exhibit self-destructive and withdrawn behavior as well as bizarre responses. As a new member of the health team, the nurse knows that the first goal is to

1. Set limits on their behavior so the children will perceive the nurse as an authority figure.
2. Assess each child's individual developmental level so the nurse will have the data for realistic care plans.
3. Understand that the children must be protected from self-destructive behavior.
4. Establish some method of relating to the children, either verbal or nonverbal.

44. A client is admitted to the surgical unit for a scheduled above-the-knee amputation with a delayed prosthesis fitting. Preoperatively, the nurse can best assist the client by instructing him to do

1. Sit-up exercises.
2. Upper body strengthening exercises.

3. Strengthening exercises with his other leg.
4. No exercises until the postoperative period.

45. The results from a client's fasting blood glucose (FBG) are being evaluated. The nurse understands that to make the diagnosis of diabetes mellitus, the results of at least two separate FBG tests would need to be over

1. 100 mg/dL.
2. 125 mg/dL.
3. 140 mg/dL.
4. 180 mg/dL.

46. Following delivery of a healthy baby, the nurse completes a postpartum assessment of the new mother. Which of the following symptoms would be indicative of a full bladder?

1. Increased uterine contractions.
2. Decreased lochia.
3. Fundus 2F above umbilicus.
4. Pulse 52 beats/min.

47. A 22-month-old child has just been admitted to the pediatric unit for a fractured right femur. Observing Bryant's traction to determine if it is properly assembled, the nurse will expect to see the

1. Moleskin taut and placed on either side of the lower leg to provide traction.
2. Weights attached to a pin that is inserted in the femur.
3. Pin site and weights aligned in a horizontal position.
4. Weights attached to skin traction and hung freely from the crib.

48. A client involved in a knifing was admitted through the emergency room and is now in the ICU. His admission assessment reveals shallow and rapid respirations, paradoxical pulse, CVP 15 cm H_2O, BP 90 mm Hg systolic, skin cold and pale, urinary output 70 mL over the last 2 hours. From these findings, the nurse concludes that he may be developing

1. Hypovolemic shock.
2. Cardiac tamponade.
3. Sepsis.
4. Atelectasis.

49. A client, Mr. Erikson, has IV orders for 3 bags of 1000 mL for the next 24 hours.
Bag 1: 1000 mL D5%/0.45 NS with 1 amp Solu B with C
Bag 2: 1000 mL D5%/0.45 NS
Bag 3: 1000 mL D5%/0.45 NS with 30 mEq KCl

You set the controller to deliver _____ drops/minute if the administration set delivers 15 gtts/mL.

50. A 35-year-old client is 36 weeks pregnant and has been admitted to the obstetrical unit for continuous close observation. She confides to the nurse that she doesn't think she will ever be a mother and begins to cry. The best nursing response is to

   1. Reassure her that advanced medical knowledge will detect any problems that may be present with this pregnancy.
   2. Sit quietly with her and follow her cues.
   3. Suggest that she discuss her fears with her physician.
   4. Gently change the subject to something more positive.

51. A client, 36 weeks pregnant, is induced with oxytocin (Pitocin). One of the most important observations is the duration of the resting phase between the end of one contraction and the beginning of the next. The nurse knows that a resting phase should not be less than

   1. 15 seconds.
   2. 30 seconds.
   3. 45 seconds.
   4. 60 seconds.

52. A client has been admitted to the hospital with symptoms of weakness, weight loss, and anorexia. The provisional diagnosis is cancer of the colon. The nurse observes that the client has remained very quiet. The nurse understands that her actions are probably due to

   1. Trying to be a good client.
   2. Denying the situation.
   3. Shyness and fear of asking questions.
   4. Feeling anger toward the hospital staff.

53. A client with a Sengstaken–Blakemore tube begins to wheeze and cough and becomes dusky in color. The immediate nursing action is to

   1. Deflate the esophageal balloon.
   2. Check the pressure in the gastric balloon.
   3. Irrigate the stomach with iced saline.
   4. Start low-flow oxygen by nasal cannula.

54. A 16-year-old client is hospitalized for adolescent adjustment problems. After assessing her, the nurse's first objective is to establish a nurse–client relationship. The next day, the nurse is late for the appointment. Knowing that the client has difficulty assuming responsibility for her own behavior, the nurse would like to use this situation as an opportunity for role

modeling. The most appropriate statement the nurse could make is

   1. "I'm late. I apologize."
   2. "Thank goodness you are still here; I just had a flat tire."
   3. "Oh, you are here. I thought we'd be arriving at the same time."
   4. "What do you mean you are angry with me? I bet you keep people waiting."

55. The nurse is assigned to do a home visit for a new mother 1 week postpartum. In the assessment, leg edema and a slight fever are noted. Aside from advising her to see the physician immediately, the nurse would tell her that she should *not*

   1. Elevate the leg.
   2. Apply warmth to the leg.
   3. Decrease leg movement.
   4. Gently massage the painful area of the leg.

56. The nurse is caring for a client who is 1 day postop for an open thoracotomy. This client has a benign neoplasm of the left lung. The client is receiving oxygen mist at 40 percent. The O_2 saturation measured by pulse oximiter was 83. ABG results are: pH 7.31, PO_2 93 mm Hg, PCO_2 50 mm Hg, HCO_3 25 mEq/L. Which of the following nursing actions would be a priority for this client?

   1. Switch to O_2 with a rebreathing bag.
   2. Increase O_2 to 70 percent.
   3. Position the client in high-Fowler's, and encourage use of incentive spirometer and coughing.
   4. Place the client in the prone position and have the respiratory therapist do postural drainage.

57. At morning report in the step-down unit, the nurse receives the following client assignments and information. The following four questions refer to this information. Client A, 80 years old, Type 2 diabetic, two days postop, is complaining of pain at his mid-line incision site and asking for ordered pain medication. Client B, a 65-year-old client with a fever, was admitted last night to rule out pneumonia. Client B slept poorly due to frequent bouts of coughing, which produced blood-streaked sputum. Client C is 90 years old, has COPD and is short of breath. His O_2 stats = 83 percent on 2 L of oxygen. He is a CO_2 retainer and his status is DNR. Client D, 55 years old, is scheduled for an arteriogram this morning. The cath lab has just called to notify you that she is next on the schedule. In which order will the nurse complete initial assessments and/or provide appropriate care?

1. Client D, C, B and A.
2. Client A, B, C and D.
3. Client C, D, A and B.
4. Client B, D, A and C.

58. Client D needs to be prepared and premedicated for an arteriogram. Which one of the following activities would *not* be part of the pretest procedure?

1. Remove undergarments, jewelry and wig.
2. Give soap suds enema and shave insertion site.
3. Remove dentures and partials, hearing aids and other prostheses.
4. Have her void, check for a signed consent form and give ordered "on call" medications.

59. As the nurse assesses client C, the nurse recognizes that his SOB is increasing. The nurse would do which of the following before notifying his physician of his current status and to obtain orders?

1. Check his chart for O_2 stats, breathing treatments, and ABG results within the last 24 hours.
2. Put him in high-Fowler's position and increase his oxygen to 6 L.
3. Change his diet to low carbohydrate, high fat and protein, and force fluids.
4. Check his intake and output for the past 24 hours and prepare to start TPN in anticipation of an order.

60. Client C's situation worsens. The supervisor sends a CNA to assist the nurse. Which of the following clients and procedures would the nurse assign the CNA to do?

1. Carry out pretest procedures and go to the cath lab with client D.
2. Vital signs and AM care for client A and client B.
3. Posttest care for client D.
4. None of the above. These clients are too sick for a CNA to provide care.

61. Following a cystoscopy, it was determined that a client with benign prostatic hypertrophy would be admitted for a transurethral resection (TUR). Preoperative nursing care includes   .

1. Discussing the surgical intervention and the fact that it causes impotence.
2. Decreasing fluid intake for at least 2 days to prevent bladder irritability.
3. Keeping the client NPO for at least 18 hours to prevent bowel evacuation during the surgical procedure.
4. Discussing hygienic care of the penis before surgery.

62. An elderly female client with newly diagnosed osteoporosis requires counseling prior to discharge. The most important component of the discharge plan is

1. Instruction in safety factors to prevent injury.
2. Monitoring medications.
3. Instruction in regular exercise and diet.
4. Appropriate use of body mechanics.

63. A client with an obstruction just proximal to her old ileostomy stoma is admitted to the hospital. She has had the ileostomy for 6 months. Which one of the following conditions is considered a major complication and should be anticipated in the client's care plan?

1. Infection.
2. Diarrhea.
3. Fluid and electrolyte imbalance.
4. Constipation.

64. A dietary goal for a client postsurgery is to support tissue repair. The nurse will know the client understands dietary principles to achieve this goal when she increases her intake of

1. Fats.
2. Carbohydrates.
3. Incomplete proteins.
4. Glucose.

65. A young male, age 11 months, has been a robust, thriving boy. Recently, his appetite has been poor, and he has vomited frequently. He is admitted to the unit after his parents brought him to the hospital following an episode when he suddenly shrieked loudly, pulled his knees to his chest, and seemed to be in acute pain. The nurse should assess for

1. Poisoning.
2. Presence of parasites.
3. Acute appendicitis.
4. Intussusception.

66. A 72-year-old client diagnosed with Ménière's disease has been admitted to the medical–surgical unit. He asks the nurse if he can get up and go to the bathroom any time he needs to. The most appropriate response is

1. "Yes, whenever you wish, you may go."
2. "No, you are on strict bedrest."
3. "Please ring for assistance when you wish to get out of bed."
4. "We will have to check with the physician."

67. A client is admitted with the diagnosis of glomerulonephritis. He was initially treated with dietary fluid

and electrolyte restrictions, but now has recurrent hypertension and edema. Analyzing the client's lab results in relationship to his disease process, the nurse would expect to find increased

1. Serum sodium.
2. Red blood cells.
3. BUN.
4. White blood cells.

68. For a client with severe cirrhosis, the physician orders lactulose 30 mL via nasogastric tube. After administering the lactulose, the nurse will assess for an increase in

1. Constipation.
2. Diarrhea.
3. Nausea.
4. Urine output.

69. A client with cirrhosis has blood test results returned that indicate a prothrombin time of 30 seconds. The nurse would expect the physician to order

1. Vitamin K.
2. Heparin.
3. Coumadin.
4. Ferrous sulfate.

70. A client with cirrhosis has ascites that has diminished, but he complains that he cannot sleep well and asks the nurse for a sedative. The best nursing response is to say

1. "Sedatives are processed in the liver and, because your liver is affected by your condition, they would be dangerous to take."
2. "I'll notify your physician."
3. "Sedatives are contraindicated because they could depress your respirations."
4. "I'll see what I can do to get you a medication to help you sleep."

71. When a client with severely decreased liver function due to cirrhosis selects a snack, the choice that indicates he understands his dietary requirements is a

1. Peanut butter sandwich.
2. Banana.
3. Hard-boiled egg.
4. Portion of cheese and crackers.

72. You are measuring and monitoring central venous pressure (CVP). From the diagram below, you will observe the meniscus at which number? _____.

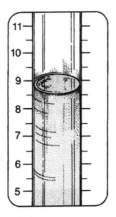

73. A 56-year-old male client is in the ICU and is being prepared to have a CVP inserted. As the physician attaches IV tubing to the hub of the needle, the nurse instructs the client to perform the Valsalva maneuver. The purpose of this procedure is to

1. Avoid infiltration of the vein.
2. Alleviate pain during the procedure.
3. Prevent an air embolism from occurring.
4. Assist with catheter advancement.

74. The nurse is monitoring the client when there is a sudden change in the CVP reading. The first nursing action is to

1. Check whether the client's position has changed.
2. Take the client's vital signs.
3. Have the client do the Valsalva maneuver.
4. Call the physician immediately.

75. A 69-year-old retired client has gouty arthritis and his physician has ordered a medication protocol of colchicine and steroids. During an acute attack, the client will be taking colchicine

1. Until the steroids reach a therapeutic level to reduce the inflammation.
2. For 12 hours until he is switched to allopurinol.
3. Every hour until pain subsides or he experiences nausea, vomiting, or diarrhea.
4. Every hour for 24 hours.

COMPREHENSIVE TEST 2

Answers with Rationale

1. (3) Ritodrine acts on type II beta-adrenergic receptors, resulting in uterine muscle relaxation. Cardiovascular complications can occur; therefore, the client should be closely assessed for signs of tachycardia and an irregular pulse. The fetus may also have a period of tachycardia, so frequent FHTs are important.

   NP:I; CN:PH; CA:M; CL:A

2. (4) The normal fibrinogen level for males is 180–340 mg/dL. Any level below 100 mg/dL is considered critical. In DIC, the fibrinogen level is used up during the blood clotting process. Therefore, a level of 85 mg/dL would concern the nurse and must be reported to the physician.

   NP:A; CN:PH; CA:S; CL:AN

3. (4) Seeking permission for simple tasks indicates dependent functioning. Forgetting where things are indicates persisting confusion, disorientation, and need for structure. He is obviously not ready for discharge (1), nor is he functioning independently (3).

   NP:AN; CN:PS; CA:P; CL:AN

4. (4) Elevation of the legs promotes circulation and prevents venous stasis and more clot formation. Nursing measures aim at preventing further thrombi from forming and the already present thrombus from detaching. Elastic hose (2) are necessary when the client is up walking again. Placing a pillow under the limb (1) could cause a bend at the groin, with resulting decreased circulation. The client must be kept on bedrest until the danger of emboli passes (4 to 7 days).

   NP:P; CN:PH; CA:S; CL:A

5. (3) Lasix promotes diuresis by preventing sodium and chloride reabsorption in the kidney tubules. Potassium and water loss occurs as well. The potassium loss could cause muscle weakness. Only if there were an excessive water loss would the client become

tachycardic (2) and have a headache (4). Dyspnea (1) is not associated with the use of Lasix.

   NP:A; CN:PH; CA:M; CL:A

6. The answer is 1 and 2. S_2 sounds are heard best over the aortic and pulmonic areas.

   NP:A; CN:PH; CA:M; CL:A

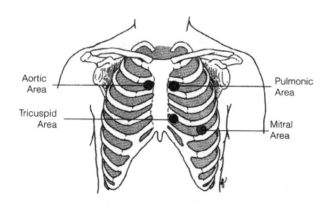

7. (2) While all of the symptoms may be present, the characteristic problem with this condition is that of emboli. If emboli arise in the right heart chambers, they will terminate in the lungs; left chamber emboli may travel anywhere in the arterial tree.

   NP:A; CN:PH; CA:M; CL:A

8. (2) The physician should be notified immediately. A suspected Wilms' tumor should never be palpated more than necessary because of the potential for metastasis and should be treated immediately following discovery. It is really not a nursing responsibility to assess for lymph node enlargement.

   NP:I; CN:PH; CA:P; CL:A

9. (3) At 12 months, the child should be starting to walk. A hospitalization at this time could delay this

---

Coding for Questions/Answers Abbreviations: **Nursing Process: NP,** Assessment: A, Analysis: AN, Planning: P, Implementation: I, Evaluation: E; **Client Needs: CN,** Safe, Effective Care Environment: S, Health Promotion and Maintenance: H, Psychosocial Integrity: PS, Physiological Integrity: PH; **Clinical Area: CA,** Medical Nursing: M, Surgical Nursing: S, Maternal/Newborn Nursing: MA, Pediatric Nursing: P, Psychiatric Nursing: PS; **Cognitive Level: CL,** Knowledge: K, Comprehension: C, Application: A, Analysis: AN.

developmental stage. The child should sit (4) by 6 months and should already be crawling (1) by 1 year of age.

NP:P; CN:S; CA:P; CL:C

10. (4) The affected leg should always be kept at an angle of at least 20 degrees from the bed. Weights are never lifted up; this action could undo all of the reduction that has already occurred.

NP:P; CN:PH; CA:S; CL:C

11. (2) Oxygen concentrations above 40 percent may cause damage to the retinas, which later may lead to severe sight limitation or blindness. Oxygen levels must be monitored carefully and the infant should not receive a higher concentration than necessary.

NP:P; CN:H; CA:M; CL:A

12. (1) Respiratory acidosis is specifically due to retention of carbon dioxide. This is a result of inadequate pulmonary ventilation caused by atelectasis, which results when the hyaline membrane develops in the bronchial tree.

NP:AN; CN:H; CA:MA; CL:C

13. (1) Placental insufficiency is a primary cause of SGA. It may result from an embryonic placental deficiency, hypertension, maternal smoking, maternal malnutrition, aging, and other associated causes.

NP:I; CN:H; CA:MA; CL:C

14. (3) Determining what the client knows about the surgical procedure and expects to happen will give you data about how to intervene. Fear of the unknown increases anxiety and stress. The first two interventions will close off communication, and answer (4) is too direct and may result in a negative response.

NP:I; CN:PS; CA:PS; CL:A

15. (4) The ileal conduit procedure incorporates implantation of the ureters into a portion of the ileum that has been resected from its anatomical position and now functions as a reservoir or conduit for urine. The proximal and distal ileal borders can be resumed. Feces should not be draining from the conduit. Edema (1) and a red color of the stoma (3) are expected outcomes in the immediate postoperative period, as is mucus from the stoma (2).

NP:A; CN:PH; CA:S; CL:AN

16. (3) Both eyes are bandaged to prevent movement in either eye. When one eye moves, the other eye follows. By preventing movement, the extension of com-

plications can be prevented. Positioning of clients is usually done with the area of detachment in a dependent position. Deep-breathing is done, but coughing increases intraocular pressure and should be discouraged or prevented by use of antitussives.

NP:P; CN:PH; CA:S; CL:C

17. The answer is ⅛ grain. Half of a grain ¼ tablet would be ⅛ of a grain; that is the amount you would give the client.

NP:I; CN:S; CA:M; CL:A

18. (1) Persons predisposed to middle-age depression tend to have been rigid and self-sacrificing and spent their personal time meeting other people's needs. When there is no longer a focus for their self-sacrifice, depression may ensue. They probably did not have a long history of depression or suicidal thoughts (3).

NP:AN; CN:PS; CA:PS; CL:C

19. (4) Caring is conveyed through acknowledgment. Asking the client if she would like to talk allows her the choice of whether to discuss the suicide attempt at this time. Revealing personal feelings (3) is inappropriate, and ignoring the attempt (1, 2) will close off communication.

NP:I; CN:PS; CA:PS; CL:A

20. (3) The priority intervention is to place the client on bedrest and assess for signs of shock. The physician should be notified (1) after the client is positioned. Depending on the severity of the condition, a cesarean section (2) may be imminent. Pelvic exams (4) are to be avoided to prevent additional bleeding.

NP:I; CN:H; CA:MA; CL:A

21. (2) Diarrhea is a common side effect of NG formula infusion due to the high-protein composition. Diluting the formula will decrease the diarrhea. The other answers are not side effects of diluting the formula.

NP:E; CN:PH; CA:M; CL:A

22. (1) It is important to decrease intracranial pressure (head of bed elevated) and to allow for drainage (head turned to left). All of the other responses are incorrect because the position would not facilitate cerebral drainage or ear drainage.

NP:I; CN:PH; CA:M; CL:AN

23. (4) Ringer's lactate is the fluid replacement of choice. Five percent dextrose solutions (1, 2) are not given in the first 24 hours because a stress-induced pseudo-

diabetes often occurs after major burns. Administration of more dextrose would increase the possibility of hyperosmolar disease. Many physicians do not order colloids to be given in the first 24 hours because the burn causes generalized increased capillary permeability. The colloids leak out of the burn area into areas such as the pulmonary interstitial spaces and may cause pulmonary edema.

NP:P; CN:PH; CA:M; CL:K

24. (1)　Upper airway burns (to the head, neck or chest) cause local edema, which may produce mechanical occlusion of the airway manifested by hoarseness and stridor. Smoke inhalation can cause parenchymal changes from superheated gases and/or toxic chemicals. The parenchyma (2) is generally unaffected in upper airway burns.

NP:A; CN:PH; CA:M; CL:C

25. (4)　While regulating or even touching an IV is definitely not within the scope of behaviors that an NA can legally perform (1), both teaching and clarification of duties are needed in this situation. Before accusing the NA, a nonpunitive environment should be created so teaching of both the LVN and the NA can occur, and this action will not happen again. Unless too much medication was given, an incident report does not need to be filled out (2). Confronting the team members in a staff meeting (3) would not be following good management principles.

NP:I; CN:S; CA:M; CL:AN

26. (1)　Hemorrhage is the major early complication due to the manipulation by the instrument in resecting away the prostatic tissue. The use of continuous drainage assists in preventing hemorrhage. Observation of the type of drainage facilitates early detection of excessive bleeding.

NP:E; CN:PH; CA:S; CL:A

27. (2)　The function of the lens is that of accommodation, the focusing of near objects on the retina by the lens; therefore, only the remaining lens will function in this capacity, depending on whether a cataract is present.

NP:P; CN:PH; CA:S; CL:A

28. (3)　The suture area must be kept clean to prevent infection. Strain on the sutures must always be prevented by using a Logan bar. The infant will be fed with a rubber-tipped medicine dropper on the unoperated side. Elbow restraints (4) will be used with supervised rest periods to protect the suture area.

NP:P; CN:PH; CA:S; CL:A

29. (2)　After 7 days, the sutures have probably been removed. The presence of serosanguineous wound drainage lasting a few hours to several days is nearly always a sign of impending dehiscence.

NP:E, CN:PH; CA:S; CL:A

30. (4)　The current guidelines suggest administering compressions "hard and fast," at a rate of about 100 per minute, with a 30:2 ratio. The first action is to check responsiveness and get help, then get the AED (1). You must start CPR within 3 minutes, because brain damage could occur after 4 minutes (3).

NP:AN; CN:PH; CA:M; CL:C

31. (3)　Contact either the poison control center or the emergency department at a local hospital. The child will most likely be given water to dilute the ferrous sulfate tablets and activated charcoal. Syrup of ipecac is not currently given to induce vomiting.

NP:I; CN:PH; CA:P; CL:C

32. (2)　A regular diet with moderate sodium is suggested for children who are in acute glomerulonephritis. If the client's condition progresses to renal failure, sodium, potassium, and protein are restricted.

NP:P; CN:PH; CA:P; CL:K

33. (1)　Hydrops fetalis occurs when large quantities of the Rh-positive antibodies attach to the fetal hemoglobin and massive hemolysis results. If the infant is delivered alive, it will require an exchange transfusion.

NP:I; CN:H; CA:MA; CL:C

34. (2)　Nausea, vomiting, and twitching are indicative of disequilibrium syndrome. They occur as a result of the rapid shift of fluids, pH, and osmolarity between fluid and blood that occurs during the dialysis treatment. In addition, it is thought that a rapid decrease in BUN levels during hemodialysis causes cerebral edema, which leads to increased intracranial pressure.

NP:E; CN:PH; CA:M; CL:AN

35. (4)　A Swan–Ganz catheter is inserted into the pulmonary artery to closely monitor a client's cardiovascular function and hydration status. It is commonly used for monitoring clients during and following major surgery, as well as for clients who are critically ill.

NP:P; CN:PH; CA:S; CL:C

36. (4)　Assertion of automony is seen in 2- to 2½-year-old toddlers as they begin their language and social development. The stage of initiative versus guilt (2) is

more common in the preschool-age child, 3 to 6 years. At 3 to 4 years of age, children have imaginary playmates (1).

NP:AN; CN:H; CA:P; CL:C

37. (2) When the S₃ heart sound is heard at the apex of the heart, it signifies cardiac decompensation. Hearing the S₃ heart sound at the upper left sternal border is indicative of cardiac disease. This sound does not signify closure of the aortic or pulmonic valve.

NP:AN; CN:S; CA:M; CL:C

38. (2) Conversion disorder symptoms are unconsciously triggered by the client as a way of dealing with high levels of anxiety. The client's aphasia may be (but is not always) symbolic of a basic problem (3). The level of affect the client displays (4) is not relevant to this disorder.

NP:AN; CN:PS; CA:PS; CL:K

39. (2) The family needs to be given honest information in words they can understand. Above all, they need to know the nurse is aware of them and will keep them in mind. Answer (1) gives conflicting messages. Answer (3) may also be true but it is very clinical and will frighten the family more than necessary. Answer (4) is a statement made without sufficient knowledge.

NP:I; CN:PS; CA:PS; CL:C

40. (2) Analysis of the data suggests that the client may be experiencing an air embolism. Positioning on the left side with the head down may help keep the air in the right atrium, where it can be absorbed, rather than going into the pulmonary or systemic circulation, where it could produce fatal results.

NP:I; CN:PH; CA:M; CL:AN

41. (2) Myxedema, or hypothyroidism, is caused by a decrease in thyroid hormone production. Symptoms are related to a generalized decrease in the metabolic rate. Hypothermia and constipation are associated with a decreased metabolic rate. Bradycardia, constipation, and cold intolerance are additional symptoms associated with myxedema.

NP:A; CN:PH; CA:M; CL:C

42. (2) To change behavior, there must be an understanding of the need or reason to change. Assuming that the team members do not fully understand the underlying principles of asepsis and germ transmission would be the first approach. Teaching how important it would be not to contaminate other surfaces or to keep transmission of contaminants to a mini-

mum by placing the bedsheets in a closed basket for delivery to the laundry would be safe nursing practice. This is also an example of good management principles, unlike answers (1), (3), and (4).

NP:I; CN:H; CA:M; CL:A

43. (4) Before the nurse can implement any care plan that might include setting limits or integrating the child into the group, the nurse would need to establish a relationship, through either verbal or nonverbal communication. After establishing a relationship, the nurse will assess each child.

NP:P; CN:H; CA:PS; CL:C

44. (2) In this instance, it would be most beneficial to strengthen the client's arm muscles to help him when walking with the crutches.

NP:I; CN:PH; CA:S; CL:C

45. (3) The normal FBG can range from 70 to 115 mg/dL in an adult. Elevations above 125 mg/dL (obtained on two separate occasions) are considered diagnostic for diabetes, as per criteria established currently by the American Diabetes Association.

NP:AN; CN:PH; CA:M; CL:K

46. (3) If the bladder is full, it will push the uterus up out of the pelvis above the umbilicus. The uterus will not contract sufficiently, which could lead to increased bleeding.

NP:AN; CN:H; CA:MA; CL:C

47. (4) Bryant's traction is a form of skin traction and, therefore, does not require a pin insertion. Moleskin is frequently used as the stabilizing material for traction application. The child's hips are flexed at a 90-degree angle with the legs suspended by pulleys and weights. The weights must hang freely from the crib to maintain alignment and decrease the fracture. This type of traction is used for children under the age of 2.

NP:E; CN:PH; CA:S; CL:A

48. (2) All of the client's signs and symptoms are found in both cardiac tamponade and hypovolemic shock except the urinary output and CVP. In shock, urinary output decreases to less than 30 mL/hr, and the CVP would be below 5 cm H₂O pressure; thus these symptoms would distinguish hypovolemic shock from cardiac tamponade. The client would be likely to also exhibit tachycardia, hypertension, and restlessness.

NP:AN; CN:PH; CA:M; CL:AN

49. The answer is *32 gtts/minute*. Calculate 2 steps for the answer.

1.
$$\frac{\text{Total solution}}{\text{Number of hours to run}} = \text{mL/hr}$$

$$\frac{1000 \text{ mL}}{8 \text{ hours}} = 125 \text{ mL/hr}$$

2.
$$\frac{\text{mL/hr} \times \text{drop factor}}{60 \text{ minutes}} = \text{gtts/min}$$

$$\frac{125 \text{ mL/hr} \times 15 \text{ gtts/mL}}{60 \text{ minutes}} = 32 \text{ gtts/min}$$

NP:I; CN:S; CA:M; CL:A

50. (2) The client has indicated a need to talk and explore her feelings. Sitting with her and following her cues is the most therapeutic response. This action will assist in developing a relationship.

NP:I; CN:H; CA:M; CL:C

51. (2) A prolonged uterine contraction of more than 90 seconds or a resting phase of less than 30 seconds is dangerous, and the safety intervention is to turn off the Pitocin drip. Sixty seconds is an acceptable resting phase between contractions.

NP:A; CN:H; CA:MA; CL:C

52. (2) Denial is a normal reaction when a client is suddenly faced with a life-threatening illness. Anger (4) may occur later. The nurse should determine if she is shy and afraid to ask questions (3), as this can happen.

NP:AN; CN:PS; CA:PS; CL:C

53. (1) The client is manifesting airway obstruction, which may be caused by the upward displacement of the Sengstaken–Blakemore tube. The priority intervention is to maintain a patent airway. Deflating the esophageal balloon will relieve the airway obstruction.

NP:I; CN:PH; CA:M; CL:A

54. (1) Assuming responsibility for one's behavior includes acknowledging the behavior and may include a statement of one's current status. It does not include making excuses (2), focusing outside of oneself (3), or blaming another (4).

NP:I; CN:PS; CA:PS; CL:A

55. (4) The client has all the signs of thrombophlebitis. To massage the area might cause a blood clot to become dislodged. The other actions would be included in the treatment plan.

NP:I; CN:PH; CA:M; CL:C

56. (3) The client has respiratory acidosis from decreased ventilation. A rebreathing bag (1) is used for respiratory alkalosis. Increasing the O_2 (2) is not necessary because the O_2 level is within normal limits. Positioning the client to improve gas exchange by deep-breathing, coughing, and removal of secretions may resolve the problem. Placing the client in prone position (4) is not beneficial.

NP:I; CN:PH; CA:S; CL:AN

57. (3) The correct order of intervention is this: Client C can be repositioned in mid-Fowler's and helped to breathe more slowly and exhale using the pursed lip method. These comfort measures take very little time and will probably reduce his anxiety. Client D must be premedicated for her arteriogram, so that the cath lab schedule will not be delayed. The incision site of client A should be checked next for signs of evisceration or infection and his position changed to determine if that is sufficient to ease his pain. If not, he should receive the medication according to the doctor's orders. Client B's vital signs should be taken next and her current sputum characteristics noted.

NP:P; CN:S; CA:M; CL:AN

58. (2) There is no reason to give an enema and the insertion site will be shaved in the cath lab. All the other activities are appropriate.

NP:P; CN:PH; CA:M; CL:A

59. (1) The first step in providing care for clients is assessment. The other three answers are inappropriate for this COPD client.

NP:I; CN:PH; CA:M; CL:AN

60. (2) CNAs are trained to provide hygiene and comfort measures for clients.

NP:P; CN:S; CA:M; CL:AN

61. (4) Usually a shower with detergent soap is taken the night before and morning of surgery. Particular attention should be paid to cleansing around the glans to rid it of microorganisms. An increased fluid intake and a good diet are essential to prevent urinary tract infections postop. Clients are not necessarily impotent following surgery.

NP:P; CN:PH; CA:S; CL:A

62. (3) Because this is a new diagnosis, regular exercise (especially weight bearing) and a diet high in protein, calcium, and vitamin D with avoidance of alcohol and coffee are the most important components of the plan to prevent extension of the condition.

NP:P; CN:S; CA:M; CL:A

63. (3) Due to the extreme loss of fluids from the high colon interruption, fluid and electrolyte imbalance is the most common complication. The lower colon reabsorbs a major portion of the fluid, whereas the upper colon does not have this function. A great potassium loss also occurs, as it is found in large amounts in the upper colon. The other answers are not expected complications.

NP:E; CN:PH; CA:S; CL:C

64. (2) Carbohydrates are protein-sparing food sources. When present, they provide for energy and allow the proteins to be used for tissue repair. The diet should also include adequate protein, not incomplete protein.

NP:E; CN:PH; CA:S; CL:A

65. (4) The client's behavior, especially indications of acute pain, is typical of a child with intussusception. Other signs may be vomiting and bloody mucus in the stool. Appendicitis would evidence pain in the right lower quadrant of the abdomen. Neither poisoning nor parasites would present with this symptom pattern.

NP:AN; CN:PH; CA:P; CL:A

66. (3) The client may be on bedrest (although not strict) due to the extreme vertigo he may experience. Because of the dizziness, he should ring for assistance if he does wish to get up to go to the bathroom. This is a safety intervention to prevent the client from falling.

NP:I; CN:S; CA:M; CL:A

67. (3) The potassium and BUN are increased due to the kidney's decreased ability to secrete these materials. Red blood cells are decreased due to the decreased production of erythropoietin, the factor that stimulates production of erythrocytes. Sodium is restricted but if diuresis is great, sodium replacement may be required.

NP:AN; CN:PH; CA:M; CL:AN

68. (2) Lactulose is a synthetic disaccharide that the small intestine cannot utilize. It causes diarrhea by lowering the pH so that the bacterial flora are changed in the bowel. The bacteria responsible for producing ammonia by acting on proteins are absent, so the ammonia level decreases.

NP:E; CN:PH; CA:M; CL:A

69. (1) A prothrombin time of 30 seconds indicates the clotting time is prolonged and bleeding could occur. The normal prothrombin time is 12 to 15 seconds. A vitamin K injection will increase the synthesis of prothrombin by the liver.

NP:P; CN:PH; CA:M; CL:C

70. (1) While answer (3) is true, the best response is (1), giving him the facts. Sedatives are metabolized by the liver. The client cannot tolerate these drugs because of his defective hepatic function. He would have very high levels of the drug in his blood for a prolonged period of time. Other options, such as relaxation techniques, are important to try before resorting to drugs.

NP:I; CN:PH; CA:M; CL:AN

71. (2) Carbohydrates are one of the mainstays of the cirrhotic client's diet. The liver can metabolize only very small amounts of protein, so usually only 50 grams of protein is allowed per day (normal diet is 80 grams per day). All of the other choices contain protein.

NP:E; CN:PH; CA:M; CL:C

72. The number you will read at the meniscus is *8.5*, because the CVP reading is at the base of the meniscus and at the end of expiration (on highest fluctuation).

NP:I; CN:H; CA:M; CL:A

73. (3) The rationale for a Valsalva procedure is to prevent air from entering the catheter, thus reducing the risk of an air embolism. None of the other answers is accurate.

NP:AN; CN:PH; CA:M; CL:K

74. (1) If the client's position has recently changed, it could alter the CVP reading. The first nursing action is to check for this and repeat the reading. Depending on the source of the reading change, the nurse would then notify the physician.

NP:I; CN:PH; CA:M; CL:A

75. (3) Colchicine is an antigout medication with parasympathetic-stimulating properties. It is given until these side effects occur, the pain subsides, 8 to 10 doses maximum have been given, or therapeutic blood levels have been reached. Allopurinol is usually started following colchicine.

NP:P; CN:PH; CA:M; CL:C

COMPREHENSIVE TEST 3 QUESTIONS

1. A 56-year-old male client is admitted to the coronary care unit. The diagnosis is myocardial infarction. The client is placed on a cardiac monitor and an IV of D_5W is infusing at a "keep open" rate. The nurse's priority concern is to assess for

   1. Apical pulse rate.
   2. Chest pain.
   3. Respiratory rate.
   4. Blood pressure increase.

2. The physician orders laboratory tests for a client with a suspected myocardial infarction. The lab finding that would indicate that there has been myocardial damage is a(n)

   1. Elevated CK-MB.
   2. Decreased CK and SGOT.
   3. Elevated total CK and elevated SGOT.
   4. Elevated SGOT and LDH.

3. A physician orders 2 mg per minute of lidocaine for a client. Using 500 mL D_5W and 2 g lidocaine, the nurse will administer _____ milliliters per minute.

4. A low-sodium diet is ordered for a client. The nurse will know he understands his low-sodium diet restrictions when he chooses a menu of

   1. Smoked turkey, mashed potatoes, spinach, and apple juice.
   2. Crab on rice, green beans, and decaffeinated coffee.
   3. Lamb chop, mint jelly, rice, beets, and low-fat milk.
   4. Roast beef, baked potato, squash, and decaffeinated coffee.

5. An 81-year-old client has right-sided heart failure and is confined to bed. Which of the following assessments by the nurse would indicate a deterioration in this client's condition?

   1. Clear lung sounds.
   2. Pitting edema of the sacral area.
   3. Stating, "I don't want breakfast today."
   4. Weight loss.

6. Before administering an immunization to a child, the nurse will assess for a primary contraindication, which is

   1. Impetigo.
   2. Failure to thrive.
   3. Congenital heart disease.
   4. Cystic fibrosis.

7. Identify the name of the arrhythmia in the following rhythm strip.

   1. PVCs.
   2. Ventricular fibrillation.
   3. Third-degree heart block.
   4. Ventricular tachycardia.

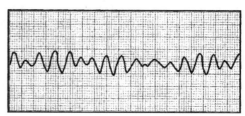

8. As you identify the rhythm in Question 7, the priority intervention is to

   1. Do nothing because it is a normal sinus rhythm.
   2. Call for the code team to start defibrillating the client.
   3. Continue to monitor the client.
   4. Repeat checking out the ECG strip to verify the rhythm.

9. Which of the following clinical manifestations would indicate that a client has developed a complication following a cystoscopy?

   1. Difficulty voiding.
   2. Pink-tinged urine.
   3. Burning on urination.
   4. Development of a chill.

10. A newly pregnant client is unsure of the date of her last menstrual period (LMP). Means other than Nägele's rule will be used to determine the estimated date of delivery. The nurse would expect the physician to estimate the date by

   1. Hearing the first audible fetal heart tone with a fetoscope.
   2. Serial estriols.
   3. Ultrasonography.
   4. The nonstress test.

11. When assessing for domestic violence or abuse, the most important question to ask the client is

1. "How are things going at home?"
2. "Is there anything you would like to tell me?"
3. "Are you now or have you been a victim of abuse?"
4. "How are you feeling right now?"

12. When a toddler is hospitalized, age-appropriate toys would include which of the following? List all that apply: _____ .

1. Music boxes.
2. Pull wooden animal.
3. Push mini-vacuum.
4. Small blocks for building.
5. Wind-up toys.
6. Colorful mobiles.

13. During the preoperative period before surgery for Hirschsprung's disease, a priority nursing intervention will focus on

1. Maintaining the child's attachment to his parents.
2. Demonstrating correct administration of tap-water enemas to his parents.
3. Providing a high-calorie diet.
4. Promoting adequate rest and sleep.

14. A female client, age 36, states she has been depressed and anxious. Her mood is one of sadness and gloom and she is requesting medication. During the admission interview, the priority assessment is the client's

1. Living situation.
2. Coping mechanisms.
3. Suicide potential.
4. Support systems.

15. To develop a working relationship with a client in a psychiatric setting, the nurse knows that goal setting is vital. To ensure that the goal is attainable, it must

1. Be mutually set by the client and the nurse.
2. Have observable outcomes.
3. Be flexible and changeable as appropriate to the situation.
4. Be set by the nurse and agreed to by the client.

16. A depressed client tells the nurse that most of the time she has no anger toward her husband and rarely says anything negative, but he is always angry with her. She may be using the defense mechanism of

1. Denial.
2. Sublimation.

3. Projection.
4. Fantasizing.

17. A male client, age 44, has recurring abscesses and recent weight loss despite a healthy appetite. What history information will be most important to elicit from this client?

1. Family history of blood disorders.
2. Family history of Type 1 diabetes.
3. Presence of pruritus and muscle cramps.
4. Presence of nocturia and excessive fatigue.

18. During a pregnant client's visit, the nurse assesses her for signs of increasing eclampsia or pregnancy-induced hypertension (PIH). If it is present, the nurse will observe

1. Edema of the hands, feet, and face.
2. Glycosuria.
3. Tachycardia.
4. Polyuria.

19. Assessing a cardiac client, the nurse will know that a normal PR interval is no more than _____ seconds.

20. The nurse notices that a client on a medical unit is alone in his room and crying. The most therapeutic nursing approach would be to say,

1. "Don't cry—you'll just feel worse."
2. "Cheer up now—crying can make you feel more sad."
3. "Spending so much time alone makes one feel lonely—let's go out on the unit."
4. "I'll get a tissue, then come back and sit with you."

21. The physician determines that a client with Type 1 diabetes requires a subtotal gastric resection. In planning his postoperative care, the nurse will take into account

1. A disruption in metabolic control.
2. An increased need for insulin.
3. An increased need for carbohydrates.
4. The onset of long-term complications.

22. The mother of a 1-month-old infant comes to the well-baby clinic. During a counseling session, the nurse learns that the mother often props the baby's bottle because the baby wiggles a lot. An appropriate response would be

1. "It is probably a good idea to prop the bottle until you feel more comfortable holding the baby."

2. "It is not a good idea to do this because the baby could choke on the formula."
3. "Do you have a fear of dropping the baby?"
4. "You need to hold the baby when you are feeding her."

23. A 57-year-old male is admitted for an endocrine work-up. The provisional diagnosis is Cushing's syndrome. Among the tests scheduled are fasting blood glucose, electrolytes, plasma ACTH level, and urinary 17-ketosteroids. Considering the lab tests that were ordered, the nurse would expect to assess the client and find

    1. Nervous exhaustion, hypertension, diaphoresis, heat intolerance.
    2. Moon face, hirsutism, emotional lability, weight gain.
    3. Increased cardiac output, heat intolerance, muscle fatigue, weight loss.
    4. Hypothermia, inactivity, weight gain, constipation.

24. A client is scheduled for a unilateral adrenalectomy. In developing goals for postoperative care, the nurse would

    1. Instruct him in daily steroid administration.
    2. Teach him signs and symptoms of hypoglycemia.
    3. Plan a diet low in protein and sodium.
    4. Maintain skin integrity.

25. The nurse is assessing a normal infant. A Moro reflex, present at birth, is described as

    1. Sudden, generalized, symmetrical movement with the legs drawn up together.
    2. Rapid movement of the arm and leg on the side opposite the stimulation.
    3. Slow, generalized, random activity of the whole body followed by a rigid positioning of the extremities.
    4. Rapid movement of all the extremities with no fixed pattern.

26. A new mother asks the nurse about nutrition instructions for breast-feeding. The nurse explains that the diet should include

    1. Four to five glasses of milk per day.
    2. Restricted salt intake.
    3. Low-calorie foods.
    4. Restricted fat intake.

27. The nurse is supervising a student nurse giving an IM injection to a client with right hip arthroplasty. The nurse will know the SN requires further instruction if she

1. Administers the injection in the left deltoid muscle.
2. Turns the client on her right hip to administer the injection.
3. Keeps the abduction pillow in place and turns the client 10 degrees to administer the injection on the unaffected side.
4. Administers the injection after turning the client to her left thigh, keeping the abduction pillow in place.

28. A client tells the nurse that she missed one menstrual cycle and her next cycle resulted in a slight amount of flow. She has not been pregnant before, but has had several sexual partners over the last year. Considering the history of her menstrual cycle, the nurse suspects she may have a tubal pregnancy. What is the appropriate intervention?

    1. Ask the physician to see the client immediately.
    2. Ask her if there is a familial history of tubal pregnancies.
    3. Examine her abdomen to determine if there is unilateral pelvic pain over a mass.
    4. Take her vital signs to determine if there are any abnormalities present.

29. Three of the following measures are necessary for a young child to maintain the desired effect of Bryant's traction. Which of the following is unnecessary?

    1. Restraining the child's upper torso.
    2. Immobilizing the child's elbow joints.
    3. Inspecting the child's leg bandages at regular intervals.
    4. Keeping the child's buttocks suspended above the mattress.

30. A wife will be involved in providing nursing care for her husband, who has had multiple sclerosis for 20 years. Which of the following nursing care measures would be most appropriate to include in the teaching sessions?

    1. Exercises that promote muscle strengthening and decrease tremors.
    2. Instruction in weight control.
    3. Side effects of routine medications.
    4. Importance of regular bowel and bladder evacuation.

31. Which of the following clients would the RN assess first after morning report?

    1. Client A, 38 years of age, motor vehicle accident (MVA) with fractured left humerus and internal injuries. He is second-day post-op splenectomy, liquids increasing to soft diet as tolerated.

2. Client B, age 74, third-day post-op RLL lobectomy, bilateral crackles, IPPB QID, antibiotics IVq6h, regular diet, encourage fluids.
3. Client C, age 51, GI bleeding, NPO, NG tube, IV Ringer's lactate 100 mL/hr, repeat Hgb, Hct in AM.
4. Client D, 88 years of age, ventral hernia repair scheduled for 11 AM, NPO, hold medications except digoxin. Anesthetist will order preoperative medication.

32. A 51-year-old client is admitted with temperature 40°C (104°F), pulse 120, respirations 30. His wife states he has had a cold for several days and yesterday was "seeing bugs on the wall." He is disoriented in all three spheres, and the neurological examination is negative for increased intracranial pressure. Throat and blood cultures are positive for hemolytic streptococci. In planning his care, the nurse recognizes that his acute reversible brain syndrome is most likely the result of

1. Dehydration.
2. Elevated temperature.
3. Disoriented brain.
4. Infectious organisms.

33. A male client admitted himself to the alcoholic treatment unit because he is having blackout spells when he drinks. He is 47 years of age, lives alone, and has a history of early cirrhosis of the liver. In planning for his care the priority nursing activity is to

1. Monitor dietary selections and appetite.
2. Observe for withdrawal symptoms.
3. Institute 24-hour suicide precautions.
4. Measure abdominal girth daily.

34. A schizophrenic client becomes more withdrawn and suspicious of other clients. He constantly tries to argue with the nursing staff that several of the clients are "out to get him." The best nursing response to this behavior is to

1. Ignore the behavior and it will diminish.
2. Disagree with the client so that his fears won't be confirmed.
3. Avoid disagreeing with the client and get him involved with an activity.
4. Attempt to move rapidly into a nurse–client relationship to establish trust.

35. A 65-year-old male client with Parkinson's disease is being treated with L-dopa. The nurse will know he understands restrictions associated with the drug when he says that he avoids food rich in

1. Vitamin B_{12}.
2. Vitamin B_6.
3. Vitamin A.
4. Vitamin E.

36. A client with alcoholic cirrhosis with ascites and portal hypertension is to receive neomycin. The desired effect of this drug is to

1. Sterilize the bowel.
2. Reduce abdominal distention.
3. Decrease the serum ammonia.
4. Prevent infection.

37. The priority nursing intervention for a child with meningitis is to

1. Frequently take vital signs and perform neuro checks.
2. Encourage fluids.
3. Administer antibiotics as ordered according to schedule.
4. Maintain respiratory isolation.

38. Your client has an arterial line inserted and you are assessing the waveform pattern. Fill in the blank with the number (1 or 2) of the waveform image that indicates damping has occurred in an arterial line: _____.

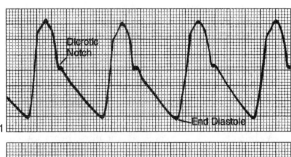

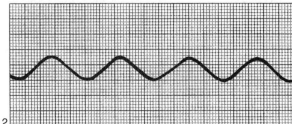

39. Appropriate toys for a 3-month-old infant would include

1. Soft, colorful squeeze toys and teething toys.
2. Teething toys with small, removable parts.
3. Push and pull toys, and pounding toys.
4. Balls and toys that stimulate the senses.

40. A client, age 11, is brought to the hospital by his parents and receives a diagnosis of acute rheumatic fever.

While the nurse is assessing his heart sounds, she keeps in mind that the cardiac structure most susceptible to damage is the

1. Ventricle.
2. Atrium.
3. Tricuspid valve.
4. Mitral valve.

41. A client on the unit becomes agitated and assaultive when stressed. The nurse learns in report that his family did not visit him, and when making rounds finds him with clenched fists, pacing the hall. The best strategy for dealing with his behavior would be to first

    1. Discuss with the client how he feels about his family not coming to visit him.
    2. Ask the client to come to the dayroom where you can better observe him in case he becomes more agitated.
    3. Invite the client to join you in an activity that you know he finds relaxing.
    4. Ignore the body language of anger and allow the client to pace off his anxiety.

42. You are assigned to complete a physical assessment of a newly admitted client. You are assessing heart sounds. The position where you will detect S_1 heart sounds is over the

    1. Fifth intercostal space, mid-clavicular line, and left sternal border.
    2. Second intercostal space, left sternal border.
    3. Lower left sternal border.
    4. Second intercostal space, right sternal border.

43. While eating in the cafeteria, the nurse hears someone yell, "Help! My husband is choking!" The first intervention is to

    1. Give him an abdominal thrust.
    2. Give him a back blow.
    3. Establish an airway.
    4. Ask him, "Can you talk?"

44. Reviewing the chart before sending a surgical client to the operating room, nursing responsibilities would include notifying the physician if the

    1. Erythrocyte count is 6 million/mm³.
    2. Leukocyte count is 5500/mm³.
    3. Hemoglobin is 14 g/dL.
    4. Platelet count is 100,000/mm³.

45. A client was admitted to the hospital 4 hours ago with a head injury, incurred when he fell off a ladder. The nurse observes his restlessness and understands that it is probably caused by

1. Decreased intracranial pressure.
2. Cerebral anoxia.
3. Dehydration.
4. Pain.

46. Which of the following clinical manifestations is a late indication that a client is developing increased intracranial pressure (ICP) following a head injury?

    1. Restlessness.
    2. Increased blood pressure.
    3. Decreased pulse rate.
    4. Widened pulse pressure.

47. A 63-year-old female client is admitted to the hospital. Her chart states that she has had a myocardial infarction that has progressed to cardiogenic shock. Which of the following parameters would indicate that cardiogenic shock is developing?

    1. A widening pulse pressure.
    2. Slow respiratory rate.
    3. Bradyarrhythmias.
    4. Decreasing arterial blood pressure.

48. Which one of the following conditions is a common cause of cardiogenic shock?

    1. Fluid overload.
    2. Electrolyte imbalance.
    3. Left ventricular failure.
    4. Constrictive pericarditis.

49. When caring for a client with acute pancreatitis, which of the following drugs, if ordered, would it be important to question?

    1. Opiates.
    2. Meperidine (Demerol).
    3. Antibiotics.
    4. Anticholinergies.

50. An 18-year-old client is admitted to a psychiatric unit with a tentative diagnosis of antisocial personality. He recently physically assaulted his 16-year-old girlfriend when she wanted to break up with him. Assessing him, the nurse knows that a person with antisocial personality disorder can be described as

    1. An individual of high intelligence who attempts to cope through manipulation.
    2. A person with good superego development who manipulates others for the fun of it.

3. A person who appears very reasonable but who is highly manipulative.

4. A person who manipulates out of fear of punishment.

51. The major goal of therapy when dexamethasone (Decadron) is ordered for a client is to

1. Replace adrenocorticoids in clients following adrenalectomy.
2. Decrease inflammation in cerebral edema.
3. Reverse signs and symptoms of septic shock.
4. Delay complications of hepatic coma in cirrhosis clients.

52. The importance of providing instructions to women on self-examination of the breast is best reflected in which of the following statements?

1. The majority of breast abnormalities are first discovered by women.
2. Once a lesion has been discovered, the informed client may monitor the progress of the abnormality herself.
3. Breast cancer occurs much more often in women than men and is a major cause of death in women.
4. The high mortality rate of breast cancer can be most effectively reduced by early detection and adequate surgical treatment.

53. The client is transferred back to the unit immediately following a stapedectomy. The priority nursing action is to

1. Turn and deep-breathe the client.
2. Put the siderails up.
3. Check for drainage.
4. Test hearing capability.

54. Morphine sulfate is an agent used for patient-controlled analgesia (PCA). The usual concentration available in a vial injector is 1 mg/mL or _____ mg/mL. Fill in the blank with the correct number of milligrams.

55. A 47-year-old client is admitted to the hospital with a 3-day history of severe, burning abdominal pain in the left epigastric area. His admitting diagnosis is suspected peptic ulcer disease. Based on nursing knowledge, which of the following questions will reveal the most information concerning the source of the pain?

1. How long does the pain last?
2. Does exercise bring on the pain?
3. Do certain foods cause the pain?
4. When does the pain occur?

56. A client is scheduled for a gastroduodenoscopy, and the nurse will prepare him for this procedure. Preprocedure instructions would include information that during the procedure he will be

1. Heavily sedated.
2. Given a local anesthetic to ease the discomfort.
3. Asked to assist by coughing.
4. Asked to assist by performing a Valsalva maneuver.

57. An elderly client with infectious hepatitis (hepatitis A) and his family are being instructed by the nurse in prevention techniques. The single most important action to prevent this disease is

1. Not to eat out in public places.
2. Good personal hygiene.
3. Thorough handwashing.
4. Active immunization.

58. Nursing care in the first 24 hours following skin grafting will include

1. Maintaining a pressure dressing on the grafted area.
2. Monitoring continuous antibiotic irrigations to the grafted area.
3. Changing the dressings every 4 hours using sterile technique.
4. Irrigating the drains placed in the burn area every 4 hours with sterile saline solution.

59. A client has been brought to the immediate treatment center by the police for attacking his neighbor with a knife. His admitting diagnosis was schizophrenia. Beginning the admission process, the first nursing action would be to

1. Search the client for concealed weapons.
2. Ask the client how he is feeling.
3. Introduce herself to the client.
4. Get the client settled on the unit.

60. Indicate the point by choosing the correct number at which you would place your stethoscope as you start auscultating breath sounds: _____ .

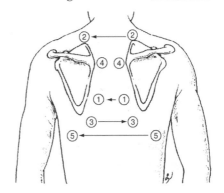

61. A client with coronary artery disease has an LDL cholesterol level of 200 mg/dL. His physician has recommended that he start on Mevacor to lower the level and slow the progression of atherosclerosis. In counseling the client, the nurse should emphasize

    1. Taking this medication with niacin to lower the LDL level.
    2. Notifying the physician if the client's gums begin to bleed.
    3. Reporting a rash, myalgia, or blurred vision.
    4. The photosensitization effects of the drug, and hence the need for sunscreen and protective clothing.

62. Oxygen is ordered for a 70-year-old client hospitalized for congestive heart failure. Which of the following methods of administration will deliver the highest concentration of oxygen?

    1. Venturi mask.
    2. Nasal prongs.
    3. Oxygen catheter.
    4. Mask with reservoir bag.

63. A client with damaged or impaired lungs cannot remove all of the CO_2 from the body. When the excess CO_2 combines with H_2O, it will form

    1. H_2CO_3.
    2. HCO_3
    3. H^+.
    4. CO_2.

64. Which one of the following rules for charting narrative notes does not fit into acceptable charting procedures?

    1. Each entry should be signed with the nurse's name and professional status.
    2. Objective facts are more relevant than nursing interpretation.
    3. Behaviors rather than feelings should be charted.
    4. Use of the word *client* or *patient* is important to designate particular entries.

65. Before a client who suffered an attack of gout is discharged from the hospital, it is important to evaluate his knowledge of dietary management. Which one of the following diet choices would indicate to the nurse that he understands his dietary restrictions?

    1. Liver, potato and spinach.
    2. Crab cakes, rice and peas.
    3. Antipasto salad, beans, rice, and asparagus.
    4. Steak, baked potato and green salad.

66. A 3-year-old child who is semiconscious with a low-grade fever is brought to the emergency room. The physician suspects a severe case of lead poisoning. The nurse expects that the child will be treated with

    1. Calcium disodium edetate (EDTA).
    2. Erythromycin.
    3. Activated charcoal.
    4. Syrup of ipecac.

67. A client has a 1000-mL bag of D5/0.45 NS hung at 10 AM/1000 hrs. His 24-hour IV orders are for 3 bags of 1000 mL. What time should the second bag be hung? _____ PM.

68. A female client has been hospitalized for 2 days with chronic congestive heart failure. Her physician has written orders that include Lasix IV and oxygen. The client suddenly complains of breathing difficulty. The immediate assessment indicates that she has bi-basilar rales, increased pulse and blood pressure, and a frequent moist cough. The first nursing intervention is to

    1. Give Lasix IV push according to standing orders.
    2. Apply rotating tourniquets according to standing orders.
    3. Place the client in high-Fowler's position.
    4. Call the physician and inform him of the change in her condition.

69. When caring for a client diagnosed with pulmonary edema who is receiving oxygen, the nurse observes that she frequently removes her oxygen mask even though she is dyspneic. The appropriate nursing intervention is to

    1. Change from O_2 mask to O_2 cannula.
    2. Increase the liter flow of O_2 to 10 L/min.
    3. Tighten the strap on the O_2 mask.
    4. Change O_2 administration to a Venturi mask.

70. When a cardiac client is brought to the emergency room with ventricular arrhythmias, the drug of choice is

    1. Digoxin.
    2. Inderal.
    3. Lidocaine.
    4. Morphine sulfate.

71. The nurse explains to a client with a duodenal ulcer that his ulcer diet will most likely include

    1. Six small feedings of regular food.
    2. Milk or cream every 2 hours.
    3. A regular diet without milk.
    4. A high-fiber diet without spices.

72. A client is diagnosed as schizophrenic, catatonic type, and has been in the hospital for 3 weeks. The client has just been told that her father was in a bad automobile accident and is critically ill in the hospital. Her response is to smile and ask what time lunch is served. This response is an example of

   1. Lack of affect.
   2. Inappropriate affect.
   3. Disturbed association of ideas.
   4. Primary disturbance.

73. The appropriate nursing response to a client's question asking when lunch will be served after the nurse tells her that a family member is in the hospital, critically ill, would be

   1. "Did you hear what I said?"
   2. "Your father is critically ill. Don't you want to talk about it?"
   3. "You are blocking, and I think you need to talk about your feelings."
   4. "I told you your father was critically ill, and you asked what time lunch would be served."

74. A client has been diagnosed as having early-stage cancer of the transverse colon. The physician has explained to the client that she needs to have part of her colon removed (partial colectomy). Knowing this, the nurse would explain to the client that postoperatively the elimination process will be done through

   1. An ileostomy for elimination.
   2. Normal elimination.
   3. A temporary colostomy for elimination.
   4. A permanent colostomy for elimination.

75. On the images below, identify the two areas preferred for insulin injections.

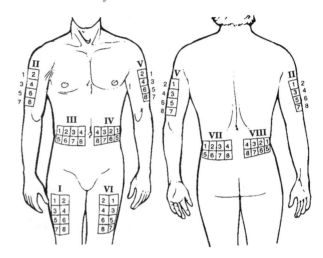

   1. I and II.
   2. II and V.
   3. I and VI.
   4. III and IV.

COMPREHENSIVE TEST 3

Answers with Rationale

1. (2) The nurse's priority is to assess the client for pain. The presence of chest pain can cause the pulse rate to increase and blood pressure to drop. It can also increase client anxiety. The client is on a cardiac monitor; therefore, an apical pulse (1) is not the priority action. Once his comfort has been established, apical pulse, blood pressure (4), and heart sound determinations are appropriate.

   NP:A; CN:PH; CA:M; CL:A

2. (1) Elevated CK-MB, which rises within 6 hours after an MI has occurred, is indicative of myocardial damage. SGOT is not specific to heart disease alone and LDH is not as specific as answer (1) in the diagnosis of myocardial infarction, even though the level rises in 6 to 8 hours and persists longer.

   NP:AN; CN:PH; CA:M; CL:C

3. The answer is *0.50 mL* per minute. Each 500 mL of IV fluid contains 2000 mg of lidocaine. One mL of IV fluid contains 4 mg; therefore, the client will receive 0.5 mL per minute.

   NP:I; CN:PH; CA:M; CL:A

4. (4) This menu provides the lowest amount of sodium. Turkey, spinach, shellfish, and beets are high in sodium, and thus would not be included in a low-sodium diet.

   NP:E; CN:PH; CA:M; CL:C

5. (2) Right-sided heart failure manifests systemic symptoms rather than respiratory involvement. Symptoms include weight gain and edema of the dependent parts of the body. Although anorexia may be a symptom, skipping one meal is not indicative of anorexia and is not as significant as the sacral edema.

   NP:A; CN:PH; CA:M; CL:A

6. (1) Children with active infections, such as impetigo, should not be immunized.

   NP:A; CN:H; CA:P; CL:A

7. (2) The strip shows ventricular fibrillation, which means that the ventricles of the heart are quivering with no audible heartbeat or pulse. The client must be defibrillated.

   NP:A; CN:S; CA:M; CL:AN

8. (2) Ventricular fibrillation means the heart is quivering and not pumping effectively. The intervention is to call the code team to begin defibrillating the client. Doing nothing, continuing to monitor, or repeating checking out the rhythm strip will be dangerous because the client should be defibrillated immediately.

   NP:I; CN:S; CA:M; CL:AN

9. (4) Cold chills could indicate the spread of infection throughout the urinary tract. Answers (2) and (3) might be present after the procedure, as would difficulty in voiding (1).

   NP:E; CN:PH; CA:M; CL:C

10. (3) Ultrasonography is the most accurate test of those listed for determining pregnancy, and can now be used as early as 5 weeks. Hearing the fetal heart tone (1) is the safest means to determine EDD (previously called EDC). However, the heart rate cannot be heard until 20 weeks' gestation. Serial estriols (2) and the non-stress test (4) are done later in pregnancy as methods of determining fetal status or fetal well-being.

    NP:AN; CN:H; CA:MA; CL:C

11. (3) The single most important question is to ask directly and specifically if the client has been abused. A direct question is more apt to elicit an honest and direct

---

Coding for Questions/Answers Abbreviations: **Nursing Process: NP,** Assessment: A, Analysis: AN, Planning: P, Implementation: I, Evaluation: E; **Client Needs: CN,** Safe, Effective Care Environment: S, Health Promotion and Maintenance: H, Psychosocial Integrity: PS, Physiological Integrity: PH; **Clinical Area: CA,** Medical Nursing: M, Surgical Nursing: S, Maternal/Newborn Nursing: MA, Pediatric Nursing: P, Psychiatric Nursing: PS; **Cognitive Level: CL,** Knowledge: K, Comprehension: C, Application: A, Analysis: AN.

response. Always do this privately so that the client will feel free to speak and will not be intimidated.

NP:A; CN:PS; CA:M; CL:A

12. The answer is *2 and 3*. Upper airway obstruction is a major problem in small children, because toys with small parts could cause a toddler to choke. Most toddlers are engrossed in large-motor activity, and they love imaginative toys that utilize large muscle groups. Fine-motor skills are more appropriate for preschoolers and older children. Colorful mobiles are appropriate for infants.

NP:P; CN:H; CA:P; CL:C

13. (3) The child will be given a low-residue, high-calorie diet. Children with aganglionic disease tend to be thin and undernourished, despite their large and distended abdomens. Improving the child's nutritional status before surgery is very important. (1) is always true, but not the best answer. Tap-water enemas can cause water intoxication.

NP:I; CN:PH; CA:S; CL:A

14. (3) It is of primary importance to assess the suicide potential of clients presenting symptoms of depression. The client is asking for medication that could be used to overdose, so suicide potential is crucial to assess. The other factors are also important to assess, but are not the priority.

NP:A; CN:PS; CA:PS; CL:C

15. (1) To ensure that goals are attainable, they must be set by both nurse and client. The other answers are important but cannot be achieved without the mutually agreed-upon goals. All outcomes must be measurable to determine whether they have been achieved.

NP:P; CN:PS; CA:PS; CL:K

16. (3) The client may be denying the feelings that belong to her and projecting them onto her husband. Depressed clients often cannot express anger directly and either repress it, project it to others, or deny these feelings.

NP:AN; CN:PS; CA:PS; CL:C

17. (2) The onset of insulin-dependent diabetes mellitus Type 1 is often insidious, becoming manifest only after some metabolic stress, such as infection.

NP:A; CN:PH; CA:M; CL:C

18. (1) Edema, proteinuria, and hypertension are the three cardinal signs of preeclampsia. Normal urine output or oliguria occurs rather than polyuria (4).

NP:A; CN:H; CA:MS; CL:C

19. The answer is *0.20 second*. The PR interval represents the time it takes for the impulse to traverse the atria to the AV node. The normal range is 0.12 to 0.20 second.

NP:AN; CN:H; CA:M; CL:C

20. (4) The most therapeutic response is to acknowledge that the client is upset and offer the opportunity to discuss these feelings. The other responses close off communication.

NP:I; CN:PS; CA:PS; CL:A

21. (1) This is the most comprehensive answer. In addition to gastric resections, clients with a radical mastectomy, thoracotomy, or abdominal perineal resection experience extensive metabolic disturbances. The metabolic disturbance is related to the effects of total stress the client is experiencing.

NP:P; CN:PH; CA:S; CL:A

22. (3) Before explaining the importance of holding the baby to develop the mother–child relationship, it is necessary to find out how the mother is feeling and to identify her fears. All of the other responses close off communication.

NP:I; CN:H; CA:P; CL:A

23. (2) Cushing's syndrome is characterized by exaggeration of normal physiological conditions generally shown by weight gain and protein wasting. Answer (1) is caused by adrenal medulla disease. Answer (3) is caused by hyperthyroidism.

NP:A; CN:PH; CA:M; CL:A

24. (1) Adrenalectomy necessitates replacement therapy with both glucocorticoids and mineralocorticoids for up to 6 months. Teaching the client about steroid administration before the surgery will help achieve goals after the surgery.

NP:P; CN:PH; CA:S; CL:C

25. (1) This reflex is termed the Moro reflex, also termed the startle reflex. This reflex is present at birth, is symmetrical, and disappears around 4 months of age.

NP:A; CN:H; CA:MA; CL:C

26. (1) Lactating mothers need four to five glasses of milk a day. They should never be advised to restrict any nutrient or attempt to diet during lactation.

NP:I; CN:H; CA:MA; CL:K

27. (2) Because the most common complication of total joint replacement is dislocation, correct positioning is important. Turning the client on either side without keeping the abduction pillow in place could lead to dislocation of the new prosthesis.

    NP:E; CN:S; CA:M; CL:A

28. (3) The triad associated with early ruptured extrauterine pregnancy includes the menstrual cycle history, unilateral pelvic pain, and presence of a cul-de-sac mass.

    NP:I; CN:PH; CA:MA; CL:A

29. (2) It is not necessary to immobilize the child's elbow joints. The other interventions are necessary to maintain the appropriate traction.

    NP:E; CN:PH; CA:P; CL:C

30. (4) Bowel and bladder retention or incontinence is a major problem with clients who have multiple sclerosis; therefore, establishing a good routine for evacuation is essential. Weight control is usually not a problem. While exercising (1) is important, specific exercises for muscle strengthening or decreasing tremors are not effective. Multiple sclerosis clients do not take medication routinely (3).

    NP:P; CN:S; CA:M; CL:C

31. (3) Client C—the nurse should first assess the most acute client, which is the client with GI bleeding. Client A (1) is second-day post-op so he can wait, as can client B (2). The nurse would assess client D (4) next, because he is scheduled for surgery and should be NPO except for meds.

    NP:A; CN:PH; CA:M; CL:AN

32. (4) The primary cause of his neurological symptoms would be bacterial infection.

    NP:A; CN:PH; CA:M; CL:A

33. (2) The nurse's priority is to observe for symptoms of withdrawal. Although nursing activities may include monitoring diet (1) and measuring abdominal girth (3), there is no need for suicide precautions at this time.

    NP:P; CN:PH; CA:M; CL:A

34. (3) The best choice is to encourage the client to become involved in an activity to get his mind off the paranoid thoughts. The nurse would also avoid power struggles (as this increases anxiety). Answer (4) is wrong because proceeding with nursing therapy too rapidly will cause a suspicious client to be more distrustful.

    NP:I; CN:PS; CA:PS; CL:A

35. (2) Foods rich in vitamin B_6 block the desired effects of L-dopa; therefore, they need to be omitted from the diet. Examples of foods to be avoided include meat, especially organ meats; whole-grain cereals; peanuts; and wheat germ. Vitamin A (3) or beta-carotene (found in fruits and vegetables) does not need to be limited.

    NP:E; CN:PH; CA:M; CL:A

36. (3) Neomycin does sterilize the bowel (1), but the rationale for use or desired outcome of this medication is to reduce ammonia production by enteric bacteria. It is not a systemic antibiotic.

    NP:E; CN:PH; CA:M; CL:C

37. (3) Even though all interventions will be carried out, administering antibiotics is the priority. Antibiotics are started after the lumbar puncture is done and the organism is identified.

    NP:I; CN:PH; CA:P; CL:A

38. (2) Waveform (2) shows that damping has occurred. The flattened arterial waveform indicates damping, which results from obstruction in the arterial line or imbalance of the transducer.

    NP:A; CN:PH; CA:M; CL:AN

39. (1) Toys should be visually appealing without small parts (2) that could choke an infant. Exploration through the mouth begins at 3 months. Push and pull toys (3) and balls (4) are appropriate for the mobile, older baby.

    NP:P; CN:H; CA:P; CL:K

40. (4) The mitral and aortic valves are most susceptible to damage as a result of this inflammatory disease.

    NP:AN; CN:PH; CA:P; CL:C

41. (1) Helping the client verbalize will reduce his tension. Later, or in addition, engaging him in an activity that he finds relaxing (3) will help prevent possible assaultive behavior, because stress reduction and assaultive behavior are incompatible. The body language (4) is an important cue, and it is important to pick it up.

    NP:P; CN:PS; CA:PS; CL:A

42. (1) Using the diaphragm of the stethoscope, S_1 sounds are best heard over mitral and tricuspid areas, fifth in-

tercostal space, mid-clavicular line. S_2 sounds are heard over the pulmonic valve (2) and the aortic valve (4). S_3 sounds are heard over the left sternal border.

NP:P; CN:PH; CA:M; CL:A

43. (4) By asking, "Can you talk?" the nurse establishes that the person has something in his airway. If he is able to answer, he is not choking. A person is unable to talk when choking.

NP:I; CN:PH; CA:M; CL:A

44. (4) All of the other reports are within normal range. The low platelet count signifies thrombocytopenia. Bleeding can result from this low platelet count and the cause should be researched before surgery. Normal platelet count is 150,000 to 450,000/mm^3.

NP:I; CN:PH; CA:S; CL:A

45. (2) Cerebral anoxia occurs frequently in severe trauma to the brain. A blood clot or edema can cause an interruption of the blood circulation, which alters oxygen supply to the tissue. Reduced oxygen causes anoxia.

NP:AN; CN:PH; CA:M; CL:C

46. (4) Widened pulse pressure is a late sign. Restlessness (1) is the earliest sign of increased intracranial pressure and is due to compression of the brain from edema or hemorrhage (or both) causing hypoxia. Blood pressure (2) and pulse changes (3) are not the earliest clinical manifestation of increased intracranial pressure.

NP:A; CN:PH; CA:M; CL:C

47. (4) As the left ventricle fails in its pumping action, the blood pressure will fall. A widened pulse pressure (1) (the difference between systolic and diastolic pressures) is indicative of decreased peripheral vascular resistance. As the heart fails, the pulse increases in an attempt to circulate more blood, and the respiratory rate (2) increases in an effort to take in more oxygen.

NP:E; CN:PH; CA:M; CL:A

48. (3) When the pump of the heart (left ventricle) is damaged, it cannot eject a normal cardiac output and the circulatory system begins to fail. Fluid overload (1) would cause a weak left ventricle to fail, but a normal myocardium would stretch and contract with increased force to handle the increased fluid. Electrolyte imbalances (2) can cause cardiac decompensation by way of arrhythmias (potassium) and decreased force of contraction (calcium).

NP:AN; CN:PH; CA:M; CL:C

49. (1) Opiates are contraindicated, as they may produce spasm of the biliary–pancreatic ducts. Thus it would be important to notify the physician and question the order. Synthetic narcotics (Demerol) are the drugs of choice for pain control.

NP:P; CN:PH; CA:M; CL:A

50. (3) The client's ability to behave within normal standards and yet be highly manipulative is characteristic of the antisocial personality. This makes it difficult not only to work with the client, but at times to diagnose him. His superego (2) is poorly developed. He may or may not have a high IQ (1).

NP:AN; CN:PS; CA:PS; CL:C

51. (2) Decadron decreases inflammation by stabilizing leukocyte lysosomal membranes. It also suppresses the immune response, so it is contraindicated in clients with infection, cirrhosis, and debilitating disease.

NP:P; CN:PH; CA:M; CL:C

52. (4) Health professionals have the responsibility to provide clear guidelines focused on the prevention and early treatment of breast cancer. Self-examinations following menstruation coupled with annual screening examination by the physician are very effective in detecting early breast cancer.

NP:AN; CN:H; CA:M; CL:K

53. (2) The issue is safety; thus the siderails should be up. Clients can sometimes experience vertigo and could fall from bed. Finally, clients should not be turned postoperatively unless there is a specific order to do so.

NP:I; CN:PH; CA:S; CL:A

54. The answer is *5*. Morphine sulfate 1 mg/mL or *5 mg/mL* can be used for PCA.

NP:P; CN:S; CA:S; CL:C

55. (4) The symptoms of peptic ulcers are due to mucosal inflammation. There is usually pain when the stomach is empty: 1 to 3 hours after meals in gastric ulcers and 3 to 4 hours after meals in duodenal ulcers. The other questions already make the assumption that the client has ulcer disease. The pattern of the pain will help to determine whether he has ulcer disease.

NP:A; CN:PH; CA:M; CL:C

56. (2) A gastroduodenoscopy is the visualization of the esophagus, stomach, and duodenum through a flexible tube inserted orally. The exam is not a comfortable

one because the muscles of the gastrointestinal tract have spasms as the tube is passed. This causes difficulty swallowing. The client is usually given a local anesthetic to the posterior pharynx to reduce the discomfort during the passage of the tube. He will not be heavily sedated (1) because he must be able to assist by swallowing. Coughing (3) or performing a Valsalva maneuver (4) would impede the passage of the tube.

NP:I; CN:PH; CA:S; CL:C

57. (3) Thorough handwashing is the most important action to prevent the transmission of hepatitis A. Good personal hygiene (2) is also important, but it does not replace handwashing. Contaminated food is a mode of transmission. Passive immunization is prevention.

NP:P; CN:H; CA:M; CL:C

58. (1) The pressure dressing is used to prevent fluid accumulation under the graft site as well as to promote immobilization of the affected area. Drains are frequently placed under the skin flap to promote drainage. The drains are attached to suction; they are not irrigated.

NP:I; CN:PH; CA:M; CL:C

59. (3) It is important for the nurse to introduce herself and make contact, rather than search the client for weapons (1), ask how he is feeling (2), or get the client settled (4). Introduction is acknowledgment and the first step in establishing a relationship.

NP:I; CN:PS; CA:PS; CL:A

60. (2) You would start auscultating at the top of the lungs and move down according to the numbers on the diagram shown below.

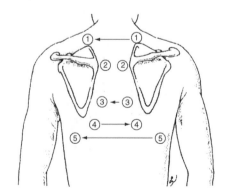

NP:I; CN:PH; CA:M; CL:A

61. (4) The LDL is high (normal is 60–100). Photosensitization is a risk for clients taking hepatic hydroxymethylglutaryl coenzyme A (HMG-COA) reductase

inhibitors (Mevacor). Niacin is usually given with bile acid sequestrants because they work synergistically (1). Bleeding from the gums (2) or rectum is a sign of vitamin K deficiency from bile acid sequestrants (Questran). Rash, myalgia, and blurred vision (3) are adverse effects of fibric acid derivatives, which are not very effective in lowering LDL.

NP:I; CN:PH; CA:M; CL:A

62. (4) A flow of 8 to 10 L will provide an FIO_2 of 70 to 100 percent. The reservoir bag contains a high level of oxygen. As the client inhales, oxygen is taken in from the bag. The Venturi mask (1) delivers a fixed FIO_2, usually 24 to 35 percent. A 38 to 44 percent FIO_2 is the maximum amount of oxygen delivered through prongs (2).

NP:P; CN:PH; CA:M; CL:C

63. (1) Excess CO_2 in the blood, when combined with H_2O, forms H_2CO_3—carbonic acid. Depending on the amount of acid in the blood, the lungs will increase or decrease ventilation to remove excess CO_2. The kidneys can excrete or retain H^+ and HCO_3, so the equation representing homeostasis is

$$CO_2 + H_2O = H_2CO_3 = H^+ = HCO_3$$
$$\text{(Lungs)} \qquad\qquad \text{(Kidney)}$$

NP:A; CN:PH; CA:M; CL:AN

64. (4) The word *patient* or *client* should not be used, as the chart belongs to the client; thus adding it to the chart is redundant.

NP:P; CN:S; CA:M; CL:K

65. (4) Steak is the best choice because foods highest in purine are shellfish, liver, chicken, beans, asparagus and various vegetables. The appropriate diet will include high carbohydrates with calorie control.

NP:E; CN:S; CA:M; CL:A

66. (1) Calcium disodium edetate, or EDTA, is a chelating agent that promotes the excretion of lead from the body by attaching to the lead and carrying it out through the kidneys.

NP:P; CN:PH; CA:P; CL:K

67. The answer is *6 PM* to hang the second bag. Each bag will cover 8 hours of a 24-hour order.

NP:P; CN:PH; CA:M; CL:A

68. (3) It is best to first do the nursing intervention that immediately helps the client's condition while the

nurse is preparing more definitive therapy. High-Fowler's position decreases venous return to the heart. Lasix would then be given and the physician notified.

NP:I; CN:S; CA:M; CL:A

69. (1) Clients often feel that they cannot breathe when experiencing pulmonary edema. A mask may increase this feeling. A cannula is often better tolerated and should be used in this case.

NP:I; CN:S; CA:M; CL:A

70. (3) Lidocaine is the drug of choice because it depresses ventricular irritability. Inderal is contraindicated as it is a beta-adrenergic inhibitor. It also depresses cardiac function. For a client who already has a compromised cardiac status, this could be fatal. Morphine reduces anxiety, but will not prevent arrhythmias. Digoxin is used to strengthen ventricular contraction.

NP:P; CN:PH; CA:M; CL:C

71. (3) Most physicians now prescribe a regular three-meal routine, eliminating roughage, gas-forming foods, highly spiced foods, and gastric acid stimulants such as caffeine, alcohol and smoking. In the past, milk and cream were the mainstays of dietary ulcer therapy. They were taken every hour, with antacids in between. Currently, it is believed that this regimen increases gastric acid secretion. A bland diet has no ef-

fect on peptic ulcer disease. Some physicians do prescribe six small feedings of bland food to keep food in the stomach.

NP:P; CN:H; CA:M; CL:C

72. (2) The client's response is inappropriate to the situation and is an example of inappropriate affect. Lack of affect is when there is no response (including facial expression). Both are indicative of a schizophrenic reaction.

NP:AN: CN:PS; CA:PS; CL:K

73. (4) The client's response is inappropriate to the situation and is an example of inappropriate affect. Lack of affect is when there is no response (including facial expression). Both are indicative of a schizophrenic reaction.

NP:AN; CN:PS; CA:PS; CL:C

74. (2) A partial colectomy is removal of a portion of the colon and reanastamosis of the remaining ends; therefore, elimination will occur normally.

NP:I; CN:PH; CA:S; CL:K

75. (4) The area preferred is around the umbilicus in the abdominal area because absorption is quickest and most reliable. Other sites are acceptable but not preferred.

NP:P; CN:PH; CA:M; CL:A

Alabama Board of Nursing
770 Washington Avenue
Montgomery, Alabama 36130
(334) 242-4060

Alaska Board of Nursing
550 West Seventh Avenue, Suite 1500
Anchorage, Alaska 99501
(907) 269-8161

Health Services Regulatory Board
LBJ Tropical Medical Center
Pago Pago, American Samoa 96799
(684) 633-1222

Arizona State Board of Nursing
1651 East Morten, Suite 150
Phoenix, Arizona 85020
(602) 889–5150

Arkansas State Board of Nursing
1123 South University, Suite 800
Little Rock, Arkansas 72204
(501) 686-2700

California Board of Registered Nursing
400 R Street, Suite 4030
Sacramento, California 95814
(916) 322-3350

Colorado Board of Nursing
1560 Broadway, Suite 880
Denver, Colorado 80202
(303) 894-2430

Connecticut Board of Examiners for Nursing
Department of Public Health
410 Capitol Avenue MS# 13PHO
Hartford, Connecticut 06134
(860) 509-7624

Delaware Board of Nursing
861 Silver Lake Boulevard
Dover, Delaware 19904
(302) 739-4522

District of Columbia
Department of Health, Board of Nursing
825 North Capitol Street NE, 2nd Floor
Washington, DC 20002
(202) 442-4778

Florida State Board of Nursing
4052 Bald Cypress Way, BIN CO2
Tallahassee, Florida 32399
(850) 245-4125

Georgia Board of Nursing
237 Coliseum Drive
Macon, Georgia 31217
(478) 207-1640

Guam Board of Nurse Examiners
P.O. Box 2816
Hagatna, Guam 96932
(671) 735-7406

Hawaii Board of Nursing
335 Merchant Street, 3rd Floor
Honolulu, Hawaii 96813
(808) 586-3000

Idaho State Board of Nursing
280 North 8th Street, Suite 210
Boise, Idaho 83720
(208) 334-3110

Illinois Department of Professional Regulations
100 West Randolph, Suite 9-300
Chicago, Illinois 60601
(312) 814-2715

Indiana State Board of Nursing
402 West Washington Street, Room W066
Indianapolis, Indiana 46204
(317) 234-2043

Iowa Board of Nursing
400 SW 8th Street, Suite B
Des Moines, Iowa 50309
(515) 281-3255

Kansas State Board of Nursing
900 SW Jackson Street, Suite 551S
Topeka, Kansas 66612
(785) 296-4929

Kentucky Board of Nursing
312 Whittington Parkway, Suite 300
Louisville, Kentucky 40222
(502) 329-7000

Louisiana State Board of Nursing
3010 North Causeway Boulevard, Suite 501
Metairie, Louisiana 70003
(504) 838-5332

Maine State Board of Nursing
158 State House Station
Augusta, Maine 04333
(207) 287-1133

Maryland Board of Nursing
4140 Patterson Avenue
Baltimore, Maryland 21215
(410) 585-1900

Massachusetts Board of Registration in Nursing
239 Causeway Street
Boston, Massachusetts 02114
(617) 727-9961

Michigan CIS/Office of Health Services
611 West Ottawa
Lansing, Michigan 48933
(517) 335-0918

Minnesota Board of Nursing
2829 University Avenue SE, Suite 500
Minneapolis, Minnesota 55414
(612) 617-2270

Mississippi Board of Nursing
1935 Lakeland Drive, Suite B
Jackson, Mississippi 39216
(601) 987-4188

Missouri State Board of Nursing
3605 Missouri Boulevard
Jefferson City, Missouri 65102
(573) 751-0681

Montana State Board of Nursing
301 South Park
Helena, Montana 59620
(406) 841-2340

Nebraska Health and Human Services Board
301 Centennial Mall South
Lincoln, Nebraska 68509
(402) 471-4376

Nevada State Board of Nursing
4330 South Valley View Boulevard, Suite 106
Las Vegas, Nevada 89103
(702) 486-5800

New Hampshire Board of Nursing
78 Regional Drive, Building B
Concord, New Hampshire 03302
(603) 271-2323

New Jersey Board of Nursing
124 Halsey Street, 6th Floor
Newark, New Jersey 07101
(973) 504-6586

New Mexico Board of Nursing
4206 Louisiana Boulevard NE, Suite A
Albuquerque, New Mexico 87109
(505) 841-8340

New York State Board of Nursing
89 Washington Avenue
2nd Floor, West Wing
Albany, New York 12234
(518) 474-3817, ext. 120

North Carolina Board of Nursing
3724 National Drive, Suite 201
Raleigh, North Carolina 27612
(919) 782-3211

North Dakota Board of Nursing
919 South 7th Street, Suite 504
Bismarck, North Dakota 58504
(701) 328-9777

Ohio Board of Nursing
17 South High Street, Suite 400
Columbus, Ohio 43215
(614) 466-3947

Oklahoma Board of Nursing
2915 North Classen Boulevard, Suite 524
Oklahoma City, Oklahoma 73106
(405) 962-1800

Oregon State Board of Nursing
800 NE Oregon Street, Suite 465
Portland, Oregon 97232
(503) 731-4745

Pennsylvania State Board of Nursing
124 Pine Street
Harrisburg, Pennsylvania 17101
(717) 783-7142

Council on Higher Education of PR
P.O. Box 23305, University Station
Rio Piedras, Puerto Rico 00931
(787) 725-7506

Rhode Island Board of Nursing
105 Cannon Building
3 Capitol Hill
Providence, Rhode Island 02908
(401) 222-5700

South Carolina State Board of Nursing
110 Centerview Drive, Suite 202
Columbia, South Carolina 29210
(803) 896-4550

South Dakota Board of Nursing
4300 South Louise Avenue, Suite C-1
Sioux Falls, South Dakota 57106
(605) 362-2760

Tennessee State Board of Nursing
426 Fifth Avenue North
Nashville, Tennessee 37247
(615) 532-5166

Texas Board of Nurse Examiners
333 Guadalupe, Suite 3-460
Austin, Texas 78701
(512) 305-7400

Utah State Board of Nursing
160 East 300 South, 4th Floor
Salt Lake City, Utah 84111
(801) 530-6628

Vermont State Board of Nursing
81 River Street
Montpelier, Vermont 05609
(802) 828-2396

Virgin Islands Board of Nurse Licensure
P.O. Box 4247
St. Thomas, Virgin Islands 00803
(340) 776-7397

Virginia State Board of Nursing
6603 West Broad Street, 5th Floor
Richmond, Virginia 23230
(804) 662-9909

Washington State Nursing Care
    Quality Assurance Commission
310 Israel Road SE
Tumwater, Washington 98501
(360) 236-4700

West Virginia Board of Examiners
    for Registered Professional Nurses
101 Dee Drive
Charleston, West Virginia 25311
(304) 558-3596

Wisconsin Department of Regulation & Licensing
1400 East Washington Avenue, Room 173
Madison, Wisconsin 53708
(608) 266-0145

Wyoming State Board of Nursing
2020 Carey Avenue, Suite 110
Cheyenne, Wyoming 82002
(307) 777-7601

BIBLIOGRAPHY

CHAPTER 1 THE NCLEX-RN AND TEST-TAKING STRATEGIES

Bloom, BS. (Ed.). (1956). *Taxonomy of educational objectives: the classification of educational goals, Handbook I.* New York: David Mckay.

National Council of State Boards of Nursing. (1998). *Model nursing practice act.* Chicago: Author.

National Council of State Boards of Nursing. (2007). *Test plan for the national council licensure examination for registered nurses (NCLEX-RN® examination).* Chicago: Author.

Report of Findings from the 2005 RN Practice Analysis. (2005). *Linking the NCLEX-RN national licensure examination to practice: practice analysis of newly licensed registered nurses in the US.* Chicago: National Council of State Boards of Nursing, Inc.

CHAPTER 2 MANAGEMENT PRINCIPLES AND LEGAL ISSUES

American Hospital Association. (2001). *A patient's bill of rights.* Chicago: AHA.

American Nurses' Association. (1997). *Unlicensed assistive personnel legislation.* Washington, DC: ANA.

American Nurses' Association. (2001). *Code of ethics for nurses with interpretive statements.* Washington, DC: ANA.

American Nurses' Association. (2004). *Standards of clinical nursing practice* (3rd ed.). Washington, DC: ANA.

Bernzweig, E. (1996). *The nurse's liability for malpractice.* (6th ed.). St. Louis: Mosby.

Boucher, MA. (1998, February). Delegation alert. *American Journal of Nursing, 98*(2), 26–32.

Brent, N. (2004). *Nurses and the law: a guide to principles and applications* (3rd ed.). Philadelphia: Saunders.

California Board of Registered Nursing. (1997). *Nursing practice act: rules and regulations.* Sacramento, CA.

Canavan, K. (1997, May). Combating dangerous delegation. *American Journal of Nursing, 97*(5), 57–58.

Gerber-Zimmerman, P. (1997, May). Delegating to unlicensed assistive personnel. *Nursing 97, 27*(5), 71.

Guido, G. (1998). *Legal issues in nursing: a source book for practice* (2nd ed.). Norwalk, CT: Appleton & Lange.

Kany, K. (1999, October). Working with UAPs. *American Journal of Nursing, 99*(10), 71.

LeMone, P, Burke, K. (2004). *Medical surgical nursing: critical thinking in client care* (3rd ed.). Upper Saddle River, NJ: Prentice Hall Health.

Parkman, C, Calfee, B. (1997, April). Advance directives: honoring your patient's end-of-life wishes. *Nursing 97, 98*(4), 48–53.

Sheehan, J. (2001, November). Delegating to UAPs. *RN Magazine, 64*(11), 65–66.

Smith, S. (1998, July). RNs and UAPs: not much difference? *RN Magazine, 62*(7), 37–38.

Smith, S, Duell, D, Martin, B. (2008). *Clinical nursing skills* (7th ed.). Upper Saddle River, NJ: Prentice Hall Health.

Ventura, M. (1999, February). Staffing issues. *RN Magazine, 62*(2), 26–30.

Ventura, M. (1996, September). Workload, UAPs and you. *RN Magazine, 59*(9), 41–45.

CHAPTER 3 NURSING CONCEPTS

American Psychiatric Association. (2000). *Diagnostic and statistical manual of mental disorders* (text revision—4th ed.). Washington, DC: Author.

Ball, J, Bindler, R. (2007). *Pediatric nursing* (4th ed.). Norwalk, CT: Appleton & Lange.

Bandura, A. (1986). *Social foundations of thought and action: a social cognitive theory.* Upper Saddle River, NJ: Prentice Hall Health.

Blais, K, Hayes, J, Kozier, B, Erb, G. (2001). *Professional nursing practice: concepts and perspectives* (4th ed.). Upper Saddle River, NJ: Prentice Hall Health.

Board of Registered Nursing. (2003). *Pain assessment: the fifth vital sign.* State of California.

Engle, G. (1964). Grief and grieving. *American Journal of Nursing, 64*(9), 93–98.

Erickson, E. (1963). *Childhood and society* (2nd ed.). New York: Norton.

Fogel, C, Lauver, D. (1990). *Sexual health promotion.* Philadelphia: Saunders.

Furman, J. (2001, April). Living with dying: how to help the family caregiver. *Nursing 2001, 31*(4), 36.

Kübler-Ross, E. (1993). *Death and dying.* New York: Macmillan.

Lark, S. (2004). *The estrogen decision.* Berkeley, CA: Celestial Arts.

McCaffery, M. (2001, April). Overcoming barriers to pain management. *Nursing 2001, 31*(4), 18.

McCaffery, M. (1999, July). Assessing pain in a confused, nonverbal patient. *Nursing 99, 29*(7), 18.

McCaffery, M, Pasero, C. (2000, September). Pain control. *Nurseweek,* Sunnyvale, CA.

McCaffery, M, Pasero, C. (2001, July). Assessment and treatment of patients with mental illness: implementing the JCAHO pain management standards. *American Journal of Nursing, 101*(7), 69.

CHAPTER 3 (Continued)

Metules, T, Unkle, DW. (2000, April). Spinal cord injury falls into two categories. *RN Magazine, 63*(4), 85.

Pagana, K, Pagana, T. (2002). *Mosby's manual of diagnostic and laboratory tests* (2nd ed.). St. Louis: Mosby.

Piaget, J. (1973). *Origins of intelligence in children.* New York: Norton.

Selye, H. (1974). *Stress without distress.* New York: Signet Books.

Selye, H. (1976). *The stress of life.* New York: McGraw-Hill.

Stuart, G, Laraia, M, Sundeen, S. (2004). *Principles and practice of psychiatric nursing* (8th ed.). St. Louis: Mosby.

Taylor, C, Lillis, C, LeMone, P. (2001). *Fundamentals of nursing: the art and science of nursing care* (4th ed.). Philadelphia: Lippincott.

Wong-Baker, D. (2000). *Choosing a FACES pain scale*, revised. www.painsourcebook.ca/pdfs/pps92.

CHAPTER 4 NUTRITIONAL MANAGEMENT

Brown, J. (2002). *Nutrition now* (3rd ed.). Belmont, CA: Wadsworth Group.

Eisenberg, P. (1994, November). Gastrostomy and jejunostomy tubes. *RN Magazine, 57*(11), 54–59.

Loan, T, Magnuson, B, Williams, S. (1998, August). Debunking six myths about enteral feeding. *Nursing 98, 28*(8), 43–48.

Metheny, W, Wiersema, M, Clark, J. (1998, January). pH, color and feeding tubes. *RN Magazine, 61*(1), 25–27.

US Department of Agriculture. (2005). *Dietary guidelines for Americans.* Washington, DC: USDA/HNIS.

Whitney, E, Cataldo, C, Rolfes, S. (2002). *Understanding normal and clinical nutrition* (6th ed.). St. Paul, MN: West Publishing.

Williams, M. (2002). *Nutrition for health, fitness, and sport.* Boston: McGraw-Hill.

Williams, SR. (2001). *Basic nutrition & diet therapy* (11th ed.). St. Louis: Mosby.

CHAPTER 5 PHARMACOLOGY

Abrams, AC. (2006). *Clinical drug therapy: rationales for nursing practice* (7th ed.). Philadelphia: Lippincott.

Adams, M, Josephon, D, Holland, L. (2005). *Pharmacology for nurses—a pathophysiologic approach.* Upper Saddle River, NJ: Prentice Hall Health.

Boyer, MJ. (2002). *Math for nurses: a pocket guide to dosage calculations and drug preparations* (5th ed.). Philadelphia: Lippincott.

Chase, S. (1997, March). Pharmacology in practice. *RN Magazine, 60*(3), 22–24.

Cobb, MD. (1990, March). Dealing fairly with medication errors. *Nursing 90, 20*(3), 42–43.

Craven, R, Hirmle, C. (2000). *Fundamentals of nursing: human health and function* (3rd ed.). Philadelphia: Lippincott.

Deglin, J, Vallerand, A. (2003). *Davis's drug guide for nurses* (7th ed.). Philadelphia: Davis.

Grajeda-Higley, L. (2000). *Pharmacology: a physiology approach.* Upper Saddle River, NJ: Prentice Hall Health.

Hodgen, B. (2002). *Saunders nursing drug handbook.* Philadelphia: Saunders.

Karch, A, Karch, F. (2001). Take part in the solution: how to report medication errors. *American Journal of Nursing, 101*(10), 25.

Kuhn, M. (1998). *Pharmacotherapeutics: a nursing process approach.* Philadelphia: Davis.

Leahy, J, Kizilay, P. (1998). *Foundations of nursing practice: a nursing process approach.* Philadelphia: Saunders.

Malseed, R, Goldstein, F, Baldon, N. (1995). *Pharmacology: drug therapy and nursing considerations* (4th ed.). Philadelphia: Lippincott.

Phillips, L. (1997). *Manual of IV therapeutics* (2nd ed.). Philadelphia: Davis.

Physicians' desk reference to pharmaceutical specialties and biologicals (60th ed.). (2006). Montvale, NJ: Medical Economics.

Wilburn, S. (2000, February). Preventing needlesticks in your facility. *American Journal of Nursing, 100*(2), 96.

Wilson, B, Shannon, M. (2005). *Dosage calculation* (5th ed.). Upper Saddle River, NJ: Prentice Hall Health.

Wilson, B, Shannon, M, Stang, C. (2000). *Nurses drug guide.* Upper Saddle River, NJ: Prentice Hall Health.

CHAPTER 6 INFECTION CONTROL

Abrutyn, E, Goldman, DA, Scheckler, WE, Biello, L. (2001). *Saunders infection control reference service.* Philadelphia: Saunders.

Beezhold, T, et al. (1996). Latex allergy can induce clinical reaction to specific foods. *Clinical and experimental allergy, 26,* 416–422.

Black, J, Matassarin-Jacobs, E. (2001). *Medical–surgical nursing: clinical management for continuity of care* (6th ed.). Philadelphia: Saunders.

Borton, D. (1996, September). Gloves: on or off? *Nursing 96, 26*(9), 46–47.

Borton, D. (1997, January). Isolated precautions. *Nursing 97, 27*(1) 49–51.

Calianno, C. (1996, May). Nosocomial pneumonia. *Nursing 96, 26*(5), 34–39.

Carroll, P. (1998, June). Preventing nosocomial pneumonia. *RN Magazine, 68*(6), 44–47.

Centers for Disease Control and Prevention. (2002). Recommendations for prevention of HIV transmission in healthcare settings. *MMWR, 36*(suppl 25).

Chettle, C. (2005, November). Will avian flu mutate into a pandemic? *Nurseweek,* 21–22.

Decennial International Conference on Nosocomial and Healthcare Associated Infections.

Doenges, M, Moorhouse, M. (2002). *Nurse's pocket guide: diagnosis, interventions, and rationales* (7th ed.). Philadelphia: Davis.

Emerging Infectious Diseases. (1998). Using nurse hotline calls for disease surveillance. www.cdc.gov/nicdod/eid/vol4no2/rodman.htm.

Friedman, M. (2000, February). Improving infection control in home care: from ritual to science-based practice. *Home Healthcare Nurse, 18*(2), 99.

Gritter, M. (1998, September). The latex threat. *American Journal of Nursing, 98*(9), 26–32.

Larson, E. (1995). APIC guideline for handwashing and hand anasepsis in health care settings. *American Journal of Infection Control, 23,* 251–269.

Marthalwe, M, Keresztes, P, Tazbir, J. (2003, August). SARS—What have we learned? *RN Magazine, 66*(8), 58–62.

Sheff, B. (1999, February). Minimizing the threat of *C. difficile. Nursing 99, 29*(5), 33–38.

Sheff, B. (2005, September). Avian influenza: are you ready for a pandemic? *Nursing 2005, 35*(9), 26–27.

Smeltzer, S, Bare, B. (2000). *Brunner & Suddarth's textbook of medical–surgical nursing.* Philadelphia: Lippincott.

CHAPTER 7 DISASTER NURSING: BIOTERRORISM

Armstrong, J. (2002, April). Chemical warfare. *RN Magazine, 65*(4), 32–39.

Fell-Carlson, D. (2003, January). Terrorist Danger. *Nurseweek California,* Sunnyvale, CA.

Fell-Carlson, D. (2003, January). The nurse's role in managing threat. *Nurseweek California,* Sunnyvale, CA.

Henderson, D. (1999, February). The looming threat of bioterrorism. *American Association for Advancement of Science, 283*(5406), 1279–1282.

Hoffman, R, Norton, J. (2000, December). Lessons learned from a full-scale bioterrorism exercise. *Emerging Infectious Diseases, 6*(6), 652–653.

Keefe, S. (2006, January). Responding to disaster. *Advance for Nurses, 8*(2), 37.

Kilpatrick, J. (2002, May). Nuclear attacks. *Nurseweek California,* Sunnyvale, CA, 47–51.

Langan, J, James, D. (2005). *Preparing nurses for disaster management.* Upper Saddle River, NJ: Prentice Hall Health.

Maniscalco, P, Christem, H. (2002). *Understanding terrorism and managing the consequences.* Upper Saddle River, NJ: Pearson Education.

Nicolson, G. (2001, December). Protection from biological warfare agents. *Townsend Letter for Doctors & Patients,* Port Townsend, WA, 62–67.

Salvucci, A. (2002, October). Bioterrorism safeguards. *Bottom Line,* Stamford, CT: Boardroom.

Steinhauer, R. (2002, May). Bioterrorism. *RN Magazine, 65*(3), 48–54.

Steinhauer, R. (2002, June). The emergency management plan. *RN Magazine, 72*(6).

References Found on the Internet

American College of Emergency Physicians. (2002). NBC Task Force; Office of Emergency Preparedness, Final Report: Resources for Dealing with Stress Brought on by Recent Terrorist Attacks. www.acep.org/Government & Advocacy.

American Hospital Association. (2002). Chemical & Biological Terrorism Preparedness Checklist; Policy Forum, Hospital Preparedness for Mass Casualties. www.hospitalconnect.com/ahapolicyforum/resources/ disaster.

Army Regulation 40-13 Medical Services. (1985). Medical Support—Nuclear, Chemical Accidents & Incidents. www.cdc.gov/nuclear.

Association for Professionalism Infection Control and Epidemiology, Inc., Mass Casualty Disaster Plan Checklist: A Template for Healthcare Facilities. www.apic.org/bioterror/checklist.doc.

Center for Strategic and International Studies. Combating chemical, biological, radiological, and nuclear terrorism. www.cis.org/home/and/reports contactchembiorad.

Centers for Disease Control and Prevention. (2000). Biological & Chemical Terrorism: Strategic Plan for Preparedness and Response. www.cdc.gov/mmwr/preview/mmwrht/rr4901 al.htm.

Centers for Disease Control and Prevention. Emerging Infectious Diseases. (2002, September). Preparing at the Local Level for Events Involving Weapons of Mass Destruction. www.cdc.gov/nicdod/EID/vol8no9/01-0520.htm.

Centers for Disease Control and Prevention. Interim Recommendations for the Selection & Use of Protective Clothing and Respirators Against Biological Agents. cdc.gov/niosh/unp-intrecppe.html.

CHAPTER 7 *(Continued)*

Centers for Disease Control and Prevention. Issues in Health-care Settings, Part II. Recommendations for Isolation Precautions in Hospitals. cdc.gov/nicdod/hip/isolat/isopart2.htm.

Centers for Disease Control and Prevention. National Center for Community Emergency Response Team (CERT). Training: Participant handbook. www.cert-la.com/manuals/tc & intro.pwf.

Centers for Disease Control and Prevention. National Center for Infectious Diseases. www.cdc.gov/ncidod/publicat.htm.

Centers for Disease Control and Prevention. National Institute for Occupational Safety and Health. Chemical protective clothing. www.cdc.gov/niosh/npptl/chemprcloth.html.

Centers for Disease Control and Prevention. (2004–2005). Natural disasters—emergency preparedness and response. www.bt.cdc.gov/disasters.

Centers for Disease Control and Prevention. Office of Communication. CDC Radiation Studies, Nuclear Terrorism & Health Effects. www.cdc.gov/od/oc/media/9-11 pk.html.

Centers for Disease Control and Prevention. Public Health Emergency Preparedness & Response FAQS about Anthrax. www.cdc.gov/documentsapp/faqanthrax.asp#Qr001.

Centers for Disease Control and Prevention. Strategic Planning Workgroup. (2002). Biological & Chemical Terrorism: Strategic Plan for Preparedness Response. www.cdc.gov/mmwr/preview/mmwrhtml/rr 4904al.htm.

Centers for Disease Control and Prevention. Trends. www.cdc nac.org/geneva98/trends/trends_6.htm.

Electronic Journal of Biotechnology. (1999). Biological warfare, bioterrorism, biodefence and the biological antitoxin weapons convention. www.ejb.org/content/vol2/issue 3/full.

Emergency Weapons of Mass Destruction Responses. (2001). Emergency decontamination triage and treatment. www.2.sbccom.army.mil/hid.

Emerging Infectious Diseases. (1998). Using Nurse Hotline Calls for Disease Surveillance. www.cdc.gov/nicdod/eid/vol4o2/rodman.htm.

Federal Emergency Management Agency. (FEMA). 2001. Federal Response Plan-ESF#8. www.fema.gov/rrr/frpesf8.shtm.

Guidance for Radiation Accident Management. (2002). Managing radiation emergencies. www.orau.gov/reacts/syndrome.htm.

Guidance for Radiation Accident Management. (2002). Oak Ridge Associated Universities Basics of Radiation Safety Around Radiation Sources. www.orau.gov/reacts/guidance.htm.

JCAHO Standards, Security Management Plan. Occupational Safety & Health Administration. (1999, April). Technical information—rubber latex gloves & other natural rubber products. www.osha.gov/as/opa/fol9/TIB 19990412-html.

Recommendations for Chemical Protective Clothing Database. www.cdc.gov/niosh/nepc/ncpc2.html.

Smallpox and Smallpox Vaccines: Adverse Reactions—Think-twice, Smallpox. www.thinktwice.com/smallpox.htm.

Weapons of mass destruction, information for EMS first responders. www.oswegocountyems.org/WMD%20sheet%2ohtml.html.

CHAPTER 8 MEDICAL–SURGICAL NURSING

Abrams, AC. (2006). *Clinical drug therapy: rationales for nursing practice* (7th ed.). Philadelphia: Lippincott.

Abrutyn, E, Goldmann, DA, Scheckler, WE, Biello, L. (2001). *Saunders infection control reference service.* Philadelphia: Saunders.

Acello, B. (2000, March). Meeting JCAHO standards for pain control. *Nursing 2000, 30*(3), 52–54.

Ackley, BJ, Ladwig, GB. (2002). *Nursing diagnosis handbook: a guide to planning care* (5th ed.). St. Louis: Mosby.

Acute Pain Management. (1999). University of Iowa Gerontological Nursing Interventions Center, April 6, p. 37.

Ahmed, D. (2000). It's not my job. *American Journal of Nursing, 100*(6), 25.

Alfaro-LeFevre, R. (1998). *Critical thinking in nursing: a practical approach* (2nd ed.). Philadelphia: Saunders.

American Diabetes Association Clinical Practice Recommendations. (2002). *Journal of Clinical and Applied Research and Education 25* (suppl 1).

American Diabetes Association Position Statement. (1998, January). Insulin administration. *Diabetes Care, 21.*

American Heart Association: ACLS for Healthcare Providers. (2005). Chicago: AHA.

Amsterdam, E, et al. (1997, March 15). Chest pain with normal coronary arteries. *Patient Care, 43.*

Arnolds, S. (1997). What you should know about cardiac stress testing. *Nursing 97, 37*(1), 58–61.

Back, J. (1999, January). Clinical practice guidelines for chronic nonmalignant pain syndrome. *Musculoskeletal Rehabilitation, 13,* 47–58.

Barker, E. (1998, February). The xenon CT: a new neuro tool. *RN Magazine, 61*(2), 22–26.

Barker, E. (1999, May). Brain attack!: a call to action. *RN Magazine, 62*(5), 54.

Bates, B. (2004). *Guide to physical examination and history taking* (9th ed.). Philadelphia: Lippincott Williams & Wilkins.

Beare, P, Myers, J. (1998). *Adult health nursing* (3rd ed.). St. Louis: Mosby.

Beers, M, Berkow, R. (2006). *The Merck manual of diagnosis and therapy.* Whitehouse Station, NJ: Merck Research Laboratories.

Beezhold, T, et al. (1996). Latex allergy can induce clinical reaction to specific foods. *Clinical and Experimental Allergy, 26,* 416–422.

Black, J, Hawkes, J, Keene, A. (2005). *Medical–surgical nursing: clinical management of positive outcomes* (7th ed.). Philadelphia: Saunders.

Bozinko, C, Lowe, K, Reigart, C. (1998, November). A new option for burn victims. *RN Magazine, 61*(11), 37–39.

Burrell, L, Gerlach, M, Pless, B. (2001). *Foundations of contemporary nursing practice* (3rd ed.). Upper Saddle River, NJ: Prentice Hall Health.

Cantwell-Gab, K. (1996). Identifying chronic peripheral arterial disease. *American Journal of Nursing, 96*(7), 40–46.

Carroll, P. (1998, May). Closing in on safer suctioning. *RN Magazine, 61*(5), 22–26.

Carroll, P. (1999, January). Chest injuries. *RN Magazine, 62*(1), 36–40.

Chiocca, E. (1997, September). Actionstat. *Nursing 97, 27*(9), 33.

Cooper, C. (2000). Reducing the use of physical restraints in nursing homes. *Postgradutae Medicine, 107*(2), 15–16, 21–22, 24.

Corbett, J. (2004). *Laboratory tests and diagnostic procedures* (6th ed.). Stamford, CT: Appleton & Lange.

Crumlish, C, et al. (2000). When time is muscle. *American Journal of Nursing, 100*(1), 26–31.

Cutler, J, et al. (1998, February 28). Preventing hypertension. *Patient Care, 32*(4), 64–77.

D'Amico, D, Barbarito, C. (2007). *Health and physical assessment in nursing.* Upper Saddle River, NJ: Prentice Hall Health.

Deedwania, P, LaRosa, J, Superko, H. (1999, Spring). Managing dyslipidemia. *Patient Care.*

Deglin, J, Vallerand, A. (2003). *Davis's drug guide for nurses* (7th ed.). Philadelphia: Davis.

Dibartolo, V. (1998, December). 9 steps to effective restraint use. *RN Magazine, 61*(12), 23–26.

Doenges, M, Moorhouse, M, Geissler-Murr, A. (2002). *Nurse's pocket guide: diagnosis, interventions, and rationales* (8th ed.). Philadelphia: Davis.

Finkelman, A. (2001, January). *Managed Care: a nursing perspective.* Upper Saddle River, NJ: Prentice Hall Health.

Fischbach, F. (2005). *Nurses' quick reference to common laboratory and diagnostic tests* (4th ed.). Philadelphia: Lippincott Williams & Wilkins.

Garza, A, Forshner, H. (1997, December). Hepatitis update. *RN Magazine, 60*(12), 39.

Gorski, L. (2001, January). TPN update: making each visit count. *Home Healthcare Nurse, 19*(1), 15.

Gritter, M. (1998, September). The latex threat. *American Journal of Nursing, 98*(9), 26–32.

Guyton, AC. (2006). *Textbook of medical physiology* (11th ed.). Philadelphia: Saunders.

Habel, M. (2006, June). Fibromyalgia—looking good and feeling awful. *Nurseweek,* 19–20.

Habel, M, Strong, MA. (1997, January). Providing excellent care for patients with post-polio syndrome. *Nurseweek,* 10–11.

Hayes, D. (1997). Mitral valve prolapse revisited. *Nursing 97, 27*(10), 34–39.

Health Insurance Portability and Accountability Act (HIPAA). (2003, April). *The privacy rule.* Washington, DC: U.S. Department of Health and Human Services.

Heffernan, L. (1998, February). Organ donation: the legal aspects. *RN Magazine, 61*(2), 51–52.

Heslin, J. (1997, January). Peptic ulcer disease. *Nursing 97, 27*(1), 34–36.

Hickey, JV. (2002). *Clinical practice of neurological and neurosurgical nursing* (5th ed.). Philadelphia: Lippincott Williams & Wilkins.

Hilton, G. (2001, September). Acute head injury: distinguishing subdural from epidural hematoma. *American Journal of Nursing, 101*(9), 51.

Hudak, C, Gallo, B, Morton, P. (2001). *Critical care nursing: a holistic approach* (8th ed.). Philadelphia: Lippincott.

Hurley, M. (1998). New hypertension guidelines. *RN Magazine, 61*(3), 25–28.

Hutcherson, C. (1998, May). What five regulatory trends mean to you. *Nursing 98, 28*(5), 54–57.

CHAPTER 8 (Continued)

Ignatavicius, D, Workman, L, Mishler, M. (2007). *Medical–surgical nursing across the health care continuum* (5th ed.). Philadelphia: Saunders.

Iomko, J. (2000). Demystifying cardiac markers. *American Journal of Nursing, 100*(1), 36–40.

Joint Commission on Accreditation of Healthcare Organization (JCAHO). (2006). *Comprehensive accreditation manual for hospitals.* Oakbrook Terrace, IL: JCAHO.

Joint Commission for the Accreditation of Hospitals. (2002, February). *Comprehensive accreditation manual for hospitals: the official handbook.* Sentinel Events. Chicago: JCAHO.

Kuhn, M. (2002). *Pharmacotherapeutics* (5th ed.). Philadelphia: Davis.

LeMone, P, Burke, K. (2008). *Medical–surgical nursing: critical thinking in client care* (4th ed.). Upper Saddle River, NJ: Prentice Hall Health.

Lewis, A. (1999, October). Neurologic emergency. *Nursing 99, 29*(10), 33, 54–55.

Lewis, S, Heitkemper, M, Dirksen, S. (2008). *Medical–surgical nursing* (7th ed.). St. Louis: Mosby.

Little, C. (2000). Renovascular hypertension. *American Journal of Nursing, 100*(2), 46–51.

Louden, K. (2007, November). Transient ischemic attack. *Nurseweek*, 17–20.

Mancini, M, Kaye, W. (1999). AEDs: changing the way you respond to cardiac arrest. *American Journal of Nursing, 99*(5), 26–30.

McCaffery, M. (1999, July). Assessing pain in a confused, nonverbal patient. *Nursing 99, 29*(7), 18.

McCaffery, M, Pasero, C. (2000, September). Pain control. *Nurseweek*, Sunnyvale, CA.

McCance, K, Huether, S. (2006). *Pathophysiology* (5th ed.). St. Louis: Mosby.

McConnell, EA. (1999, January). Myths and facts . . . about fractures. *Nursing 99, 29*(1), 17.

McGrath, D. (1997). Mitral valve prolapse. *American Journal of Nursing, 97*(5), 40.

McKee, R. (1999, May). Clarifying advance directives. *Nursing 99, 29*(5), 52–53.

Meissner, J. (1997, October). Caring for patients with pancreatitis. *Nursing 97, 27*(10), 50–51.

Metules, T. (2002, April). Stroke prevention depends on skilled assessment. *RN Magazine, 65*(4), 66.

Metules, T. (2005, February). Unstable angina. *RN Magazine, 68*(2), 23–28.

Miller, C, Holden, P. (1999, June). Women and asthma; facts about the disease. *Nurseweek*, 14–15.

Monahan, F, Sands, J, Neighbors, M, Marek, J. (2007). *Phipps' medical–surgical nursing: concepts and clinical practice* (8th ed.). St. Louis: Mosby.

NeHina, S. (2006). *Lippincott manual of nursing practice* (8th ed.). Philadelphia: Lippincott Williams & Wilkins.

O'Donnell, L. (1996). Complications of MI. *American Journal of Nursing, 96*(9), 24–30.

Oertel, L. (1999, November). Monitoring warfarin therapy. *Nursing 99, 29*(11), 41–44.

Packer, M, Cohn, J. (1999, January 21). Consensus recommendations for the management of chronic heart failure. *American Journal of Cardiology, 83,* A1–A38.

Pettinicchi, T. (1998, March). Troubleshooting chest tubes. *RN Magazine, 28*(3), 58–60.

Phillips, J. (1998). Abdominal aortic aneurysm: confronting a compound problem. *Nursing 98, 28*(5), 34–39.

Porth, C. (2004). *Pathophysiology: concepts of altered health states* (7th ed.). Philadelphia: Lippincott.

Puhl, R. (2006, July). The stigma of obesity. *Advance for Nurses,* 31–33.

Rice, K. (1998). Peripheral arterial occlusive disease, Part I. *Nursing 98, 28*(2), 33–38.

Riley, M. (1997). Elective cardioversion. *RN Magazine, 60*(5), 27–29.

Rockett, J. (1999). Endothelial dysfunction and the promise of ACE inhibitors. *American Journal of Nursing, 99*(10), 44–45.

Shelton, B. (1998, December). Mounting an offense against lobar pneumonia. *Nursing 98, 28*(12), 42–46.

Smeltzer, S, Bare, B. (2004). *Brunner & Suddarth's textbook of medical–surgical nursing* (10th ed.). Philadelphia: Lippincott.

Smith, S, Duell, D, Martin, B. (2008). *Clinical nursing skills* (7th ed.). Upper Saddle River: Prentice Hall Health.

Stockert, P. (1999, March). Getting UTI patients back on track. *RN Magazine, 62*(3), 49–51.

Taber's cyclopedic medical dictionary. (2005). Philadelphia: Davis.

Taylor, E. (2002). *Spiritual care.* Upper Saddle River, NJ: Prentice Hall Health.

Taylor, N. (2006, January). This just in: for new CPR guidelines, think 30. *Nursing 2006 Critical Care, 1*(1), 56.

Thelan, L, Urden, L, Lough, M, Stacy, K. (2002). *Critical care nursing: diagnosis and management* (4th ed.). St. Louis: Mosby.

Tierney, L, McPhee, S, Papadakis, M. (2006). *Current medical diagnosis and treatment* (45th ed.). New York: Lange Medical Books/McGraw-Hall.

US Department of Health and Human Services, Public Health Service. (1992, February). *Acute pain management: operative or medical procedures and trauma.* USDHHS, Pub. No. 920032.

Urben, L, Lough, M, Stacy, K. (1996). *Priorities in critical care nursing* (2nd ed.). St. Louis: Mosby.

Walsh, E. (1998). Peripheral arterial occlusive disease, Part II. *Nursing 98, 28*(2), 39–44.

Warmkessel, J. (1997, June). Caring for patients with non-Hodgkin's lymphoma. *Nursing 97, 27*(6), 48–49.

Warren, C. (1999). What is homocysteine? *American Journal of Nursing, 99*(10), 39–41.

Willson, P. (2006, January). Metabolic syndrome. *Advance for Nurses,* 30–32.

CHAPTER 9 ONCOLOGY NURSING

Bence, Sharlene A. (2000, April). Stop cervical cancer in its tracks. *Nursing 2000, 30*(4).

Brown, CG, Yoder, LH. (2002, April). Stomatitis: an overview. *American Journal of Nursing,* 102(4).

Brown, K, Esper, P, et al. (Eds.). (2001). *Chemotherapy and biotherapy guidelines and recommendations for practice.* Pittsburgh: Oncology Nursing Press.

Carr, B, Burke, C. (April, 2001). Outpatient chemotherapy: hypersensitivity and anaphylaxis. *American Journal of Nursing, 101*(4), 27–30.

Carr, B, Burke, C. (US Preventive Services Task Force). (May, 2003). Chemoprevention of breast cancer: recommendations and rationale. *American Journal of Nursing, 103*(5), 107–114.

Connor, TH. (2002). *Occupational hazards related to antineoplastic agents.* University of Texas–Houston Health Science Center. www.uth.tmc.edu/schools/sph/an_agents/index.htm.

Del Gaudio, D, Menonna-Quinn, D. (1998, November). Chemotherapy: potential occupational hazards. *American Journal of Nursing, 98*(11), 59.

Engstrom, PF. (2000, May). Cancer prevention: from concept to practice. *Career.*

Goldsmith, C, Coleman, C. (2004, April). Breast cancer. *Nurseweek,* Mt. View, CA.

Held-Warmkessel, J. (1998, April). Chemotherapy complications. *Nursing 98, 28*(4), 41–45.

Hinson-Smith, V. (2000). Breast cancer survivors: learning from the faces of hope. *Nursing 2000.*

Kazda, R. (2001, April). Coming out on top: one woman coping with chemotherapy-induced alopecia finds strength in humor. *American Journal of Nursing, 101*(4), 24KK–24LL.

Lewis, S, Heitkemper, M, Dirksen, S. (2000). *Medical–surgical nursing assessment and management of clinical problems.* St. Louis: Mosby.

Lewis, S, Heitkemper, M, Dirksen, S. (2002, December). Low- versus high-dose radiation therapy. (Horizons). *Journal of Neuroscience Nursing.*

Machia, J, Napoli, M. (2001, April). Breast cancer: risk, prevention, and tamoxifen. *American Journal of Nursing, 101*(4), 26–34.

Myers, J. (2000, April). Emergency: chemotherapy-induced hypersensitivity reaction. *American Journal of Nursing, 100*(4), 53–56.

Napoli, M. (April, 2000). The lingo of chemo: how language misleads patients with cancer. *American Journal of Nursing, 100*(4), 13–14.

National Cancer Institute. http://cis.nci.nih.gov/fact/5_9.htm

National Institutes of Health, Division of Safety, Clinical Center Pharmacy Department and Cancer Nursing Service. (2002, January). *Recommendations for the safe handling of cytotoxic drugs.* www.nih.gov/od/ors/ds/pubs/cyto/index.htm

Navarro, T. (1998, November). Chemotherapy extravasation. *American Journal of Nursing, 98*(11), 38.

Nielsen, E, Brant, J. (2002, April). Chemotherapy-induced neurotoxicity: assessment and interventions for patients at risk. *American Journal of Nursing, 102*(4), 16–19.

Occupational Safety and Health Administration. (1999). *Controlling occupational exposure to hazardous drugs.* OSHA technical manual. www.osha-slc.gov/dts/osta/otm/otm_vi/otm_vi_2.html (31 Jan. 2002).

Oncology Nursing Society. www.ons.org.

Sitton, E. (2000, August). Beaming in on radiation therapy. *Nursing 2000, 30*(8).

Sitton, E. (2001, October). Support for preventive mastectomies. *Nursing 2000, 31*(10).

Wakeling, K. (1999, July). The latest weapon in the war against cancer. *RN Magazine, 62*(7), 58–60.

Welch, J, Silveira, J. (Eds.). (1997). *Safe handling of cytotoxic drugs: an independent study module* (2nd ed.). Pittsburgh: Oncology Nursing Press.

CHAPTER 10 EMERGENCY NURSING

Asselin, M, Cullen, H. (2001, March). New guidelines for BLS and ACLS. *Nursing 2001, 31*(3), 48–50.

Bailey, M. (1996, March). Emergencies handbook. *Nursing 96, 26*(3), 61–64.

Black, J, Hawkes, J, Keen, A. (2005). *Medical-surgical nursing* (7th ed.). Philadelphia: Saunders.

Glazer, J. (2005). Management of heatstroke and heat exhaustion. *American Family Physician, 71*(11), 2133.

Harwood, S. (1997, February). Anaphylaxis. *Nursing 97, 27*(2), 33.

LeMone, P, Burke, K. (2007). *Medical-surgical nursing: critical thinking in client care* (4th ed.). Upper Saddle River, NJ: Prentice Hall Health.

Lewis, S, Heitkemper, M, Dirkson, M. (2008). *Medical-surgical nursing: assessment and management of clinical problems* (7th ed.). St. Louis: Mosby.

Phipps, W, Sands, J, Marek, J. (2007). *Medical-surgical nursing: concepts and clinical practice* (8th ed.). St. Louis: Mosby.

Porth, C. (2002). *Pathophysiology: concepts of altered health states* (6th ed.). Philadelphia: Lippincott.

Sheehy, G. (2003). *Sheehy's emergency nursing: principles and practice* (5th ed.). St. Louis: Mosby.

Smeltzer, S, Bare, B. (2004). *Brunner & Suddarth's textbook of medical-surgical nursing* (10th ed.). Philadelphia: Lippincott.

Smith, S, Duell, D, Martin, B. (2008). *Clinical nursing skills* (8th ed.). Upper Saddle River, NJ: Prentice Hall Health.

Taylor, N. (2006, January). This just in: for new CPR guidelines, think 30. *Nursing 2006 Critical Care, 1*(1), 56.

Veronesi, J. (2005). Heat emergencies. *RN Magazine, 68*(6), 46.

CHAPTER 11 LABORATORY TESTS

Carroll, P. (1997, September). Clarifying the CBC. *RN Magazine, 60*(9), 47–50.

Carroll, P. (1997, November). Analyzing the Chem 7. *RN Magazine, 60*(11), 32–36.

Chernecky, C, Berger, B. (2001). *Laboratory tests and diagnostic procedures* (3rd ed.). Philadelphia: Saunders.

Corbett, J. (2004). *Laboratory tests and diagnostic procedures with nursing diagnoses* (6th ed.). Upper Saddle River: Prentice Hall Health.

Fischbach, F. (2005). *Nurses' quick reference to common laboratory and diagnostic tests* (4th ed.). Philadelphia: Lippincott Williams & Wilkins.

Frizzell, J. (1998, February). Avoiding lab test pitfalls. *American Journal of Nursing, 98*(2), 34–37.

Gaedeke, MK. (2000). *Laboratory and diagnostic handbook*. Menlo Park: Addison-Wesley.

Gibbar Clements, T, et al. (1997, July). PT and APTT: seeing beyond the numbers. *Nursing 97, 27*(7), 49–51.

Kee, J. (2006). *Laboratory and diagnostic tests with nursing implications* (7th ed.). Upper Saddle River: Prentice Hall Health.

Pagana, K, Pagana, T. (2006). *Mosby's manual of diagnostic and laboratory tests* (3rd ed.). St. Louis: Mosby.

Tasota, F, Wesmiller, S. (1998, December). Keeping blood pH in equilibrium. *Nursing 98, 28*(12), 35–40.

CHAPTER 12 MATERNAL–NEWBORN NURSING

American Academy of Pediatrics, American Heart Association. (2000). *Textbook of neonatal resuscitation* (4th ed.). Elk Grove Village, IL: Authors.

Bernstein, J. (1995). Ectopic pregnancy: a nursing approach to excess risk among minority women. *JOGNN 24*(9), 803–810.

Bougere, M. (1998). Abruptio placentae. *Nursing 98, 28*(2), 47.

Carr, D, Gabbe, S. (1998). Gestational diabetes: detection, management, and implications. *Clinical Diabetes* [Online] *16*(1), 4. www.diabetes.org.clinicaldiabetes/v16n1j-f98/pg4.htm.

Gilbert, E, Harmon, J. (1998). *Manual of high-risk pregnancy and delivery* (2nd ed.). St. Louis: Mosby.

Hockenberry, MJ, Wilson, D, Winkelstein, ML, Kline, NE. (2003). *Wong's nursing care of infants and children* (7th ed.). St. Louis: Mosby.

Letko, M. (1996). Understanding the Apgar score. *JOGNN, 25*(4), 299–303.

Lowdermilk, DL, Perry, SE, Bobak, IM. (2004). *Maternity and women's health care nursing* (8th ed.). St. Louis: Mosby.

Lucas, L, Jordan, E. (1997). Phenytoin as an alternative treatment for preeclampsia. *JOGNN, 26*(3), 263–269.

Mandeville, L, Troiano, N. (1998). *High-risk and critical care intrapartum nursing*. Philadelphia: Lippincott Williams & Wilkins.

Olds, S, London, M, Ladewig, P. (2004). *Maternal–newborn nursing: a family and community-based approach* (7th ed.). Upper Saddle River, NJ: Prentice Hall.

Oliveto, TM. (1997). Emergency! Severe preeclampsia. *American Journal of Nursing, 97*(7), 47.

Persson, B, Hanson, U. (1998). Neonatal morbidities in gestational diabetes mellitus. *Diabetes Care* [Online] 21(2). www.diabetes.org/diabetescare/supplement298/b79.htm.

Schnare, S, Matsoda, K. (1997). Today's contraceptive choices. *RN Magazine, 60*(12), 30–37.

Tomlinson, P, Bryan, A. (1996). Family centered intrapartum care: revisiting an old concept. *JOGNN, 25*(4), 331–337.

White, J. (2007, October). Late preterm infants need special care. *Nurseweek*, 14–16.

CHAPTER 13 PEDIATRIC NURSING

American Academy of Pediatrics. (2003). Recommended childhood immunization schedule—United States, January–December 2003. Available from AAP Web site: www.aap.org.

American Academy of Pediatrics. (2003). *Car safety seats: a guide for families*. Elk Grove Village, IL: Authors.

Ball, J, Bindler, R. (2003). *Pediatric nursing* (3rd ed.). Upper Saddle River, NJ: Prentice Hall Health.

Bates, B. (2004). *A guide to physical examination history taking* (9th ed.). Philadelphia: Lippincott.

Bazinski, M. (1999). *Manual of pediatric critical care*. St. Louis: Mosby.

Betz, C, Hunsburger, M, Wright, S. (Eds.). (1994). *Family-centered nursing care of children* (2nd ed.). Philadelphia: Saunders.

Buck, M. (2001). Pediatric vaccine update. *Pediatric Pharmacotherapy* 7(3).

Centers for Disease Control and Prevention. (2000). *Attention deficit/hyperactivity disorder*. Division of Birth Defects, Child Development and Disability and Health, Development Disabilities Branch. Available from CDC Web site: www.cdc.gov.

Centers for Disease Control and Prevention. (2003, May). *Childhood injury fact sheet*. National Center for Injury Prevention and Control. Available from CDC Web site: www.cdc.gov.

Centers for Disease Control and Prevention. (2003, May). *10 Leading causes of death, United States, 2000, all races, both sexes*. National Center for Injury Prevention and Control. Available from CDC Web site: www.cdc.gov.

Curley, M, Smith, J, Moloney-Harmon, P. (1996). *Critical care nursing of infants and children*. Philadelphia: Saunders.

Estrada, B. (2000, May). Pediatric bulletin: what's new in varicella vaccine? *Infections in Medicine*, 17(3). Available from Infections in Medicine®.

Garfunkel, L, Kaszorous, J, Christy, C. (2003). *Mosby's pediatric clinical advisor*. St. Louis: Mosby Yearbook.

Gern, J. (1999). *Diagnosis and treatment of childhood asthma: geographic and socioeconomic variables*. Proceedings from the American Lung Association/ American Thoracic Society

CHAPTER 13 *(Continued)*

International Conference, April 25, 1999. As published on Medscape©.

Gern, J. (1999). *Pediatric asthma: risk factors and clinical implications.* Proceedings from the American Lung Association/American Thoracic Society International Conference, April 25, 1999. As published on Medscape©.

Gibson, E, Dembofsky, CA, Rubin, S, Greenspan, JS. (2000, May). Infant sleep practices two years into the "Back to Sleep" campaign. *Clinical Pediatrics, 39*(5), 285–289.

Green, M. (Ed.). (1994). *Bright futures, guidelines of health supervision of infants, children and adolescents.* Arlington, VA: National Center of Education in Maternal and Child Health.

Lewis, D, Shala, A. (1999, April). Syncope in the pediatric patient, the cardiologist's perspective. *Pediatric Clinics of North America, 46*(2), 205–219.

Melish, M. (1996, May). Kawasaki syndrome. *Pediatrics in Review, 17*(5), 153–162.

Morris, C. (2000, May). Pediatric iron poisonings in the United States. *South Med Journal, 93*(4), 351–358.

National Center for Injury Prevention and Control. (2003). *Child maltreatment prevention.* http://www.cdc.gov/ncipe/dvp/CMP/default.htm

Paoletti, J. (2007, November). Tipping the scales: what nurses need to know about the childhood obesity epidemic. *RN Magazine, 70*(11), 35–39.

Patel, SR, Benjamin, RS. (2000, May). *Sarcomas of soft tissue and bone.* Harrison's Online, The McGraw-Hill Company, 2000. Available from Medscape©.

Shiminski-Maher, T, Shields, M. (1995, October). Pediatric brain tumors: diagnosis and management. *Journal of Pediatric Oncology Nursing, 12*(4), 188–198.

Siegler, R. (1995, December). The hemolytic uremic syndrome. *Pediatric Clinics of North America, 42*(6), 1505–1522.

Tumiston, S. (2003). A practical guide to using the new combination vaccines. *Contemporary Pediatrics, 20*(2), 36–53.

US Department of Health and Human Services. (2002). *Child maltreatment 2000: reports from the states to the national child abuse and neglect data system.* Washington, DC: US Government Printing Office.

Veasy, G, et al. (1987, February). Resurgence of acute rheumatic fever in the intermountain area of the United States. *New England Journal of Medicine, 316,* 421–427.

Velasco-Whetsell, M, et al. (2001). *Pediatric nursing.* New York: McGraw-Hill Nursing Care Services.

Welch, M. (1999). *Pediatric asthma: new options for young children.* Proceedings from the American Lung Association/American Thoracic Society International Conference April 25, 1999. As published on Medscape©.

Wong, D. (2005). *Whaley & Wong's essentials of pediatric nursing* (7th ed.). St. Louis: Mosby.

Wubbel, DO, McCracken, G. (1998, March). Management of bacterial meningitis: 1998. *Pediatrics in Review, 19*(3), 78–84.

CHAPTER 14 PSYCHIATRIC NURSING

Aguilera, DC. (1998). *Crisis intervention and methodology* (8th ed.). St. Louis: Mosby.

American Psychiatric Association. (2000). *Diagnostic and statistical manual of mental disorders* (4th ed.). Washington, DC: Author.

Fontaine, K. (2003). *Mental health nursing* (5th ed.). Upper Saddle River, NJ: Prentice Hall Health.

Geldmucher, DM. (2004). *Alzheimer's dementia (contemporary diagnosis and management).* Newtown, PA: Handbooks in Health Care.

Haber, J, Krainovich-Miller, B, McMahon, AL, Price-Hoskins, P. (2001). *Comprehensive psychiatric nursing* (6th ed.). St. Louis: Mosby.

Kneisl, C, Wilson, H, Trigoboff, E. (2004). *Contemporary psychiatric–mental health nursing.* Upper Saddle River, NJ: Pearson Education Inc.

Physicians' desk reference (2006). Montvale, NY: Medical Economics Company.

Stuart, G, Laraia, M. (2002). *Principles and practice of psychiatric nursing* (7th ed.). St. Louis: Mosby.

Sundeen, S, et al. (1998). *Nurse–client interaction: implementing the nursing approach* (6th ed.). St Louis: Mosby.

Varcarolis, EM. (1998). *Foundations of psychiatric mental health nursing.* Philadelphia: Saunders.

CHAPTER 15 GERONTOLOGICAL NURSING

Staff. (2003, March). Acute confusion in the elderly: assessment at admission can uncover risk factors. *American Journal of Nursing 103*(3), 21.

Staff. (2003, June). American's life expectancy reaches record high. *RN, 66*(6), 93.

Ayello, E, Braden, B. (2001, November). Why is pressure ulcer risk assessment so important? *Nursing, 31*(11), 74.

Bauer, J. (2003, June). "Silent" strokes increase elderly patients' risk of developing dementia. *RN, 66*(6), 23.

Boyd, L, Bauer, J. (2001, November). Study: Medicaid shortchanges nursing home care. *RN, 64*(11), 16.

Brody, J. (2007, September). The "poisonous cocktail" of multiple drugs. *New York Times*, p. D9.

Centers for Disease Control and Prevention. (2003, March). Deaths: Preliminary data for 2001. *National Vital Statistics Report, 51*(5). www.cdc.gov/nchs/data/nvsr/nvsr51/nvsr51_05.pdf.

Chelewski, P, Forsythe, J. (2002, November). How to streamline your risk assessment form. *Nursing, 32*(11), 66.

Clark, B, Halm, MA. (2003, May). Postprocedural acute confusion in the elderly: assessment tools can minimize this common condition. *American Journal of Nursing, 103*(5), 64.

Cohen, MR. (2002, February). Hold that juice (drug–nutrient interactions). *Nursing, 32*(2), 28.

Finch, M. (2003, April). Assessment of skin in older people. *Nursing Older People, 15*(2), 29.

Gallagher, B. (2001, August). Managing pain in elderly patients at home. *Nursing, 31*(8), 18.

Garrison, J. (2003, May). Heart failure and older people. *Nursing Older People, 15*(3), 38.

Gill, TM, Baker, DI, et al. (2002). A program to prevent functional decline in physically frail, elderly persons who live at home. *New England Journal of Medicine, 347*(14), 10.

Gray-Vickrey, P. (2001, October). Protecting the older adult. *Nursing Management, 32*(10), 37.

Haban, S. (2000, November). Elder abuse and neglect. *American Journal of Nursing, 100*(11), 49.

Heath, H. (2003, May). Sharp vision blunted by frontline reality. *Nursing Older People, 15*(3), 3.

Henry, M. (2002, March). Descending into delirium; confusion, isolation, forgetfulness, lethargy. *American Journal of Nursing, 102*(3), 49.

Herr, K. (2002, December). Pain assessment in cognitively impaired older adults: new strategies and careful observation help pinpoint unspoken pain. *American Journal of Nursing, 102*(12), 65.

Higginbotham, E. (2003, March). The misuse of psychotropics in the elderly. *RN, 66*(13), 67–68.

Karch, FE, Karch, AM. (2003, June). It was a shock: food allergies and some drugs don't mix well. *American Journal of Nursing, 103*(6), 27.

Lekan-Rutledge, D. (2003, March). Preventing progression to frailty: for the elderly, care planning can be the difference between home and nursing home. *American Journal of Nursing, 103*(3), 40.

Lekan-Rutledge, D, Colling, J. (2003, March). Urinary incontinence in the frail elderly: even when it's too late to prevent a problem, you can still slow its progress. *American Journal of Nursing, 103*(3), 36.

Lewis, L. (2003, March). Managing incontinence at home: the right instructions can make all the difference for caregivers. *American Journal of Nursing, 103*(3), 41.

Lewis, SM, Heitkemper, MM, Dirksen, SR. (2000). *Medical surgical nursing: assessment and management of clinical problems.* St. Louis: Mosby.

Lueckenotte, AG. (1998). *Pocket guide to gerontologic assessment* (3rd ed.). St. Louis: Mosby.

Luxton, T, Riglin, J. (2003, April). Preventing falls in older people: a multi-agency approach: falls among older people are common, disabling and often fatal. *Nursing Older People, 15*(2), 18.

Metules, T. (2000, April). Tips for keeping the elderly well hydrated. *RN, 63*(4), 86.

Missildine, K, Harvey, S. (2000, June). Restraints rock. *Nursing Management, 31*(6), 44.

Moore, AS. (2000, March). How to prevent contractures in the foot. *RN, 63*(3), 75.

Moore, AS. (2003, January). "Prehabilitation" for frail elderly at home: exercise may slow decline in physical function. *American Journal of Nursing, 103*(1), 20.

Stanly, M, Beare, PG. (1999). *Gerontological nursing* (2nd ed.). Philadelphia: Davis.

Tabloski, P. (2006). *Gerontological nursing.* Upper Saddle River, NJ: Prentice Hall Health.

Vernaree, E. (2003, June). Help reduce adverse drug events in elderly outpatients. *RN, 66*(6), 95.

Wallis, MA. (2000, September). Looking at depression through bifocal lenses. *Nursing, 30*(9), 58.

Whetstone, G, Boswell, S. (2002, September). The geriatric heart: nurses need to be aware of how aging and disease affect the myocardium. *American Journal of Nursing, 102*(9), 22.

Zhan, C. (2002, March). One in five elderly is prescribed inappropriate medications: safety is a major concern. *American Journal of Nursing, 102*(3), 18.

Zulkowski, K. (2003, January). Protecting your patient's aging skin. *Nursing, 33*(1), 84.

INDEX

Note: Page numbers with f and t indicate figures and tables respectively.

A

abdomen
  newborn assessment, 584t
  normal/abnormal findings, 530t
  pediatric assessment of, 636t
  during pregnancy, 527
abducens nerve, 170
ABO blood grouping, 398t, 505
abortions, 49–50, 535t, 541, 603–604
abruptio placentae, 544
absence seizures, 180, 650
absorption of drugs, 84–85
accessory organs, 60
accessory organs of the GI tract, 281–282
accidental injuries. *See* trauma
ACE inhibitors, 226, 235, 236–237
acetaminophen poisoning, 720
acid–base balance/imbalance, 323–324,
    324–330, 328–329t, 505
acid-fast bacilli, 509–510
acidifiers, 88
acne vulgaris, 382–383, 704
acoustic nerve, 170
acquired immunodeficiency syndrome
    (AIDS), 122–127
acromegaly (anterior pituitary
    hyperfunction), 414–415
activated partial thromboplastin time
    (APTT), 506
activity levels, 64, 646–647
acupuncture, 51
acute diarrhea (gastroenteritis), 679–680
acute gastritis, 292
acute glomerulonephritis (AGN),
    688–689
acute lymphocytic leukemia (ALL),
    405–406
acute myeloid leukemia (AML), 405
acute otitis media (AOM), 669
acute pulmonary edema, 227
acute radiation syndrome, 146–147
acute renal failure, 338–339
acute respiratory distress syndrome
    (ARDS), 261, 453
acute tumor lysis syndrome (ATLS), 711
acyanotic heart defects, 657t, 659–660
adaptation factors of age, 34
adaptive processes of labor/delivery,
    556–557
Addisonian crisis, 417

Addison's disease (adrenocortical
    insufficiency), 416–418
adenoiditis, 668–669
ADHD (attention deficit-hyperactivity
    disorder), 723–724
administration of drugs. *See also*
    vaccines/vaccine administration
  to children, 730
  guidelines for, 90–91
  intravenous (IV), 90
  legal issues of, 23–24
  metabolism and, 84
  narcotics, 93
  Nurse Practice Act guidelines for, 90
  oral, 89, 90, 92
  parenteral, 89–90, 93–95
  patient-controlled analgesia, 93
  rectal, 89
  Six Rights of Medication
    Administration, 91
adolescents/adolescence. *See also*
    pediatrics
  acne vulgaris, 704
  concept of death in, 45
  general assessment of, 639
  growth/development during, 629
  impact of hospitalization on, 643
  physical growth during, 623
  pregnancy in, 554
  suicide in, 725
adrenal cortex disorders, 416–418
adrenalectomies, 419
adrenal glands, 412, 413t
adrenal medulla disorders, 418–419
adrenergic class of drugs, 87
adrenocortical hyperfunction (Cushing's
    syndrome), 417–418, 419
adrenocortical insufficiency (Addison's
    disease), 416–418
adulthood
  developmental tasks of, 39
  major health problems of, 40
  nursing management of dying adults,
    45
  parenting, 39
  physiological changes in, 39–40
  psychosocial changes in, 40
advance directives, 22–23
AED operation, 492
AFP (alpha-fetoprotein), 539
African American culture, 42t
age-related macular degeneration
    (ARMD), 203–204
AGN (acute glomerulonephritis),
    688–689

agranulocytosis, 400–401
AHA (American Heart Association)
  BLS ABCD maneuvers, 493t
  CPR (cardiopulmonary resuscitation),
    490, 491f
AIDS. *See also* HIV
  characteristics of/assessment for,
    553–554
  in children, 694
  immunosuppression and, 122, 123–127
  in newborns, 589–590
  transmission via blood transfusions,
    399
airborne precautions, 113, 115
airway. *See also* respiratory (pulmonary)
    system
  assessing, 482
  lower, 247
  obstructions, 492, 666t
  resistance, 248
  upper, 247
akinetic (atonic) seizures, 180, 650
alcohol use, 87
alkaline phosphate, 510
alkalinizers, 88
ALL (acute lymphocytic leukemia),
    405–406
allergens, 86
allergic responses
  anaphylactic shock, 489
  to blood transfusions, 398t, 399
  skin, 385
all-or-none principle (cardiac muscle
    contraction), 213–214
alpha-fetoprotein (AFP), 539
ALS (amyotrophic lateral sclerosis), 199
altered blood supply to brain, 190–193
alternative/complementary therapies
  acupuncture, 197
  herb–drug interactions, 96–99
  summary of various, 51
alveolar ventilation, 249
ambiguous genitalia, 47
ambulatory exercise electrocardiography
    (ECG or EKG), 218
amenorrhea, 37, 347
American Academy of Pediatrics
    recommendations, 647
American Heart Association (AHA)
  BLS ABCD maneuvers, 493t
  cardiopulmonary resuscitation (CPR),
    490, 491f
AML (acute myeloid leukemia), 405
ammonia levels, 510
amniotic fluid, 524, 532t, 538, 543